BATES'

Guide to

Physical Examination

and History Taking

Second South Asian Edition

As per the Indian Competency-Based Medical Curriculum

BATES' Guide to Physical Examination and History Taking

Second South Asian Edition

As per the Indian Competency-Based Medical Curriculum

SAE Editor

Dharma Rao V., MBBS, MD (General Medicine)
Professor and Additional Medical Superintendent
Gayatri Vidya Parishad Institute of Healthcare and Medical Technology
Visakhapatnam, Andhra Pradesh

International Editors

Lynn S. Bickley, MD, FACP
Clinical Professor of Internal Medicine
School of Medicine
University of New Mexico
Albuquerque, New Mexico

Peter G. Szilagyi, MD, MPH
Professor of Pediatrics and Executive Vice-Chair
Department of Pediatrics
University of California at Los Angeles (UCLA)
Los Angeles, California

Richard M. Hoffman, MD, MPH, FACP
Professor of Internal Medicine and Epidemiology
Director, Division of General Internal Medicine
University of Iowa Carver College of Medicine
Iowa City, Iowa

This second South Asian edition is an adaptation of the *Bates' Guide to Physical Examination and History Taking, Thirteenth Edition*. Authorized for sale only in South Asia.

Wolters Kluwer

Publishing Manager: Dr. Vandana Mittal
Development Editor: Ms. Megha Saini
Production Editor: Ms. Pooja Chauhan
Asstt. Manager Manufacturing: Mr. Sumit Johry

3rd Floor, Tower B, Building No. 10, Phase – II, DLF Cyber City
Gurgaon, Haryana - 122002

First South Asian Edition, 2019
Second South Asian Edition, 2023

ISBN: 978-93-93553-36-2

Authorised for sale only in South Asia

Published by Wolters Kluwer (India) Pvt. Ltd., New Delhi
Compositor: Design Modus, New Delhi (www.designmodus.in)
Printed and bound at SDR Printers, Trans Delhi Signature City, Ghaziabad (U.P.)

For product enquiry, please contact– Marketing Department (marketing@wolterskluwerindia.co.in) or log on to our website www.wolterskluwerindia.co.in.

Preface*

Bates' Guide to Physical Examination and History Taking, now in its thirteenth international edition, spans an evolution of five decades. Drs. Barbara Bates and Robert Hoekelman launched the first edition in 1974 as a hands-on manual for medical and advanced practice nursing students learning the techniques of regional examination for adults and children. They devised the classic format of the Bates' Guide—black explanatory text in the major column, examples of abnormalities in red in the minor column, and comparative tables of abnormalities at the end of each chapter.

The second South Asian edition carries forward the legacy of *Bates' Guide to Physical Examination and History Taking* and explores the intricacies of a history taking session, meticulousness of physical examination, and sincerity of planning a workup for a case. The content has been reorganized into system-based chapters to suit the needs of Indian medical graduates. This edition addresses the *competency-based medical education* curriculum currently adopted by *National Medical Commission* for the medical undergraduate students.

New Content and Features

The second South Asian edition has new and expanded content as well as unique features to facilitate student learning and clinical skills education.

- In this edition, system-based approach is adopted to help students focus on the competencies aligning with the current curriculum while learning the skills. As a result, new chapters are either created from existing chapters or combined together.
- The opening chapter focuses on the patient encounter, including critical elements such as the use of preferred names, gender pronouns, the approach to special populations including persons who are differently abled, and discussions of LGBTQ health medical ethics and racism in health care.
- Frameworks of advance communication and interpersonal skills are expanded, including communicating difficult news using SPIKES and Ask-Tell-Ask methods; motivational interviewing and teach-back methods in patient communication; and the SBAR method for interprofessional communication.
- A stepwise approach to the process of clinical reasoning includes an emphasis on the use of illness scripts and semantic qualifiers and the development of summary statements with illustrative examples.
- A key regional chapter, *Beginning the Physical Examination: General Survey, Vital Signs, and Pain* is replaced by *General Examination*. Pallor, cyanosis, jaundice, clubbing, edema, and lymph node are now part of this chapter. Information on vital signs is also revised and expanded.
- Another key regional chapter, *Head and Neck,* is subdivided into smaller chapters for a more focused understanding of its component organ systems and their pathophysiologic interconnectedness.
- General health maintenance screening and counseling topics are organized into a single chapter for easy access that includes informative tables of updated recommendations.
- All regional chapters follow a uniform template that facilitates locating critical information including the methodology of *Focused Physical Examination* approach.
- Summary checklists of key physical examination steps are included in the regional examination chapters for review purposes.

**Derived from the Preface to the Thirteenth International Edition.*

Organization

The book comprises four units: Foundations of Health Assessment, Regional Examinations, Special Populations, and Case-Based Learning.

Unit 1, Foundations of Health Assessment, consists of chapters that follow a logical sequence beginning with an overview of the components of the history taking, followed by important concepts in assessment of clinical evidence and clinical decision making.

Unit 2, Regional Examinations, covers the regional examinations from head to toe. The 15 chapters in this unit were reorganized and thoroughly updated. They contain a review of anatomy and physiology, the common symptoms encountered in the health history, detailed descriptions and images of techniques of examination, a sample written record, and comparative tables of abnormalities. Important topics for health promotion and counseling were moved to the end of the chapter for a more focused understanding of these complex topics.

Other notable features include discussion of updated screening guidelines for breast cancer, prostate cancer, and colon cancer as well as updated information on sexually transmitted infections and their prevention.

Unit 3, Special Populations, includes chapters covering stages in the life cycle—infancy through adolescence, pregnancy, and aging.

Unit 4, Case-Based Learning, includes common case vignettes encountered in clinical practice with question–answer format. For a student, these cases are a learning resource for approaching a whole series of clinical problems. This section will help them approach common clinical scenarios and, perhaps more importantly, learn how to analyze a clinical setting and efficiently extract the information necessary for diagnosis and the initiation of management which in turn help them to score better in exams.

Additional Resources

Videos are a key adjunct for mastering the many techniques of physical examination. This edition features 20 Objective Structured Clinical Examination (OSCE) videos of Physiology along with 16 OSCE videos of Medicine History Taking. We encourage students to study the written chapters and videos in tandem, often numerous times.

For students preparing for clinical testing, the 36 OSCE videos show students evaluating patients with common clinical problems in standard OSCE formats, interspersed with questions to guide learning key points.

Closing Note

It is our hope and expectation that the content, style, and organization of this second South Asian edition will be helpful to those students who want to become skilful, thoughtful readers and to those wishing to enhance their clinical performance.

Dharma Rao V.

Acknowledgments

My experience with the second South Asian edition of *Bates' Guide to Physical Examination and History Taking* has been both arduous and rewarding. I would like to start by thanking my team of contributors for a wonderful collaboration, sprinkled with compassion and constructive criticism, right from reviewing early scribblings to contemporizing the final drafts.

Words shall fall short to acknowledge the generous support and encouragement of Prof. P. Somaraju, Secretary, GVP Society. I also express my deepest appreciation for Prof. A. Ranga Rao, Prof. U. S. N. Murthy, Prof. K. L. N. Raju, Dr. Naruttam Sonowal, Dr. M. Akhilesh, Dr. M. Harika Chowdary, Dr. A. Sam Rao, Dr. O. Mrunalini, Dr. K. Gopa Naik, Mr. S. Jayabalakrishnan, Dr. T. Pujitha, Dr. K Vishnu Chaitanya, Dr. G. Geetha Madhuri, Dr. Ratna Harika, and Ms. P. M. Sucharita who shared their gift of valuable time, enthusiasm, and dynamism for videos and illustrations.

I would like to recognize the unhesitating assistance of Mr. Lovaraju, Mr. Satya, and Mrs. Bhagyalakshmi for the provision of instruments and ambience during the video recordings. I would not miss the opportunity to compliment and congratulate the technical team at Wolters Kluwer (India), especially Dr. Vandana Mittal, Ms. Pooja Chauhan, and Ms. Megha Saini, for their tireless contribution in the form of priceless patience, editorial help, and ingenious suggestions. I am also thankful for the insightful comments from peer reviewers who helped me to improvise the content. The list shall be incomplete without special mention of Mr. Chandan Kumar and Mr. Saravanan Somasundaram for their involvement during the initial phases of this project.

I am eternally grateful and indebted to all the patients for their gracious support and co-operation to accomplish the conception of videos for better learning.

A special thanks to my dear students who always inspire and motivate me and keep me going.

At this juncture, I would reminisce about my parents who are the source of impetus and guidance in whatever I pursue in my life. I gratefully acknowledge the love and full-time supportiveness of my in-laws for taking care of my wonderful children, Ishaana and Riyansh.

I am deeply indebted with humbleness and gratitude to everyone, all named and unnamed, for their suggestions and facilitation to give a concrete shape to this endeavor.

Dharma Rao V.

Contributors and Reviewers

Contributors

Himavathy K Gara
Associate Professor
Department of Physiology
Gayatri Vidya Parishad Institute of Healthcare & Medical Technology
Visakhapatnam, Andhra Pradesh

A S Veeramani Kartheek
Assistant Professor
Department of General Medicine
Government Medical College
Srikakulum, Andhra Pradesh

Reviewers

Faculty

Aiswarya M Nair
Professor
Department of Medicine
Sri Ramachandra Medical College and Research Institute
Chennai, Tamil Nadu

Amit Aggarwal
Senior Specialist
Department of Medicine
ABVIMS & Dr Ram Manohar Lohia Hospital
New Delhi

C Raghavendra
Associate Professor
Department of Respiratory Medicine
Gayatri Vidya Parishad Institute of Healthcare & Medical Technology
Visakhapatnam, Andhra Pradesh

Prashanth Kumar M
Vice-Principal, Professor and HOD
Department of Physiology
Dr. Chandramma Dayananda Sagar Institute of Medical Education & Research
Bengaluru, Karnataka

Pushpa K
Assistant Professor
Department of Physiology
Chikkaballapur Institute of Medical Sciences
Chikkaballapur, Karnataka

Rajeev Bandhu
Professor and Head
Department of Physiology
Lady Hardinge Medical College
New Delhi

Ravi Kaushik
Associate Professor
Department of Physiology
Maulana Azad Medical College
New Delhi

Suchitra Sachin Palve
Professor and Head
Department of Physiology
Symbiosis Medical College for Women
Pune, Maharashtra

Sudhakar H H
Professor
Department of Physiology
Kempegowda Institute of Medical Sciences
Bengaluru, Karnataka

Surendra S Shivalkar
Professor
Department of Physiology
Grant Government Medical College
Mumbai, Maharashtra

Thejaswini K O
Professor and HOD
Department of Physiology
Sri Siddhartha Institute of Medical Sciences and Research Centre
Bengaluru, Karnataka

Upendra Baitha
Associate Professor
Department of Medicine
All India Institute of Medical Sciences
New Delhi

Varuni S J
Professor
Department of Kriya Shareera
Sri Sri College of Ayurvedic Science and Research
Bengaluru, Karnataka

Senior Resident

Anjuman Fayaz
Senior Resident
Department of Medicine
School of Medical Sciences and Research
Greater Noida, Uttar Pradesh

Students

Aadesh K Garg
Intern
School of Medical Science and Research
Greater Noida, Uttar Pradesh

Adarsh Pal
PG (Medicine), First Year
Department of Medicine
All India Institute of Medical Sciences
New Delhi

Aisiri Deepak
MBBS Student, Third Year
BGS Global Institute of Medical Sciences
Bengaluru, Karnataka

Akshay Kumar Gupta
PG (Medicine), First Year
ABVIMS and Dr RML Hospital
New Delhi

Arun S Doddannavar
MBBS Student, Third Year
East Point College of Medical Sciences
Bengaluru, Karnataka

Ayesha Abdullah
MBBS Student, Third Year
East Point College of Medical Sciences
Bengaluru, Karnataka

Ayush Agarwal
PG (Medicine), Third Year
All India Institute of Medical Sciences
New Delhi

Bharat Saini
MBBS Student, Final Year
Maulana Azad Medical College
New Delhi

Bhumika C
MBBS Student, Third Year
BGS Global Institute of Medical Sciences
Bengaluru, Karnataka

Deena Mariyam
Intern
Vice President, South Indian Medical Student's Association
Kempegowda Institute of Medical Science
Bengaluru, Karnataka

Deepika H S
MBBS Student, Third Year
Bangalore Medical College and Research Centre
Bengaluru, Karnataka

Divyanshi Makhija
MBBS Student, Final Year
Ramaiah Medical College
Bengaluru, Karnataka

Himanshu Kaushik
MBBS Student, Third Year
SGT Medical College
Gurgaon, Haryana

Ignatius Roshan R
Compulsory Rotatory Residential Internship
Muthukumaran Medical College and Hospital
Chennai, Tamil Nadu

Jagadeeswar Reddy
PG (Medicine), Third Year
Chettinad Health and Research Institute
Chennai, Tamil Nadu

Kanav Khanna
PG (Medicine), Third Year
Postgraduate Institute of Medical Education and Research
Chandigarh

Pragya Mitra
MBBS Student, Final Year
University College Medical Sciences and GTB Hospital
New Delhi

Prashant Kumar
PG (Medicine), Third Year
University College Medical Sciences and GTB Hospital
New Delhi

Priyanshu Kumar
PG (Medicine), Third Year
ABVIMS & Dr RML Hospital
New Delhi

Raghunandan Ramanathan
Compulsory Rotatory Residential Internship
Tagore Medical College and Hospital
Chennai, Tamil Nadu

Rohil Jain
PG (Medicine), Third Year
Vardhaman Mahavir Medical College and SJH Hospital
New Delhi

Sajith K M
Compulsory Rotatory Residential Internship
Sri Ramachandra Medical College & Research Institute
Chennai, Tamil Nadu

Sanil Karanth
MBBS Student, Final Year
St. Johns Medical College and Hospital
Bengaluru, Karnataka

Saurabh Sangam
MBBS Student, Third Year
Sri Siddhartha Institute of Medical Sciences and Research Center
Bengaluru, Karnataka

Sharanu Rajole
MBBS Student, Final Year
Joint Secretary, BMCRI Students' Association
Bangalore Medical College and Research Institute
Bengaluru, Karnataka

Shimoni Jain
MBBS Student, Final Year
General Secretary, BMCRI Students' Association
Bangalore Medical College and Research Institute
Bengaluru, Karnataka

Shobith M A
MBBS Student, Final Year
Cultural Secretary, BMCRI Students' Association
Bangalore Medical College and Research Institute
Bengaluru, Karnataka

Shushrutha K
MBBS Student, Final Year
MVJ Medical College and Research Hospital
Bengaluru, Karnataka

Sindhu S
MBBS Student, Final Year
MVJ Medical College and Research Hospital
Bengaluru, Karnataka

Sourabh Singh
Intern
VMMC and Safdarjung Hospital
New Delhi

Sushrut Agrawal
MBBS Student, Final Year
Maulana Azad Medical College
New Delhi

Suvarna Sharma
MBBS Student, Third Year
Sri Siddhartha Institute of Medical Sciences and Research Center
Bengaluru, Karnataka

Tanvi Deshpande
MBBS Student, Final Year
St. Johns Medical College and Hospital
Bengaluru, Karnataka

Tanya Avis Cherian
MBBS Student, Final Year
Kempegowda Institute of Medical Sciences
Bengaluru, Karnataka

Umme Shifa
MBBS Student, Final Year
Kempegowda Institute of Medical Sciences
Bengaluru, Karnataka

Vaibhav Wali
MBBS Student, Third Year
Bangalore Medical College and Research Centre
Bengaluru, Karnataka

Veerapaneni Kiran
Compulsory Rotatory Residential Internship
ACS Medical College and Hospital
Chennai, Tamil Nadu

How To Use

Bates' Guide to Physical Examination and History Taking

The second South Asian edition of *Bates' Guide to Physical Examination and History Taking* is your comprehensive guide to learning to effectively conduct the health interview and physical examination. This section introduces you to the features and learning tools that will lead to successful health assessments, regional examinations, and working with special patient populations.

Key Terms—NEW!

These terms, highlighted in **bold text,** are frequently asked in clinical rounds and rotations and worth remembering. These "must-know" definitions are also compiled in a glossary section available at the end of the book.

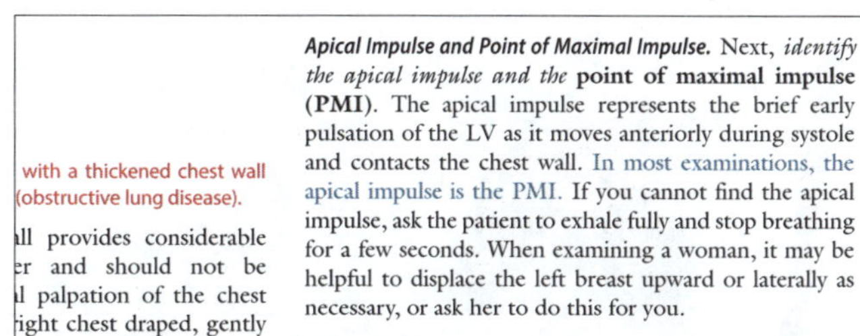

with a thickened chest wall (obstructive lung disease).

ll provides considerable
er and should not be
l palpation of the chest
ight chest draped, gently

Apical Impulse and Point of Maximal Impulse. Next, *identify the apical impulse and the* **point of maximal impulse (PMI)**. The apical impulse represents the brief early pulsation of the LV as it moves anteriorly during systole and contacts the chest wall. In most examinations, the apical impulse is the PMI. If you cannot find the apical impulse, ask the patient to exhale fully and stop breathing for a few seconds. When examining a woman, it may be helpful to displace the left breast upward or laterally as necessary, or ask her to do this for you.

Clinical Pearls

Be sure to pay special attention to the clinical pearls, printed in blue. These clinical comments provide practical "pearls" that enhance your understanding of the assessment techniques.

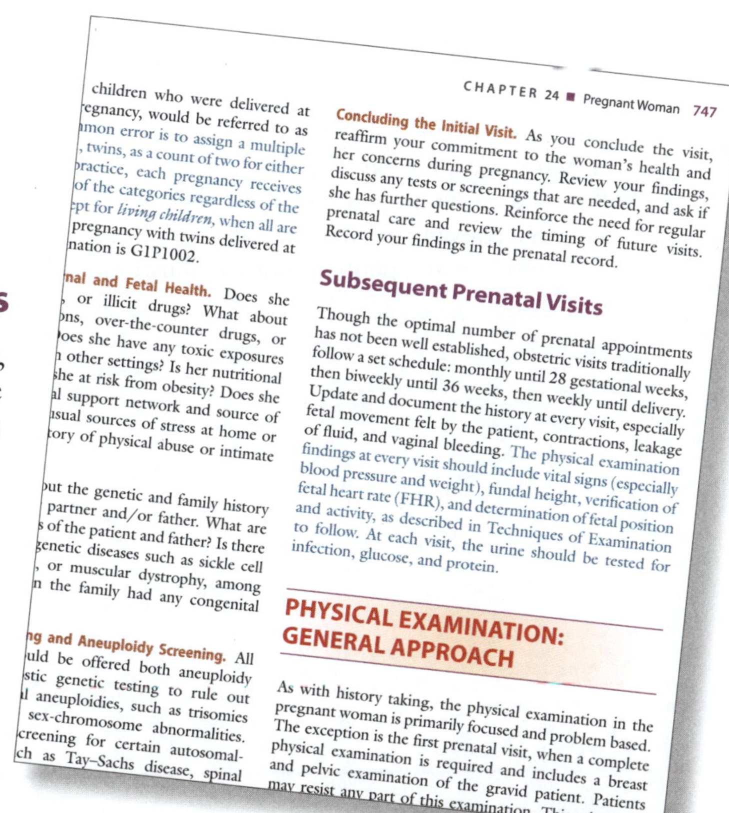

CHAPTER 24 ■ Pregnant Woman 747

children who were delivered at
regnancy, would be referred to as
mon error is to assign a multiple
, twins, as a count of two for either
practice, each pregnancy receives
of the categories regardless of the
ept for *living children*, when all are
pregnancy with twins delivered at
nation is G1P1002.

nal and Fetal Health. Does she
, or illicit drugs? What about
ons, over-the-counter drugs, or
oes she have any toxic exposures
n other settings? Is her nutritional
she at risk from obesity? Does she
al support network and source of
usual sources of stress at home or
tory of physical abuse or intimate

out the genetic and family history
partner and/or father. What are
s of the patient and father? Is there
genetic diseases such as sickle cell
, or muscular dystrophy, among
n the family had any congenital

ng and Aneuploidy Screening. All
uld be offered both aneuploidy
stic genetic testing to rule out
l aneuploidies, such as trisomies
sex-chromosome abnormalities.
creening for certain autosomal-
ch as Tay–Sachs disease, spinal

Concluding the Initial Visit. As you conclude the visit, reaffirm your commitment to the woman's health and her concerns during pregnancy. Review your findings, discuss any tests or screenings that are needed, and ask if she has further questions. Reinforce the need for regular prenatal care and review the timing of future visits. Record your findings in the prenatal record.

Subsequent Prenatal Visits

Though the optimal number of prenatal appointments has not been well established, obstetric visits traditionally follow a set schedule: monthly until 28 gestational weeks, then biweekly until 36 weeks, then weekly until delivery. Update and document the history at every visit, especially fetal movement felt by the patient, contractions, leakage of fluid, and vaginal bleeding. The physical examination findings at every visit should include vital signs (especially blood pressure and weight), fundal height, verification of fetal heart rate (FHR), and determination of fetal position and activity, as described in Techniques of Examination to follow. At each visit, the urine should be tested for infection, glucose, and protein.

PHYSICAL EXAMINATION: GENERAL APPROACH

As with history taking, the physical examination in the pregnant woman is primarily focused and problem based. The exception is the first prenatal visit, when a complete physical examination is required and includes a breast and pelvic examination of the gravid patient. Patients may resist any part of this examination. This reluctance

Examples of Abnormalities

As your skills progress, study the abnormal variants of common physical findings in red to deepen your knowledge of important clinical conditions.

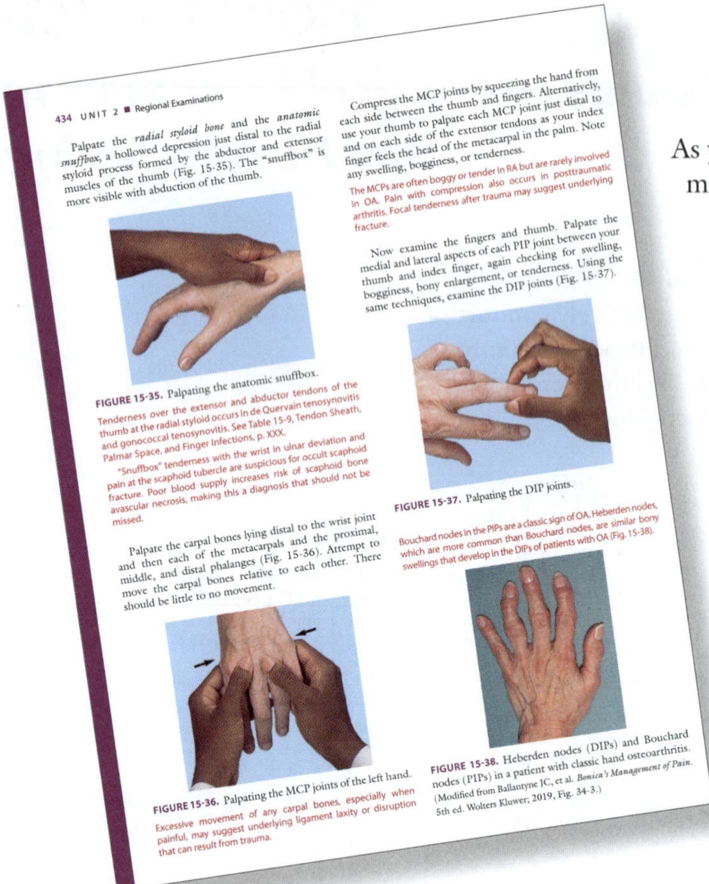

434 UNIT 2 ■ Regional Examinations

Palpate the *radial styloid bone* and the *anatomic snuffbox*, a hollowed depression just distal to the radial styloid process formed by the abductor and extensor muscles of the thumb (Fig. 15-35). The "snuffbox" is more visible with abduction of the thumb.

FIGURE 15-35. Palpating the anatomic snuffbox.

Tenderness over the extensor and abductor tendons of the thumb at the radial styloid occurs in de Quervain tenosynovitis and gonococcal tenosynovitis. See Table 15-9, Tendon Sheath, Palmar Space, and Finger Infections, p. XXX.

"Snuffbox" tenderness with the wrist in ulnar deviation and pain at the scaphoid tubercle are suspicious for occult scaphoid fracture. Poor blood supply increases risk of scaphoid bone avascular necrosis, making this a diagnosis that should not be missed.

Palpate the carpal bones lying distal to the wrist joint and then each of the metacarpals and the proximal, middle, and distal phalanges (Fig. 15-36). Attempt to move the carpal bones relative to each other. There should be little to no movement.

FIGURE 15-36. Palpating the MCP joints of the left hand.

Excessive movement of any carpal bones, especially when painful, may suggest underlying ligament laxity or disruption that can result from trauma.

Compress the MCP joints by squeezing the hand from each side between the thumb and fingers. Alternatively, use your thumb to palpate each MCP joint just distal to and on each side of the extensor tendons as your index finger feels the head of the metacarpal in the palm. Note any swelling, bogginess, or tenderness.

The MCPs are often boggy or tender in RA but are rarely involved in OA. Pain with compression also occurs in posttraumatic arthritis. Focal tenderness after trauma may suggest underlying fracture.

Now examine the fingers and thumb. Palpate the medial and lateral aspects of each PIP joint between your thumb and index finger, again checking for swelling, bogginess, bony enlargement, or tenderness. Using the same techniques, examine the DIP joints (Fig. 15-37).

FIGURE 15-37. Palpating the DIP joints.

Bouchard nodes in the PIPs are a classic sign of OA. Heberden nodes, which are more common than Bouchard nodes, are similar bony swellings that develop in the DIPs of patients with OA (Fig. 15-38).

FIGURE 15-38. Heberden nodes (DIPs) and Bouchard nodes (PIPs) in a patient with classic hand osteoarthritis. (Modified from Ballantyne JC, et al. *Bonica's Management of Pain*. 5th ed. Wolters Kluwer; 2019, Fig. 34-3.)

To further sharpen your clinical acumen, turn to the end-of-chapter *Tables of Abnormalities*, which allow you to compare and contrast clinical conditions in a convenient table format with accompanying photographs and illustrations.

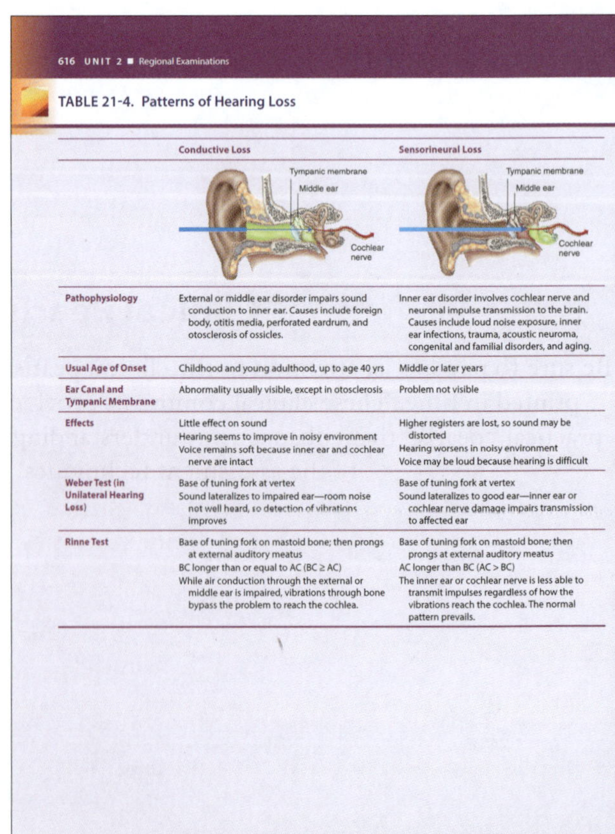

616 UNIT 2 ■ Regional Examinations

TABLE 21-4. Patterns of Hearing Loss

	Conductive Loss	Sensorineural Loss
	Tympanic membrane; Middle ear; Cochlear nerve	Tympanic membrane; Middle ear; Cochlear nerve
Pathophysiology	External or middle ear disorder impairs sound conduction to inner ear. Causes include foreign body, otitis media, perforated eardrum, and otosclerosis of ossicles.	Inner ear disorder involves cochlear nerve and neuronal impulse transmission to the brain. Causes include loud noise exposure, inner ear infections, trauma, acoustic neuroma, congenital and familial disorders, and aging.
Usual Age of Onset	Childhood and young adulthood, up to age 40 yrs	Middle or later years
Ear Canal and Tympanic Membrane	Abnormality usually visible, except in otosclerosis	Problem not visible
Effects	Little effect on sound Hearing seems to improve in noisy environment Voice remains soft because inner ear and cochlear nerve are intact	Higher registers are lost, so sound may be distorted Hearing worsens in noisy environment Voice may be loud because hearing is difficult
Weber Test (in Unilateral Hearing Loss)	Base of tuning fork at vertex Sound lateralizes to impaired ear—room noise not well heard, so detection of vibrations improves	Base of tuning fork at vertex Sound lateralizes to good ear—inner ear or cochlear nerve damage impairs transmission to affected ear
Rinne Test	Base of tuning fork on mastoid bone; then prongs at external auditory meatus BC longer than or equal to AC (BC ≥ AC) While air conduction through the external or middle ear is impaired, vibrations through bone bypass the problem to reach the cochlea.	Base of tuning fork on mastoid bone; then prongs at external auditory meatus AC longer than BC (AC > BC) The inner ear or cochlear nerve is less able to transmit impulses regardless of how the vibrations reach the cochlea. The normal pattern prevails.

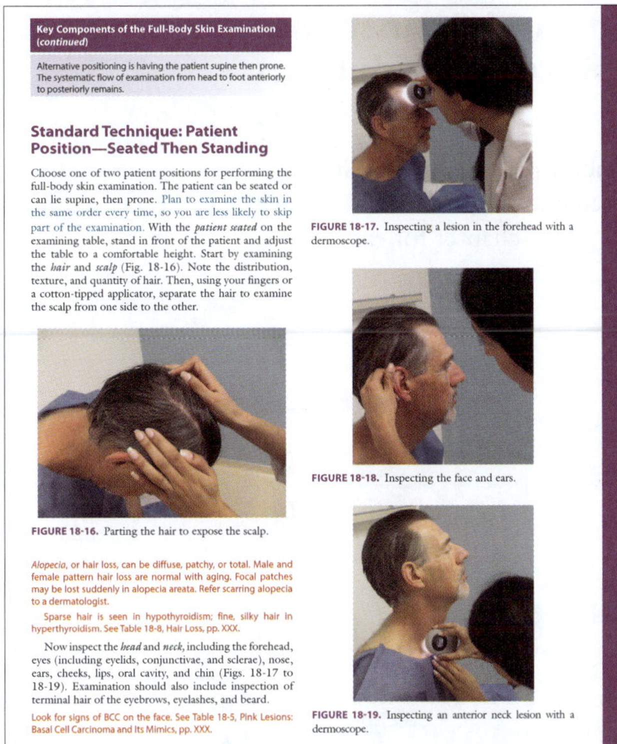
Key Components of the Full-Body Skin Examination (*continued*)

Alternative positioning is having the patient supine then prone. The systematic flow of examination from head to foot anteriorly to posteriorly remains.

Standard Technique: Patient Position—Seated Then Standing

Choose one of two patient positions for performing the full-body skin examination. The patient can be seated or can lie supine, then prone. Plan to examine the skin in the same order every time, so you are less likely to skip part of the examination. With the *patient seated* on the examining table, stand in front of the patient and adjust the table to a comfortable height. Start by examining the *hair* and *scalp* (Fig. 18-16). Note the distribution, texture, and quantity of hair. Then, using your fingers or a cotton-tipped applicator, separate the hair to examine the scalp from one side to the other.

FIGURE 18-16. Parting the hair to expose the scalp.

Alopecia, or hair loss, can be diffuse, patchy, or total. Male and female pattern hair loss are normal with aging. Focal patches may be lost suddenly in alopecia areata. Refer scarring alopecia to a dermatologist.

Sparse hair is seen in hypothyroidism; fine, silky hair in hyperthyroidism. See Table 18-8, Hair Loss, pp. XXX.

Now inspect the *head* and *neck*, including the forehead, eyes (including eyelids, conjunctivae, and sclerae), nose, ears, cheeks, lips, oral cavity, and chin (Figs. 18-17 to 18-19). Examination should also include inspection of terminal hair of the eyebrows, eyelashes, and beard.

Look for signs of BCC on the face. See Table 18-5, Pink Lesions: Basal Cell Carcinoma and Its Mimics, pp. XXX.

FIGURE 18-17. Inspecting a lesion in the forehead with a dermoscope.

FIGURE 18-18. Inspecting the face and ears.

FIGURE 18-19. Inspecting an anterior neck lesion with a dermoscope.

Techniques of Examination

This section is where you will learn the crucial and relevant examinations you will perform every day.

Key Components of the Examination Checklists—NEW!

The *Techniques of Examination* sections are now preceded by a listing of the *Key Components of the Examination* to serve as a checklist and guide.

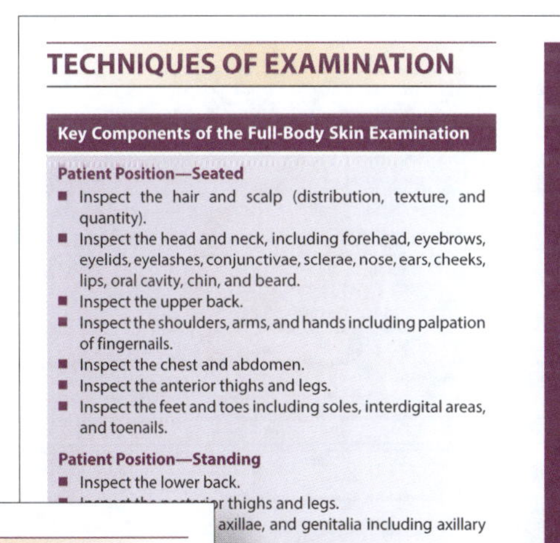
TECHNIQUES OF EXAMINATION

Key Components of the Full-Body Skin Examination

Patient Position—Seated
- Inspect the hair and scalp (distribution, texture, and quantity).
- Inspect the head and neck, including forehead, eyebrows, eyelids, eyelashes, conjunctivae, sclerae, nose, ears, cheeks, lips, oral cavity, chin, and beard.
- Inspect the upper back.
- Inspect the shoulders, arms, and hands including palpation of fingernails.
- Inspect the chest and abdomen.
- Inspect the anterior thighs and legs.
- Inspect the feet and toes including soles, interdigital areas, and toenails.

Patient Position—Standing
- Inspect the lower back.
- ...r thighs and legs.
- ... axillae, and genitalia including axillary

Special Techniques

Additional *Special Techniques* offer the examination approach for more uncommon conditions and special circumstances.

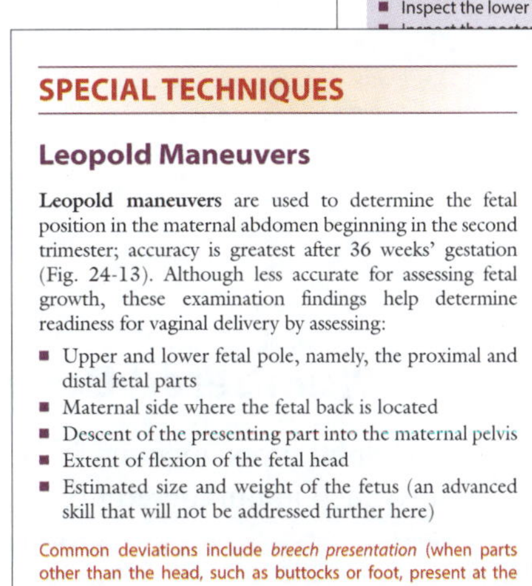
SPECIAL TECHNIQUES

Leopold Maneuvers

Leopold maneuvers are used to determine the fetal position in the maternal abdomen beginning in the second trimester; accuracy is greatest after 36 weeks' gestation (Fig. 24-13). Although less accurate for assessing fetal growth, these examination findings help determine readiness for vaginal delivery by assessing:

- Upper and lower fetal pole, namely, the proximal and distal fetal parts
- Maternal side where the fetal back is located
- Descent of the presenting part into the maternal pelvis
- Extent of flexion of the fetal head
- Estimated size and weight of the fetus (an advanced skill that will not be addressed further here)

Common deviations include *breech presentation* (when parts other than the head, such as buttocks or foot, present at the

HEALTH PROMOTION AND COUNSELING: EVIDENCE AND RECOMMENDATIONS

Important Topics for Health Promotion and Counseling

- Viral hepatitis
- Colon cancer

Viral Hepatitis

Hepatitis A. HAV infection is rarely fatal; it does not cause a chronic hepatitis, and deaths usually occur only in those with other liver diseases. Viral transmission is primarily person to person through the fecal–oral route and can be reduced by handwashing with soap and water after using the bathroom or changing diapers and before preparing or eating food.

The Advisory Committee on Immunization Practices (ACIP) recommends hepatitis A vaccination for all children at age 1 year, for persons with chronic liver

Health Promotion and Counseling: Evidence and Recommendations Sections

General health maintenance screening, counseling, and immunization topics occur as the last section in each chapter for easy access.

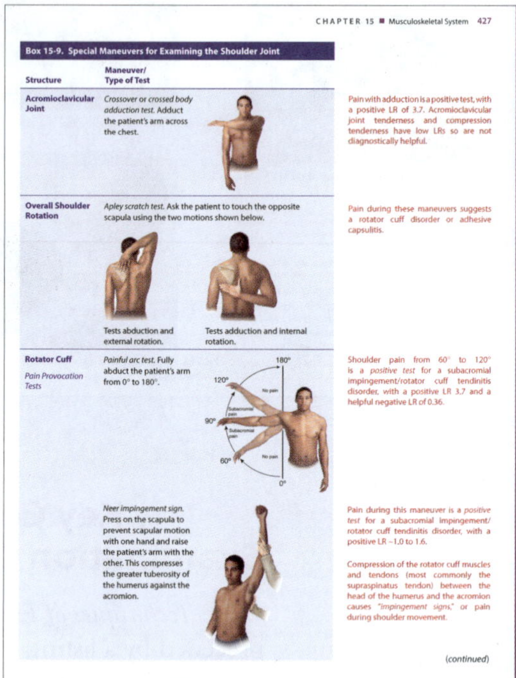

CHAPTER 15 ■ Musculoskeletal System 427

Box 15-9. Special Maneuvers for Examining the Shoulder Joint

Structure	Maneuver/ Type of Test	
Acromioclavicular Joint	*Crossover or crossed body adduction test.* Adduct the patient's arm across the chest.	Pain with adduction is a positive test, with a positive LR of 3.7. Acromioclavicular joint tenderness and compression tenderness have low LRs so are not diagnostically helpful.
Overall Shoulder Rotation	*Apley scratch test.* Ask the patient to touch the opposite scapula using the two motions shown below. Tests abduction and external rotation. Tests adduction and internal rotation.	Pain during these maneuvers suggests a rotator cuff disorder or adhesive capsulitis.
Rotator Cuff *Pain Provocation Tests*	*Painful arc test.* Fully abduct the patient's arm from 0° to 180°.	Shoulder pain from 60° to 120° is a *positive test* for a subacromial impingement/rotator cuff tendinitis disorder, with a positive LR 3.7 and a helpful negative LR of 0.36.
	Neer impingement sign. Press on the scapula to prevent scapular motion with one hand and raise the patient's arm with the other. This compresses the greater tuberosity of the humerus against the acromion.	Pain during this maneuver is a *positive test* for a subacromial impingement/rotator cuff tendinitis disorder, with a positive LR ~1.0 to 1.6. Compression of the rotator cuff muscles and tendons (most commonly the supraspinatus tendon) between the head of the humerus and the acromion causes *"impingement signs,"* or pain during shoulder movement.

(*continued*)

Photographs and Illustrations

The art program includes detailed, full-color photographs, drawings, and diagrams, some new or revised, to further illustrate key points in the text. They will enhance your learning potential by providing accurate and realistic representations.

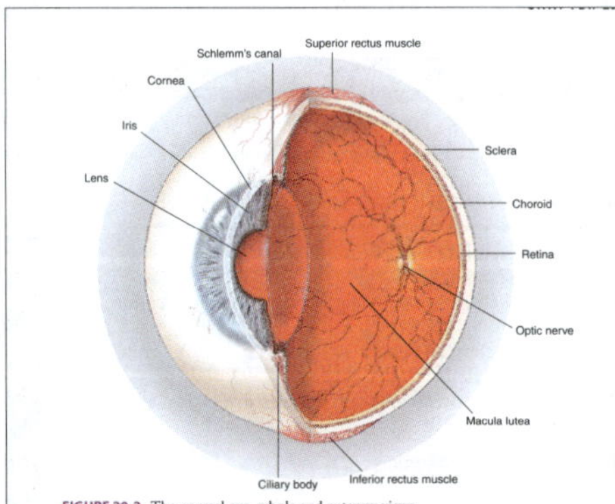

FIGURE 20-2. The normal eye, whole and cutaway views.

Each figure has a figure number and caption to make the figures easier to find and understand.

Numbered Boxes—NEW!

Helpful supplementary information is now provided in numbered boxes for easier location and reference.

Box 25-7. Exercise Recommendations for Older Adults

Adults need at least:

- 2 hours and 30 minutes (150 minutes) of moderate-intensity aerobic activity (i.e., brisk walking) every week **and**
- muscle-strengthening activities on two or more days a week that work all major muscle groups (legs, hips, back, abdomen, chest, shoulders, and arms)

OR

- 1 hour and 15 minutes (75 minutes) of vigorous-intensity aerobic activity (i.e., jogging or running) every week **and**
- muscle-strengthening activities on two or more days a week that work all major muscle groups (legs, hips, back, abdomen, chest, shoulders, and arms)

OR

- an equivalent mix of moderate- and vigorous-intensity aerobic activity **and**
- muscle-strengthening activities on two or more days a week that work all major muscle groups (legs, hips, back, abdomen, chest, shoulders, and arms)

Videos

Videos are a key adjunct for mastering the many techniques of physical examination. This edition includes 20 Objective Structured Clinical Examination (OSCE) videos of Physiology along with 16 OSCE videos of Medicine History Taking. We encourage students to study the written chapters and videos in tandem, often numerous times.

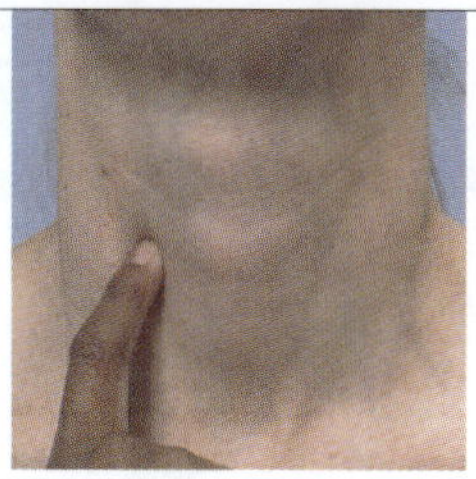

FIGURE 10-25. Palpating the trachea.

Physiology OSCE Video:
Palpation of Trachea

- Identify any *tender areas*

Tender pectoral muscles or costal cartilages suggest, but do not prove, that chest pain has a localized musculoskeletal origin.

- Assess for the presence of *bruising, sinus tracts*, or other *skin changes*.
- Assess *chest expansion*. Place your thumbs along each

Physiology OSCE Video:
Chest Movements

- Assess *tactile fremitus*. If needed, compare both sides of the chest, using the ball or ulnar surface of your hand. Fremitus is usually decreased or absent over the precordium. When examining a woman, gently displace the breasts as necessary (Fig. 10-27).

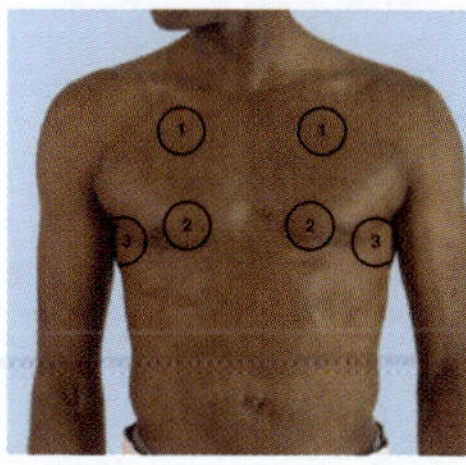

FIGURE 10-27. Locations for palpating tactile fremitus in the anterior chest.

Recording the Physical Examination of the Pregnant Woman

"32-year-old G3P1102 at 18 weeks' gestation by LMP presents to establish prenatal care. Pregnancy complicated by closely spaced pregnancies, prior iatrogenic preterm birth for preeclampsia, and prior cesarean delivery. Patient does not yet note fetal movement; denies contractions, vaginal bleeding, and leakage of fluids. On external examination, low-transverse cesarean scar is evident; fundus is palpable just below umbilicus. On internal examination, cervix is open to fingertip at the external os but closed at the internal os; cervix is 3 cm long; uterus enlarged to size consistent with 18-week gestation. Speculum examination shows leukorrhea with positive Chadwick sign. FHR by Doppler is between 140 and 145 BPM."

These findings describe the examination of a healthy pregnant woman at 18 weeks' gestation.

OR

"21-year-old G1P0 at 33 weeks' gestation as determined by 19-week ultrasound presents with chief complaint of decreased fetal movement. Pregnancy complicated by rare prenatal visits and homelessness. Patient reports minimal fetal movement over the last 24 hours; denies contractions, vaginal bleeding, or leakage of fluid. On external exam, a nontender gravid abdomen with no scars is noted; fundus is measured at 32 cm; fetus is vertex but not engaged in pelvis by Leopold maneuvers. On internal examination, cervix is closed, long, and high; speculum examination shows thin gray discharge with clue cells on wet mount. FHT by Doppler are between 155 and 160 BPM."

These findings describe the examination of a more complex presentation of a pregnant woman at 33 weeks' gestation.

Recording Your Findings

A well-organized clinical record must clearly display important clinical information and your clinical reasoning and plan. You will gain this skill and learn the descriptive vocabulary of physical findings in the *Recording Your Findings* section of each of the regional examination and special populations' chapters.

Suggested Readings

Consult the chapter-wise *Suggested Readings* given online to deepen your knowledge of important clinical conditions. The habit of searching the clinical literature will serve you and your patients well throughout your career.

Suggested Readings

Chapter 1—Approach to the Clinical Encounter

1. Athreya BH. *Handbook of Clinical Skills: A Practical Manual.* New Jersey: World Scientific; 2010.
2. Students TFotCSEoM. Recommendations for Clinical Skills Curricula for Undergraduate Medical Education. Association of American Medical Colleges. Available at https://members.aamc.org/eweb/upload/Recommendations%20for%20Clinical%20Skills%20Curricula%202005.pdf. Published 2005. Updated November 2005. Accessed March 29, 2019.
3. Fortin AV, Dwamena FC, Frankel RM, Smith RC. *Smith's Patient-Centered Interviewing: An Evidence-Based Method*; 2012.
4. Smith RC. An evidence-based infrastructure for patient- centered interviewing. In: Frankel RM, Quill TE, McDaniel SH, eds. *The Biopsychosocial Approach: Past, Present, and Future.* Rochester, NY: University of Rochester Press; 2003:148.
5. Kleinman A, Eisenberg L, Good B. Culture, illness, and care: clinical lessons from anthropologic and cross-cultural research. *Ann Intern Med.* 1978;88:251–258.
6. Mauksch L, Farber S, Greer HT. Design, dissemination, and evaluation of an advanced communication elective at seven U.S. medical schools. *Acad Med.* 2013;88:843–851.
7. Haidet P, Paterniti DA. "Building" a history rather than "taking" one: a perspective on information sharing during the medical interview. *Arch Intern Med.* 2003;163:1134–1140.
8. Stewart M. *Patient-Centered Medicine: Transforming the Clinical Method.* Abingdon, U.K.: Radcliffe Medical Press; 2003. Print.
9. Atlas SJ, Grant RW, Ferris TG, et al. Patient-physician connectedness and quality of primary care. *Ann Intern Med.* 2009;150:325–335.
10. Kurtz S, Silverman J, Benson J, et al. Marrying content and process in clinical method teaching: enhancing the Cal-

17. Matthews DA, Suchman AL, Branch WT. Making "connexions": enhancing the therapeutic potential of patient-clinician relationships. *Ann Intern Med.* 1993;118:973–977.
18. Larson EB, Yao X. Clinical empathy as emotional labor in the patient-physician relationship. *JAMA.* 2005;293:1100–1106.
19. Krasner MS, Epstein RM, Beckman H, et al. Association of an educational program in mindful communication with burnout, empathy, and attitudes among primary care physicians. *JAMA.* 2009;302:1284–1293.
20. Deutsch MB, Buchholz D. Electronic health records and transgender patients—practical recommendations for the collection of gender identity data. *J Gen Intern Med.* 2015; 30(6):843–847.
21. Makoul G, Zick A, Green M. An evidence-based perspective on greetings in medical encounters. *Arch Intern Med.* 2007;167:1172–1176.
22. Meiri N, Ankri A, Hamad-Saied M, et al. The effect of medical clowning on reducing pain, crying, and anxiety in children aged 2–10 years old undergoing venous blood drawing—a randomized controlled study. *Eur J Pediatr.* 2016;175(3): 373–379.
23. Meiri N, Ankri A, Ziadan F, et al. Assistance of medical clowns improves the physical examinations of children aged 2–6 years. *Isr Med Assoc J.* 2017;19(12):786–791.
24. Damm L, Leiss U, Habeler U, et al. Improving care through better communication: understanding the benefits. *J Pediatr.* 2015;166(5):1327–1328.
25. Drutz JE. The Pediatric Physical Examination: General Principles and Standard Measurements. UpToDate. Available at www.uptodate.com/contents/the-pediatric-physical-examination-general-principles-and-standard-measurements?search=pediatric%2Bphysical%2Bexam&source=search_result&selectedTitle=1~150&usage_type=default&display_rank=1. Published 2019.
26. Berlan ED, Bravender T. Confidentiality, consent, and caring

Table of Contents at a Glance

Detailed Table of Contents

CHAPTER **16**

Peripheral Vascular System 480

CHAPTER **17**

Breasts and Axillae 500

CHAPTER **18**

Skin, Hair, and Nails 512

CHAPTER **19**

Head and Neck 556

UNIT 4

Case-Based Learning 790

List of Tables

CHAPTER 13 Nervous System 300

CHAPTER 14 Genitourinary System 368

CHAPTER 15 Musculoskeletal System 413

CHAPTER 16 Peripheral Vascular System 480

CHAPTER 17 Breasts and Axillae 500

CHAPTER 18 Skin, Hair, and Nails 512

CHAPTER 19 Head and Neck 556

CHAPTER 20 Eyes 568

CHAPTER 21 Ears and Nose 600

CHAPTER 22 Throat and Oral Cavity 617

CHAPTER 23 Children: Infancy through Adolescence 634

CHAPTER 24 Pregnant Woman 741

CHAPTER 25 Older Adult 763

List of Videos

CBME Topics*

Competency-Based Undergraduate Curriculum Topics: Chapter-Wise Coverage

Competency Number	Description	Chapter No.
IM1.10	Elicit document and present an appropriate history that will establish the diagnosis, cause and severity of heart failure including: presenting complaints, precipitating and exacerbating factors, risk factors exercise tolerance, changes in sleep patterns, features suggestive of infective endocarditis	11
IM1.11	Perform and demonstrate a systematic examination based on the history that will help establish the diagnosis and estimate its severity including: measurement of pulse, blood pressure and respiratory rate, jugular venous forms and pulses, peripheral pulses, conjunctiva and fundus, lung, cardiac examination including palpation and auscultation with identification of heart sounds and murmurs, abdominal distension and splenic palpation	8, 11
IM1.12	Demonstrate peripheral pulse, volume, character, quality and variation in various causes of heart failure	8, 11
IM1.13	Measure the blood pressure accurately, recognise and discuss alterations in blood pressure in valvular heart disease and other causes of heart failure and cardiac tamponade	8, 11
IM1.14	Demonstrate and measure jugular venous distension	11
IM1.15	Identify and describe the timing, pitch quality conduction and significance of precordial murmurs and their variations	11
IM1.16	Generate a differential diagnosis based on the clinical presentation and prioritise it based on the most likely diagnosis	5
IM1.26	Develop document and present a management plan for patients with heart failure based on type of failure, underlying etiology	11
IM1.29	Elicit document and present an appropriate history, demonstrate correctly general examination, relevant clinical findings and formulate document and present a management plan for an adult patient presenting with a common form of congenital heart disease	8, 11
IM2.6	Elicit document and present an appropriate history that includes onset evolution, presentation risk factors, family history, comorbid conditions, complications, medication, history of atherosclerosis, IHD and coronary syndromes	11
IM2.7	Perform, demonstrate and document a physical examination including a vascular and cardiac examination that is appropriate for the clinical presentation	11
IM2.8	Generate document and present a differential diagnosis based on the clinical presentation and prioritise based on "cannot miss", most likely diagnosis and severity	11
IM2.24	Counsel and communicate to patients with empathy lifestyle changes in atherosclerosis/post coronary syndromes	11
IM3.4	Elicit document and present an appropriate history including the evolution, risk factors including immune status and occupational risk	11

*Reference: National Medical Commission. Competency Based Undergraduate Curriculum for the Indian Medical Graduate, Vol. 2 (2018), pages 60 to 142. Available at https://www.nmc.org.in/wp-content/uploads/2020/01/UG-Curriculum-Vol-II.pdf

AN = Human Anatomy; AS = Anesthesiology, CM = Community Medicine, CT = Respiratory Medicine, DR = Dermatology, Venereology, and Leprosy, IM = General Medicine, OG = Obstetrics and Gynaecology, PE = Pediatrics, PS = Psychiatry, PY = Physiology, SU = General Surgery.

Competency Number	Description	Chapter No.
IM3.5 (Pneumonia)	Perform, document and demonstrate a physical examination including general examination and appropriate examination of the lungs that establishes the diagnosis, complications and severity of disease	8, 10
IM3.6 (Pneumonia)	Generate document and present a differential diagnosis based on the clinical features, and prioritise the diagnosis based on the presentation	10
IM3.18 (Pneumonia)	Communicate and counsel patient on family on the diagnosis and therapy of pneumonia	10
IM3.19 (Pneumonia)	Discuss, describe, enumerate the indications and communicate to patients on pneumococcal and influenza vaccines	6
IM4.9	Elicit document and present a medical history that helps delineate the etiology of fever that includes the evolution and pattern of fever, associated symptoms, immune status, comorbidities, risk factors, exposure through occupation, travel and environment and medication use	8
IM4.10	Perform a systematic examination that establishes the diagnosis and severity of presentation that includes: general skin mucosal and lymph node examination, chest and abdominal examination (including examination of the liver and spleen)	8, 12
IM4.25 (Fever and febrile syndromes)	Communicate to the patient and family the diagnosis and treatment	3
IM5.9 (Liver disease)	Elicit document and present a medical history that helps delineate the etiology of the current presentation and includes clinical presentation, risk factors, drug use, sexual history, vaccination history and family history	12
IM5.10	Perform a systematic examination that establishes the diagnosis and severity that includes nutritional status, mental status, jaundice, abdominal distension ascites, features of portosystemic hypertension and hepatic encephalopathy	12
IM5.11	Generate a differential diagnosis and prioritise based on clinical features that suggest a specific etiology for the presenting symptom	3, 5
IM5.17	Enumerate the indications, precautions and counsel patients on vaccination for hepatitis	12
IM6.7 (HIV)	Elicit document and present a medical history that helps delineate the etiology of the current presentation and includes risk factors for HIV, mode of infection, other sexually transmitted diseases, risks for opportunistic infections and nutritional status	6
IM6.8 (HIV)	Generate a differential diagnosis and prioritise based on clinical features that suggest a specific etiology for the presenting symptom	5
IM6.19	Counsel patients on prevention of HIV transmission	6
IM6.20	Communicate diagnosis, treatment plan and subsequent follow up plan to patients	6
IM6.21	Communicate with patients on the importance of medication adherence	3
IM7.12	Perform a systematic examination of all joints, muscle and skin that will establish the diagnosis and severity of disease	15
IM7.13	Generate a differential diagnosis and prioritise based on clinical features that suggest a specific etiology	5, 15
IM8.10 (Hypertension)	Perform a systematic examination that includes: an accurate measurement of blood pressure, fundus examination, examination of vasculature and heart	8, 11, 16
IM8.10 (Hypertension)	Perform a systematic examination that includes: an accurate measurement of blood pressure, fundus examination, examination of vasculature and heart	8, 11
IM8.16 (Hypertension)	Develop and communicate to the patient lifestyle modification including weight reduction, moderation of alcohol intake, physical activity and sodium intake	6, 8
IM9.3 (Anemia)	Elicit document and present a medical history that includes symptoms, risk factors including GI bleeding, prior history, medications, menstrual history, and family history	3, 12
IM9.4 (Anemia)	Perform a systematic examination that includes : general examination for pallor, oral examination, DOAP session of hyper dynamic circulation, lymph node and splenic examination	8, 12

Competency Number	Description	Chapter No.
IM9.5 (Anemia)	Generate a differential diagnosis and prioritise based on clinical features that suggest a specific etiology	8
IM9.14	Describe the national programs for anemia prevention	6
IM9.20	Communicate and counsel patients with methods to prevent nutritional anemia	6
IM10.12 (Acute Kidney Injury and Chronic renal failure)	Elicit document and present a medical history that will differentiate the etiologies of disease, distinguish acute and chronic disease, identify predisposing conditions, nephrotoxic drugs and systemic causes	12
IM10.13 (Acute Kidney Injury and Chronic renal failure)	Perform a systematic examination that establishes the diagnosis and severity including determination of volume status, presence of edema and heart failure, features of uremia and associated systemic disease	8, 12
IM10.14 (Acute Kidney Injury and Chronic renal failure)	Generate a differential diagnosis and prioritise based on clinical features that suggest a specific etiology	12
IM10.24	Counsel patients on a renal diet	12
IM11.7 (Diabetes Mellitus)	Elicit document and present a medical history that will differentiate the etiologies of diabetes including risk factors, precipitating factors, lifestyle, nutritional history, family history, medication history, comorbidities and target organ disease	12
IM11.8 (Diabetes Mellitus)	Perform a systematic examination that establishes the diagnosis and severity that includes skin, peripheral pulses, blood pressure measurement, fundus examination, detailed examination of the foot (pulses, nervous and deformities and injuries)	8, 12
IM12.5 (Thyroid dysfunction)	Elicit document and present an appropriate history that will establish the diagnosis cause of thyroid dysfunction and its severity	19
IM12.6 (Thyroid dysfunction)	Perform and demonstrate a systematic examination based on the history that will help establish the diagnosis and severity including systemic signs of thyrotoxicosis and hypothyroidism, palpation of the pulse for rate and rhythm abnormalities neck palpation of the S SH Y Bed side clinic, DOAP session Skill assessment General Surgery the pulse for rate and rhythm abnormalities, neck palpation of the thyroid and lymph nodes and cardiovascular findings	8, 19
IM12.7	Demonstrate the correct technique to palpate the thyroid	19
IM12.8 (Thyroid dysfunction)	Generate a differential diagnosis based on the clinical presentation and prioritise it based on the most likely diagnosis	19
IM13.9	Demonstrate in a mannequin the correct technique for performing breast exam, rectal examination and cervical examination and pap smear.	17
IM14.6 (Obesity)	Elicit and document and present an appropriate history that includes the natural history, dietary history, modifiable risk factors, family history clues for secondary causes and motivation to lose weight	6
IM14.7 (Obesity)	Perform, document and demonstrate a physical examination based on the history that includes general examination, measurement of abdominal obesity, signs of secondary causes and comorbidities	6, 8
IM14.8 (Obesity)	Generate a differential diagnosis based on the presenting symptoms and clinical features and prioritise based on the most likely diagnosis	6
IM14.11 (Obesity)	Communicate and counsel patient on behavioural, dietary and lifestyle modifications	6

Competency Number	Description	Chapter No.
IM14.12 (Obesity)	Demonstrate an understanding of patient's inability to adhere to lifestyle instructions and counsel them in a non - judgemental way	6
IM15.4 (GI bleeding)	Elicit and document and present an appropriate history that identifies the route of bleeding, quantity, grade, volume loss, duration, etiology, comorbid illnesses and risk factors	12
IM15.5 (GI bleeding)	Perform, demonstrate and document a physical examination based on the history that includes general examination, volume assessment and appropriate abdominal examination	8, 12
IM15.6 (GI bleeding)	Distinguish between upper and lower gastrointestinal bleeding based on the clinical features	12
IM15.7 (GI bleeding)	Demonstrate the correct technique to perform an anal and rectal examination in a mannequin or equivalent	12
IM15.8 (GI bleeding)	Generate a differential diagnosis based on the presenting symptoms and clinical features and prioritise based on the most likely diagnosis	12
IM15.18 (GI bleeding)	Counsel the family and patient in an empathetic non-judgmental manner on the diagnosis and therapeutic options	12
IM16.4 (Diarrheal disorder)	Elicit and document and present an appropriate history that includes the natural history, dietary history, travel, sexual history and other concomitant illnesses	12
IM16.5 (Diarrheal disorder)	Perform, document and demonstrate a physical examination based on the history that includes general examination, including an appropriate abdominal examination	8, 12
IM16.6 (Diarrheal disorder)	Distinguish between diarrhoea and dysentery based on clinical features	12
IM16.7 (Diarrheal disorder)	Generate a differential diagnosis based on the presenting symptoms and clinical features and prioritise based on the most likely diagnosis	12
IM16.15 (Diarrheal disorder)	Distinguish based on the clinical presentation Crohn's disease from Ulcerative Colitis	12
IM17.2 (Headache)	Elicit and document and present an appropriate history including aura, precipitating aggravating and relieving factors, associated symptoms that help identify the cause of headaches	13
IM17.4 (Headache)	Perform and demonstrate a general neurologic examination and a focused examination for signs of intracranial tension including neck signs of meningitis	13
IM17.5 (Headache)	Generate document and present a differential diagnosis based on the clinical features and prioritise the diagnosis based on the clinical features, and prioritise the diagnosis based on the presentation	13
IM17.14 (Headache)	Counsel patients with migraine and tension headache on lifestyle changes and need for prophylactic therapy	13
IM18.3 (cerebrovascular accident)	Elicit and document and present an appropriate history including onset, progression, precipitating and aggravating relieving factors, associated symptoms that help identify the cause of the cerebrovascular accident	13
IM18.5 (cerebrovascular accident)	Perform, demonstrate & document physical examination that includes general and a detailed neurologic examination as appropriate, based on the history	13
IM18.6 (cerebrovascular accident)	Distinguish the lesion based on upper vs lower motor neuron, side, site and most probable nature of the lesion	13
IM18.7 (cerebrovascular accident)	Describe the clinical features and distinguish, based on clinical examination, the various disorders of speech	9, 13

Competency Number	Description	Chapter No.
IM18.17 (cerebrovascular accident)	Counsel patient and family about the diagnosis and therapy in an empathetic manner	1, 13
IM19.3 (Movement disorders)	Elicit and document and present an appropriate history including onset, progression precipitating and aggravating relieving factors, associated symptoms that help identify the cause of the movement disorders	13
IM19.4 (Movement disorders)	Perform, demonstrate and document a physical examination that includes a general examination and a detailed neurologic examination using standard movement rating scales	8, 13
IM19.5 (Movement disorders)	Generate document and present a differential diagnosis and prioritise based on the history and physical examination	13
IM19.6 (Movement disorders)	Make a clinical diagnosis regarding on the anatomical location, nature and cause of the lesion based on the clinical presentation and findings	13
IM24.2	Perform multidimensional geriatric assessment that includes medical, psycho-social and functional components	25
IM26.9	Identify, discuss and defend medicolegal, sociocultural, economic and ethical issues as it pertains to rights, equity and justice in access to health care	1
IM26.10	Identify, discuss and defend medicolegal, socio-cultural and ethical issues as it pertains to confidentiality in patient care	1
IM26.16	Identify, discuss and defend medicolegal, socio-cultural, professional and ethical issues as it pertains to the physician patient relationship (including fiduciary duty)	1
IM26.20	Demonstrate ability to communicate to patients in a patient, respectful, non threatening, non judgemental and empathetic manner	1
IM26.21	Demonstrate respect to patient privacy	1, 2
IM26.22	Demonstrate ability to maintain confidentiality in patient care	1
IM26.23	Demonstrate a commitment to continued learning	7
IM26 25	Demonstrate responsibility and work ethics while working in the health care team	1
IM26.26	Demonstrate ability to maintain required documentation in health care (including correct use of medical records)	1
IM26.27	Demonstrate personal grooming that is adequate and appropriate for health care responsibilities	1
IM26.32	Demonstrate appropriate respect to colleagues in the profession	1
IM26.33	Demonstrate an understanding of the implications and the appropriate procedures and response to be followed in the event of medical errors	1
IM26.34	Identify conflicts of interest in patient care and professional relationships and describe the correct response to these conflicts	1
IM26.35	Demonstrate empathy in patient encounters	1
IM26.36	Demonstrate ability to balance personal and professional priorities	1
IM26.37	Demonstrate ability to manage time appropriately	1
IM26.38	Demonstrate ability to form and function in appropriate professional networks	1
IM26.39	Demonstrate ability to pursue and seek career advancement	1
IM26.40	Demonstrate ability to follow risk management and medical error reduction practices where appropriate	1
IM26.41	Demonstrate ability to work in a mentoring relationship with junior colleagues	1
IM26.48	Demonstrate altruism	1
IM26.49	Administer informed consent and appropriately address patient queries to a patient being enrolled in a research protocol in a simulated environment	1

Competency Number	Description	Chapter No.
Human Anatomy		
AN24.2	Identify side, external features and relations of structures which form root of lung & bronchial tree and their clinical correlation	10
AN25.9	Demonstrate surface marking of lines of pleural reflection, Lung borders and fissures, Trachea	10
AN25.9	Demonstrate surface marking of Heart borders, Apex beat & Surface projection of valves of heart	11
AN35.5	Applied anatomy of cervical lymph nodes	8
Physiology		
PY4.10	Demonstrate the correct clinical examination of the abdomen in a normal volunteer or simulated environment	12
PY5.12	Record blood pressure & pulse at rest and in different grades of exercise and postures in a volunteer or simulated environment	8
PY5.15	Demonstrate the correct clinical examination of the cardiovascular system in a normal volunteer or simulated environment	11
PY6.9	Demonstrate the correct clinical examination of the respiratory system in a normal volunteer or simulated environment	10
PY10.11	Demonstrate the correct clinical examination of the nervous system: Higher functions, sensory system, motor system, reflexes, cranial nerves in a normal volunteer or simulated environment	13
PY10.20	Demonstrate (i) Testing of visual acuity, colour and field of vision in volunteer/simulated environment	20
PY10.20	Demonstrate (i) hearing and (ii) Testing for smell in volunteer/simulated environment	21
PY10.20	Demonstrate taste sensation in volunteer/simulated environment	22
PY11.13	Obtain history and perform general examination in the volunteer/simulated environment	8
Community Medicine		
CM7.6	Enumerate and evaluate the need of screening tests	7
Dermatology, Venereology & Leprosy		
DR5.2	Identify and differentiate scabies from other lesions	18
DR6.2	Identify and differentiate pediculosis from other skin lesions	18
Anesthesiology		
AS7.3	Observe and describe the management of an unconscious patient	13
AS8.2	Elicit and determine the level, quality and quantity of pain and its tolerance in patient or surrogate	8
Psychiatry		
PS3.5	Perform, demonstrate and document a mini-mental examination	9
Obstetrics & Gynaecology		
OG8.3	Describe, demonstrate, document and perform an obstetrical examination including a general and abdominal examination and clinical monitoring of maternal and foetal well-being;	24
OG17.2	Counsel in a simulated environment, care of the breast, importance and the technique of breastfeeding	17, 24
OG18.2	Demonstrate the steps of neonatal resuscitation in a simulated environment	24
OG19.2	Counsel in a simulated environment, contraception and puerperal sterilisation	24
OG35.4	Demonstrate interpersonal and communication skills befitting a physician in order to discuss illness and its outcome with patient and family	24
OG35.5	Determine gestational age, EDD and obstetric formula	24
OG35.7	Obtain informed consent for any examination/procedure	24
OG35.8	Write a complete case record with all necessary details	24
OG35.11	Demonstrate the correct use of appropriate universal precautions for self-protection against HIV and hepatitis and counsel patients	24

Competency Number	Description	Chapter No.
OG35.12	Obtain a PAP smear in a stimulated environment	24
Pediatrics		
PE1.4	Perform Anthropometric measurements, document in growth charts and interpret	23
PE1.6	Discuss the methods of assessment of development	23
PE1.7	Perform Developmental assessment and interpret	23
PE2.2	Assessment of a child with failing to thrive including eliciting an appropriate history and examination	23
PE2.5	Assessment of a child with short stature: Elicit history, perform examination, document and present	23
PE3.3	Assessment of a child with developmental delay - Elicit document and present history	23
PE3.4	Counsel a parent of a child with developmental delay	23
PE3.7	Visit a Child Developmental Unit and observe its functioning	23
PE6.9	Perform routine Adolescent Health check-up including eliciting history, performing examination including SMR (Sexual Maturity Rating), growth assessments (using Growth charts) and systemic exam including thyroid and Breast exam and the HEADSS screening	23
PE7.5	Observe the correct technique of breast feeding and distinguish right from wrong techniques	23
PE7.7	Perform breast examination and identify common problems during lactation such as retracted nipples, cracked nipples, breast engorgement, breast abscess	17, 23
PE7.8	Educate mothers on antenatal breast care and prepare mothers for lactation	23
PE7.9	Educate and counsel mothers for best practices in Breast feeding	23
PE7.10	Respects patient privacy	1, 23
PE7.10	Respects patient privacy	4
PE8 4	Elicit history on the Complementary Feeding habits	23
PE8.5	Counsel and educate mothers on the best practices in Complementary Feeding	23
PE9.4	Elicit document and present an appropriate nutritional history and perform a dietary recall	23
PE9.5	Calculate the age-related calorie requirement in Health and Disease and identify gap	23
PE9.6	Assess and classify the nutrition status of infants, children and adolescents and recognize deviations	23
PE10.3	Assessment of a patient with SAM and MAM, diagnosis, classification and planning management including hospital and community-based intervention, rehabilitation and prevention	23
PE11.3	Assessment of a child with obesity with regard to eliciting history including physical activity, charting and dietary recall	23
PE11.4	Examination including calculation of BMI, measurement of waist hip ratio, identifying external markers like acanthosis, striae, pseudogynecomastia, etc	23
PE11.5	Calculate BMI, document in BMI chart and interpret	23
PE12.3	Identify the clinical features of dietary deficiency/excess of Vitamin A	23
PE12 8	Identify the clinical features of dietary deficiency of Vitamin D	23
PE12.17	Identify the clinical features of Vitamin B complex deficiency	23
PE12.18	Diagnose patients with Vitamin B complex deficiency and plan management	23
PE12.21	Identify the clinical features of Vitamin C deficiency	23
PE18.3	Conduct Antenatal examination of women independently and apply at-risk approach in antenatal care	24
PE18.4	Provide antenatal care and conduct a normal Delivery in a simulated environment	24
PE18.6	Perform Postnatal assessment of newborn and mother, provide advice on breastfeeding, weaning and on family planning	23
PE18.6	Perform Postnatal assessment of newborn and mother, provide advice on breastfeeding, weaning and on family planning	24

Competency Number	Description	Chapter No.
PE19.6	Assess patient for fitness for immunisation and prescribe an age-appropriate immunisation schedule	23
PE19.7	Educate and counsel a patient for immunisation	23
PE19.11	Document Immunisation in an immunisation record	23
PE19.14	Practice Infection control measures and appropriate handling of the sharps	23
PE19.15	Explain the term implied consent in Immunisation services	23
PE20.4	Assessment of a normal neonate	23
PE20.6	Explain the follow up care for neonates including Breastfeeding, temperature maintenance, immunisation, importance of growth monitoring and red flag	6, 24
PE21.8	Elicit, document and present a history pertaining to diseases of the Genitourinary tract	23
PE21.9	Identify external markers for kidney disease, like Failing to thrive, hypertension, pallor, Ichthyosis, anasarca	23
PE21.10	Analyse symptom and interpret the physical findings and arrive at an appropriate provisional/ differential diagnosis	23
PE23.7	Elicit appropriate history for a cardiac disease, analyse the symptoms e.g., breathlessness, chest pain, tachycardia, feeding difficulty, failing to thrive, reduced urinary output, swelling, syncope, cyanotic spells, Suck rest cycle, frontal swelling in infants. Document and present	23
PE23.8	Identify external markers of a cardiac disease e.g., Cyanosis, Clubbing, dependent edema, dental caries, arthritis, erythema rash, chorea, subcutaneous nodules, Osler's node, Janeway lesions and document	23
PE23.9	Record pulse, blood pressure, temperature and respiratory rate and interpret as per the age	8, 23, 24
PE23.10	Perform independently examination of the cardiovascular system – look for precordial bulge, pulsations in the precordium, JVP and its significance in children and infants, relevance of percussion in Paediatric examination, Auscultation and other system examination and document	23
PE24.9	Elicit, document and present history pertaining to diarrheal diseases	23
PE24.10	Assess for signs of dehydration, document and present	8, 23
PE26.5	Elicit document and present the history related to diseases of Gastrointestinal system	23
PE26.6	Identify external markers for GI and Liver disorders e.g., Jaundice, Pallor, Gynaecomastia, Spider angioma, Palmar erythema, Ichthyosis, Caput medusa, Clubbing, failing to thrive, Vitamin A and D deficiency	8, 23
PE26.7	Perform examination of the abdomen, demonstrate organomegaly, ascites etc.	23
PE26.8	Analyse symptoms and interpret physical signs to make a provisional/differential diagnosis	23
PE27.22	Assess level of consciousness & provide emergency treatment to a child with convulsions/coma - Position an unconscious child - Position a child with suspected trauma - Administer IV/per rectal Diazepam for a convulsing child in a simulated environment	23
PE27 23	Assess for signs of severe dehydration	8, 23
PE27.27	Assess for hypothermia and maintain temperature	8, 23
PE27.31	Assess child for signs of abuse	23
PE27.32	Counsel parents of dangerously ill/terminally ill child to break bad news	23
PE27.33	Obtain Informed Consent	23
PE28.9	Elicit, document and present age-appropriate history of a child with upper respiratory problem including Stridor	23
PE28.10	Perform otoscopic examination of the ear	23
PE28.11	Perform throat examination using tongue depressor	23
PE28 12	Perform examination of the nose	23
PE28.13	Analyse the clinical symptoms and interpret physical findings and make a provisional/differential diagnosis in a child with ENT symptoms	23

Competency Number	Description	Chapter No.
PE29.11	Identify external markers for haematological disorders e.g.. Jaundice, Pallor, Petechiae purpura, Ecchymosis, Lymphadenopathy, bone tenderness, loss of weight, Mucosal and large joint bleed	8, 23
PE29.12	Perform examination of the abdomen, demonstrate organomegaly	23
PE29.13	Analyse symptoms and interpret physical signs to make a provisional/differential diagnosis	23
PE29.19	Counsel and educate patients about prevention and treatment of anemia	23
PE30.17	Elicit document and present an age-appropriate history pertaining to the CNS	23
PE30.18	Demonstrate the correct method for physical examination of CNS including identification of external markers. Document and present clinical findings	23
PE30.19	Analyse symptoms and interpret physical findings and propose a provisional/differential diagnosis	23
PE33.7	Perform genital examination and recognize Ambiguous Genitalia and refer appropriately	23
PE33.9	Perform Sexual Maturity Rating (SMR) and interpret	23
PE33.10	Recognize precocious and delayed Puberty and refer	23
PE33.11	Identify deviations in growth and plan appropriate referral	23
PE34.5	Able to elicit, document and present history of contact with tuberculosis in every patient encounter	23
General Surgery		
SU22.3	Demonstrate and document the correct clinical examination of thyroid swellings and discus the differential diagnosis and their management	19
SU25.5	Demonstrate the correct technique to palpate the breast for breast swelling in a mannequin or equivalent	17
SU27.2	Demonstrate the correct examination of the vascular system and enumerate and describe the investigation of vascular disease	16
SU27.5	Describe the applied anatomy of venous system of lower limb	16
SU27.6	Describe pathophysiology, clinical features, Investigations and principles of management of DVT and Varicose veins	16
SU27.8	Demonstrate the correct examination of the lymphatic system	16
SU28.2	Demonstrate the correct technique to examine the patient with hernia and identify different types of hernias.	12
SU28.9	Demonstrate the correct technique of examination of a patient with disorders of the stomach	12
SU28.18	Describe and demonstrate clinical examination of abdomen. Order relevant investigations. Describe and discuss appropriate treatment plan	12
Physical Medicine & Rehabilitation		
PM4.5	Demonstrate correct assessment of muscle strength and range of movements	15
PM7.4	Assess bowel and bladder function and identify common patterns of bladder dysfunction	12
Respiratory Medicine		
CT2.21	Describe discuss and counsel patients appropriately on smoking cessation	6

UNIT 1

Foundations of Health Assessment

CHAPTER 1

Approach to the Clinical Encounter

> *"The ritual of one individual coming to another and telling him things that she would not tell her preacher or rabbi; and then, incredibly, on top of that, disrobing and allowing touch…I think our skills in examining a patient have to be worthy of that kind of trust."*
>
> ~Abraham Verghese, MD, A Doctor's Touch, TEDGlobal, 2011.

FOUNDATIONAL SKILLS ESSENTIAL TO THE CLINICAL ENCOUNTER

As you embark on clinical training, you will acquire a growing array of time-honored skills that deepen your patient relationships and acumen in patient care. A *clinical skill* is any discrete act within the overall process of patient care. Clinical skills are the singular elements that constitute clinical competence. The purposeful selection and integration of this set of individual skillful acts during the patient encounter lay the foundation for clinical care. These skills evolve with each patient as you develop your professional relationship, take the clinical history, perform a mental and physical examination, initiate clinical tests or procedures, and undertake diagnostic and therapeutic interventions.

The acquisition and effective implementation of clinical skills is fundamentally developmental in nature and grows over time. To become a skilled clinician, you need to integrate contemporary biomedicine in a professional manner into the care of your patients within their personal, cultural, and social life context. As a student, you acquire these clinical skills as you move to active patient assessment, gradually at first, but then with growing confidence and expertise, and ultimately clinical competence. In doing so, you must commit to ongoing practice and honesty in self-assessment.

The initial chapters in this unit will introduce you to the essentials of the clinical encounter, especially establishing trust—the foundation of your therapeutic alliance with patients (Fig. 1-1). At first, you will focus on gathering information, but with experience and empathic listening, you will allow the patient's story to unfold in its most authentic and detailed form. From mastery of these skills and the mutual trust and respect of caring patient relationships, emerge the timeless rewards of the clinical professions. These are the fundamental features of all clinical care.

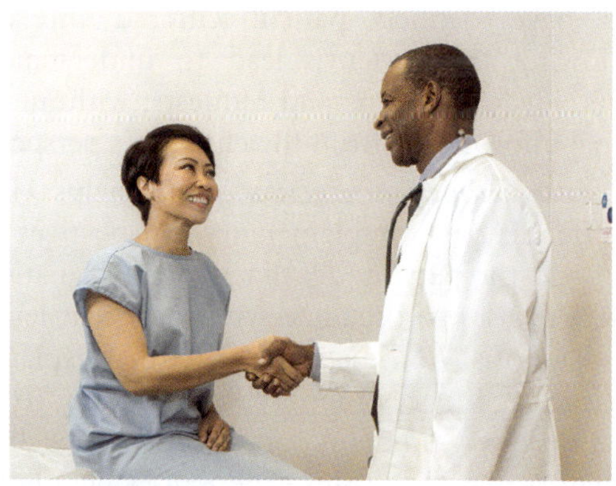

FIGURE 1-1. Therapeutic alliance between clinician and patient.

APPROACH TO THE CLINICAL ENCOUNTER

The approach to a clinical encounter is *both* clinician-centered and patient-centered. In the more symptom-focused *clinician-centered* approach, the clinician "takes charge of the interaction to meet his or her own need to acquire the symptoms, their details, and other data that will help him or her identify a disease," which, if used exclusively, can often bypass the personal dimensions of the

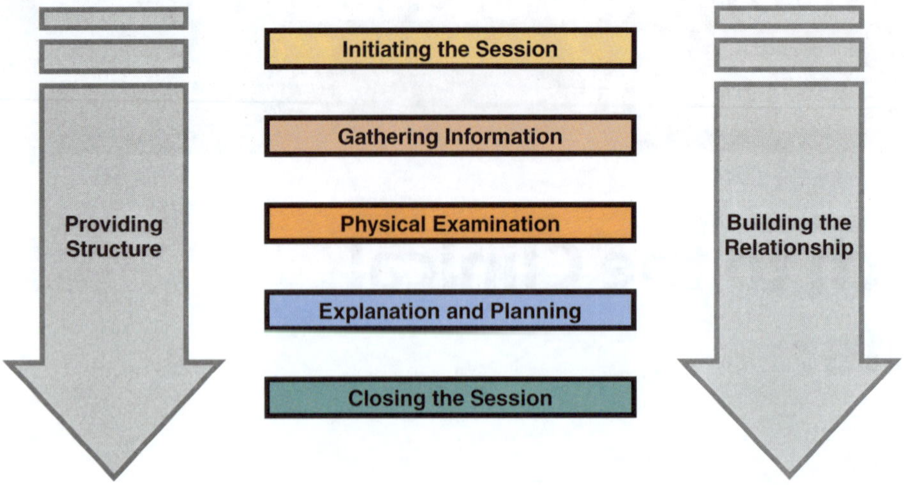

FIGURE 1-2. Enhanced Calgary–Cambridge Guides. Enhanced Calgary-Cambridge Guides: Structure and timeline of the clinical encounter. (Reproduced from Kurtz S et al. *Acad Med.* 2003;78(8):802–809.)

illness. This framework emphasizes the features of disease at the expense of needs and perspectives of the patient. As a consequence, information required to understand and manage patients' problems may never be elicited.

In contrast, the *patient-centered* approach "recognizes the importance of patients' expressions of personal concerns, feelings, and emotions" and evokes "the personal context of the patient's symptoms and disease." Experts have defined patient-centered interviewing as "following the patient's lead to understand their thoughts, ideas, concerns and requests, without adding additional information from the clinician's perspective."

The *disease/illness distinction model* helps elucidate these different yet complementary perspectives of the clinician and the patient. *Disease* is the explanation that the *clinician* uses to organize symptoms that leads to a clinical diagnosis. *Illness* is a construct that explains how the *patient* experiences the disease, including its effects on relationships, function, and sense of well-being. Many factors may shape this experience, including prior personal or family health, its impact on everyday life, the patient's outlook, style of coping, and expectations about care. The clinical interview needs to incorporate both the clinician's and the patient's views of reality, disease, and illness.

For example, if you are seeing a patient with a sore throat, you may focus on specific points in the history that differentiate streptococcal pharyngitis from other etiologies, or on your patient's questionable history of allergy to penicillin. However, your patient may in fact be worried about pain and difficulty swallowing, missing time from work, or a cousin who had sore throat and was later diagnosed to have throat cancer. As you can see, even a straightforward symptom like sore throat can illustrate these divergent concerns. Therefore an effective and skilled patient–clinician encounter merges both the patient-centered and clinician-centered approaches.

Evidence suggests that integrating these approaches leads to a more complete picture of the patient's illness and allows clinicians to more fully convey the caring attributes of "respect, empathy, humility, and sensitivity." Evidence also shows that this merged approach is not only more satisfying for the patient and the clinician, but also more effective in achieving desired health outcomes. Using both approaches in your clinical encounters results in looking at patients' problems from two perspectives: your own as well as theirs. The balance between these two essential components results in an effective clinical interview in a patient encounter.

An illustrative example of this framework is the enhanced *Calgary–Cambridge Guides* (Fig. 1-2) which describe the structure and timeline of the clinical encounter and highlight the need to elicit information regarding both the biomedical disease process and the patient's perspective. They also include a place for the physical examination. The structure includes five major steps: *initiating the session, information gathering, the physical examination, explaining and planning*, and *closing the session*.

STRUCTURE AND SEQUENCE OF THE CLINICAL ENCOUNTER

In general, an effective clinical encounter moves through a logical sequence (Box 1-1). In this chapter we focus on the behaviors related to the initiation and closure of the clinical encounter as well as the exploration of the patient's perspectives of his or her illness. The succeeding

Box 1-1. General Structure and Sequence of the Clinical Encounter

1. Initiating the encounter
   - Setting the stage/preparation
   - Greeting the patient and establishing initial rapport
2. Gathering information
   - Initiating information gathering
   - Exploring patient's perspective of illness
   - Exploring biomedical perspective of disease including relevant background and context
3. Performing the physical examination
4. Explaining and planning
   - Provide correct amount and type of information
   - Negotiate plan of action
   - Shared decision making
5. Closing the encounter

Note: Two additional frameworks occur as continuous threads throughout the sequence—namely, building the relationship and structuring the interview (see Fig. 1-2).

Source: Adapted from Kurtz S et al. *Acad Med.* 2003;78(8):802–809; van de Poel K et al. *Communication Skills for Foreign and Mobile Medical Professionals.* Springer; 2013:xvii, 145; de Haes et al. *Patient Educ Couns.* 2009;74:287–294.

chapters will focus on behaviors that explore the clinician's perspective of disease including relevant patient background and context (Chapter 3), the physical examination (Chapter 4) and the explanation of the differential diagnosis and plan (Chapter 5). The wide variety of verbal and nonverbal communication skills and general strategies which contribute to enhance your clinical encounters are detailed in Chapter 2.

Stage 1: Initiating the Encounter

This is the stage of relationship building with your patient. Fostering the patient–clinician relationship is critical because without a good relationship none of the other goals of the clinical encounter can be pursued in an optimal manner. Respect trust, and rapport are necessary components of a therapeutic relationship that is just beginning.

Set the Stage. Prepare for the interview. Check your appearance. Make sure the patient is comfortable and the environment is conducive to the very personal information soon to be shared. You will find that each interview has its own rhythm and sequence. Master the steps described. Finally, the interview has important societal dimensions. Reflect on any biases you have that color your reactions to the patient and the therapeutic alliance you need to create.

Adjust the Environment. Make the interview setting as private and comfortable as possible. You may have to talk with the patient in surroundings like a two-bedded hospital room or the corridor of a busy emergency department. Making the environment as confidential as possible improves communication. If there are privacy curtains, try to pull them shut. Suggest moving to an empty room instead of talking in a waiting area. If possible, adjust the room temperature for the patient's comfort. *As the clinician, it is part of your role to make the patient more comfortable.* These efforts are always worth the time.

Consider the best way to *arrange the room* and how close you should be to the patient. Remember that many factors may influence preferences about interpersonal space such as cultural background and individual taste. Choose a distance that facilitates conversation and allows good eye contact. You should probably be within several feet, close enough to hear and be heard clearly. Pull up a chair and, if possible, sit at eye level with the patient. Move physical barriers like bed railings or bedside tables out of the way (Fig. 1-3). In an outpatient setting, sitting on a rolling stool, for example, allows you to change distances in response to patient cues. Avoid arrangements that convey disrespect, like interviewing a woman already positioned for a pelvic examination or with your back facing the patient while washing your hands. Position a computer monitor so as not to obstruct your view of the patient or hide your face from the patient. Also position the monitor so you can easily swivel its base if necessary, to show information on the screen such as a radiographic image or laboratory result value. Lighting also makes a difference. If you sit between a patient and a bright light or window the patient may have to squint to see you, lending the interaction an air of interrogation.

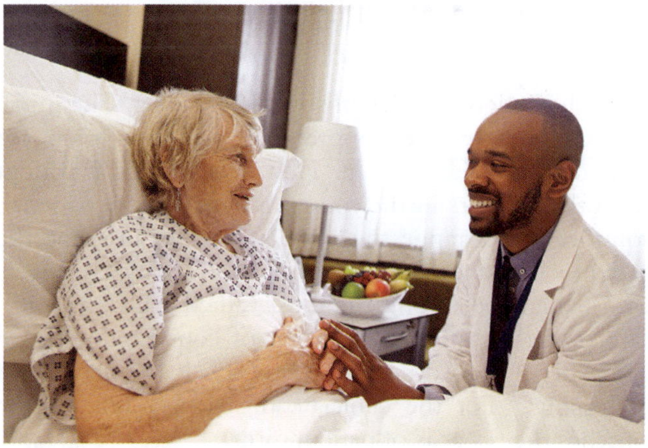

FIGURE 1-3. Move physical barriers out of the way and sit at eye level. (Used with permission from Shutterstock. By Monkey Business Images.)

Review the Clinical Record. Before seeing the patient, *review the clinical record* (Fig. 1-4). This provides important background information and suggests areas you need to explore. Review identifying data such as

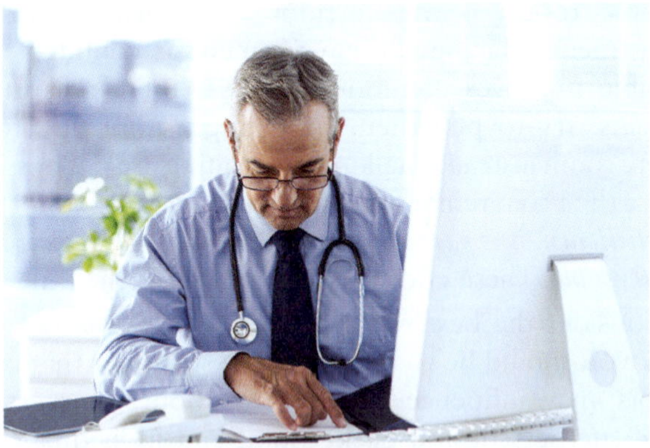

FIGURE 1-4. Review the health record before the clinical encounter. (Used with permission from Shutterstock. By wavebreakmedia.)

age, gender, address, and insurance. Review the patient's medications and allergies. Even though the clinical record usually contains past diagnoses and treatments, you need to make your own assessment based on what you learn from the visit ahead.

Set Your Agenda. Before you talk with the patient, clarify your goals for the interview. As a student, your primary purpose may be to complete a comprehensive history required for your rotation. As an advanced trainee or practicing clinician, your goals can range from assessing a new concern, to treatment follow-up, to completing forms. The clinician must balance these provider-centered goals with patient-centered goals. Weighing multiple agendas arising from the needs of the patient, the patient's family, and health care agencies and facilities. Taking a few minutes to think about your goals makes it easier to align your priorities with the patient's agenda.

Greet the Patient and Establish Initial Rapport. The initial moments of your encounter lay the foundation for your ongoing relationship. How you greet the patient and other visitors in the room, provide for the patient's comfort, and arrange the physical setting, all shape the patient's first impressions (Fig. 1-5). Relating effectively with patients is among the most valued skills of clinical care. For the patient, "a feeling of connectedness… of being deeply heard and understood… is the very heart of healing." For the clinician, this deeper relationship enriches the rewards of patient care.

As you begin, *welcome the patient by introducing yourself*, giving your own first and last name. If possible, shake hands with the patient. If this is the first time you are seeing the patient, explain your role, your status as a student or trainee, and how you will be involved in their care.

Identify Patient Title, Name, and Preferred Gender Pronoun. As much as possible, let the patient dictate how they would like to be addressed (Box 1-2). Clinicians should ask all patients their *preferred name* and *gender pronouns*, ideally at the beginning of the visit and/or on an intake questionnaire. This includes formal titles such as Mr., Mrs., Ms. or honorifics such as Professor or Doctor. This not only provides valuable information about the patient's identity but is also important in establishing rapport and showing respect, especially if you are seeing the patient for the first time. This promotes a welcoming environment, especially those individuals whose preferred titles or names do not conform to societal norms.

The *preferred name* may be a nickname (e.g., "Raju" for "Rajesh"), use of a middle name, or some other name altogether. After stating your name, ask the patient what name they would like to be called. If you are unsure how to pronounce the patient's name, don't be afraid to ask. You can say, "I am afraid of mispronouncing your name. Could you say it for me?" Then repeat it to make sure that you heard it correctly. For transgender and gender nonbinary patients, the preferred name may match their affirmed gender and also be recognizable as a different gender than the name assigned at birth.

Except with children or adolescents, avoid first names until you have specific permission. Calling a patient *"dear," "sweetie"* or overly familiar names can depersonalize and demean.

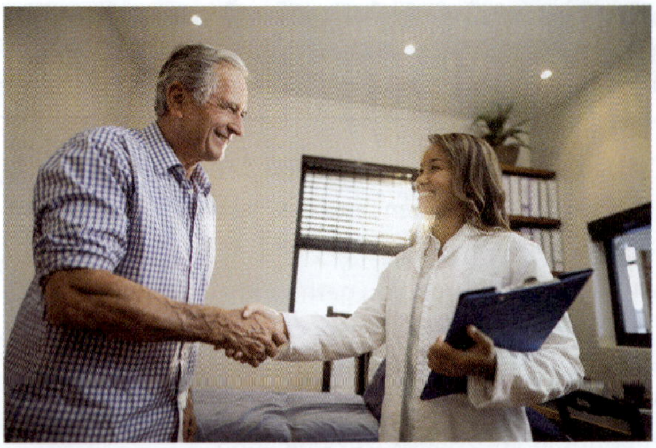

FIGURE 1-5. Greeting the patient and establishing rapport. (Used with permission from Shutterstock. By wavebreakmedia.)

Box 1-2. Obtaining Patients' Preferred Method of Address

Example:

Student: *"Good morning. I am Susanth Gupta, a third-year medical student. I am part of the clinical team taking care of you. I am here to assist them figure out how we can best help you. Are you Ramesh Shetty?"*

Patient: *"Yes."*

Student: *"How would you like me to address you?"*

Patient: *"You can call me Mr. Ramesh."* Or, *"Shetty is also fine."*

Box 1-3. Obtaining Patients' Gender Pronoun

Example:
Student: *"Good morning. I am Susanth Gupta, a third-year medical student. I am part of the clinical team taking care of you and will assist them figure out how we can best help you. Are you Ramesh Shetty?"*
Patient: *"Yes."*
Student: *"How would you like me to address you?"*
Patient: *"You can call me Mr. Ramesh."* Or, *"Shetty is also fine."*
Student: *"It is a pleasure to meet you, Mr. Ramesh. Please call me Susanth. May I ask you a few more background questions before we start?"*
Patient: *"Sure."*
Student: *"In our effort to promote an inclusive and respectful environment, we use pronouns that are right for us. The pronouns I prefer when others talk about me are 'she' and' 'her.' How about you? What pronouns do you prefer?"*
Patient: *"I use 'he' and 'him', I guess."*

The concept of gender is evolving, and therefore so are gender identities. All patients, regardless of gender identity, have *pronouns*. When asking patients about their pronouns, it can be helpful to share your own pronouns with patients, asking: "Which gender pronouns do you use?" (Box 1-3). For example, "I use... he and him/she and hers/they and theirs." Some of your patients may use nontraditional pronouns.

It is important to then use the title, name, and pronoun the patient has provided, both with the patient but also when talking about the patient to other clinicians and staff. Referring to a patient with the wrong name or pronoun, can make them feel disrespected, invalidated, dismissed, alienated, or dysphoric.

It is not always possible to avoid making mistakes and simple apologies can go a long way. If you do slip, you can say something like: "I apologize for using the wrong pronoun or preferred name. I did not mean to disrespect you." It can be tempting to overstate how badly you feel about making a mistake, but that would only make the mis-gendered patient feel more awkward and inclined to comfort you, which is not appropriate.

Approach to Establishing Rapport with Specific Populations

Newborns and Infants. It is obvious that newborns (birth to 30 days) and infants (1 month to 1 year) will not be able to communicate like older children, but that does not mean that building rapport is any less important. Never forget that having a baby is a major milestone in many people's lives; congratulate the family on the new baby if appropriate for the circumstances. Encourage the caregivers to feed the baby either while you are talking or before the encounter begins to help keep the baby calm and relaxed. This will also naturally lead into a good feeding history. Although newborns may not be able to talk with you, they will still react to the emotional and physical cues that you convey, so keep your voice calm. Encourage caregivers to hold the baby wherever they are most comfortable for as much of the encounter as possible. It is often helpful to begin a newborn or infant encounter by focusing on the caregivers and asking about their well-being. This makes it obvious that you are caring as much for them as their child and typically helps them feel at ease, while allowing you to introduce quick screening questions about family health topics.

Young and School-Aged Children. Young (1 to 4 years) and school-aged children (5 to 10 years) can be among the most challenging patients. The school-aged years are characterized by increasing feelings of autonomy, socialization, and curiosity, all things to which you as a clinician will need to be sensitive (Fig. 1-6). For a young child, you may come into a room and find your patient in a tantrum before you even begin. Distraction and mood management are essential. Beginning the encounter from a place of play is a great way to build rapport with the child and the parents. Luckily many of the important milestones to assess in this age group are typical ways of playing, that is, jumping, drawing, imitation, and throwing a ball. Begin the encounter by introducing yourself to the patient first and then to the family. While the child is scribbling, playing with a stuffed animal or drawing, take this opportunity to obtain the health history from the caregiver. When possible, pull the school-aged child into the interview by asking age-appropriate questions. You should ask caregivers to confirm or elaborate as needed. A final tip for this age group and for school-aged children is to brush up on your "kid culture." Correctly identifying a character on a piece of clothing or backpack can do wonders for your relationship with a child.

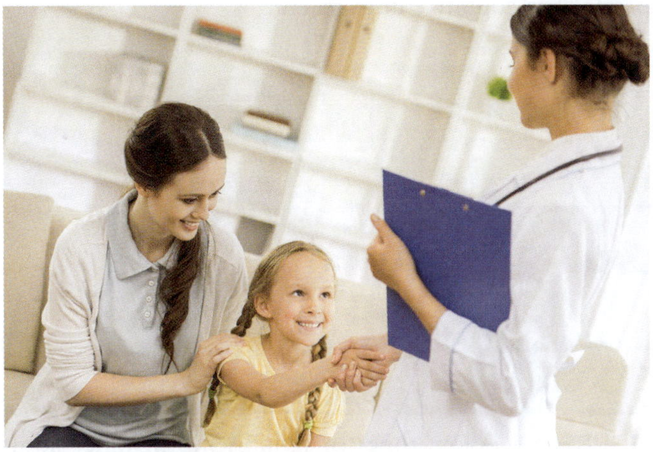

FIGURE 1-6. Establishing rapport with child and parent. (Used with permission from Shutterstock. By VGstockstudio.)

Adolescents. Adolescents generally want to be treated as adults and to be given respect and choices. Commonly, the most challenging part of this encounter for clinicians is balancing the needs of the family and the autonomy of the adolescent. It is important that you direct questions to and obtain responses from your adolescent patient while at the same time ensuring that family members and caregivers feel comfortable and that their concerns are heard. Sometimes it is helpful to delineate those expectations at the start of the encounter. Let the family know that they will have the opportunity to speak with you; however, you would like to hear from your adolescent patient first. Provide ample opportunity for the adolescent to share questions or concerns with you through the use of broad open-ended questions. Additionally, a significant part of these clinical encounters is the increasing amount of time you will spend with your adolescent patient alone without any family members present. During this time, it is critical that you acknowledge the confidentiality and trust inherent to that space.

Older Adults. As a student, you are likely to be much younger than patients in this age group (Fig. 1-7). Be sure to elicit from older patients their preferred way of being addressed. As mentioned earlier, calling an older adult patient overly familiar names can be perceived as depersonalizing and demeaning. Take the time to adjust the environment of the office, hospital, or nursing home to put your older adult patient at ease. Recall the physiologic changes in aging. Provide a well-lit, moderately warm setting with minimal background noise, chairs with arms, and access to the examining table. Provide enough space in the examination room for the older adult to safely navigate especially if ambulating with an assistive device such as a cane or a walker. Allow time for open-ended questions and reminiscing; include family and caregivers when indicated, especially if the patient has cognitive impairment.

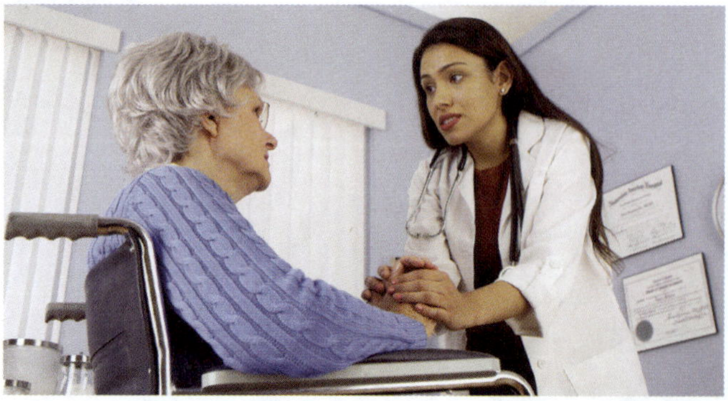

FIGURE 1-7. Allow time for reminiscing in older adult patient encounters. (Used with permission from Shutterstock. By Rocketclips, Inc.)

Patients with Physical and Sensory Disabilities. Use "people-first" language especially when referring to patients with disabilities (e.g., person who is blind, person who uses a wheelchair, person with hearing loss) unless the patient asks to be referred to in another manner. Always presume that patients with physical and/or sensory disabilities are competent to handle their own medical care. It is important to avoid making assumptions about what assistance the patient needs. Ask how you can help and respect their answers. You should always speak directly with the patient with and not to an aide companion. If a patient came into the room alone, do not ask whether they are accompanied. Box 1-4 provides guidelines on establishing rapport with patients with disabilities.

Box 1-4. Establishing Rapport with Patients with Physical and Sensory Disabilities

- Based on 2010 global population estimates more than a billion people (15% of the world's population) are estimated to live with some form of disability.

Patients Who Are Blind or Have Low Vision

- Always verbally identify yourself when you approach and introduce other people in the room.
- Do not leave without letting the patient know.
- Ask before you help. Always ask how the patient would like to be assisted.
- Be prepared to provide written materials in an auditory, tactile, or electronic format of the patient's preference (audio file, Braille, large print).
- Explain what is about to happen before beginning the encounter and ask if the patient has any questions.
- Tell the patient where personal effects (clothes and other belongings) are in the room and do not move them without telling the patient.
- Staff should be welcoming and describe the physical environment (doors, steps, ramps, bathroom location, etc.).
- Never distract or touch a service animal without asking the owner.

Patients Who Are Hard of Hearing

- Ask how best to communicate.
- Be prepared to give written materials as long as they are not the primary form of communication.
- Inform patients that sign language interpreting and real-time captioning services are available.
- If requested, promptly provide sign language interpreting or real-time captioning service for effective communication.
- Do not talk at a distance from the patient or from another room.
- Look directly at the patient when speaking so your mouth is visible.
- Speak normally and clearly. Do not shout, exaggerate mouth movements, or speak rapidly.
- Minimize background noise and glare.

(continued)

Box 1-4. Establishing Rapport with Patients with Physical and Sensory Disabilities (*continued*)

Patients Who Are Deaf

- Ask how best to communicate.
- Inform patients that sign language interpreting and real-time captioning services are available.
- If requested, promptly provide sign language interpreting or real-time captioning service for effective communication.
- Family members should not be used to interpret.
- Address the patient, not the interpreter.
- Be prepared to give written materials as long as they are not the primary form of communication.

Patients Who Use Wheelchairs

- Make sure there is a path of access to the room.
- Respect personal space, including wheelchair and assistive devices.
- Do not propel the wheelchair unless asked to do so.
- Provide accessible equipment as needed.
- Provide assistance as needed, such as by clearing obstacles from the path of travel or helping patients transfer to equipment if accessible equipment is unavailable.
- Do not separate patients from their wheelchairs.

Source: Reprinted with permission from Access to Medical Care: Adults with Physical Disabilities. Berkeley: World Institute on Disability; 2016. Available at: https://worldinstituteondisabilityblog.files.wordpress.com/2016/01/access-to-medical-care-curriculum-pdf-format.pdf. Accessed April 30, 2019.

Lesbian, Gay, Bisexual, and Transgender Adults. During clinical encounters, LGBT and sexual minority patients often experience significant anxiety related to fears of being accepted; they may be uncomfortable disclosing their sexual behaviors and may still be fluctuating in their sexual identity (Fig. 1-8). When they experience bias or discrimination, they are unlikely to reveal their sexual identity or health concerns. Furthermore, reports indicate that clinicians are often unprepared to respond to questions about fertility and transgender issues like hormonal therapy and gender-affirming procedures. Expand your knowledge and clinical skills about gay, lesbian, and transgender health as you talk with your patients and pursue the many resources available (Box 1-5).

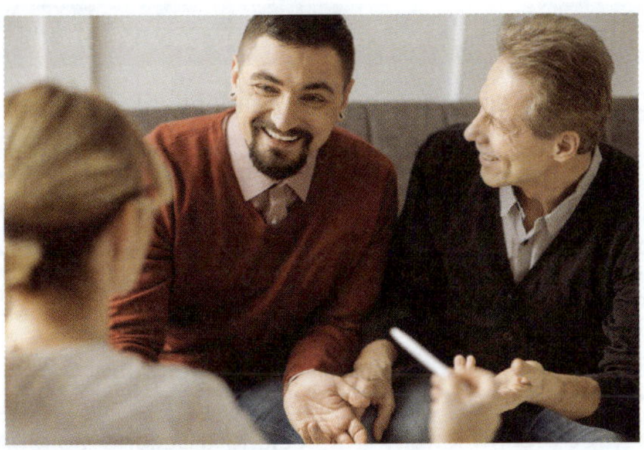

FIGURE 1-8. Create a welcoming environment for LGBTQ patients. (Used with permission from istockphoto. By yacobchuk.)

Box 1-5. Lesbian, Gay, Bisexual, and Transgender Health

Several recent surveys provide some of the first national data sets on the lesbian, gay, bisexual, and transgender (LGBT) population.

- For the first time, in 2013, the National Health Interview Survey included a measure of sexual orientation: in a sample of more than 34,000 adults, 1.6% identified as gay or lesbian, 0.7% identified as bisexual, and 1.1% responded either other or did not know. Most gay and lesbian respondents were between the ages of 18 and 64 years, with a higher percentage of bisexual respondents between 18 and 44 years.
- LGBT patients have higher rates of depression, suicide, anxiety, drug use, sexual victimization, and risk of infection with HIV and STIs.
- One-third (33%) of transgender people who saw a health care provider in the past year reported having at least one negative experience related to being transgender, such as "being refused treatment, verbally harassed, or physically or sexually assaulted, or having to teach the provider about transgender people in order to get appropriate care, with higher rates for people of color and people with disabilities."
- The Institute of Medicine has stated that barriers to accessing quality health care for LGBT adults are "a lack of providers who are knowledgeable about LGBT health needs as well as a fear of discrimination in health care settings."

Stage 2: Gathering Information

This stage has two functions: *gathering* and *providing information*. Clinicians gather information from their patients about symptoms, experience and expectations for establishing a diagnosis and treatment plan. Patients, on the other hand, need information that clarifies their health problems, reduces possible uncertainties, and supports their coping efforts. This stage is also the b4asis for shared decision making later in the clinical encounter.

Initiate Information Gathering. Once you have established rapport, you are ready to pursue the patient's reason for seeking care, traditionally called the *chief complaint*. In the ambulatory setting, where there are often three or four reasons for the visit, the phrase *presenting problem(s)* may be preferable. One benefit to this phrase is that it does not characterize the patient as a complainer. This may also be the time to keep track of your patient's responses to your questions. As a novice, you may need to write down much of what you learn during the interview

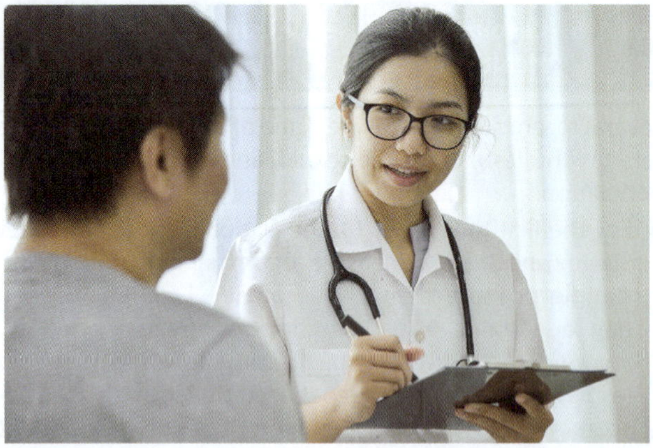

FIGURE 1-9. Maintain good eye contact. (Used with permission from Shutterstock. By eggeegg.)

Box 1-6. A Note about Taking Notes

- Jot down or type short phrases, specific dates, or words; but do not let note-taking or the keyboard and computer screen distract you from the patient.
- Maintain good eye contact. If the patient is talking about sensitive or disturbing material, put down your pen or move away from the keyboard.
- For patients who find note taking uncomfortable, explore their concerns and explain your need to make an accurate record.
- When using an electronic health record, face the patient directly as you elicit the patient's story, maintaining good eye contact and observing nonverbal behaviors; turn to the screen only after engaging the patient in the goals for the visit.
- Look up at the patient as often as possible, readjusting your screen and position if needed.

(Fig. 1-9). Experienced clinicians usually recall much of the interview without any notes, but few remember all the details of a comprehensive history (Box 1-6).

Establish the Agenda for the Patient Encounter. Begin with open-ended questions that allow full freedom of response: "What are your special concerns today?", "How can I help you?", or "Are there specific concerns that prompted your appointment today?" These questions encourage the patient to talk about *any* kinds of concerns, not just clinical ones. Note that the first problem the patient mentions may not be the one that is most important. Often, patients give one reason for the visit to a member of the clinical care team, and another to you. For some visits, patients do not have a specific concern and only want a "check-up."

Identifying all the concerns at the outset allows you and the patient to decide which ones are most pressing and which ones can be postponed to a later visit. Questions such as "Is there anything else?", "Have we discussed everything?", or "Is there anything we missed?" help you uncover the patient's full agenda and "the true reason" for the visit. You may want to address different goals, like discussing an elevated blood pressure or an abnormal test result. Identifying the full agenda protects time for the most important issues. However, even negotiating the agenda at the outset does not avert "oh by the way" concerns that suddenly emerge at the end of the visit.

Invite the Patient's Story. Once you have prioritized the agenda, invite the patient's story by asking about the foremost concern, *"Tell me more about..."* Encourage patients to tell their stories in their own words, using an open-ended approach. Avoid biasing the patient's story—do not inject new information or interrupt. Instead, use active listening skills: lean forward as you listen; add continuers such as nodding your head and phrases like "uh huh," "go on," or "I see." Train yourself to follow the patient's leads. If you ask specific questions prematurely, you risk suppressing details in the patient's own words. Studies show that clinicians wait only 18 seconds before they interrupt. Once interrupted, patients usually do not resume their stories. After the patient's initial description, explore the patient's story in more depth. Ask, "How would you describe the pain?", "What happened next?", or "What else did you notice?" so that the patient enriches important details.

Gather Information about the Patient's Perspective of Illness. Patients do not seek a clinician with just a symptom. Rather, your patients come with ideas about their symptoms shaped by their own concepts of health and frames of reference. You, as their clinician, also have your own frame of reference. Like that of your patients, it is shaped by your family values, cultural background, and personal experiences. Because our frames of reference differ from our patients', exploring their perspectives of their illness prevents misinterpretation or miscommunication. Clues during the clinical encounter can illuminate their perspectives (Box 1-7).

Box 1-7. Clues to the Patient's Perspective on Illness

- Direct statement(s) by the patient of explanations, emotions, expectations, and effects of the illness
- Expression of feelings about the illness without naming the illness
- Attempts to explain or understand symptoms
- Speech clues (e.g., repetition, prolonged reflective pauses)
- Sharing a personal story
- Behavioral clues indicative of unidentified concerns, dissatisfaction, or unmet needs such as reluctance to accept recommendations, seeking a second opinion, or early return appointment

Source: Lang F et al. *Arch Fam Med.* 2000;9:222.

Box 1-8. Exploring the Patient's Perspective (F-I-F-E)

- The patient's **F**eelings, including fears or concerns, about the problem
- The patient's **I**deas about the nature and the cause of the problem
- The effect of the problem on the patient's life and **F**unction
- The patient's **E**xpectations of the disease, of the clinician, or of health care, often based on prior personal or family experiences

To explore the patient's perspective, use different types of questions. A mnemonic for the patient's perspective on the illness is *FIFE—**F**eelings, **I**deas, effect on **F**unction, and **E**xpectations* (Box 1-8). The combination of concerns and expectations has been shown to have a major influence on the patient's decision to seek help from a clinician.

To uncover the patient's feelings, ask, "What concerns you most about the pain?" or "How has this been for you?"

For views about the cause of the problem, ask, "Why do you think you have this [stomachache]?" You might ask, "What have you tried to help?" since these choices suggest how the patient perceives the cause. Some patients worry that their pain is a symptom of serious disease. Others just want relief.

To determine how the illness affects the patient's lifestyle, particularly if the illness is chronic, ask, "What did you do before that you can't do now? How has your [backache, shortness of breath, etc.] affected you? Your life at home? Your social activities? Your role as a parent? Your function in intimate relationships? The way you feel about yourself as a person?"

To find out what the patient expects from you or from the encounter in general, consider asking, "I am glad the pain is almost gone, how specifically can I help you now?" Even if the pain is gone, the patient may still need a work excuse to take to an employer.

Identify and Respond to the Patient's Emotional Cues. Illness is often accompanied by emotional distress; 30% to 40% of patients have anxiety and depression in primary care practices. Visits tend to be longer when clinicians miss emotional clues. Patients may withhold their true concerns in up to 75% of acute care visits even though they give clues to these concerns that are direct, indirect, verbal, nonverbal, or disguised as related ideas or emotions. Check on these clues and feelings by asking, "How did you feel about that?" or "Many people would be frustrated by something like this." See Box 1-9 for suggested techniques.

Gather Information by Exploring the Biomedical Perspective. The *health history format* is a structured framework for organizing patient information in written or verbal form. This format focuses your attention on the specific kinds of information you need to obtain, facilitates clinical reasoning, and standardizes communication to other health care providers involved in the patient's care.

Box 1-9. Responding to Emotional Cues Using NURSE Statements

Learn to respond attentively to emotional cues using techniques like reflection, feedback, and "continuers" that convey support. A mnemonic for responding to emotional cues is NURSE:

Name: *"That sounds like a scary experience"*
Understand or legitimize: *"It's understandable that you feel that way"*
Respect: *"You've done better than most people would with this"*
Support: *"I will continue to work with you on this"*
Explore: *"How else were you feeling about it?"*

Gather Important Background Information and Context. The past medical history, family history, personal and social history, and review of systems give shape and depth to the patient's story. The personal and social history is an opportunity for the clinician to see the patient as a person and gain deeper understanding of the patient's outlook and background. Learning about the patient's life circumstances, emotional health, perception of health care, health behaviors, and access to and utilization of health care strengthens your therapeutic alliance and improves health outcomes.

Stage 3: Performing the Physical Examination

The physical examination also enhances your relationship with the patient (Fig. 1-10). Physical findings denote the presence or absence of disease and an opportunity for you to learn more about your patient's outlook

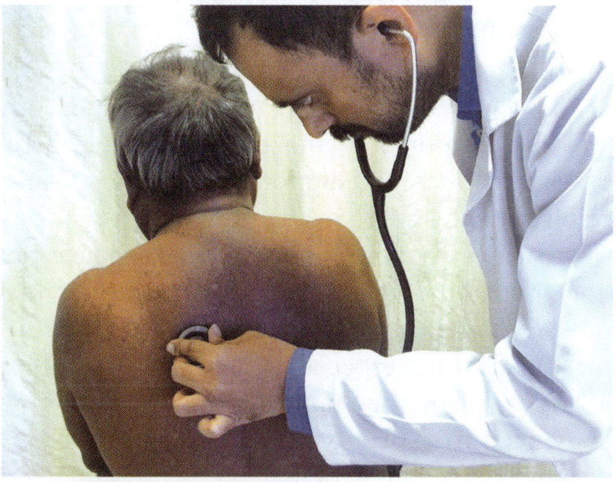

FIGURE 1-10. Performing the physical examination.

and condition. Since the physical examination almost always follows the history, it provides an avenue for the patient to talk about deeper fears or more serious issues. Maintain your patient's comfort throughout, avoid embarrassment, and demonstrate facility with the skills of physical examination to enhance the patient's satisfaction with the clinical encounter.

Stage 4: Explaining and Planning

This stage includes the elaboration of the patient's chief complaints from the disease and illness perspectives. Your goal is to assess and respond to the patient's needs for information. To achieve a shared understanding, it is important to make it easy for the patient to understand and remember your explanations and to encourage mutual discussion rather than one-way communication. This will allow your patients to understand shared clinical decision making, determine how much they want to be involved, and hopefully increase their commitment to the plans made.

Provide Useful Information and Verify Patient Understanding. Studies have shown that 40% to 80% of the clinical information patients receive during office visits is forgotten immediately, and nearly half of the information retained is incorrect. A useful technique to assess the patient's understanding is to "*teach back*," whereby you invite the patient to tell you, in his or her own words, the plan of care (Box 1-10). Keep in mind "teach back" is not a test of the patient's knowledge. It is a test of how well you explained things in a manner your patient understands. The related *"show-me"* method allows staff to confirm that patients are able to follow specific instructions (e.g., how to use an inhaler).

Negotiate the Plan of Action through Shared Decision Making. Interactive history taking allows you and the patient to create a shared picture of the patient's problems. This multifaceted picture then forms the basis for planning further evaluation and negotiating a treatment plan.

Shared decision making has been called the pinnacle of patient-centered care. Experts recommend a three-step process: introducing choices and describing options using patient decision support tools when available; exploring patient preferences; and moving to a decision, checking that the patient is ready to make a decision and offering more time, if needed. Shared decision making promotes optimal therapy, adherence to treatment, and patient satisfaction, especially since there is often no single "right" plan, but a range of variations and options. You may need to explain your recommendations several times to make sure the patient agrees to and understands what lies ahead.

Box 1-10. Teach-Back Method

- **Plan your approach.** Think about how you will ask your patient to teach back the information. An example would be: "We covered a lot today and I want to make sure that I explained things clearly. So, let's review what we discussed. Can you please describe the 3 things you agreed to do to help you control your diabetes?"
- **"Chunk and Check."** Don't wait until the end of the visit to initiate teach-back. Chunk out information into small segments and have your patient teach it back. Repeat several times during a visit.
- **Clarify and check again.** If teach-back uncovers a misunderstanding, explain things again using a different approach. Ask patients to teach-back again until they are able to correctly describe the information in their own words. If they parrot your words back to you, they may not have understood.
- **Start slowly and use consistently.** At first, you may want to try teach-back with the last patient of the day. Once you are comfortable with the technique, use teach-back with everyone, every time!
- **Practice.** It will take a little time, but once it is part of your routine, teach-back can be done without awkwardness and does not lengthen a visit.
- **Use the *show-me* method.** When prescribing new medicines or changing a dose, research shows that even when patients correctly say when and how much medicine they will take, many will make mistakes when asked to demonstrate the dose.
- **Use handouts along with teach-back.** Write down key information to help patients remember instructions at home. Point out important information by reviewing written materials to reinforce your patients' understanding. You can allow patients to refer to handouts when using teach-back, but make sure they use their own words and are not reading the material back verbatim.

Source: Use the Teach-Back Method: Tool #5. Content last reviewed February 2015. Agency for Healthcare Research and Quality, Rockville, MD. Available at http://www.ahrq.gov/professionals/quality-patient-safety/quality-resources/tools/literacy-toolkit/healthlittoolkit2-tool5.html. Accessed March 30, 2019.

Stage 5: Closing the Encounter

You may find that ending the interview, and later concluding the encounter, are difficult. Patients often have many questions, and if you have done your job well, they feel engaged and affirmed as they talk with you. Let the patient know that the end of the interview or the visit is approaching to allow time for any final questions.

Although the patient should have a chance to ask any final questions, the last few minutes are not a good time to bring up new topics. If this happens and the concern is not life threatening, simply assure the patient of your interest and make plans to address the problem at a future time. "That knee pain sounds concerning. Why don't you make an appointment for next week so we can discuss it?" Reaffirming your ongoing commitment to the patient's health shows your involvement and esteem.

Make sure the patient is aware of the mutual plans you have developed. For example, before gathering your papers or standing to leave the room, you can say, "We need to stop now. Do you have any questions about what we've covered?" As you close, summarizing plans for future evaluation, treatments, and follow-up is helpful.

Taking Time for Self-Reflection. The role of self-reflection, or mindfulness, in developing clinical empathy cannot be overemphasized. *Mindfulness* refers to the state of being "purposefully and nonjudgmentally attentive to [one's] own experience, thoughts, and feelings." As you encounter people of diverse ages, gender identities, social class, race, and ethnicity, being consistently respectful and open to individual differences is an ongoing challenge of clinical care. Because we bring our own values, assumptions, and biases to every encounter, we must look inward to see how our own expectations and reactions affect what we hear and how we behave. Self-reflection is a continual part of professional development in clinical work. It brings a deepening personal awareness to our work with patients. This personal awareness is one of the most rewarding aspects of patient care.

DISPARITIES IN HEALTH CARE

Disparities in risks of disease, morbidity, and mortality are marked and broadly documented across different population groups, reflecting inequities in health care access, income level, type of insurance, educational level, language proficiency, and provider decision making. This section focuses on important factors that potentiate unequal treatment in the clinical encounter and approaches to help mitigate them.

Disparities in Health Care

- Social Determinants of Health
- Racism and Bias
- Cultural Humility

Social Determinants of Health

There is a growing understanding of the remarkable sensitivity of health to the social environment and to what have become known as the *social determinants of health (SDOH)*. The World Health Organization (WHO) defines social determinants of health (Fig. 1-11) as "the conditions in which people are born, grow, work, live, and age, and the wider set of forces and systems shaping the conditions of daily life. These forces

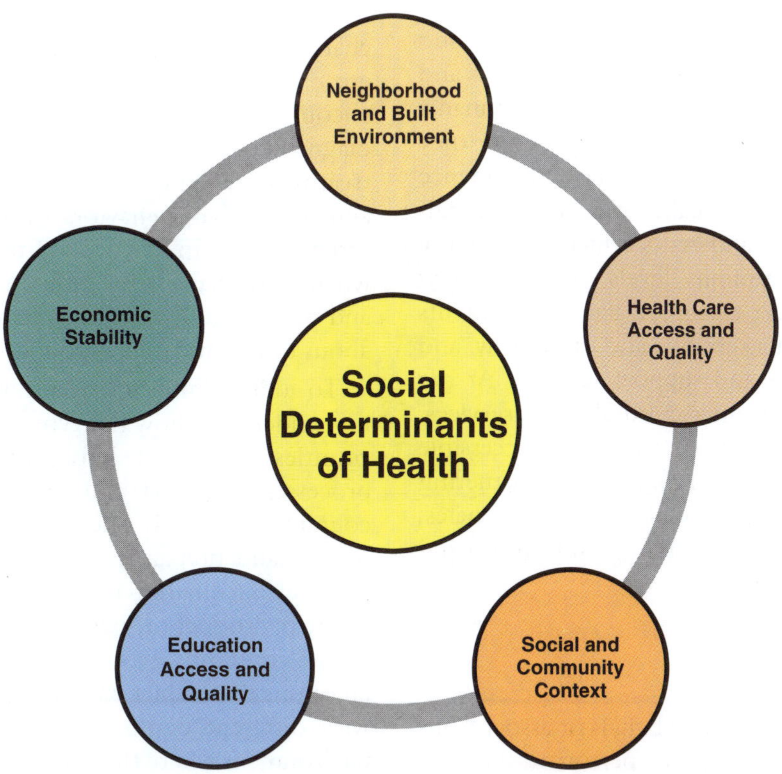

FIGURE 1-11. Social Determinants of Health. (Adapted from HealthyPeople2030 at https://www.healthypeople.gov.)

Box 1-11. Key Social Health Determinants

- Economic stability (employment, food insecurity, housing instability, poverty)
- Education (early childhood education and development, enrollment in higher education, high school graduation, language and literacy)
- Social and community context (civic participation, discrimination, incarceration, social cohesion)
- Health and health care (access to health care, access to primary care, health literacy)
- Neighborhood and built environment (access to foods that support healthy eating, patterns, crime and violence, environmental conditions, quality of housing)

Source: Secretary's Advisory Committee on Health Promotion and Disease Prevention Objectives for 2020. Healthy People 2020: An Opportunity to Address the Societal Determinants of Health in the United States. July 26, 2010. Available at http://www.healthypeople.gov/2010/hp2020/advisory/SocietalDeterminantsHealth.htm. Accessed: March 30, 2019.

and systems include economic policies and systems, development agendas, social norms, social policies and political systems." Simply, these are the social, economic, and political conditions that influence the health of individuals and populations (Box 1-11). You will quickly learn that, far more common than their individual genetic susceptibilities, your patient's health is strongly influenced by social determinants of health such as stress, early life, social exclusion, working conditions, unemployment, social support, addiction, healthy food, and transport policy.

Although challenging for both decision makers and public health advocates, the "development of policies and action for health needs to address the social determinants of health, attacking the causes of ill health before they can lead to problems." An increasing body of evidence guides clinicians and other health care professionals to improve patient health and reduce inequities at the patient, practice and community levels. At the *patient level*, clinicians can be alert to clinical flags, ask patients about social challenges in a sensitive and caring way, and help them access benefits and support services. At the *practice level*, clinicians can offer culturally safe services, use patient navigators, and ensure that care is accessible to those most in need. At the *community level*, partnering with local organizations and public health agencies, getting involved in health planning, and improving environments for health is possible.

Racism and Bias

Implicit bias is a set of unconscious beliefs or associations that lead to a negative evaluation of a person on the basis of their perceived group identity. Research has shown that implicit clinician biases can have a negative effect on the patient encounter, and more broadly, contribute to health care disparities among various demographic groups. A patient assuming a female doctor is a nurse upon meeting or a doctor audibly sighing in frustration about a patient's substance use disorder are examples of implicit bias. These examples reveal unconscious stereotypes generated by the knowledge, beliefs, and expectations of that individual. These unconscious biases can permeate the patient encounter through nonverbal behaviors such as poor eye contact, speech errors, and other subtle avoidance behaviors that convey distrust or dislike. More importantly, while they may appear minimal in scale, the aggregation of these implicit biases, and others like it, can lead to a structural system of privilege (*institutional bias*) that leads to a misallocation of care, particularly for the most marginalized demographic groups. Thus, in order to address these disparities, we must investigate the role implicit bias plays in our patient care.

One of the challenges to addressing implicit bias in health care is its relation to explicit bias. *Explicit bias* is the conscious or deliberate decisions or preferences founded on beliefs, stereotypes or associations on the basis of a perceived group identity. A patient who refuses to see a South Indian doctor because they "want a qualified doctor" or a clinician who believes that all gay males are at risk of HIV are examples of explicit bias. Although implicit bias lies within the subconscious of the subject, explicit bias can be acted on consciously.

A growing body of literature illustrates how patient characteristics (race, gender, sexual orientation, age, etc.) can influence various aspects of the patient encounter such as: questions within the clinical interview, diagnostic decision making, symptom management, treatment recommendations, referral to specialty care, and nonverbal behaviors (poor eye contact, speech errors, etc.). In particular, this becomes problematic when physicians use different communication styles and provide different information reflecting their biases about different patient groups.

To address implicit bias in clinical encounters, we must first understand how this type of bias arises. As we process countless pieces of information, unconscious mental processes help sort and organize patterns to improve cognitive efficiency. These unconscious processes help us predict and prepare for whatever encounters may arise from the information that is processed. Thus, implicit bias is one byproduct of such a cognitive system. As a society, we are constantly exposed to imagery, values, media, and emotions that depict wide-ranging stereotypes associated with different demographic groups. Particularly in an environment where this is commonplace, it is not difficult to see how these implicit biases are formed.

Box 1-12. Skills and Practices to Mitigate Bias in Your Clinical Encounters

Reflect on patterns of emotion and behavior.	Pay attention to how you feel and how you behave around patients of different identities. The patterns you recognize may reflect biases that impact your interactions with patients as well as your clinical reasoning. Being aware of these biases is the first step in reducing their impact on patient care.
Pause before starting an encounter and prepare for potential triggers of bias	Once you are aware of your potential biases, pay attention to situations that may trigger them. Simply being aware of a bias can help minimize its effect. You may take deliberate actions to reduce the impact of your biases.
Generate alternative hypotheses for biases anchored in behavior	Many biases are anchored in clinician assumptions about observed patient behavior (nonadherence, substance use, etc.). Make it a habit to consider what structural forces (socioeconomic status, race/racism, homophobia, etc.) impact patient behaviors, and how they can challenge assumptions you make about patients.
Practice universal communication and interpersonal skills	Often, clinicians will not recognize when a bias is at play in a clinical encounter. The foundational communication and interpersonal skills described in this book (see Chapter 2) can reduce the impact of such truly unconscious biases on the way you interact with patients.
Explore your patients' identities	Many biases are anchored in clinician assumptions about patient identities. By simply asking patients to clarify what their identities mean to them, clinicians can dismantle their assumptions and better understand their patients. Many approaches to exploring patient identities are presented in this book.
Explore your patients' experiences of bias	Clinical encounters are influenced by patients' prior experiences of implicit and explicit bias in their health care. Exploring and understanding these experiences can help you be a better partner with your patients. "Unfortunately, many of my patients have had negative experiences with health care. What have been your experiences with health care?"

There are several skills that clinicians can use to mitigate the impact of bias in their clinical encounters (Box 1-12).

Cultural Humility

The practice of cultural humility helps mitigate implicit bias, promotes empathy, and aids clinicians in acknowledging and respecting patients' individuality. *Cultural humility* is defined as a "process that requires humility as individuals continually engage in self-reflection and self-critique as lifelong learners and reflective practitioners" in an effort to address power imbalances and to advocate for others. It is a process that includes "the difficult work of examining cultural beliefs and cultural systems of both patients and providers to locate the points of cultural dissonance or synergy that contribute to patients' health outcomes." It has been proposed that to moderate disparities in health care, clinicians should engage in self-reflection, critical thinking, and cultural humility as they experience diversity in their clinical practices. This process calls for clinicians to "bring into check the power imbalances that exist in the dynamics of (clinician)–patient communication" and maintain mutually respectful and dynamic partnerships with patients and communities (Box 1-13).

Box 1-13. Three Dimensions of Cultural Humility

1. **Self-awareness.** Learn about your own biases; we all have them.
2. **Respectful communication.** Work to eliminate assumptions about what is "normal." Learn directly from your patients; they are the experts on their culture and illness.
3. **Collaborative partnerships.** Build your patient relationships on respect and mutually acceptable plans.

Self-Awareness. Cultural humility starts by exploring your own cultural identity. How do you describe yourself in terms of ethnicity, class, region or country of origin, religion, and political affiliation? Don't forget the characteristics we often take for granted—gender identity, life roles, sexual orientation, physical ability, and racial identity—especially if we belong to majority groups. What aspects of your family of origin do you identify with, and how are you different from your family of origin? How do these identities influence your beliefs and behaviors?

A more challenging task is to bring our own values and biases to a conscious level. *Values* are the standards we use to measure our own and others' beliefs and behaviors. *Biases* are the attitudes or feelings that we attach to perceived differences. Being attuned to difference is normal; in

Box 1-14. The 5Rs of Cultural Humility

	Aim	Ask
Reflection	Clinicians will approach every encounter with humility and understanding that there is always something to learn from everyone.	What did I learn from each person in that encounter?
Respect	Clinicians will treat every person with the utmost respect and strive to preserve dignity at all times.	Did I treat everyone involved in that encounter respectfully?
Regard	Clinicians will hold every person in their highest regard, be aware of, and not allow unconscious biases to interfere in any interactions.	Did unconscious biases drive this interaction?
Relevance	Clinicians will expect cultural humility to be relevant and apply this practice to every encounter.	How was cultural humility relevant in this encounter?
Resiliency	Clinicians will embody the practice of cultural humility to enhance personal resiliency and global compassion.	How was my personal resiliency affected by this interaction?

Source: The 5Rs of Cultural Humility. Reprinted with permission from Society of Hospital Medicine. Available at https://www.hospitalmedicine.org/practice-management/the-5-rs-of-cultural-humility/. Accessed May 10, 2019.

fact, in the distant past, reacting to differences may have ensured survival. Instinctively knowing members of one's own group is a survival skill that we may have outgrown as a society, but that is still actively at work.

Respectful Communication. Given the complexities of global society, no one can possibly know the health beliefs and practices of every culture and subculture. Let your patients be the experts on their own unique cultural perspectives. Even if patients have trouble describing their values or beliefs, they can often respond to specific questions. Find out about the patient's cultural background. Maintain an open, respectful, and inquiring attitude. "What did you hope to get from this visit?" If you have established rapport and trust, patients will be willing to teach you. Be aware of questions that contain assumptions. And always be ready to acknowledge your areas of ignorance or bias.

Learning about the patient's specific culture broadens the areas you, as a clinician, need to explore. Do some reading about the life experiences of individuals in ethnic or racial groups who live in your area. There may be historic reasons for loss of trust in clinicians or health care. Learn about the explicit health agendas of different consumer groups. Talk with different kinds of healers and learn about their practices. Most importantly, be open to learning from each patient. Do not assume that your impressions about a given cultural group apply to the individual before you.

Collaborative Partnerships. Through continual work on self-awareness and seeing through the "lens" of others, the clinician lays the foundation for the collaborative relationship that best supports the patient's health. Communication based on trust, respect, and your own willingness to re-examine assumptions allows patients to be more open to expressing views that diverge from the dominant culture. They may have strong feelings such as anger or shame. You, the clinician, must be willing to listen to and validate these emotions, and not let your own feelings of discomfort or time pressure prevent you from exploring painful areas. Be willing to re-examine your beliefs about the "right approach" to clinical care in a given situation. Make every effort to be flexible as you develop shared plans that reflect patients' knowledge about their best interests that are congruent with both their beliefs and effective clinical care. Remember that if the patient stops listening, fails to follow your advice, or does not return, your care has not been successful.

The 5Rs of Cultural Humility *(reflection, respect, regard, relevance, and resiliency)* is a coaching tool (Box 1-14) that provides clinicians with a concise framework with specific aims and asks incorporate skills identified at reducing implicit biases in health care.

OTHER MAJOR CONSIDERATIONS

Other Major Considerations

- Spirituality
- Medical Ethics
  - Decisional Capacity
  - Approach to a Clinical Ethical Dilemma
- Clinical Documentation including the EHR

Spirituality

The terms spirituality and religion are sometimes used synonymously. It is helpful, however, to distinguish the two. *Spirituality* encompasses religion, but is broader, focusing on larger universal themes such as meaning and purpose, transcendence (both transpersonal and intrapersonal), and connection with others. It is the aspect of humanity that refers to the way individuals seek and express meaning and purpose and the way they experience their connectedness to the moment, to self, to others, to nature, and to the significant and sacred. *Religion* includes specific beliefs, practices, texts, and rituals, common to a community and in relationship to something larger than themselves (God, the holy, the transcendent, a higher power, etc.).

Paying attention to your patients' religion and spirituality are aspects of cultural competence in health care (Box 1-15). It is important not to make several assumptions about your patients.

- *Don't assume that patients are religious.* Many patients may find meaning, purpose, and/or connection through nonreligious beliefs, practices, and communities. For example, a patient may find her life purpose in taking care of her grandchildren or through connection and commitment to a fitness organization such as The Art of Living.
- *Don't assume that patients are not religious.* Many Indians identify as religious, with the majority identifying as Hindus.
- *Don't assume that if a patient does identify as religious or spiritual you know exactly what that means to that particular patient.* Despite how patients identify, individuals tend to customize their religious or spiritual practices and beliefs, which is one reason why it is important to take a spiritual history.
- *Don't assume that religion or spirituality has a neutral or no effect on health.* Religion and spirituality are considered *social determinants of health* which may contribute to negative or positive health outcomes. For example, Seventh-Day Adventists, who typically embrace a vegetarian diet for religious reasons, may live an average of 10 years longer than most Americans. Conversely, medically ill older adult patients who believe God has abandoned them have an increased risk of death.

Box 1-15. Guiding Questions in Assessing the Role of Spirituality in Your Patient

- What values guide your patient's health care decisions?
  - Does your patient consult a religious/spiritual leader before making important health care decisions?
  - Does your patient have particular religious/spiritual concerns about blood products or porcine implants?
- How do patient spiritual beliefs and practices influence how they cope with their illness and care for themselves?
  - Is there a significant community involved who may aid them while they are sick?
  - Is there a spiritual practice such as yoga or meditation that may aid them in their healing?
- Does your patient have spiritual struggle or distress and need a referral to a chaplain?
  - *Spiritual struggle* is defined as "…tensions, conflicts, and questions over sacred matters within oneself, with others, and with God." Examples include feeling abandoned by God or one's religious community, a belief that the universe is out to get you, or doubts about one's fundamental beliefs and values.
  - Spiritual struggle has been shown to increase depressive symptoms, emotional distress, and risk of mortality while decreasing physical health, quality of life, and recovery of independence in daily activities.

Medical Ethics

Although clinicians often know how to act ethically, the complexity and uncertainty of many clinical situations mean that they cannot rely on common sense morality to direct them. Although often your sense of right and wrong may be all that you need, even as students, you will face decisions that call for the application of ethical principles (Box 1-16).

Medical ethics, a subdiscipline of applied ethics, which is itself a subdiscipline of philosophy, is the system of norms that guide the practice and support clinician decision making. It has an ancient heritage typically dated to Hippocrates, namely, beneficence, confidentiality, and nonmaleficence that can be found in the Hippocratic Oath. Hippocratic medicine was paternalistic, and this ethical orientation remained dominant with the professionalization of medicine in the 18th century, when University of Edinburgh–trained physicians, John Gregory and Thomas Percival, contributed to the development of a professional ethic dedicated to prioritizing patients' welfare, and the public good.

In the 20th century, medicine's dominant ethic of paternalism was challenged. Court decisions like Schloendorff vs. Society of New York Hospital established that clinicians must elicit *informed consent* for treatment from patients. In the mid-20th century, revelations of physician misconduct, like that of the Nazi doctors and the U.S. Tuskegee Syphilis study, and the development of technology like mechanical ventilation, which could support people with irreversible comas indefinitely, generated the need to further reassess medical ethics. The American Medical Association's limited response and the absence of ethics from school curricula led to a

Box 1-16. Core Values of Medical Ethics

- ***Nonmaleficence*** *("first, do no harm")* directive that health care professionals should avoid causing harm to patients and minimize the negative effects of treatments.
- ***Beneficence*** dictum that clinicians are to act for the patients' good by preventing or treating disease.
- ***Respect for autonomy*** commitment to accept the choices patients with decisional capacity make about which treatments to undergo, including to reject treatment. The addition of this value to medical ethics changed the clinician–patient relationship from a paternalistic one to a more collaborative one.
- ***Decisional capacity*** ability to make an autonomous choice that clinicians should respect.
- ***Confidentiality*** duty to prevent the disclosure of patients' personal information to parties who are not authorized to learn that information.
- ***Informed consent*** principle that clinicians must elicit patients' voluntary and informed authorization to test or treat them for illness or injury. Because patients cannot consent to treatment without knowing what they are being treated for, this principle also encompasses the responsibility to inform patients of diagnoses, prognoses, and treatment alternatives.
- ***Truth telling*** value that clinicians should disclose information beyond that required by informed consent that may be relevant to patients (e.g., the number of similar procedures a physician has performed).
- ***Justice*** value that all patients with similar medical needs should receive similar medical treatment and should be treated fairly by clinicians.

"bioethics revolution" by philosophers and theologians that retained Hippocratic and professional values, while establishing *respect for autonomy* among the core values of medicine. The effect was to empower patients to make health choices that do reflect their own view of what is good for them. Respect for autonomy, in addition to the older principles of beneficence, nonmaleficence, and justice were established as the common core of health care ethics and became incorporated into most professional codes for health care providers.

Decisional Capacity. *Capacity* is a clinical designation and can be assessed by clinicians, whereas *competence* is a judicial determination and can only be decided by a court. Some patients can provide a history but lack the ability to make informed health care decisions. You then need to determine whether a patient has *decisional capacity*. The elements that constitute decisional capacity are the capability to communicate a choice; understand the relevant information; appreciate the situation and its consequences; and reason about treatment options (Box 1-17).

If a patient lacks capacity to make a health care decision, then identify the health care proxy or the agent

Box 1-17. Elements of Decisional Capacity

Patients must have the ability to:

- Understand the relevant information about proposed diagnostic tests or treatment
- Appreciate their situation (including their underlying values and current clinical situation)
- Use reason to make a decision
- Communicate their choice

Source: Sessums LL et al. *JAMA*. 2011,306:420.

with power of attorney for health care. If the patient has not identified a surrogate decision maker, then that role may shift to a spouse or family member. It is critical to remember that decisional capacity is both "temporal and situational." It can fluctuate depending on the condition of the patient and the complexity of the decision involved. A patient who is quite ill may be unable to make decisions about care but can regain capacity with clinical improvement. A patient may be unable to make a complex decision, but still able to make simple decisions.

The Aid to Capacity Evaluation (ACE) is an instrument that has been validated against a gold standard, is free and available online, can be performed in less than 30 minutes, and uses the patient's actual clinical scenario in the evaluation.

Approach to a Clinical Ethical Dilemma. Medical ethics plays a role in all clinical encounters with patients, even though you may not have to explicitly consider the ethics of each clinical situation. As students, you are exposed to ethical challenges that you will encounter later as practicing clinicians. Through training, acting according to these values becomes a natural part of being a clinician, but some patients' care is so complex that determining the ethical thing to do requires explicit, critical reflection. In situations where you need to explicitly consider the ethical aspects of the clinical situation, there are heuristics that provide guidance for how to reason through an ethical dilemma (Box 1-18). This practical method is not guaranteed to be optimal or perfect but instead sufficient for reaching an immediate goal. Where finding an optimal solution is impossible or impractical, heuristic methods can be used to speed up the process of finding a satisfactory solution.

Step 1: Clearly State the Ethical Question. This step asks clinicians to formulate an ethics question that summarizes the challenge they face in an ethically complex clinical situation. Because ethics is principally concerned about what constitutes right and wrong conduct, the question ought to be formulated as a question about what a person should do in the situation. For example: Should a nurse accept a patient's request to postpone a dressing change to a time that is less convenient for the nurse?

Box 1-18. How to Resolve a Clinical Ethical Dilemma

1. Clearly state the ethical question
2. Collect relevant information
   - Medical facts
   - Patient preferences and interests (e.g., culture, religion, social support, financial concerns, quality of life)
     - Does the patient have capacity?
     - Does the patient have advance directives or a surrogate?
   - Other parties' preferences
3. Identify ethical principles and guidelines
   - Are there legal guidelines that apply to the case?
   - Are there institutional guidelines that apply to the case?
   - What ethical values are relevant to the case?
4. Delineate and relate options to values and principles
   - Identify course of action by prioritizing each of the ethical values.
   - If principle X is primary, then course of action Y is justified, etc.
5. Evaluate the different options
   - Formulate justification for best course of action by identifying the dominant principle based on legal, institutional, and ethical guidelines.
6. Make an action plan

Step 2: Collect Relevant Information. It is not possible for clinicians to determine how to resolve a complex situation with insufficient information. This step asks clinicians to collect all of the information that they believe is relevant to the case. This includes clinical information relevant to the patient—diagnosis, prognosis, benefits and risks of treatment alternatives, including not treating. Facts about the patient and the patient's preferences and interests are also pertinent. You would want to know what the patient's goals are for care; for example, a patient with a terminal illness may prefer a treatment that will preserve an active lifestyle over a treatment that extends life with side effects. Moreover, patients may have cultural or religious commitments that influence their choices. Jehovah Witnesses are well known to refuse even lifesaving blood transfusions because of religious convictions. Patients also may or may not have the financial resources to support a treatment option they prefer. The interests and concerns of other stakeholders such as family members and caregivers can also be important. For example, a patient who needs rehabilitative care may wish to be discharged home with outpatient rehabilitation, but this treatment plan is not feasible if the spouse or child is unwilling or unable to assist the patient at home. It can require creative thinking to identify all of the relevant information.

Step 3: Identify Ethical Principles and Guidelines. Society grants professions broad discretion to regulate their practice and their members, but they are still subject to the law which usually sets a floor for acceptable conduct. Institutions also have policies and guidelines which set expectations for their members that prescribe or proscribe conduct. Health care professionals should obey the law and the policies of their institutions, so they must take these into account when reflecting on an ethically complex situation. While the law and institutional polices typically establish what health care professionals *cannot* choose to do, ethics aims to help guide them to make the best choice from their options. To determine this, one should brainstorm what the relevant ethics concepts might be.

Step 4: Delineate and Relate Options to Values and Principles. In this step, the clinicians should reflect on how the relevant principles identified in the prior step would guide their conduct in the case. This step helps to clarify just why the situation is ethically complex. Often, the source of this complexity is that the relevant ethical concepts provide the clinician with conflicting guidance. Confidentiality might guide a clinician not to disclose a minor patient's sexual activity to the parents but minimizing harm might be interpreted to support the disclosure if the physician suspects the patient is acting out sexually because of personal difficulties. Sometimes this step can reveal that there is no ethical dilemma because once the guidance of the ethical concepts is established, it becomes clear that there is only one potential course of action.

Step 5: Evaluate the Different Options. Clinicians must ultimately act, and resolving a clinical situation that poses an ethical dilemma means that they must decide which ethical concept is the most important in the case and follow its guidance. Clinicians must attend to facts about the case and reflect on the relative significance of the ethical concepts in conflict and explain how they support the prioritization of one ethical value over another.

Step 6: Make an Action Plan. Once clinicians have decided what the ethical course of action is, they must decide how to go about acting—they must do the right thing in the right way. This will involve planning how to communicate a decision about what to do that may not be welcomed by patients, families, or colleagues. If it is anticipated that the decision may not be accepted positively, it is advisable that the clinician enlist institutional support from an ethics consultant or committee. If the patient will need extensive support services, social work services may be needed.

Review an example of an ethical dilemma you may encounter in your clinical training (Box 1-19). Reflect on how you would approach this dilemma. An approach to resolving this issue using the previously described heuristics is also provided.

Box 1-19. Ethics Case Analysis

Clinical Case Description

You are in your clinical rotation and your supervising clinician requested that you see RG. He is a 30-year-old man who came to the clinic for follow-up after being discharged from the hospital 2 months ago for a surgical repair of his torn rotator cuff. RG reports that he feels well, has stopped taking any pain medications, and is doing well in physical therapy. While at home, RG complains of occasional visual symptoms that remind him of hallucinations he had when experimenting with hallucinogenic drugs in high school. During the health history interview, RG enthusiastically describes his symptoms and unabashedly recounts his history of drug use, which included multiple experiences with LSD, psilocybin, ayahuasca, ketamine, and phencyclidine. Your examination does not reveal any neurologic abnormality, and you doubt that RG's prior drug use is a cause of the visual symptoms, but you cannot rule it out either. At the end of your examination, RG tells you that he does not want any of his history of drug use documented in his electronic health record. He says that he has not experimented with drugs since high school over a decade ago, and he is planning to apply for a position in the local police department. RG is afraid past his drug use will disqualify him, and he is paranoid that the local police department will access his electronic health record by hacking into it, which would be illegal.

What is your course of action?

Ethical Analysis of Clinical Case

Step 1: Clearly state the ethical question: Should you record RG's report of drug experimentation in your note in his health record despite his request that you not do so?

Step 2: Collect relevant information: The case description summarizes the relevant medical facts. The patient's preference is to exclude his history of drug experimentation from his health record, and his reason for this appears to be a fear of financial loss from not gaining his preferred form of employment. The patient may overestimate the risk that his health record will be compromised, but this should not undermine the presumption that he has decisional capacity. Clinicians who will treat RG in the future have an interest in a complete, accurate health history for developing differential diagnoses for RG, especially if RG is not able to describe his past medical history.

Step 3: Identify ethical principles and guidelines: Patients have the right to get a copy of their health records and to request corrections to inaccurate information. However, it does not establish that patients have a right to control the content of their health records. Health records can be subpoenaed under certain circumstances and can serve as legal documents in legal proceedings. A general rule is that if something is not documented, then it did not happen. In addition, insurance reviewers depend on the completeness and accuracy of a health record to determine if billed services are consistent with a patient's health insurance coverage. Some of the medical ethics principles that apply to this case include *beneficence*, *confidentiality* and *respect for autonomy*.

Step 4: Delineate and relate options to values and principles: Documenting RG's drug history in his health record is supported by the ethical concept of *beneficence*. Patients benefit when their health care professionals have a complete, accurate record of their health history to support clinical decision making. Patients may not always remember past details of their health history or know which details are relevant to their care. In addition, illness can compromise patients' ability to supply their health history, which their record can provide. *Confidentiality* may be construed to require you not to record RG's drug history to ensure that this information is only known to RG and to you. And, *respect for autonomy* may be interpreted to permit RG to make decisions about what information he wants included in his record. If confidentiality or respect for autonomy are determined to be the primary values in this case, then you should not document RG's drug history in his record, but if beneficence is paramount, then you should document it.

Step 5: Evaluate the different options: The resolution of this dilemma primarily depends on an accurate understanding of the scope of both confidentiality and respect for autonomy. The interpretation of how confidentiality in Step 4 would make confidentiality incompatible with the collaborative, team-based nature of contemporary clinical practice. Interdisciplinary teams depend on the accuracy of their colleagues' entries into the health record when developing an appropriate treatment plan. All of the health care professionals caring for a patient operate within a circle of confidentiality that authorizes them to access this information. They and their institutions are responsible for ensuring that the health record is secure against unauthorized access; and, those clinicians not caring for the patient have a duty not to access the record. Respect for autonomy is not a concept that licenses patients to make clinical judgments about their care. Instead, it empowers an informed patient to decide which of a clinician's treatment recommendations best supports the patient's goals. Health care professionals are still obliged to consult evidence-based health care and standards of care when making recommendations for treatment to patients, so patients cannot request interventions that lie outside of those parameters.

These considerations indicate that confidentiality and respect for autonomy are not values that play an operative role in this case. The ethical value of beneficence is the pertinent one in this case, and the student should document RG's drug history in the record. Moreover, the potential for the health record to serve as a legal document and institutional policy are also compelling expectations for complying with thorough documentation.

Step 6: Make an action plan: You should then document RG's drug history in the health record, and you should also tell RG. You should acknowledge RG's concern about unauthorized access to his electronic health record, but also explain the security protocols the clinic has in place for preventing this from occurring. In addition, you should remind RG it would be illegal for a local police department to hack any electronic health record. Finally, you should enlist your supervising clinician in this conversation for support, since your supervising clinician has ultimate responsibility to ensure the accuracy of RG's health record.

Documenting the Clinical Encounter

A clear, well-organized health record is one of the most important adjuncts to patient care. Your goal is a clear, concise, but comprehensive report that documents key findings and communicates your assessment in a succinct format to clinicians, consultants, and other members of the health care team. It serves a dual purpose—it reflects your analysis of the patient's health status, tracking their progress and it documents the unique features of the patient's history, examination, laboratory and test results, assessment, and plan in a formal written format. The patient record facilitates clinical reasoning, promotes communication and coordination among the professionals who care for your patient, and documents the patient's problems and management for medicolegal purposes.

See Tables 1-1 and 1-2 for examples of clinical documentation. The discussions of its components are in Chapters 3, 4, and 5. Other examples are in the "Recording Your Clinical Findings" sections in all regional examination chapters.

Regardless of your experience, adopting certain principles will help you organize a good record. Think especially about the *order and clarity* of the record and the *amount of detail* needed. How much detail to include often varies at different points in training. As a student, you may wish (or be required) to be quite detailed. This builds your descriptive skills, vocabulary, and speed. Later, the pressures of workload and time management will lead to less but more focused detail. A good record always provides sufficient evidence from the history, physical examination, and laboratory findings to support all the problems or diagnoses identified.

Compose the clinical record as soon after seeing the patient as possible, before your findings fade from memory. At first you may take written notes but work toward recording each segment of the health history during the interview, leaving spaces for filling in details later. Jot down or type in the EHR the blood pressure, heart rate, and key abnormal findings to prompt your recall when you complete the record later.

Almost all clinical information is subject to error. Patients forget to mention symptoms, confuse the events of their illness, avoid recounting embarrassing facts, and may slant their stories to what they believe the clinician wants to hear. Clinicians misinterpret patient statements, overlook information, fail to ask "the one key question," jump prematurely to conclusions and diagnoses, or forget an important part of the examination, such as the funduscopic examination in a woman with headache, leading to diagnostic errors. You can avoid some of these errors by acquiring the habits summarized in Box 1-20.

See Chapter 5 for common diagnostic errors in clinical care, p. 87.

Documenting Clinical Information in the Electronic Health Record. Clinicians today have come a long way from the days of documenting clinical encounters on paper. Gone

Box 1-20. Checklist to Ensure a Quality Clinical Record

Is the Organization Clear?

Organization is imperative. Make sure that readers can easily find specific points of information. Keep the *subjective* items of the history, for example, in the history; do not let them stray into the physical examination. Did you:

- Make the headings clear?
- Accent your organization with indentations and spacing?
- Arrange the *History Present Illness* in chronologic order, starting with the current episode, then filling in relevant background information?

Does the Included Information Contribute Directly to the Assessment?

Spell out the supporting evidence, both positive and negative, for each problem or diagnosis. Make sure there is sufficient detail to support your differential diagnosis and plan.

Are Pertinent Negatives Specifically Described?

Often, portions of the history or examination suggest that an abnormality might exist or develop in that area. For example, for the patient with notable bruises, record the *"pertinent negatives,"* such as the absence of injury or violence, familial bleeding disorders, or medications or nutritional deficits that might lead to bruising. For the patient who is depressed but not suicidal, recording both facts are important. In the patient with a transient mood swing, on the other hand, a comment on suicide is unnecessary.

Are There Overgeneralizations or Omissions of Important Data?

Remember that any information not recorded is information lost. No matter how vividly you can recall clinical details today, you will probably not remember them in a few months. The phrase "neurologic examination negative," even in your own handwriting, may leave you wondering in a few months' time, *"Did I really check the reflexes?"*

Is There Too Much Detail?

Is there excess information or redundancy? Is important information buried in a mass of detail, to be discovered by only the most persistent reader? Make your descriptions concise. *"Cervix pink and smooth"* indicates you saw no redness, ulcers, nodules, masses, cysts, or other suspicious lesions, but this description is shorter and more easily read. You can omit unimportant structures even though you examined them, such as normal eyebrows and eyelashes. *Concentrate on major negative findings* such as "no heart murmurs" rather than negative findings unrelated to the patient's complaints or specific exclusions in your differential diagnosis.

(continued)

Box 1-20. Checklist to Ensure a Quality Clinical Record (*continued*)

Is the Written Style Succinct? Are Phrases, Short Words, and Abbreviations Used Appropriately? Is Data Unnecessarily Repeated?

Using words or brief phrases instead of whole sentences is common, but abbreviations and symbols should be used only if they are readily understood. Use shorter words when possible such as *"felt"* for *"palpated"* or *"heard"* for *"auscultated."* Omit unnecessary words, such as those in parentheses in the examples below. This saves valuable time and space. For example, *"Cervix is pink* (in color)." *"Lungs are resonant* (to percussion)." *"Liver is tender* (to palpation)." *"Both* (right and left) *ears with cerumen." "II/IV systolic ejection murmur* (audible)." *"Thorax symmetric* (bilaterally)." Describe what you observed, not what you did. *"Optic discs seen"* is less informative than *"disc margins sharp."*

Are Clear Descriptions or Images Included Whenever Possible?

To ensure accurate evaluations and future comparisons, describe findings fully. Use measurements in centimeters, not in fruits, nuts, or vegetables.

- *"1 × 1 cm lymph node"* versus a *"pea-sized lymph node…"*
- Or *"2 × 2 cm mass on the left lobe of the prostate"* versus a *"walnut-sized prostate mass."*

Images add greatly to the clarity of the record. If possible, take a picture or scan an image of the finding then upload to the patient's electronic health record.

Is the Tone of the Write-Up Neutral and Professional?

It is important to be objective. Hostile or disapproving comments have no place in the patient's record. Never use inflammatory or demeaning words or punctuation.

Comments such as *"Patient DRUNK and LATE TO CLINIC AGAIN!!"* are unprofessional and set a bad example for other clinicians reading the chart. They also might prove difficult to defend in a legal setting.

are the days of clinicians frustratingly searching for paper charts and files, patient orders left in patient charts for an extended period of time waiting to be read and acted upon, illegible handwriting of health care team documentation and orders which have led to communication issues and increased medical errors, as well as work flow delays that has led to inefficient use of time and resources impacting patient care. The ubiquitous use of electronic health records (EHRs) in health institutions nowadays has certainly led to numerous opportunities to improve patient care and increase the accuracy of communication. Its use has facilitated the improvement of quality, safety, and efficiency of patient care. It has also improved the privacy of health information and allows greater patient access to their own health records (Fig. 1-12).

The EHR has included numerous functions designed to assist clinicians achieve patient care efficiency (e.g., check boxes, automated history/physical examination functions, pre-worded phrases, templates, copying and pasting, and "note forwarding"). These functions also have the potential to be abused. As a novice student, you should be careful in utilizing these functions not only due to the potential liability risks but also because these functions may ultimately impact the care you and your team provide for your patient and can lead to harm. For example, using templates that automatically populate fields that you have not used during the encounter is misleading; copying and pasting information from a prior encounter may not accurately reflect the current status of the patient. Try to work on a set of identified EHR-related skills that could effectively enhance your use of the EHR for clinical care (Box 1-21).

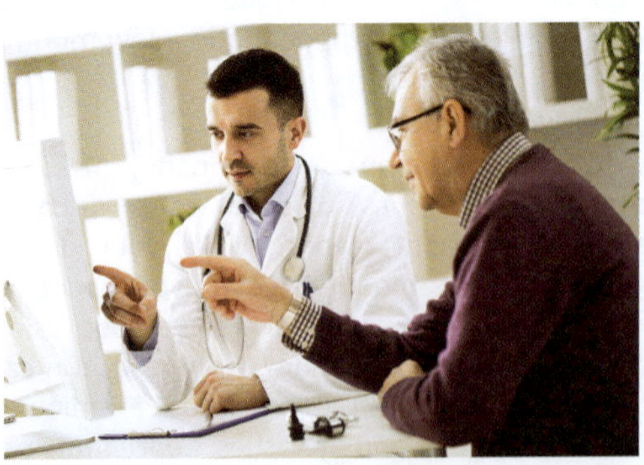

FIGURE 1-12. Maintaining patient-centeredness while using the EHR. (Used with permission from Shutterstock. By didesign021.)

See Chapter 2 for maintaining patient-centeredness during the clinical encounter with the EHR, pp. 41–42.

Box 1-21. Skills Required for Effective Use of the EHR

- Mastery of key elements of traditional patient encounter documentation, including familiarity with use of templates and checklists
- Comprehensive understanding of key/critical elements of order entry, including familiarity with use of order sets and pharmacy/prescription entries
- Familiarity with medication reconciliation and how/when it must be done
- Familiarity with how to access basic laboratory and radiologic data
- Familiarity with how to locate and interpret ancillary staff entries including vital signs, inputs/outputs, and nursing/allied health documentation
- Ability to locate and review historical data from prior hospitalizations or ambulatory visits including progress notes, admission note, consultation reports, procedure notes, and discharge summaries
- Familiarity with how to identify patient demographics including contact information

Source: From Hammoud MM et al. *Teach Learn Med.* 2012;24(3):257–266. Reprinted by permission of Taylor & Francis Ltd, http://www.tandfonline.com.

TABLE 1-1. Example of a Comprehensive Clinical Record: The Case of Patient MN

8/25/20 11:00 AM
MN, 54 years old, salesperson
Source and Reliability.
Self-referred; reliable.

Chief Complaint
"My head has been aching for the past 3 months."

History of Present Illness
MN is a 54-year-old salesperson with a remote history of intermittent headaches who states that her "head has been aching for the past 3 months." She was in good health until 3 months prior to consultation when she started experiencing episodes of headache. These episodes occur on both sides of the front of her head without any radiation. They are described as throbbing and mild to moderately severe in intensity (rated as 3 to 6 out of 10 in the 10-point pain scale). The headaches usually last 4–6 hours and started as one to two episodes a month but now average once a week. The episodes are usually related to stress. The headaches are relieved with sleep and placing a damp cool towel over her forehead. There is little relief from acetaminophen.

MN has missed work on several occasions because of associated nausea and occasional vomiting during the episodes. There are no associated visual changes, motor-sensory deficits, loss of consciousness or paresthesias. She had headaches with nausea and vomiting beginning at age 15 years. These recurred throughout her mid-20s, then decreased to one every 2 or 3 months, and almost disappeared. She thinks her headaches may be like those in the past but wants to be sure because her mother had a headache just before she died of a stroke. She is concerned because her headaches interfere with her work and make her irritable with her family. She reports increased pressure at work from a demanding supervisor as well as being worried about her daughter. She eats three meals a day and drinks three cups of coffee a day and tea at night. Due to the increasing frequency of the headaches, she decided to come to the clinic today.

Allergies: Ampicillin causes rash. No environmental or food allergies

Medications: Acetaminophen, 1 to 2 tablets every 4 to 6 hours as needed.

Past Medical History

Childhood Illnesses: Measles, chickenpox. No scarlet fever or rheumatic fever.

Adult Illnesses: *Medical:* Pyelonephritis, 2016, with fever and right flank pain; treated with ampicillin; developed generalized rash with itching several days later; no recurrence of infection. Last dental visit 2 years ago. *Surgical:* Tonsillectomy, age 6; appendectomy, age 13. Sutures for laceration, 2012, after stepping on piece of glass. *Ob/Gyn:* G3P3 (3–0–0–3), with normal vaginal deliveries. Three living children. Menarche age 12. Last menses 6 months ago. *Psychiatric:* None.

Health Maintenance: *Immunizations:* Age-appropriate immunizations up to date as per immunization registry. *Screening tests:* Last Pap smear, 2018, normal. Mammogram, 2019, normal.

Family History
Father died at age 43 years in a train accident. Mother died at age 67 years from stroke; had varicose veins, headaches.
One brother, age 61 years, with hypertension, otherwise well; one brother, age 58 years, well except for mild arthritis; one sister, died in infancy of unknown cause.
Husband died at age 54 of heart attack.
Daughter, age 33 years, with migraine headaches, otherwise well; son, age 31 years, with headaches; son, age 27 years, well.
No family history of diabetes, heart or kidney disease, cancer, epilepsy, or mental illness.

Personal and Social History
Born and raised in Indore, was assigned female sex at birth, and currently identifies as female, finished high school, married at age 19 years. Worked as a salesperson for 2 years, then moved with her husband to Pune, had three children. Returned to work as a salesperson 15 years ago to improve family finances. Children all married. Four years ago, her husband died suddenly of a heart attack, leaving little savings. MN has moved to a small apartment to be near daughter, Rinku. Rinku's husband, Kiran, has an alcohol problem. MN's apartment is now a haven for Rinku and her two children, Kavita, age 6 years, and Durga, age 3 years. MN feels responsible for helping them; she feels tense and nervous but denies feeling depressed. She has friends, but rarely discusses family problems: "I'd rather keep them to myself. I don't like gossip." During the FICA assessment she reports being raised as a Catholic, but that she stopped attending church after the death of her husband. Although she states her faith is still important to her now describes having no faith community or spiritual support system. She feels this has contributed to her sense of anxiety and agrees to meet with a chaplain. She is typically up at 7:00 AM, works 9:00 AM to 5:30 PM, and eats dinner alone.

(continued)

TABLE 1-1. Example of a Comprehensive Clinical Record: The Case of Patient MN *(Continued)*

Exercise and diet. Gets little exercise. Diet high in carbohydrates.

Safety measures. Uses seat belt regularly. Uses sunblock. Medications kept in an unlocked medicine cabinet. Cleaning solutions in unlocked cabinet below sink. Handgun stored in unlocked dresser in bedroom.

Tobacco. About 1 pack of cigarettes per day since age 18 (36 pack-years).

Alcohol/drugs. Wine on rare occasions. No illicit drugs.

Sexual history. Little interest in sex, and not sexually active. Her deceased husband was her only sexual partner. Never had STIs before. Could not recall if she has had testing done for STIs before. No concerns about HIV infection.

Review of Systems

General: Has gained 5 kg in the past 4 years.

Skin: No rashes or other changes.

Head, Eyes, Ears, Nose, Throat (HEENT): See ***Present Illness. Head:*** No history of head injury. ***Eyes:*** Reading glasses for 5 years, last checked 1 year ago. No symptoms. ***Ears:*** Hearing good. No tinnitus, vertigo, infections. ***Nose, sinuses:*** No hay fever, sinus trouble. ***Throat*** (or mouth and pharynx): No tooth pain or gum bleeding.

Neck: No lumps, goiter, pain. No swollen glands.

Breasts: No lumps, pain, discharge.

Respiratory: No cough, wheezing, shortness of breath.

Cardiovascular: No dyspnea, orthopnea, chest pain, palpitations.

Gastrointestinal: Appetite good; no nausea, vomiting, indigestion. Bowel movement about once daily, though sometimes has hard stools for 2 to 3 days when especially tense; no diarrhea or bleeding. No pain, jaundice, gallbladder or liver problems.

Urinary: No frequency, dysuria, hematuria, or recent flank pain; occasionally loses urine when coughing.

Genital: No vaginal or pelvic infections. No dyspareunia.

Peripheral vascular: No history of phlebitis or leg pain.

Musculoskeletal: Mild low backaches, often at the end of the workday; no radiation into the legs; used to do back exercises, but not now. No other joint pain.

Psychiatric: No history of depression or treatment for psychiatric disorders.

Neurologic: No fainting, seizures, motor or sensory loss. No memory problems.

Hematologic: No easy bleeding or bruising.

Endocrine: No known heat or cold intolerance. No polyuria, polydipsia.

Physical Examination

General Examination: MN is a short, overweight, middle-aged woman, who is animated and responds quickly to questions. Her hair is well groomed. Her color is good, and she lies flat without discomfort.

Skin: Palms cold and moist, but color good. Scattered cherry angiomas over upper trunk. Nails without clubbing, cyanosis.

Head, Eyes, Ears, Nose, Throat (HEENT): Head: Hair of average texture. Scalp without lesions, normocephalic/atraumatic (NC/AT). ***Eyes:*** Vision 20/30 in each eye. Visual fields full by confrontation. Conjunctiva pink; sclera white. Pupils 4 mm constricting to 2 mm, round, regular, equally reactive to light. Extraocular movements intact. Disc margins sharp, without hemorrhages, exudates. No arteriolar narrowing or A-V nicking. ***Ears:*** Cerumen partially obscures right tympanic membrane (TM); left canal clear, TM with good cone of light. Acuity good to whispered voice. Weber midline. AC > BC. ***Nose:*** Mucosa pink, septum midline. No sinus tenderness. ***Mouth:*** Oral mucosa pink. Dentition good. Tongue midline. Tonsils absent. Pharynx without exudates.

Neck: Neck supple. Trachea midline. Thyroid isthmus barely palpable, lobes not felt.

Lymph nodes: No cervical, axillary or epitrochlear nodes.

Extremities: Warm and without edema. Calves supple, nontender.

Vital signs: Height (without shoes) 157 cm (5′2″). ***Weight*** (dressed) 65 kg. ***BMI*** 26 kg/m2. ***BP:*** 164/98 right arm, supine; 160/96 left arm, supine; 152/88 right arm, supine with wide cuff. ***Pulse:*** 88/min, regular, normal volume and character. Arterial wall slightly palpable. ***Respiration:*** 18/min, abdominothoracic. ***Temperature (oral):*** 98.6°F.

Respiratory: Thorax symmetric with good excursion. Lungs resonant on percussion. Breath sounds vesicular with no added sounds. Diaphragms descend 4 cm bilaterally.

Cardiovascular: Jugular venous pressure 1 cm above the sternal angle, with head of examining table raised to 30 degrees. Carotid upstrokes brisk, without bruits. Apical impulse discrete and tapping, barely palpable in the 5th left interspace, 8 cm lateral to the midsternal line. Good S_1, S_2; no S_3 or S_4. A II/VI medium-pitched midsystolic murmur at the 2nd right interspace; does not radiate to the neck. No diastolic murmurs.

(continued)

TABLE 1-1. Example of a Comprehensive Clinical Record: The Case of Patient MN *(Continued)*

Breasts: Pendulous, symmetric. No masses; nipples without discharge.

Abdomen: Protuberant. Well-healed scar, right lower quadrant. Bowel sounds active. No tenderness or masses. Liver span 7 cm in right midclavicular line; edge smooth, palpable 1 cm below right costal margin (RCM). Spleen not felt. No costovertebral angle tenderness (CVAT). No external hemorrhoids, with tight sphincter tone, rectal vault without masses. Stool brown, negative for occult blood.

Genitourinary: External genitalia without lesions. Mild cystocele at introitus on straining. Vaginal mucosa pink. Cervix pink, parous, and without discharge. Uterus anterior, midline, smooth, not enlarged. Adnexa not palpated due to obesity and poor relaxation. No cervical or adnexal tenderness. Pap smear taken. Rectovaginal wall intact.

Peripheral vascular: Trace edema at both ankles. No varicosities in lower extremities. No stasis pigmentation or ulcers. Pulses (2+ = brisk, or normal):

	Radial	Femoral	Popliteal	Dorsalis Pedis	Posterior Tibial
RT	2+	2+	2+	2+	2+
LT	2+	2+	2+	2+	2+

Musculoskeletal: No joint deformities or swelling on inspection and palpation. Good range of motion in hands, wrists, elbows, shoulders, spine, hips, knees, ankles.

Neurologic: *Mental Status:* Alert and cooperative. Thought processes are coherent and insight is good. Oriented to person, place, and time. *Cranial nerves:* II to XII intact. *Motor:* Good muscle bulk and tone. *Strength:* 5/5 bilaterally in deltoids, biceps, triceps, hand grips, iliopsoas, hamstrings, quadriceps, tibialis anterior and gastrocnemius. *Cerebellar:* Rapid alternating movement (RAMs) and point-to-point movements intact. Gait stable, fluid. *Sensory:* Pinprick, light touch, position sense, vibration, and stereognosis intact. Romberg negative. *Reflexes:*

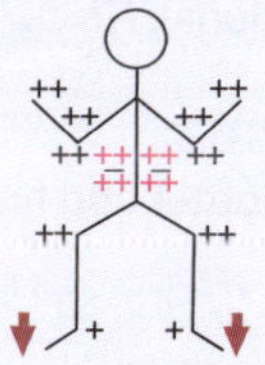

Assessment and Plan

MN is a 54-year-old salesperson with a history of migraines since childhood presenting with chronic intermittent, progressive pulsatile headaches which are similar in nature to prior attacks and precipitated by current life stressors. The headaches are accompanied by nausea and vomiting. On examination has elevated blood pressure but otherwise a normal cardiovascular and nonfocal neurologic examination.

1. **Headaches:**
   The differential diagnosis includes the following.
   a. Migraine headache is most likely as the patient has a history of migraine headaches and describes her current headaches as of a similar quality. The pulsatile quality, duration between 4 and 72 hours, associated nausea and vomiting and disability intensity all support this diagnosis, as does the normal neurologic examination.
   b. Tension headache is also a possibility as the headaches are bilateral, which is less common in migraine headaches. A 54-year-old woman with migraine headaches since childhood, with a throbbing vascular pattern and frequent nausea and vomiting. Headaches are associated with stress and relieved by sleep and cold compresses. There is no papilledema, and there are no motor or sensory deficits on the neurologic examination.
   c. Other dangerous conditions are less likely. There are no fever, stiff neck, or focal findings to suggest meningitis, and the lifelong recurrent pattern makes subarachnoid hemorrhage unlikely (usually described as "the worst headache of my life"). A normal neurologic and funduscopic examination make a space-occupying lesion such as tumor less likely as well.

   Plan:
   - Discuss features of migraine versus tension headaches with the patient. Also discuss warning signs that would prompt urgent re-evaluation.
   - Discuss biofeedback and stress management.
   - Advise patient to avoid caffeine, including coffee, colas, and other carbonated beverages.
   - Start nonsteroidal anti-inflammatory drugs (NSAIDs) for headache, as needed.
   - If needed next visit, begin prophylactic medication if headaches are occurring more than 2 days a week or 8 days a month.

(continued)

TABLE 1-1. Example of a Comprehensive Clinical Record: The Case of Patient MN *(Continued)*

2. **Elevated blood pressure:** Elevated systolic and diastolic blood pressure are noted. The patient denies chest pain and shortness of breath and is not symptomatic at the time of the interview, making hypertensive urgency unlikely.
   Plan:
   - Discuss standards for assessing blood pressure.
   - Check a hemoglobin A_{1C} to assess for diabetes, which would impact the target blood pressure.
   - Recheck blood pressure in 2 weeks.
   - Discuss weight reduction and exercise programs (see #4).
   - Reduce salt intake.
3. **Cystocele with occasional stress incontinence:** Cystocele on pelvic examination, probably related to bladder relaxation. Patient is perimenopausal. Incontinence reported with coughing, suggesting alteration in bladder neck anatomy. No dysuria, fever, flank pain. Not taking any contributing medications. Usually involves small amounts of urine, no dribbling, so doubt urge or overflow incontinence.
   Plan:
   - Explain cause of stress incontinence.
   - Review urinalysis.
   - Recommend Kegel exercises.
   - Consider topical estrogen cream to vagina during next visit if no improvement.
4. **Overweight:** Patient 5′2″, weighs 143 lb; BMI is ~26.
   Plan:
   - Explore diet history, ask patient to keep food intake diary.
   - Explore motivation to lose weight, set target for weight loss by next visit.
   - Schedule visit with dietitian.
   - Discuss exercise program, specifically, walking 30 minutes most days a week.
5. **Stress and Housing insecurity:** Son-in-law with alcohol problem; daughter and grandchildren seeking refuge in patient's apartment, leading to tensions in these relationships. Patient also has financial constraints and describes spiritual duress with lack of social and spiritual support. Stress currently situational. No current evidence of depression (PHQ2 = 0).
   Plan:
   - Explore patient's views on strategies to cope with stress.
   - Explore sources of support, including Al-Anon for daughter and financial counseling for patient. Refer to social work and discuss in interdisciplinary team meeting.
   - Refer to chaplain to discuss spiritual support systems.
   - Continue to monitor for possible signs of depression.
6. **Occasional musculoskeletal low back pain:** Usually with prolonged standing. No history of trauma or motor vehicle accident. Pain does not radiate; no tenderness or motor-sensory deficits on examination. Doubt disc or nerve root compression, trochanteric bursitis, sacroiliitis.
   Plan:
   - Review benefits of weight loss and exercises to strengthen low back muscles.
7. **Tobacco misuse:** 1 pack per day for 36 years. No signs of oral cancer on examination today. Seems pre-contemplative for smoking cessation in setting of multiple life stressors and progressive headaches.
   Plan:
   - Check peak flow or FEV_1/FVC on office spirometry to assess for obstructive lung disease.
   - Discuss low-dose CT for lung cancer screening
   - Pre-contemplative at this point, but offered ongoing support moving forward should she change her mind and provided information resources regarding nicotine replacement therapy and oral medications to review. Can re-address after improvement of life stressors and relief from headaches.
8. **Murmur:** A II/IV midsystolic murmur was appreciated on examination. Given its location in the aortic position and the patient's age this most likely represents aortic sclerosis or stenosis. The patient has no shortness of breath, chest pain or syncope to suggest severe aortic stenosis. Will monitor symptoms examination and consider a transthoracic echocardiogram if the murmur changes in intensity or if she develops any symptoms.
9. **Health maintenance:** Last Pap smear 2018; Mammogram, 2019; has never had a colonoscopy.
   Plan:
   - Referred for colonoscopy, prescribed prep medications and discussed use. Provided hand out with instructions and discussed using teach-back technique.
   - Referred to dentist for oral cancer screening in light of smoking.
   - Advise patient to move medications and caustic cleaning agents to locked cabinet above shoulder height. Urge patient to store handgun in a secured locked location, unloaded with trigger lock, and to store ammunition in a separate locked location.

TABLE 1-2. Example of a Focused Clinical Record: The Case of Patient XY

4/10/2022 11:00 am
XY, 56 years old, housewife
Source and Reliability.
Self-referred; reliable.

Chief Complaint
"I am having chest pain for the last 1 week."

History of Present Illness
XY presented to the emergency department with chest pain for the past 1 week. She was in good health until 1 week prior to admission. At that time, she noticed that the chest pain was abrupt in onset (over a few seconds to a minute). She described the chest pain as dull and aching in character. The pain began in the left parasternal area, radiating up to the left side of the neck and the jaw. It was mild to moderate in intensity (rated as 3 to 6 out of 10 in the 10-point pain scale), lasted approximately 10 to 15 minutes, and subsided with rest. The pain occurred when XY was doing her household work in the morning. She states that she was working for about 30 minutes before she felt tired and started having pain. The chest discomfort was accompanied by mild shortness of breath but no nausea, vomiting, or sweating.

XY had two more episodes of pain, similar in quality and site to the first episode. This morning, she had an episode of pain while she was washing her clothes, lasting more than half an hour. She did not take any specific measures to relieve her pain. She only took rest. She did not have any other associated symptoms during this episode of pain. She thinks that her chest pain is not normal and is occurring more frequently while she does any physical activity. She is concerned because chest pain is interfering with her day-to-day activities.

Allergies: Ampicillin, experienced rash and hives in 1974.

Medications: None.

Past Medical History

Medical: Diagnosed with type 2 diabetes mellitus in 2017 and began an unknown medication.

Surgical: Total abdominal hysterectomy and bilateral oophorectomy for dysfunctional uterine bleeding (DUB) in 2015.

Family History
- Mother, age 83 years, alive and well.
- Father died at the age of 65 years from heart attack.
- One younger brother, age 49 years, with hypertension, otherwise well.

Personal and Social History
Married and housewife; she is a science graduate. One son and one daughter who live nearby. She neither smokes nor takes alcohol.

Review of Systems
General: Has gained 2 kg in the past 5 years.
Skin: No rashes or other changes.
Head, Eyes, Ears, Nose, Throat (HEENT): No complaints of headache, change in vision, nose or ear problems, or sore throat.
Neck: No lumps, goiter, pain. No swollen glands.
Breasts: No lumps, pain, discharge.
Respiratory: No cough, wheezing, shortness of breath.
Cardiovascular: No exertional dyspnea, orthopnea, or paroxysmal nocturnal dyspnea.
Gastrointestinal: No dysphagia, nausea, vomiting, or change in stool pattern, consistency, or color. XY complains of epigastric pain, burning in quality, occasionally one to two times a month, especially on an empty stomach.
Genitourinary: No complaints of dysuria, nocturia, polyuria, hematuria, or vaginal bleeding.
Peripheral vascular: No history of phlebitis or leg pain.
Musculoskeletal: XY complains of lower back pain, aching in quality, once or twice a month if she does more work than usual. This pain is usually relieved with diclofenac gel. No other joint pain.

(continued)

TABLE 1-2. Example of a Focused Clinical Record: The Case of Patient XY *(Continued)*

Neurologic: No fainting, seizures, motor or sensory loss. No memory problems.

Hematologic: No easy bleeding or bruising.

Endocrine: No known heat or cold intolerance. No polyuria, polydipsia.

Physical Examination

General Examination: XY is an obese, middle-aged woman. Her hair is well groomed. She is dark colored and lies flat without discomfort. She appears alert, oriented, and cooperative.

Skin, Hair, and Nails: Palms cold and moist, but color good. Nails without clubbing, cyanosis. No evidence of pallor or jaundice. Capillary refill is normal.

Normal facial expressions. No bad odor from the body or breath.

Height (without shoes) 157 cm (5′2″). ***Weight*** (dressed) 65 kg (143 lb). ***BMI*** is 26.

Vital signs: BP: 164/98 right arm, supine; 160/96 left arm, supine; 152/88 right arm, supine with wide cuff. ***Pulse:*** 88 beats/min, regular, normal volume and character. All the peripheral pulses are felt and are symmetrical. Arterial wall is not palpable. ***Respiratory rate (RR):*** 18/min and abdominothoracic. ***Temperature (oral):*** 98.6°F.

Hydration: No evidence of dehydration or edema.

Eyes: Vision 6/6 in each eye. Visual fields full by confrontation. Conjunctiva pink; sclera white. Pupils equally round, 4 mm, reactive to light and accommodation, sclera and conjunctiva normal. Fundoscopic examination reveals normal vessels without hemorrhage. No arteriolar narrowing or A-V nicking. ***Ears:*** Right and left canals clear, TM with good cone of light. Acuity good to whispered voice. Weber midline. AC > BC. ***Nose:*** Mucosa pink, septum midline. No sinus tenderness. ***Mouth:*** Oral mucosa pink. Dentition good. Tongue midline. Tonsils absent. Pharynx without exudates.

Neck: Neck supple. Trachea midline. Thyroid isthmus barely palpable, lobes not felt.

Lymph nodes: No cervical, axillary, or epitrochlear nodes.

Extremities: Warm and without edema. Calves supple, nontender.

Speech and language: Normal. No dysarthria.

Cognitive functions: Normal.

Gait: Normal.

System or Region Examination

Cardiovascular: Jugular venous pressure 8 cm above the sternal angle, with the head of the examining table raised to 30 degrees. Carotid upstrokes brisk, without bruits. Apical impulse discrete and tapping, barely palpable in the 5th left interspace, 8 cm lateral to the midsternal line. Good S1, S2; a third heart sound is heard at the apex. No fourth heart sound or rub is heard. A 2/6 medium-pitched mid-systolic decrescendo murmur at the 2nd right interspace which radiates to the neck. No diastolic murmurs.

Respiratory: Chest symmetric with good excursion. Lungs resonant on percussion. Breath sounds vesicular with no added sounds. Diaphragms descend 4 cm bilaterally.

Abdomen: The abdomen is symmetrical without distention; bowel sounds are normal in quality and intensity in all areas. No tenderness or masses. Liver span 7 cm in the right midclavicular line; edge smooth, palpable 1 cm below the right costal margin (RCM). Spleen not felt. No costovertebral angle tenderness (CVAT).

Neurological: Cranial nerves II to XII are normal. Motor and sensory examination of the upper and lower extremities is normal. Cerebellar function is also normal. Reflexes are normal and symmetrical bilaterally in both extremities.

Note: Please refer to Table 1-1 for assessment and plan.

CHAPTER

2

Interviewing, Communication, and Interpersonal Skills

You may have many reasons for choosing to enter the healthcare professions, but building effective and healing relationships is undoubtedly paramount. This chapter describes the fundamental techniques of therapeutic interviewing, the timeless skills you will continually polish as you care for patients. These skills require practice and feedback from your teachers so that you can monitor your progress. Over time, you will learn to select the techniques best suited to the everchanging dynamics of human behavior in your patient relationships.

As discussed in Chapter 1, the *interviewing process* during a clinical encounter is more than just a series of questions; it requires a highly refined sensitivity to the patient's feelings and behavioral cues (Fig. 2-1). This process generates a patient's story that is fluid and draws on various relational skills to respond effectively to patient cues, feelings, and concerns. The previous chapter also emphasized that the skills required during this process are quite different from the *format of the health history*. The health history format provides an essential framework for organizing the patient's story into various categories pertinent to the patient's present, past, and family health. The interview process and the health history format have distinct but complementary purposes. Keep these differences in mind as you learn the techniques of skilled interviewing in this chapter.

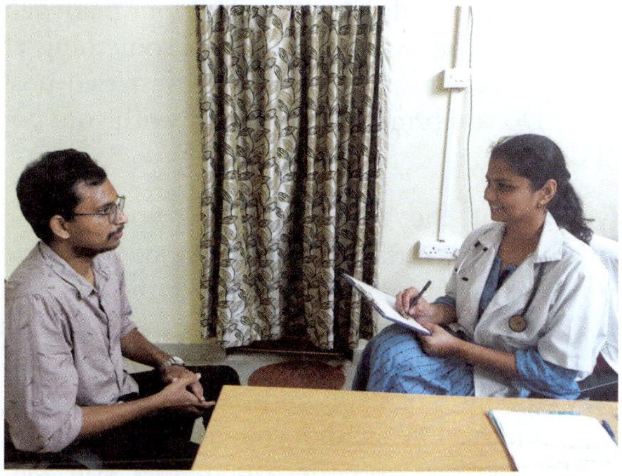

FIGURE 2-1. The interviewing process using effective communication skills.

FUNDAMENTALS OF SKILLED INTERVIEWING

You may recall that the clinical encounter has a structure and sequence: *initiating the session, information gathering, the physical examination, explaining and planning*, and *closing the session*. In this section, we will highlight the global communication and interpersonal techniques that can be utilized across all stages of the clinical encounter (Box 2-1).

Box 2-1. Skilled Interviewing Techniques

- Active or attentive listening
- Guided questioning
- Empathic responses
- Summarization
- Transitions
- Partnering
- Validation
- Empowering the patient
- Reassurance
- Appropriate verbal communication
- Appropriate nonverbal communication

Active or Attentive Listening

Active listening or *attentive listening* lies at the heart of the patient interview. It involves a number of different, specific skills that help facilitate, direct and structure your interaction with your patient. It means carefully attending to what the patient is communicating, connecting to the patient's emotional state, and using verbal and nonverbal skills to encourage the patient to expand on his or her feelings and concerns. Active listening allows you to relate to those concerns at multiple levels of the patient's experience. This takes practice. It is easy to drift into thinking about your next question or possible diagnoses and lose your concentration on the patient's story. Focus on what the patient is telling you, both verbally and nonverbally. Sometimes one's body language tells a different story from one's words.

Guided Questioning

There are several ways to elicit more information without changing the flow of the patient's story. Your goal is to facilitate full communication, in the patient's own words, without interruption. Guided questions show your sustained interest in the patient's feelings and deepest disclosures (Box 2-2). They help you avoid questions that prestructure or even shut down the patient's responses. A series of "yes-no" questions makes the patient feel more restricted and passive, leading to significant loss of detail. Instead, use guided questioning to absorb the patient's full story.

Box 2-2. Techniques of Guided Questioning

- Moving from open-ended to focused questions
- Using questioning that elicits a graded response
- Asking a series of questions, one at a time
- Offering multiple choices for answers
- Clarifying what the patient means
- Encouraging with continuers
- Using echoing/repetition

Moving from Open-Ended to Focused Questions. Your questions should flow from general to specific. Think about a cone, open at the top, then tapering to a focal point (Fig. 2-2). Start with the most general questions

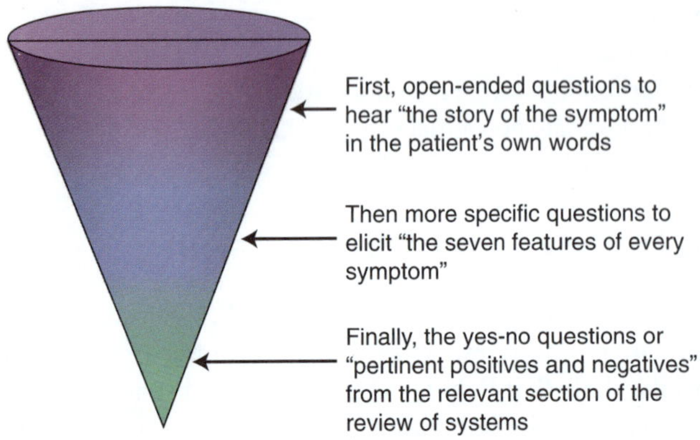

FIGURE 2-2. Guided questioning from open-ended to more focused questions.

like, "How can I help?" or "What brings you in today?" Then move to still open, but more focused, questions like, "Can you tell me more about what happened when you took the medicine?" Then pose closed questions like, "Did the new medicine cause any problems?"

Begin with a truly open-ended question that does not prefigure an answer. A possible sequence might be:

> "Tell me about your chest discomfort." (Pause)
> "What else?" (Pause)
> "Where did you feel it?" (Pause) "Show me."
> "Anywhere else?" (Pause) "Did it travel anywhere?" (Pause) "To which arm?"

Avoid *leading questions* that already contain an answer or suggested response like: "Has your pain been improving?" or "You don't have any blood in your stools, do you?" If you ask, "Is your pain like a pressure?" and the patient answers yes, the patient's response is truncated instead of including details about what he or she experienced. Adopt the more neutral "Please describe your pain."

Questioning That Elicits a Graded Response. Ask questions that require a graded response rather than a yes-no answer. "How many steps can you climb before you get short of breath?" is better than "Do you get short of breath climbing stairs?"

Asking a Series of Questions, One at a Time. Be sure to ask one question at a time. "Any tuberculosis, diabetes, asthma, heart condition, or high blood pressure in the family?" may prompt "No" out of sheer confusion. Try "Do you have any of the following problems?" Be sure to pause and establish eye contact as you list each problem.

Offering Multiple Choices for Answers. Sometimes, patients need help in describing their symptoms. To minimize bias, offer multiple-choice answers: "Which of the following words best describes your pain: aching, sharp, pressing, burning, shooting, or something else?" Almost any specific question can contrast two possible answers. "Do you bring up any phlegm with your cough, or is it dry?"

Clarifying What the Patient Means. Sometimes the patient's history is difficult to understand. It is better to acknowledge confusion than to act like the story makes sense. To understand what the patient means, you need to *request clarification*, as in "Tell me exactly what you mean by 'the flu'" or "You said you were behaving just like your mother. What did you mean?" Taking time for clarification reassures the patient that you want to understand his or her story and builds your therapeutic relationship.

Encouraging with Continuers. Without even speaking, you can use posture and gestures (nonverbal encouragements) or words (neutral utterances) to encourage the patient to say more. Pausing and nodding your head or remaining silent, yet attentive and relaxed, is a *cue for the patient to continue.* Leaning forward, making eye contact, and using phrases like "Uh-huh," or "Go on," or "I'm listening" all enhance the flow of the patient's story.

Echoing (Repetition). Simply repeating the patient's last words, or *echoing,* encourages the patient to elaborate on details and feelings. Echoing also demonstrates careful listening and a subtle connection with the patient by using the same words. For example:

Patient: "The pain got worse and began to spread." (Pause)
Response: "Spread?" (Pause)
Patient: "Yes, it went to my shoulder and down my left arm to the fingers. It was so bad that I thought I was going to die." (Pause)
Response: "Going to die?"
Patient: "Yes, it was just like the pain my father had when he had his heart attack, and I was afraid the same thing was happening to me."

This reflective technique helped to reveal not only the location and severity of the pain but also its meaning to the patient. It did not bias the story or interrupt the patient's train of thought.

Empathic Responses

Empathic responses are vital to patient rapport and healing. *Empathy* has been described as "the capacity to identify with the patient and feel the patient's pain as your own, then respond in a supportive manner." Empathy "requires a willingness to suffer some of the patient's pain in the sharing of suffering that is vital to healing." As patients talk with you, they may convey, in their words or facial expressions, feelings they have not consciously acknowledged. These feelings are crucial to understanding their illnesses.

To express empathy, you must first recognize the patient's feelings, then actively move toward and elicit emotional content. At first, exploring these feelings may make you feel uncomfortable, but your empathic responses will deepen mutual trust. When you sense unexpressed feelings from the patient's face, voice, behavior or words, gently ask: "How do you feel about that?" or "That seems to trouble you, can you say more?"

Sometimes a patient's response may not correspond to your initial assumptions. Responding to a patient that the death of a parent must be upsetting, when in fact the death relieved the patient of a heavy emotional burden, reflects your interpretation, not what the patient feels. Instead, you can ask: "You have lost your father. What has that been like for you?" It is better to ask the patient to expand or clarify a point than assume you understand. Empathy may also be nonverbal—placing your hand on the patient's arm or offering tissues when the patient is crying. Unless you affirm your concern, important dimensions of the patient's experience may go untapped.

Once the patient has shared these feelings, reply with understanding and acceptance. Your responses may be as simple as: "I cannot imagine how hard this must be for you" or "That sounds upsetting" or "You must be feeling sad." For a response to be empathic, it must convey that you feel what the patient is feeling.

Summarization

Giving a capsule summary of the patient's story during the course of the interview serves several purposes. It communicates that you have been listening carefully. It identifies what you know and what you don't know. "Now, let me make sure that I have the full story. You said you've had a cough for three days, that it's especially bad at night, and that you have started to bring up yellow phlegm. You have not had a fever or felt short of breath, but you do feel congested, with difficulty breathing through your nose." Following with an attentive pause or asking, "Anything else?" allows the patient to add other information and correct any misunderstandings.

You can use summarization at different points in the interview to structure the visit, especially at times of transition. This technique also allows you to organize your clinical reasoning and convey your thinking to the patient, making the relationship more collaborative. It also helps learners when they draw a blank on what to ask next.

Transitions

Patients may be apprehensive during a healthcare visit. To put them more at ease, tell them when you are changing directions during the interview. Just like signs along the highway, *"signposting"* transitions help prepare patients for what comes next. As you move through the history and on to the physical examination, orient the patient with brief transitional phrases like "Now I'd like to ask some questions about your past health." Make clear what the patient should expect or do next. "Before we move on to reviewing all your medications, was there anything else about past health problems?" "Now I would like to examine you. I will step out for a few minutes. Please undress and put on this gown."

Partnering

When building rapport with patients, express your commitment to an ongoing relationship. Make patients feel that no matter what happens, you will continue to provide care. Even as a student, especially in a hospital setting, this support can make a big difference.

Validation

Another way to affirm the patient is to validate the legitimacy of his or her emotional experience. A patient caught in a car accident, even if uninjured, may still feel very distressed. Saying something like, "Your accident must have been terrifying. Car accidents are always unsettling because they remind us how vulnerable we are. Perhaps that explains why you still feel upset," validates the patient's response as legitimate and understandable.

Empowering the Patient

The clinician–patient relationship is inherently unequal. Your feelings of inexperience as a student predictably change over time as you grow in clinical experience. Patients, however, have many reasons to feel vulnerable. They may be in pain or worried about a symptom. They may feel overwhelmed by even scheduling a visit, a task you might take for granted. Differences of gender, ethnicity, race, or socioeconomic status contribute to the power asymmetry of the relationship. Ultimately, however, patients are responsible for their care. When you empower patients to ask questions, express their concerns, and probe your recommendations, they are most likely to adopt your advice, make lifestyle changes, or take medications as prescribed.

Listed in Box 2-3 are techniques for sharing power with your patients. Although many have already been discussed, reinforcing patients' responsibility for their health is fundamental and worth summarizing here.

Box 2-3. Empowering the Patient: Techniques for Sharing Power

- Evoke the patient's perspective.
- Convey interest in the person, not just the problem.
- Follow the patient's leads.
- Elicit and validate emotional content.
- Share information with the patient, especially at transition points during the visit.
- Make your clinical reasoning transparent to the patient.
- Reveal the limits of your knowledge.

Reassurance

When patients are anxious or upset, it is tempting to provide reassurance like "Don't worry. Everything is going to be all right." Although this is common in social interactions, for clinicians, such comments may be premature and counterproductive. Depending on the actual situation, they may even be misleading and block further disclosure. The patient may sense that you are uncomfortable handling anxiety or fail to appreciate the depth of the distress.

The first step to effective reassurance is simply identifying and acknowledging the patient's feelings. For example, you might say, "You seem upset today." This promotes a sense of connection. Meaningful reassurance comes later after you have completed the interview, the physical examination, and perhaps some laboratory tests. At that point, you can explain what you think is happening and deal openly with any concerns. Reassurance is more appropriate when the patient feels that problems have been fully understood and are being addressed.

APPROPRIATE VERBAL COMMUNICATION

As a clinician, it is important that we are careful in *what* we say, but equally important we should also be cautious as to *how* we say things. The effectiveness of the clinical encounter rests on the use of appropriate language. This can also enhance patient rapport and lead to a satisfying clinician–patient relationship.

Use Understandable Language

Understandable language uses simple, recognizable and clear words. It is an essential communication technique for speaking to patients, regardless of their level of health literacy. It is critical to use short sentences and words and only communicate essential information. Simple words avoid the use of medical jargon, abbreviations or any complex words or phrases. Avoid saying "Does the pain radiate?" Simply say "Does the pain move anywhere?" If you catch yourself using medical jargon or complex words, apologize for it and explain it immediately to your patient using simpler, less complex words or phrases that the patient knows. Also use clear and concrete words or phrases, rather than vague ones such as "a little bit," "common," "possible," "rare." It is crucial to practice communicating to all patients with plain language, regardless of a person's education, socioeconomic status or cultural background.

Even when using plain language, your patients can still sometimes get overwhelmed when given too much information at once. Ideally, your patient encounters should focus on one to three key points, and you as the clinician should repeat the points often. One way to narrow in on the key message is with the "Ask Me Three" approach. This approach is intended to help patients become more active members of their healthcare team. It encourages patients to ask—and clinicians to answer—three main questions during each clinical encounter.

1. What is my main problem?
2. What do I need to do?
3. Why is it important for me to do this?

Modifying this approach to "Tell Them Three" can also help clinicians keep their message focused and simple. Another approach to make sure your patient understands you is the teach-back method. Again, keep in mind "teach back" is not a test of the patient's knowledge but a test of how well you explained things in a manner your patient understands.

Use Nonstigmatizing Language

On occasion, one may unintentionally use words or phrases during the clinical interview which could be perceived by the patient as dehumanizing, perpetuate stigma, and tend to marginalize rather than support them. The language we use to reference people should reflect their full identities and acknowledge their capacity to change and grow. Unintentionally stigmatizing language can distance and traumatize patients, create barriers to patients seeking help or accessing treatment, and perpetuate negative stereotypes. For example, avoid saying: "Do you still consider yourself a drug addict?" or "Are you wheelchair bound?" but instead say "Do you still consider yourself a person with an addiction to drugs?" or "Are you a person who uses a wheelchair daily?"

A step to avoid stigmatizing language includes the use of *"people-first" language*. For example, saying *"drug abuser"* can imply that the person is the problem. Instead, say *"person who uses drugs"* or *"person with a substance use disorder"* which suggests that the person might have a particular condition or chronic illness, but it does not define them completely. See Box 2-4.

Box 2-4. Examples of Stigmatizing and Corresponding Nonstigmatizing Language

What You Should AVOID Saying...	What You Should Say...
Ex-offender, thug, criminal, ex-felon, ex-con, convict, inmate, offender, felon, prisoner	Person who was/is incarcerated, formerly incarcerated person
Parolee, probationer	Person on parole, a person on probation
Drug abuser, addict, junkie	Person who uses/injects drugs, a person with an addiction
Schizophrenic, depressive	Person who has been diagnosed with schizophrenia or depression
AIDS or HIV patient, suffering from HIV, AIDS victim	Person living with HIV, a person living with AIDS
Prostitute, hooker, street walker	Sex worker, a person who is involved in transactional or survival sex
Rape victim	Sexual assault survivor, a rape survivor
The handicapped, the disabled	People with disabilities
Normal, healthy, whole or typical people	People without disabilities
Dwarf, a midget	Person of short stature, little person
Confined to a wheelchair; wheelchair bound	Person who uses a wheelchair or a mobility chair

Source: People First Language. Texas Council for Developmental Disabilities. Available at http://www.tcdd.texas.gov/resources/people-first-language/. Accessed March 30, 2019.

APPROPRIATE NONVERBAL COMMUNICATION

Just as you carefully observe the patient, the patient will be watching you. Consciously or not, you send messages through both your words and your behavior. Posture, gestures, eye contact, and tone of voice all convey the extent of your interest, attention, acceptance, and understanding (Fig. 2-3).

The skilled interviewer seems calm and unhurried, even when time is limited. Patients sense when you are preoccupied. It is essential to learn to focus and give the patient your full attention. Patients are also sensitive to any implied disapproval, embarrassment, impatience, or boredom and to behaviors that condescend, stereotype, criticize, or belittle. Professionalism requires

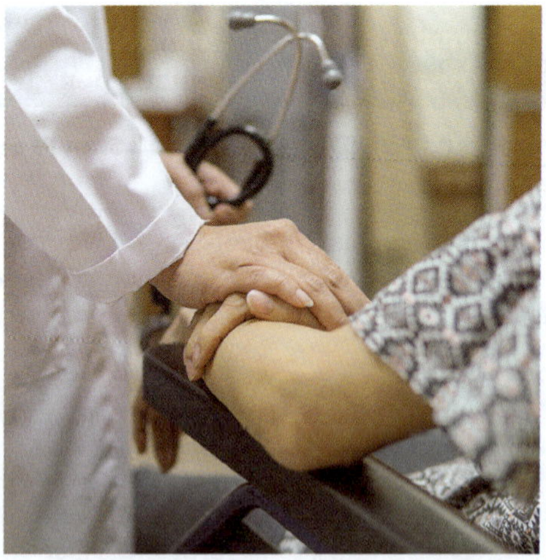

FIGURE 2-3. Nonverbal behaviors can convey empathy. (Used with permission from Shutterstock. By nuiza11.)

equanimity and "unconditional positive regard" to nurture healing relationships.

Both clinicians and patients continuously display nonverbal communication that provides vital clues to our underlying feelings. Being sensitive to nonverbal cues allows you to "read the patient" more effectively and send messages of your own. Pay close attention to eye contact, facial expression, posture, head position and movement such as shaking or nodding, interpersonal distance, and placement of the arms or legs—crossed, neutral, or open. Be aware that some forms of nonverbal communication are universal, but many are culturally bound.

Just as mirroring your posture shows the patient's sense of connection, matching your position to the patient's can transmit increased rapport. Moving closer or making physical contact like placing your hand on the patient's shoulder can convey empathy and can help the patient gain control of upsetting feelings. In fact nonverbal behavior might be more important than verbal messages in the communication of empathy and serves as the primary vehicle for expressing emotions. The first step to using this valuable technique is to notice nonverbal behaviors and bring them to a conscious level. See Box 2-5.

Box 2-5. Forms of Nonverbal Communication

- Body orientation toward and physical proximity to patient*
- Gaze orientation (eye contact) toward patients*
- Head nodding with facial animation*
- Head nodding with gesture*
- Posture
- Tone and use of voice
- Use of silence
- Use of touch (*haptics*)

*Found in studies to be correlated with increasing patient rapport with clinician.

OTHER CONSIDERATIONS IN COMMUNICATION AND INTERPERSONAL SKILLS

Broaching Sensitive Topics

You will learn in the following chapters that clinicians talk with patients about many sensitive topics. These discussions can be awkward when you are inexperienced or assessing patients you do not know well. Even seasoned clinicians are inhibited by societal constraints when discussing certain subjects: abuse of alcohol or drugs, sexual practices, death and dying, financial concerns, racial and ethnic bias, domestic violence, psychiatric illness, physical deformity, bowel function, and others. Many of these topics trigger strong personal responses related to family, cultural, and societal values. Several basic principles can help guide your response to sensitive topics.

Look into strategies that help make you more comfortable when discussing sensitive areas (Box 2-6). These include reading about these topics in clinical and lay literature; talking with colleagues and teachers about your concerns; taking courses that help you explore your feelings and reactions; and ultimately, reflecting on your own life experience. Take advantage of all these resources. If possible, listen to experienced clinicians as they approach these issues with patients, then practice similar techniques in your discussions. Over time, your level of comfort will grow and expand.

Box 2-6. Guidelines for Broaching Sensitive Topics

- The single most important rule is to be nonjudgmental. Your role is to learn from the patient and help the patient achieve better health. Acceptance is the best way to reach this goal.
- Explain why you need to know certain information. This makes patients less apprehensive. For example, say to patients, *"To help me take better care of you, I need to ask you some questions about your sexual health and practices."*
- Find opening questions for sensitive topics and learn the specific kinds of information needed for your shared assessment and plan.
- Consciously acknowledge whatever discomfort you are feeling. Denying your discomfort may lead you to avoid the topic altogether.

Informed Consent

A patient's consent to a procedure or treatment is more than simply signing a form. *Informed consent* is a communication process in which a clinician educates a patient about the risks, benefits, and alternatives of a given procedure or intervention.

The following are the required elements for documentation of the informed consent discussion:

- Nature of the procedure or treatment
- Risks and benefits of the procedure or treatment
- Reasonable alternatives
- Risks and benefits of alternatives
- Assessment of the patient's understanding of the first four elements

Clinicians have a legal and ethical duty to follow the process of obtaining consent without leaving out any of the core elements.

Obtaining informed consent will vary from patient to patient. It will be obvious to you that each patient has their own set of circumstances which will affect their ability to make informed decisions. Ensure that your patient has the *decisional capacity*. If not, then discuss with the person whom the patient has designated as the *healthcare proxy*. You must take into consideration all of the aspects of your patient's life and the best way to communicate with them. Use understandable language that is not condescending and avoid medical jargon. You may want to use the teach-back method to assess how well you explained the information to the patient. If possible, provide other sources of information for your patient to research on their own, such as a brochure, website, or video. Ask: "What questions do you have for me?" and remain available to answer any questions after the initial conversation. Every patient with decisional capacity has the right to consent or decline procedures or treatments after they have been properly informed.

Working with a Medical Interpreter

A few words in the language that is most comfortable for your patient may enhance rapport, but they are no substitute for the full story. Even if you are fluent, you may miss important nuances in the meanings of certain words. Recruiting family members as translators is equally hazardous—it may violate confidentiality, and information may be incomplete, misleading, or harmful. Lengthy patient explanations may be telescoped into a few words, omitting significant details. The ideal interpreter is a "cultural navigator" who is neutral and trained in both languages and cultures. However, even trained interpreters may be unfamiliar with the various subcultures in many societies.

When you work with an interpreter, begin by establishing rapport and reviewing the information that will be most useful (Box 2-7). Ask the interpreter

Box 2-7. Guidelines for Working with an Interpreter: "INTERPRET"

I	**Introductions:** Make sure to introduce all the individuals in the room. During the introduction, include information as to the roles individuals will play.
N	**Note Goals:** Note the goals of the interview. What is the diagnosis? What will the treatment entail? Will there be any follow-up?
T	**Transparency:** Let the patient know that everything said will be interpreted throughout the session.
E	**Ethics:** Use qualified interpreters (not family members or children) when conducting an interview. Qualified interpreters allow the patient to maintain autonomy and make informed decisions about his or her care.
R	**Respect Beliefs:** Patient with limited English proficiency (LEP) may have cultural beliefs that need to be taken into account as well. The interpreter may be able to serve as a cultural broker and help explain any cultural beliefs that may exist.
P	**Patient Focus:** The patient should remain the focus of the encounter. Providers should interact with the patient and not the interpreter. Make sure to ask and address any questions the patient may have before ending the encounter. If you don't have trained interpreters on staff, the patient may not be able to call in with questions.
R	**Retain Control:** It is vital as the provider that you remain in control of the interaction and not let the patient or the interpreter take over the conversation.
E	**Explain:** Use simple language and short sentences when working with an interpreter. This will ensure that comparable words can be found in the second language and that all the information can be conveyed clearly.
T	**Thanks:** Thank the interpreter and the patient for their time. On the chart, note that the patient needs an interpreter and who served as an interpreter this time.

Source: Administration for Children and Families. U.S. Department of Health and Human Services. INTERPRET tool: working with interpreters in cultural settings. Available at https://www.acf.hhs.gov/sites/default/files/otip/hhs_clas_interpret_tool.pdf. Accessed March 30, 2019.

to translate everything, not to condense or summarize. Make your questions clear, short, and straightforward. Help the interpreter by outlining your goals for each segment of the history. After going over your plans, arrange the seating so that you have easy eye contact with the patient. Then speak directly to the patient, "How long have you been sick?" rather than "How long has the patient been sick?" Having the interpreter sit close to the patient, or even behind you, keeps you from turning your head back and forth.

Advance Directives

In general, it is important to encourage any adult, but especially adults who are older or chronically ill, to have an *advance directive* and establish a *healthcare proxy* or *healthcare power of attorney* who can act as the patient's health decision maker. This part of the interview can be a "values history" that identifies what is important to the patient and makes life worth living, and when living would no longer be worthwhile. Ask how patients spend their time every day, what they enjoy, and what they look forward to. Make sure to clarify the meaning of statements like, "You said that you don't want to be a burden to your family. What exactly do you mean by that?" Ask, "I wonder if you have concerns about your illness? your pain? your preferences for treatment?" Provide the information requested and demonstrate your commitment to support and coordinate the patient's care throughout the illness. Explore the patient's religious or spiritual beliefs so that you and the patient can make the most appropriate decisions about health care.

Dying patients rarely want to talk about their illnesses at each encounter, nor do they wish to confide in everyone they meet. If they wish to stay at a social level, respect their preferences. A smile, a touch, an inquiry about a family member, a comment on the day's events, or even gentle humor conveys your concern and responsiveness.

Clarifying the patient's wishes about treatment at the end of life is an important responsibility. Failing to facilitate end-of-life decision-making is widely viewed as a flaw in clinical care. The health status of the patient and the healthcare setting often determine what needs to be discussed.

For patients who are acutely ill and, in the hospital, discussions about how to respond to a cardiac or respiratory arrest are usually mandatory. Asking about *Do Not Resuscitate (DNR)* or *allow natural death status* is often difficult if you have not had a previous relationship with the patient or are unsure of the patient's understanding of the illness. The media give many patients an unrealistic view of the effectiveness of resuscitation. Explore, "What experiences have you had with the death of a close friend or relative?" "What do you know about cardiopulmonary resuscitation (CPR)?" Educate patients about the likely success of CPR, especially if they are chronically ill or advanced in age. Assure them that relieving pain and taking care of their spiritual and physical needs will be a priority.

Disclosing Serious News

The complex task of disclosing serious news to patients such as illnesses with poor survival outcomes, disease recurrence or failure of treatments requires advanced communication skills. In addition to the verbal component of actually giving the serious news, it also requires responding to patients' emotional reactions, shared decision-making, the stress created by patients' expectations, the involvement of multiple family members, and how to provide hope despite a situation that is bleak. The SPIKES protocol for disclosing serious news has been recommended to guide clinicians due to the complexity of these interactions that can often create serious communication issues. The 6-step protocol: **S**etting up the interview, assessing the patient's **P**erception, obtaining the patient's **I**nvitation, giving **K**nowledge and information to the patient, addressing the patient's **E**motions with empathic responses and **S**trategy and **S**ummary (Box 2-8).

Box 2-8. SPIKES: The Six-Step Protocol for Delivering Bad News

Steps	Information
1: **S**etting up the interview	Arrange for some privacy Involve significant others Sit down Make a connection with the patient Manage time constraints and interruptions *"Let me take a minute to make sure I've got what I need."*

(continued)

Box 2-8. SPIKES: The Six-Step Protocol for Delivering Bad News (*continued*)

Steps	Information
2: Assessing the patient's **P**erception	The clinician uses open-ended questions to create a reasonably accurate picture of how the patient perceives the medical situation Examples: *"What thoughts have you had since the biopsy?" "What is your understanding of the reasons we did the MRI?"*
3: Obtaining the patient's **I**nvitation	Find out how much the patient wants to know. In any conversation about bad news the real issue is not "do you want to know?" but "at what level do you want to know?" *"If this turns out to be something serious are you the kind of person who likes to know exactly what's going on."*
4: Giving **K**nowledge and information to the patient	Present information based on the assessed level of patient's understanding, compliance, and wishes for disclosure. Start with a warning message *("Unfortunately I've got some bad news to tell you" or "I'm sorry to tell you that…")* Pause after sharing the primary information before proceeding further. Avoid jargon
5: Addressing the patient's **E**motions with **E**mpathic responses	Expect the patient's first response to be an emotion Be prepared to acknowledge the emotion explicitly. Examples: *"I can see how upsetting this is to you." "I can tell you weren't expecting to hear this." "I'm sorry to have to tell you this." "I was also hoping for a better result."*
6: **S**trategy and **S**ummary	Ensure that the patient understands the information that has been provided first before discussing the next steps If they are prepared for such a discussion: Examples: *"Is there anything I could do to make this a little easier?"* *"I want you to be prepared for the next step. Can I explain…"*

Sources: Baile WF et al. *Oncologist*. 2000,5(4):302–311. VitalTalk. Serious News. Available at https://www.vitaltalk.org/guides/serious-news/. Accessed April 3, 2019.

Motivational Interviewing

Many of your patient visits will close with a discussion of behavior changes needed to optimize health or treat illness. These could include a change in diet, exercise habits, cessation of smoking or drinking, adherence to medication regimens, or self-management strategies, among others. Motivational interviewing is a set of well-documented techniques that improve health outcomes, especially for patients with substance abuse. It encourages you to help your patients discover their interest in considering and making a change in their behaviors. Helpful reminders for clinicians regarding self-awareness of their attitudes, thoughts, and communication and interpersonal styles are suggested in Box 2-9.

See Table 2-1, Motivational Interviewing.

Interprofessional Communication

As a trainee in the clinical environment, you will often find yourself caring for patients with other trainees and clinicians from various fields such as medicine, nursing, dentistry, advance practice nursing, social work, podiatry, and rehabilitation therapists (Fig. 2-4). Without a doubt, working as a team using effective communication is key in providing efficient, quality care that leads to excellence in patient outcomes.

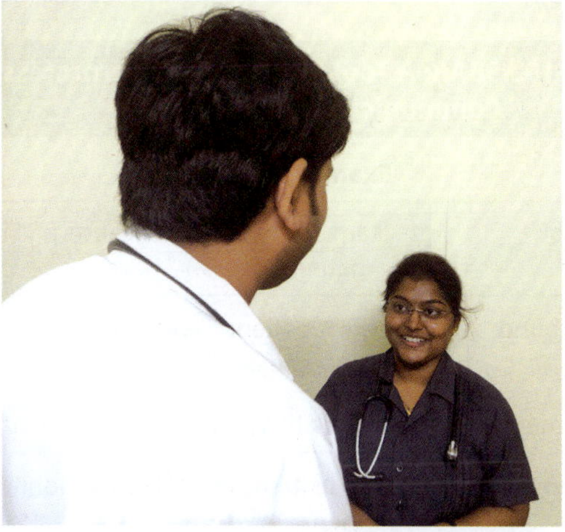

FIGURE 2-4. Effective communication between disciplines is key to patient safety.

Box 2-9. Motivational Interviewing: Am I Doing This Right?

- Do I listen more than I talk?
  Or am I talking more than I listen?
- Do I keep myself sensitive and open to this patient's issues, whatever they may be?
  Or am I talking about what I think the problem is?
- Do I invite this patient to talk about and explore his/her own ideas for change?
  Or am I jumping to conclusions and possible solutions?
- Do I encourage this person to talk about his/her reasons for not changing?
  Or am I forcing him/her to talk only about change?
- Do I ask permission to give my feedback?
  Or am I presuming that my ideas are what he/she really needs to hear?
- Do I reassure this patient that ambivalence to change is normal?
  Or am I telling him/her to take action and push ahead for a solution?
- Do I help this patient identify successes and challenges from his/her past and relate them to present change efforts?
  Or am I encouraging him/her to ignore or get stuck on old stories?
- Do I seek to understand this patient?
  Or am I spending a lot of time trying to convince him/her to understand me and my ideas?
- Do I summarize for this patient what I am hearing?
  Or am I just summarizing what I think?
- Do I value this patient's opinion more than my own?
  Or am I giving more value to my viewpoint?
- Do I remind myself that this patient is capable of making his/her own choices?
  Or am I assuming that he/she is not capable of making good choices?

Source: The Institute for Research, Education and Training in Addictions (IRETA). MI Reminder Card (Am I Doing This Right?) Available at https://www.centerforebp.case.edu/client-files/pdf/miremindercard.pdf. Accessed May 7, 2019.

Collaboration between disciplines is also critical in minimizing the risk of errors in patient care. However, many barriers can obstruct this team-based approach. These barriers include different skill sets, knowledge, and professional identities, lack of interprofessional cultural competence, perceived power differentials, and profession-centric role models. Mutual respect is essential for interprofessional communication because it helps facilitate a positive environment for setting shared goals, creating collaborative plans, making decisions, and sharing responsibilities.

One of the frameworks to improve interprofessional communication and teamwork is the SBAR (**S**ituation-**B**ackground-**A**ssessment-**R**ecommendation), a shared mental model which provides a clear, concise, and organized framework for communication between clinicians. This framework facilitates active listening (Box 2-10) and provides all interprofessional team members a constructive and standardized approach to openly discuss patient issues they may have especially around patient safety.

Box 2-10. SBAR: A Tool to Facilitate Interprofessional Communication

SBAR	Examples
Situation	"I am…I am calling because…" "I have a patient who is…"
Background	"The patient was admitted on… because of…"
Assessment	"I think this patient is likely having a…"
Recommendation	"Let us transfer…" "Let us monitor and then…"

Source: Agency for Health Research and Quality (AHRQ). TeamSTEPPS. Available at http:// teamstepps.ahrq.gov/. Accessed May 8, 2019.

See Table 2-2, SBAR: A Tool for Interprofessional Communication.

CHALLENGING PATIENT SITUATIONS AND BEHAVIORS

- Silent
- Talkative
- With confusing narrative
- With altered state or cognition
- With emotional lability
- Angry or aggressive
- Flirtatious
- Discriminatory
- With hearing loss
- With low or impaired vision
- With limited intelligence
- Burdened by personal problems
- Nonadherent
- With low literacy
- With low health literacy
- With limited language proficiency
- With terminal illness or dying

As you spend time inviting patient stories, you will find that some patients are more difficult to interview than others. For some clinicians, a patient who is silent might seem complicated, for others, a patient who is more assertive. Being aware of your reactions helps develop your clinical skills. Your success in eliciting the history from different types of patients grows with experience, but takes into account your own stressors, such as fatigue, mood, and overwork. Self-care is also vital in caring for others. Even if a patient is challenging, *always remember the importance of listening to the patient and clarifying his or her concerns.*

Patient Who Is Silent

Novice interviewers often feel uncomfortable with periods of silence and try to keep the conversation going. Silence has many meanings. Patients fall silent to collect their thoughts, remember details, or decide if they can trust you with certain information. Periods of silence usually seem longer to the clinician than the patient. Be attentive and respectful and encourage the patient to continue when ready such as "You are quiet...What are you thinking about?" Watch the patient closely for nonverbal cues, such as difficulty controlling emotions. Being comfortable with periods of silence may be therapeutic, prompting the patient to reveal more profound feelings.

At times, silence may be the patient's response to how you are asking questions. Are you asking too many short-answer questions in rapid succession? Have you offended the patient by showing disapproval or criticism? Have you failed to recognize an overwhelming symptom such as pain, nausea, or shortness of breath? If so, you may need to ask the patient directly, "You seem very quiet. Have I said something that has upset you?"

Patient Who Is Talkative

A patient who may be garrulous and rambling is also challenging. Faced with limited time to "get the whole story," you may grow impatient, even exasperated. Although this problem has no perfect solution, several techniques are helpful. Give the patient free reign for the first 5 or 10 minutes, while listening carefully. Perhaps the patient simply needs a good listener and is expressing pent-up concerns, or enjoys telling stories. Does the patient seem obsessively detailed? Is the patient unduly anxious or apprehensive? Is there a flight of ideas or a disorganized thought process that suggests a thought disorder?

Focus on what seems most important to the patient. Show your interest by asking questions in those areas. Interrupt only if necessary but be courteous. Learn to set limits when needed, since part of your task is structuring the interview to gain valuable information about the patient's health. A brief summary may help you change the subject yet validate any concerns. "Let me make sure that I understand. You have described many concerns. In particular, I heard about two different kinds of pain, one on your left side that goes into your groin and is fairly new, and one in your upper abdomen after you eat that you have had for months. Let's focus just on the side pain first. Can you tell me what it feels like?" Alternatively, you can ask the patient, "What is your number one concern today?"

Finally, avoid showing impatience. If time runs out, explain the need for a second visit and prepare the patient by setting a time limit. "I know we have much more to talk about. Can you come again next week? We will have a 30-minute visit then."

Patient with Confusing Narrative

Some patient stories are confusing and do not seem to make sense. Just as you develop a differential diagnosis from the symptoms of the Present Illness, keep several possibilities in mind as you assess why the story is confusing. It may be the patient's style, and by using your skills of guiding questions, clarification, and summarizing, you can put together a coherent story. Watch for an underlying issue; however, that is interfering with communication.

Some patients present a confusing array of *multiple symptoms.* They seem to have every symptom that you ask about, or "a positive review of systems." With these patients, focus on the context of the symptom, emphasizing the patient's perspective, and guide the interview into a psychosocial assessment.

At other times, you may feel baffled and frustrated because the history is vague, and ideas are poorly connected and hard to follow. Even with careful wording, you cannot prompt clear answers to your questions. The patient may seem peculiar, distant, aloof, or inappropriate. Symptoms may seem bizarre: "My fingernails feel too heavy" or "My stomach knots up like a snake." Perhaps there is a mental status change like psychosis or delirium, a mental illness such as schizophrenia, or a neurologic disorder. Consider an acute confusional state or delirium in acutely ill or intoxicated patients and dementia in the older adult patient. Their histories are inconsistent, and dates are hard to follow. Some may even confabulate to fill in the gaps in their memories.

If you suspect a psychiatric or neurologic disorder, gathering a detailed history can tire and frustrate both you and the patient. Shift to the mental status examination, focusing on the level of consciousness, orientation, memory, and capacity to understand. You can ease this transition by asking questions like "When was your last appointment at the clinic? Let's see... that was about how long ago?" "Your address now is...?... and your phone number?" You can confirm these responses in the chart or ask permission to speak with family members or friends to obtain their perspectives.

Patient with Altered State or Cognition

Some patients cannot provide their own histories because of delirium, dementia, or mental health conditions. Others are unable to remember certain parts of the history, such as events related to a febrile illness or a seizure. Under these circumstances, you will need to obtain historical information from other sources such as family members or caregivers. Always seek the best-informed source. Apply the basic principles of interviewing to your conversations with relatives or friends. Find a private place to talk. Introduce yourself, state your purpose, inquire how they are feeling under the circumstances, and recognize and acknowledge their concerns. As you listen to their accounts, assess their credibility in light of the quality of their relationship with the patient. Establish how they know the patient. For example, when a child is brought in for health care, the accompanying adult may not be the parent, but just the most available person to accompany the child to the visit. Remember that while you are gathering information about the history, you should not disclose information about the patient unless the informant is the healthcare proxy or has a durable power of attorney for health care, or you have permission from the patient. Some patients can provide a history but cannot make informed health care decisions. You then need to determine whether a patient has "decision-making capacity," which is the ability to understand information related to health, weigh choices and their consequences, reason through the options, and communicate a choice.

Patient with Emotional Lability

Crying signals strong emotions, ranging from sadness to anger or frustration. Pausing, gentle probing, or responding with empathy gives the patient permission to cry. Usually crying is therapeutic, as is your quiet acceptance of the patient's distress. Offer a tissue and wait for the patient to recover. Make a supportive remark like "I am glad you were able to express your feelings." Most patients will soon compose themselves and resume their story. Crying makes many clinicians uncomfortable. If this is true for you, learn how to accept displays of emotion so you can support patients at these moving and significant times.

Patient Who Is Angry or Aggressive

Many patients have reasons to be angry: They are ill, they have suffered a loss, they have lost control of their health, or they feel overwhelmed by the healthcare system. They may direct this anger toward you. It is possible that their anger at you is justified... were you late for your appointment, inconsiderate, insensitive, or angry yourself? If so, acknowledge the situation and try to make amends. More often, however, patients displace their anger onto the clinician as a reflection of their frustration or pain.

Learn to accept angry feelings from patients without getting angry in return or retreating from the patient's affect. Avoid reinforcing criticism of other clinicians, the clinical setting, or the hospital, even if you feel sympathetic. You can validate patients' feelings without agreeing with their reasons (Fig. 2-5). "I understand that you felt frustrated by answering the same questions over and over. Repeating the same information to everyone on the team can seem unnecessary when you are sick." After the patient has calmed down, help the patient to work through his or her angry feelings and move on to other concerns.

Some angry patients become overtly disruptive, belligerent, or out of control. Before approaching such patients, alert the security staff; ensuring a safe environment is one of your responsibilities. Stay calm and avoid being confrontational. Keep your posture relaxed and nonthreatening. At first, do not try to make disruptive patients lower their voices or stop threatening you or the staff. Listen carefully. Try to understand what they are saying. Once you have established rapport, gently suggest moving to a more private location.

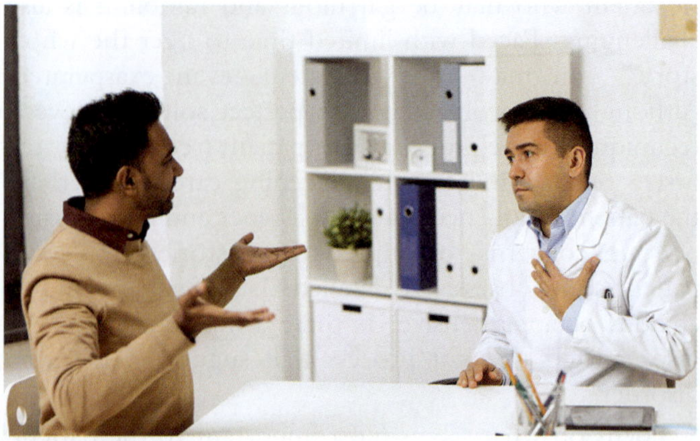

FIGURE 2-5. Validate the patient's feelings. (Used with permission from Shutterstock. By Syda Productions.)

Patient Who Is Flirtatious

Clinicians occasionally find themselves physically attracted to their patients. Similarly, patients may make sexual overtures or exhibit flirtatious behavior. The emotional and physical intimacy of the clinician–patient relationship can lend itself to these sexual feelings. If you become aware of such feelings, bring them to a conscious level to keep them from affecting your professional behavior. Denial can heighten the risk of responding inappropriately. *Any sexual contact or romantic relationship with patients is unethical;* keep your relationship with the patient within professional bounds and seek help if you need it.

When patients are flirtatious, you may be tempted to ignore their behavior because you are not sure it happened, or you are just hoping it will go away. Calmly but firmly set clear limits that your relationship is professional, not personal. If necessary, leave the room and find a chaperone before you continue the visit. Think carefully about your own behavior. Has your clothing or demeanor been inappropriate? Have you been overly warm with the patient? It is your responsibility to evaluate and avoid sending any misleading signals to the patient.

Patient Who Is Discriminatory

When encountering racist-based or other discriminatory mistreatment by a patient, you may be conflicted about your course of action due to your duty to care for patients, your obligation as a clinician to your hospital or clinic, and your duty to take care of yourself. Discriminatory patient behavior should be named and processed appropriately, since such interactions with patients can undermine one's resilience. However, clinicians and especially trainees may be reluctant to discuss concerns regarding mistreatment and discrimination due to fear of being labeled as "overly sensitive" and nonempathetic. Furthermore, reporting a discriminatory interaction to a supervisor can be stressful and discourage reporting itself. The cumulative effect of unacknowledged discriminatory behaviors toward trainees and clinicians can lead to increased anxiety, avoidance of certain patients, and a change in career interests. Developing a personal action plan when confronted with such patient behavior requires institutional support and the availability of supervisors identified as mentors, with whom you can debrief. Be familiar with the faculty education and programs at your institution for identifying, anticipating, and debriefing discriminatory patient encounters with medical trainees.

Strategies for addressing racist and discriminatory patient behavior against students and clinicians have been identified.

- First, you should *assess the illness acuity* of the patient. Is the encounter one of "high stakes" (e.g., does the patient need your assistance, do you need to acquire certain information in order to treat the patient, or is the encounter being evaluated?)? Options include continuing care for your patient, reaching out to another team member for assistance, or removing yourself from the situation entirely. You should be empowered to state your discomfort with continuing an encounter with a discriminatory patient to your supervisor.
- Next, you can seek to *cultivate a therapeutic alliance* with your patient. If your plan is to continue caring for the patient, you should engage your patient by asking about their concerns. This is best done with the assistance of a supervising clinician. As a trainee, in the presence of a supervisor you are empowered to state, "I work as part of your medical team . . ." when engaging the patient. The patient's discriminatory behavior may be due to the patient's illness, underlying delirium, or lack of control. Acknowledging these factors does not make the behavior acceptable or easier to manage. A supervising clinician should *name the behavior* with the patient, "Are you discriminating against this trainee because of his/her skin color/gender/religion/other?"
- Finally, it is the role of your supervising clinician to *establish a supportive learning environment* for you on the clinical team. After such an encounter, you should receive additional training as to how and to whom to report further incidents, and come up with next steps or ideal responses, should you encounter further discrimination when caring for your patients.

Patient with Hearing Loss

According to the World Health Organization (WHO), >5% of the world's population (466 million) has *disabling hearing loss* defined as hearing loss >40 dB in the better hearing ear in adults. This population "is a heterogeneous group that includes persons who have varying degrees of hearing loss, use multiple languages, and belong to different cultures. Solutions to providing health care to one group from one population do not necessarily apply to other groups. Factors that must be considered with this population include the degree of hearing loss, age of onset of loss, preferred language, and psychological issues." Communication and trust are particular challenges, and the risk of miscommunication is high. Even hearing-impaired patients who use English may not follow standard English usage.

Find out the patient's preferred method of communication. Learn whether the patient belonged to the deaf culture or the hearing culture when the hearing loss occurred relative to the development of speech and language as well as the kinds of schools the patient attended. Review responses to written questionnaires. Patients may use varying combinations of signs and speech. If working with an interpreter, adopt the principles identified earlier. Alternatively, time-consuming handwritten questions and answers may be the only solution.

Partial hearing deficits vary. If the patient has a hearing aid, find out if the patient is using it. Make sure it is working. For patients with unilateral hearing loss, sit on the hearing side. A person who is *hard of hearing* may not be aware of the problem, a situation you will have to address tactfully. Eliminate background noise from the television or hallway. Face patients who can read lips directly, in good light. Patients should put on their glasses to see cues that help them understand you. Speak at a normal volume and rate. Avoid letting your voice trail off at the ends of sentences, covering your mouth, or looking down at papers while speaking. Emphasize key points first. Even the best lip readers comprehend only a part of what you say, so asking them to "teach back" is essential. When closing, write out your instructions for them to take home.

Patient with Low or Impaired Vision

With patients who have low or impaired vision, shake hands to establish contact and explain who you are and why you are there. If the room is unfamiliar, orient the patient to the surroundings and report if anyone else is present. If helpful, adjust the light. Encourage visually impaired patients to wear glasses whenever possible. Spend more time on verbal explanations because postures and gestures are unseen.

Patient with Limited Intelligence

Patients of moderately limited intelligence can usually give adequate histories. If you suspect a disability, pay special attention to the patient's school record and ability to function independently. How far have such patients gone in school? If they didn't finish, why not? What kinds of courses have they taken? How did they do? Has any testing been done? Are they living alone? Do they need assistance with activities like transportation or shopping? Sexual history is equally important and often overlooked. Find out if the patient is sexually active and provide information about pregnancy or sexually transmitted infections (STIs) if needed.

If you are unsure about the patient's level of intelligence, transition to the mental status examination and assess simple calculations, vocabulary, memory, and abstract thinking. For patients with severe mental retardation, turn to family or caregivers for the history, but always show interest in the patient first. Establish rapport, make eye contact, and engage in simple conversation. As with children, avoid "talking down" or behavior that may be condescending. The patient, family members, caregivers, or friends demand your respect.

Patient Burdened by Personal Problems

Patients may ask you for advice about personal problems that fall outside the range of your clinical expertise. Should the patient quit a stressful job, for example, or move out of state? Instead of responding, ask about what alternatives that the patient has considered, related pros and cons, and others who have provided advice. Letting the patient talk through the problem with you is more therapeutic than giving your own opinions.

Patient Who Is Nonadherent

The term *adherence* is preferred over *compliance* because when a patient does not cooperate with suggested therapy, it is not fair to assume that the patient is always at fault. Studies show that several factors lead to patient nonadherence, including patient cognitive abilities, emotional status, socioeconomic conditions, cultural attitudes and beliefs as well as their disease condition, therapy, and systems of delivery of medical care. Strategies for better adherence include the use of informational handouts; cues and reminders using e-mails or form letters; positive feedback to the patient; steps to minimize discomfort and inconvenience such as simplifying dosing schedule; disease monitoring to alter management; and obtaining counseling, if appropriate.

Patient with Low Literacy

Before giving written instructions, assess the patient's *ability to read*. Low literacy may explain why the patient has not taken medications or followed your recommendations.

To detect low literacy, you can ask about years completed in school, or "How is your reading?" You can ask "How comfortable are you with filling out health forms?" or check how well the patient reads written instructions. One rapid screen is to hand the patient a written text upside down—most patients will turn the page around immediately. Many patients are embarrassed about reading poorly. Be sensitive to their quandary, and do not confuse their degree of literacy with the level of intelligence. Explore the reasons for impaired literacy—language barriers, learning disorders, poor vision, or level of education.

Patient with Low Health Literacy

Health literacy goes beyond just reading. It includes the practical skills the patient needs to navigate the healthcare environment: print literacy, or the ability to interpret information in documents; numeracy, or the ability to use quantitative information for tasks like understanding food labels or adhering to medication regimens; and oral literacy, or the ability to speak and listen effectively.

Patient with Terminal Illness or Who Is Dying

There is a growing and important emphasis in healthcare education on improving care for dying patients and their families (Fig. 2-6). Even as beginning students, working through your own feelings about death and dying and acquiring necessary skills to ensure excellent communication are essential, as you will come into contact with patients of all ages near the end of their lives.

Studies show that clinicians are still not communicating effectively with patients and families about how to manage symptoms and their preferences for care. Clinician interventions that improve symptoms and avoid hospitalization reduce grief and bereavement, improve outcomes and quality of care, reduce costs, and sometimes even prolong survival. For those facing death and their survivors, there are overlapping and sometimes prolonged phases of anticipatory grief and bereavement. Kübler–Ross provided the classical description of the stages in our response to loss or the anticipatory grief of impending death: *denial and isolation, anger, bargaining, depression or sadness,* and *acceptance.* These stages may occur sequentially or in any order or combination. Offer openings for patients and family members to talk about their feelings and ask questions. As defined by the WHO, your goal is "the prevention and relief of suffering by means of early identification and impeccable assessment and treatment of pain and other problems, physical, psychosocial, and spiritual."

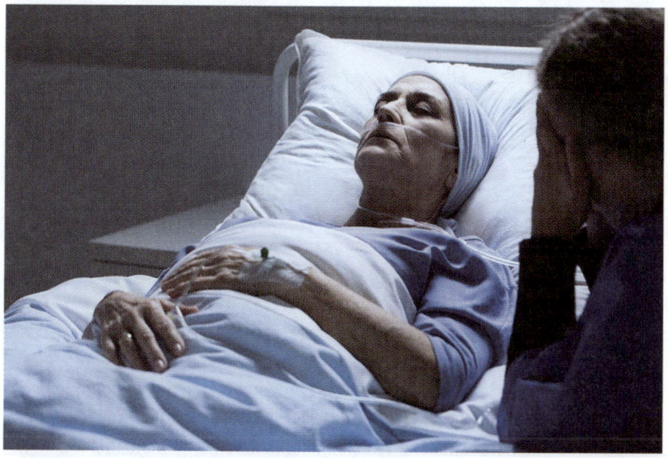

FIGURE 2-6. Learn how to improve the care of dying patients. (Used with permission from Shutterstock. By Photographee.eu.)

BEING PATIENT-CENTERED IN COMPUTERIZED CLINICAL SETTINGS

One of the most ubiquitous changes in general clinical practice is the introduction of the electronic health record (EHR). It has previously been argued that the presence of a computer during a clinical interview changes the dyadic patient–clinician interaction into a triadic interaction (Fig. 2-7).

As a novice, you may find it particularly challenging to engage patients at the same time you are trying to make the record accurate and compliant with information safety. Potentially negative communication behaviors with EHR use include interrupted patient and clinician speech patterns, increased gaze shifts and episodes of multitasking, and low rates of sharing the computer screen with patients. However, effective EHR use has also been shown to facilitate the process of communication, clarification, and discussion as well as some potentially patient-centered communication behaviors (e.g., screen sharing, signposting, cessation of typing during sensitive discussions). Many studies describe strategies and techniques to help you maintain your rapport with your patients and minimize the negative impact of the EHR on communication in computerized settings (Box 2-11).

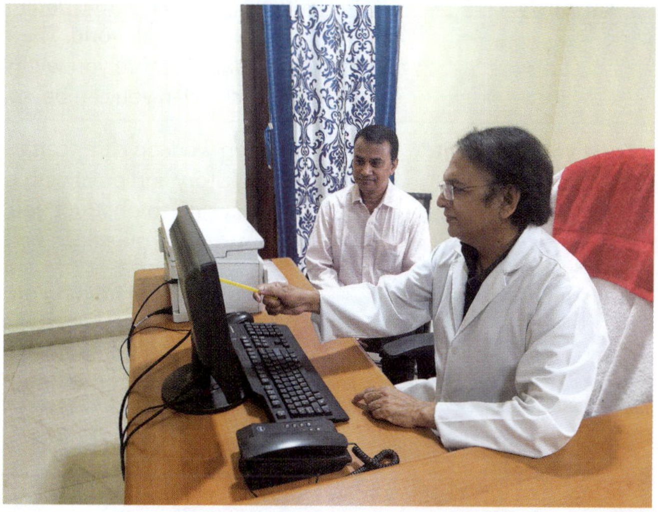

FIGURE 2-7. Visually sharing EHR information using the screen with the patient.

Box 2-11. Strategies to Maintain Patient-Centeredness in Computerized Clinical Settings

- Review the patient's medical record before calling the patient in.
- Start the visit by asking about the patient's concerns and building rapport before turning to computer.
- Move the computer or change the patient's location to facilitate communication as you use the EHR (i.e., construct a clinician/patient/computer triangle) (see Fig. 2-7).
- Maintain your body orientation toward the patient; maintain consistent eye contact with the patient despite using the EHR.
- Talk while working on the computer to remain engaged with the patient and break long silences.
- Explain computer use (e.g., the purpose for using it) and describe your actions on the computer (e.g., describe what you are looking for); read out loud while typing.
- Visually or verbally share the screen and EHR information with the patient (see Fig. 2-7); involve the patient in building their chart.
- Separate communication with the patient from using the screen, especially when building rapport or discussing treatment options; verbalize or use gestures to indicate switches in attention between the patient and the computer.
- Use gaps [illegible] the interaction with the patient for computer work (e.g., when the patient is dressing up after a physical examination).
- Document the patient encounter in the patient's electronic health record after the visit.

Sources: Crampton NH et al. *J Am Med Inform Assoc*. 2016;23(3):654–665; Biagioli FE et al. *Acad Med*. 2017;92(1):87–91.

LEARNING COMMUNICATION SKILLS FROM STANDARDIZED PATIENTS

Sir William Osler famously said in 1905 that *"it is a safe rule to have no teaching without a patient for a text, and the best teaching is that taught by the patient himself."* Although clinical training has traditionally relied on patient contact, often alternative approaches to using "real" patients augment clinical learning for many reasons: patients with conditions required for learning who are unavailable, patients with unpredictable behavior, or patients in situations that may be inappropriate. The concept of standardized patients (SPs) for teaching, learning, and assessment is predicated on their reliable, repeatable portrayals of a broad range of clinical cases with predictable behaviors where students can practice skills in a safe learning environment. In addition to providing examples for teaching and assessment, SPs can also be trained to assess a student's performance and provide feedback. They are of most value in training students in simple and complex communication skills (Box 2-12).

Box 2-12. Tips for Making the Most Out of Learning from Standardized Patients

Take the SP encounter seriously.	Although the standardized patient (SP) is an actor playing a made-up scenario, treat the SP as you would treat an actual patient. The goal of these encounters is to help you provide better patient care in the real world. The more you are able to see the SP in the scenario as a patient and a person, the more you will gain from the experience. SPs are dedicated to helping you become best clinician you can be, so respect their efforts.
Trust your "patient."	SPs often work on case scenarios for hours or even days at a time. They are responsible for creating a backstory and practicing how they will answer questions in a standardized fashion. SPs are not attempting to obstruct you with their responses, but rather they are guiding you and helping you structure questions better and boost your critical thinking skills.
Ask specific questions.	The faculty at your training program want you to ask questions a particular way. As a result, your SP will often give vague answers when you ask general questions. Practice phrasing questions in a more specific manner before and during interviews. This will help you get through assessments faster and more efficiently.
Make your "patient" comfortable.	Practice putting SPs at ease as you would with real patients. This will be helpful when you encounter real patients who may be embarrassed or uncomfortable with the interview or examination. Ask the SP for permission if you need to move or lower their clothing, be gentle while performing examinations, and display kindness throughout the process.

(*continued*)

Box 2-12. Tips for Making the Most Out of Learning from Standardized Patients (*continued*)

Build a connection.	Patience, empathy, and the ability to connect with people are crucial for successful patient encounters. To interact with SPs more effectively, try to relax and be yourself. This encourages the SPs to open up and engage with you on a personal level during interviews, which leads to a more rewarding experience.
Keep your cool.	From time to time, SPs will test your ability to deal with challenging patient situations. For instance, they might act confused, suspicious, or even antagonistic; this behavior may make you feel stressed, anxious or confused. Learning to remain calm and keep your emotions under control, and being assertive rather than aggressive, will often defuse the situation.
Summarize the encounter.	In general, try wrapping up the interview with a quick summary of key points you discussed. It shows that you have attentively listened during the interview. It also allows the SP to fill in gaps or correct mistakes during your questioning.
Enjoy the experience.	It is important to enjoy these SP encounters. These exercises give you the chance to try new things in a safe and controlled setting. They offer a unique opportunity to learn from mistakes before you work with actual patients.

Source: Modified from: Brown E. Eight Tips for Standardized Patient Encounters. Available at https://www.codeblueessays.com/standardized-patient/. Accessed April 19, 2019.

TABLE 2-1. Motivational Interviewing: A Clinical Example

The typical psychiatric approach to this problem would be a combination of education and confrontation; the psychiatrist would explain the dangers of alcoholism to the patient and encourage her to seek treatment, handing her a list of alcohol treatment centers.

In contrast, the actual motivational interviewing (MI) conversation proceeded like this:

The police brought a 40-year-old woman to the psychiatric emergency room because while intoxicated she threatened to kill her partner and herself. She had no history of violence or of legal or psychiatric problems. When she became sober the next day, she reported calmly that she was an "alcoholic" and was not violent and had no intention of hurting herself. She wanted to be discharged.

Patient: I am an alcoholic and don't want to change. I am not dangerous; just let me go home now.

Psychiatrist: OK, that's what we'll do. We can't force you to change. Can I just ask you a few questions and then we'll let you out of here?

MI: Respect for autonomy—the psychiatrist respects the individual's right to change or not make a change; collaboration—the psychiatrist is equal to the patient in power and asks permission for further inquiry.

Patient: OK.

Psychiatrist: I am interested in learning a little about your drinking. I understand you don't want to change. So, I am assuming that the alcohol is mostly a good thing in your life. I am wondering if there is anything not so good about the alcohol in your life?

MI: Elicit ambivalence.

Patient: Well, they said my liver is not so good anymore. It's going to fail if I don't stop drinking.

Psychiatrist: OK, so that sounds like one part of the drinking that is not so good.

MI: Explore ambivalence.

Patient: Right.

Psychiatrist: But it doesn't sound important enough to make you want to change. I'm guessing that you don't care so much whether your liver fails or not.

MI: Not at all sarcastic here; really respecting her autonomy.

Patient: Well, I can't live without a liver.

Psychiatrist: OK. Then it sounds like you don't care much whether you live or die.

MI: Again, not at all sarcastic; simply reflecting content and respecting autonomy.

Patient: No way! I love life!

Psychiatrist: Well, I'm not sure I understand then. On the one hand, you are very sure that you are not going to stop drinking, yet you also say you love life and don't want your liver to fail.

MI: Develop discrepancy. Elicit change talk.

Patient: Well, I know I'm going to have to cut down or stop sometime. This is just not the time.

Psychiatrist: OK. I hear what you are saying. You want to stop drinking at some point, to save your liver and save your life—it's just not the right time now.

MI: Listen, understand, express empathy, and reflect feelings; respect autonomy.

Patient: Right.

Psychiatrist: OK. Can I ask another question or two? If you do think you're going to stop at some point, I wonder what thoughts you've had about when and how you would like to stop drinking? Would you want or need any help if and when you decided to cut down or stop drinking?

MI: Open questions for understanding; encourage change talk.

Source: Cole S et al. *Focus IX.* 2011:42–52.

TABLE 2-2. SBAR: A Tool for Interprofessional Communication

Situation-Background-Assessment-Recommendation (SBAR)

This technique provides a framework for communication between members of the health care team about a patient's condition. SBAR is an easy-to-remember, concrete mechanism useful for framing any conversation, especially critical ones, requiring a clinician's immediate attention and action. It allows for an easy and focused way to set expectations for what will be communicated and how between members of the team, which is essential for developing teamwork and fostering a culture of patient safety.

This tool includes:

- SBAR Guidelines ("Guidelines for Communicating with Physicians Using the SBAR Process"): Explains in detail how to implement the SBAR technique
- SBAR Worksheet: A worksheet/script that a provider can use to organize information in preparation for communicating with a physician about a critically ill patient

Guidelines for Communicating with Physicians Using the SBAR Process

1) Use the following modalities according to physician preference, if known.
   - Direct page (if available)
   - Physician's Call Service
   - During weekdays, the physician's office directly
   - On weekends and after hours during the week, physician's home phone
   - Cell phone

   Start by defining the first and the last step in the process—so that everyone has a shared understanding of where the process you're working on begins and ends.
2) Prior to calling the physician, follow these steps:
   - Have I seen and assessed the patient myself before calling?
   - Has the situation been discussed with resource nurse or preceptor?
   - Review the chart for appropriate physician to call.
   - Know the admitting diagnosis and date of admission.
   - Have I read the most recent MD progress notes and notes from the nurse who worked the shift ahead of me?
   - Have available the following when speaking with the physician:
     - Patient's chart
     - List of current medications, allergies, IV fluids, and labs
     - Most recent vital signs
     - Reporting lab results: provide the date and time test was done and results of previous tests for comparison
     - Code status
3) When calling the physician, follow the SBAR process:

   (S) Situation: What is the situation you are calling about?
   - Identify self, unit, patient, ward/room number.
   - Briefly state the problem, what is it, when it happened or started, and how severe.

   (B) Background: Pertinent background information related to the situation could include the following:
   - The admitting diagnosis and date of admission
   - List of current medications, allergies, IV fluids, and labs
   - Most recent vital signs
   - Lab results: provide the date and time test was done and results of previous tests for comparison
   - Other clinical information
   - Code status

   (A) Assessment: What is the nurse's assessment of the situation?

   (R) Recommendation: What is the nurse's recommendation or what does he/she want?

   Examples:
   - Notification that patient has been admitted
   - Patient needs to be seen now
   - Order change

(continued)

TABLE 2-2. SBAR: A Tool for Interprofessional Communication *(Continued)*

4) Document the change in the patient's condition and physician notification.

Example 1: SBAR Report to Physician about a Critical Situation	
S	**Situation** Dr. Jones, this is Sharon Smith calling from the CCU. I have Mr. Holloway in Room 217, a 55-year-old man who looks pale and sweaty, feels confused and weak, and is complaining of chest pressure.
B	**Background** ■ He has a history of HTN. ■ He was admitted for a GI bleed, received 2 units. ■ His last crit two hours ago was 31. ■ His vital signs are BP 90/50, pulse 120
A	**Assessment** I think he's got an active bleed and we can't rule out an MI, but we don't have a troponin or a recent H&H.
R	**Recommendation** I'd like to get an EKG and labs, and I need for you to evaluate him right away.

Source: Institute for Healthcare Improvement. SBAR Tool: Situation-Background-Assessment-Recommendation. Reprinted from www.IHI.org with permission of the Institute for Healthcare Improvement, ©2019.

CHAPTER 3

Health History

HEALTH HISTORY

The clinical interview in a patient encounter is a conversation with a purpose, undertaken with a set of goals and priorities (Fig. 3-1). In Chapter 1, we discussed how each stage of the clinical encounter has a corresponding purpose and unfolds in a logical sequence. Then in Chapter 2, we focused on describing the fundamental communication and interpersonal techniques you can use throughout the interview to achieve therapeutic alliance with the patient (the *process*, or flow of the patient's history). In this chapter, we will focus on how to structure the *content*, starting with the *format of the health history*.

It is intentional that we have introduced you to the process for eliciting historical information before focusing on the specific information you need to gather in the clinical encounter. Often, especially for a novice student, pursuing specific information about the patient's symptoms, from the presenting complaint to the wider circle of the patient's social and occupational history, leads to sacrificing the relational skills that respond effectively to patient cues, feelings, and concerns. So be mindful of keeping your interview patient-centered as you learn and practice obtaining the information related to the format of the health history.

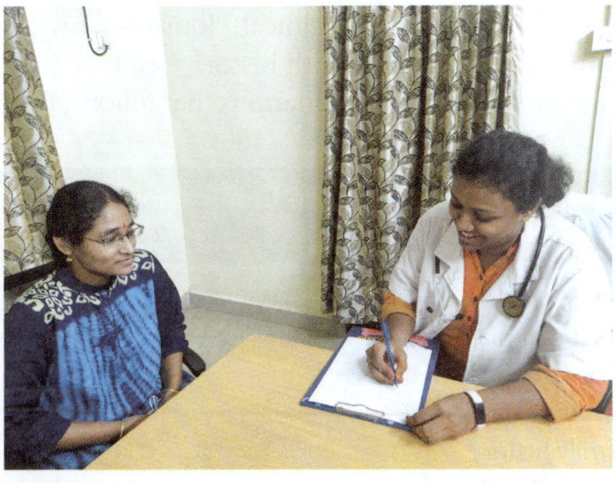

FIGURE 3-1. The clinical interview is a conversation with a purpose.

Different Kinds of Health Histories

The scope and detail of the history depends on the patient's needs and concerns, your goals for the encounter, and the clinical setting (inpatient or outpatient, the amount of time available, primary care or subspecialty).

- For new patients, in most settings, you will do a *comprehensive health history*.
- For patients seeking care for specific concerns, for example, cough or painful urination, a more limited interview tailored to that specific problem may be indicated; this is sometimes known as a *focused* or *problem-oriented history*.
- For patients seeking care for ongoing or chronic problems, focusing on the patient's self-management, response to treatment, functional capacity, and quality of life is most appropriate.
- Patients frequently schedule health maintenance visits with the more focused goals of keeping up screening examinations or discussing concerns about smoking, weight loss, or sexual behavior.
- A specialist may need a more comprehensive history to evaluate a problem with numerous possible causes.

Determining the Scope of Your Patient Assessment: Comprehensive or Focused?

At the outset of each clinical encounter, you will face the common questions, "How much should I do?" and "Should my assessment be comprehensive or focused?" For patients you are seeing for the first time in the office or hospital, you will usually choose to conduct a *comprehensive assessment*, which includes all the elements of the health history and the complete physical examination. In many situations, a more flexible *focused* or *problem-oriented assessment* is appropriate, particularly for patients you know well returning for routine care, or those with specific "urgent care" concerns like sore throat or knee pain. You will adjust the scope of your history and physical

Box 3-1. Patient Assessment: Comprehensive or Focused?

Comprehensive Patient Assessment	Focused Patient Assessment
■ Is appropriate for new patients in the office or hospital ■ Provides fundamental and personalized knowledge about the patient ■ Strengthens the clinician–patient relationship ■ Helps identify or rule out physical causes related to patient concerns ■ Provides a baseline for future assessments ■ Creates a platform for health promotion through education and counseling ■ Develops proficiency in the essential skills of physical examination	■ Is appropriate for established patients, especially during routine or urgent care visits ■ Addresses focused concerns or symptoms ■ Assesses symptoms restricted to a specific body system ■ Applies examination methods relevant to assessing the concern or problem as thoroughly and carefully as possible

examination to the situation at hand, keeping several factors in mind: the magnitude and severity of the patient's problems; the need for thoroughness; the clinical setting—inpatient or outpatient, primary or subspecialty care; and the time available (Tables 1-1 and 1-2). Skill in all the components of a comprehensive assessment allows you to select the elements that are most pertinent to the patient's concerns yet meet clinical standards for best practice and diagnostic accuracy.

As outlined in Box 3-1, the *comprehensive patient assessment* does more than assess body systems. It is a source of fundamental and personalized knowledge about the patient that strengthens the clinician–patient relationship. Most people seeking care have specific worries or symptoms. The comprehensive examination provides a more complete basis for assessing these concerns and answering patient questions. For the *focused patient assessment,* you will select the methods relevant to thorough assessment of the targeted problem. The patient's symptoms, age, and health history help determine the scope of the focused examination, as does your knowledge of disease patterns.

Subjective Versus Objective Data

As you acquire the techniques of history taking and physical examination, remember the important differences between *subjective information* and *objective information.* Subjective information includes *symptoms* which are health concerns that the patient tells you. Examples include complaints of a sore throat, headache, or pain. It also includes feelings, perceptions, and concerns obtained from the clinical interview. One type of objective information is the physical examination findings or *signs* you detect during the examination. All laboratory and diagnostic testing results are also considered objective information. For example, "chest pain" is subjective information while "tenderness on palpation of anterior chest" is an objective one. The clinical record from the Chief Complaint (CC) through the Review of Systems is considered subjective information, whereas all physical examination, laboratory information and test data are objective information.

COMPREHENSIVE ADULT HEALTH HISTORY

This section will highlight the key components related to your patient's health history (Box 3-2). For certain components such as the History of Present Illness (HPI) and Past Medical History (PMH), we provide clarifying examples of how you would synthesize and properly document this information in the clinical record.

As you learned in Chapter 1, when you talk with patients, the health history rarely emerges in this order. The interview is more fluid; you will closely follow the patient's cues to elicit the patient's narrative of illness, provide empathy, and strengthen rapport. You will quickly learn where to fit different aspects of the patient's story into the more formal format of the oral presentation and written record. You will transform the patient's language and story into the components of the health history familiar to all members of the healthcare team. This restructuring organizes your clinical reasoning and provides a foundation for your expanding clinical expertise.

As you begin your clinical journey, review the components of the adult health history (see Box 3-2), then study the more detailed explanations that follow (Box 3-3).

Box 3-2. Components of the Comprehensive Adult Health History

- Initial information
- Chief complaint(s)
- History of present illness
- Past medical history
- Family history
- Personal and social history
- Review of systems

Box 3-3. Details of the Components of the Adult Health History

Identifying Patient Information	■ *Identifying data*—such as patient's initials, age and gender
Source/Reliability	■ *Source of the history*—usually the patient, but can be a family member, caregiver or friend, or the clinical record ■ *Reliability* varies according to the patient's memory, trust, and mood
Chief Complaint(s)	■ The primary symptom or concern causing the patient to seek care. It may be one or two concerns and rarely more than that
History of Present Illness	■ Amplifies the *Chief Complaint;* describes the chronology of events as to how each symptom developed ■ Includes patient's thoughts and feelings about the illness ■ Pulls in relevant portions of the *Review of Systems,* called "pertinent positives and negatives" (see p. 86)
Past Medical History	■ Lists *adult illnesses* with dates for events in at least four categories: medical, surgical, obstetric/gynecologic, and psychiatric ■ May list *childhood illnesses* ■ Includes *health maintenance practices* such as immunizations, screening tests, lifestyle issues, and home safety ■ May include *medications* and *allergies*
Family History	■ Outlines or diagrams age and health, or age and cause of death, of siblings, parents, and grandparents ■ Documents presence or absence of specific illnesses in family, such as hypertension, diabetes, or type of cancer
Personal and Social History	■ Includes any history of *tobacco, alcohol,* or *recreational drug use* ■ Describes *sexual history* ■ Describes *educational level, family of origin, current household, personal interests,* and *lifestyle*
Review of Systems	■ Documents presence or absence of common symptoms related to each of the major body systems

Initial Information

Date and Time of History. The date is always important. Be sure to take note of the time you evaluate the patient, especially in urgent, emergent, or hospital settings.

Identifying Data. These include age and gender. The patient's name is frequently abbreviated as initials.

Source of Information and Reliability. The *source of information* can be the patient, a family member or friend, a consultant, or the clinical record. Document the patient's *reliability*, if relevant. This judgment reflects the quality of the information provided by the source and is usually made at the end of the interview. For example, *"The patient is vague when describing symptoms, and the details are confusing"* or, *"The patient's spouse is a reliable historian."*

Chief Complaint

Gathering Information. The *CC* or *presenting complaint* is the term used to describe the primary problem or condition of the patient prompting the clinician visit (reason for visit). Some prefer the more neutral term *"chief complaint."*

The CC is the starting point that triggers the beginning of information gathering by the clinician. Ask "What problem brings you in today?" There is usually one primary complaint with other accompanying minor symptoms. For example, a patient may complain of chest pain with accompanying palpitations and shortness of breath.

Documentation. When documenting the CC, make every attempt to quote the patient's own words especially if it is descriptive, unusual, or unique. For example, you may document, "My stomach hurts and I feel awful." or "My urine is darkly colored and smells funny." or "I feel like an elephant is sitting on my chest." For those with multiple complaints, one of them may predominate. In the previous example, the "chest pain" can be documented as the CC and will be elaborated fully in the History of Present Illness (HPI) section. The "palpitations" and "shortness of breath" may be included in the HPI but as accompanying symptoms. If there are multiple presenting problems of equal importance, then the CC documentation will list the multiple problems and then each one will be fully described and elaborated in the HPI. If patients have no specific complaints, report their reason for the visit, such as "I have come for my regular checkup."

History of Present Illness

Gathering Information. The *HPI* is a concise, clear, and chronologic description of the problems prompting the patient's visit, including the onset of the problem, the setting in which it developed, its manifestations, and any treatments to date. The HPI in its most basic form is the story of the patient's problem. It should reveal the patient's responses to his or her symptoms and what effect the illness has had on the patient's life. Always remember, the information flows spontaneously from the patient, but the task of oral and written organization is yours.

The HPI is where you characterize the CC fully by describing its attributes (Box 3-4). This set of attributes works particularly well for pain-based symptoms, but

Box 3-4. Attributes of a Symptom

Attribute	Description	Examples
Location	Where in/on the body the problem, symptom, or pain occur or move to other areas	■ "Where did the pain start?" ■ "Does your pain move anywhere?"
Quality	An adjective describing the type of problem, symptom, or pain	■ "Can you describe the pain for me?" ■ "Tell me how you feel when you… (use the patient's words about the quality of the pain)"
Quantity or severity	Patient's nonverbal actions or verbal description as to the degree or extent of the problem, symptom, or pain: pain scale 0–10, comparison of the current problem, symptom, or pain to previous experiences	■ "On a scale of 1–10, with 10 being the worst possible pain, how would you rate your pain? At its worst? At its best?" ■ "How would you characterize the severity of your shortness of breath—mild, moderate, or severe?" ■ "Overall, has the pain been getting better, worse, or staying the same?"
Timing including:	Describes when the symptom or pain started	
■ **Onset**	Setting in which it occurs, what actions or circumstances cause the problem, symptom, or pain to occur, worsen, or improve	■ "When did this start?" "Tell me what you were doing when this started?" "Was anything unusual going on in your life when this started?"
■ **Duration**	How long the problem, symptom, or pain have been present or how long the problem, symptom, or pain last	■ "How long does the headache last?"
■ **Frequency**	How often the problem, symptom, or pain occur	■ "How often did you vomit yesterday?" ■ "Is the dizziness more frequent today?"
Modifying factors	Actions or activities taken to improve the problem, symptom, or pain and their outcome	■ "Does anything make it worse? ■ "Does anything make it better?"
Associated manifestations	Other signs or symptoms that occur when the problem, symptom, or pain occur	■ "Do you get nauseous when you are dizzy?" ■ "Are there any other things that happen when you are experiencing this problem?"

Box 3-5. Helpful Mnemonics for Characterizing the Chief Complaint

OPQRST	OLD CARTS
■ **O**nset	■ **O**nset
■ **P**recipitating and **P**alliating factors	■ **L**ocation
■ **Q**uality	■ **D**uration
■ **R**egion or **R**adiation	■ **C**haracter
■ **S**everity	■ **A**ggravating or Alleviating factors
■ **T**iming or **T**emporal characteristics	■ **R**adiation
	■ **T**iming
	■ **S**etting

may also be used, with some modification, to describe CCs such as shortness of breath, cough, or diarrhea.

There are also helpful mnemonics to assist you in remembering these attributes (Box 3-5).

It is also important to ask about the presence or absence of additional symptoms or other relevant information—such as risk factors for coronary artery disease in patients with chest pain, or current medications in patients with syncope—that may help you generate a list of possible causes (*differential diagnosis*) to explain the patient's problem or condition. This list will include the *most likely* and, at times, the *most serious* causes, even if less likely. When clinicians obtain a history, they are continually generating possible explanations in their minds, allowing the patient's answers to direct the logical use of additional probing questions. This process of probing with questions is similar to testing a hypothesis. With each question, the list of probable diagnoses (or hypotheses) is pared down until a few likely choices are left from a formerly longer list of diagnostic possibilities.

You may find this stage of gathering "clinician" information to be challenging because it requires experience and exposure as well as clinical knowledge. In due time, you will learn the appropriate lines of questioning pertinent for a particular CC and their more commonly occurring causes.

Documentation. Structuring how to document the HPI in the clinical record is one of the most daunting tasks for any beginning student. You should learn how to document the patient's story from the information you have gathered and chronologically organize the events leading up to your clinical interview in a concise and clear manner. Box 3-6 suggests a framework that could guide you in structuring this section of the documentation.

Opening Statement. Opening statements for the health history documentation provide a foundation for the reader to begin to think of possible causes for the patient's condition (Box 3-7). This first statement should be the CC stated within the patient's clinical context (e.g., critical historical elements most related to the CC that hints to possible causes of the patient's condition).

Box 3-6. Suggested Steps in Documenting the HPI

- ■ Start with an opening statement
- ■ Further characterize the chief complaint with attention to chronology of events
- ■ Then describe accompanying symptoms and their pertinence, called pertinent positives
- ■ Include absent symptoms and their pertinence, called pertinent positives
- ■ Add information from other parts of the health history that are relevant

Box 3-7. HPI Documentation Example Part 1: Opening Statement

MN is a 54-year-old female with a remote history of intermittent headaches who states that her "head has been aching for the past 3 months."

For example: "JM is a 48-year-old male with poorly controlled diabetes mellitus presenting with 3 days of fever." This example alerts the clinician that the fever may have some connection to the patient's diabetes. It reminds the clinician to think of common possible causes of fever, most likely due to an infection, that typically happen in a patient with diabetes.

Another example is, "RP is a 23-year-old male with recent travel to Nepal presenting with 1 month of low-grade fever and night sweats." This statement again hints at possible causes of fever and night sweats in a patient who recently traveled to Nepal. The reader of this documentation may start thinking of infectious etiologies endemic to that region pertinent to this patient's symptoms just by reading the Opening Statement.

Elaboration of Chief Complaint with Attention to Chronology. In the HPI, the CC should be documented and well characterized by its attending attributes as described earlier. Based on the patient's responses to your questions, document the information, paying particular attention to the clarity of the story. This section should be a chronologic account of events as well, so pay attention to the timing of symptoms (Box 3-8).

1. **Location**—Examples: area of body, bilateral, unilateral, left, right, anterior, posterior, upper, lower, diffuse or localized, fixed or migratory, radiating to other areas
2. **Quality**—Examples: dull, sharp, throbbing, constant, intermittent, itching, stabbing, acute, chronic,

Box 3-8. HPI Documentation Example Part 2: Elaboration of Chief Complaint

MN is a 54-year-old female with a remote history of intermittent headaches who states that her "head has been aching for the past 3 months."

She was in her usual good health until 3 months prior to consultation when she started experiencing episodes of headache. These episodes occur on both sides of the front of her head without any radiation. They are throbbing and mild to moderately severe in intensity (rated as 3 to 6 out of 10 in the 10-point pain scale). The headaches usually last 4–6 hours, started as one to two episodes a month but now average once a week. The episodes are usually related to stress. The headaches are relieved by sleep and placing a damp cool towel over her forehead. There is little relief from acetaminophen.

improving or worsening, red or swollen, cramping, shooting, scratchy

3. **Quantity or severity**—Examples: 8/10 on the pain scale, moderately dizzy, approximately half a cup of bloody urine
4. **Timing including:**
   a. Onset—Examples: this morning, last night, 6 days ago
   b. Duration—Examples: since last night, for the past week, until today, it lasted for 2 hours
   c. Frequency—Examples: every 6 hours, daily, comes and goes
5. **Setting in which it occurs**—Examples: worse when standing, improved with sitting, aggravated by eating, fell going down the stairs, during a football game
6. **Modifying factors**—Examples: relieved with acetaminophen, no relief with ibuprofen, it felt better/worse when I....
7. **Associated manifestations**—Examples: generalized symptoms (constitutional), frequency and urgency with urination, headache with blurred vision, back pain leads to numbness and tingling down the leg.

One method to maintain clarity of the patient's story is to anchor each event to a timeline or its chronology. For example: "Two days prior to hospitalization, the patient developed multiple episodes of watery nonbloody diarrhea followed a day later by two episodes of nonbloody vomiting. Six hours prior to hospitalization, the patient developed severe epigastric pain...." Try to avoid common mistakes such as inconsistent time anchors: "On June 12, the patient started to develop...then 3 days prior to admission...then on Monday...." Try to keep the time anchors consistent to make it easier to follow each event's timeline.

Pertinent Accompanying Symptoms and Absent Symptoms. In this section, you should describe any symptoms brought up during the encounter that you believe may be related to the CC, termed *pertinent positives* (Box 3-9). Pertinent positives are "symptoms or signs that you would expect to find if a possible cause for a patient's problem were true, which then supports this diagnosis." For example, in a patient presenting with shortness of breath: "...The patient also had an episode of palpitations described as her 'heart racing really fast' for approximately less than a minute followed by intense facial flushing."

Box 3-9. HPI Documentation Example Part 3: Pertinent Positive and Negative Symptoms

MN is a 54-year-old female with a remote history of intermittent headaches who states that her "head has been aching for the past 3 months." She was in her usual good health until 3 months prior to consultation when she started experiencing episodes of headache. These episodes occur on both sides of the front of her head without any radiation. They are described as throbbing, and mild to moderately severe in intensity (rated as 3 to 6 out of 10 in the 10-point pain scale). The headaches usually last 4–6 hours, started as one to two episodes a month but now average once a week. The episodes are usually related to stress. The headaches are relieved by sleep and placing a damp cool towel over her forehead. There is little relief from acetaminophen.

MN has missed work on several occasions because of associated nausea and occasional vomiting during the episodes. There are no associated visual changes, motor-sensory deficits, loss of consciousness, or paresthesia.

You also note the absence of any symptoms related to your differential diagnosis, termed *pertinent negatives.* Pertinent negatives are "expected symptoms or signs that are not present, facts that you would expect to find if a possible cause for a patient's problem were true, which then weaken this diagnosis by their absence." In this same example regarding a patient with shortness of breath: "...There was no fever, cough with sputum production, chest pain, nausea or vomiting. He has no prior history of coronary artery disease or anxiety." Historical information that may be possible causes of shortness of breath to consider in this example is lung infections (fever, cough with sputum production), heart attack (history of coronary artery disease, chest pain), and anxiety. The pertinent positives and especially the negatives clarify the possible causes of the patient's condition as well as eliminate other less likely possibilities based on the patient's story.

Additional Pertinent Information. Here you should note any additional facts pertinent to the CC, regardless of where they are typically documented (Box 3-10). For example, if your patient has a fever and cough whom you believe has pneumonia, you may want to include the patient's smoking history in the HPI. For a patient with fever and weight loss whom you think may have tuberculosis, you may want to include a history of living in a homeless shelter

Box 3-10. HPI Documentation Example Part 4: Additional Pertinent Information

MN is a 54-year-old female with a remote history of intermittent headaches who states that her "head has been aching for the past 3 months." She was in her usual good health until 3 months prior to consultation when she started experiencing episodes of headache. These episodes occur on both sides of the front of her head without any radiation elsewhere. They are described as throbbing, and mild to moderately severe in intensity (rated as 3 to 6 out of 10 in the 10-point pain scale). The headaches usually last 4–6 hours, started as one to two episodes a month but now average once a week. The episodes are usually related to stress. The headaches are relieved by sleep and placing a damp cool towel over her forehead. There is little relief from acetaminophen. MN has missed work on several occasions because of associated nausea and occasional vomiting during the episodes. There are no associated visual changes, motor-sensory deficits, loss of consciousness, or paresthesia.

She had headaches with nausea and vomiting beginning at age 15 years. These recurred throughout her mid-20s, then decreased to one every 2 or 3 months, and almost disappeared. She thinks her headaches may be like those in the past but wants to be sure because her mother had a headache just before she died of a stroke. She is concerned because her headaches interfere with her work and make her irritable with her family. She reports increased pressure at work from a demanding supervisor as well as being worried about her daughter. She eats three meals a day and drinks three cups of coffee a day and tea at night. Due to the increasing frequency of the headaches, she decided to come to the clinic today.

and possible close contact with persons with pulmonary TB. These two facts would typically be documented in the social history, but for these examples they are included in the HPI because they may have an impact on the evolving list of possible causes of the CC. Do not document these items twice. For example, for the patient who smokes in the example above, when you get to smoking in the social history, you can simply write "as per HPI" unless you are providing additional information.

Often, it is helpful to end your HPI by documenting how and why the patient came to seek medical attention. This concluding statement in the HPI gives insight into the severity of the condition, as well as the patient's motivations for seeking care. For example: "He went to his primary doctor when the fevers did not resolve with acetaminophen." or "He was brought to the ER by ambulance when he nearly passed out on the subway."

See Table 3-1, Suggested Templates for Documenting the History of Presenting Illness.

Past Medical History

Gathering Information. The PMH includes all medical problems of the patient whether they are currently active or remote. It should include *childhood illnesses, adult illnesses* and its four areas: *medical, surgical, psychiatric, obstetric/gynecologic* health information. Also ask for information regarding the patient's immunizations, and age-appropriate preventive measures such as colonoscopy and mammography are also included in this section. A statement of the patient's general state of health may also be included in this section. You may ask: "Over your lifetime, how would you describe your health status?"

Childhood Illnesses: Ask patients about illnesses such as measles, rubella, mumps, whooping cough, chickenpox, rheumatic fever, scarlet fever, and polio. Also included are any chronic childhood illnesses such as asthma or diabetes mellitus.

Adult Illnesses: Ask the patient to provide information in each of the four areas:

- *Medical:* Ask about illnesses such as diabetes, high blood pressure, heart attack, hepatitis, asthma, and human immunodeficiency virus (HIV), seizures, arthritis, tuberculosis, and cancer as well as time frame and hospitalizations.
- *Surgical:* Ask dates and types of operations or procedures. If they are unable to recall the name of the operation or procedure, ask for the reason why it was performed (indication).
- *Obstetric/Gynecologic:* Ask about obstetric history, menstrual history, methods of contraception, and sexual function.
- *Psychiatric:* Ask patient for any illnesses such as depression, anxiety, suicidal ideations/attempts; including time frame, diagnoses, hospitalizations, and treatments (Box 3-11).
- *Health Maintenance:* Ask about immunizations and screening tests. For *immunizations,* find out whether the patient has received vaccines for tetanus, pertussis, diphtheria, polio, measles, rubella, mumps, influenza, varicella, hepatitis B virus (HBV), human papillomavirus (HPV), meningococcal disease, *Haemophilus influenzae* type B, pneumococci, and herpes zoster. For *screening tests,* review tuberculin tests, Pap smears, mammograms, stool tests for occult blood, colonoscopy and cholesterol tests, together with results and when they were last performed.

Documentation. The information gathered from the PMH is typically documented under separate headings: *Past Medical History* (which includes child and adult illnesses), *Past Surgical History, Obstetrics and Gynecologic History,* and *Psychiatric History.* For example:

Childhood Illnesses: Measles, chickenpox. No scarlet fever or rheumatic fever.

Adult Illnesses: Medical: Pyelonephritis, 2016, with fever and right flank pain; treated with ampicillin;

Box 3-11. Mental Health

Cultural constructs of mental and physical illness vary widely, leading to differences in social acceptance and attitudes. Think how easy it is for patients to talk about diabetes and take insulin compared with discussing schizophrenia and using psychotropic medications. Ask open-ended questions initially. *"Have you ever had any problem with emotional or mental illnesses?"*

Then move to more specific questions such as *"Have you ever seen a counselor or psychotherapist?" "Have you ever taken medication for a mental health condition?" "Have you ever been hospitalized for an emotional or mental health problem?" "What about members of your family?"*

For patients with depression or thought disorders such as schizophrenia, take a careful history of their symptoms and course of illness. Watch for mood changes or symptoms such as fatigue, unusual tearfulness, appetite or weight changes, insomnia, and vague somatic complaints.

Two validated screening questions for depression are: *"Over the past 2 weeks, have you felt down, depressed, or hopeless?"* and *"Over the past 2 weeks, have you felt little interest or pleasure in doing things?"*

If the patient seems depressed, always ask about suicide: *"Have you ever thought about hurting yourself or ending your life?"* As with chest pain, you must evaluate severity—both depression and angina are potentially lethal.

Many patients with psychotic disorders like schizophrenia are living in the community and can tell you about their diagnoses, symptoms, hospitalizations, and current medications. Investigate whether their symptoms and level of function are stable and review their support systems and plan of care.

developed generalized rash with itching several days later; no recurrence of infection. Last dental visit 2 years ago. *Surgical:* Tonsillectomy, age 6; appendectomy, age 13. Sutures for laceration, 2012, after stepping on piece of glass. *Ob/Gyn:* G3P3 (3-0-0-3), with normal vaginal deliveries. Three living children. Menarche age 12. Last menses 6 months ago. *Psychiatric:* None.

Gravida (G)—Number of pregnancies; Parity (P)—Number of deliveries (term, preterm, abortions [spontaneous abortions and terminated pregnancies], and living children); see Chapter 26, Pregnant Woman, p. 1091.

Health Maintenance: Immunizations: Oral polio vaccine, year uncertain; tetanus shots × 2, 1982, followed with booster 1 year later; flu vaccine, 2000, no reaction. *Screening tests:* Last Pap smear, 2018, normal. Mammograms, 2019, normal.

Information regarding the patient's immunizations and age-appropriate preventive measures, such as screening tests, are included in this section under the heading *Health Maintenance.*

Allergies. Ask about *specific reactions* to each medication. Also ask allergies to foods, insects, or environmental factors. Try to differentiate the terms adverse drug reaction, allergic reaction, and side effect of a medication. An *adverse drug reaction* is any "noxious and unintended response to a drug which occurs at doses normally used in humans for prophylaxis, diagnosis, or therapy of disease or for the modification of physiologic function." An *allergy* is an adverse drug reaction mediated by an immune response (e.g., generalized rash, wheezing, or appearance of hives). A *side effect* is an expected and known effect of a drug that is not the intended therapeutic outcome (e.g., nausea, constipation). Often, your patient may report an "allergy" to a medication when it was instead a side effect. For example, a patient may relate a penicillin allergy that was actually nausea after taking a penicillin-based antibiotic in the past. This may have untoward consequences on future decisions about administering antibiotics by limiting possible alternatives.

Medications. Medications should be carefully documented, including name, dose, route, and frequency of use. Also list nonprescription or over-the-counter (OTC) medications, vitamins, mineral or herbal supplements, eye drops, ointments, oral contraceptives, home remedies, and medicines borrowed from family members or friends. Ask patients to bring in all medications, so that you can see exactly what they take (Fig. 3-2).

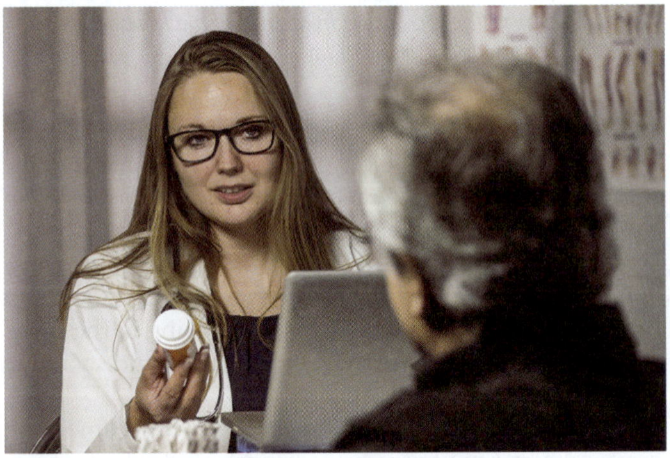

FIGURE 3-2. Reviewing and reconciling patient's medications. (Used with permission from Shutterstock. By Burlingham.)

Family History

The *Family History* is a record of health information about the patient and his or her immediate relatives. It lists the age and health, or age and cause of death, of each immediate relative including parents, grandparents, siblings, children, and grandchildren. Review each of the following conditions and record whether they are present or absent in the family: hypertension, coronary artery disease, elevated cholesterol levels, stroke, diabetes, thyroid or renal disease, arthritis, tuberculosis, asthma or lung disease, headache, seizure disorder, mental illness, suicide, substance abuse, and allergies, as well as symptoms reported by the patient. Ask about any history of breast, ovarian, colon, or prostate cancer. Although diagrammatic representation or a medical family tree clearly illustrates genetically inherited conditions, this may not be possible in the advent of the use of the EHR for clinical documentation.

Personal and Social History

The *Social History* includes the patient's *Personal History* which captures their personality and interests, their coping style, strengths, and concerns. It attempts to personalize your relationship with the patient and builds rapport. This personal history includes their *sexual orientation* and *gender identification (SOGI)*, place of birth, and personal environmental map; *occupation and education*; significant *relationships* including *safety* in those relationships; *home environment* including family and household composition; important *life experiences* such as military service, job history, financial situation, and retirement; *leisure activities*; *sexuality, spirituality*; and *social support systems*. Baseline *level of function*, that is, activities of daily living (ADLs) is particularly important in older adults or patients with disabilities (Box 3-12).

Other parts of the *Social History* include *tobacco, illicit drug, and alcohol use*. It also includes *lifestyle habits that promote health* or *create risk*: exercise and nutrition including frequency of exercise, usual daily food intake, dietary supplements or restrictions, and use of coffee, tea, and other caffeinated beverages; safety measures including use of seat belts, bicycle helmets, sunblock, smoke detectors, firearm and other devices related to specific hazards.

Box 3-12. Basic and Instrumental Activities of Daily Living

Basic ADLs	Instrumental ADLs
■ Ambulating	■ Using the telephone
■ Feeding	■ Shopping
■ Dressing	■ Preparing food
■ Toileting	■ Housekeeping
■ Bathing	■ Doing laundry
■ Transferring	■ Using transportation
	■ Taking medicine
	■ Managing money

Sexual Orientation and Gender Identity. Discussing sexual orientation and gender identity (SOGI) touches a vital and multifaceted core of your patients' lives (Box 3-13). Reflect on any biases you may have so that they do not interfere with professional responses to your patients' disclosures and concerns. A supportive nonjudgmental approach is essential for exploring your patients' health and well-being. Asking patients their SOGI will enable

Box 3-13. Terminology and Definitions

Term	Definition
Assigned sex	Biologic sex designated at birth, usually based only on the appearance of genitalia
Sexual orientation	Person's physical, romantic, and/or emotional attraction to another person
Gender identity	Individual's internal sense of being male, female, or something else; this is not necessarily visible to others
Gender expression	External manifestations of gender, expressed through a person's name, pronouns, clothing, haircut, behavior, voice, and/or body characteristics
Transgender (trans)	Person whose gender identity, expression, or behavior is different from those typically associated with assigned sex at birth
Transgender man (transman)	Individual who currently identifies as a man but was assigned female at birth
Transgender woman (transwoman)	Individual who currently identifies as a woman but was assigned male at birth
Cisgender	Person whose gender identity, expression, or behavior is the same as those typically associated with assigned sex at birth
Gender nonbinary/ genderqueer	Individual who identifies as neither entirely male nor entirely female
Transition	Period when a person begins living as the gender with which they identify rather than the gender they were assigned at birth, which often includes changing their first name and dressing and grooming differently; transitioning may or may not also include medical and legal aspects, including taking hormones, having surgery, or changing identity documents

Adapted with permission from the National Center for Transgender Equality. Available at: https://transequality.org/issues/resources/tips-journalists. Accessed April 23, 2019.

you to provide relevant, specific, and compassionate care that is patient centered and grounded in appropriate language.

Some questions may need to be asked at every visit, as SOGI can be fluid, especially in adolescents, and clinicians should recall that many patients may have sexual encounters that may not be predicted by their declared orientation. Clinicians should not assume the sexual orientation or gender identity of patients is the same as prior visits or is based on behavior, appearance, or genders of partners. For example, many males do not identify as gay but have same-sex partners, and one study found that 81% of females with same-sex attraction also report having sexual experiences with males. Instead, you should ask open-ended questions and use language that is inclusive, allowing your patient to decide when and what to disclose:

Sample questions:

- "How would you describe your sexual orientation?" The range of responses can include heterosexual or straight, lesbian, gay, bisexual, pansexual, queer, and questioning, among others.
- Continue with "How would you describe your gender identity?" Responses include male, female, transgender, transmale, transfemale, genderqueer, gender nonbinary, unsure or questioning, or even "prefer not to answer."
- "What is the sex on your original birth certificate?" This question helps elicit further gender history when asked as a follow-up to gender identity and will give the clinician a sense of which organs the patient may have in order to help guide STI and cancer screening recommendations.

Familial and Social Relationships. Social relationships have short- and long-term effects on mental health, health behavior, and physical health. Many studies provide evidence that social ties influence health behaviors that promote health and prevent illness (e.g., exercise, consuming nutritionally balanced diets, adherence to medical regimens) and those that undermine health (e.g., smoking, excessive weight gain, drug abuse, heavy alcohol consumption). Ask about parents, children, partners, friends, acquaintances, and distant relatives. Seek those that your patient identifies as providing *social support*, which refers to the emotionally sustaining qualities of relationships, or to those who provide a sense that the patient is loved, cared for, and listened to.

Detecting Threatening Relationships. While social relationships are the central source of emotional support for most patients, they can also be stressful, overburdened, strained, conflicted, or abusive, which then undermine the patient's health (Box 3-14). Experts recommend beginning with normalizing statements such as "Because abuse is common in many of my patients' lives, I've begun to ask about it routinely." Disclosure is more likely when probing questions lead and then in-depth direct questions follow. "Are you in a relationship where you have been hit or threatened?" with a pause to encourage the patient to respond. If the patient says no, continue with "Has anyone ever treated you badly or made you do things you don't want to do?" or "Is there anyone you are afraid of?" or "Have you ever been hit, kicked, punched, or hurt by someone you know?" Following disclosure, empathic validating and nonjudgmental responses are critical, but currently occur less than half the time.

Box 3-14. Clues to Physical and Sexual Abuse

- Injuries that are unexplained, seem inconsistent with the patient's story, are concealed by the patient, or cause embarrassment
- Delay in getting treatment for trauma
- History of repeated injuries or "accidents"
- Presence of alcohol or drug abuse in patient or partner
- Partner tries to dominate the visit, will not leave the room, or seems unusually anxious or solicitous
- Pregnancy at a young age; multiple partners
- Repeated vaginal infections and sexually transmitted infections (STIs)
- Difficulty walking or sitting due to genital/anal pain
- Vaginal lacerations or bruises
- Fear of the pelvic examination or physical contact
- Fear of leaving the examination room

When you suspect abuse, it is important to spend part of the visit alone with the patient. You can use the transition to the physical examination as a reason to ask others to leave the room. If the patient is also resistant, do not force the situation, potentially placing the patient, who may be a survivor, in jeopardy.

Alcohol History. It is important to learn about your patient's *patterns* of alcohol consumption, not just their average levels of consumption. *"Tell me about your use of alcohol"* is an opening query that avoids the easy yes-no response. Positive answers to two additional questions are highly suspicious for problem-drinking: "Have you ever had a drinking problem?" and "When was your last drink?", especially if the night before.

The most widely used screening questions are the ***CAGE*** questions about ***C***utting down, ***A***nnoyance when criticized, ***G***uilty feelings, and ***E***ye openers. Two or more affirmative answers to the CAGE Questionnaire suggest lifetime alcohol abuse and dependence alcohol use disorders (AUDs) A more preferred well-validated short screening test is the Alcohol Use Disorders

Identification Test-Concise (AUDIT-C). It identifies not just the harmful drinkers detected by the CAGE, but also hazardous drinkers, who have not yet reached that level of harm and who may respond better to interventions aimed at reducing their consumption.

If you detect misuse, ask about blackouts (loss of memory about events during drinking), seizures, accidents or injuries while drinking, job problems, and conflict in personal relationships.

Tobacco Use History. Determine tobacco use, including the type (smoking, chewing). Examples: "Do you smoke?" "Have you ever smoked?" "What do you smoke?" "How many cigarettes per day? For how many years?" "Do you chew tobacco?" Cigarettes are often reported in pack-years. It is a way to measure the amount a person has smoked over a period of time. It is calculated by multiplying the number of packs of cigarettes smoked per day by the number of years the person has smoked. For example, a person who has smoked 1½ packs a day for 12 years has an 18–pack-year history. If someone has quit, note for how long and note as a former smoker.

Illicit Drug Use History. The National Institute on Drug Abuse recommends first asking a highly sensitive and specific single question: "How many times in the past year have you used an illegal drug or used a prescription medication for nonclinical reasons?" If the response is positive, ask specifically about nonclinical use of illicit and prescription drugs: "In your lifetime, have you ever used marijuana; cocaine; prescription stimulants; methamphetamines; sedatives or sleeping pills; hallucinogens like lysergic acid diethylamide (LSD), ecstasy, or mushrooms; street opioids like heroin or opium; prescription opioids like fentanyl, oxycodone, or hydrocodone; or other substances?" For those answering yes, a series of further questions is recommended.

Sexual History. Exploring the sexual history can be lifesaving. Sexual behaviors determine risks for pregnancy, STIs, and HIV; good interviewing helps prevent or reduce these risks and promote and maintain health. Sexual practices may be directly related to the patient's symptoms and integral to both diagnosis and treatment. Many patients express their concerns more freely when you ask about sexual health. In addition, sexual dysfunction may result from medications or clinical issues that can be readily corrected.

Answering questions about sexual health may be uncomfortable for some patients, particularly if they have experienced judgment or discrimination. Acknowledging and validating these feelings and experiences and providing reassurance that all patients are asked these questions, can help build an environment of understanding and respect.

You can elicit the sexual history at multiple points in the interview. If the CC involves genitourinary symptoms, include questions about sexual health as part of expanding and clarifying the patient's story. For patients with vaginas, you can ask these questions during the Obstetric/Gynecologic section of the PMH. You can include the sexual history in discussions about Health Maintenance, or in the Social History as you explore lifestyle issues and important relationships. In a comprehensive history, you can also ask about sexual practices during the Review of Systems. Do not forget to cover the sexual history in older patients and patients living with disabilities or chronic illnesses.

An orienting sentence or two are often helpful. "To help me take better care of you, I need to ask you some questions about your sexual health and practices" or "I routinely ask all patients about their sexual function." For more specific complaints you might state, "To figure out why you have this discharge and what we should do, I need to ask some questions about your sexual activity." If you are straightforward, the patient is more likely to follow your lead.

In order to broach this sensitive topic using appropriate, direct but also sensitive questioning, it is often helpful to use a sexual history script that includes questions about sexual problems or concerns. Students have reported that having a written script improves ease of learning sexual history–taking skills. The most common sexual history script is the 5 Ps (*partners, practices, protection from STIs, past history of STIs,* and *prevention of pregnancy*) from the Centers for Disease Control and Prevention (CDC) that outlines the important elements of a sexual risk assessment (Box 3-15). It has been recommended that a sixth "P" for "plus" be added. The "plus" should encompass an assessment of trauma, violence, sexual satisfaction, sexual health concerns/problems, and support for gender identity and sexual orientation.

These questions are designed to help patients reveal their concerns. Note that these questions make no assumptions about marital status, sexual orientation, or attitudes about pregnancy or contraception. Listen to each of the patient's responses, and invite additional history as indicated. To elicit information about sexual behaviors, you will need to ask more specific and focused questions.

Use specific language. Refer to genitalia with explicit words. Choose words that are understandable and explain what you mean. Be aware to avoid referring to body parts with language that might increase a patient's discomfort with how they now identify, especially for transgender and gender nonbinary patients. For example, transmasculine patients may use the term *"front hole"* or *"bottom"* to describe the vagina and *"chest"* rather than breasts. You should attempt to refer to body parts with

Box 3-15. Sexual History: The Five Ps+

General	■ *"Do you have any specific concerns or questions we can start with, about your sexual health or sexual practices?"*
Partners	■ *"When was the last time you had intimate physical contact with someone?" "Did that contact include sexual intercourse?"* The term "sexually active" can be ambiguous. Patients have been known to reply, *"No, I just lie there."* ■ *"What are the genders of your sexual partners?"* Asking broad open-ended questions with gender-neutral terms validates the wide diversity of sex and gender and allows the patient to provide a more accurate representation of their history, instead of asking *"Do you have sex with men, women, or both?"* Patients may have same-sex partners, yet not consider themselves gay, lesbian, or bisexual. Some gay and lesbian patients have had opposite-sex partners. ■ *"How many sexual partners have you had in the last 6 months? In the last 5 years? In your lifetime?"* These questions make it easy for the patient to acknowledge multiple partners. ■ Ask, *"Have you had any new partners in the past 6 months?"* If patients question why this information is important, explain that new partners or multiple partners over a lifetime can raise the risk for STIs.
Practices	■ *"How do you have sex?"* or *"What kinds of sex are you having?* (e.g., oral sex, vaginal sex, anal sex, sharing sex toys)*"* ■ *"What parts of your body do you use for sex?"* or *"What body parts go where, when you are sexually active?"* (penis, mouth, anus, vagina, hands, toys and other objects)
Protection from STIs	■ *"What do you do to protect yourself from HIV and STIs ?"* ■ Ask about routine use of condoms. *"Can you tell me when you use condoms? With which partners?"* are open-ended questions that do not presume an answer. If never: *"There are a lot of reasons why people don't use condoms. Can you tell me why you are not using them for sex?"* ■ It is important to ask all patients, *"Do you have any concerns about HIV infection or AIDS?"* since infection can occur in the absence of risk factors.
Past history of STIs	■ *"Have you ever had a sexually transmitted infection* (e.g., gonorrhea, chlamydia, herpes, genital warts, syphilis)?*"* If yes: *"What kind have you had?" "When did you have it?" "How were you treated/what medications did you take?"* ■ *"Have you ever been tested for any (other) STIs?"* If yes: *"When and what were the test results?"*
Pregnancy plans	■ For all patients: *"Do you have any plans or desires to have (more) children?"* ■ For opposite sex partners: *"Are you concerned about getting pregnant or getting your partner pregnant?" "Are you doing anything to prevent yourself or your partner from getting pregnant?" "Do you want information on birth control?" "Do you have any questions or concerns about pregnancy prevention?"*
Plus	■ The "plus" should encompass an assessment of trauma, violence, sexual satisfaction, sexual health concerns/problems, and support for sexual orientation and gender identity (SOGI).

Sources: U.S. Department of Health and Human Services: Centers for Disease Control and Prevention. *Taking a Sexual History: A Guide to Taking a Sexual History. CDC Publication 99–8445.* Centers for Disease Control and Prevention; 2005. Available at https://www.cdc.gov/std/treatment/sexualhistory.pdf. Accessed April 30, 2019; National LGBT Health Education Center. Taking routine histories of sexual health: a system-wide approach for health centers. Available at https://www.lgbthealtheducation.org/publication/taking-routine-histories-of-sexual-health-a-system-wide-approach-for-health-centers. Accessed April 30, 2019; and Rubin ES et al. *J Sex Med.* 2018;15:1414–1425.

gender-neutral language whenever possible or better yet, ask the patient what terms they use for their own body parts and then use those terms throughout the visit. Inquire about the use of toys or other objects for sex. If a patient is engaging in anal sex, a clinician should clarify if they are engaging in insertive ("top") or receptive ("bottom") penetration or both.

Spiritual History. Taking a spiritual history is a process of interviewing patients to better understand their spiritual and/or religious needs and resources. Many patients would like their clinicians to ask about their religious and/or spiritual beliefs, yet many do not. Inquiring about a patient's spirituality can convey compassion and hope and increase a patient's sense of being understood by their clinicians.

Your role is to conduct a spiritual history as part of your comprehensive health history in the personal and social history portions. A spiritual history may be taken as part of a new patient visit, annual examination, or a follow-up visit. Keep it patient centered and listen actively. Several formats for spiritual histories exist including FICA, HOPE, and

Box 3-16. FICA Spiritual Tool

Faith or Beliefs	■ *What is your faith or belief?* ■ *Do you consider yourself spiritual or religious?* ■ *What things do you believe in that give meaning to your life?* If the patient responds *"No,"* then you might ask, *"What gives your life meaning?"* ■ Sometimes patients respond with answers such as family, career, or nature. The question of meaning should also be asked even if people answer yes to spirituality.
Importance and **I**nfluence	■ *Is it important in your life?* ■ *What importance does your spirituality have in your life?* ■ *Has your spirituality influenced how you take care of yourself, your health?* ■ *What influence does it have on how you take care of yourself?* ■ *How have your beliefs influenced your behavior during this illness?* ■ *Does your spirituality influence you in your healthcare decision making (e.g., advance directives, treatment, etc.)?* ■ *What role do your beliefs play in regaining your health?*
Community	■ *Are you part of a spiritual or religious community? Is this a support to you and how?* ■ *Is there a group of people you really love or who are important to you?*
Address	■ *How would you like me, your healthcare provider, to address these issues in your health care?*

Source: Borneman T et al. *J Pain Symptom Manage.* 2010;40(2):163–173; Puchalski C, Romer AL. *J Palliat Med.* 2000;3(1):129–137. Reprinted with permission from Christina Puchalski, MD.

Open Invite. The most widely used is the FICA Spiritual Tool, which is an acronym for **F**aith or Beliefs, **I**mportance and **I**nfluence, **C**ommunity and **A**ddress (Box 3-16). Use FICA as a guide for opening up a discussion about spiritual issues. It typically only takes about 2 minutes.

Summary of Social History. Box 3-17 summarizes several questions you can ask your patient regarding the various sections of the Social History. In time, you will learn to intersperse these questions throughout the interview to make the patient feel more at ease and enhance rapport.

Box 3-17. Social History: Sample Questions

Social History Domain	Sample Questions
Sexual orientation and gender identity	■ How would you describe your sexual orientation? ■ How would you describe your gender identity? ■ What is the sex on your original birth certificate?
Personal geographic map	■ Where were you born? ■ How long have you lived in the United States? In New York? ■ Where do you currently live?
Significant relationships	■ Do you have a life partner, spouse, significant other? ■ Do you have any children? ■ Are there times in your relationship that you felt afraid or unsafe?
Local support systems	■ Who lives with you at home? ■ Are there friends or family nearby? ■ With whom do you spend your day?
Work History/ Occupation	■ Are you currently working? ■ What kind of jobs have you had in the past? ■ Have you ever held more than one job at a time? ■ What did you do before you retired? Is that what you have always done? ■ Tell me what that job is like for you. What are your hours like? ■ Do you feel secure in your job? ■ Do you think anything at work is making you feel sick or affecting your symptoms?

(continued)

Box 3-17. Social History: Sample Questions (*continued*)

Social History Domain	Sample Questions
Education	■ What is the highest level of school that you have completed? ■ Where did you go to school?
Lifestyle	■ What do you do when you are not working or going to school? ■ Can you walk me through a typical day? ■ Do you travel?
Activities of daily living	■ How do you get around the house? ■ Do you need help with dressing or bathing? ■ How do you travel outside of your home?
Nutrition	■ Tell me about your eating habits. ■ Do you eat fresh fruits and vegetables? ■ Do you maintain the same weight? ■ Are you happy with your weight? ■ What do you eat on a typical day? ■ Do you cook at home? Do you eat out?
Exercise	■ Do you get a chance to exercise? ■ Do you exercise regularly? ■ How often do you exercise? ■ What form of exercise do you enjoy?
Alcohol use	■ Tell me about your use of alcohol. ■ Have you ever had a drinking problem? ■ When was your last drink?
Tobacco use	■ Do you smoke? ■ Have you ever smoked? ■ What do you smoke? ■ How many cigarettes per day? For how many years? Do you chew tobacco?
Illicit drug use	■ How many times in the past year have you used an illegal drug or used a prescription medication for nonclinical reasons?
Safety measures	■ Have you ever been seriously injured? (How)? How about anyone that you know? ■ Do you always wear a seat belt? ■ Do you own a firearm? Does someone you live with own a firearm? How do you keep it safely stored? ■ Where do you keep your medications? Cleaning materials? ■ How do you protect yourself from the sun?
Spirituality	■ What is your faith or belief? ■ Do you consider yourself spiritual or religious? ■ What things do you believe that give your life meaning and purpose? ■ Are you active in your faith community? ■ Are you a part of a religious or spiritual community? Do you have access to what you need/want to apply your faith/beliefs? ■ Do any of your beliefs conflict with your medical treatments?
Sexual history	■ Do you have any specific concerns or questions we can start with, about your sexual health or sexual practices? ■ When was the last time you had intimate physical contact with someone? ■ How do you have sex? ■ What are the genders of your sexual partners?

Review of Systems

The *Review of Systems* questions may uncover problems or symptoms that you or the patient may have overlooked, particularly in areas unrelated to the HPI. This is an inquiry method called *scanning* in which you ask patients questions regarding dysfunctions in different organ systems. These "yes-no" questions should come at the end of the interview. This section of the health history is useful when your clinical reasoning process has run aground. By going over the Review of Systems, you may uncover supporting facts that may generate new possibilities for your patient's problems.

It is helpful to prepare the patient by saying, "The next part of the history may feel like a lot of questions, but it is important to make sure we have not missed anything. I would just like you to answer yes or no to each question." Think about asking a series of questions going from "head to toe." Start with a fairly general question as you address each of the different systems, then shift to more specific questions about systems that may be of concern. Examples of starting questions are, "How are your ears and hearing?" "How about your lungs and breathing?" "Any trouble with your heart?" "How is your digestion?" "How about your bowels?"

Understanding and using Review of Systems questions (Box 3-18) may seem challenging at first. Keep your technique flexible. The need for additional questions will vary depending on the patient's age, complaints, and general state of health and your clinical judgment. Remember that major symptoms discovered during the Review of Systems which may be related to the patient's CC (pertinent positives) should be moved to the History Present Illness in your write-up.

Box 3-18. Review of Systems

For each regional system, ask: *"Have you ever had any . . .?"*

- **General:** Usual weight, recent weight change; weakness, fatigue, or fever.
- **Skin:** Rashes, lumps, sores, itching, dryness, changes in color; changes in hair or nails; changes in size or color of moles.
- **Head, Eyes, Ears, Nose, Throat (HEENT):**
    - *Head*: Headache, head injury, dizziness, lightheadedness. *Eyes*: Vision, glasses or contact lenses, pain, redness, excessive tearing, double or blurred vision, spots, specks, flashing lights, glaucoma, cataracts. *Ears*: Hearing, tinnitus, vertigo, earaches, infection, discharge. If hearing is decreased, use or nonuse of hearing aids. *Nose and sinuses*: Frequent colds, nasal stuffiness, discharge, or itching, hay fever, nosebleeds, sinus trouble. *Throat (or mouth and pharynx)*: Condition of teeth and gums, bleeding gums, dentures, if any, and how they fit, sore tongue, dry mouth, frequent sore throats, hoarseness.
- **Neck:** "Swollen glands," goiter, lumps, pain, or stiffness in the neck.
- **Breasts:** Lumps, pain, or discomfort, nipple discharge.
- **Respiratory:** Cough, sputum (color, quantity; presence of blood or *hemoptysis*), shortness of breath (*dyspnea*), wheezing, pain with a deep breath (*pleuritic pain*).
- **Cardiovascular:** "Heart trouble"; high blood pressure; rheumatic fever; heart murmurs; chest pain or discomfort; palpitations; shortness of breath; need to use pillows at night to ease breathing (*orthopnea*); need to sit up at night to ease breathing (*paroxysmal nocturnal dyspnea*); swelling in the hands, ankles, or feet (*edema*).
- **Gastrointestinal:** Trouble swallowing, heartburn, appetite, nausea. Bowel movements, stool color and size, change in bowel habits, pain with defecation, rectal bleeding or black or tarry stools, hemorrhoids, constipation, diarrhea. Abdominal pain, food intolerance, excessive belching or passing of gas. Jaundice, liver, or gallbladder trouble.
- **Peripheral Vascular:** Intermittent leg pain with exertion (*claudication*); leg cramps; varicose veins; past clots in the veins; swelling in calves, legs, or feet; color change in fingertips or toes during cold weather; swelling with redness or tenderness.
- **Urinary:** Frequency of urination, polyuria, nighttime urination (*nocturia*), urgency, burning or pain during urination, blood in the urine (*hematuria*), urinary infections, kidney or flank pain, kidney stones, ureteral colic, suprapubic pain, incontinence; in males, reduced caliber or force of the urinary stream, hesitancy, dribbling.
- **Genital:**
    - *Male:* Hernias, discharge from or sores on the penis, testicular pain or masses, scrotal pain or swelling, history of sexually transmitted infections and their treatments. Sexual interest (*libido*), function, satisfaction.
    - *Female:* Menstrual regularity, frequency, and duration of periods, amount of bleeding; bleeding between periods or after intercourse, dysmenorrhea, premenstrual tension. Menopausal symptoms, postmenopausal bleeding. Vaginal discharge, itching, sores, lumps, sexually transmitted infections and treatments. Sexual interest, satisfaction, any problems, including pain during intercourse (*dyspareunia*).

(*continued*)

Box 3-18. Review of Systems (*continued*)

- **Musculoskeletal:** Muscle or joint pain, stiffness, arthritis, gout, backache. If present, describe location of affected joints or muscles, any swelling, redness, pain, tenderness, stiffness, weakness, or limitation of motion or activity; include timing of symptoms (e.g., morning or evening), duration, and any history of trauma. Neck or low back pain. Joint pain with systemic symptoms such as fever, chills, rash, anorexia, weight loss, or weakness.
- **Psychiatric:** Nervousness, tension, mood, including depression, memory change, suicidal ideation, suicide plans or attempts.
- **Neurologic:** Changes in mood, attention, or speech; changes in orientation, memory, insight, or judgment; headache, dizziness, vertigo, fainting, blackouts; weakness, paralysis, numbness or loss of sensation, tingling or *"pins and needles,"* tremors or other involuntary movements, seizures.
- **Hematologic:** Anemia, easy bruising or bleeding.
- **Endocrine:** Heat or cold intolerance, excessive sweating, excessive thirst (*polydipsia*), hunger (*polyphagia*), or urine output (*polyuria*).

Some experienced clinicians ask questions of the Review of Systems during the physical examination, asking about the ears, for example, as they examine them. If the patient has only a few symptoms, this combination can be efficient. If there are multiple symptoms, however, this can disrupt the flow of both the history and the examination, and necessary note taking becomes awkward.

RECORDING YOUR FINDINGS

Recall that your goal is to produce a clear, concise, but comprehensive report that documents key findings and communicates your assessment in a succinct format to clinicians, consultants, and other members of the healthcare team (review Box 1-20). In Box 3-19, scrutinize the documentation of the health history information.

Box 3-19. The Case of Patient MN: Health History

8/25/20 11:00 AM

MN, 54 years old, female

Source and Reliability

Self-referred; reliable.

Chief Complaint

"My head has been aching for the past 3 months."

History of Present Illness

MN is a 54-year-old female with a remote history of intermittent headaches who states that her "head has been aching for the past 3 months." She was in her usual state of health until 3 months prior to consultation when she started experiencing episodes of headache. These episodes occur on both sides of the front of her head without radiation elsewhere. They are described as throbbing, and mild to moderately severe in intensity (rated as 3 to 6 out of 10 in the 10-point pain scale). The headaches usually last 4–6 hours, started as one or two episodes a month but now average once a week. The episodes are usually related to stress. The headaches are relieved with sleep and placing a damp cool towel over her forehead. There is little relief from acetaminophen.

MN has missed work on several occasions because of associated nausea and occasional vomiting during the episodes. There are no associated visual changes, motor-sensory deficits, loss of consciousness, or paresthesia. She had headaches with nausea and vomiting beginning at age 15 years. These recurred throughout her mid-20s, then decreased to one every 2 or 3 months, and almost disappeared. She thinks her headaches may be like those in the past but wants to be sure because her mother had a headache just before she died of a stroke. She is concerned because her headaches interfere with her work and make her irritable with her family. She reports increased pressure at work from a demanding supervisor as well as being worried about her daughter. She eats three meals a day and drinks three cups of coffee a day and tea at night. Due to the increasing frequency of the headaches, she decided to come to the clinic today.

Allergies: Ampicillin causes rash. No environmental or food allergies

Medications: Acetaminophen, 1–2 tablets every 4–6 hours as needed.

Past Medical History

Childhood Illnesses: Measles, chickenpox. No scarlet fever or rheumatic fever.

Adult Illnesses: Medical: Pyelonephritis, 2016, with fever and right flank pain; treated with ampicillin; developed generalized rash with itching several days later; no recurrence of infection. Last dental visit 2 years ago. *Surgical:* Tonsillectomy, age 6; appendectomy, age 13. Sutures for laceration, 2012, after stepping on piece of glass. *Ob/Gyn:* G3P3 (3-0-0-3), with normal vaginal deliveries. Three living children. Menarche age 12. Last menses 6 months ago. *Psychiatric:* None.

Health Maintenance: Immunizations: Age-appropriate immunizations up to date as per immunization registry.

(continued)

Box 3-19. The Case of Patient MN: Health History (*continued*)

Screening tests: Last Pap smear, 2018, normal. Mammograms, 2019, normal.

Family History

Father died at age 43 years in a train accident. Mother died at age 67 years from stroke; had varicose veins, headaches.

One brother, age 61 years, with hypertension, otherwise well; one brother, age 58 years, well except for mild arthritis; one sister—died in infancy of unknown cause.

Husband died at age 54 of heart attack.

Daughter, age 33 years, with migraine headaches, otherwise well; son, age 31 years, with headaches; son, age 27 years, well.

No family history of diabetes, heart or kidney disease, cancer, epilepsy, or mental illness.

Family History can be recorded as a diagram or a narrative. The diagram is more helpful for tracing genetic disorders although its use has declined due to the use of the EHR. The negatives from the family history should follow either format.

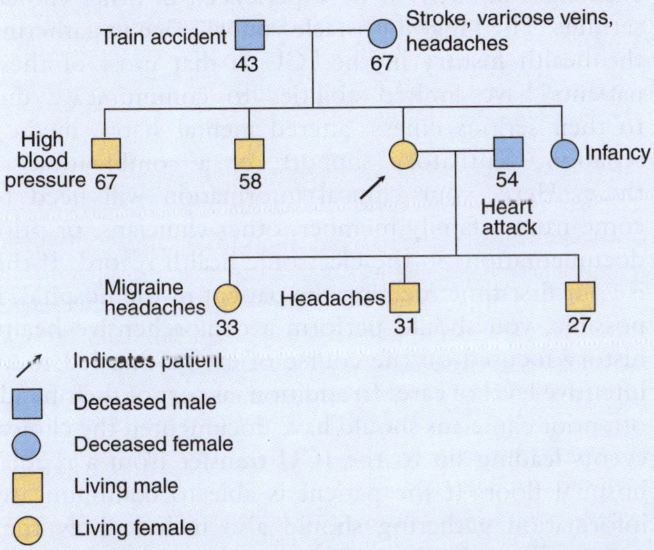

Personal and Social History

Born and raised in Las Cruces, was assigned female sex at birth, and currently identifies as female, finished high school, married at age 19 years. Worked as a salesclerk for 2 years, then moved with her husband to Española, had three children. Returned to work as a salesclerk 15 years ago to improve family finances. Children all married. Four years ago, her husband died suddenly of a heart attack, leaving little savings. MN has moved to a small apartment to be near daughter, Isabel. Isabel's husband, John, has an alcohol problem. MN's apartment is now a haven for Isabel and her two children, Kevin, age 6 years, and Lucia, age 3 years. MN feels responsible for helping them; she feels tense and nervous but denies feeling depressed. She has friends, but rarely discusses family problems: "I'd rather keep them to myself. I don't like gossip." During the FICA assessment, she reports being raised as a Catholic, but that she stopped attending church after the death of her husband. Although she states her faith is still important to her, she now describes having no faith community or spiritual support system. She feels this has contributed to her sense of anxiety and agrees to meet with a chaplain. She is typically up at 7:00 AM, works 9:00 AM to 5:30 PM, and eats dinner alone.

Exercise and diet: Gets little exercise. Diet high in carbohydrates.

Safety measures: Uses seat belt regularly. Uses sunblock. Medications kept in an unlocked medicine cabinet. Cleaning solutions in unlocked cabinet below sink. Handgun stored in unlocked dresser in bedroom.

Tobacco: About 1 pack of cigarettes per day since age 18 (36 pack-years).

Alcohol/drugs: Wine on rare occasions. No illicit drugs.

Sexual history: Little interest in sex, and not sexually active. Her deceased husband was her only sexual partner. No history of sexually transmitted infection. No concerns about HIV infection.

Review of Systems

General: Has gained 10 lb in the past 4 years.

Skin: No rashes or other changes.

Head, Eyes, Ears, Nose, Throat (HEENT): See *Present Illness*. *Head:* No history of head injury. *Eyes:* Reading glasses for 5 years, last checked 1 year ago. No symptoms. *Ears:* Hearing good. No tinnitus, vertigo, infections. *Nose, sinuses:* No hay fever, sinus trouble. *Throat* (or mouth and pharynx): No tooth pain or gum bleeding.

Neck: No lumps, goiter, pain. No swollen glands.

Breasts: No lumps, pain, discharge.

Respiratory: No cough, wheezing, shortness of breath.

Cardiovascular: No dyspnea, orthopnea, chest pain, palpitations.

Gastrointestinal: Appetite good; no nausea, vomiting, indigestion. Bowel movement about once daily, though sometimes has hard stools for 2 to 3 days when especially tense; no diarrhea or bleeding. No pain, jaundice, gallbladder or liver problems.

Urinary: No frequency, dysuria, hematuria, or recent flank pain; occasionally loses urine when coughing.

Genital: No vaginal or pelvic infections. No dyspareunia.

Peripheral vascular: No history of phlebitis or leg pain.

Musculoskeletal: Mild low backaches, often at the end of the workday; no radiation into the legs; used to do back exercises, but not now. No other joint pain.

Psychiatric: No history of depression or treatment for psychiatric disorders.

Neurologic: No fainting, seizures, motor or sensory loss. No memory problems.

Hematologic: No easy bleeding or bruising.

Endocrine: No known heat or cold intolerance. No polyuria, polydipsia.

MODIFICATION OF THE CLINICAL INTERVIEW FOR VARIOUS CLINICAL SETTINGS

You will encounter patients in a variety of clinical settings ranging from ambulatory clinics to inpatient wards to busy emergency rooms. So far we have discussed conducting health history interviews in ideal situations: quiet, with unlimited time, and with minimal distractions. As you may know, the realities of patient encounters are far from ideal. In this section, we will focus on how to modify and tailor your health history taking in various clinical care sites.

Ambulatory Care Clinic

The clinic is probably one of the most ideal clinical settings for conducting a health history, especially for beginning clinicians as examination rooms tend to be quiet, private, and have minimal distractions. Patients are also most likely to be mobile and independent with CCs of low acuity such as a headache, skin rash, cough, or a sore throat. Patients may also provide clinical information more readily than hospitalized patients. Since patients are seen on a regular basis in the ambulatory setting, focus your information gathering not only on the CC (if there is one) but also chronic health issues and any changes to them since their last visit. You should also ask about routine health care maintenance, especially in an ambulatory setting with a primary care focus.

Emergency Care

The emergency department can be a daunting place to take a medical history, even for the experienced clinician because of the acuity of the patients, its fast pace, and its round-the-clock nature. You should ensure that your patient is clinically stable before initiating a detailed but focused interview (Fig. 3-3). Ask about symptoms related to possible causes of the patient's problem to quickly rule out life-threatening illnesses. Your information gathering may be intermittently interrupted (e.g., if the patient needs to be taken temporarily for testing) so that you may have to complete your interview at a later time. In certain scenarios, patients may be incapable of providing information due to confusion or change in mental status. In these cases, you should obtain the health history from family members, caregivers, other clinicians, emergency medical providers, or the patient's clinical records if available.

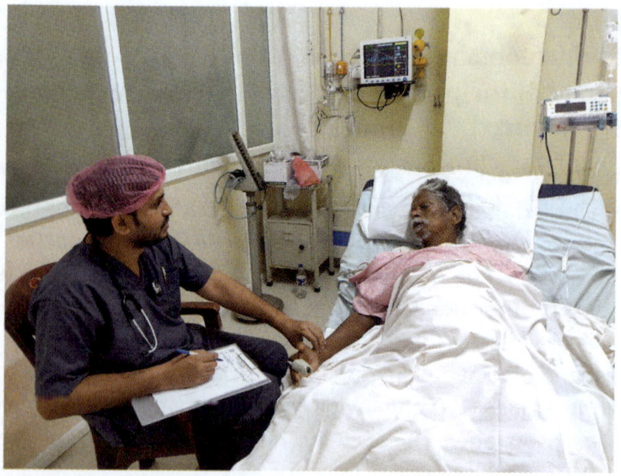

FIGURE 3-3. Modifying the health interview in an emergent clinical setting.

Intensive Care Unit

The intensive care unit (ICU) setting has many unique challenges unlikely to be experienced in other clinical settings. The biggest obstacle you will face in gathering the health history in the ICU is that most of these patients have limited abilities to communicate due to their serious illness, altered mental states, medical sedation, ventilatory support, or a combination of these. Here, your clinical information will need to come from a family member, other clinicians, or prior documentations in the electronic health record. If this is your first time meeting the patient in the hospital, if possible, you should perform a comprehensive health history focused on the course of events that led to an intensive level of care. In addition, as part of their hand-off, prior clinicians should have documented the clinical events leading up to the ICU transfer from a regular hospital floor. If the patient is able to communicate, information gathering should also include how they wish to direct their care. This requires asking a series of questions regarding preferences about treatment as well as resuscitation and use of life-sustaining interventions if required.

Nursing Home

The first change you will notice in the nursing home is that the patients are called *residents*, as they live there temporarily or permanently. Residents may be undergoing rehabilitation with the goal of returning home after improvement and others may be long-term residents who are unable to live independently in the community due to requirements of partial to full assistance for day-to-day tasks. Dementia, hearing loss, and vision loss are also common. You should always attempt to obtain history from the resident first. If you suspect that the patient may have cognitive dysfunction, you may need to confirm certain information with family or the clinical staff. Always include information as to how well they can care for themselves—their *activities of daily living (ADLs)* and *instrumental activities of daily living (IADLs)*. ADLs focus on basic needs like feeding, dressing, and toileting, while IADLs focus on independence in activities like grocery shopping, laundry, cooking, using a telephone, bills, or driving. Getting a detailed history that covers not only medical but functional and social can be taxing on these frail residents. Do not feel pressured to get every part of the history on a single occasion. As the residents live in the facility, you can always return, even over the course of a few days, to get a more comprehensive history.

Home

When obtaining the health history, try to focus on level of function. A patient's ability to function at home has a profound impact on overall health status. Evaluate the environment. Upon entering a patient's home, many environmental details become evident, including environmental hazards, level of cleanliness or upkeep, presence of available food, and medication status. It is also useful to know whether your patient has friends or family nearby who may be helpful resources for a variety of needs.

TABLE 3-1. Suggested Templates for Documenting the History of Present Illness

The following are suggestions on how to structure the History of Present Illness (HPI). The templates emphasize clarity of the story in the HPI as well as provide clues to the reader as to possible causes of the patient's problems. It is understood that variations of these suggested templates may occur. Examples for each template are also provided.

HPI Template (Basic—one chief complaint):

- Opening statement: Chief complaint in light of the patient's clinical context
- Elaborate description of the chief complaint
- Accompanying symptomatology
- Absent pertinent symptomatology
- Pertinent past medical history, family history, or social history
- Concluding statement: How the patient got to the care site

CC: "I have been having chest pain for the past 3 hours."

HPI: FS is a 58-year-old male with hypertension and 30–pack-year smoking history presenting with episodes of chest pain for the past 3 hours. He was in his usual state of health when 3 hours prior to consultation, he started to develop pain in the front of his chest while watching TV. He describes the initial episode of chest pain as sudden and unprecipitated, squeezing in quality, 7/10 in severity, and with radiation to the left arm. It lasted 1–2 minutes and was alleviated with rest. He has never experienced anything like this before. He had episodes with the same characteristics four more times. His most recent chest pain episode an hour ago was accompanied by mild shortness of breath and feeling flushed. There was no nausea, palpitation, diaphoresis, or headache. He was diagnosed with hypertension 2 years ago and is currently on hydrochlorothiazide. His father died at 48 years old from an apparent heart attack. Due to the recurrence of the episodes, he decided to drive to the hospital to seek help.

HPI Template (Chief complaint that represents a symptom of an exacerbation of the patient's chronic illness):

- Opening statement: Chief complaint in light of the patient's clinical context
- Description of condition and symptom control of the chronic illness
  - Diagnosis or symptom
  - When diagnosed
  - Complications
  - Treatments
  - Recent symptom control prior to this exacerbation
- Elaborate description of the chief complaint
- Accompanying symptomatology
- Absent pertinent symptomatology
- Pertinent past medical history, family history, or social history
- Concluding statement: How the patient got to the care site

CC: "I have had difficulty breathing since this morning."

HPI: AJ is a 28-year-old female with bronchial asthma presenting with shortness of breath since this morning. AJ was diagnosed with bronchial asthma at age 8 years and usually gets asthma attacks every 2–3 months triggered by exposure to allergens such as dust and smoke. Sometimes, changes in temperature also precipitate an attack. Each attack is characterized by sudden-onset shortness of breath described as "gasping for air." During attacks, she takes her bronchodilator inhaler and the attacks almost always subside. In addition to the bronchodilator inhaler, she also uses a steroid inhaler. She is not on chronic systemic steroids. She has not been to the emergency room or intubated for her asthma attacks. This morning, while visiting a client at her home, she suddenly felt short of breath similar to prior asthma attacks. AJ said she felt like she was gasping for air and her breathing felt labored. She also noticed that her client has cats as pets. She excused herself so she could take her inhalers. After several attempts the shortness of breath persisted and actually became worse. She denies any fever, runny nose, palpitations, or chest pain. She asked her client to call emergency services and was promptly brought in via ambulance to the emergency room.

(continued)

TABLE 3-1. Suggested Templates for Documenting the History of Present Illness *(Continued)*

HPI Template (No chief complaint)

- Opening statement: Simple statement of the patient and medical problems
- Status report of the patient's chronic conditions/illnesses
  - Pertinent symptoms—present and absent
  - Current treatment and response
  - Prior relevant labs/studies
- Concluding statement: How the patient got to the care site

CC: "I am here for my checkup"

HPI: EL is a 72-year-old female with hypertension, osteoarthritis, and constipation presenting to the clinic for follow-up. She was last seen 3 months ago and today reports no complaints. She has hypertension diagnosed 12 years ago and controlled well on hydrochlorothiazide. She has not had any myocardial infarctions or strokes in the past. Her average blood pressure at home is approximately 110/80 mm Hg. She reports that she does not have any chest pain, palpitations, headaches, loss of consciousness, dizziness, or leg swelling.

She also has osteoarthritis diagnosed 10 years ago involving her shoulders and knees. She takes acetaminophen on occasion for pain with prompt relief. She also does yoga at a local yoga center and says that it also helps with the pain. Her last lumbosacral x-ray, taken after her fall after slipping while trying to get on a bus 3 years ago, showed diffuse osteoarthritic changes. She reports that she has not fallen recently or had any pain elsewhere.

EL also has constipation and takes senna on occasion. She usually has regular bowel movements daily without any straining or blood in the stools. The patient was called in to come to the clinic for her regularly scheduled follow-up visit.

CHAPTER

4

Physical Examination

ROLE OF THE PHYSICAL EXAMINATION IN THE ERA OF TECHNOLOGY

Careful physical examination together with skilled health history taking have long been the cornerstones of clinical practice (Fig. 4-1). Historically, the patient's story and physical examination findings have been the primary means for discerning the causes of a patient's symptoms. This is often true today in emergencies and in resource-poor clinical settings.

The emergence of new resources and technologies has redefined clinical practice. They have enhanced and sometimes appeared to replace the classic clinical skills. Diagnostic technologies have expanded our ability to define anatomic and physiologic abnormalities and have deepened our clinical capabilities. But, even these advanced surrogates should not replace careful physical examination to reach a diagnosis. Information from these technologies should be merged with findings from the physical examination if clinicians are to maximize diagnosis. Overreliance on tests can compromise patient care in the same way as overreliance on bedside evaluation. The question is not whether physical examination alone is better than technology, but whether clinicians combining both approaches deliver better patient outcomes than using one approach alone.

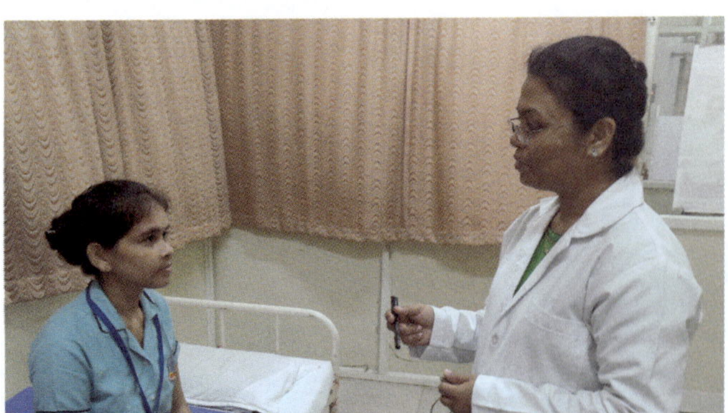

FIGURE 4-1. Art of the physical examination.

DETERMINING SCOPE OF THE PHYSICAL EXAMINATION: COMPREHENSIVE OR FOCUSED?

The decision to perform a comprehensive or focused physical examination depends on many factors including the patient's concerns, the information you have gathered from the interview, and time. The *comprehensive examination* is a basic "head-to-toe-examination" but does more than assess body systems. It is a source of fundamental and personalized knowledge about the patient that strengthens the clinician–patient relationship. Most people seeking care have specific worries or symptoms. The comprehensive examination provides a more complete basis for assessing these concerns and answering patient questions. For the *focused examination*, you will select the methods relevant to a thorough assessment of the targeted problem. The patient's symptoms, age, and health history help determine the scope of the focused examination, as does your knowledge of disease patterns (Tables 1-1 and 1-2).

Comprehensive Adult Physical Examination

Before you begin the adult physical examination, take time to prepare for the tasks ahead (Box 4-1). Think through your approach to the patient, your professional demeanor, and how to make the patient feel comfortable and relaxed. Review the measures that promote the patient's physical comfort and make any adjustments needed in the environment.

Box 4-1. Steps in Beginning the Physical Examination

1. Reflect on your approach to the patient.
2. Adjust the lighting and the environment.
3. Check your equipment.
4. Make the patient comfortable.
5. Observe standard and universal precautions.
6. Choose the sequence, scope, and positioning of examination.

Reflect on Your Approach to the Patient. As you greet the patient, identify yourself as a student. Appear calm and organized even when you feel inexperienced. It is common to forget part of the examination, especially at first. Simply examine that area out of sequence. It is not unusual to go back to the patient later and ask to check one or two items that you might have overlooked.

Beginners need to spend more time than seasoned clinicians on selected portions of the examination, such as the funduscopic examination or cardiac auscultation. To avoid alarming the patient, warn the patient ahead of time by saying, for example, "I would like to spend extra time listening to your heart and the heart sounds, but this doesn't mean I hear anything wrong."

Many patients view the physical examination with some anxiety. They feel vulnerable, physically exposed, apprehensive about possible pain, and uneasy about what the clinician may find. At the same time, they appreciate your concern about their health and respond to your attention. With this in mind, the skillful clinician is thorough without wasting time, systematic but flexible and gentle, yet not afraid to cause discomfort should this be required. The skillful clinician examines each region of the body, and at the same time senses the whole patient, notes the wince or worried glance, and shares information that calms, explains, and reassures.

As a beginner, avoid interpreting your findings. You do not have the final responsibility for the patient, and your views may be premature or wrong. As you grow in experience and responsibility, sharing findings will become more appropriate. If the patient has specific concerns, discuss them with your teachers. At times, you may discover abnormalities such as an ominous mass or a deep ulceration. Always avoid showing distaste, alarm, or other reactions that may be negatively perceived by the patient.

Adjust the Lighting and the Environment. Several environmental factors affect the caliber of your examination. For the best results, it is important to "set the stage" so that both you and the patient are comfortable. Awkward positioning makes assessing physical findings more difficult for both you and the patient. Take the time to adjust the bed to a convenient height (but be sure to lower it when finished), and ask the patient to move toward you, turn over, or shift position whenever this makes the examination of selected areas of the body easier.

Good lighting and a quiet environment are keys for successful patient encounters but may be hard to arrange. Do the best you can. Make sure that the patient can adequately see you and that you can see the patient during the interview. Turn on the overhead or bedside light sources or open curtains and blinds to ensure adequate visualization for the physical examination. If needed, use an additional source such a penlight for more focused and directed lighting of a body part such as the mouth or looking for neck vein distention. If a television interferes with auscultating heart sounds, politely ask the nearby patient to lower the volume, and remember to thank the patient as you leave.

Check Your Equipment. Equipment necessary for performing the physical examination are shown in Box 4-2. Additional equipment and supplies for specialized examination are also listed.

Make the Patient Comfortable

Ensuring Patient Privacy and Comfort. Your access to the patient's body is a unique and time-honored privilege of your role as a clinician. Showing sensitivity to privacy and patient modesty must be ingrained in your professional behavior and conveys respect for the patient's vulnerability. Close nearby doors, draw the curtains in the hospital or examining room, and wash your hands carefully before the examination begins.

During the examination, be aware of the patient's feelings and any discomfort. Respond to the patient's facial expressions and even ask, "Are you okay?" or "Is this painful?" to elicit unexpressed worries or sources of pain. Adjusting the angle of the bed or examining table, rearranging the pillows, or adding blankets for warmth demonstrates that you are attentive to the patient's well-being.

Positioning and Draping the Patient. Properly positioning your patient will aid greatly in examining each region of the body and assist your physical comfort as examiner. Box 4-3 shows patient positions during the physical examination and selected procedures (e.g., indwelling catheter insertion, administration of rectal medications, or performing a Pap smear). It also shows how to adjust the bed and patient position for different examinations or procedures.

As you learn each segment of the examination in the chapters ahead, you will also acquire the proper

Box 4-2. Tools of the Trade: Instruments and Supplies for the Physical Examination

- **Stethoscope (A)** with the following characteristics:
  - Ear tips that fit snugly and painlessly. To get this fit, choose ear tips of the proper size, align the earpieces with the angle of your ear canals, and adjust the spring of the connecting metal band to a comfortable tightness.
  - Thick-walled tubing as short as feasible to maximize the transmission of sound: ~30 cm (12 in), if possible, and no longer than 38 cm (15 in)
  - A bell and a diaphragm with a good change over mechanism
- **Sphygmomanometer (B)**
- **Ophthalmoscope (C)**
- **Visual acuity card or chart (D)**
- **Otoscope (E).** If you are examining children, the otoscope should allow pneumatic otoscopy.
- **Tuning forks (F),** 128 Hz and 256 Hz
- **Thermometer (G)**
- **Neurologic reflex or percussion hammer (H)**
- **Vaginal speculum (I)**
- **Dermoscope (J)**
- Sampling equipment for cytologic and bacteriologic studies
- Cotton swabs, safety pins, or other disposable objects for testing light touch sensation and two-point discrimination
- Tongue depressor
- Ruler or a flexible tape measure, preferably marked in centimeters
- Disposable face mask
- Disposable gown
- Gloves and lubricant for oral, vaginal, and rectal examinations
- Light source
- A timepiece with second hand (timer)
- Hand sanitizer
- Paper and pen or pencil
- Handheld ultrasound
- Access via desktop or laptop computer to the electronic health record

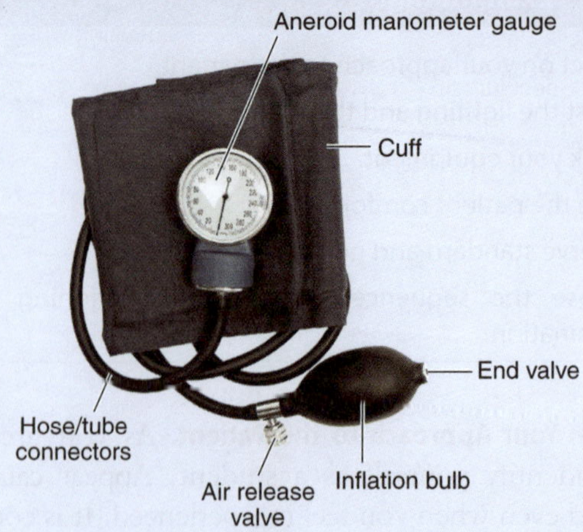

B. Aneroid sphygmomanometer and parts.

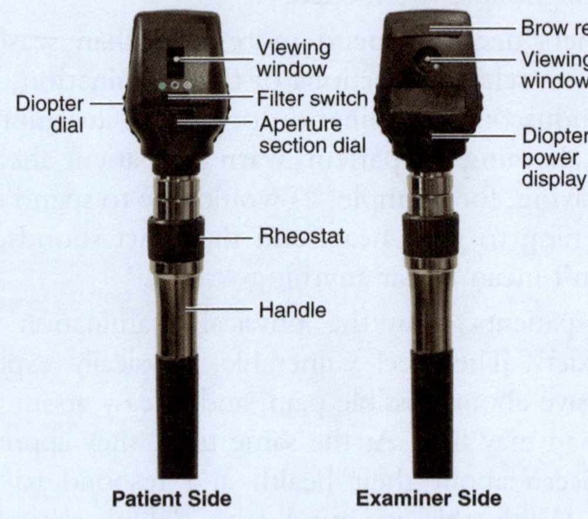

C. Ophthalmoscope and parts.

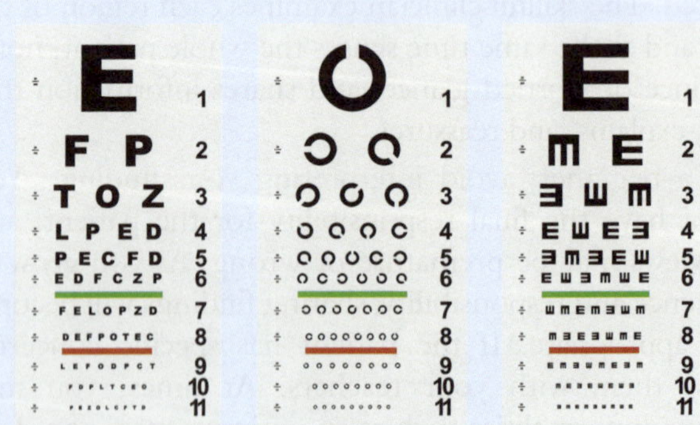

D. Snellen chart.

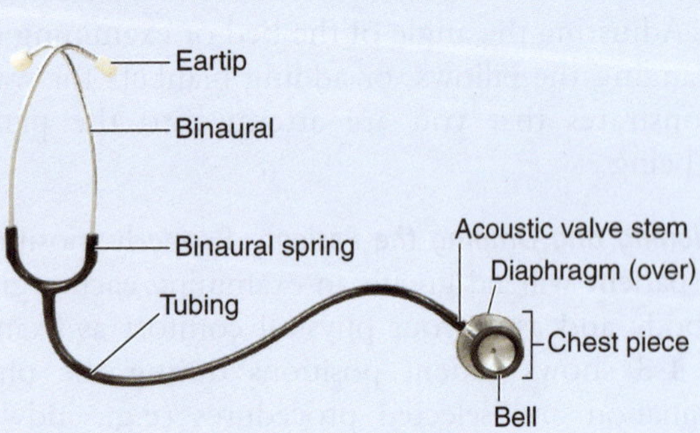

A. Stethoscope and parts.

(continued)

Box 4-2. Tools of the Trade: Instruments and Supplies for the Physical Examination (*continued*)

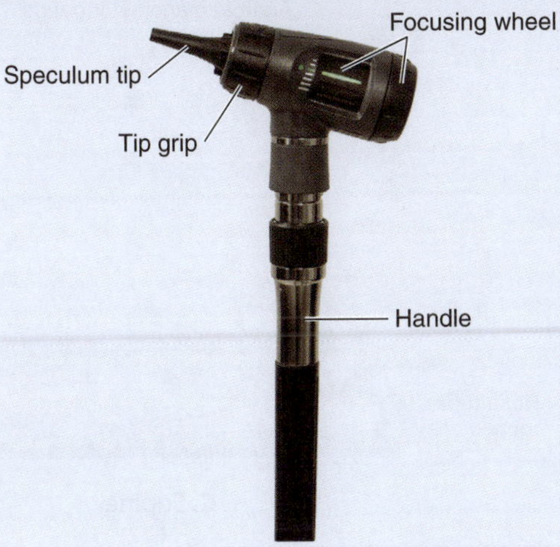

E. Otoscope and parts.

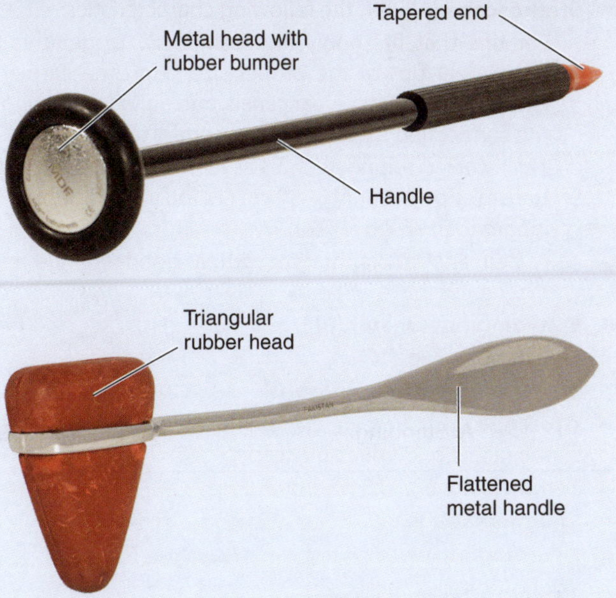

H. Reflex hammers and parts.

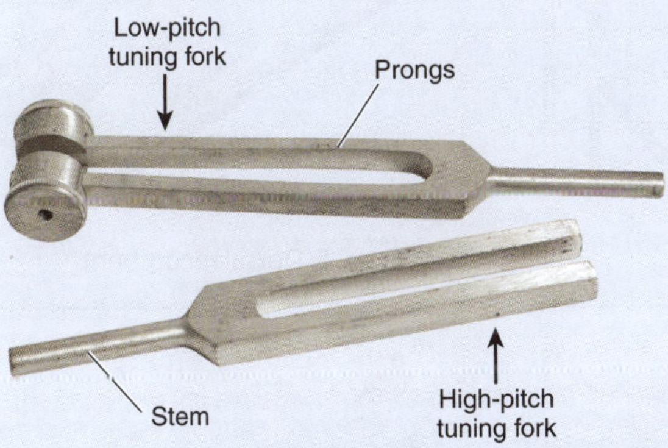

F. Tuning forks and parts.

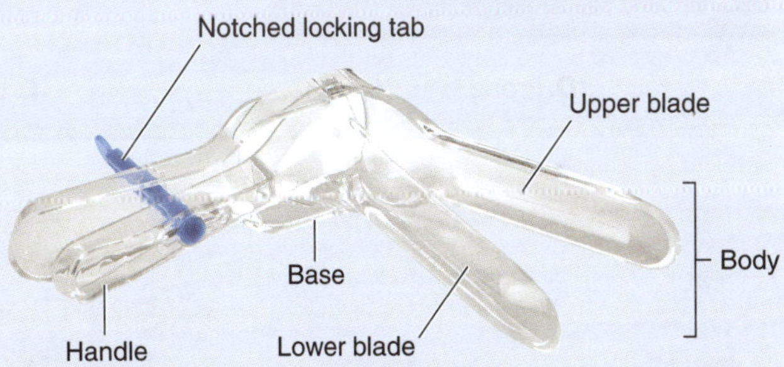

I. Vaginal speculum and parts.

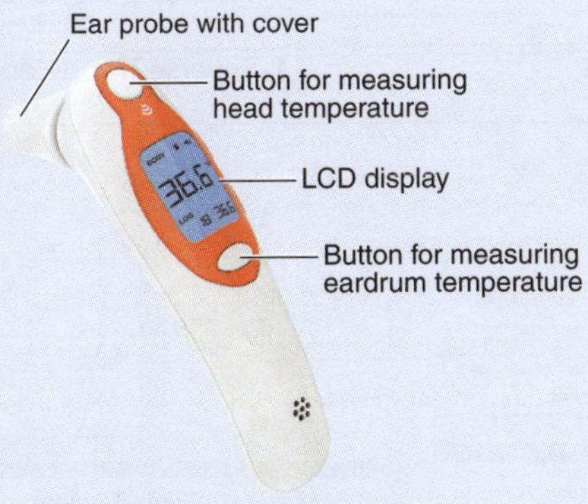

G. Thermometers.

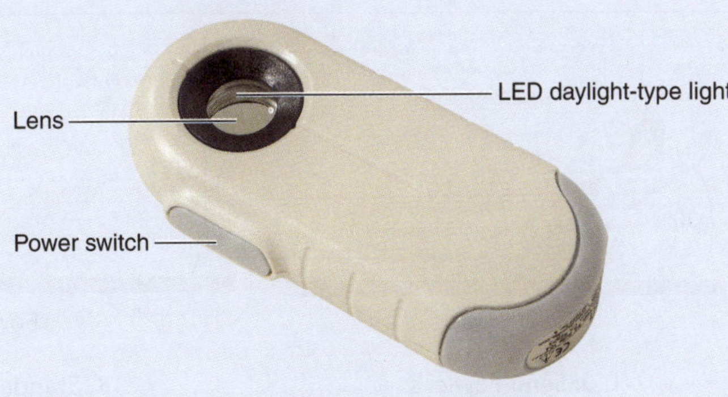

J. Dermoscope and parts.

Source of images A–G, I: Used with permission from Shutterstock. A, by Paul Maguire; B, by LeventeGyori; D, by tuulijumala; F, by Duntrune Studios; G, by doomu; I, by New Africa.

Box 4-3. Common Patient Positioning for Physical Examinations and Procedures

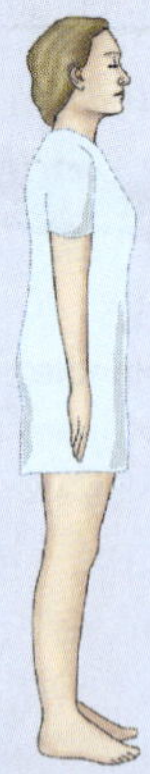

A. Standing.

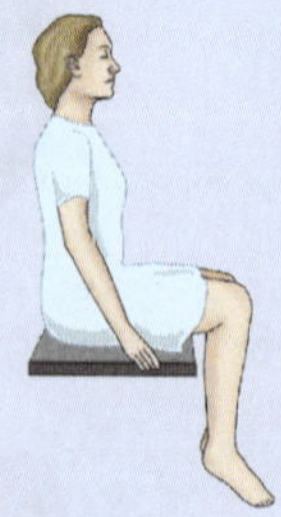

B. Sitting.

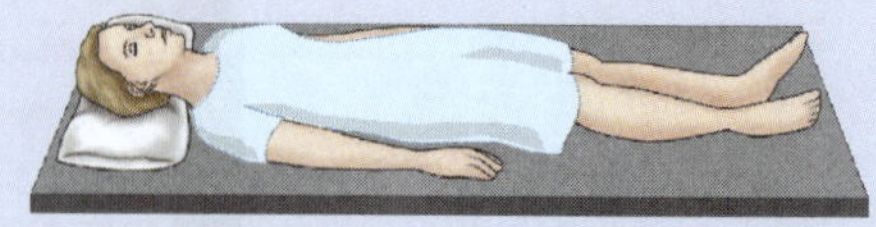

C. Supine.

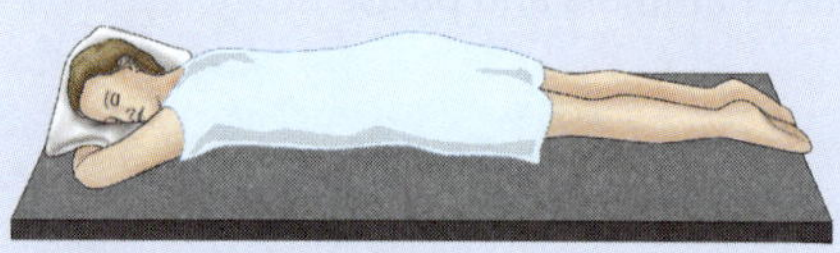

D. Prone.

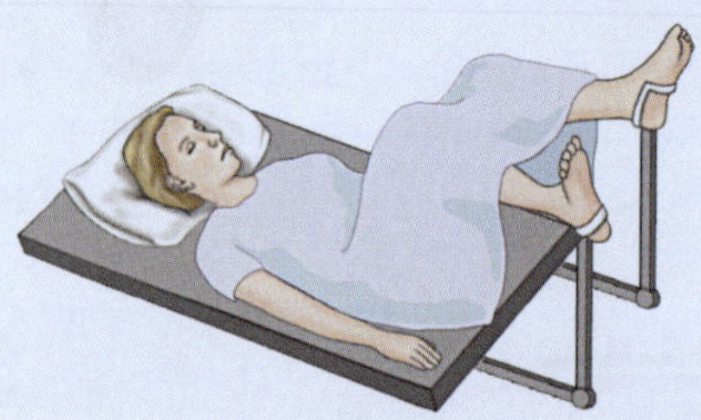

E. Lithotomy.

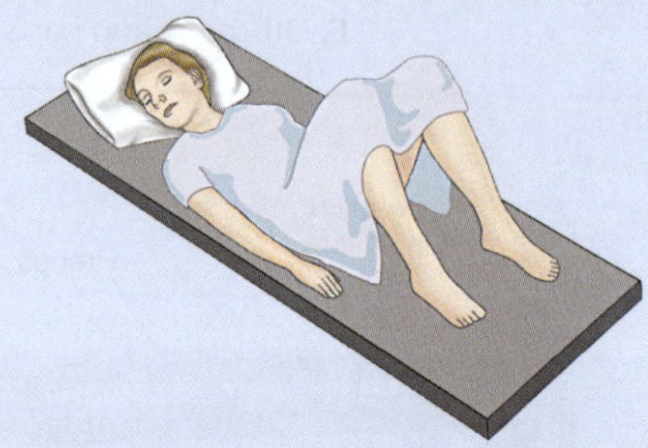

F. Dorsal recumbent.

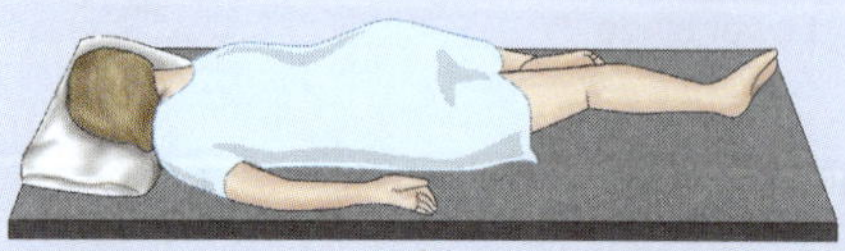

G. Lateral recumbent (Sims).

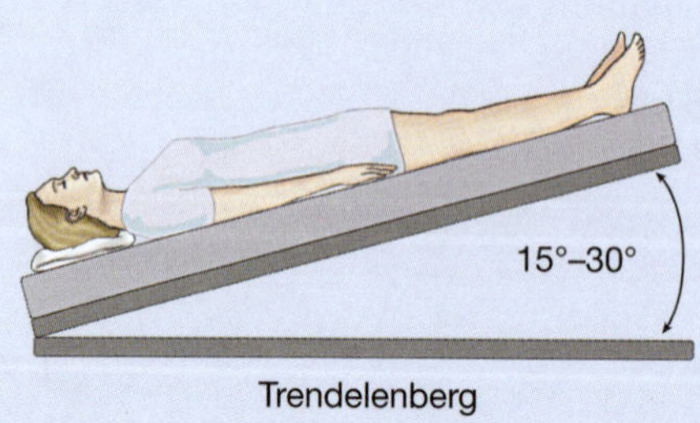

H. Trendelenburg.

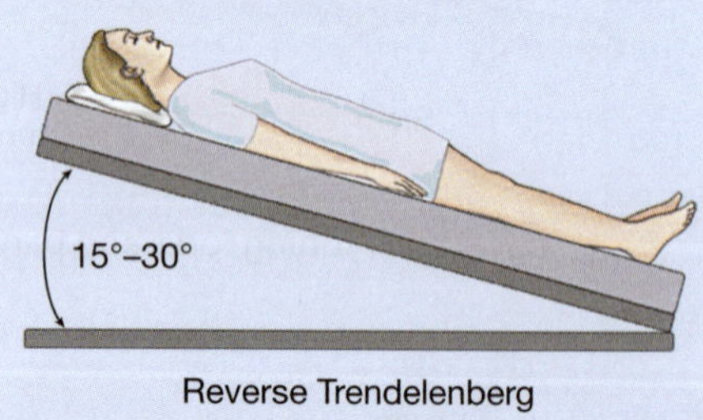

I. Reverse Trendelenburg.

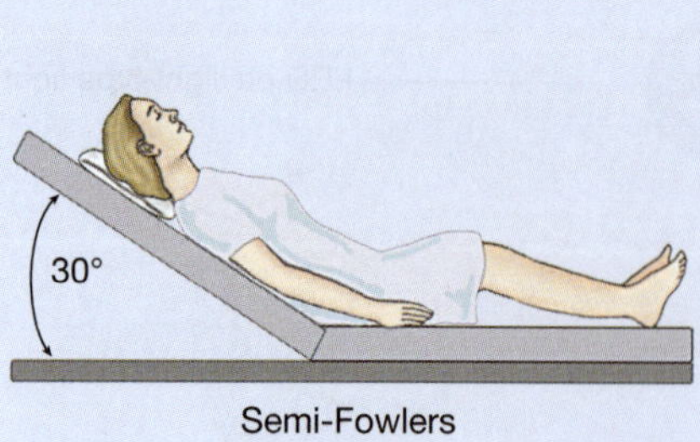

J. Semi-Fowler's.

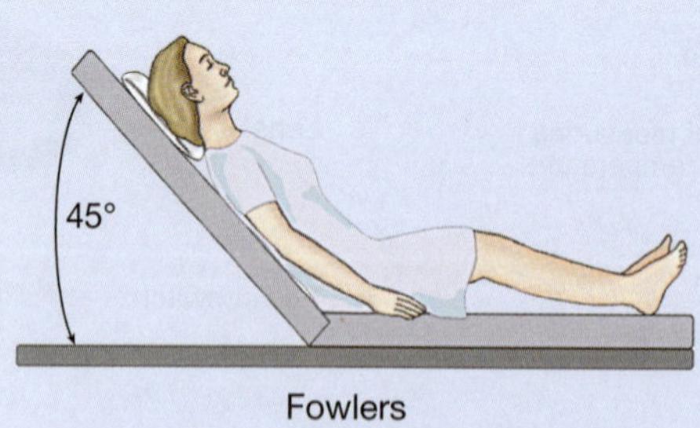

K. Standard Fowler's.

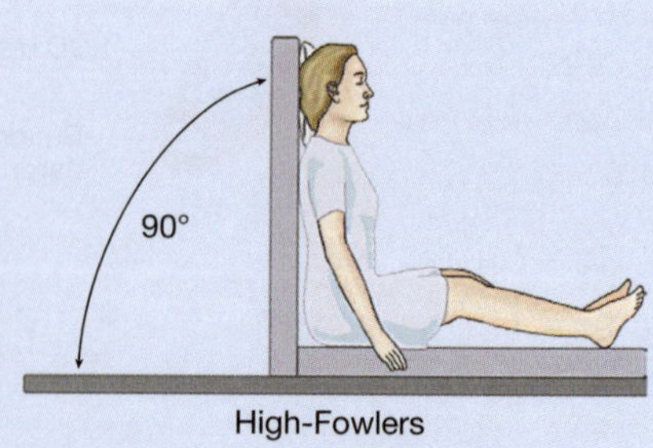

L. High Fowler's.

Source of images A–G: Modified from Taylor C et al. *Fundamentals of Nursing: The Art and Science of Person-Centered Care.* 8th ed. Wolters Kluwer; 2015, Figs. 25-2-1 through 25-2-7.

Note: The patient drape has been omitted from the images to show body positioning.

Box 4-4. Tips for Draping the Patient

- Thoughtful draping preserves the patient's modesty and helps you focus on the area being examined.
- With the patient sitting, for example, untie the gown in back to better listen to the lungs.
- For the breast examination, with the patient supine, uncover the right breast but keep the left chest draped. Drape the right chest again, then uncover the left chest and proceed to examine the left breast and heart.
- For the abdominal examination, only the abdomen should be exposed. Adjust the gown to cover the chest and place the sheet or drape at the inguinal level. To help the patient prepare for potentially awkward segments of the examination, briefly describe your plans before starting, for example, *"Now I am going to move your gown so I can check the pulse in your groin area,"* or *"Because you mentioned irritation, I am going to inspect your perirectal area."*

technique of draping a patient with the gown or a draw sheet (Box 4-4). Your task is to visualize one area of the body at a time, maximizing patient comfort without compromising your diagnostic goals.

Providing Courteous Clear Instructions. Make sure your instructions to the patient at each step in the examination are courteous and clear. For example, "I would like to examine your heart now, so please lie down," or "Now I am going to check your abdomen." Let the patient know if you anticipate embarrassment or discomfort

Keeping the Patient Informed. As you proceed with the examination, talk with the patient to see if he or she wants to know about your findings. Is the patient curious about the lung findings or your method for assessing the liver or spleen?

Concluding the Examination. When you have completed the examination, consider telling the patient your general impressions and what to expect next once your knowledge and skills advance. For hospitalized patients, make sure the patient is comfortable and rearrange the immediate environment to the patient's satisfaction. Be sure to lower the bed to avoid risk of falls and raise the bedrails. As you leave, wash your hands, clean your equipment, and dispose of any waste materials.

Observe Standard and Universal Precautions. The Centers for Disease Control and Prevention (CDC) has issued several guidelines to protect patients and examiners from the spread of infectious disease. All clinicians examining patients are advised to study and observe these precautions at the CDC websites. Advisories for standard and methicillin-resistant *Staphylococcus aureus* (MRSA) precautions and for universal precautions are summarized below.

Standard and MRSA Precautions. Standard precautions are based on the principle that all blood, body fluids, secretions, excretions (except sweat), nonintact skin, and mucous membranes may contain transmissible infectious agents. Standard precautions apply to all patients in any setting. They include hand hygiene (Fig. 4-2); use of personal protective equipment (gloves; gowns; and mouth, nose, and eye protection) (Fig. 4-3); safe injection practices; safe handling of contaminated equipment or surfaces; respiratory hygiene and cough etiquette; patient isolation criteria; and precautions relating to equipment, toys, solid surfaces, and laundry handling. White coats, scrub suits, and stethoscopes also harbor bacteria and should be cleaned frequently. Because hand hygiene practices have been shown to reduce the transmission of multidrug-resistant organisms, especially MRSA and vancomycin-resistant enterococcus (VRE), the CDC hygiene recommendations are reproduced in Box 4-5.

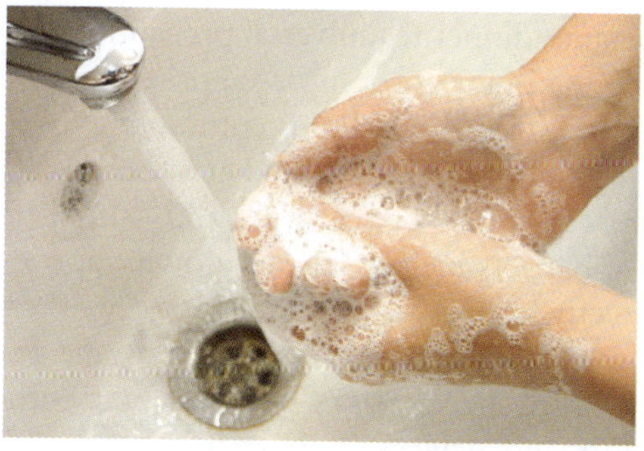

FIGURE 4-2. Observing proper standard precaution with handwashing.

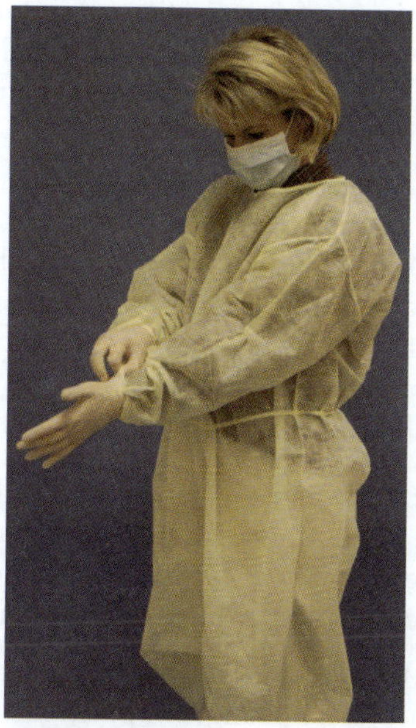

FIGURE 4-3. Personal protective equipment (PPE).

Box 4-5. CDC Recommendations for Hand Hygiene

Use an Alcohol-Based Hand Sanitizer	Wash with Soap and Water
■ Immediately before touching a patient ■ Before performing an aseptic task (e.g., placing an indwelling device) or handling invasive medical devices ■ Before moving from work on a soiled body site to a clean body site on the same patient ■ After touching a patient or the patient's immediate environment ■ After contact with blood, body fluids, or contaminated surfaces ■ Immediately after glove removal	■ When hands are visibly soiled ■ After caring for a person with known or suspected infectious diarrhea ■ After known or suspected exposure to spores (e.g., *Bacillus anthracis, Clostridioides difficile* outbreaks)

Source: CDC. *Introduction to Hand Hygiene*. April 29, 2019. Available at https://www.cdc.gov/handhygiene/providers/index.html. Accessed May 10, 2019.

Universal Precautions. Universal precautions are a set of guidelines designed to prevent parenteral, mucous membrane, and noncontact exposures of health care workers to bloodborne pathogens, including HIV and Hepatitis B virus (HBV). Immunization with the HBV vaccine for health care workers with exposure to blood is an important adjunct to universal precautions (Box 4-6). The following fluids are considered potentially infectious: all blood and other body fluids containing visible blood, semen, and vaginal secretions and cerebrospinal, synovial, pleural, peritoneal, pericardial, and amniotic fluids. Protective barriers include gloves, gowns, aprons, masks, and protective eyewear. All health care workers should follow the precautions for safe injections and prevention of injury from needlesticks, scalpels, and other sharp instruments and devices. Report to your health service immediately if such injury occurs.

Choose the Sequence, Scope, and Positioning of Examination

Cardinal Techniques of Examination. As you begin the examination, study the four cardinal techniques of examination. Plan your sequence and scope of examination and how you will position the patient.

The physical examination relies on four classic techniques: inspection, palpation, percussion, and auscultation (Box 4-7). You will learn in later chapters about additional maneuvers that are important in amplifying physical diagnosis, such as having the patient lean forward to better detect the murmur of aortic regurgitation or balloting the patella to check for joint effusion.

Sequence of Examination. The key to a thorough and accurate physical examination is developing a systematic sequence of examination. Organize your comprehensive or focused examination around three general goals:

- Maximize the patient's comfort.
- Avoid unnecessary changes in position.
- Enhance clinical efficiency.

We recommend examining the patient from the patient's right side, moving to the opposite side or foot of the bed or examining table as necessary. This is the standard position for the physical examination and has several advantages compared with the left side: Estimates of jugular venous pressure are more reliable, the palpating hand rests more comfortably on the apical impulse, the right kidney is more frequently palpable than the left, and examining tables are frequently positioned to accommodate a right-handed approach.

Students who are left-hand dominant are encouraged to adopt right-sided positioning if possible, even it may seem awkward. The left hand can still be used for percussing or for holding instruments such as the otoscope or reflex hammer. Review the proposed physical examination sequence in Box 4-8, which meets the three goals of patient comfort, minimal changes in positioning, and efficiency.

In a comprehensive examination, in general, move from head to toe. Avoid examining the patient's feet, for example, before checking the face or mouth. You will quickly see that some segments of the examination are best assessed when the patient is sitting, such as examination of the head and neck and the thorax and lungs, whereas others are best obtained with the patient supine, such as the cardiovascular and abdominal examinations.

As you review the following pages, note that clinicians vary in where they place different segments of the examination, especially examinations of the musculoskeletal system and the nervous system. Some of these options are indicated in red in the right-hand column. Suggestions for patient positioning during the different segments of the examination are also indicated in the right-hand column in red.

With practice, you will develop your own sequence of examination, keeping the need for thoroughness and patient comfort in mind. At first, you may need notes to remind you what to look for, but over time, this

Box 4-6. Transmission-Based Precautions in Patient Care Facilities

Type of Precaution	Description	Type of Personal Protective Equipment Required			
		Gloves	Gown	Mask	Respirator Mask
Contact precautions	Conditions that can be contracted through touching or contact such as MRSA and *C. difficile.*	✓	✓		
Droplet precautions	Conditions that can be spread through contact with secretions from the mouth, nose, and lungs, especially when a patient coughs or sneezes. Droplets usually travel only ~3 ft. (e.g., influenza, whooping cough); COVID-19 droplets can travel up to 6 ft.	✓	✓	✓	
Airborne precautions	Conditions that can spread through the air over long distances such as tuberculosis and chickenpox. Patients are also placed in a *negative pressure room* designed to prevent the air from flowing into the hallways.	✓	✓		✓
Reverse isolation	To protect the patient from any germs the staff or visitors are carrying. Patients who have a decreased immune system, usually from chemotherapy, may be placed in reverse isolation.	✓	✓	✓	

Source: CDC. *Guideline for Isolation Precautions: Preventing Transmission of Infectious Agents in Healthcare Settings* (2007). Updated November 14, 2018. Available at https://www.cdc.gov/infectioncontrol/pdf/guidelines/isolation-guidelines-H.pdf. Accessed April 4, 2019.

Box 4-7. Cardinal Techniques of Examination

Technique	Description
Inspection	Close observation of the details of the patient's appearance, behavior, and movement such as facial expression, mood, body habitus and conditioning, skin conditions such as petechiae or ecchymoses, eye movements, pharyngeal color, symmetry of thorax, height of jugular venous pulsations, abdominal contour, lower extremity edema, and gait.
Palpation	Tactile pressure from the palmar fingers or fingerpads to assess areas of skin elevation, depression, warmth, or tenderness, lymph nodes, pulses, contours and sizes of organs and masses, and crepitus in the joints.
Percussion	Use of the striking or *plexor finger,* usually the third, to deliver a rapid tap or blow against the distal *pleximeter finger,* usually the distal third finger of the left hand laid against the surface of the chest or abdomen, to evoke a sound wave such as resonance or dullness from the underlying tissue or organs. This sound wave also generates a tactile vibration against the pleximeter finger.
Auscultation	Use of the diaphragm and bell of the stethoscope to detect the characteristics of heart, lung, and bowel sounds, including location, timing, duration, pitch, and intensity. For the heart, this involves sounds from closure of the four valves, extra sounds from blood flow into the atria and ventricles, and murmurs. Auscultation also permits detection of bruits or turbulence over arterial vessels.

Box 4-8. Physical Examination: Suggested Sequence and Positioning

- General survey
- Vital signs
- Skin: upper torso, anterior and posterior
- Head and neck, including thyroid and lymph nodes
- *Optional:* nervous system (mental status, cranial nerves, upper extremity motor strength, bulk, tone, cerebellar function)
- Thorax and lungs
- Breasts
- Musculoskeletal as indicated: upper extremities
- Cardiovascular, including jugular venous pressure (JVP), carotid upstrokes and bruits, point of maximal impulse (PMI), S_1, S_2; murmurs, extra sounds
- Cardiovascular, for S_3 and murmur of mitral stenosis
- Cardiovascular, for murmur of aortic insufficiency
- *Optional:* thorax and lungs—anterior
- Breasts and axillae
- Abdomen
- Peripheral vascular
- *Optional:* skin—lower torso and extremities
- Nervous system: lower extremity motor strength, bulk, tone, sensation; reflexes; Babinski reflex
- Musculoskeletal, as indicated
- *Optional:* skin, anterior and posterior
- *Optional:* nervous system, including gait
- *Optional:* musculoskeletal, comprehensive
- *Women:* pelvic and rectal examination
- *Men:* prostate and rectal examination

Key to the Symbols for the Patient's Position

- Sitting
- Lying supine, with head of bed raised 30 degrees
- Same, turned partly to left side
- Sitting, leaning forward
- Lying supine
- Standing
- Lying supine, with hips flexed, abducted, and externally rotated, and knees flexed (lithotomy position)
- Lying on the left side (left lateral decubitus)

Each symbol pertains until a new one appears. Two symbols separated by a slash indicate either or both positions.

sequence will become habitual and remind you to return to segments of the examination you may have skipped, helping you to be complete.

HEAD-TO-TOE PHYSICAL EXAMINATION

General Survey

Observe the patient's general state of health, build, and sexual development. Obtain the patient's height and weight. Note posture, motor activity, and gait; dress, grooming, and personal hygiene; and any odors of the body or breath. Watch the patient's facial expressions and note manner, affect, and reactions to people and the environment. Listen to the patient's speech and note the state of awareness or level of consciousness.

Close observation begins at the outset of the patient encounter and continues throughout the history and physical examination.

Vital Signs

Measure the blood pressure. Count the pulse and respiratory rate. If indicated, measure the body temperature.

The **patient is sitting** on the edge of the bed or examining table. Stand in front of the patient, moving to either side as needed.

Skin

Observe the skin of the face and its characteristics. Assess skin moisture or dryness and temperature. Identify any lesions, noting their location, distribution, arrangement, type, and color. Inspect and palpate the hair and nails. Study both surfaces of the patient's hands. Continue your assessment of the skin as you examine the other body regions.

Head, Eyes, Ears, Nose, Throat

Head: Examine the hair, scalp, skull, and face. ***Eyes:*** Check visual acuity and screen the visual fields. Note the position and alignment of the eyes. Observe the eyelids and inspect the sclera and conjunctiva of each eye. With oblique lighting, inspect each cornea, iris, and lens. Compare the pupils, and test their reactions to light. Assess the extraocular movements. With an ophthalmoscope, inspect the ocular fundi. ***Ears:*** Inspect the auricles, canals, and drums. Check auditory acuity. If acuity is diminished, check lateralization (Weber test) and compare air and bone conduction (Rinne test). ***Nose and sinuses:*** Examine the external nose; using a light and a nasal speculum, inspect the nasal mucosa, septum, and turbinates. Palpate for tenderness of the frontal and maxillary sinuses. ***Throat (or mouth and pharynx):*** Inspect the lips, oral mucosa, gums, teeth, tongue, palate, tonsils, and pharynx. You may wish to assess the cranial nerves during this portion of the examination.

The room should be darkened for the ophthalmoscopic examination. This promotes pupillary dilation and improved visibility of the fundi.

Neck

Inspect and palpate the cervical lymph nodes. Note any masses or unusual pulsations in the neck. Feel for any deviation of the trachea. Observe the sound and effort of the patient's breathing. Inspect and palpate the thyroid gland.

Move behind the sitting patient to feel the thyroid gland and to examine the back, posterior thorax, and lungs.

Back

Inspect and palpate the spine and muscles of the back. Observe shoulder height for symmetry.

Posterior Thorax and Lungs

Inspect and palpate the spine and muscles of the *upper* back. Inspect, palpate, and percuss the chest. Identify the level of diaphragmatic dullness on each side. Listen to the breath sounds; identify any adventitious (or added) sounds, and, if indicated, listen to the transmitted voice sounds.

A Note on the Musculoskeletal System. By this time, you have made preliminary observations of the musculoskeletal system. You have inspected the hands and surveyed the upper back. If indicated, *with the patient still sitting,* examine the hands, arms, shoulders, neck, and temporomandibular joints. Inspect and palpate the joints and check their range of motion. You may choose to examine upper extremity muscle bulk, tone, strength, and reflexes at this time, or wait until later.

Breasts and Axillae

In a woman, inspect the breasts with the arms relaxed, then elevated, and then with the hands pressed on the hips. In either sex, inspect the axillae and feel for the axillary nodes.

The patient is **still sitting**. Move to the front again.

Palpate the breasts, while at the same time continuing your inspection.

The patient position is supine. Ask the patient to lie down. You should stand at the *right side* of the patient's bed.

Anterior Thorax and Lungs

Inspect, palpate, and percuss the chest. Listen to the breath sounds, any adventitious sounds, and, if indicated, transmitted voice sounds.

Cardiovascular System

Observe the jugular venous pulsations and measure the jugular venous pressure in relation to the sternal angle. Inspect and palpate the carotid pulsations. Listen for carotid bruits.

Elevate the head of the examining table or bed to ~30 degrees for the cardiovascular examination, adjusting as necessary to see the jugular venous pulsations.

Inspect and palpate the precordium. Note the location of the apical impulse. Attempt to note its diameter, amplitude, and duration. Listen at each auscultatory area with the diaphragm of the stethoscope. Listen at the apex and the lower sternal border with the bell. Listen for the first and second heart sounds and for physiologic splitting of the second heart sound. Listen for any abnormal heart sounds or murmurs.

If indicated, ask the patient to roll partly onto the left side while you listen at the apex for an S_3 or ***mitral stenosis***. The patient should sit, lean forward, and exhale while you listen for the murmur of *aortic regurgitation*.

Abdomen

Inspect, auscultate, then percuss the abdomen. Palpate lightly, then deeply. Assess the liver and spleen by percussion and then palpation. Attempt to palpate the kidneys. Try to palpate the aorta and its pulsations. If you suspect inflammation of the kidney from infection, percuss posteriorly over the costovertebral angles (CVAs).

Lower the head of the bed to the flat position. **The patient should be supine.**

Lower Extremities

Examine the legs, assessing three systems while the patient is still supine. Each of these three systems can be further assessed when the patient stands.

- *Peripheral vascular system.* Palpate the femoral pulses and, if indicated, the popliteal pulses. Palpate the inguinal lymph nodes. Inspect for lower extremity edema, discoloration, or ulcers. Palpate for pitting edema. Inspect for varicose veins.

  The patient is **supine.**

- *Musculoskeletal system.* Note any deformities or enlarged joints. If indicated, palpate the joints, check their range of motion, and, if necessary, perform any special maneuvers.
- *Nervous system.* Assess lower extremity muscle bulk, tone, and strength; also assess sensation and reflexes. Observe any abnormal movements. Observe the patient's gait and ability to walk heel-to-toe, walk on the toes, walk on the heels. Do a Romberg test.
- *Musculoskeletal system.* Examine the alignment of the spine and its range of motion, the alignment of the legs, and the feet.

  The patient is **standing.**

Nervous System

The complete examination of the nervous system can also be done at the end of the examination. It consists of the five segments: *mental status, cranial nerves* (including funduscopic examination), *motor system, sensory system,* and *reflexes.*

The patient is **sitting or supine**.

Mental Status. If indicated and not done during the interview, assess the patient's orientation, mood, thought process, thought content, abnormal perceptions, insight and judgment, memory and attention, information and vocabulary, calculating abilities, abstract thinking, and constructional ability.

Cranial Nerves. If not already examined, check sense of smell, strength of the temporal and masseter muscles, corneal reflexes, facial movements, gag reflex, and strength of the trapezia and sternocleidomastoid muscles. Perform funduscopic examination if not done yet.

Motor System. Assess muscle bulk, tone, and strength of major muscle groups. *Cerebellar function:* rapid alternating movements (RAMs), point-to-point movements, such as finger-to-nose (F → N) and heel-to-shin (H → S), gait.

Sensory System. Assess pain, temperature, light touch, vibration, and discrimination. Compare right with left sides and distal with proximal areas on the limbs.

Reflexes. Including biceps, triceps, brachioradialis, patellar, Achilles deep tendon reflexes; also plantar reflexes or Babinski response (see p. 133).

Additional Examinations

The *rectal* and *genital* examinations are often performed at the end of the physical examination. Patient positioning is as indicated.

Genital and Rectal Examination in Men. Inspect the sacrococcygeal and perianal areas. Palpate the anal canal, rectum, and prostate. Examine the penis and scrotal contents and check for indirect hernias. If the patient cannot stand, examine the genitalia before doing the rectal examination.

The patient is **lying on his left side** (lateral recumbent or Sims position, p. 119) for the rectal examination (or standing and bending forward).

Genital and Rectal Examinations in Women. Examine the external genitalia, vagina, and cervix, with a chaperone when needed. Obtain a Pap smear. Palpate the uterus and adnexa bimanually. Perform the rectal examination if indicated.

The patient is **supine in the lithotomy position** (p. 119). You should be seated during examination with the speculum, then standing during bimanual examination of the uterus, adnexa (and rectum as indicated).

ADULT-FOCUSED PHYSICAL EXAMINATION

The focused physical examination is usually limited to one or two systems or regions, and it is largely based on the nature of the patient's presenting complaint(s). While choosing to perform a focused examination, consider the differential diagnosis of the presenting complaint and rule out the various medical conditions.

See Box 4-9, Sequence of Adult-Focused Physical Examination.

By considering your differential diagnosis, you can select a particular region or body system to assess in greater detail. It makes sense while performing focused physical examination to consider adjacent regions or body systems as well. Also, a patient's symptoms may help in determining whether or not to also assess a region adjacent to the area of primary interest.

Box 4-9. Sequence of Adult-Focused Physical Examination

General Examination

- General survey
  - Apparent state of health
  - Level of consciousness
  - Apparent state of discomfort or distress
- Skin, hair, and nails
  - Look for any changes in skin color, scars, plaques, or nevi.
  - Look for signs of pallor.
  - Look for cyanosis.
  - Look for jaundice.
  - Inspect and palpate the fingernails. Note their color, shape, and any lesions.
  - Look for clubbing and capillary refill.
- Dress, grooming, and personal hygiene
- Facial expression
- Odors of the body and breath
- Posture, gait, and motor activity
- Height and weight measurement, and calculation of BMI
- Vital signs
  - Blood pressure
  - Pulse
  - Temperature
  - Respiration
- Hydration
  - Look for evidence of dehydration or edema.
- Eyes
  - Inspect for symmetry, swelling, and redness of the eyes and eyelids. If the patient reports a change in vision, pursue the related details. Note pupils' size and reaction to light. Observe extraocular eye movements. Note any strabismus and nystagmus.
- Face
  - Palpate the sinuses and observe for any tenderness or swelling.
- Nose
  - Inspect the nasal mucosa, nasal septum, and any abnormalities.
- Mouth and oral cavity
  - Inspect the lips, oral mucosa, gums and teeth, roof of the mouth, tongue and the floor of the mouth, and pharynx.
- Ears
  - Note any discharge, redness, cerumen, swelling, tenderness, or abnormalities.
- Neck
  - Inspect the neck; note its symmetry and any masses or scars. Palpate the trachea and note any deviation.
- Lymph nodes
  - Palpate the lymph nodes. Note size, shape, mobility, and consistency of the lymph nodes, and any tenderness.
- Thyroid gland
  - Note size, swelling, and tenderness of the thyroid gland, its symmetry, and any mass.
- Extremities
  - Inspect for alterations and bilateral inconsistencies in color, warmth, movement, swelling, tenderness, and sensation. Note edema of lower legs and feet, and presence of superficial distended veins.
- Speech and language
- Cognitive functions
- Gait and posture

System or Region Examination

- Appropriate system(s) examination is performed based on symptoms/condition (refer to chief complaint or present illness) and understanding of anatomy and physiology.
  - Respiratory (thorax and lungs)
  - Cardiovascular (heart and peripheral vessels)
  - Gastrointestinal (abdomen, anus, and rectum)
  - Genitourinary (genitalia, prostate in males)
  - Nervous
  - Musculoskeletal
- Do not narrow your examination prematurely: "Confirming what is not wrong may be as important as what is wrong."

ADAPTING THE PHYSICAL EXAMINATION: SPECIFIC PATIENT CONDITIONS

As you progress through your training, you may need to modify your physical examination due to the patient's clinical status, which in turn may dictate changes in your sequence of examination. These situations include patients who are:

- Bedbound
- Wheelchair bound
- Postprocedure
- Obese
- In pain
- On special precautions

Patient on Bedrest

Patients on bedrest are often required to abstain from weightbearing or certain activities as a precaution after an injury or surgical procedure. Often, this only allows examination of the anterior head, neck, and chest with the patient lying supine. If it is safe for the patient to roll over on the bed, you will be able to perform an examination of the posterior region such as auscultation of the posterior chest. Since patients on bedrest are at risk of developing pressure injuries, rolling the patient to one side also allows you to examine the entire skin in the back, especially the area that is in constant contact with the bed surface such as the sacral area.

Patient Using a Wheelchair

Certain examination maneuvers like the head and neck, cardiovascular, and pulmonary exams can be easily performed with the patient sitting in the wheelchair and leaning forward if necessary. However, some maneuvers, like the abdominal exam, must be done in the supine position, so the patient must transfer from the wheelchair to the examination table or bed. Have the patient position the wheelchair parallel and up against the table or bed. Then, if possible, have the patient stand up and pivot toward the bed. Provide assistance if needed. Since these patients often spend considerable amounts of time sitting in their wheelchairs, pursue detailed skin examination to look for pressure injuries. The major areas to look for these injuries are pressure points in the sacrum, heels, calves, elbows, and spine.

Patient Who Is Postprocedure

Examining patients after a surgical procedure can be puzzling for novice examiners. Often, the patient may still be recovering from the effects of anesthesia, thus making following commands difficult. Patients may also be on certain restrictions, limiting your performance of certain examination maneuvers. Before examining a patient postprocedure, confirm any restrictions of movement from the supervising clinician. These restrictions are most common after spinal and orthopedic surgeries and procedures performed using vascular access in which the patient must be in the supine position for up to 4 hours after the procedure. Pay particular attention to the surgical site and its dressing; the abdomen for return of bowel function; and, depending on the operation, peripheral vascular or neurologic examinations. These exams, though brief, are routinely done to monitor the patient's recovery. Inspect the current dressing to ensure that it is clean and dry. You should also inspect the wound under the dressing, if possible, to check for good wound healing via primary or secondary intention. Also inspect for signs of continued bleeding from the surgery or infection like erythema, warmth, wound discharge, or excessive drainage. Also assess drains, lines, and tubes such as chest tubes, indwelling catheters, and large intravenous lines.

Patient Who Is Obese

Obesity is a common disorder that threatens patients with significant morbidity and mortality. Patients who are obese provide unique challenges during a physical examination due to adipose tissue obscuring certain areas of examination and palpation of underlying structures. When examining patients, note the patient's fat distribution. If it is centered around the abdomen rather than the pelvis, the patient is at higher risk for metabolic syndrome disorders such as cardiovascular disease and diabetes mellitus. When examining the skin, you should examine within body folds. Since these areas are usually moist, warm, and often missed in daily hygiene, they are prone to skin breakdown and infection. Also inspect the lower extremities for any signs of skin breakdown, swelling, or vascular changes, which are all chronic signs of obesity. In addition, disorders like breast cancer (from increased adipose tissue conversion into estrogen), heart failure, and hypoventilation are associated with obesity, so complete breast (including men), cardiovascular, and pulmonary examinations are crucial.

Patient in Pain

Patients in pain present a challenge to the beginning student because you must balance the need to assess important physical findings with the possibility that the maneuvers themselves can exacerbate the patient's pain. Therefore, the first step in examining a patient in pain is observation. Look for signs of distress like an increased respiratory rate, sweating, tearing, and facial expressions such as grimacing or biting. In addition, assess the patient's vital signs, as pain commonly elevates blood pressure and heart rate. If the patient is in pain prior to examination, or a critical examination is expected to exacerbate the pain, consider controlling the pain before starting the examination. If your patient cannot perform a certain maneuver, use other characteristics of the pain to help determine possible causes. Patients who are nonverbal or in a coma can still experience pain, especially if they are postprocedure, bedbound, or in the intensive care setting. Note their vital signs, facial expressions, signs of agitation, and withdrawal to guide your pain assessment and subsequent management.

Patient on Special Precautions

You must wear special personal protective equipment (PPE) when examining a patient who has an infection or at risk for developing an infection. Using protective equipment may present a barrier for certain parts of the examination. For example, if the infectious precautions require a self-contained head cover, you will be prevented from doing auscultation using a stethoscope. You may be unable to palpate the patient's skin if you are required to wear gloves. Omit this part of the examination and document accordingly.

RECORDING YOUR FINDINGS

Recall that your goal is to produce a clear, concise, but comprehensive report that documents key findings and communicates your assessment in a succinct format to clinicians, consultants, and other members of the health care team (review Box 1-20). Study Box 4-10 and scrutinize the documentation of the physical examination findings. Note the standard format of the clinical record from General Survey to Neurological Examination. Additional sample documentation can also be found in each of the regional chapters.

Box 4-10. The Case of Patient MN—Physical Examination

Physical Examination

General Survey: MN is a short, overweight, middle-aged female, who is animated and responds quickly to questions. Her hair is well groomed. Her color is good, and she lies flat without discomfort.

Vital signs: Ht (without shoes) 157 cm (5′2″). Wt (dressed) 65 kg (143 lb). BMI 26. BP 164/98 right arm, supine; 160/96 left arm, supine; 152/88 right arm, supine with wide cuff. Heart rate (HR) 88 and regular. Respiratory rate (RR) 18. Temperature (oral) 98.6 °F.

Skin: Palms cold and moist, but color good. Scattered cherry angiomas over upper trunk. Nails without clubbing, cyanosis.

Head, Eyes, Ears, Nose, Throat (HEENT): Head: Hair of average texture. Scalp without lesions, normocephalic/atraumatic (NC/AT). *Eyes:* Vision 20/30 in each eye. Visual fields full by confrontation. Conjunctiva pink; sclera white. Pupils 4 mm constricting to 2 mm, round, regular, equally reactive to light. Extraocular movements intact. Disc margins sharp, without hemorrhages, exudates. No arteriolar narrowing or A-V nicking. *Ears:* Cerumen partially obscures right tympanic membrane (TM); left canal clear, TM with good cone of light. Acuity good to whispered voice. Weber midline. AC > BC. *Nose:* Mucosa pink, septum midline. No sinus tenderness. *Mouth:* Oral mucosa pink. Dentition good. Tongue midline. Tonsils absent. Pharynx without exudates.

Neck: Neck supple. Trachea midline. Thyroid isthmus barely palpable, lobes not felt.

Lymph nodes: No cervical, axillary or epitrochlear nodes.

Thorax and lungs: Thorax symmetric with good excursion. Lungs resonant on percussion. Breath sounds vesicular with no added sounds. Diaphragms descend 4 cm bilaterally.

Cardiovascular: Jugular venous pressure 1 cm above the sternal angle, with head of examining table raised to 30 degrees. Carotid upstrokes brisk, without bruits. Apical impulse discrete and tapping, barely palpable in the 5th left interspace, 8 cm lateral to the midsternal line. Good S_1, S_2; no S_3 or S_4. A II/VI medium-pitched midsystolic murmur at the 2nd right interspace; does not radiate to the neck. No diastolic murmurs.

Breasts: Pendulous, symmetric. No masses; nipples without discharge.

Abdomen: Protuberant. Well-healed scar, right lower quadrant. Bowel sounds active. No tenderness or masses. Liver span 7 cm in right midclavicular line; edge smooth, palpable 1 cm below right costal margin (RCM). Spleen not felt. No costovertebral angle tenderness (CVAT).

Genitalia: External genitalia without lesions. Mild cystocele at introitus on straining. Vaginal mucosa pink. Cervix pink, parous, and without discharge. Uterus anterior, midline, smooth, not enlarged. Adnexa not palpated due to obesity and poor relaxation. No cervical or adnexal tenderness. Pap smear taken. Rectovaginal wall intact.

Rectal: No external hemorrhoids, with tight sphincter tone, rectal vault without masses. Stool brown, negative for occult blood.

Extremities: Warm and without edema. Calves supple, nontender.

Peripheral vascular: Trace edema at both ankles. No varicosities in lower extremities. No stasis pigmentation or ulcers. Pulses (2+ = brisk, or normal):

	Radial	Femoral	Popliteal	Dorsalis Pedis	Posterior Tibial
RT	2+	2+	2+	2+	2+
LT	2+	2+	2+	2+	2+

Musculoskeletal: No joint deformities or swelling on inspection and palpation. Good range of motion in hands, wrists, elbows, shoulders, spine, hips, knees, ankles.

Neurologic: Mental Status: Alert and cooperative. Thought processes are coherent and insight is good. Oriented to person, place, and time. *Cranial nerves:* II to XII intact. *Motor:* Good muscle bulk and tone. *Strength:* 5/5 bilaterally in deltoids, biceps, triceps, hand grips, iliopsoas, hamstrings, quadriceps, tibialis anterior, and gastrocnemius. *Cerebellar:* Rapid alternating movement (RAMs) and point-to-point movements intact. Gait stable, fluid. *Sensory:* Pinprick, light touch, position sense, vibration, and stereognosis intact. Romberg negative. *Reflexes:*

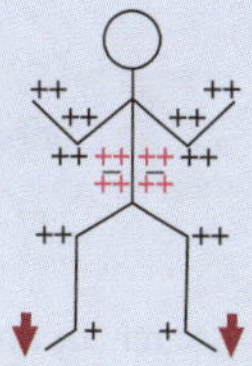

CHAPTER 5

Clinical Reasoning, Assessment, and Plan

After completing the history and physical examination, you reach the critical step of formulating a *differential diagnosis*. Using sound clinical reasoning, you must analyze your findings and identify a list of potential causes for the patient's problems. The length of the list will reflect your uncertainty about the possible explanation for a given problem. It will start with the most likely explanation but will also include other plausible diagnoses, particularly those that have serious consequences if undiagnosed and untreated. You will assign probabilities to the various diagnoses that correspond to how likely you consider them to as explanations for your patient's problem.

As you gain experience, your clinical reasoning will begin at the outset of the patient encounter, not at the end. Think about these steps as you see your first patients. As with all patients, focus on determining "What explains this patient's concerns?" and "What are the findings, problems, and diagnoses?"

CLINICAL REASONING: PROCESS

Kahneman describes two different thought processes when making decisions, a theory known as "*dual processing*." *System 1* or the *intuitive system* is fast and an automatic reaction to information that functions on mental shortcuts called *heuristics*, which are formulaic response patterns based on formed habits. These are difficult to change or manipulate. *System 2* or the *hypotheticodeductive system* is a more tempered, controlled thought process. It is subject to conscious judgments and attitudes and uses logic and probabilities to come to a conclusion. This process is time and resource intensive and requires more cognitive effort. These methods are not mutually exclusive, and clinicians rely on different blends of clinical reasoning approaches in different scenarios (Fig. 5-1).

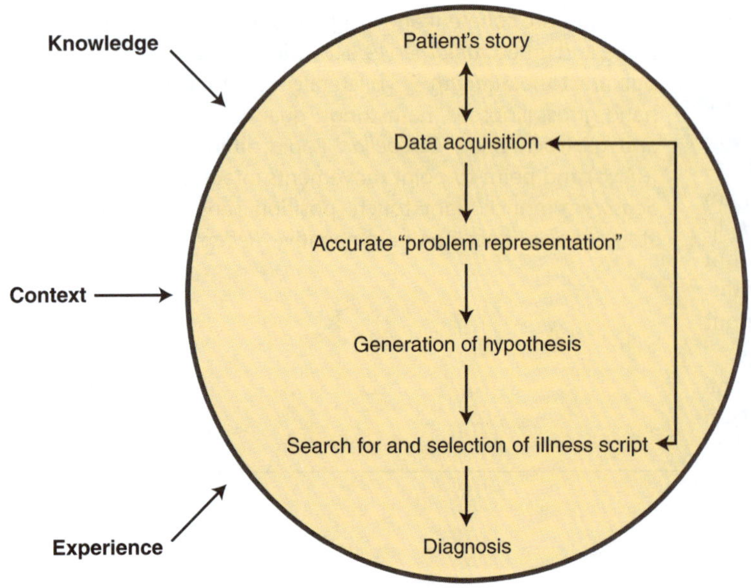

FIGURE 5-1. Key elements of the clinical diagnostic reasoning process. (From Bowen JL. *N Engl J Med.* 2006;355(21):2217–2225. Copyright © 2006 Massachusetts Medical Society. Reprinted with permission from Massachusetts Medical Society.)

Basic Structure of the Clinical Reasoning Process

The basic process of clinical reasoning (Box 5-1) starts with the information you have gathered from your patient. This data includes historical information, findings from your physical examination, and any preliminary diagnostic and laboratory testing. These may also include information you have obtained from other clinicians and from your review of the patient's prior health records. These have been discussed extensively in previous chapters. The next step is to organize and interpret these sets of information with the goal of creating a concise and appropriate *problem representation* (documented in the clinical record as the *summary statement*). From this problem representation, generate, prioritize, and test a list of possible diagnosis until you have selected a *working diagnosis*—one that fits your patient's problem best. Your working diagnosis will then be your basis for selecting your patient's treatment plan.

Box 5-1. Basic Structure of the Clinical Reasoning Process

- Gathering initial patient information (health history and physical examination)
- Organizing and interpreting information to synthesize the problem (problem representation)
- Generating hypotheses (differential diagnosis) for patient's problem
- Testing hypotheses until a working diagnosis is selected
- Planning the diagnostic and treatment strategy

Gathering Initial Patient Information (Health History and Physical Examination). The process of gathering information from the health interview and physical examination has been extensively discussed in Chapters 3 and 4 Additional information may also be available to you before and after the clinical encounter, such as prior health records and comments from family members, caregivers, health care providers, or any person with knowledge of the patient. This includes the patient's *symptoms* elicited during the history, the *signs* you observed during the physical examination, and any laboratory and other reports available to you. Be methodical and organized to make sure that all abnormal and unexpected findings are identified. As you progress in your clinical reasoning skills, this process will increasingly occur during the patient encounter, in real time. However, it is always good practice to revisit your data at the conclusion of the encounter to ensure no abnormal findings were missed. Once you have a list of abnormal findings, you can begin to organize them in a way that helps narrow the list of possible causes of these findings.

Organizing and Interpreting Clinical Information. It is often challenging to decide whether clinical data fit into one problem or several problems. If there is a relatively long list of symptoms and signs, and an equally long list of potential explanations, one approach is to *tease out separate clusters of observations and analyze one cluster at a time*. Several identifying differentiating and key clinical features may help.

Anatomic Location. You can organize your information by clustering your findings *anatomically*, which could point to a potential source of the problem. The symptom of a scratchy throat and the sign of an erythematous inflamed posterior pharynx, for example, clearly localize the problem to the pharynx. A complaint of headache leads you quickly to the structures of the skull and brain. Other symptoms, however, may present greater difficulty. Chest pain, for example, can originate in the coronary arteries, the stomach and esophagus, or the muscles and bones of the thorax. If the pain is exertional and relieved by rest, either the heart or the musculoskeletal components of the chest wall may be involved. If the patient notes pain only when carrying groceries with the left arm, the musculoskeletal system becomes the likely culprit. When localizing findings, be as specific as your data allow; however, you may have to settle for a body region, such as the chest, or a body system, such as the musculoskeletal system. On the other hand, you may be able to define the exact structure involved, such as the left pectoral muscle. Some symptoms and signs are constitutional and cannot be localized, such as fatigue or fever. Furthermore, some groups of signs and symptoms, such as those caused by endocrine disorders or exposures to toxins, may not be anatomically related despite their common cause.

Age. The patient's *age* may help; younger and otherwise healthy patients are more likely to have a single disease, whereas older patients tend to have multiple diseases.

Timing of Symptoms. The *timing* of symptoms is often useful. For example, an episode of pharyngitis 6 weeks ago is probably unrelated to the fever, chills, pleuritic chest pain, and cough that prompted a clinic visit today. To use timing effectively, you need to know the natural history of various diseases and conditions. A yellow penile discharge followed 3 weeks later by a painless penile ulcer suggests two problems: gonorrhea and primary syphilis. In contrast, a penile ulcer followed in 6 weeks by a maculopapular skin rash and generalized lymphadenopathy suggests two stages of the same problem: primary and secondary syphilis.

Involvement of Different Body Systems. Involvement of the *different body systems* may help group clinical data. If symptoms and signs occur in a single system, one disease may explain them. Problems in different, apparently unrelated, systems often require more than one explanation. Again, knowledge of disease patterns is necessary. For example, you might decide to group a patient's high blood pressure and sustained apical impulse together with flame-shaped retinal hemorrhages, place them in the cardiovascular system, and label the constellation "hypertensive cardiovascular disease with hypertensive retinopathy." You would develop another explanation for the patient's mild fever, left lower quadrant tenderness, and diarrhea.

Multisystem Conditions. With experience, you will become increasingly adept at recognizing *multisystem conditions* and building plausible explanations that link manifestations that are seemingly unrelated. To explain cough, hemoptysis, and weight loss in a 60-year-old plumber who has smoked cigarettes for 40 years, you would rank lung cancer high in your differential diagnosis. You might support your diagnosis with your observation of the patient's cyanotic nailbeds. With experience and continued reading, you will recognize that his other symptoms and signs fall under the same diagnosis. Dysphagia would reflect extension of the cancer to the esophagus, pupillary asymmetry would suggest pressure on the cervical sympathetic chain, and jaundice could result from metastases to the liver. In another example of multisystem disease, a young man who presents with odynophagia, fever, weight loss, purplish skin lesions, leukoplakia, generalized lymphadenopathy, and chronic diarrhea is likely to have acquired immune deficiency syndrome (AIDS). Related risk factors should be explored promptly.

Synthesizing Clinical Information and Developing the Problem Representation. As clinical information is gathered and organized during a patient encounter, the clinician simultaneously *synthesizes* this information to form a *problem representation*—a clinician's evolving sense of the clinical picture. It usually contains the *patient's initial information* (chief complaint, epidemiology, and risk factors), *key features in the history and physical examination*, and *results of diagnostic testing*. In your clinical documentation, the problem representation is called the *Summary Statement*. The problem representation becomes more and more detailed as additional data is collected as exemplified in the unfolding clinical case in Box 5-2.

This is an important step in the clinical reasoning process. The development of a well-developed and concise problem representation guides a clinician to generating a hypothesis and developing the differential diagnosis. This summary rarely contains unnecessary data and rarely leaves out any significant data. An accurate problem representation also helps activate appropriate illness scripts (see Box 5-5, p. 142).

Box 5-2. Case Example: Development of a Problem Representation

Part 1: A 57-year-old male comes to the emergency room with a chief complaint of pain in his chest for the past 2 hours.

The first step in synthesizing this information and formulating your problem representation is to identify the *salient* patient information. Your initial problem representation may be: *"A 57-year-old male with acute onset of chest pain."*

Part 2: He says that he was shoveling snow from his driveway when he suddenly developed a moderately severe pain in the center of his chest right behind the sternum. The pain lasted for approximately 1–2 minutes and did not move anywhere else. He said that the pain was accompanied by shortness of breath. He has smoked one pack of cigarettes per day for the last 35 years and has a history of congestive heart failure.

As you gather more information from the patient and synthesize the information further, adding now the additional salient history and clinical findings in the physical examination may yield the following problem representation: *"A 57-year-old male with congestive heart failure and a 35 pack-year smoking history presenting with acute, severe, exertional, retrosternal pain and associated shortness of breath."*

Part 3: His physical examination is notable for cardiovascular findings of an S_3 gallop that is new, chest findings showing crackles in both lung bases, and swelling of both of his legs.

Your resulting problem representation for the case could be: *"A 57-year-old man with congestive heart failure and a 35 pack-year smoking history presenting with acute, severe, exertional, retrosternal pain and associated shortness of breath. His examination is notable for a new S_3 gallop, bibasilar crackles, and bilateral lower extremity edema."*

Generating Hypotheses by Searching for the Probable Cause of the Findings. For early learners, or for clinicians encountering a new or challenging set of clinical problems, an organized, stepwise approach is critical to avoid cognitive errors (Box 5-3). For each identified problem or cluster of problems you will generate a clinical hypothesis. Draw on the full range of your knowledge and experience and read widely. It is at this point that reading about diseases and abnormalities is most useful. By consulting the clinical literature, you embark on the lifelong goal of evidence-based decision making and clinical practice. At first, your hypotheses may not be highly specific, but proceed as far as your knowledge and available data allow.

Box 5-3. Approaches to Searching for Probable Causes of the Findings

- Generate an exhaustive list
- Match findings against all conditions that can produce them
- Eliminate diagnostic possibilities that fail to explain the findings
- Weigh competing possibilities and select the most likely diagnosis
- Give special attention to potentially life-threatening conditions

Generate an Exhaustive List. As a novice clinician, this is what you are most likely to be familiar with. This approach is based on understanding the underlying mechanisms of the disease process in question. This is where every possible question is asked, and every piece of available information is collected and organized to help arrive at the diagnosis. You can list pathologic processes involving diseases of a body system or structure or pathophysiologic processes reflecting derangements of biologic functions, such as heart failure or migraine headache. Still other problems are psychopathologic, such as disorders of mood like depression or headache as an expression of a somatic symptom disorder. Box 5-4 describes helpful diagnostic development tools for this method.

Select the Most Specific and Critical Findings to Support Your Hypothesis. Look for clues that can help generate a differential diagnosis and distinguish between diseases with shared characteristics. These could be descriptors that are characteristic of the diagnoses (*defining features*) or features unique to disease (*discriminating feature*) and therefore useful for distinguishing the diagnoses from one another (Fig. 5-2).

For example, if the patient reports *"the worst headache of her life,"* nausea, and vomiting, and you find altered mental status, papilledema, and meningismus, build your hypothesis around elevated intracranial pressure rather than gastrointestinal disorders.

Match Findings Against All Causative Conditions (Illness Scripts). In this method, a pattern of clues or clinical characteristics (*illness script*) trigger a memory response to a clinician's previously learned information (Box 5-5). The clinician tries to see if the patient's problem can match one of these patterns during the clinical encounter. Typically, as a novice learner, your illness scripts will consist of prototypical or "textbook" characteristic presentations of diseases. You will then refine this over time with increasing clinical experience and further learning from experienced clinicians and experts.

Box 5-4. Memory Aids for Generating Differential Diagnosis (Exhaustive Method)

Tom G. Prince, MD, Psychiatrist, General Hospital

Toxin/**T**rauma including medications
Oncologic
Musculoskeletal/Rheumatologic
Gastrointestinal
Pulmonary
Renal
Infectious
Neurologic
Cardiovascular
Endocrine
Metabolic/Genetic
Dermatologic
Psychiatric
Genitourinary/Gynecologic
Hematologic

VINDICATE

Vascular
Infectious
Neoplastic
Drug related
Inflammatory/**I**diopathic/**I**atrogenic
Congenital
Autoimmune/**A**llergic
Trauma/**T**oxic
Endocrine/Metabolic

An everyday example can be used to illustrate this process. If someone asks you to visualize a typical fire truck in your mind, you will likely be imagining a large, red truck, with lights, a ladder, and a hose. This is a typical, textbook "script" for fire trucks based on books, media, and real-life experiences. Even most children would be able to describe this and recognize a fire truck on the street. However, most adults, with more real-world experience, would also recognize a large yellow truck with a hook and a ladder as a fire truck—a less common presentation of a very common vehicle.

Even early in your clinical training, you have already developed illness scripts for common conditions. Consider a patient with acute appendicitis—picture this patient in your mind, in an emergency room. How old is the patient? What symptoms is the patient complaining? When did these symptoms start? How does the patient appear, and what key physical examination findings would you expect? Most people will imagine a young patient, with abdominal pain, and perhaps with nausea and vomiting. The abdominal pain probably started a day or two ago as opposed to last month. The patient would

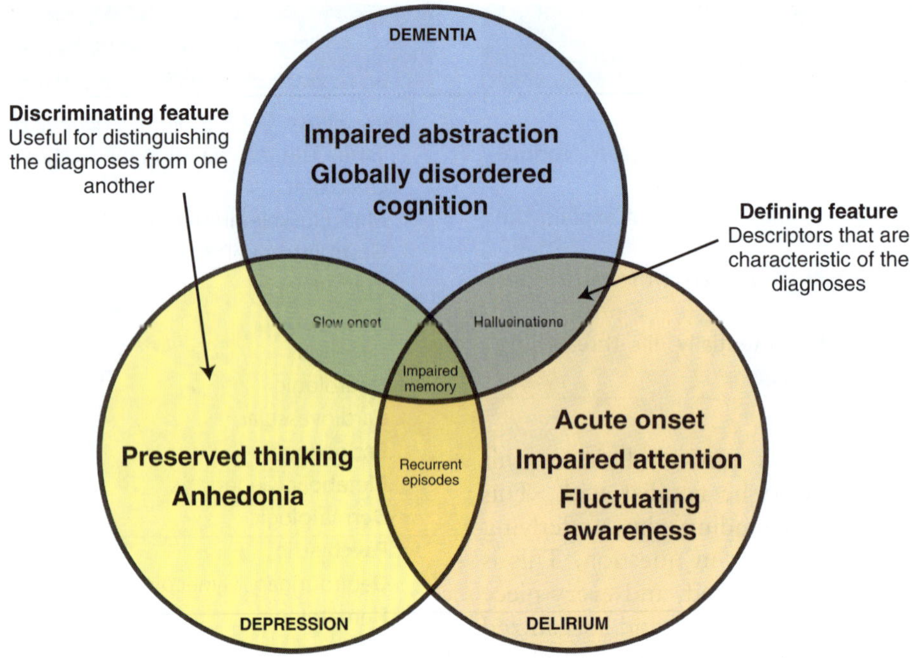

FIGURE 5-2. Defining and discriminating features: memory impairment.

Box 5-5. Example: Illness Script for Acute Coronary Syndrome

	Acute Coronary Syndrome
Epidemiology/ Pathophysiology	Older age, risk factors include diabetes, hypertension, dyslipidemia, family history, tobacco use
Time course	Acute onset, not necessarily preceded by exertional angina
Clinical presentation	Chest pain, with crescendo to maximal pain; often dull and substernal, radiating to arms/ shoulders; diaphoresis; dyspnea; nausea/vomiting, diaphoresis; tachycardia on examination
Diagnostic studies	Elevated cardiac biomarkers; ST elevation/depression, T-wave changes on ECG; regional wall motion abnormality on echocardiogram

probably be uncomfortable and have a tender abdomen on physical examination.

Knowledge recalled as illness scripts has a predictable structure: the predisposing conditions, the pathophysiologic insult, and the clinical consequences. In concrete terms, the elements of an illness script often include a disease's pathophysiology, epidemiology, time course, salient symptoms and signs, diagnostics, and treatment. Box 5-5 provides an example of a basic illness script that represents the most common historical information of a patient presenting with acute coronary syndrome.

As you progress through your training and gain clinical experience your illness scripts will increase in number, detail, and nuance. Not only will you get better at recognizing common diseases more quickly, but you will able to appreciate the subtle nuances of a disease's characteristics including an awareness of less common ways that disease can manifest in a given patient.

Eliminate Diagnostic Possibilities That Fail to Explain the Findings. For example, you might consider cluster headache as a cause of Patient MN's headaches (see Box 5-10), but eliminate this hypothesis because it fails to explain the patient's throbbing bifrontal localization with associated nausea and vomiting. Also, the pain pattern is atypical for cluster headache—it is not unilateral, boring, or occurring repetitively at the same time over a period of days, nor is it associated with lacrimation or rhinorrhea.

Weigh Competing Possibilities and Select the Most Likely Diagnosis. Look for a close match between the patient's clinical presentation and a typical case of a given condition. Other clues help in this selection. The statistical probability of a given disease in a patient of this age, sex, ethnic group, habits, lifestyle, and locality should greatly influence your selection.

For example, you should consider the possibilities of osteoarthritis and metastatic prostate cancer in a 70-year-old male with back pain, but not in a 25-year-old female with the same complaint. The *timing* of the patient's illness also makes a difference. Headache in the setting of fever, rash, and stiff neck that develops suddenly over 24 hours suggests quite a different problem than recurrent headache over a period of years associated with stress, visual scotoma, and nausea and vomiting relieved by rest.

Giving Special Attention to Potentially Life-Threatening Conditions. One rule of thumb is to always include "the worst-case scenario" in your differential diagnosis and make sure you have ruled out this possibility based on your findings and patient assessment. Your goal is to minimize the risk of missing unusual or infrequent conditions such as meningococcal meningitis, bacterial endocarditis, pulmonary embolus, or subdural hematoma that are particularly ominous.

Testing Hypotheses and Establishing a Working Diagnosis. Now that you have made a hypothesis about the patient's problem, you are ready to *test your hypothesis*. You are likely to need further history, additional maneuvers on physical examination, or laboratory studies or x-rays to confirm or rule out your tentative diagnosis or to clarify which of two or three possible diagnoses are most likely. When the diagnosis seems clear-cut—a simple upper respiratory infection or a case of hives, for example—these steps may not be necessary.

Establish a working definition of the problem at the highest level of explicitness and certainty that the data allow. You may be limited to a symptom, such as "tension headache, cause unknown." At other times, you can define a problem more specifically based on its anatomy, disease process, or cause. Examples include "bacterial meningitis, pneumococcal," "subarachnoid hemorrhage, left temporoparietal lobe," or "hypertensive cardiovascular disease with left ventricular dilatation and heart failure." Although most diagnoses are based on the identification of abnormal structures, disease processes, and clinical syndromes, patients frequently have clinically unexplained symptoms. You may not be able to move beyond simple descriptive categories such as "fatigue" or "anorexia." Other problems relate to stressful events in the patient's life such as losing a job or a family member that increase the risk for subsequent illness. Identifying these events and helping the patient develop coping strategies are just as important as managing a headache or a duodenal ulcer.

Planning the Diagnostic and Treatment Strategy. Planning the diagnostic and treatment strategy flows logically from the working diagnosis you have identified. These steps are often wide ranging and incorporate the diagnostic and therapeutic interventions that you recommend, patient education, changes in medications, needed tests, referrals to other clinicians, and return visits for counseling and support. However, a plan does more than just describe the approach to the patient's problem. Developing an effective plan requires good interpersonal skills and sensitivity to the patient's goals, economic means, competing responsibilities, and family structure and dynamics. It is critical to obtain both the patient's agreement and their participation in decision making whenever possible. These discussions should use evidence-based medicine, which exists at the intersection of the best available evidence, clinician judgment, and patient values. These practices promote optimal therapy, adherence to treatment, and patient satisfaction, especially since there is often no single "right" plan, but a range of variations and options. It is important to discuss your assessment with the patient before finalizing the *Plan* and proceeding with further testing or evaluation, ensuring the patient's active participation in the plan of care.

Clinical Diagnostic Errors

While learning the process of clinical reasoning, it is also important to consider common sources of error in this process. Box 5-6 describes common sources of cognitive error in clinical reasoning.

An awareness of the cognitive processes used to make decisions can reduce the likelihood of poor decisions. You should be vigilant for these errors and follow several general rules to improve your decision-making process (Box 5-7).

CLINICAL REASONING: DOCUMENTATION

While all of your clinical documentation of the health history and physical examination is a reflection of your data gathering skills, the *Summary Statement, Assessment*, and *Plan* represent the most robust reflection of your clinical reasoning and data synthesis skills. The *subjective data* of the health history and the *objective data* from the physical examination and testing are primarily descriptive and factual. As you move to *Assessment*, you go beyond description and observation to analysis and interpretation. You select and cluster relevant pieces of information, analyze their significance, and try to explain

Box 5-6. Common Types of Clinical Cognitive Errors

Cognitive Error	Description	Vignette
Anchoring bias	Tendency to perceptually lock onto salient features in the patient's initial presentation too early in the diagnostic process and failure to adjust in light of later information	A clinician "locks onto" a patient's description of an aura that precedes her headaches as indicative of a migraine and fails to recognize red flags of increased intracranial pressure that should prompt neuroimaging for this patient
Availability heuristic	Assumption that a diagnosis is more likely, or more frequently occurring, if it more readily comes to mind	A clinician who has recently seen several patients with acute appendicitis does not consider ovarian torsion in an adolescent girl presenting with acute right lower quadrant abdominal pain
Confirmation bias	Seeking supportive evidence for a diagnosis at the exclusion of more persuasive information refuting it	A clinician makes a presumptive diagnosis of an upper respiratory infection in a well-appearing patient presenting with cough, rhinorrhea, and fever, and does not consider pneumonia even after finding asymmetric chest wall excursion and dullness to chest percussion on examination
Diagnostic momentum	Prioritizing a diagnosis made by prior clinicians, discounting evidence of alternative explanations	A clinician does not consider acute myocardial infarction in a patient who was recently diagnosed with acid reflux in the setting of similar symptoms
Framing effect	Interpretation of information is influenced heavily by the way in which information about the problem are presented (*framed*)	A patient is presented as having "frequent emergency room visits for asthma exacerbation in the setting of medication noncompliance." The clinician fails to explore structural forces that drive medication adherence and fails to explore alternative causes of the current exacerbation
Representation error	Failure to take prevalence into account when estimating the probability of a diagnosis	Clinician who often sees older patients places diverticular bleed high on her differential diagnosis when evaluating rectal bleeding in an adolescent patient
Visceral bias	Visceral arousal (negative and positive feelings toward patients) lead to poor diagnostic decisions	Clinician assumes that a patient who is homeless will not be able to manage a complicated treatment plan and prescribes a simpler, less optimal plan, without discussing the options with the patient

Sources: Croskerry P. *Acad Med*. 2003;78(8):775–780; Weinstein A et al. *MedEdPORTAL*. 2017;13:10650.

Box 5-7. Suggested Rules for Good Decision Making

- Slow down.
- Be aware of base rates for your differentials.
- Consider what data is truly relevant.
- Actively seek alternative diagnoses.
- Ask questions to disprove, rather than confirm, your current hypothesis.
- Remember you are often wrong. Consider the immediate implications of this.

them logically using principles of biopsychosocial and biomedical science. Your clinical reasoning process is pivotal to how you interpret the patient's history and physical examination, single out problems identified in the Assessment, and move from each problem to its action plan. Not only does you record facilitate clinical reasoning, but it also promotes communication and coordination among the professionals who care for your patient and documents the patient's problems and management for medicolegal purposes.

Document the Problem Representation (Summary Statement)

The problem representation is a synthesis and distillation of the salient information which "makes a case" for your working diagnosis. This is written in your patient's health record as the *summary statement* and often starts the Assessment section of the clinical record. A summary statement should not simply be a recitation of the facts. The elements of an effective summary statement include a restated patient's chief complaint and its clinical context with the salient historical information, physical examination findings, and study data results. There is a direct correlation between the summary statement and the illness script for the leading item on your differential diagnosis—the goal is for the summary statement to elicit this diagnosis in the mind of the reader by aligning with the illness script.

A summary statement:

- Is the chief complaint placed in context of patient's overall health status
- Includes pertinent parts of the history, physical examination, and lab data
- Is succinct and short (no more than two to three sentences)
- Demonstrates your clinical reasoning skills
- Should make a case for the diagnosis
- Is a distillation of your understanding of the case

For example: "A 57-year-old male with congestive heart failure and a 35 pack-year smoking history presenting with acute, severe, exertional, retrosternal pain and associated shortness of breath. His examination is notable for a new S_3 gallop, bibasilar crackles, and bilateral lower extremity edema."

A well-developed summary statement often contains important qualifying adjectives called *semantic qualifiers*. Semantic qualifiers are qualitative terms that are binary in nature (opposing descriptors) that can be used to compare and contrast diagnostic considerations (Box 5-8).

Box 5-8. Examples of Semantic Qualifiers

- Acute, chronic
- At rest, with activity (*exertional*)
- Constant, intermittent
- Diffuse, localized
- Mild, severe
- Old, new
- Sharp, dull
- Unilateral, bilateral
- Young, old

In the previous example, "A 57-year-old male with congestive heart failure and a 35 pack-year smoking history presenting with acute, exertional, retrosternal pain, and associated shortness of breath. His examination is notable for a new S_3 gallop, bibasilar crackles, and bilateral lower extremity edema," you will notice that the problem representation contained several semantic qualifiers including *"acute," "severe," "exertional," "new," "bibasilar,"* and *"bilateral."* These semantic qualifiers tend to focus the list of possible hypotheses (differential diagnosis) to those that relate directly to these terms. Studies have shown that successful clinicians use semantic qualifiers more frequently, which is associated with strong clinical reasoning.

Assessment and Plan

Following the summary statement, you should make a list of all of the patient's problems addressed during the clinical encounter. This list should include known diagnoses, symptoms, abnormalities, and psychosocial concerns. It is related to the initial list of abnormalities you have made at the start of the clinical reasoning process; however, it reflects how those observations are analyzed and synthesized.

As such, the Problem List:

- Is a synthesis of all abnormal and unexpected findings during an encounter
- Includes known diagnoses and new/undiagnosed symptoms/signs
- Includes significant social factors that impact health such as food or housing insecurity
- Is prioritized, with the patient's chief complaint on top

In a well-constructed record, the *Assessment* and *Plan* section stems from this list of problems addressed in the clinical encounter. Each problem is listed in order of priority and expanded with an explanation of supporting findings and a differential diagnosis, followed by a plan for addressing that problem. In general, an assessment and plan can be *diagnostic*, *therapeutic*, or both (Box 5-9). If one of your problems in your list is a symptom without a known cause (e.g., anorexia or fatigue), your assessment will include a brief description of the potential causes (your *differential diagnosis*), and your plan will describe your diagnostic steps in reaching a diagnosis. Some elements of management or therapy may also be included. For known diagnoses and chronic conditions your assessment will describe the current status of that condition, and your plan will describe your management moving forward. The status may include symptom or disease control, complications, and current management with adherence to treatment or any adverse effects.

Box 5-9. Annotated Example of Diagnostic and Therapeutic Assessment and Plan

Assessment/Plan: A 62-year-old male with diabetes mellitus and hypertension, on a recent long-haul flight presents with an acute exertional chest pain. On examination, the patient is tachycardic but without leg edema.

This is the summary statement.

1. Chest pain

   The patient's known cardiovascular risk factors of hypertension and diabetes mellitus, and the acute onset and exertional nature of the chest pain make this diagnosis most likely. Pulmonary embolism is less likely as the patient has no evidence of shortness of breath or unilateral leg swelling; however, the patient has tachycardia and recently took a long flight.

   An example of a *diagnostic assessment*. You should provide supporting evidence for the likelihood of each item in your differential diagnosis.

   Plan:

   - Request for an EKG and serial troponin levels to evaluate acute coronary syndrome.
   - Request for d-dimer. As this patient has low probability for a pulmonary embolism, a negative d-dimer would likely rule out this diagnosis as the cause of the patient's chest pain.

   This is an example of a *diagnostic plan*. You should provide rationale for evaluating each item in your differential diagnosis.

2. Diabetes mellitus, type 2

   The diabetes is currently poorly controlled, with a hemoglobin A_1C of 9.0%, on metformin 1,000 mg twice a day. He reports excellent adherence to this medication without any side effects.

   This is an example of a *therapeutic assessment*. You should provide the clinical status of the chronic condition or a known diagnosis.

   Plan:

   - After discussing with the patient, a long-acting insulin will be started, as the addition of a second oral agent is unlikely to bring his hemoglobin A_1C to goal. Educate patient on the use of the insulin pen and possible complications. Excellent teach-back.

   This is an example of a *therapeutic plan*. You should provide rationale for the management of chronic condition or known diagnosis moving forward.

Another increasingly prominent item on problem lists is *Health Maintenance*. Routinely listing Health Maintenance helps you track several important health concerns more effectively: immunizations, screening tests such as mammograms or colonoscopies, instructions regarding nutrition or testicular self-examinations, recommendations about exercise or use of seat belts, and responses to important life events. See Box 5-10 for an example of a Health Maintenance section of the Assessment and Plan.

Box 5-10. The Case of Patient MN: Summary Statement, Assessment, and Plan

Summary Statement: MN is a 54-year-old female with a history of migraines since childhood presenting with chronic intermittent, progressive pulsatile headaches which are similar in nature to prior attacks and precipitated by current life stressors. The headaches are accompanied by nausea and vomiting. On examination, she has elevated blood pressure but otherwise a normal cardiovascular and nonfocal neurologic examination.

The key characteristics included are the patient information (age) and the chief complaint (duration, quality, associated symptoms). Only the salient characteristics are included. For example, the chronic duration of 3 months rules out many acute life-threatening processes such as meningitis, subarachnoid hemorrhage, and stroke. The clinical context here is her history of migraines since childhood.

Assessment and Plan:

1. Headaches:

   The differential diagnosis includes:

   (a) Migraine headache—this is most likely as the patient has a history of migraine headaches and describes her current headaches as of a similar quality. The pulsatile quality, duration between 4 and 72 hours, associated nausea and vomiting, and disability intensity all support this diagnosis, as does the normal neurologic examination.

   (b) Tension headaches—this is also a possibility as the headaches are bilateral, which is less common in migraine headaches; a 54-year-old female with migraine headaches since childhood, with a throbbing vascular pattern and frequent nausea and vomiting. Headaches are associated with stress and relieved by sleep and cold compresses. There is no papilledema, and there are no motor or sensory deficits on the neurologic examination.

The key parts of the physical examination include pertinent positives (elevated blood pressure that might be related to hypertensive causes of headaches) and pertinent negatives (normal neurologic examination) that make serious space-occupying lesions causing increased intracranial pressure less likely.

(*continued*)

Box 5-10. The Case of Patient MN: Summary Statement, Assessment, and Plan (*continued*)

(c) Other dangerous conditions are less likely. There is no fever, stiff neck, or focal findings to suggest meningitis, and the lifelong recurrent pattern makes subarachnoid hemorrhage unlikely (usually described as "the worst headache of my life"). A normal neurologic and fundoscopic examination make a space-occupying lesion such as tumor less likely as well.

Plan:

- Discuss features of migraine versus tension headaches with the patient. Also discuss warning signs that would prompt urgent reevaluation.
- Discuss biofeedback and stress management.
- Advise patient to avoid caffeine, including coffee, colas, and other carbonated beverages.
- Start nonsteroidal anti-inflammatory drugs (NSAIDs) for headache, as needed.
- If needed next visit, begin prophylactic medication if headaches are occurring more than 2 days a week or 8 days a month.

Nausea and vomiting are discussed under "headache" on the problem list. Despite their different anatomic location, they are recognized as part of a cluster of clinical findings that are all related to a common diagnosis.

2. Elevated blood pressure: Elevated systolic and diastolic blood pressure are noted. The patient denies chest pain and shortness of breath and is not symptomatic at the time of the interview, making hypertensive urgency unlikely.

   Plan:

   - Discuss standards for assessing blood pressure.
   - Check a hemoglobin A1C to assess for diabetes, which would impact the target blood pressure.
   - Recheck blood pressure in 2 weeks.
   - Discuss weight reduction and exercise programs (see #4).
   - Reduce salt intake.

A single elevated blood pressure reading does not qualify as a diagnosis of hypertension. Therefore, this abnormal physical examination finding is reported as "elevated blood pressure" in the problem list.

3. Cystocele with occasional stress incontinence: Cystocele on pelvic examination, probably related to bladder relaxation. Patient is perimenopausal. Incontinence reported with coughing, suggesting alteration in bladder neck anatomy. No dysuria, fever, flank pain. Not taking any contributing medications. Usually involves small amounts of urine, no dribbling, so doubt urge or overflow incontinence.

   Plan:

   - Explain cause of stress incontinence.
   - Review urinalysis.
   - Recommend Kegel exercises.
   - Consider topical estrogen cream to vagina during next visit if no improvement.

Most likely the patient symptom of stress incontinence and the physical examination finding of cystocele are discussed together under a single diagnosis, as they are causally related.

4. Overweight: Patient 5'2", weighs 143 lb. BMI is ~26.

   Plan:

   - Explore diet history, ask patient to keep food intake diary.
   - Explore motivation to lose weight, set target for weight loss by next visit.
   - Schedule visit with dietitian.
   - Discuss exercise program, specifically, walking 30 minutes most days a week.

5. Stress and housing insecurity: Son-in-law with alcohol problem; daughter and grandchildren seeking refuge in patient's apartment, leading to tensions in these relationships. Patient also has financial constraints and describes spiritual duress with lack of social and spiritual support. Stress currently situational. No current evidence of depression (PHQ2 = 0).

   Plan:

   - Explore patient's views on strategies to cope with stress.
   - Explore sources of support, including Al-Anon for daughter and financial counseling for patient. Refer to social work and discuss in interdisciplinary team meeting.
   - Refer to chaplain to discuss spiritual support systems
   - Continue to monitor for possible signs of depression.

(*continued*)

Box 5-10. The Case of Patient MN: Summary Statement, Assessment, and Plan (*continued*)

6. Occasional musculoskeletal low back pain: Usually with prolonged standing. No history of trauma or motor vehicle accident. Pain does not radiate; no tenderness or motor-sensory deficits on examination. Doubt disc or nerve root compression, trochanteric bursitis, sacroiliitis.
   Plan:
   - Review benefits of weight loss and exercises to strengthen low back muscles.
7. Tobacco misuse: One pack per day for 36 years. No signs of oral cancer on examination today. Seems precontemplative for smoking cessation in setting of multiple life stressors and progressive headaches.
   Plan:
   - Check peak flow or FEV_1/FVC on office spirometry to assess for obstructive lung disease.
   - Discuss low-dose CT for lung cancer screening.
   - Precontemplative at this point, but offered ongoing support moving forward should she change her mind and provided information resources regarding nicotine replacement therapy and oral medications to review. Can readdress after improvement of life stressors and relief from headaches.
8. Murmur: A II/IV midsystolic murmur was appreciated on examination. Given its location in the aortic position and the patient's age this most likely represents aortic sclerosis or stenosis. The patient has no shortness of breath, chest pain, or syncope to suggest severe aortic stenosis. Will monitor symptoms' examination and consider a transthoracic echocardiogram if the murmur changes in intensity or if she develops any symptoms.
9. Health maintenance: Last Pap smear 2018; mammogram, 2019; has never had a colonoscopy.
   Plan:
   - Referred for colonoscopy, prescribed prep medications and discussed use. Provided hand out with instructions and discussed using teach-back technique.
   - Referred to dentist for oral cancer screening in light of smoking.
   - Advise patient to move medications and caustic cleaning agents to locked cabinet above shoulder height. Urge patient to store handgun in a secured locked location, unloaded with trigger lock, and to store ammunition in a separate locked location.

RECORDING YOUR FINDINGS

Recall that your goal is to produce a clear, concise, but comprehensive report that documents key findings and communicates your assessment in a succinct format to clinicians, consultants, and other members of the health care team. Study Box 5-10 and scrutinize the documentation of the physical examination findings. Note the standard format of the clinical record from *Summary Statement* to *Assessment and Plan* including *Health Maintenance*. Recall that the summary statement is the documented problem representation described previously in p. 89. Also remember that how you organize your clinical data into the problem list is a result of your clinical reasoning. This was based on your differential diagnoses developed by considering the anatomic location, clustering of symptoms, time course, and patient characteristics. This section also provides how the list of problems in the Assessment is generated from the initial clinical information gathered during first step of the clinical reasoning process described previously on p. 89.

PROGRESS NOTE AND PATIENT PROBLEM LIST IN THE ELECTRONIC HEALTH RECORD

The format of the clinic or hospital progress note is quite variable, but it should meet the same standards as the initial assessment. The note should be clear, sufficiently detailed, and easy to follow. It should reflect your clinical reasoning and delineate your assessment and plan. Be sure to learn the documentation standards for billing in your institution, because this can affect the detail and type of information needed in your progress notes. The progress note often follows the SOAP format: **S**ubjective, **O**bjective, **A**ssessment, and **P**lan.

See Table 5-1, Example of a Progress Note: The Case of Patient MN: Follow-Up Clinic Visit 1 Mo Later, for an example of a progress note of a follow-up clinic visit.

Patient Problem List

After you complete the clinical record for the current patient encounter, it is good clinical practice to generate a *Patient Problem List* that summarizes the patient's problems to be included on the patient's summary page in the electronic health record (EHR). This list lives outside of any particular clinical note and includes *all of the patient's significant problems.* In contrast, the *problem list* documented with the assessment and plan for a particular encounter includes only those problems identified or addressed then. When constructing a Patient Problem List, *list the most active and serious problems first and record their date of onset.* Some clinicians make separate lists for active and inactive problems; others make one list in order of priority. A good Patient Problem List helps you to individualize the patient's care.

On follow-up visits, the Patient Problem List provides a quick summary of the patient's clinical history and a reminder to review the status of problems the patient may not mention. An accurate Patient Problem List allows better population management of patients, by using EHRs to track patients with specific problems, recall patients who are behind on appointments, and follow up on specific issues. The Patient Problem List also allows other members of the health care team to learn about the patient's health status at a glance.

A sample Patient Problem List for Patient MN is provided in Box 5-11. You may wish to number each problem and use the number to refer to specific problems in subsequent notes.

Problems can be symptoms, signs, past health events such as a hospital admission or surgery, or diagnoses. Good lists vary in emphasis, length, and detail, depending on the clinician's philosophy, specialty, and role as a provider.

The list illustrated in Box 5-11 includes problems that need attention now, like Patient MN's headaches, as well as problems that need future observation and attention, such as her blood pressure and cystocele. Listing the allergy to ampicillin reminds you not to prescribe antibiotics in the penicillin family. Some symptoms do not appear on this list because they are minor concerns and do not require attention during this visit. Problem lists with too many relatively insignificant items are distracting. If these symptoms increase in importance, they can be added at a later visit.

Box 5-11. Patient Problem List: The Case of Patient MN

Date	Problem No.	Problem
8/25/20	1	Headaches probably migraine
	2	Elevated blood pressure
	3	Cystocele with occasional stress incontinence
	4	Overweight
	5	Social stress with housing insecurity
	6	Low back pain
	7	Tobacco use since age 18 years
	8	Murmur
	9	Allergy to ampicillin
	10	Health maintenance

ORAL PRESENTATION

The *oral presentation* is a structured, accurate, and tailored account of the patient and the patient's clinical his story. It serves as a primary means of communication between clinicians and the patient's other clinical teams. When done well, oral presentations can improve efficiency of patient care and serve as a forum for group learning. Oral presentations should also be an expression of your clinical reasoning. The included information should inform the listener about your thinking process and differential diagnosis.

During your encounter with the patient, you will gather more data than necessary for your written note. The oral presentation further reduces information from your write-up to include only what is most relevant to your differential diagnosis and management of the patient's chief complaint. The oral presentation represents a distillation of the information in the written patient note (Fig. 5-3).

You should always obtain a comprehensive health history for the written note of a new patient in an inpatient clinical setting. However, any clinical information obtained that is not relevant to explaining your differential diagnosis, you should omit it in the oral presentation, or you can simply report that these sets of information are "noncontributory." The review of systems in particular should not be included in the oral presentation, as any relevant symptoms should already have been presented as pertinent positive symptoms within the History of Present Illness section of the oral

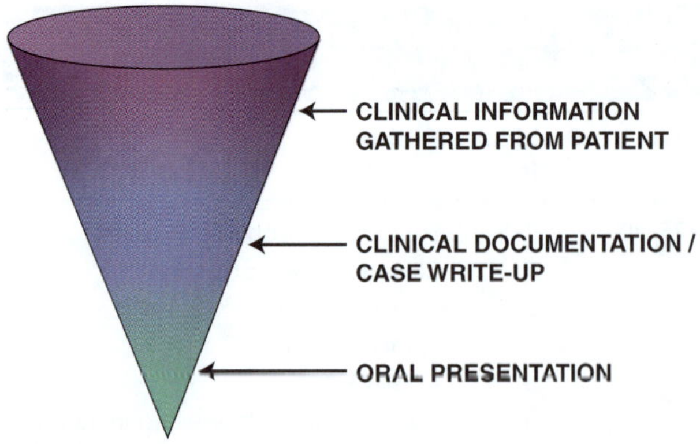

FIGURE 5-3. Reducing information to the essentials.

presentation. Also note that oral presentations will vary based on the expectations of the specific clinical audience, the amount of time available, the clinical service (e.g., medical vs. surgical), and the clinical setting. A suggested framework of a comprehensive oral presentation of a new patient is shown in Box 5-12.

This framework is best applied to a comprehensive oral presentation of a new patient. The types of information and level of detail in other oral presentations, however, will vary depending on the context. For example, an oral presentation made on daily work rounds would focus on overnight events and key updates, followed by that day's physical examination and any new diagnostic data, and finally an updated summary statement with assessment and plan. An oral presentation of a patient in the emergency room would focus almost exclusively on their chief complaint. A presentation made to a consulting clinician would focus on the specific question being asked of the consultant. In each case the structure of the oral presentation stems directly from its function.

Box 5-12. Guideline for Oral Patient Presentation: New Patient

Make a convincing case for the important problems, the differential, and the plan. Make it structured, organized, and targeted, as it should take only 3–5 minutes.

Opening Statement

- Briefly state the chief complaint and why patient was admitted.
- Include pointed and relevant historical information.

Source

- If indicated, briefly note if/why the patient cannot give reliable history.
- Note any information sources besides the patient.
- Unless you comment on the source, the patient will be assumed to be reliable.

Present Illness

- Use your differential diagnosis as a guide for what to include.
- Consider starting with: *"... usual state of health until ...."*
- Be chronologically organized and clear without analyzing.
- Remember the attributes of a chief complaint.
- Include elements of past history (with supporting studies and therapeutic interventions), medications, family history, social history (including psychosocial factors) that specifically contribute to the Present Illness.
- Include pertinent positives and negatives so the listener better understand your differential diagnosis.
- Only include ER course if it significantly affects/alters triage or immediate treatment decisions prior to the patient's coming to your care.

Other History

- Include important Past Medical History (with supporting history/data).
- Exclude minor diagnoses without impact on current care.
- Include important meds with doses of relevant ones. Omit unimportant medications.
- List allergies.
- Include focused Family History/Social History/Review of Systems. Do not repeat previously stated information.

Physical Examination

- Always include general appearance and specific vitals.
- Include pertinent elements of examination and any abnormal findings.
- Note the remainder as "unremarkable."

Labs/Data

- Include pertinent or otherwise significant labs/studies.
- Start with basic blood tests first.
- It is appropriate to mention other tests as being "normal."

Synthesis

- Consider beginning with: *"And in summary, ..."*
- Assess and synthesize, avoid regurgitating information.
- Demonstrate your thinking about the patient-specific differential diagnosis.
- If multiple issues present, weave together or discuss lesser issues in problem list.

Enumerated Problem List

- Start with most important problem first.
- Use most specific label for the problem you can.
- Avoid labeling a problem solely by its organ system.
- Include your understanding of the cause of the *problem.*
- *Include a diagnostic and/or therapeutic specific plan for addressing it.*

Source: Modified from Green EH et al. *Teach Learn Med.* 2005;17(3):263–267. Reprinted by permission of Taylor & Francis Ltd, http://www.tandfonline.com.

TABLE 5-1. Example of a Progress Note: The Case of Patient MN: Follow-Up Clinic Visit 1 Mo Later

10/25/20 1:00 PM

Source and Reliability:

Patient; excellent.

Chief Complaint:

Follow-up of migraine headaches.

MN is a 54-year-old female with a history of migraine headaches who returns after being seen a month ago with symptoms attributed to a recurrence of her migraine headaches. She was advised to cut back on caffeine and adopt stress-reduction techniques. She has had fewer headaches since reducing caffeine. She is now drinking decaffeinated coffee and has stopped drinking tea. She has joined a support group and started exercising to reduce stress. She is still having one to two headaches a month with some nausea, but they are less severe and generally relieved with 400 mg of ibuprofen. She denies any fever, stiff neck, associated visual changes, motor-sensory deficits, or paresthesias.

For her elevated blood pressure, she has been checking her blood pressure at home. It is running about 150/90. She is walking 30 minutes three times a week in her neighborhood and has reduced her daily caloric intake. She has been unable to stop smoking. She has been doing the Kegel exercises, but still has some leakage with coughing or laughing.

Medications: Ibuprofen 400 mg up to three times daily as needed for headache.

Allergies: Ampicillin causes rash.

Tobacco: One pack per day since age 18 years.

Physical Examination:

General Appearance: Overweight, middle-aged woman, who appears alert and somewhat deconditioned.

Vitals: Ht 157 cm (5′ 2″). Wt 63 kg. BMI 26. BP 150/90. HR 86 and regular. RR 16. Temp 36.8°C.

Skin: No suspicious nevi. *HEENT:* Normocephalic, atraumatic. Pharynx without exudates. Funduscopic examination without papilledema *Neck:* Supple, without thyromegaly. *Lymph nodes:* No lymphadenopathy. *Lungs:* Resonant and clear to auscultation bilaterally. *CV:* carotid upstrokes brisk, no bruits. Good S_1, S_2. No murmurs heard today. No S_3, S_4. *Abdomen:* Active bowel sounds. Soft, nontender, no hepatosplenomegaly. *Extremities:* Without edema. *Neuro:* Cranial nerves II–XII grossly intact.

Labs: Basic metabolic panel and urinalysis from 8/25/20 unremarkable. Hemoglobin A_{1C} 5.5%, and urine microalbumin/creatinine ratio of 15.

Assessment and Plan:

1. Migraine headaches—improved with reduction to one to two per month due to decreased caffeinated beverages and stress. Headaches are responding to ibuprofen.
   - Will defer daily prophylactic medication for now because patient is having fewer than three headaches per month and feels better.
   - Affirm need to stop smoking and to continue exercise program.
   - Affirm patient's participation in support group to reduce stress.
2. Hypertension—second measurement with elevation above goal at 150/90.
   - Discussed recommendation to start medication, as her blood pressure remained elevated despite improved exercise.
   - Will start with a calcium channel blocker as no indication for an ACE inhibitor, and a thiazide diuretic may worsen her urinary symptoms.
   - Patient to take blood pressure three times a week at home and bring recordings to next office visit.
3. Cystocele with occasional stress incontinence—stress incontinence improved with Kegel exercises but still with some urine leakage. Urinalysis from last visit without signs of infection of hematuria.
   - Continue Kegel exercises and refer to gynecology to discuss additional options.
4. Overweight—has lost ~2 kg.
   - Continue exercise.
   - Review diet history; affirm weight reduction.

(continued)

TABLE 5-1. Example of a Progress Note: The Case of Patient MN: Follow-Up Clinic Visit 1 Mo Later *(Continued)*

5. Stress and housing insecurity: She describes reductions in stress since joining her support group and expressed appreciation for the assistance of the chaplain and team social worker.
   - Continue to monitor for possible signs of depression.
6. Occasional low back pain
   - No complaints today.
7. Tobacco abuse—she did not review materials provided last visit and remains precontemplative.
   - Has pulmonary function test scheduled.
   - Has agreed to low-dose CT for lung cancer screening, referral placed.
8. Health maintenance
   - Last Pap smear 2019 normal cytology.
   - Mammogram, 2019 BiRads2 (benign findings).
   - Colonoscopy scheduled for next month.
   - Has dental appointment.

CHAPTER 6

Health Maintenance and Screening

CONCEPT OF PREVENTIVE CARE

Advances in preventive health care in the past 50 years have resulted in a tremendous decline in the incidence of debilitating common illnesses. Increasing knowledge and acceptance of health maintenance and disease prevention measures by patients have greatly facilitated and improved healthcare delivery by clinicians. As you proceed through your training, you will soon realize that many clinical conditions are largely preventable. Counseling your patients to eat a healthy diet, to exercise regularly, to avoid tobacco, and to receive preventive services such as cancer screenings, preventive visits, and vaccinations are just a few examples of ways you can help them maintain and promote their overall health and well-being. The promotion of health, as the World Health Organization has stated in its *Ottawa Charter for Health Promotion*, "enables patients to increase their control over, and improve, their health."

SCREENING

Basic Approach to Screening

Screening involves testing to identify asymptomatic patients with early-stage disease or precursors to disease who could benefit from early treatment. Some of the criteria for considering whether to implement a screening program, based on a monograph by the World Health Organization and subsequently modified by others, are shown in Box 6-1. Most screening programs target common diseases that have substantial morbidity and mortality, such as cancers, diabetes, chronic viral infections, substance abuse, and cardiovascular disease

Box 6-1. When Does It Make Sense to Consider Screening for a Disease or Condition?

- When a disease or condition causes substantial public health burden.
- When the natural history is well understood and there is a recognized latent or early symptomatic stage.
- When screening tests are available, acceptable, and accurate.
- When treatment for patients with clinically detected disease is available, acceptable, and more effective when delivered at the time of screening diagnosis.
- When screening programs are cost-effective.
- When net health benefits of screening outweigh the harms.

(CVD). However, sometimes screening programs target a rare disease, such as phenylketonuria in newborns, because detection is based on a simple blood test and avoiding products with phenylalanine can prevent disease complications. There should be a sufficiently long period when disease can be detected at an early stage and when treatment can be more effective and/or easy to deliver compared to when the disease is clinically detected. Screening tests should be widely available; acceptable to patients in terms of safety, convenience, and cost; and be accurate. Effective treatments for clinically detected disease should be widely available and acceptable.

In determining whether to recommend a screening program in India, organizations such as the Indian Council of Medical Research (ICMR) will weigh the evidence for benefit and harm (Box 6-2). The strongest evidence comes from randomized trials where patients are randomly assigned to receive either screening or usual care and followed—often for many years—to look for differences in disease survival (Fig. 6-1).

Box 6-2. Benefits and Harms of Screening

Benefits	Harms
■ Mortality reduction ■ Morbidity reduction ■ Reassurance	■ False-positive results that can cause anxiety and lead to additional testing ■ Overdiagnosis of low-risk disease that will never cause any clinical problems but may lead to overtreatment ■ False reassurance from false-negative tests ■ Pain or discomfort from diagnostic tests ■ Incidental findings leading to additional tests and treatments ■ Complications from treating disease

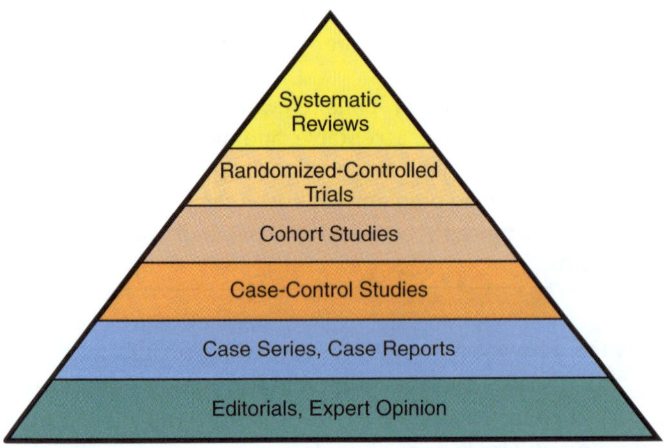

Systematic Reviews
Randomized-Controlled Trials
Cohort Studies
Case-Control Studies
Case Series, Case Reports
Editorials, Expert Opinion

FIGURE 6-1. Evidence pyramid showing strength of study types. (Adapted from Sackett DL et al. *Evidence-Based Medicine: How to Practice and Teach EBM.* 2nd ed. Churchill Livingstone; 2000. Copyright © 2000 Elsevier. With permission.)

Box 6-3. Potential Biases with Studies Evaluating Screening

Bias	Explanation of Bias
Selection bias	People who voluntarily undergo screening may be different from those who do not. These people may be healthier than the general population and likely to have better survival even without screening ("healthy volunteers").
Lead-time bias	Occurs when a screening test finds a disease at an early stage, but early treatment does not actually prolong life expectancy. The "survival" benefit is an artifact of earlier detection.
Length-time bias	Occurs because screening preferentially detects asymptomatic patients with slower-growing disease while patients with faster-growing disease are more likely to present with clinical symptoms. In comparing outcomes, the patients with screening-detected disease, which are likely to be less aggressive than diseases found during clinical care, will appear to have a better survival.

Observational studies, which compare outcomes between patients who receive screening and those who do not, are subject to important biases (Box 6-3).

BEHAVIORAL COUNSELING

One of the most important skills of an effective clinician is being able to help patients make behavioral changes. You can support a healthy lifestyle by counseling patients to exercise and follow healthy diets and to avoid unhealthy habits related to tobacco, alcohol, drugs, and unsafe sexual practices. However, changing behaviors is difficult and an important first step is to understand where patients are in terms of thinking about change. A useful model characterizing patients who should be adopting healthy behaviors or stopping unhealthy behaviors is the Prochaska and DiClemente *Transtheoretical* or *Stages of Behavioral Change Model*, as shown in Box 6-4. In this model, behavior change is conceptualized as a process that unfolds over time and involves progression through a series of five stages: *precontemplation*, *contemplation*, *preparation*, *action*, and *maintenance* (Fig. 6-2). Patients do not always move through the stages of change in a linear manner and may recycle depending on their level of motivation and self-efficacy. For example, patients in the maintenance stage work hard to practice a new and healthier behavior but may revert back to their old behaviors (*relapse*). Try to identify where your patient is in this continuum and tailor your interventions to your patient's readiness and self-efficacy to make lifestyle changes.

Box 6-4. Transtheoretical Model for Behavioral Change

Stage	Description	Statement
Precontemplation	Patients have no intention to change behavior in the foreseeable future. They are often unaware of their problems.	*"I do not think that I need to change any behaviors"*
Contemplation	Patients are aware that a problem exists and are seriously thinking about overcoming it. No commitment has been made to take action.	*"I'm concerned about my behavior, but not ready to make any changes now"*
Preparation	Patients have expressed intention to take action soon and are reporting small behavioral changes.	*"I'm ready to change my behavior now"*
Action	Patients modify their behavior to overcome their problems.	*"I'm changing my behavior now"*
Maintenance	Patients continue their action for behavioral change and work to prevent relapse.	*"I've changed my behavior"*
Relapse*	Cessation of behavioral changes and patients revert to old behavior.	*"I've returned to my old behavior"*

*Not a stage in itself but rather the "return from action or maintenance to an earlier stage."

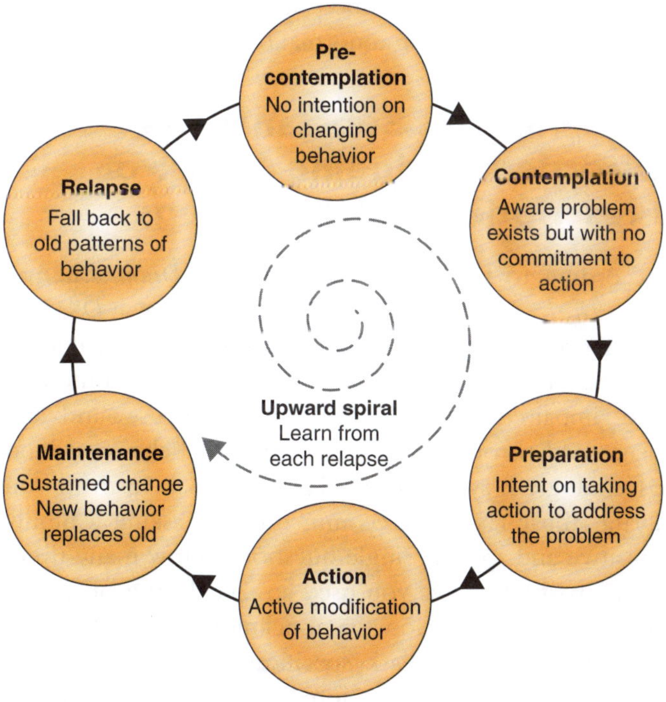

FIGURE 6-2. Transtheoretical Model for Behavioral Change. (Adapted with permission from Prochaska JO, DiClemente CC. *J Consult Clin Psychol.* 1983;51(3):390–395. Copyright © 1983 American Psychological Association.)

Motivational Interviewing

An effective strategy for patients in the precontemplative or contemplative stages is *motivational interviewing*. As defined by its originators, "motivational interviewing is a collaborative conversation style for strengthening a person's own motivation and commitment to change." This approach can effectively support behavioral changes to improve health outcomes such as glucose control, weight management, and physical activity, and particularly in the area of substance use disorders. Motivational interviewing is a "person-centered counseling style for addressing the common problem of ambivalence about change." Motivational interviewing acknowledges that persons are the experts on themselves and seeks to understand their perspectives about a given behavior in order to evoke their motivation and to arrive at an agenda for making positive behaviors changes. The style of motivational interviewing is guiding and collaborative, and "lies between and incorporates elements of *directing* and *following* styles." Box 6-5 highlights some of the core skills for drawing out your patients' ideas and solutions.

Box 6-5. Guiding Style of Motivational Interviewing

- **"Ask"** open-ended questions—invite the patient to consider how and why they might change
- **"Listen"** to understand your patient's experience—"capture" their account with brief summaries or reflective listening statements such as "quitting smoking feels beyond you at the moment"; this expresses empathy, encourages the patient to elaborate, and is often the best way to respond to resistance
- **"Inform"**—by asking permission to provide information, and then asking what the implications might be for the patient.

Specific communication and interpersonal techniques utilized in basic motivational interviewing such as the use of open-ended questions, reflective listening, use of empathic statements, and summarizing are discussed in Chapter 2. Advanced motivational interviewing techniques are beyond the scope of this book.

IMMUNIZATIONS

Vaccines are a cornerstone of public health and their use has significantly contributed to the prevention and control of infectious diseases everywhere. *Immunization* denotes the process of inducing or providing immunity by administering an immunobiologic. Immunization can be active or passive. Although often used interchangeably, the terms vaccination and immunization are not synonymous. The administration of an immunobiologic cannot be equated automatically with development of adequate immunity. Benefits of immunization are not limited to the vaccinated individual but also include promotion of *herd immunity* for the population at large, including nonimmunized persons and those with waning immunity or who may not have fully responded to prior vaccination.

SCREENING GUIDELINES FOR ADULTS

Screening guidelines for adults include:

- Unhealthy weight and diabetes mellitus
- Substance use disorders, including misuse of prescription and illicit drugs
- HIV infection
- Screening for intimate partner violence (IPV), elder abuse, and abuse of vulnerable adults

Screening for Unhealthy Weight and Diabetes Mellitus

The body mass index (BMI), which is a person's weight divided by the square of their height, is routinely measured at primary care visits. BMI is often used to screen for being overweight (Box 6-6).

Box 6-6. Classification of Weight by Body Mass Index (BMI) (kg/m^2)

	WHO (BMI)	Asia-Pacific (BMI)
Underweight	<18.5	<18.5
Normal	18.5–24.9	18.5–22.9
Overweight	25–29.9	23–24.9
Obese	≥30	≥25

Although BMI does not directly measure body fat, it is correlated with percentage of body fat and body fat mass as determined by more direct measures. Furthermore, a high BMI is associated with sleep apnea, nonalcoholic fatty liver disease, osteoarthritis, CVD, and metabolic disorders, including dyslipidemia and type 2 diabetes. Because diabetes is an important modifiable risk factor for CVD, overweight or obese adults aged 40 to 70 years should be screened for abnormal blood glucose.

Screening for Substance Use Disorders, Including Misuse of Prescription and Illicit Drugs

According to the Fifth Edition of the *Diagnostic and Statistical Manual of Mental Disorders* (*DSM-5*), substance use disorders are characterized by "clinically significant impairments in health, social function, and impaired control over substance use and are diagnosed through assessing cognitive, behavioral, and psychological symptoms." The National Institute on Drug Abuse (NIDA) recommends first asking a highly sensitive and specific single question: "How many times in the past year have you used an illegal drug or used a prescription medication for nonclinical reasons?" If the response is positive, ask specifically about nonclinical use of illicit and prescription drugs: "In your lifetime have you ever used: marijuana; cocaine; prescription stimulants; methamphetamines; sedatives or sleeping pills; hallucinogens like lysergic acid diethylamide (LSD), ecstasy, mushrooms…; street opioids like heroin or opium; prescription opioids like fentanyl, oxycodone, hydrocodone…; or other substances." For those answering yes, a series of further questions is recommended.

Once you identify substance abuse, probe further with questions like, "Are you always able to control your use of drugs?" "Have you had any bad reactions?" "What happened…Any drug-related accidents, injuries, or arrests? Job or family problems?" "Have you ever tried to quit? Tell me about it." Depending upon their risk level, patients may require referral for further treatment.

Screening for IPV, Domestic Violence, Elder Abuse, and Abuse of Vulnerable Adults

IPV and abuse of older or vulnerable adults are common problems in India, though often undetected. *Intimate partner violence* is defined as the "physical violence, sexual violence, psychological aggression (including coercive tactics, such as limiting access to financial resources), or stalking by a romantic or sexual partner, including spouses, boyfriends, girlfriends, dates, and casual 'hookups.'" The term *elder abuse* refers to "acts" whereby a trusted person (e.g., a caregiver) causes or creates risk of harm to an older adult. *Vulnerable adult* is generally defined as "a person who is or may be mistreated and who, because of age, disability, or both, is unable to protect himself or herself."

Screening for IPV can begin with general "normalizing" questions: "Because abuse is common in many lives of my patients, I've begun to ask about it routinely." "Are there times in your relationships that you feel unsafe or afraid?" "Have you ever been hit, kicked, punched, or hurt by someone you know?"

Several screening instruments are recommended, including the Humiliation, Afraid, Rape, Kick (HARK); Hurt, Insult, Threaten, Scream (HITS); Extended-HITS (E-HITS); Partner Violence Screen (PVS); and Woman Abuse Screening Tool (WAST). The sensitivity of these tests ranged from 64% to 87% while specificity ranged from 80% to 95%. Effective interventions following screen-detected IPV include ongoing delivery of support services, including counseling and home visits.

COUNSELING GUIDELINES FOR ADULTS

Counseling guidelines for adults include:

- Weight loss
- Healthful diet and physical activity

Weight Loss

Intensive, multicomponent behavioral interventions prevent cardiovascular disease (CVD) in adults with a BMI ≥30 and adults with a BMI 25 to <30 with CVD risk factors (hypertension, dyslipidemia, abnormal blood glucose levels) (Box 6-7). These interventions, which often lasted for 1 to 2 years, commonly included elements of self-monitoring weight, tools to support and maintain weight loss (e.g., pedometers, food scales, or exercise videos), and motivational counseling sessions.

Box 6-7. USPSTF Recommendations for Behavioral Counseling for Weight Loss

BMI (kg/m^2)	No Hypertension, Dyslipidemia, or Abnormal Blood Glucose Levels	Hypertension, Dyslipidemia, or Both	Abnormal Blood Glucose Levels or Diabetes
Comorbidity			
Normal weight (BMI 18.5 to <25)	Individualize the decision to provide or refer to behavioral counseling	Individualize the decision to provide or refer to behavioral counseling	Provide or refer to intensive behavioral counseling
Overweight (BMI 25 to <30)	Individualize the decision to provide or refer to behavioral counseling	Provide or refer to intensive behavioral counseling	Provide or refer to intensive behavioral counseling
Obese (BMI ≥30)	Provide or refer to intensive behavioral counseling	Provide or refer to intensive behavioral counseling	Provide or refer to intensive behavioral counseling

Source: U.S. Preventive Services Task Force; et al. *JAMA*. 2018;320(11):1163–1171.

To promote optimal patient weight and nutrition, adopt the approach outlined in Box 6-8.

Box 6-8. Steps to Promote Optimal Weight

1. Measure BMI and waist circumference:
   - Adults with a BMI ≥25 kg/m^2, men with waist circumferences >40 in, and women with waist circumferences >35 in are at increased risk for heart disease and obesity-related diseases.
   - Measuring the waist-to-hip ratio (waist circumference divided by hip circumference) may be a better risk predictor for individuals older than 75 years. Ratios >0.95 in men and >0.85 in women are considered elevated.
2. Determine additional risk factors for cardiovascular diseases, including smoking, high blood pressure, high cholesterol, physical inactivity, and family history.
3. Assess dietary intake.
4. Assess the patient's motivation to change.
5. Provide counseling about nutrition and exercise.

A key element of effective counseling is working with the patient to set reasonable goals (Box 6-9). A 5% to 10% weight loss is realistic and proven to reduce risk of diabetes and other obesity-associated health problems. Educate your patients about common roadblocks to sustained weight loss: hitting a plateau due to feedback physiologic systems that maintain body homeostasis; poor adherence to diet due to increasing hunger over time as weight declines; and inhibition of leptin, a protein cytokine secreted and stored in fat cells that modulates hunger. A safe goal for weight loss is 0.25 to 1 kg per week.

Box 6-9. Strategies That Promote Weight Loss

- The most effective diets combine realistic weight loss goals with exercise and behavioral reinforcements.
- Encourage patients to walk 30 to 60 minutes 5 or more days a week, or a total of at least 150 minutes a week.
- The total calorie deficit goal, usually 500 to 1,000 kilocalories a day, is more important than the type of diet. Since many types of diets have been studied and appear to confer similar results, support the patient's preferences as long as they are reasonable.
- Encourage proven behavioral habits such as portion-controlled meals, meal planning, food diaries, and activity records.
- Follow professional guidelines for pharmacologic therapies and surgical procedures in patients having high weights and morbidities who do not respond to conventional treatment.
- Reducing weight by even 5% to 10% can improve blood pressure, lipid levels, and glucose tolerance, and reduce the risk of diabetes or hypertension.

Healthful Diet and Physical Activity

In order to help reduce the risk for cardiovascular disease (CVD), clinicians should offer behavioral counseling to promote a healthful diet and physical activity to adults who are overweight or obese and who have at least one other known risk factor for CVD. Clinicians, however, should individualize the decision to offer behavioral counseling to nonobese patients without specific risk factors for CVD.

Healthful Diet. You should be well informed about diet and nutrition as you counsel patients who are overweight, especially in light of the many and often contradictory diet options in the popular press. A heart-healthy diet is rich in vegetables, fruits, fiber, and whole grains and is low in salt, red and processed meats, and saturated fats. Key recommendations to help clinicians and patients address the obesity epidemic more effectively include:

- Limiting sodium intake to <2,300 mg/day since excess sodium intake can lead to hypertension, a major risk factor for CVD.
- Limiting added sugars and saturated fats each to ≤10% of total calories.
- Alcohol, if consumed, should be consumed in moderation.

The "10 Tips: Choose MyPlate" by the U.S. Department of Agriculture may provide additional dietary guidance (Box 6-10 and Fig. 6-3).

Box 6-10. 10 Tips: Choose MyPlate

1. Find your healthy eating style
2. Make half your plate fruits and vegetables
3. Focus on whole fruits
4. Vary your veggies
5. Make half your grains whole grains
6. Move to low-fat or fat-free milk or yogurt
7. Vary your protein routine
8. Drink and eat beverages and foods with less sodium, saturated fat, and added sugars
9. Drink water instead of sugary drinks
10. Everything you eat and drink matters

Source: ChooseMyPlate. USDA Center for Nutrition Policy & Promotion. Available at https://www.choosemyplate.gov/. Accessed May 10, 2019.

Physical Activity. The benefits of physical activity include reducing risks for early death, CVD, hypertension, type 2 diabetes, breast and colon cancer, obesity, osteoporosis, falls, and depression (Box 6-11). Physical activity also helps improve cognition and functional capacity in older adults.

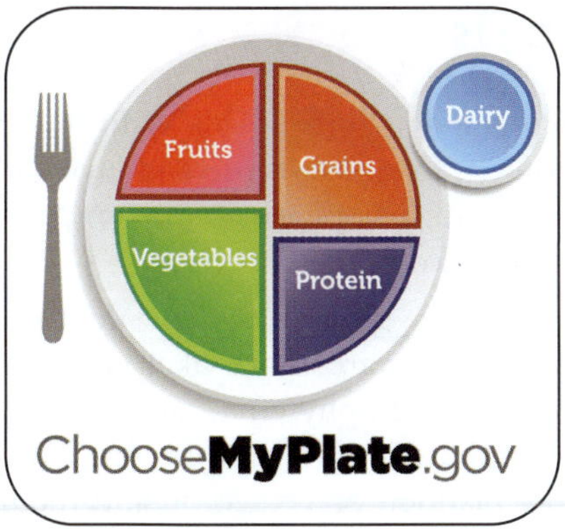

FIGURE 6-3. Rate your plate. (From choosemyplate.gov.)

Box 6-11. Physical Activity Guidelines for South Asians

- Adults should do at least 150 to 300 minutes of moderate-intensity aerobic activity or 75 to 150 minutes of vigorous-intensity aerobic activity each week.
- Moderate- or greater-intensity *muscle-strengthening activity* that involves all major muscle groups on 2 or more days a week.
- Greater health benefits can be achieved by increasing the frequency, duration, and/or intensity of physical activity.
- Adults should avoid being sedentary; doing any amount of moderate-to-vigorous intensity physical activity has health benefits.
- Older adults should also engage in balance training activities.

Sedentary people should gradually build up their activity level, starting with even brief episodes of exercise such as climbing a few flights of stairs or parking further away from their place of work or shopping. Inactive adults should start with lower-intensity activities and gradually increase how often and how long they perform these activities—*"start low and go slow."* Clinicians should assess patients with chronic pulmonary, cardiac, or musculoskeletal conditions to determine the appropriate types and amounts of activity.

Refer adults with a body mass index of 30 or more to intensive, multicomponent behavioral interventions. However, individualization about referring adults without cardiovascular risks for behavioral counseling to promote physical activity may be beneficial for persons motivated to make behavioral changes (see Box 6-4).

SCREENING AND COUNSELING GUIDELINES FOR ADULTS

Screening and counseling guidelines for adults include:

- Unhealthy alcohol use
- Tobacco misuse
- Sexually transmitted infections (STIs) (chlamydia, gonorrhea, and syphilis)
- HIV/AIDS

Unhealthy Alcohol Use

Alcohol: Screening. Because early detection of at-risk behaviors may be challenging, screen for risky or hazardous alcohol use and implement brief behavioral counseling interventions when indicated *for all adults in primary care settings*, including pregnant women.

If your patient reports drinking alcoholic beverages, you can begin to assess for unhealthy alcohol use (Box 6-12) by asking some simple screening questions. The Single Alcohol Screening Question (SASQ) asks "How many times in the past year have you had five or

Box 6-12. Unhealthy Alcohol Use

Standard Drink Equivalents: One standard drink is equivalent to 12 oz of regular beer or wine cooler, 8 oz of malt liquor, 5 oz of wine, or 1.5 oz of 80-proof spirits.

Definitions of Drinking Levels for Adults—National Institute of Alcohol Abuse and Alcoholism

	Women	Men
Moderate drinking	≤1 drink/day	≤2 drinks/day
Unsafe drinking levels (increased risk for developing an alcohol use disorder)[a]	>3 drinks/day and >7 drinks/week	>4 drinks/day and >14 drinks/week
Binge drinking[b]	≥4 drinks on one occasion	≥5 drinks on one occasion

[a]Pregnant women and those with health problems that could be worsened by drinking should not drink any alcohol.

[b]Brings blood alcohol level to 0.08%, usually within 2 hrs.

more drinks in a day (men) or four or more drinks in a day (women)." The SASQ has a sensitivity ranging from 0.73 to 0.88 for detecting unhealthy alcohol use with a specificity ranging from 0.74 to 1.00. The Alcohol Use Disorders Identification Test-Consumption (AUDIT-C) questionnaire asks about how often the person drinks alcohol, how many standard alcohol drinks are consumed on a typical day, and how often the person consumes six or more drinks on one occasion. The AUDIT-C, which is scored from 0 to 12, has sensitivities ranging from 0.73 to 1.00 using cutoffs of ≥3 (women) or ≥4 (men). The corresponding specificities range from 0.28 to 0.94. The widely used CAGE tool, which asks about **C**utting down, **A**nnoyance when criticized, **G**uilty feelings, and **E**ye-openers, is best at detecting alcohol dependence.

Patients with positive screens for unhealthy alcohol use should be further assessed, including asking about blackouts (loss of memory for events during drinking), seizures, accidents or injuries while drinking, job loss, marital conflict, legal problems, and drinking while driving or operating machinery. Clinicians will need to address the appropriate care strategies for patients with confirmed unhealthy alcohol use.

Alcohol: Counseling. Primary care clinicians should provide behavioral counseling interventions to adults with unhealthy alcohol use. The screening tools described above can be used to identify adults with at-risk or hazardous alcohol use. A number of effective behavioral interventions, which vary by elements (feedback, motivational interviewing, drinking diaries, cognitive behavioral therapy, and action plans on alcohol use), delivery method (in person, web based, one on one, group), frequency (most involved at least four sessions), and intensity (most involved ≤2 hours of contact time) can be used.

One commonly used approach that has been shown to effectively reduce alcohol use and alcohol-related complications is the Screening, Brief Intervention, and Referral to Treatment (SBIRT) program. This program is designed to be administered in a series of encounters conducted by practitioners who are not experts in substance abuse to reduce and prevent harms for those with nondependent alcohol use. Brief interventions target people at low risk for unhealthy alcohol use by educating them about the harms of exceeding drinking limits and, if applicable, identifying any links between alcohol use and other health problems. Motivational techniques are used to help those at moderate to high risk for unhealthy alcohol use to reduce their alcohol intake or to seek additional treatment, particularly those with a high-risk screening result.

Tobacco Use

Tobacco: Screening. Screen all adults, particularly pregnant women, for tobacco use and provide behavioral interventions and/or pharmacotherapy for tobacco cessation to all who are using tobacco.

Teens are more susceptible to nicotine addiction than adults. Smokers are more likely than nonsmokers to develop CVD, emphysema, and lung cancer. In addition to respiratory tract cancers, smoking can cause cancers of the bladder, cervix, colon and rectum, kidney, oropharynx, larynx, esophagus, stomach, liver, and pancreas as well as acute myeloid leukemia. Half of all long-term smokers die of smoking-related diseases, losing an average of 10 years of life. Smoking is associated with developing diabetes, cataracts, and rheumatoid arthritis and increases risk of infertility, preterm birth, low birth weight, and sudden infant death syndrome.

Questions one may ask at every visit include "Have you ever used tobacco (smoke, chew, e-cigarettes) or vapor products?" For nonsmokers, ask about exposure to secondhand smoke and tobacco use by other persons in the household or workplace.

Tobacco: Counseling. Ask all adult patients about tobacco use, advise tobacco cessation for tobacco users, and then offer behavioral support and pharmacotherapy. Pregnant women should be similarly screened and advised to stop using tobacco products and be offered behavioral support. Use the "5 As" framework or the stages of change model to assess readiness to quit using tobacco products (Box 6-13).

Box 6-13. Assessing Readiness to Quit Smoking: Brief Interventions Models

5 As Model	Transtheoretical or Stages of Change Model
■ **Ask** about tobacco use ■ **Advise** to quit ■ **Assess** willingness to make a quit attempt ■ **Assist** in quit attempt ■ **Arrange** follow-up	■ **Precontemplation**—"I don't want to quit." ■ **Contemplation**—"I am concerned but not ready to quit now." ■ **Preparation**—"I am ready to quit." ■ **Action**—"I just quit." ■ **Maintenance**—"I quit 6 months ago."

The most commonly used pharmacotherapies are nicotine replacement therapy (NRT), including patches, gum, lozenges, and inhalers, as well varenicline, and bupropion SR. Combining multiple types of NRT has additive benefits and combining pharmacotherapy with behavioral counseling is more effective than either modality alone. Effective behavioral interventions include minimal and intensive individual or group counseling sessions led by clinicians or other types of primary care providers, telephone counseling sessions led by trained professionals, and tailored, print-based self-help material or self-help tools delivered by apps, web, and mobile interventions (Box 6-14). Motivational interviewing techniques are also helpful for patients who are not yet ready to quit smoking. E-cigarettes may benefit adult smokers if used to completely replace the use of all tobacco products, but this remains an active area of research.

Box 6-14. Helpful Clinician Resources

- Indian Council of Medical Research, New Delhi (icmr.gov.in)
- Ministry of Health and Family Welfare, GOI (mohfw.gov.in)
- National Health Mission (nhm.gov.in)
- Cancer Prevention and Cancer Treatment in India (cancerindia.org.in)
- Directorate General of Health Services (dghs.gov.in)
- Centers for Disease Control and Prevention fact sheet on smoking cessation (https://www.cdc.gov/tobacco/data statistics/fact_sheets/cessation/quitting/index.htm)
- The U.S. Department of Health and Human Services' websites
- BeTobaccoFree (https://betobaccofree.hhs.gov/quit-now/index.html)
- SmokeFreeWomen (https://women.smokefree.gov/pregnancymotherhood)

Screening and Counseling for STIs

Chlamydia, Gonorrhea, and Syphilis: Screening. Screen sexually active women aged 24 years and younger for chlamydia and gonorrhea; the evidence is insufficient to make a recommendation for sexually active men. Screen high-risk nonpregnant adults and adolescents for syphilis infection. Risk factors include being an MSM, being infected with HIV, and having a history of incarceration or commercial sex work. Also screen all pregnant women for syphilis infection. The CDC recommends chlamydia and gonorrhea screening annually for all sexually active women aged <25 years and older and women with risk factors such as new or multiple sex partners or a sex partner infected with an STD. Chlamydia, gonorrhea, and syphilis screening are recommended at least once a year for all sexually active gay, bisexual, and other MSM. MSM who have multiple or anonymous partners should be screened more frequently for STDs (i.e., at 3- to 6-month intervals).

HIV: Screening. Despite advances in detection and treatment, HIV infection remains a significant public health threat, particularly for younger individuals, MSM, and injection drug users. Identifying early HIV infection and initiating combined ART decreases the risk of progressing to AIDS. Treatment also reduces the risk of transmitting HIV to uninfected heterosexual partners and from a pregnant mother to her child. Current screening recommendations are summarized in Box 6-15.

Box 6-15. Summary: Screening Recommendations for HIV

- The USPSTF gives a grade A recommendation for HIV screening of adolescents and adults from age 15 to 65 years and for screening all pregnant women. Screening is also recommended for younger adolescents and older adults who are at increased risk for infection.
- The CDC recommends universal HIV testing for adolescents and adults aged 13 to 64 years in healthcare settings and prenatal testing of all pregnant women.
- The CDC recommends an opt-out approach to HIV testing—notifying the patient verbally or in writing that testing will be performed unless the patient declines. Separate written consent is not required.
- Patients and prospective sex partners should be tested before beginning a new sexual relationship.
- One-time testing for low-risk patients is reasonable, but at least annual testing is recommended for high-risk groups, defined as MSM; individuals with multiple sexual partners; past or present injection drug users; persons who exchange sex for money or drugs; and sex partners of persons who are HIV infected, bisexual, or injection drug users. Patients beginning treatment for tuberculosis and those with any STI or requests for STI testing should be tested for coinfection with HIV.

Sexually Transmitted Infections Including HIV: Counseling. Behavioral counseling is recommended for all sexually active adolescents and for adults who are at increased risk for STIs, including HIV/AIDS. Adults at increased risk include those having current or previous STIs, multiple or new sex partners, a sexual partner recently treated for an STI, or sexual contact with sex workers; exchanging sex for money or drugs; currently or formerly using intravenous drugs; and inconsistently or not using condoms outside of a mutually monogamous sexual partnership. Behavioral counseling can reduce the risk of acquiring an STI, and successful interventions usually "provide basic information about STIs and STI transmission; assess risk for transmission; and provide training in pertinent skills, such as condom use, communication about safe sex, problem solving, and goal setting." The CDC recommends using condoms, reducing the number of sex partners, getting vaccinations for hepatitis B and HPV, practicing mutual monogamy, and abstinence.

Clinicians must master the skills of eliciting the sexual history and asking frank but tactful questions about sexual practices. Key information includes the number of partners in the past month, any history of past STIs, the genders of the patient's sexual partners, and which body parts they use during sex, so clinicians can base their counseling, STI screening, and prevention recommendations on sexual behaviors and not identities or assumptions (see also pp. 376–377).

For example, when compared to heterosexual patients, women who have sex with women (WSW) are almost 20 times less likely to perceive themselves at risk for STIs but are nearly as likely to have had intercourse, experience twice the rate of pregnancy, and are more likely to have had two or more pregnancies.

When discussing sexual activity, it is also important to inquire about the nature and patterns of sexual negotiation, such as communication and decision making, and about condom use and STI prevention (pre-exposure prophylaxis [PrEP]). Clinicians should also inquire about the use of toys or other objects for sex.

Patient counseling should be interactive, nonjudgmental, and combine information about general risk reduction with personalized messages based on the patient's personal risk behaviors. As you counsel patients, encourage them to seek prompt attention for any genital lesions or penile discharge. Highlight risky behaviors such as not using condoms, particularly when engaging in anal intercourse; having multiple sexual partners, concomitant use of alcohol and drugs, which may be associated with disinhibition; and engaging in sexual intercourse while being treated for an STI. Ask: "Have you ever had sex with someone when you didn't want to?", "Do you use alcohol or any drugs when you have sex?", "Have you exchanged sex for money, drugs, or a place to stay?" If the patient uses toys or other objects for sex, emphasize the importance of using condoms and appropriately cleaning them if they are sharing the sex toy with others. Ask: "How do you feel about using condoms?", "In what situations do you feel you need to use condoms?", "Tell me about the last time you had sex and didn't use a condom."

Correct use of male condoms is highly effective in preventing the transmission of HIV, HPV, and other STIs. Key instructions should include:

- Using a new condom with each sex act.
- Applying the condom before any sexual contact occurs.
- Adding only water-based lubricants.
- Immediately withdraw if the condom breaks during sexual activity and hold the condom during withdrawal to keep it from slipping off.

Standard recommendations for preventing HIV infection include choosing less risky sexual behaviors, getting treated for injection drug use and using sterile equipment, getting HIV tests with partners, and using condoms correctly. Another strategy for preventing HIV infections is PrEP, which involves taking a daily pill containing two antiretroviral drugs (tenofovir and emtricitabine). PrEP is recommended for HIV-negative people who are at risk for HIV through sexual transmission or illicit drug injection. Consistent use has been shown to reduce the risk of HIV infections.

IMMUNIZATION GUIDELINES FOR ADULTS

Immunization guidelines for adults include:

- Influenza vaccine–inactivated (IIV), recombinant (RIV), or live attenuated (LAIV)
- Pneumococcal polysaccharide vaccine (PPSV23) and pneumococcal conjugate vaccine (PCV13)
- Varicella vaccine (VAR)
- Herpes zoster vaccine–recombinant (RZV) or live (ZVL)
- Tetanus, diphtheria (Td) or tetanus, diphtheria, pertussis (Tdap) vaccine
- Human papilloma virus (HPV) vaccine
- Hepatitis A vaccine (HepA)
- Hepatitis B vaccine (HepB)

Influenza Vaccine

Provide *flu shots* to everyone aged 6 months or older and especially to those with chronic pulmonary conditions, nursing home residents, household contacts, and healthcare personnel during the flu season including pregnant women during any trimester.

The CDC Advisory Committee on Immunization Practices (ACIP) updates its recommendations for vaccination annually (Box 6-16). Two types of vaccine are available. The "flu shot" is an inactivated vaccine containing killed virus, which comes in a standard dose for those younger than 65 years and a high dose for those ≥65 years. A nasal spray vaccine, containing attenuated live viruses, is approved only for healthy people between the ages of 2 and 49 years and is not recommended every year. Because influenza viruses mutate from year to year, each vaccine contains three to four vaccine strains and is modified yearly. Note that annual vaccination is recommended for everyone age ≥6 months.

Box 6-16. Summary of 2019 CDC Influenza Vaccine Recommendations—Adults and Children

Annual vaccination is recommended for all people aged 6 months and older, especially the groups listed below:

- Adults and children with chronic pulmonary and cardiovascular conditions (except hypertension) and renal, hepatic, neurologic, hematologic, or metabolic disorders (including diabetes mellitus); persons who are immunosuppressed due to any cause; and persons who are morbidly obese
- Adults ≥50 years of age
- Women who are or will be pregnant during influenza season
- Residents of nursing homes and long-term care facilities
- American Indians and Alaska natives
- Healthcare personnel
- Household contacts and caregivers of children ≤5 years of age (especially infants ≤age 6 months) and of adults ≥50 years of age with clinical conditions placing them at higher risk for complications of influenza

Pneumococcal Vaccine

Recommend *pneumococcal vaccines* to adults 65 years and older, smokers, and those with increased risk of pneumococcal pneumonia between the ages of 19 and 64 years. Two pneumococcal vaccines are recommended. One dose of PCV13 (conjugate vaccine) followed by one dose of PPSV23 (polysaccharide vaccine).

Streptococcal pneumonia causes pneumonia, bacteremia, and meningitis.

Since 2010, infants younger than age 2 years have routinely been vaccinated with the 13-valent PCV13. In 2014, the ACIP recommended vaccinating adults aged ≥65 years using the PCV13 followed by the 23-valent inactivated PPSV23. The vaccines should not be coadministered. Adults in this age range who never received the PPSV23 should first receive the PCV13 followed 12 months later by the PPSV23. Adults aged ≥65 years previously vaccinated with PPSV23 should receive a dose of PCV13 no earlier than 1 year following the most recent PPSV23 vaccination. The ACIP recommends using PCV13 and PPSV23 for the high-risk groups listed in Box 6-17.

Box 6-17. Pneumococcal Vaccine Recommendations for High-Risk Adults

		PCV13	PPSV23	
Risk Group	**Medical Condition**	**Recommended**	**Recommended**	**Revaccination 5 Years after First Dose**
Immunocompetent persons	Chronic heart disease		✓	
	Chronic lung disease		✓	
	Diabetes mellitus		✓	
	Cerebrospinal fluid leak	✓	✓	
	Cochlear implant	✓	✓	
	Alcoholism		✓	
	Chronic liver disease, cirrhosis		✓	
	Cigarette smoking		✓	
Persons with functional or anatomic asplenia	Sickle cell disease	✓	✓	✓
	Congenital or acquired asplenia	✓	✓	✓
Immunocompromised persons	Congenital or acquired immunodeficiency	✓	✓	✓
	HIV infection	✓	✓	✓
	Chronic renal failure	✓	✓	✓
	Nephrotic syndrome	✓	✓	✓

(*Continued*)

Box 6-17. Pneumococcal Vaccine Recommendations for High-Risk Adults (*continued*)

Risk Group	Medical Condition	PCV13	PPSV23	
		Recommended	Recommended	Revaccination 5 Years after First Dose
Immunocompromised persons (*continued*)	Leukemia	✓	✓	✓
	Lymphoma	✓	✓	✓
	Hodgkin disease	✓	✓	✓
	Generalized malignancy	✓	✓	✓
	Iatrogenic immunosuppression	✓	✓	✓
	Solid organ transplants	✓	✓	✓
	Multiple myeloma	✓	✓	✓

Varicella Vaccine

Recommend VAR to adults who have not received two doses of chickenpox vaccine or never had chickenpox.

Varicella infection, or *chicken pox*, usually occurs in childhood and causes an itchy rash. Infections can also occur in adults, particularly immunocompromised patients who are at risk for disseminated disease.

A two-dose series of varicella vaccine is recommended for children under age 13 and those aged 13 and older who were previously unvaccinated and who have no evidence of immunity. Live vaccines should not be given to pregnant women or people who have a very weakened immune system, which includes people with HIV infection and a CD4 count less than 200.

Herpes Zoster Vaccine

Offer RZV vaccine (two doses, 2 to 6 months apart) to adults 50 years and older, including adults who have had shingles or received the previous shingles vaccine.

Herpes zoster, which results from reactivation of latent varicella (chicken pox) virus infection within the sensory ganglia, usually causes painful unilateral vesicular rashes in a dermatomal distribution. The lifetime risk of herpes zoster infection is about one in three, and is higher for women than for men. Up to one in four adults experience complications following infection, including postherpetic neuralgia (persistent pain in the area of the rash), bacterial skin infections, ophthalmic complications, cranial and peripheral neuropathies, encephalitis, pneumonitis, and hepatitis. Herpes zoster risk is increased in immunocompromised conditions including cancer, HIV, bone marrow or organ transplantation, and immunosuppressive therapies. Increasing age is also strongly associated with developing both herpes zoster infection and postherpetic neuralgia.

The herpes zoster vaccine effectively reduces the short-term risks for zoster and postherpetic neuralgia in adults ≥50 years. The ACIP currently recommends offering the two-dose series of RZV for immunocompetent adults aged ≥50 years. Doses should be 2 to 6 months apart.

Tetanus, Diphtheria, Pertussis Vaccine

Recommend once, regardless of last Td vaccine. Offer the Td vaccine booster every 10 years. Pregnant women also need Tdap vaccine during every pregnancy.

All adults aged 19 and older who have not previously received a Tdap vaccine should receive one dose followed by a Td booster every 10 years.

Human Papillomavirus Vaccine

Recommend HPV vaccination for females and males starting at age 11 or 12 years (as early as age 9 years); females age 13 through 26 years and for males age 13 through 21 years who have not been vaccinated previously or who have not completed the vaccination series; and MSM ages 22 through 26 or men who are immunocompromised.

HPV is associated with cervical, vulvar, and vaginal cancer in females; penile cancer in males; and anal and oropharyngeal cancer in both women and men.

ACIP recommends vaccinating all adolescents at ages 11 or 12 (though vaccination can begin at age 9) with the 9-valent HPV vaccine. Depending on age at initial vaccination, either a two-dose (ages 9 through 14) or three-dose (ages 15 and older) series will be administered within a period of 6 to 12 months. A three-dose series is recommended for those who are immunocompromised or have a history of sexual abuse or assault.

For men, the vaccine can prevent HPV-related diseases (genital warts, anal cancer, and penile cancer), lower the risk of oropharyngeal cancers, and possibly reduce HPV transmission to female sexual partners.

Hepatitis A Vaccine

Recommend a two-dose series for those at risk for hepatitis A infection including those with chronic liver disease or clotting factor disorders; MSM; injection or noninjection drug users; and people who are homeless, travel in countries with high or intermediate endemic hepatitis A, and who have close personal contact with international adoptee with high or intermediate endemic hepatitis A. Persons not at risk but wanting protection from hepatitis A infection should also receive the full two-dose series.

Hepatitis B Vaccine

Recommend a two- or three-dose series for those at risk for hepatitis B infection including those with hepatitis C virus infection, chronic liver disease, HIV infection, sexual exposure risk, current or recent injection drug use, or percutaneous or mucosal risk for exposure to blood and persons who are incarcerated or travel in countries with high or intermediate endemic hepatitis B. Persons not at risk but wanting protection from hepatitis B infection should also receive the full two- or three-dose series.

PREVENTIVE CARE IN SPECIAL POPULATIONS

Screening, counseling, and immunization recommendations for children, older adults, and pregnant women are found in Unit 3.

DISEASE-SPECIFIC RECOMMENDATIONS

To provide appropriate context, the screening and prevention recommendations for various diseases and conditions, are discussed in the individual regional examination chapters.

CHAPTER 7

Evaluating Clinical Evidence

Clinical decision making requires integrating clinical expertise, patient preferences, and the best available clinical evidence (Fig. 7-1). Acquisition of corresponding skills for each of these components is essential for excellence in patient care. You will develop your clinical expertise as you practice your clinical discipline, enabling you to more efficiently make diagnoses and identify potential interventions. You will also begin to learn how to incorporate your patients' individualized preferences, concerns, and expectations into those health decisions. Finally, you will learn to select the current best evidence from the full spectrum of studies available as the basis of your assessments and recommendations. Throughout the regional examination chapters, you will encounter current evidence for using elements of the history and physical examination to support diagnostic reasoning. This chapter provides you with foundational knowledge about the criteria for evaluating that clinical evidence.

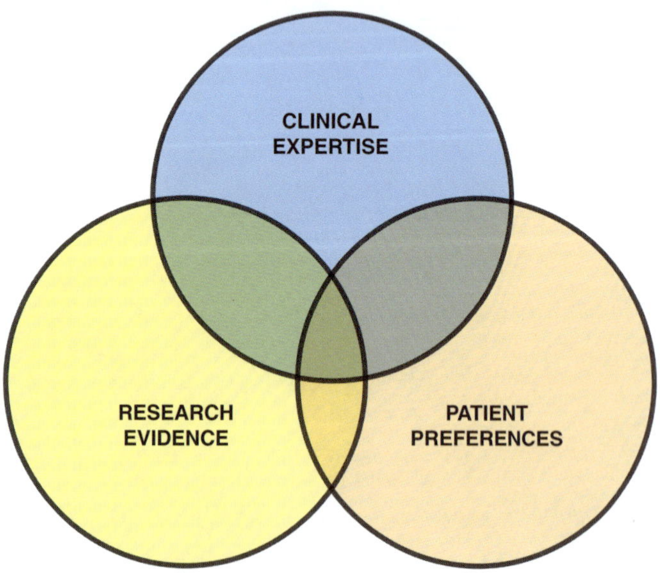

FIGURE 7-1. Evidence-based clinical practice Venn diagram. (Adapted from Haynes RB et al. *ACP J Club.* 1996;125(3): A14–A16.)

USING ELEMENTS OF THE HISTORY AND PHYSICAL EXAMINATION AS DIAGNOSTIC TESTS

As discussed in Chapter 5, the process of diagnostic reasoning begins with the generation of a list of potential causes for the patient's problems (*differential diagnosis*). As you learn more about your patient, you will assign probabilities to various diagnoses that correspond to how likely they are to explain your patient's problem with the goal of determining the need to perform additional testing or initiate treatment.

Key elements from the history, especially those discussed in the History of Present Illness (e.g., precordial chest pain, a vertiginous sensation, or orthopnea), are used in this initial step in the diagnostic reasoning process. This is also true for findings in the physical examination elicited through the classic techniques of inspection, palpation, percussion, and auscultation or through special maneuvers.

Box 7-1 illustrates how selected elements in the history and physical examination might be used to support diagnostic reasoning.

Box 7-1. Example: Use of History and Physical Examination Findings to Support Diagnostic Reasoning

The patient is a 43-year-old female who presents with an acute episode of right upper quadrant abdominal pain. The pain is steady and severe, has lasted for over 4 hours, and developed about an hour after eating a fatty meal. She reports nausea, vomiting, and anorexia.

Studies evaluating the predictive value of elements of the history suggest that the location of this patient's pain and her symptoms—often preceded by a fatty meal—increase

(Continued)

Box 7-1. Example Use of History and Physical Examination Findings to Support Diagnostic Reasoning (*continued*)

the likelihood of this being cholecystitis. However, your list of possible causes also includes diagnoses such as biliary colic, acute cholangitis, or hepatitis.

On physical examination, she has a temperature of 38°C, her blood pressure is 145/90 mm Hg, her pulse is 110 per minute, and she appears uncomfortable. She is not jaundiced but has right upper quadrant tenderness without rebound and a positive Murphy sign (suggestive of inflammatory irritation of the gallbladder).

The presence or absence of jaundice and rebound tenderness has not been consistently found to be significantly associated with acute cholecystitis. However, fever, right upper quadrant tenderness, and positive Murphy sign increase the likelihood of acute cholecystitis. Nonetheless, you still need to consider the other diagnoses in your list.

Laboratory studies show an elevated white blood cell count and normal liver function tests, including transaminases, bilirubin, and alkaline phosphatase.

These results make the diagnosis of acute hepatitis unlikely, though they do not substantially alter the likelihood of having acute cholecystitis. Indeed, no single element of the history, physical examination, or laboratory results is sufficient to help you cross the treatment threshold for acute cholecystitis. Because the suspicion for a gallbladder problem is high, the next step in this case is visually confirming abnormalities of the gallbladder with imaging.

The right upper quadrant bedside ultrasound shows gallstones and gallbladder wall thickening. The sonographic Murphy sign is positive. These results confirm the diagnosis of acute cholecystitis and the patient will be admitted for antibiotics and surgery.

EVALUATING DIAGNOSTIC TESTS

You can turn to the clinical literature to determine *quantitatively* how a diagnostic test—any information in the clinical history and physical examination, as well as laboratory tests, radiographic imaging, and procedures—has the ability to revise the probabilities of the possible causes for a patient's condition (*differential diagnosis*). Two concepts in evaluating diagnostic tests will be explored: the *validity* of the findings and the *reproducibility* of the test results.

Validity

The initial step in evaluating a diagnostic test is to determine whether it provides valid results. *Does the test accurately identify whether a patient has a disease?* This involves comparing the test against a *gold standard*—the best measure of whether a patient has a disease. This could be a biopsy to evaluate a lung nodule, a structured psychiatric examination by an expert to evaluate a patient for depression, or a colonoscopy to evaluate a patient with a positive stool blood test.

The *2 × 2 table* is the basic format for evaluating the performance characteristics of a diagnostic test, which means how much the test results revise probabilities for disease (Box 7-2). The two columns represent patients with disease present and patients with disease absent, respectively. These categorizations are based on the gold-standard test. The two rows correspond to the presence of the element of the history or physical examination of interest (positive) or its absence (negative). The four cells (a, b, c, d) would then correspond to true positives, false positives, false negatives, and true negatives, respectively.

Box 7-2. Setting up the 2 × 2 Table

History or PE Element	Gold Standard: Disease Present	Gold Standard: Disease Absent
Present (test positive)	a True positive	b False positive
Absent (test negative)	c False negative	d True negative

Sensitivity and Specificity. The first test statistics to estimate are *sensitivity* and *specificity* (Box 7-3).

Box 7-3. Sensitivity and Specificity

- **Sensitivity** is the probability that a person with disease has a positive test. This is represented as a/(a + c) in the disease present column of the 2 × 2 table.

  Sensitivity is also known as the true positive rate.
- **Specificity** is the probability that a nondiseased person has a negative test, represented as d/(b + d) in the disease absent column of the 2 × 2 table.

  Specificity is also known as the true negative rate.

Knowing the sensitivity and specificity of a test does not necessarily help you make clinical decisions because they are statistics based on knowing whether the patient has disease. However, there are two exceptions. A negative result from a test with a high sensitivity (i.e., a very low false-negative rate) usually excludes disease. This is represented by the mnemonic SnNOUT—a **S**e**n**sitive test with a **N**egative result rules **OUT** disease. Conversely, a positive result in a test with high specificity (e.g., a very low–false-positive rate) usually indicates disease. This is represented by the mnemonic SpPIN—a **S**pecific test with a **P**ositive result rules **IN** disease.

For example, if you suspect that the likely cause of a patient's low back pain is a herniated lumbosacral disc, you may want to perform physical examination maneuvers that could assist in bolstering your diagnosis. One maneuver, called the *straight-leg raise test*, has a sensitivity of about 92%. Conversely, the specificity of this maneuver is about 28%. In contrast, another maneuver, the *crossed straight-leg raise test*, has a sensitivity of only about 28% for detecting a herniated disc, but a specificity of about 80%. Thus, the presence of a positive crossed straight-leg test bolsters your confidence in diagnosing a herniated disc, while a negative straight-leg raise makes the diagnosis less likely.

Unfortunately, most single physical examination maneuvers and elements of the history lack either a high sensitivity or high specificity.

Predictive Values. The typical clinical scenario faced by clinicians involves determining whether a patient actually has disease based on a test result that is either positive or negative. *How useful is the test in telling us whether the disease is present or absent?* This is called the *predictive value* and it links the sensitivity and specificity of the test with how common the disease in question is (*prevalence*). Predictive values can be *positive* or *negative*.

- The **positive predictive value (PPV)** is the probability that a person with a positive test has the disease represented as a/(a + b) from the first (test positive) row in the 2 × 2 table.

  For example, a physical examination maneuver you can perform in adults with symptoms suspicious of carpal tunnel syndrome is the Phalen test, which has a PPV of 76%. This means that a patient with a positive Phalen test result has about a 76% probability of having carpal tunnel syndrome based on the gold-standard diagnostic test (i.e., an abnormal nerve conduction study).
- The **negative predictive value (NPV)** is the probability that a person with a negative test does not have the disease represented as d/(c + d) in the second (test negative) row in the 2 × 2 table.

  As in the previous example, the Phalen test has an NPV of 56%, which means that among adults with a *negative* Phalen test, about 56% do not have carpal tunnel syndrome based on nerve conduction testing.

Prevalence of Disease. Although the predictive value statistics seem intuitively useful, they vary substantially according to the *prevalence of disease* (i.e., the proportion of patients in the disease present column). The prevalence is based on the characteristics of the patient population and the clinical setting. For example, the prevalence of many diseases will usually be higher among older populations and among patients being seen in specialist clinics or at referral hospitals.

Let us see how variability in the prevalence of a disease modifies the predictive values of diagnostic tests. For example, consider a physical examination maneuver, which has a sensitivity of 90% and specificity of 90%. You decide to perform this examination maneuver in a patient population of 1,000 in which the disease prevalence (proportion of subjects that have the disease) is 10%. Box 7-4 shows a 2 × 2 table set up with these parameters.

Sensitivity = a/(a + c) = 90/100 or 90%;
specificity = d/(b + d) = 810/900 = 90%

Box 7-4. Predictive Values: Prevalence of 10% with Sensitivity and Specificity = 90%

	Disease Present	Disease Absent	Total
Test positive	a 90	b 90	**180**
Test negative	c 10	d 810	**820**
Total	**100**	**900**	**1,000**

The PPV calculated from the test positive row of the table would be 90/180 = 50%. This means that half of the people with a positive test have disease.

However, if the sensitivity and specificity of the diagnostic test remained the same, but prevalence of the disease was only 1%, then the cells would look very different (Box 7-5).

Sensitivity = a/(a + c) = 9/10 or 90%;
specificity = d/(b + d) = 891/990 = 90%

Box 7-5. Predictive Values: Prevalence of 1% with Sensitivity and Specificity = 90%

	Disease Present	Disease Absent	Total
Test positive	a 9	b 99	**108**
Test negative	c 1	d 891	**892**
Total	**10**	**990**	**1,000**

Now the PPV calculated from the test positive row of the table would be 9/108 = 8.3%.

The consequence is that the great majority of positive tests are false positives—meaning most subjects with positive tests will not have disease. However, to determine that nondiseased patients have false positive results, they may have to undergo further definitive (gold-standard) diagnostic tests, which are often invasive, expensive, and potentially harmful. This has implications for patient safety and resource allocation because clinicians want to limit the number of nondiseased patients who undergo gold standard tests.

However, as shown by the example, predictive values will not necessarily provide us with sufficient guidance for using diagnostic tests across populations with differing disease prevalence.

Likelihood Ratios. Fortunately, there are other ways to evaluate the performance of a diagnostic test—again elements of the clinical history and physical examination, laboratory tests, radiographic imaging, and procedures—that can account for the varying disease prevalence observed in different patient populations. One way uses *likelihood ratio* (*LR*) statistics, defined as the probability of obtaining a given test result in a diseased patient divided by the probability of obtaining a given test result in a nondiseased patient. The LR tells us how much a test result changes the probability of having the disease of interest before the diagnostic test is performed (*pre-test disease probability*) to the probability of having the disease of interest after the diagnostic test is performed and its findings known (*post-test disease probability*). In the general population, without taking a history or examining the patient, the pre-test probability is the *prevalence* of the disease in the population.

In the simplest case, we will assume that the test result is either positive or negative. Therefore, the *LR for a positive test* is the ratio of getting a positive test result in a diseased person divided by the probability of getting a positive test result in a nondiseased person. From the 2 × 2 table, we see that this is the same as saying the ratio of the true positive rate (sensitivity) over the false positive rate (1 – specificity). A higher value (much >1) indicates that a positive test is much more likely to be coming from a diseased person than from a nondiseased person, increasing our confidence that a person with a positive result has disease.

The *LR for a negative test* is the ratio of the probability of getting a negative test result in a diseased person divided by the probability of getting a negative test result in a nondiseased person. From the 2 × 2 table, we see that this is the same as saying the ratio of the false negative rate (1 – sensitivity) divided by the true negative rate (specificity). A lower value (much <1) indicates that the negative test is much more likely to be coming from a nondiseased person than from a diseased person, increasing our confidence that a person with a negative result does not have disease.

The magnitude of the LR provides an intuitive feeling for how strongly a given test result will raise (rule in) or lower (rule out) the likelihood of disease. Box 7-6 shows how to interpret LRs based on how much a test result changes the pre- to post-test probabilities for disease.

Box 7-6. Interpreting Likelihood Ratios

Likelihood Ratios[a]	Effect on Pre- to Post-Test Probability
LRs >10 or <0.1	Generate large changes
LRs 5–10 or 0.1–0.2	Generate moderate changes
LRs 2–5 and 0.5–0.2	Generate small (sometimes important) changes
LRs 1–2 and 0.5–1	Alter the probability to a small degree (rarely important)

[a]*Likelihood ratios >1* are associated with positive results and an increased probability for disease. *Likelihood ratios <1* are associated with negative results and a decreased probability of disease. A test with a *likelihood ratio of 1* provides no additional information about the probability of disease.

Applying Concepts to Evaluating Abdominal Pain. The cholecystitis example on p. 110 used general terms to describe whether an element of the history, physical examination, or laboratory or imaging finding made the diagnosis more or less likely. However, each of these elements can be evaluated for their performance as a diagnostic test. Box 7-7 shows the LRs for the presence or absence of various elements from the physical examination.

Figure 7-2 shows how the presence or absence of these physical findings can alter the probability for diagnosis. Elements of the history, laboratory, and imaging study results can also be used to revise these probabilities.

APPLYING CONCEPTS TO SCREENING TESTS

Throughout the regional examination chapters, you will find evidence-based recommendations for health promotion interventions, especially screening and prevention. These recommendations are also based on evidence from the clinical literature that can be evaluated

Box 7-7. Likelihood Ratios of Physical Examination Signs for Diagnosing Cholecystitis in Adult Patients with Abdominal Pain or Suspected Acute Cholecystitis

Finding	Sensitivity (%)	Specificity (%)	Likelihood Ratio if Finding Is	
			Present	Absent
Fever	2–44	37–83	Not significant	Not significant
RUQ tenderness	60–98	1–97	2.7	0.4
Murphy sign	48–97	48–98	3.2	0.6
RUQ mass	2–23	70–99	Not significant	Not significant

Adapted from McGee S, ed. Abdominal pain and tenderness. In: *Evidence-Based Physical Diagnosis*. 4th ed. Elsevier; 2018.

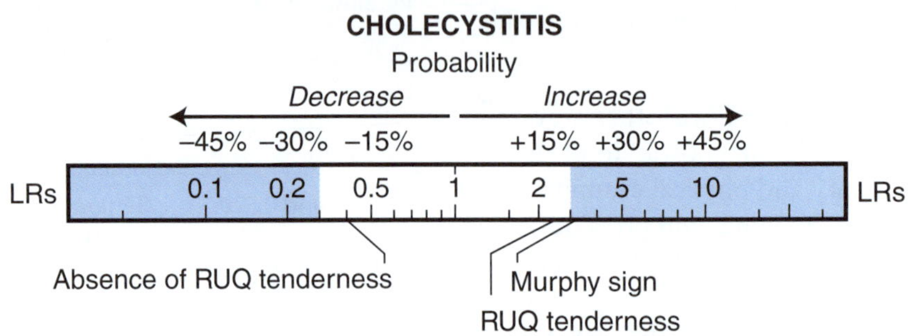

FIGURE 7-2. Revising probabilities for acute cholecystitis. (Reprinted from McGee S, ed. Abdominal pain and tenderness. In: *Evidence-Based Physical Diagnosis*. 4th ed. Elsevier; 2018:445–456.e444. Copyright © 2018 Elsevier. With permission.)

according to criteria presented in this chapter. Box 7-8 shows how LRs can be used to revise probabilities for disease with the example of breast cancer screening.

Box 7-8. How Likely Is It That a Woman with Abnormal Mammogram Has Breast Cancer?

CASE: A 57-year-old female at average risk for breast cancer has an abnormal mammogram. She wants to know the probability that she has breast cancer. The literature states that the baseline risk (prevalence) is 1%, the sensitivity of mammography is 90%, and the specificity is 91%. *What will you tell her?*

Fagan Nomogram

The Fagan nomogram provides a simple way to use LRs for revising probabilities (Fig. 7-3). With this nomogram, you read the pre-test probabilities from the line on the left, then take a straight edge and draw a line from the pre-test probability through the LR in the middle line, and then read the post-test probability on the line on the right.

Box 7-9 shows how to apply the nomogram to the abnormal mammogram.

Box 7-9. Using the Fagan Nomogram to Answer the Mammography Question

The pre-test probability (prevalence) = 1% and the likelihood ratio for a positive test (sensitivity/[1 − specificity]) = 10. The blue line corresponds to the case of a positive test with a post-test probability of about 9%. If the mammogram result was negative (red line), then the LR for a negative test ([1 − sensitivity]/specificity) = 0.11 and the post-test probability for breast cancer would be about 0.1%.

Natural Frequencies

Using frequency statements is another, perhaps more intuitive, alternative to LRs for determining how a test result will change the probability of disease (Box 7-10). *Natural frequencies* represent the joint frequency of two events, such as the number of patients with disease and the number of patients who have a positive test result.

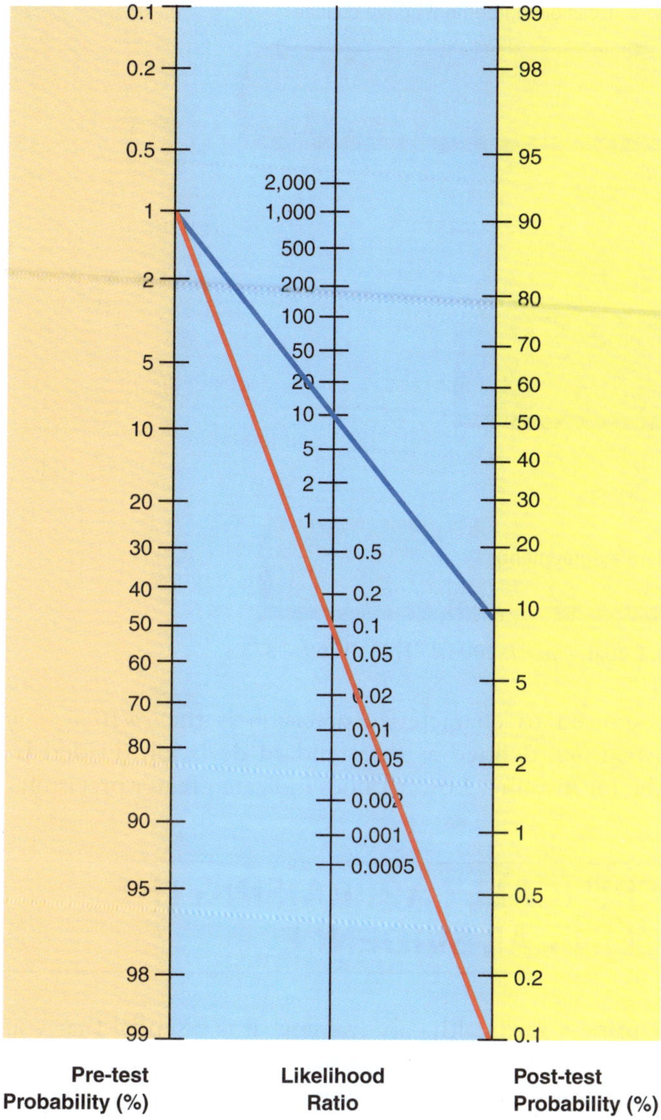

FIGURE 7-3. Fagan nomogram. (Adapted from Fagan TJ. *N Engl J Med*. 1975;293(5):257. Copyright © 1975 Massachusetts Medical Society. Reprinted with permission from Massachusetts Medical Society.)

Start by taking a large number of people (e.g., 100 or 1,000, depending on the prevalence) and break the number down into natural frequencies (i.e., how many of the people have disease, how many with disease will test positive, how many without disease will test positive).

Reproducibility

Another characteristic of a diagnostic test is *reproducibility*. An important aspect of evaluating diagnostic elements of the history or physical examination is determining the reproducibility of the findings for diagnosing a clinical disorder.

Box 7-10. Using Natural Frequencies to Answer the Mammography Question

We begin by creating a 2 × 2 table based on a population of 1,000 women. The 1% prevalence means that 10 women will have breast cancer. The sensitivity of 90% means that 9 of the women with breast cancer will have an abnormal mammogram. The specificity of 91% means that 89 of the 990 women without breast cancer will still have an abnormal mammogram. The probability that a woman with an abnormal mammogram will have breast cancer is 9/(9 + 89) = about 9%.

Mammogram Result	Breast Cancer	No Breast Cancer	Total
Positive	9	89	**98**
Negative	1	901	**902**
	10	**990**	**1,000**

Source: Data compiled from Gigerenzer G. *BMJ*. 2011;343:d6386.

When, for example, two clinicians perform the Murphy sign on a patient suspected as having acute cholecystitis, they may not always agree upon the presence of this finding. This raises the question of whether this finding is useful for diagnosing the clinical disorder of acute cholecystitis. By chance, if many patients are being examined, there will be a certain amount of agreement in the findings between the two clinicians. Understanding whether there is agreement well beyond chance, though, is important in knowing whether the finding is useful enough to support clinical decision making.

Kappa Score. The *kappa score* measures the amount of agreement that occurs beyond chance. In Figure 7-4, let us say that the agreement between observers for a given abnormal physical examination finding based on chance is 50% (i.e., observers would agree 50% of the time by chance on whether the abnormal physical examination finding is present or absent). In our example, that abnormal physical examination finding is a positive Murphy sign. If our two clinicians agree 75% of the time on whether a patient suspected of having acute cholecystitis has a positive Murphy sign, this means that the *potential* agreement beyond chance is 50% and the actual observer agreement *beyond* chance is 25%.

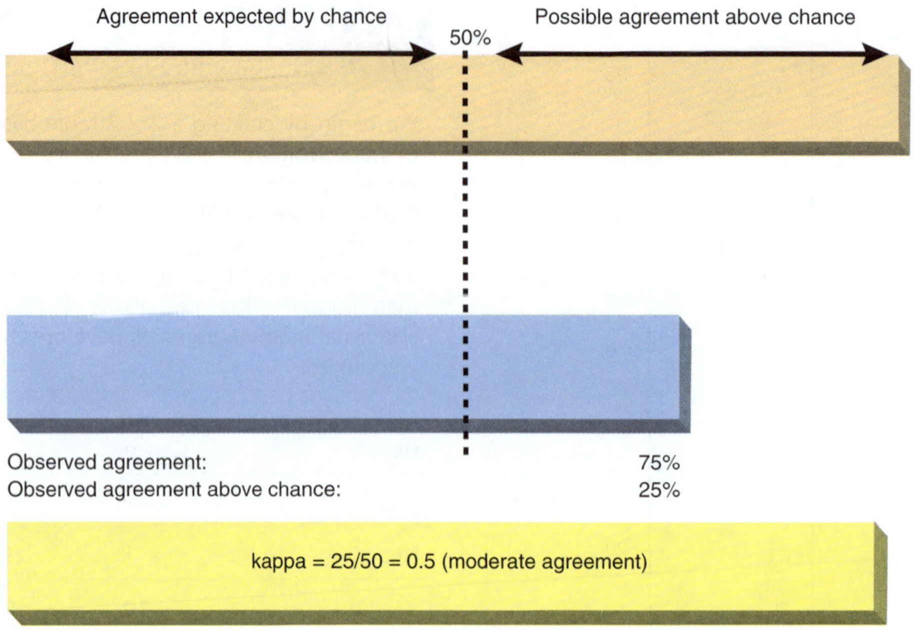

FIGURE 7-4. Kappa scores. (Reprinted with permission from McGinn T et al. *CMAJ.* 2004;171(11):1369–1373.)

The kappa level is then calculated as 25%/50% = 0.5, which indicates moderate agreement. Box 7-11 shows how to interpret kappa values.

Box 7-11. Interpreting Kappa Values

Value of Kappa	Strength of Agreement
<0.20	Poor
0.21–0.40	Fair
0.41–0.60	Moderate
0.61–0.80	Good
0.81–1.00	Excellent

The degree of agreement for routinely elicited findings can be quite variable; for example, kappa levels are 0.18 for detecting an S_3 gallop on cardiac auscultation and 0.80 in detecting palpable pulses in patients with peripheral arterial disease.

Precision. In the context of reproducibility, *precision* refers to being able to apply the same test to the same unchanged person and obtain the same results. Precision is often used when referring to laboratory tests. For example, when measuring a troponin level for cardiac ischemia, clinicians might use a particular cutoff level to decide whether to admit a patient to a coronary care unit. If the test results are imprecise, this could lead to admitting a patient without ischemic heart disease or sending a patient home with an ischemic event. A statistical test used to characterize precision is the *coefficient of variation,* defined as the standard deviation divided by the mean value. Lower values indicate greater precision.

CRITICALLY APPRAISING THE CLINICAL EVIDENCE

During your health care training, it is essential that you learn the process of *critically appraising* the clinical literature in order to be able to interpret new studies, recommendations, and guidelines as they appear throughout your professional career.

A widely accepted process for critically appraising the clinical literature appears in the Users' Guides to the Medical Literature. These experts in epidemiology, or the study of disease in populations, created a rigorous and standardized approach for evaluating studies. This approach has been applied to a wide range of clinical topics, including therapeutic and prevention trials, diagnostic tests, meta-analysis, economic analysis, and practice guidelines. This approach asks three basic questions:

1. Are the results valid (can you believe them)?
2. What are the results (magnitude and precision)?
3. How can you apply the results to patient care (generalizability)?

Are the Results Valid?

Understanding Bias. When evaluating study results, it is important to have a thorough understanding of *bias,* which is a systematic error in conducting a study that threatens the validity of the results. Studies with a low risk of bias provide the most valid evidence for clinical decision making and health promotion interventions. The key sources of bias in clinical research are selection bias, performance bias, detection bias, and attrition bias (Box 7-12).

Box 7-12. Types of Biases Affecting Evidence

Selection Bias

- Occurs when comparison groups have systematic differences in their baseline characteristics that can affect the outcome of the study
- Creates problems in interpreting observed differences in outcomes because they could result from the interventions or the baseline differences between groups
- Randomly allocating subjects to the intervention is the best approach to minimizing this bias

Performance Bias

- Occurs when there are systematic differences in the care received between comparison groups (other than the intervention)
- Creates problems in interpreting outcome differences
- Blinding subjects and providers to the intervention is the best approach to minimizing this bias

Detection Bias

- Occurs when there are systematic differences in efforts to diagnose or ascertain an outcome
- Blinding outcome assessors (ensuring that they are unaware of the intervention received by the subject) is the best approach to minimizing this bias

Attrition Bias

- Occurs when there are systematic differences in the comparison groups in the number of subjects who do not complete the study
- Failing to account for these differences can lead to incorrectly estimating the effectiveness of an intervention
- Using an intention-to-treat analysis, where all analyses consider all subjects who were assigned to a comparison group, regardless of whether they received or completed the intervention, can minimize this bias

What Are the Results?

Assessing Performance of a Treatment or Prevention Intervention. We have discussed the results found in studies of diagnostic tests. Guidelines for health promotion are usually based on clinical trials of therapy or prevention. Results from these studies are also calculated from a 2 × 2 table where the columns correspond to whether the subject developed the outcome and the rows correspond to whether the subject received (or was exposed to) the intervention (Box 7-13).

Box 7-13. 2 × 2 Table for Evaluating Studies of Treatment or Prevention

	Event Occurred	No Event	Total
Experimental group	a	b	a + b
Control group	c	d	c + d

The statistics used to characterize the performance of a treatment or prevention intervention include *relative risks*, *relative risk differences* (can be a reduction or increase, reflecting benefit or harm), *absolute risk differences* (can be a reduction or increase, reflecting benefit or harm), *numbers needed to treat*, and *numbers needed to harm (Box 7-14).*

Box 7-14. Statistics Used to Characterize the Performance of a Treatment or Prevention Intervention

- *Experimental event rate (EER),* the probability that an intervention subject had the outcome, is described by a/(a + b) from row 1 (experimental group).
- *Control event rate (CER),* the probability that a control subject had the outcome, is c/(c + d) from row 2 (control group).
- *Relative risk,* the probability of an outcome in the intervention group compared to the probability of an outcome in the control group, is expressed as the EER/CER.
- *Relative risk difference,* defined as |CER − EER|/CER × or 1 − the relative risk, which describes the proportion of baseline risk, is reduced/increased by the therapy.
- *Absolute risk difference,* the difference in outcome rates between the comparisons groups, is expressed by the |CER − EER|.
- *Number needed to treat (NNT)* is the reciprocal of the absolute risk difference (reported as a fraction) and is the number of subjects who need to be treated over a specific period of time to prevent one outcome. If the intervention actually increases the risk for a bad outcome, then this statistic becomes the *number needed to harm (NNH).*

Calculating these statistics from the 2 × 2 table begins with determining probabilities for outcomes.

An example of these calculations in Box 7-15 is based on the results from the National Lung Screening Trial, which compared two ways of detecting lung cancer in subjects who were heavy smokers ages 55 to 74: either low-dose computed tomography (LDCT)—and standard chest x-ray (CXR). The outcome of interest (event) was death from lung cancer. After three rounds of annual screening and about 7 years of follow-up, the LDCT (experimental) group had an event rate of 0.018 while the CXR (control) group had an event rate of 0.021.

Box 7-15. 2 × 2 Table for Evaluating Lung Cancer Screening

Screening Test	Lung Cancer Death	No Lung Cancer Death	Total
Low-dose computed tomography (LDCT)	18	982	1,000
Chest x-ray (CXR)	21	979	1,000

Source: National Lung Screening Trial Research Team et al. *N Engl J Med.* 2011;365(5):395–409.

The relative risk of dying from lung cancer with LDCT screening compared to CXR screening was 0.018/0.021 = 0.86. The relative risk reduction was 1 – 0.86 = 0.14, meaning that the risk of a lung cancer death among the LDCT group was 14% lower than in the CXR group. LDCT led to a reduction in lung cancer deaths, so we used the absolute risk reduction, which was reported as a decimal: 0.021 – 0.018 = 0.003. The reciprocal of this value (1/0.003) gave us a number needed to screen of 333—meaning that screening 333 patients with LDCT prevented one lung cancer death. The number needed to screen (and treat) is always based on a specific period of time, so we should say that we need to screen 333 patients three times over 3 years with LDCT to prevent one lung cancer death after 7 years.

How Can You Apply the Results to Patient Care?

Generalizability. The final point to consider when evaluating the quality of the literature is whether the results are generalizable (e.g., whether the study results can be applied to your patients). To make this determination, you need to first look at the *demographics of the study subjects* (e.g., age, gender, race/ethnicity, socioeconomic status, clinical conditions). Then, you need to determine whether the demographics are similar enough to your patient to make the results applicable. You also need to determine whether the *intervention is feasible* in your setting. *Do you have the clinical expertise, technology, and capacity to offer the intervention?* Most importantly, you need to consider the *range of potential benefits and harm* associated with the intervention and decide whether the intervention is acceptable for your patient.

COMMUNICATING CLINICAL EVIDENCE TO PATIENTS

Healthcare providers need to be able to effectively communicate evidence on prognosis, treatments, diagnostic testing, and prevention in order to help patients understand their risks and options. Often, how information is framed can lead to misleading or uninformed patient decisions. In one study, respondents were given information on three different screening tests for unspecified cancers. In fact, the benefits were identical, except that they were expressed differently. When the benefit of the test was presented in the form of relative risk reduction, 80% of people said they would likely accept the test. When the same information was presented in the form of absolute risk reduction and NNT, only 53% and 43%, respectively, would agree to testing. Clinicians must therefore present information in such a way as to reduce framing effects and encourage informed shared decision-making process. Several approaches for these discussions include the five As (ask, advise, assess, assist, and arrange) and FRAMES (feedback about personal risk, responsibility of patient, advice to change, empathetic style, promote self-efficacy). Decision aids, which provide support for patients facing treatment or prevention decisions, increase knowledge, improve communication with clinicians, and increase confidence in making a decision.

UNIT 2 Regional Examinations

CHAPTER 8

General Examination

The general examination is the first step in the physical examination process. This helps in assessing the patient's general condition and severity of the disease. This also helps in arriving at the correct diagnosis. The main components of the general examination include the general survey and the vital signs. Pain assessment is not routinely done unless patient complains of pain.

HEALTH HISTORY: GENERAL APPROACH

This chapter focuses on patient concerns that accompany many disease processes collectively known as **constitutional symptoms**. The underlying etiologies of these common manifestations (Box 8-1) are often not confined to just one specific organ system but rather broadly affecting a patient's "constitution," or his or her physical state with regard to vitality, health, and strength. These may include *fatigue, weakness, fever, chills, night sweats, weight loss or weight gain*, and *pain*. The patients should be asked on a regular basis for these symptoms so that vigorous efforts can be made to diagnose, or at least treat, their complaints. Even if it is not possible to identify etiologies for these symptoms, aggressive strategies to control them may reduce their effect on health-related quality of life.

Box 8-1. Common or Concerning Symptoms

- Fatigue and weakness
- Fever, chills, night sweats
- Weight change
- Pain

Fatigue and Weakness

Fatigue is a nonspecific symptom with many causes. It refers to a sense of weariness or loss of energy that patients describe in various ways. "I don't feel like getting up in the morning" ... "I don't have any energy" ... "I can hardly get through the day" ... "By the time I get to work, I feel as if I've already done a day's work." Because fatigue is a normal response to hard work, sustained stress, and grief, the life circumstances in which it occurs should be elicited. Fatigue unrelated to such situations requires further investigation.

Fatigue is a common symptom of depression and anxiety, but also consider infections (such as hepatitis, infectious mononucleosis, tuberculosis); endocrine disorders (hypothyroidism, adrenal insufficiency, diabetes mellitus); heart failure; chronic disease of the lungs, kidneys, or liver; electrolyte imbalance; moderate-to-severe anemia; malignancies; nutritional deficits; and medications.

Use open-ended questions to encourage the patient to fully describe what he or she is experiencing. Important clues about etiology often emerge from a good psychosocial history, exploration of sleep patterns, and a thorough review of systems.

Weakness is different from fatigue. It denotes a demonstrable loss of muscle power and will be discussed later with other neurologic symptoms (see Chapter 13, *Nervous System*, p. 300).

Weakness, especially if localized in a neuroanatomical pattern, suggests possible neuropathy or myopathy.

Fever, Chills, and Night Sweats

Fever refers to an abnormal elevation in body temperature (see p. 142 for definitions of normal). Ask about fever if the patient has an acute or chronic illness. Find out whether the patient has measured his or her temperature. Has the patient felt feverish or unusually hot, noted excessive sweating, or felt chilly and cold? Try to distinguish between feeling cold and a shaking chill with shivering throughout the body and chattering of teeth.

Recurrent shaking chills suggest more extreme swings in temperature and systemic bacteremia.

Feeling cold, goose bumps, and shivering accompany a *rising* temperature, whereas feeling hot and sweating accompany a *falling* temperature. Normally, the body temperature rises during the day and falls during the night. When fever exaggerates this swing, *night sweats* occur. Malaise, headache, and pain in the muscles and joints often accompany fever.

Feeling hot and sweating also accompany menopause. Night sweats occur in tuberculosis and malignancy.

Fever has many causes. Focus on the timing of the illness and its associated symptoms. Become familiar with patterns of infectious diseases that may affect your patient. Inquire about travel, contact with sick people, and other unusual exposures. Even medications may cause fever. By contrast, recent ingestion of aspirin, acetaminophen, corticosteroids, and nonsteroidal anti-inflammatory drugs may mask fever and affect the temperature recorded at the office visit.

In immunocompromised patients with sepsis, fever may be absent, low-grade, or drop below normal (*hypothermia*).

Medicine History Taking OSCE Video: **Fever**

Weight Change

Weight change results from changes in body tissues or body fluid. Good opening questions include, "How often do you check your weight?" "How is it compared to a year ago?" If there are changes, ask, "Why do you think it has changed?" If weight gain or loss appears to be a problem, ask about the amount of change, its timing, the setting in which it occurred, and any associated symptoms.

Rapid changes in weight, over a few days, suggest changes in body fluid, not tissue.

Weight Gain. *Weight gain* occurs when caloric intake exceeds caloric expenditure over time and typically results in increased body fat. It can also reflect abnormal accumulation of body fluids, particularly when the gain is very rapid.

Edema from extravascular fluid retention is visible in heart failure, nephrotic syndrome, liver failure, and venous stasis.

Patients with a body mass index (BMI) of ≥25 to 29 kg/m^2 are defined as *overweight;* those with a BMI ≥30 kg/m^2 are considered *obese*. For these patients, plan a thorough assessment to avert the many associated risks of morbidity and mortality.

See section on height, weight, and calculation of BMI on p. 125.

Clarify the timing and evolution of the weight gain. Was the patient overweight as a child? Are the parents overweight? Ask about weight at life milestones like birth, kindergarten, high school or college graduation, military discharge, pregnancy, menopause, and retirement. Has a recent disability or surgery affected weight? What about depression or anxiety? Is there a change in sleep pattern or daytime drowsiness suspicious for sleep apnea? Establish the level of physical activity and results of prior attempts at weight loss. Assess eating patterns and dietary preferences.

Review the patient's medications.

Many drugs are associated with weight gain, such as tricyclic antidepressants; insulin and sulfonylurea; contraceptives, glucocorticoids, and progestational steroids; mirtazapine, citalopram, and paroxetine; gabapentin and valproate; and metoprolol, atenolol, and propranolol.

Weight Loss. Explore any clinically **significant weight loss**, defined as loss of 5% or more of usual body weight over a 6-month period. Mechanisms include decreased food intake due to anorexia, depression, dysphagia, vomiting, abdominal pain, or financial difficulties; defective gastrointestinal (GI) absorption or inflammation; and increased metabolic requirements. Ask about abuse of alcohol, cocaine, amphetamines, or opiates, or withdrawal from marijuana, all associated with weight loss. Heavy smoking also suppresses appetite.

Causes of weight loss include GI diseases (Crohn's disease, ulcerative colitis); endocrine disorders (diabetes mellitus, hyperthyroidism, adrenal insufficiency); chronic infections, (HIV/AIDS); malignancy; chronic cardiac, pulmonary, or renal failure; depression; and anorexia nervosa or bulimia.

Weight loss with relatively high food intake suggests diabetes mellitus, hyperthyroidism, or malabsorption. Consider also binge eating (bulimia) with clandestine vomiting.

Assess food intake. Has it been normal, dropped, or even increased?

Pursue a thorough psychosocial history. Who cooks and shops for the patient? Where does the patient eat? With whom? Are there any problems with obtaining, storing, preparing, or chewing food? Does the patient avoid or restrict certain foods for medical, religious, or other reasons?

Poverty, old age, social isolation, physical disability, emotional or mental impairment, lack of teeth, ill-fitting dentures, alcoholism, and drug abuse increase risk of malnutrition.

Check the medication history.

Drugs associated with weight loss include anticonvulsants, antidepressants, levodopa, digoxin, metformin, and thyroid medication.

Be alert for symptoms and signs of *malnutrition*. These may be subtle and nonspecific, such as weakness, easy fatigability, cold intolerance, flaky dermatitis, and ankle swelling. Securing a good diet history of eating patterns and quantities is essential. Ask general questions about intake at different times throughout the day, such as "What do you typically eat for lunch?" "What do you eat for a snack?" "When?"

See Chapter 6, Health Maintenance and Screening, p. 97.

Pain

Pain is one of the most common presenting symptoms in office practice. The most frequent causes are low back pain, headache or migraine, and knee and neck pain; prevalence varies by ethnicity and socioeconomic status. Localizing symptoms, the "seven attributes of every symptom," and the psychosocial history are essential to your physical examination, assessment, and a comprehensive management plan (refer Chapter 3).

See section on acute and chronic pain, p. 144, for an approach to assessment.

Medicine History Taking OSCE Video:
Chest Pain, Abdominal Pain, Headache, and Back Pain

PHYSICAL EXAMINATION: GENERAL APPROACH

The skills of observation begin with the opening moments of the patient encounter. The best clinicians continually sharpen their powers of observation and description of the encounter. As you talk with and examine the patient, heighten your focus on the patient's mood, build, and behavior. These details enrich and deepen your emerging clinical impression. Your goal is to describe the distinguishing features of the patient so clearly that colleagues can spot the patient in a crowd of strangers, avoiding clichés like "middle-aged gentleman" and uninformative statements such as "in no acute distress."

TECHNIQUES OF EXAMINATION

Key Components of the General Examination

- Perform a general survey (appearance, apparent state of health, consciousness, discomfort or distress, skin color, dress, grooming and personal hygiene, facial expression, odors, posture, and gait and motor activity).
- Assess the state of nutrition, measure height and weight, and calculate BMI.

(continued)

- Examine the head and neck.
- Examine the extremities.
- Assess speech and language and cognitive functions.
- Measure blood pressure using a sphygmomanometer.
- Measure orthostatic blood pressure (if indicated).
- Examine arterial pulses.
- Observe rate, rhythm, depth, and effort of breathing.
- Measure core body temperature (oral, tympanic, rectal, or temporal).
- Assess acute and chronic pain (if indicated).

General Survey

The **general survey** begins with the opening moments of the patient encounter, but your observations of the patient's appearance often crystallize as you start the physical examination.

Many factors contribute to the patient's body habitus: socioeconomic status, nutrition, genetic makeup, physical fitness, mood state, early illnesses, gender, geographic location, and age cohort. Nutritional status affects many of the characteristics you scrutinize during the general survey: height and weight, blood pressure (BP), posture, mood and alertness, facial coloration, dentition and condition of the tongue and gingiva, color of the nail beds, and muscle bulk, to name a few. Your assessment of height, weight, BMI, and risk for obesity should be routine for each patient in your clinical practice.

Recall your observations from the first moments of the encounter that you have been refining throughout your assessment. Does the patient hear you when greeted in the waiting room or examination room? Rise with ease? Walk easily or stiffly? If hospitalized when you first meet, what is the patient doing—sitting up and watching television? … or lying in bed? … What do you see in the room—a magazine? … candy bars or chips? … photos of loved ones? … a religious image or object? … multiple beverage containers? … or nothing at all? Each observation raises questions or hypotheses to consider as your assessment unfolds.

General Appearance

Apparent State of Health. Try to make a general judgment based on observations throughout the encounter. Support it with the significant details.

Is the patient acutely or chronically ill, frail, or fit and robust?

Level of Consciousness. Is the patient awake, alert, and responsive to you and others in the environment? If not, promptly assess the level of consciousness.

See Chapter 13, *Nervous System*, Level of Consciousness, p. 336.

Apparent State of Discomfort or Distress. Does the patient show evidence of the problems listed below?

- Cardiac or respiratory distress
- Pain
- Anxiety or depression

Is there clutching of the chest, pallor, diaphoresis, labored breathing, wheezing, or coughing?

Is there wincing, diaphoresis, protectiveness of a painful area, grimacing, or an unusual posture favoring one limb or region of the body? Are there anxious facial expressions, fidgety movements, cold moist palms, inexpressive or flat affect, poor eye contact, or psychomotor slowing?

See Chapter 9, Cognition, Behavior, and Mental Status, p. 155.

Dress, Grooming, and Personal Hygiene. How is the patient dressed? Is the clothing suitable for the temperature and weather? Is it clean and appropriate to the setting?

Excess clothing may reflect the cold intolerance of hypothyroidism, hide skin rash or needle marks, mask anorexia, or signal personal lifestyle preferences.

Notice the patient's shoes. Are there cutouts or holes? Are the shoes run-down?

Holes or slippers suggest gout, bunions, edema, or other painful foot conditions. Run-down shoes can contribute to foot and back pain, calluses, falls, and infection.

Is the patient wearing unusual jewelry? Are there body piercings?

Copper bracelets and magnetic wrist straps suggest joint pain. Tattoos and piercings may be associated with risktaking behavior in adults.

Note the patient's hair, fingernails, and use of makeup. They may be clues to the patient's personality, mood, lifestyle, and self-regard.

"Grown-out" hair and nail polish suggest the length of a possible illness. Bitten fingernails may reflect stress.

Do personal hygiene and grooming seem appropriate for the patient's age, lifestyle, and occupation?

Neglected appearance may appear in depression and dementia but should be compared with the patient's norm.

Facial Expression. Observe the facial expression at rest, during conversation and social interactions, and during the physical examination. Watch closely for eye contact. Is it natural? … sustained and unblinking? … averted quickly? … absent?

Watch for the stare of hyperthyroidism, the immobile facies of parkinsonism, and the flat or sad affect of depression. Decreased eye contact may be culture-specific or suggest anxiety, fear, or sadness.

Odors of the Body and Breath. Odors can be important diagnostic clues, like the fruity odor of diabetes or the scent of alcohol.

Breath odors can reveal the presence of alcohol or acetone (diabetes), pulmonary infections, uremia, or liver failure.

Never assume that alcohol on a patient's breath explains changes in the mental status or neurologic findings.

These changes can have serious but treatable causes such as hypoglycemia, subdural hematoma, or *postictal state* (the abnormal condition occurring between the end of an epileptic seizure and the return to the baseline condition).

Skin, Nails, and Hair. Inspect for any changes in skin with the patient seated or supine, and then in the prone position. Inspect the skin in a head-to-toe sequence with the breast and genitalia examined last. Start with a general survey of the skin, including color, pigmentation, vascularity, bruising, lesions, color variations, and general hygiene.

Palpate the skin and note the temperature, texture, moisture, and turgor. Note the distribution, texture, and quantity of hair.

See Chapter 18, Skin, Hair, and Nails, p. 512.

Pallor. Pallor is the paleness of the skin and mucous membranes, usually resulting from anemia. Anemia is due to low number of circulating red cells as a result of blood loss, hemolysis, or underproduction of cells by the bone marrow. In patients with acute blood loss, the physical findings are abnormal vital signs suggestive of hypovolemia, but in patients with chronic anemia, physical findings include changes in color of the skin and conjunctiva.

In chronic anemia, there is reduced amount of red-colored oxyhemoglobin circulating in the dermal and subconjunctival capillaries and venules. This results in a pale appearance of the skin and conjunctiva. Remember, pallor does not always indicate anemia. The skin vascularity, the amount of circulating deoxyhemoglobin, and the patient's natural skin pigments determine the skin color. Cold exposure or sympathetic stimulation causes vasoconstriction which can also cause pallor. On the other hand, vasodilation due to inflammation or vascular injury from ischemia, radiation, etc., the blue color of cyanosis, or the brown pigments of dark-skinned persons may obscure the pallor of anemia.

Examine the conjunctiva, nail beds, and palms to avoid the effects of the patient's natural skin pigments.

Look for pallor in the lower palpebral conjunctiva, tip and dorsum of the tongue, soft palate, nail beds, general skin, palms, and soles. If you look for pallor only in extremities, this may be related to arterial spasm or obstruction, such as Raynaud disease and Buerger disease.

Ask the patient to look upward and gently pull the lower eyelid to expose the lower palpebral conjunctiva and observe its color. The conjunctival rim pallor is considered when the anterior rim appears pale as compared to the deeper posterior aspect of the palpebral conjunctiva. Ask the patient to protrude the tongue and observe the dorsum of the tongue for paleness. Ask the patient to show his or her palms and compare with your palm. Normal individuals have a pinkish appearance. Hyperextend the patient's fingers or by stretching the skin on either side of the creases to look for pallor in palmar creases. Inspect the nail beds for pallor.

See Table 8-1, Causes of Anemia.

Cyanosis. Cyanosis is an abnormal bluish discoloration of the skin and mucous membranes, caused by excessive amount of deoxygenated hemoglobin. Clinical cyanosis is present if oxygen saturation is less than 85%. Cyanosis may be central or peripheral. Central cyanosis is due to excessive oxygen unsaturation of the arterial blood, but peripheral cyanosis is due to pronounced oxygen unsaturation of the venocapillary and capillary blood. The arterial oxygen saturation is normal. Pseudocyanosis is permanent bluish discoloration caused by deposition of blue pigments in the skin.

In some patients, cyanosis may result from increased amounts of methemoglobin or sulfhemoglobin.

Look for cyanosis on the lips, nose, cheeks, ears, hands, feet, and mucous membranes of the oral cavity. In these areas, the overlying epidermis is thin and subepidermal vessels are abundant, and, therefore, cyanosis is best appreciated. Cyanosis is detected more easily with fluorescent lighting than with incandescent lighting or daylight.

Patients with central cyanosis have blue discoloration of the lips, tongue, and sublingual tissues, as well as of the hands and feet. Peripheral cyanosis causes blue hands and feet, although the mucous membranes of the mouth are pink. The peripheral cyanosis diminishes on warming the skin on the patient's limbs because of increased blood flow to the involved area, whereas the color of central cyanosis is unchanged or deepens after warming of the skin. In patients with pseudocyanosis, the mucous membranes of the mouth are pink, and pressure on the skin fails to blanch the abnormal color.

See Table 8-2, Causes of Cyanosis.

Medicine History Taking OSCE Video:
Cyanosis

Jaundice. *Jaundice* (or *icterus*) is a yellowish discoloration of the skin and sclerae from increased levels of *bilirubin*, a bile pigment derived chiefly from the breakdown of hemoglobin. It is usually apparent when plasma bilirubin is >3 mg/dL. The yellow color may have a greenish tinge in patients with long-standing jaundice, due to oxidation of bilirubin to biliverdin.

Carotenemia, the presence of the orange pigment *carotene* in the blood due to ingestion of carrots, presents as a yellow discoloration of the skin, especially palms and soles, but not of the sclera or mucous membranes.

Normally, the hepatocytes conjugate unconjugated bilirubin with bile salts, making the bile water soluble, to excrete the conjugated bilirubin into bile. Bile is stored in the gallbladder and secreted via the cystic duct into the common bile duct during fat digestion. The common bile duct also directly drains the hepatic ducts from the liver. More distally, the common bile duct and the pancreatic ducts converge and empty into the duodenum at the ampulla of Vater. Mechanisms of jaundice are listed in Box 8-2.

Box 8-2. Mechanisms of Jaundice

- Increased production of bilirubin
- Decreased uptake of bilirubin by the hepatocytes
- Decreased ability of the liver to conjugate bilirubin
- Decreased excretion of bilirubin into the bile, resulting in absorption of conjugated bilirubin back into the blood

Predominantly unconjugated bilirubin occurs from the first three mechanisms, as in hemolytic anemia (increased production) and Gilbert syndrome.

Impaired excretion of conjugated bilirubin is seen in viral hepatitis, cirrhosis, primary biliary cirrhosis, and drug-induced cholestasis from drugs such as oral contraceptives, methyltestosterone, and chlorpromazine.

Intrahepatic jaundice can be *hepatocellular*, from damage to the hepatocytes, or *cholestatic*, from impaired excretion as a result of damaged hepatocytes or intrahepatic bile ducts.

Extrahepatic jaundice arises from obstruction of the extrahepatic bile ducts, most commonly the common bile ducts.

Gallstones or pancreatic, cholangio-, or duodenal carcinoma may obstruct the common bile duct.

In patients with jaundice, pay special attention to the associated symptoms and setting in which the illness occurred. What was the *color of the urine and stool* as the patient became ill? When the level of conjugated bilirubin increases in the blood, it may be excreted into the urine, turning the urine a dark yellowish brown or tea color. Unconjugated bilirubin is not water soluble, so it is not excreted into urine. Is there any associated pain?

Dark urine indicates impaired excretion of bilirubin into the GI tract.

Painless jaundice points to malignant obstruction of the bile ducts, seen in duodenal or pancreatic carcinoma; painful jaundice is commonly infectious in origin, as in hepatitis A and cholangitis.

Ask also about the *color of the stools.* When excretion of bile into the intestine is completely obstructed, the stools become gray or light colored, or *acholic*, without bile.

Acholic stools may occur briefly in viral hepatitis; they are common in obstructive jaundice.

Does the skin itch without other obvious explanation? Is there any associated pain? What is its pattern? Has it been recurrent in the past?

Itching or *pruritus* occurs in cholestatic or obstructive jaundice when bilirubin levels are markedly elevated.

Ask about risk factors for liver diseases (Box 8-3).

Medicine History Taking OSCE Video: **Jaundice**

Box 8-3. Risk Factors for Liver Diseases

- ***Infectious hepatitis:*** Travel or meals in areas with poor sanitation; ingestion of contaminated water or foodstuffs *(hepatitis A)*; parenteral or mucous membrane exposure to infectious body fluids such as blood, serum, semen, and saliva, especially through sexual contact with an infected partner or use of shared needles for injection drug use *(hepatitis B)*; and illicit injection drug use or blood transfusion *(hepatitis C)*. Hepatitis B is also endemic in certain regions of the world and can present in patients with no risk factors.
- ***Nonalcoholic steatohepatitis:*** It occurs in patients with metabolic syndrome.
- ***Alcoholic hepatitis or alcoholic cirrhosis:*** Screen patients carefully about alcohol use.
- ***Toxic liver damage:*** It may occur because of medications, industrial solvents, environmental toxins, or some anesthetic agents.
- ***Gallbladder disease or prior surgery:*** It may result in extrahepatic biliary obstruction.
- ***Hereditary disorders:*** These include family history of hemolytic anemia or liver disease, such as hemochromatosis, α_1-antitrypsin deficiency, and Wilson disease.

Pigmentation. Pigmentation is the color of the skin. Normal skin color depends on the amount of melanin. Low deposits of melanin impart a fair skin tone and high deposits a darker skin tone.

Look for pigmentation on the face, inside the cheek, and creases of the palms and skin, particularly pressure points and areas exposed to light.

Malaria, leishmaniasis, cirrhosis, advanced liver cancer, acromegaly, and drugs (e.g., arsenic agent and busulfan) can cause varying degrees of skin pigmentation. Secondary hemochromatosis due to massive transfusion may cause brown or bronze skin pigmentation, which is due to the deposition of hemosiderin.

Nails. Inspect the fingernails and toenails. Note their color and shape. Nail polish should be removed. Palpate fingernails and toenails for texture and note capillary refill time.

See Table 18-9, Findings in or Near the Nails.

Nails are normally pink with white lunulae, smooth and firm in texture, rounded in shape with a 160° angle between the nail base and the skin, and are firmly attached to the nail bed. Longitudinal bands of pigment may be seen in the nails of people who have darker skin.

Clubbing. Clubbing refers to a bulbous swelling of the terminal part of the fingers and toes with an increase in the soft-tissue mass. There is an increase in anteroposterior and transverse diameter of the nails due to proliferation of subungual connective tissue (Box 8-4).

Box 8-4. Signs of Early Clubbing

Floating nail sign: Apply pressure at the root of the nail plate. Observe movement. Normally, pressure on the root produces no movement. The root of the nail plate which lies snugly against the bone of the distal phalanx is separated from bone by connective tissue and edema with the development of clubbing and moves toward the bone on applying pressure on the nail plate.

Profile sign: Normally, the angle between the nail plate and the skin overlying the proximal part of the distal phalanx is about 160° or less. In clubbing, tissue under the nail plate proliferates and causes obliteration of the angle between the nail and the nailbed. This is the earliest sign of clubbing.

Clubbing usually develops first in the thumb and forefinger, and occurs in the other fingers later.

Increased nail curvature, chronic paronychia, and abscesses of the terminal pulp space are pseudoclubbing conditions. The base angle is unaltered in these conditions. Ask the patient to perform Schamroth's maneuver. Ask the patient to hold the two thumbs back-to-back with the two fingertips and interphalangeal joints aligned. A diamond-shaped window is apparent in normal individuals and in pseudoclubbing conditions, but this window is lost in true clubbing (Box 8-5).

Medicine History Taking OSCE Video: **Clubbing**

Box 8-5. Causes of Clubbing

- Cardiac causes: Congenital cyanotic heart diseases, infective endocarditis, cardiac tumors
- Lung causes: Bronchiectasis, lung abscess, empyema, fibrocaseous type of tuberculosis, bronchogenic carcinoma
- Ulcerative colitis
- Biliary and other types of cirrhosis
- Unilateral clubbing, which may be found in presubclavian coarctation, bronchogenic carcinoma, and aneurysm of right subclavian artery
- Painful clubbing, which may be seen in bronchogenic carcinoma

Hypertrophic osteoarthropathy is usually considered as a further extension of the clubbing process, and in this, the changes are in the larger bones and joints of distal parts of limbs. See Box 8-6, Grades of Clubbing.

Box 8-6. Grades of Clubbing

Grade 1: Only increased fluctuation of the nail bed
Grade 2: Increased anteroposterior and transverse diameter
Grade 3: Increased pulp tissue
Grade 4: Subperiosteal thickening in bones of wrist and ankles

Hair. Note the quantity, distribution, texture, and pattern of loss of hair, if any. You may see loose flakes of dandruff.

See Table 18-8, Hair Loss.

Nutrition. Nutritional status is related to food intake, digestion, absorption, and metabolism, which is one of the criteria for identifying the state of health and disease. Obesity and emaciation are two abnormal states of nutrition. This is usually determined by comprehensive analysis of the skin, hair, subcutaneous fat and muscles, etc. The physical indexes that are commonly used to assess the nutritional status are as follows:

1. Height, weight, and BMI
2. Waist circumference or waist-to-hip ratio
3. Arm circumference
4. Skinfold thickness

Height and Weight. Note any changes in height or weight over time.

Is the patient unusually short or tall? Is the build slender, muscular, or stocky? Is the body symmetric? Note the general body proportions.

Watch for very short stature in Turner syndrome, childhood renal failure, and achondroplastic and hypopituitary dwarfism; long limbs in proportion to the trunk in hypogonadism and Marfan syndrome; and height loss in osteoporosis and vertebral compression fractures.

Is the patient emaciated, slender, overweight, or obese? If the patient is obese, is the fat distributed evenly, concentrated over the upper torso, or settled around the hips?

There is generalized fat distribution in simple obesity and truncal fat with relatively thin limbs in Cushing syndrome and metabolic syndrome.

Make note of any weight changes.

Causes of weight loss include malignancy, diabetes mellitus, hyperthyroidism, chronic infection, depression, diuresis, and successful dieting.

Measuring Height and Weight. Height and weight are fundamental in nutrition screening as well as interventions that may arise from treatment, including accurate drug dosage, body fluid gain or loss, and fluid requirements.

Measure the patient's height and weight to determine the BMI (Figs. 8-1 and 8-2). You should use proper technique with appropriate equipment that is regularly calibrated to ensure accuracy (Boxes 8-7 and 8-8).

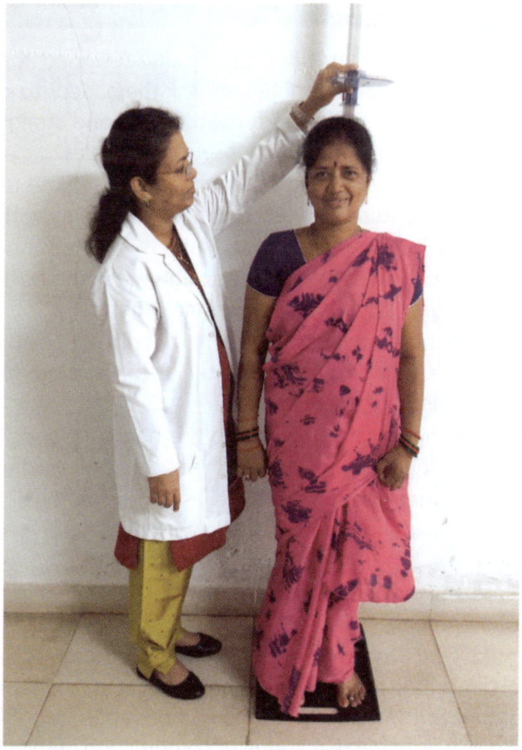

FIGURE 8-1. Measuring the height using a stadiometer.

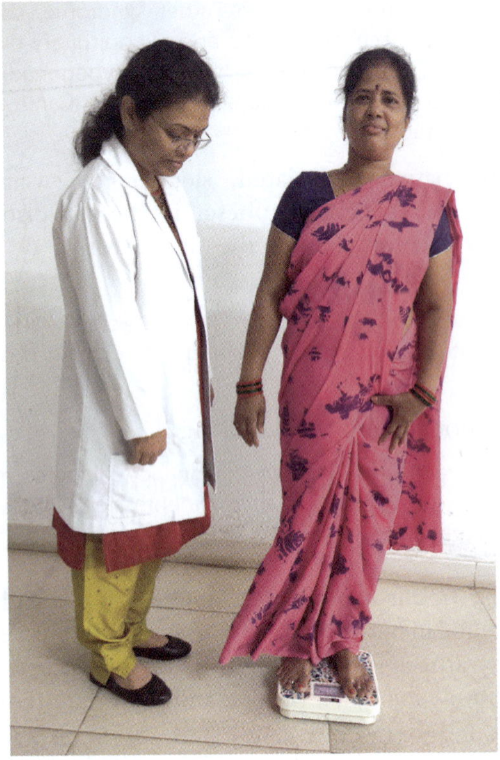

FIGURE 8-2. Measuring the weight using a weighing machine.

Box 8-7. Determining the Patient's Height

- **Stadiometers** are devices specifically designed for the accurate measurement of height. Ask the patient to stand on the stadiometer, facing forward as tall and straight as possible with arms hanging loosely at the sides.
- The patient's feet should be flat on the baseplate of the stadiometer and positioned slightly apart, in line with the hips, to aid balance.
- The patient's knees should be straight, and the buttocks and shoulders should touch the stadiometer.
- Ensure that the patient's head is in the midline position—an imaginary line from the center of the earhole to the lower border of the eye socket.
- Bring the headplate down onto the head, ensuring that it rests on the crown of the head (i.e., the top back half).
- Read the measurement. Your eyes should be level with the counter/pointer and measurement read to the nearest 1 mm.
- Record the measurement and assist the patient off the stadiometer.
- Should you be making repeated measurements on the same individual on different days, it is advisable to measure at the same time of day if possible. Throughout the day, height decreases due to compression of the spine.

Box 8-8. Determining the Patient's Weight

- Ask the patient to remove shoes and outdoor garments as appropriate. If weighing a patient with a stoma or catheter bag, ensure that it is emptied beforehand.
- Ensure that the scales are balanced, or display zero, before weighing the patient.
- The patient should remain as still as possible while being weighed. Monitor to ensure that:
  - Clothing is not touching any fixed part of the scales or surroundings.
  - Body weight is not supported on an object (e.g., a walking stick or wall) and the patient's feet are not placed on the floor (when using chair scales).
- Once the scales register a weight, record the reading on the scales in the appropriate documentation.
- Once accurate weight is recorded, assist the patient to move away from the weighing scale. Ensure that he or she is dressed appropriately and comfortable at the end of the procedure.
- When monitoring periodical weight change, ensure that the patient always wears clothing of similar weight.

Calculating the BMI. Use your measurements of height and weight to determine **BMI**. Body fat consists primarily of adipose in the form of triglycerides and is stored in subcutaneous, intra-abdominal, and intramuscular fat deposits that are difficult to measure directly. The BMI incorporates estimated but more accurate measures of body fat than weight alone. The National Institutes of Health cautions that people who are very muscular can have a high BMI, but still be healthy. Likewise, the BMI for older adults and those with low muscle mass may appear inappropriately "normal."

See Chapter 6, for discussion of optimal weight, nutrition, and diet, p. 97.

To determine the BMI, choose the method best suited to your practice. Use a standard BMI table or the electronic medical record software, which frequently shows the BMI automatically. You can also calculate the BMI as shown below with the weight in kilograms and height in meters:

$$\text{BMI} = \frac{\text{Weight (kg)}}{\text{Height (m}^2\text{)}}$$

Conversion formulas: 1 lb = 0.45 kg; 1 in = 2.54 cm; 100 cm = 1 m.

You may also use the online BMI Calculator from the National Institutes of Health—National Heart, Lung, and Blood Institute available at https://www.nhlbi.nih.gov/health/educational/lose_wt/BMI/bmicalc.htm.

Then classify the BMI according to the national guidelines (Box 8-9).

Box 8-9. Classification of Overweight and Obesity by BMI

Obesity Class		BMI (kg/m^2)
Underweight		<18.5
Normal		18.5–24.9
Overweight		25.0–29.9
Obesity	I	30.0–34.9
	II	35.0–39.9
Extreme obesity	III	≥40

BMI, body mass index.

If the BMI is *above 25 kg/m^2*, assess the patient for additional risk factors for heart disease and other obesity-related diseases: hypertension, high low-density lipoprotein (LDL) cholesterol, low high-density lipoprotein (HDL) cholesterol, high triglycerides, high blood glucose, family history of premature heart disease, physical inactivity, and cigarette smoking.

Waist Circumference. Waist circumference measures abdominal fat content. Excess abdominal fat relative to total body fat is an independent predictor of disease risk and morbidity.

See Box 8-10 for measurement of waist circumference.

Box 8-10. Instructions for Measuring Waist Circumference

- Place the measuring tape around the trunk, at a point midway between the lower costal margin and the iliac crest, while the patient is standing with feet about 25–30 cm (10–12 in) apart.
- Wrap the measuring tape around the abdomen without compressing underlying soft tissues.
- Record the waist circumference to the nearest 0.5 cm (1/4 in) at the end of a usual expiration.

Waist circumference provides additional information on health risk beyond that determined by the BMI. Measure both BMI and waist circumference if you are assessing a patient's disease risk (Box 8-11).

Box 8-11. Waist Circumference and BMI Association with Disease Risk

Waist Circumference	BMI		
	Normal	Overweight	Obesity Class I
Men ≤ 102 cm (40 in); Women: ≤ 88 cm (35 in)	Least risk	Increased risk	High risk
Men > 102 cm (40 in); Women: > 88 cm (35 in)	Increased risk	High risk	Very high risk

Mid-Upper Arm Circumference (MUAC). It is the circumference of the left upper arm and is measured at the midpoint between the tips of the shoulder and the elbow. The following steps are performed to measure MUAC:

1. Identify and mark with a skin pencil the olecranon process and acromion.
2. Mark the midpoint between these two marks.
3. With the arm hanging straight down, wrap an MUAC tape around the arm at the midpoint mark.
4. Measure to the nearest 1 mm.

MUAC is an important indicator of malnutrition.

The normal MUAC range is >23 cm in males and >22 cm in females.

Skinfold Thickness. A skinfold caliper is used to assess the skinfold thickness. This measurement is less reliable in elderly people, due to their weak skin and muscles. Four skinfolds are measured:

- Biceps skinfold (front side middle upper arm)
- Triceps skinfold (back side middle upper arm)
- Subscapular skinfold (under the lowest point of the shoulder blade)
- Suprailiac skinfold (above the upper bone of the hip)

State of Hydration. Normal hydration is important for the health and well-being and is often called *euhydration*. Dehydration can have a negative effect on muscle strength, endurance, and maximal oxygen uptake. Hydration is difficult to measure as it is a dynamic process. It is different for each individual.

Acute changes in body mass over a short period of time are commonly assumed to be due to body water loss or gain. As 1 mL of water has a mass of 1 g, changes in body mass can be used to quantify water gain or loss. Clinical assessment of dehydration is always approximate. When we talk about "5% dehydration," it means that the patient has lost an amount of fluid equal to 5% of the body weight.

Assessment of Dehydration. Take a detailed history of fluid loss including the amount and route (e.g. through gastrointestinal tract or urinary tract).

Assess the percentage of loss of fluid (Box 8-12) during physical examination. Check skin turgor on the dorsum of the hands or the abdomen; look for the state of oral mucous membranes, pulse rate, and pulse pressure; and look for evidence of shock.

Medicine History Taking OSCE Video: **Dehydration**

Box 8-12. Degree of Dehydration

- **Mild dehydration but clinically undetectable (5%):** A history of fluid loss is present but no physical findings are detectable.
- **Moderate dehydration (5% to 9%):** The patient appears to be unwell, irritable, and lethargic, and has a history of decreased urine output, dry mucous membranes, tachycardia, tachypnea, and decreased skin turgor. At this stage, pulse pressure, peripheral pulses, and capillary refill time remain normal.
- **Severe dehydration (≥10%):** The patient's level of consciousness decreases and the skin becomes pale or mottled with cold extremities. Tachycardia, tachypnea, decreased pulse pressure, weak peripheral pulses, prolonged capillary refill time, and hypotension with other signs of shock are seen.

Eyes. A basic eye examination (Box 8-13) usually consists of a series of tests for vision and inspection of the external eye, anterior segment, and internal eye.

Box 8-13. Examination of Eyes

- Test vision in each eye separately.
  - Use Snellen chart for distant vision with or without corrective lens. Test without lenses first and record readings separately.
  - Use near vision card for near vision.
  - Test peripheral vision (nasal, temporal, superior, inferior) by moving your finger into the field from outside.

(continued)

- Inspect the eyebrows for size/extension, hair texture, orbital area, eyelids for position, ability to open wide and close completely, margins, and eyelashes.
- Palpate eyelids and eyeballs.
- Pull down the lower lids and inspect the conjunctiva and sclera for color, condition, and lacrimal gland region.
- Evaluate muscle balance and movement of the eyes for six cardinal fields of gaze and corneal reflex.
- Inspect corneal clarity, irises, pupillary size/shape, pupillary response to light, accommodation, and afferent pupillary testing.
- Perform ophthalmoscopic examination.

Face. The face is "the organ of emotion," and it provides important clues to one's own feelings as well as systemic illness (Box 8-14).

Box 8-14. Examination of Face

- Inspect the face for skin color, asymmetry, scars, edema, masses, involuntary movements, or tics.
- Observe the facial expressions for signs of distress or for the appearance of abnormal facies associated with them.

Nose and Sinuses. The nose is the primary "organ of smell." It also serves as an important organ for respiration (Box 8-15).

Box 8-15. Examination of Nose and Sinuses

- Inspect the external nose for shape, size, color, and nares.
- Palpate the ridge and soft tissues of the nose.
- Check the patency of the nose.
- Inspect the nasal mucosa and nasal septum for color, shape, and condition.
- Test the sense of smell.
- Inspect the frontal and maxillary sinuses.
- Palpate the frontal and maxillary sinuses.

See Chapter 21, Ears and Nose, p. 600.

Mouth and Oral Cavity. The mouth and oral cavity include examination of the lips, organs, and tissues in the oral cavity (Box 8-16).

See Chapter 22, Throat and Oral Cavity, p. 617.

Box 8-16. Examination of Mouth and Oral Cavity

- Inspect and palpate the lips with the mouth closed for symmetry, color, and condition.
- Inspect the teeth for occlusion, color, and condition.
- Inspect the buccal mucosa for color and condition.
- Inspect and palpate the gingiva (use gloves to palpate) for color and condition.
- Inspect the tongue for size, symmetry, color, dorsal surface, ventral surface and floor of the mouth, and lateral borders.
- Palpate the tongue and floor of the mouth.
- Inspect and palpate the uvula for color, landmarks, and movements.
- Inspect the oropharynx after depressing the tongue with a tongue blade for tonsils, posterior wall, and pharynx.
- Elicit gag reflex.

Ears. The ear is the organ responsible for hearing and balance. There are three compartments: external ear, middle ear, and inner ear (Box 8-17).

See Chapter 21, Ears and Nose, p. 600.

Box 8-17. Examination of Ear

- Inspect the auricles for contour, size, position of the earlobes, and symmetry. Note any deformity, injury, scarring, redness, swelling, lumps, or fistulous tract.
- Gently pull and palpate the auricle for texture and tenderness.
- Inspect the external auditory canal for skin color and drainage.
- Gently pull the auricle upward and backward and observe the tympanic membrane. Inspect the color, transparency, and position of the tympanic membrane. Note any perforation.
- Inspect and palpate the mastoid area. Note any abnormality.
- Auditory acuity can be estimated by several screening tests. In a quiet room, ask the patient to occlude one ear. Move the fingers/watch from 1 m toward the patient's ear. Instruct the patient to acknowledge the rubbing of the examiner's fingers/watch sounds. Use the examiner's own hearing as a reference. Repeat this procedure on the opposite ear. Record the distance and compare the results of the two ears.
- If screening tests are abnormal, perform further tests for hearing evaluation.

Neck

- Inspect for symmetry and smoothness of the neck and thyroid.
- Inspect for jugular venous pressure (JVP).
- Perform active and passive range of motion. Test resistance against the examiner's hand.
- Test the strength of shoulder shrug (cranial nerve XI).
- Palpate the thyroid.
- Palpate the lymph nodes.
- Auscultate the carotid arteries and thyroid.

Axillae. The axillae are examined preferably with the patient in sitting position. Inspect the skin of each axilla, noting evidence of rash, infection, and pigmentation. Palpate the axillae for tenderness and lymph node enlargement.

See Chapter 17, Axillae, p. 500.

Thyroid Gland. Inspect the thyroid gland for swelling and asymmetry. Observe the patient swallowing. Palpate the thyroid gland for size, shape, and consistency of the gland. Identify any nodules or tenderness. Auscultate the gland for any bruit.

See Chapter 19, Thyroid Gland, p. 561.

Extremities. Observe and palpate the hands, arms, foot, thighs, skin and nails, muscle mass, muscle strength, musculoskeletal deformities, range of motion of muscles, fingers, wrist, elbow, shoulders, toes, ankles, knees, and hips. Palpate the epitrochlear nodes.

The length of both arms and arm span are compared with those of the trunk. This may help in the diagnosis of Marfan syndrome. Bony deformities such as bowing of the legs may be seen in Paget disease of bone and in rickets.

Palpate for temperature, texture, edema, and pulses (dorsalis pedis, posterior tibial, popliteal).

Edema. Edema is defined as clinically apparent accumulation of extracellular fluid as swelling, especially of the lower extremities.

Blood circulates from arteries to veins through the capillary bed (Fig. 8-3). Most filtered fluid returns to the circulation not as fluid resorbed at the venous end of the capillaries, but as lymph. The kidneys also play a role in retention of sodium and water when plasma volume goes down. Any aberration of (1) *venous capillary pressure*, (2) *capillary osmotic pressure*, or (3) *abnormal fluid balance*—either by exogenous administration or by resorption by the kidney—can cause *edema*.

Mechanisms for the development of **edema** include increased plasma volume from sodium retention, altered capillary dynamics resulting in net filtration, inadequate removal of filtered lymph fluid, lymphatic or venous obstruction, and increased capillary permeability. See Table 8-3, Types of Peripheral Edema.

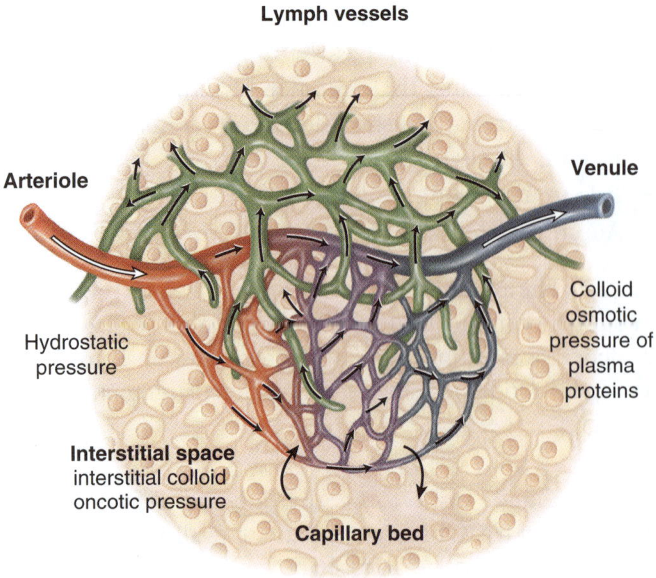

FIGURE 8-3. Capillary fluid exchange.

Edema that is *compressible*, or lessens when external pressure is applied, is known as *pitting edema*. **Lymphedema**, from obstructed lymphatic drainage, is usually not compressible.

Interstitial tissue can absorb up to 5 L of fluid, accommodating up to a 10% weight gain, before pitting edema appears. Causes vary from systemic to local. Focus on the location, timing, and setting of the swelling and on associated symptoms. "Have you had any swelling anywhere? Where? Anywhere else? When does it occur? Is it worse in the morning or at night? Do your shoes get tight?"

Causes are frequently cardiac (right or left ventricular dysfunction; pulmonary hypertension) or pulmonary (obstructive lung disease) but can also be nutritional (hypoalbuminemia), and/or positional. *Dependent edema* appears in the lowest body parts: the feet and lower legs when sitting, or the sacrum when bedridden. *Anasarca* is severe generalized edema extending to the sacrum and abdomen.

Continue with "Are the rings tight on your fingers? Are your eyelids puffy or swollen in the morning? Have you had to let out your belt?" Also, "Have your clothes gotten tight around the middle?" Consider asking patients who retain fluid to record daily morning weights because edema may not be obvious until several liters of extra fluid have accumulated; however, rapid weight gain (more than 0.5 to 1 kg/day) will occur prior to visible edema (See Box 8-18. Examination of Edema).

Look for the periorbital puffiness and tight rings of nephrotic syndrome and an enlarged waistline from ascites and liver failure.

Box 8-18. Examination of Edema

Inspect both legs from the groin to the feet and also sacrum.

Note:

- Their size and symmetry—Inspect and compare the thighs, calves, and ankles for symmetry. Note their relative size. It is wise to use a tape ruler to measure the circumference of the thighs, calves, and ankles. Normally, the difference in calf circumference is <3 cm. Measure and compare other areas of asymmetry, if needed, including the thighs and ankles.
- Any swelling or edema—Unilateral or bilateral? Extent of swelling?

If swelling or edema is present, *palpate for pitting edema*. **Press firmly but gently with your thumb for at least 20 seconds (1) over the dorsum of each foot, (2) behind each medial malleolus, and (3) over the shins** (Fig. 8-4). Look for *pitting*—a depression caused by pressure from your thumb. Normally there is none. The severity of edema is graded on a subjective four-point scale, from slight to very marked (Box 8-19).

If you detect unilateral swelling or edema, *measure the calves* 10 cm below the tibial tuberosity. Unilateral edema is mainly due to local causes such as venous obstruction, lymphatic obstruction (e.g., filariasis, metastatic carcinoma), superficial or deep tissue infections, arteriovenous aneurysms, stings and bites. Bilateral edema is present in heart failure, cirrhosis, and nephrotic syndrome. Venous distention suggests a venous cause of edema.

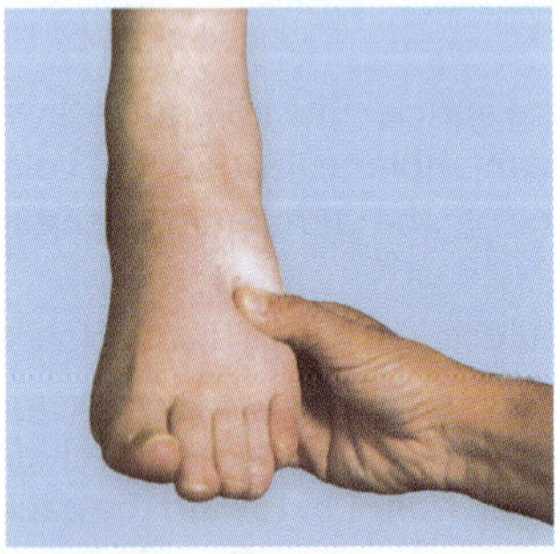

FIGURE 8-4. Palpating for pitting edema.

Box 8-19. Pitting Edema Scale

1+: Barely detectable impression when finger is pressed into skin
2+: Slight indentation; 15 seconds to rebound
3+: Deeper indentation; 30 seconds to rebound
4+: >30 seconds to rebound
Figure 8-5 shows 3+ pitting edema.

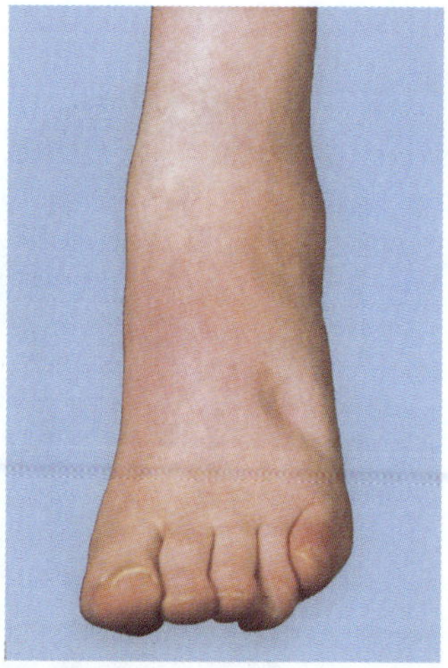

FIGURE 8-5. 3+ pitting edema.

Medicine History Taking OSCE Video: **Edema**

Speech and Language. Note the quantity, rate, loudness, clarity, and fluency of speech. If indicated, test for aphasia.

See Chapter 9, Test for Aphasia, p. 162.

Cognitive Functions. If indicated, assess the following:

- Orientation to time, place, and person
- Attention
- Remote memory
- Recent memory
- New learning abilities

See Chapter 9, Cognitive Functions, p. 155.

Posture, Gait, and Motor Activity. What is the patient's preferred posture?

Patients often prefer sitting upright in left-sided heart failure and leaning forward with arms braced (*tripod position*) in chronic obstructive pulmonary disease (COPD) or acute pericarditis.

Is the patient restless or quiet? How often does the patient change position?

Anxious patients appear agitated and restless. Patients in pain often avoid movement.

Is there any involuntary motor activity? Are some body parts immobile? Which ones?

Look for tremors, other involuntary movements, or paralysis. See Chapter 13, Nervous System, Table 13-8, Tremors and Involuntary Movements.

Does the patient walk smoothly, with comfort, self-confidence, and balance, or is there a limp, fear of falling, loss of balance, or any movement disorder?

An impaired gait increases risk of falls. See Chapter 13, Table 13-3, Abnormalities of Gait and Posture.

Lymph Nodes. Lymph nodes are round, oval, or bean-shaped structures that vary in size according to their location. Some lymph nodes, such as the preauricular nodes, if palpable at all, are typically very small. The inguinal nodes, by contrast, are relatively larger—often 1 cm in diameter and occasionally even 2 cm in an adult. Only the superficial lymph nodes are accessible to physical examination. These include the cervical nodes, the axillary nodes, inguinal nodes and nodes in the arms and legs.

See Table 8-4, Causes of Lymphadenopathy.

Cervical Lymph Nodes. The lymph nodes of the cervical region are variably classified. One classification identifies nodes based on specific names of local anatomy as shown in Figure 8-6 together with the directions of lymphatic drainage.

1. **Submental lymph node group**—in the midline a few centimeters behind the tip of the mandible
2. **Submandibular lymph node group**—midway between the angle and the tip of the mandible
3. **Preauricular lymph node group**—in front of the ear
4. **Posterior auricular lymph node group**—superficial to the mastoid process
5. **Tonsillar (jugulodigastric) lymph node group**—at the angle of the mandible

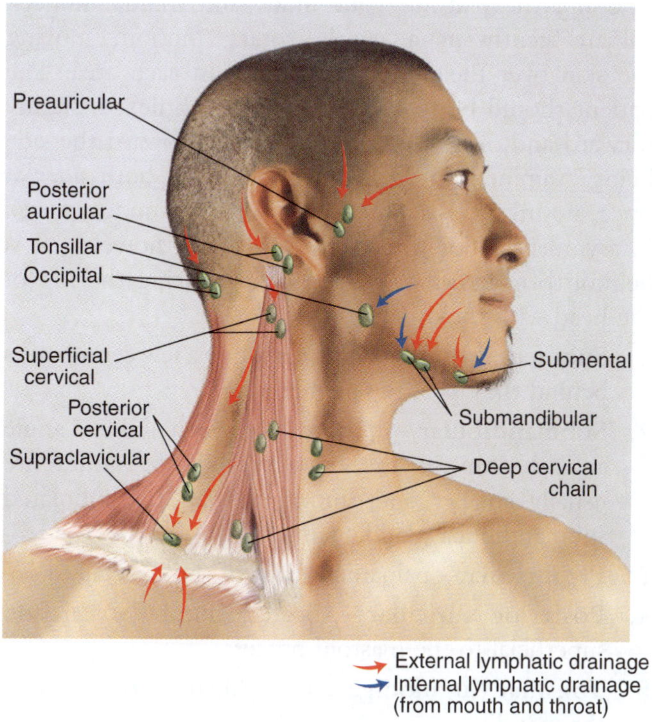

FIGURE 8-6. Lymph nodes of the neck.

6. **Occipital lymph node group**—at the base of the skull posteriorly
7. **Anterior superficial cervical lymph node group**—superficial to the SCM muscle
8. **Posterior cervical lymph node group**—along the anterior edge of the trapezius
9. **Deep cervical chain lymph node group**—deep to the SCM muscle and often inaccessible to examination
10. **Supraclavicular lymph node group**—deep in the angle formed by the clavicle and the SCM muscle

The deep cervical chain is largely obscured by the overlying SCM muscle, but at its two extremes, the tonsillar (jugulodigastric) node and supraclavicular nodes may be palpable. The submandibular nodes lie superficial to the submandibular gland and should be differentiated. Nodes are normally round or ovoid, smooth, and smaller than the submandibular gland. The gland is larger and has a lobulated, slightly irregular surface (see p. 556).

Note that the tonsillar, submandibular, and submental nodes drain portions of the mouth and throat as well as the face. Lymphatic drainage patterns are helpful when assessing possible malignancy or infection. For suspected malignant or inflammatory lesions, look for enlargement of the neighboring regional lymph nodes; when a node is enlarged or tender, look for a source in its nearby drainage area.

Using the pads of your index and middle fingers, palpate gently in a gentle rotary motion, moving the skin over the underlying tissues in each area. The patient should be relaxed, with the neck flexed slightly forward and, if needed, turned slightly toward the side being examined. You can usually examine both sides at once, noting both the presence of lymph nodes as well as asymmetry. For the submental nodes, however, it is helpful to feel with one hand while bracing the top of the head with the other.

1. **Submental**—palpate in the midline a few centimeters behind the tip of the mandible.
2. **Submandibular**—midway between the angle and the tip of the mandible. These nodes are usually smaller and smoother than the lobulated submandibular gland against which they lie.
3. **Preauricular**—palpate in front of the ear (Fig. 8-7).
4. **Posterior auricular**—palpate behind the ear and superficial to the mastoid process.
5. **Tonsillar (jugulodigastric)**—palpate at the angle of the mandible.
6. **Occipital**—palpate at the base of the skull posteriorly.

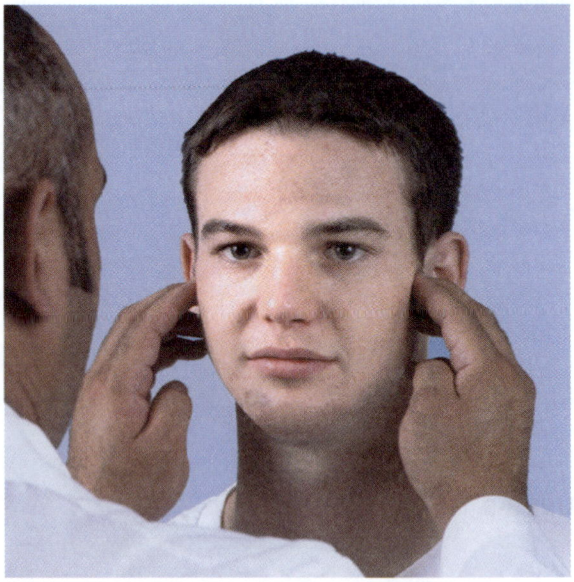

FIGURE 8-7. Palpating the preauricular nodes.

A small hard tender "tonsillar node" high and deep between the mandible and the SCM is probably an elongated temporal styloid process.

1. **Anterior superficial cervical**—palpate for these nodes anterior and superficial to the SCM muscle.
2. **Posterior cervical**—palpate along the anterior edge of the trapezius by flexing the patient's neck slightly forward toward the side being examined (Fig. 8-8).
3. **Deep cervical chain**—deep in the SCM muscle and often inaccessible to examination. Hook your thumb and fingers around either side of the SCM muscle to find them.
4. **Supraclavicular**—palpate deep in the angle formed by the clavicle and the SCM muscle (Fig. 8-9).

Enlargement of a supraclavicular node, especially on the left (**Virchow's node**), suggests possible metastasis from a thoracic or an abdominal malignancy.

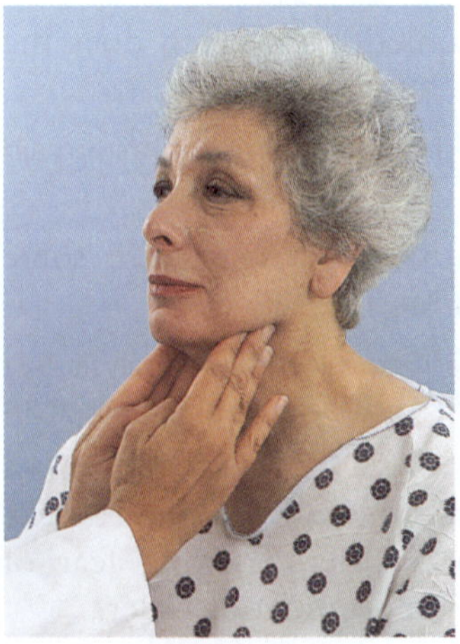

FIGURE 8-8. Palpating the submandibular nodes.

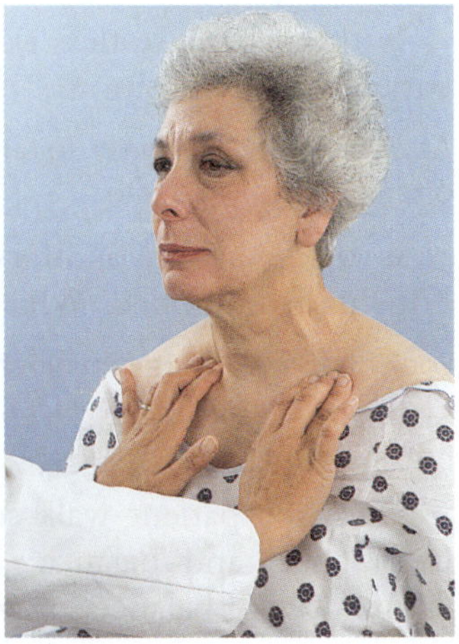

FIGURE 8-9. Palpating the supraclavicular nodes.

Note lymph node *size, shape, delimitation* (discrete or matted together), *mobility, consistency,* and any *tenderness.* Small, mobile, discrete, nontender nodes, sometimes termed **"shotty,"** are frequently found in normal people. Describe enlarged nodes in two dimensions, maximal *length* and *width,* for example, 1 cm × 2 cm.

Tender nodes suggest inflammation; hard or fixed nodes (fixed to underlying structures and not movable on palpation) suggest malignancy.

Also note any overlying *skin changes* (erythema, induration, drainage, or breakdown). Enlarged or tender nodes, if unexplained, call for (1) re-examination of the regions they drain and (2) careful assessment of lymph nodes in other regions to identify regional from generalized lymphadenopathy.

Generalized lymphadenopathy is seen in viral infections like HIV or AIDS, Infectious mononucleosis, Cytomegalovirus; Bacterial infections like tuberculosis, brucellosis, syphilis; autoimmune diseases such as systemic lupus erythromatosus, rheumatoid arthritis; toxoplasmosis, lymphoma, leukemia (acute and chronic), sarcoidosis and lipid storage diseases.

Occasionally, you may mistake a band of muscle or an artery for a lymph node. Unlike a muscle or an artery, you should be able to roll a node in two directions: up and down, and side to side. Neither a muscle nor an artery will pass this test.

Axillary Lymph Nodes. The axillary lymph nodes are arranged in six groups (Fig. 8-10). They lie along the chest wall, usually high in the axilla, midway between the anterior and posterior axillary folds. Of these, the central nodes are most likely to be palpable during physical examination.

- *Anterior (pectoral) group:* Lying along the lower border of the pectoralis minor behind the pectoralis major, these nodes receive lymph vessels from the lateral quadrants of the breast and superficial vessels from the anterolateral abdominal wall above the level of the umbilicus.
- *Posterior (subscapular) group:* Lying in front of the subscapularis muscle, these nodes receive superficial lymph vessels from the back, down as far as the level of the iliac crests.
- *Lateral (humeral or deep) group:* Lying along the medial side of the axillary vein, these nodes receive most of the lymph vessels of the upper limb (except those superficial vessels draining the lateral side).
- *Central group:* Lying in the center of the axilla in the axillary fat, these nodes receive lymph from the above three groups. Nodes are also located between the pectoralis minor and pectoralis major muscles in an area called the Rotter space (**Rotter's nodes**).
- *Apical (terminal) group:* Lying at the apex of the axilla at the lateral border of the first rib, these nodes receive the efferent lymph vessels from all the other axillary nodes. The apical nodes are the final common pathway for all of the axillary lymph nodes.
- *Infraclavicular (deltopectoral) group:* These nodes are not strictly axillary nodes because they are located outside the axilla. They lie in the groove between the deltoid and pectoralis major muscles and receive superficial lymph vessels from the lateral side of the hand, forearm, and arm.

Recall that the axillary lymph nodes drain most of the arm (Fig. 8-11). Lymphatics from the ulnar surface of the forearm and hand, the third and fourth fingers, and

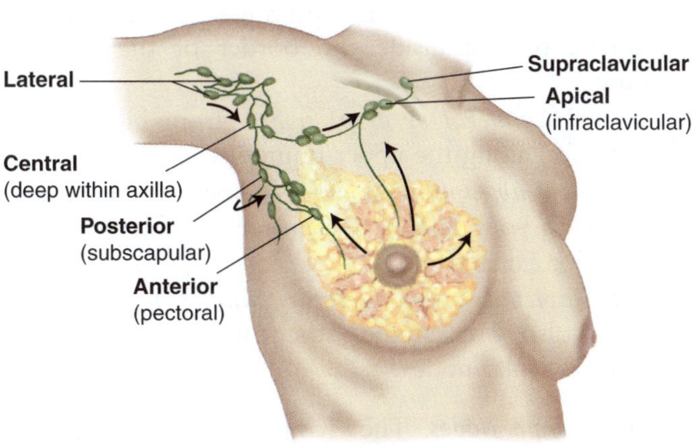

FIGURE 8-10. Direction of lymph flow.

The lymphatic drainage of the breast is of great importance in the spread of carcinoma, and about three-quarters of it is to the axillary nodes.

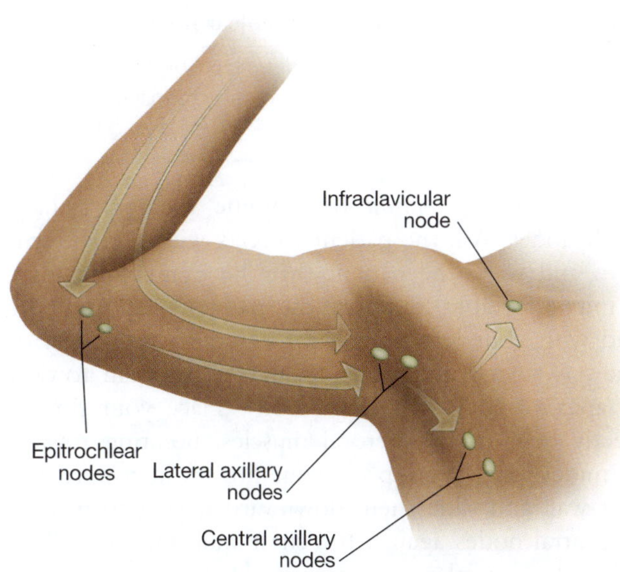

FIGURE 8-11. Lymph nodes of the arm.

the adjacent surface of the middle finger, however, drain first into the epitrochlear nodes. These are located on the medial surface of the arm approximately 3 cm above the elbow. Lymphatics from the rest of the arm drain primarily into the axillary nodes. Some lymph fluid may go directly to the infraclavicular nodes.

Palpate one or more epitrochlear nodes. With the patient's elbow flexed to about 90° and the forearm supported by your hand, reach around behind the arm and feel in the groove between the biceps and triceps muscles, about 3 cm above the medial epicondyle (Fig. 8-12). If a node is present, note its size, consistency, and tenderness. Epitrochlear nodes are usually not palpable in healthy individuals.

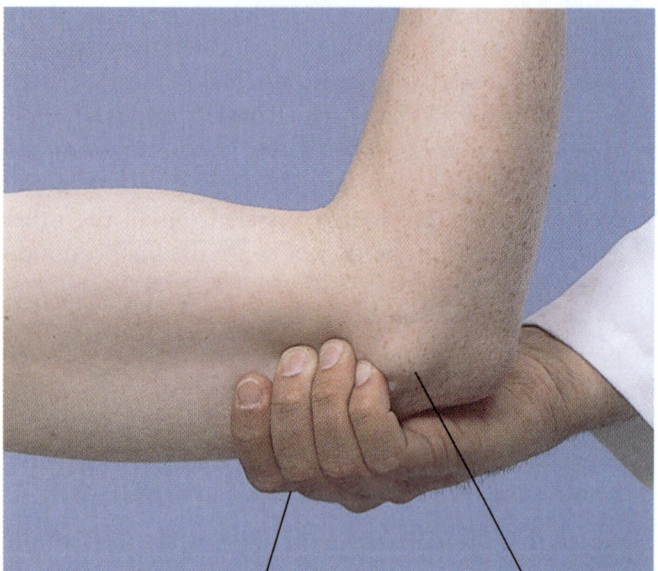

FIGURE 8-12. Palpating the epitrochlear nodes.

An enlarged epitrochlear node suggests local or distal infection or may be associated with lymphadenopathy from lymphoma or human immunodeficiency virus (HIV).

Use your *right hand* to examine the left axillary lymph nodes. Ask the patient to relax with the left arm down and warn the patient that the examination may be uncomfortable. Support the patient's left wrist or hand with your left hand. Cup together the fingers of your *right hand* and reach as high as you can toward the apex of the axilla (Fig. 8-13). Place your fingers directly behind the pectoral muscles, pointing toward the midclavicle. Now press your fingers in toward the chest wall and slide them downward, trying to palpate the central nodes against the chest wall. Of the axillary nodes, the central nodes are most likely to be palpable. One or more soft, small (<1 cm), nontender nodes are

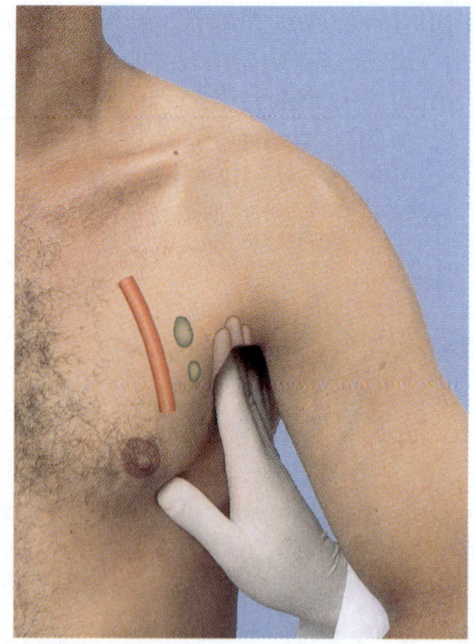

FIGURE 8-13. Palpating the left axilla.

frequently felt. Note their size, shape, delimitation, mobility, consistency, and any tenderness.

Enlarged axillary nodes may result from infection of the hand or arm, recent immunizations or skin tests, or generalized lymphadenopathy.

Use your *left hand* to examine the right axillary lymph nodes.

If the central nodes feel large, hard, or tender, or if there is a suspicious lesion in the drainage areas for the axillary nodes, palpate for the other groups of axillary lymph nodes:

Nodes that are large (≥1 to 2 cm) and firm or hard, matted together, or fixed to the skin or underlying tissues suggest malignancy.

- *Anterior (pectoral) nodes*—grasp the anterior axillary fold between your thumb and fingers, and, with your fingers, palpate inside the border of the pectoral muscle.
- *Lateral (humeral or deep) nodes*—from high in the axilla, feel along the upper humerus.
- *Posterior (subscapular) nodes*—step behind the patient, and, with your fingers, feel inside the muscle of the posterior axillary fold.
- *Infraclavicular (deltopectoral) and supraclavicular nodes*—also reexamine the infraclavicular and supraclavicular nodes.

Inguinal Lymph Nodes. The lymphatics of the lower limb, following the venous supply, consist of both deep and superficial systems. Only the superficial nodes are palpable. The superficial inguinal nodes include two groups (Fig. 8-14). The *horizontal group* lies in a chain high in the anterior thigh below the inguinal ligament. It drains the superficial portions of the lower abdomen and buttock, the external genitalia (but not the testes), the anal canal and perianal area, and the lower vagina.

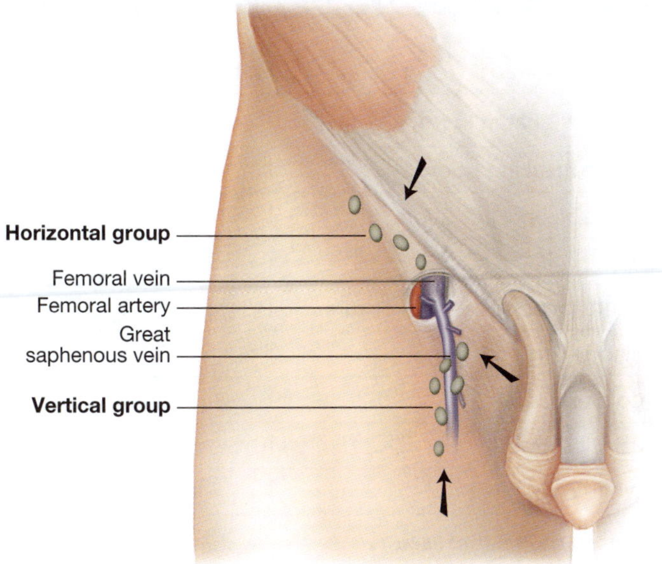

FIGURE 8-14. Superficial inguinal lymph nodes.

The *vertical group* clusters near the upper part of the saphenous vein and drains a corresponding region of the leg. By contrast, lymphatics from the portion of leg drained by the small saphenous vein (the heel and outer aspect of the foot) join the deep system at the level of the popliteal space. Lesions in this space are not usually associated with palpable inguinal lymph nodes.

Palpate the superficial inguinal nodes, including both the horizontal and the vertical groups (Fig. 8-14). Note their size, consistency, and discreteness, and note any tenderness. Nontender, discrete inguinal nodes up to 1 cm or even 2 cm in diameter are commonly palpable in healthy people.

Distinguish between local and generalized lymphadenopathy by locating either a causative lesion in the drainage area or enlarged nodes in at least two other noncontiguous lymph node regions.

Vital Signs

The vital signs—BP, pulse, respiration, and temperature—provide critical initial information that often influences the tempo and direction of your evaluation. If already recorded by office staff, review the vital signs promptly at the outset of the encounter. If the vital signs are abnormal, you will often retake them yourself during the visit. Learn the techniques that ensure accuracy when you measure the vital signs, described in the pages to follow.

Blood Pressure

Blood Pressure Measurement. The accuracy of BP measurements varies according to how these measurements are taken. Office screening with manual and automated cuffs remains common, but elevated readings increasingly require confirmation with home and ambulatory monitoring (Box 8-20).

See Out-of-Office and Self-Monitoring of Blood Pressure, p. 139.

Box 8-20. In-Office Methods for Measuring Blood Pressure

Method	Features
Auscultatory office blood pressure with aneroid or mercury blood pressure	■ Common, inexpensive ■ Subject to patient anxiety ("white coat hypertension"), observer technique, cuff recalibration every 6 months ■ Requires measurements over several visits ■ Ambulatory or home monitoring needed to detect masked hypertension ■ Single measurements with sensitivity and specificity of 75% compared to ambulatory monitoring
Automated oscillometric office blood pressure	■ Requires optimal patient positioning, cuff size and placement, and device calibration ■ Takes multiple measurements over short period ■ Requires confirmatory measurements to reduce misdiagnosis ■ Comparable sensitivity and specificity to manual measurements

Selecting the Appropriate Blood Pressure–Measuring Device (Sphygmomanometer). Measure the BP using a **sphygmomanometer**. Take the time to ensure that your BP measurement will be accurate. Proper technique is important and reduces the inherent variability arising from the patient or examiner, the equipment, and the procedure itself.

To detect BP, an accurate instrument is essential. No matter which device you use, all measuring instruments should be routinely calibrated.

Two types of measuring instruments are currently used to measure BP: manual and digital sphygmomanometers. With *manual sphygmomanometers* (either mercury or aneroid), a stethoscope is required to auscultate both the systolic and diastolic pressures. *Mercury sphygmomanometers*, although still considered the gold standard, have primarily been replaced in most clinical settings with aneroid sphygmomanometers due to safety concerns from accidental breakage of the glass column that contains the mercury. **Aneroid ("without fluid") sphygmomanometers** use mechanical parts to transmit the pressure in the cuff to a dial. These aneroid devices, however, can be knocked out of calibration more easily than mercury ones and should be recalibrated every 6 months for continued accuracy.

Digital sphygmomanometers utilize oscillometric technique to measure BP. They do not require a stethoscope. The cuff is inflated and deflated electronically, and a transducer in the device detects the pressure wave generated by the brachial arterial wall. The systolic and diastolic pressures are calculated electronically using an algorithm producing a digital BP readout.

The BP measurement techniques that follow mostly apply to the use of manual sphygmomanometers.

Preparing the Patient and the Setting. The examining room should be quiet and comfortably warm. The patient should be seated comfortably, with the back supported and legs uncrossed. The patient should avoid smoking, caffeine, or exercise for 30 minutes prior to measurement (Box 8-21). He or she should rest for 5 minutes prior to measuring the BP.

Selecting the Correct Size Blood Pressure Cuff. It is important for clinicians and patients to use a cuff that fits the patient's arm. Follow the guidelines outlined here for selecting the correct size:

- The standard cuff is 12 × 23 cm, appropriate for arm circumferences up to 28 cm.
- Width of the inflatable bladder of the cuff should be about 40% of upper arm circumference (about 12 to 14 cm in the average adult).
- Length of the inflatable bladder should be about 80% of upper arm circumference (almost long enough to encircle the arm).

If the cuff is *too small* (narrow), the blood pressure will read *high;* if the cuff is *too large* (wide), the blood pressure will read *low* on a small arm and *high* on a large arm.

For patients with *large arm circumferences,* use a cuff 16 cm in width. If the upper arm is short despite a large circumference, use a thigh cuff or a very long cuff. If the arm circumference is >50 cm and not amenable to use of a thigh cuff, wrap an appropriately sized cuff around the forearm, hold the forearm at the heart level, and feel for the radial pulse. For the patient with a *very small arm circumference,* consider using a pediatric cuff. Other options include using a Doppler probe at the radial artery or an oscillometric device.

Positioning the Arm and Cuff Appropriately. The arm selected should be free of clothing, fistulas for dialysis, or lymphedema from axillary node dissection or radiation therapy. Palpate the brachial artery to confirm a viable pulse and position the arm so that the brachial artery, at the antecubital crease, is at the heart level. If the patient is seated, rest the arm on a table a little above the patient's waist or roughly level with the fourth interspace at its junction with the sternum; if the patient is standing, try to sup-

Box 8-21. Potential Sources of Inaccuracy in the Measurement of Adult Blood Pressure in Clinical Settings

	Effect on Systolic BP	Effect on Diastolic BP
Patient-Related Factors		
Acute meal ingestion	↓	↓
Acute alcohol ingestion	↓	↓
Acute caffeine use	↑	↑
Acute nicotine use or exposure	↑	↑
Bladder distention	↑	↑
Cold exposure	↑	↑
Paretic arm	↑	↑
White coat effect	↑	↑
Procedure-Related Factors		
Insufficient rest period	↑	↑
Legs crossed at knees	↑	↑
Unsupported arm	↑	↑
Arm lower than heart level	↑	↑
Talking during measurement	↑	↑
Incorrect smaller cuff size	↑	↑
Incorrect larger cuff size	↓	↓
Stethoscope under cuff	↑	↓
Fast cuff deflation rate (>3 mm Hg/sec)	↑	↓
Unsupported back	No effect	↑
Excessive pressure on stethoscope head	No effect	↑

Other factors that may contribute to measurement errors include *device-related factors* (such as device model inaccuracy, integrity and calibration); reliance on a single measurement; interarm variability; and *observer-related factors* including observer hearing deficit, Korotkoff sound interpretation (e.g., phase IV instead of phase V, increase in DBP), and terminal digit preference for zero—a preference to round BP readings to a specific end digit, usually zero (e.g., records 120 mm Hg when the device shows a value between 117 and 122 mm Hg). *BP*, blood pressure; *DBP*, diastolic blood pressure.

port the patient's arm at the midchest level. With the arm at the appropriate level, center the inflatable bladder over the brachial artery. The lower border of the cuff should be about 2.5 cm above the antecubital crease. Secure the cuff snugly. Slightly flex the patient's arm at the elbow.

A loose cuff or a bladder that balloons outside the cuff leads to falsely high readings.

Using the Palpated Radial Pulse Obliteration Pressure to Estimate Systolic Blood Pressure. To decide how high to raise the cuff pressure, first estimate the systolic blood pressure (SBP) by palpating the radial artery. As you palpate the radial artery with the fingers of one hand, rapidly inflate the cuff until the pulse disappears. When using an aneroid device, hold the dial so that it faces you directly. Read this pressure on the manometer *and add 30 mm Hg. Remember this sum value.* Use this value as your *target level* for subsequent inflations to minimize patient discomfort from unnecessarily high cuff pressures. Deflate the cuff promptly and completely and wait for 15 to 30 seconds.

This palpatory technique also avoids the occasional error caused by an *auscultatory gap*—a silent interval that may be present between the systolic and the diastolic pressures (Fig. 8-15).

An unrecognized auscultatory gap may lead to serious underestimation of SBP (150 mm Hg instead of 200 mm Hq in the example below) or overestimation of diastolic blood pressure (DBP).

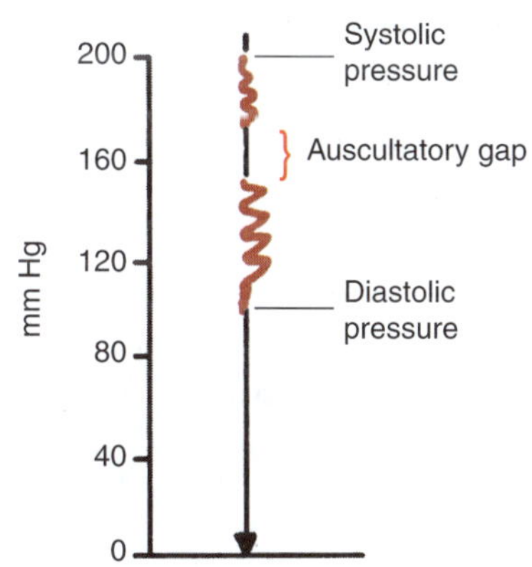

FIGURE 8-15. Auscultatory gap.

If you find an auscultatory gap, record your findings completely (e.g., 200/98 mm Hg with an auscultatory gap from 170 to 150 mm Hg).

An auscultatory gap is associated with arterial stiffness and atherosclerotic disease.

Positioning the Stethoscope Diaphragm or Bell Over the Brachial Artery. Now place the diaphragm or bell of your stethoscope lightly over the brachial artery, taking care to make an air seal with the full rim (Fig. 8-16). There should be a 2- to 3-cm space for the stethoscope between the lower end of the cuff and the antecubital fossa.

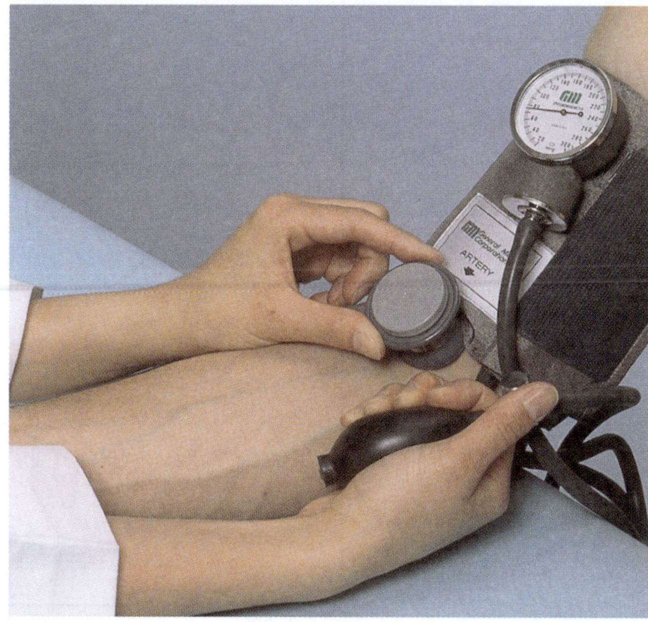

FIGURE 8-16. Properly positioned arm and stethoscope over the brachial artery.

Inflating the Cuff Rapidly to Target Level Followed by Gradual Deflation. Inflate the cuff again rapidly to the target level, and then deflate the cuff slowly at a rate no faster than 2 to 3 mm Hg per second. Avoid slow or repetitive inflations of the cuff because the resulting venous congestion can cause false readings.

By making the sounds less audible, venous congestion may produce artificially low systolic and high diastolic pressures.

Identifying the Systolic and Diastolic Blood Pressures. Note the level when you hear faint, repetitive, clear tapping **Korotkoff sounds** (*phase I*) that gradually increase in intensity for at least two consecutive beats. This is the *SBP.* Do not use the upward deflections of the needle or mercury column on the manometer to measure systolic pressure. This will be followed by a brief period (*phases II and III*) during which the sounds soften and acquire a swishing quality that may become crisper to regain, or even exceed, the intensity of phase I.

Continue to deflate the cuff slowly until the Korotkoff sounds become muffled (*phase IV*) and disappear (*phase V*). To confirm the disappearance point, listen as the pressure falls another 10 to 20 mm Hg. Then deflate the cuff rapidly to zero. The disappearance point (phase V), which is usually only a few mm Hg below the muffling point, provides the best estimate of the *DBP* (Fig. 8-17).

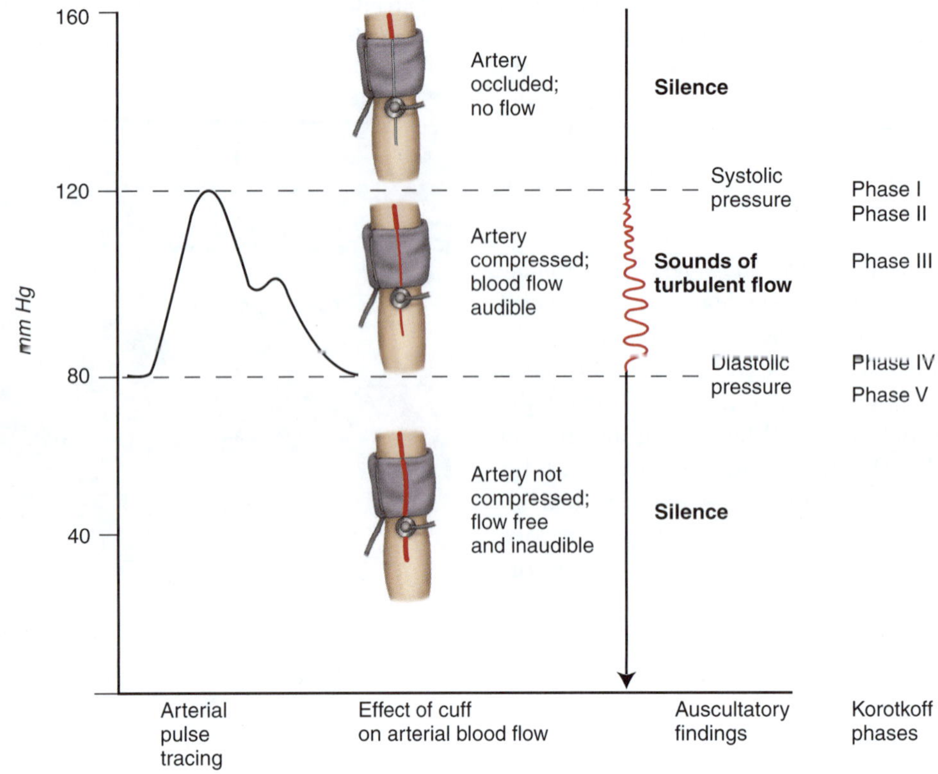

FIGURE 8-17. Auscultating systolic (phase I) and diastolic (phase V) Korotkoff sounds.

Occasionally, as in aortic regurgitation, the sounds never disappear. If the difference is 10 mm Hg or greater, record both figures (e.g., 154/80/68).

BP in adults should be categorized as normal if SBP is <120 mm Hg and DBP is <80 mm Hg.

BP 120 to 129/<80 mm Hg should be categorized as elevated, 130 to 139/80 to 89 mm Hg as stage 1 hypertension, and ≥140/90 mm Hg as stage 2 hypertension.

When you hear weak Korotkoff sounds, consider erroneous placement of your stethoscope, failure to make full skin contact with the bell, and venous engorgement of the patient's arm from repeated inflations of the cuff. If you cannot hear Korotkoff sounds at all, alternative methods using a Doppler probe or direct arterial pressure tracings may be necessary.

Also consider the possibilities of severe vascular disease or shock for inaudible Korotkoff sounds.

In rare cases, patients are pulseless due to occlusive disease in the arteries of all the limbs from Takayasu arteritis, giant cell arteritis, or atherosclerosis.

Read both the systolic and the diastolic levels. Wait for at least 1 minute and repeat. Average your readings. The first reading in a series is usually the highest. Additional readings should be taken if the difference between the first two is >5 mm Hg.

Physiology OSCE Video:
Blood Pressure

Normally, there may be a difference in pressure measurements of 5 mm Hg and sometimes up to 10 mm Hg on the arms of the same patient. Measure BP in both arms at least once. Subsequent readings for the patient should be made on the arm with the higher pressure.

A pressure difference of more than 10 to 15 mm Hg occurs in subclavian steal syndrome, supravalvular aortic stenosis, and aortic dissection and should be investigated.

Classifying Normal and Abnormal Blood Pressure. In 2013, the *Eighth Joint National Committee (JNC 8)* issued the JNC 8 report based on rigorous scientific review of clinical trial data. This guideline recommends classifying BP into four categories (Box 8-22). When the systolic and diastolic levels fall in different categories, use the higher category. For example, 170/88 mm Hg is stage 2 hypertension; 136/78 mm Hg is stage 1 hypertension.

Box 8-22. Blood Pressure Categories for Adults (JNC 8)

Category[a]	Systolic (mm Hg)		Diastolic (mm Hg)
Normal	<120	and	<80
Elevated	120–129	and	<80
Stage 1 hypertension	130–139	or	80–89
Stage 2 hypertension	≥140	or	≥90

Patients with SBP and DBP in two categories should be designated to the higher BP category. *BP*, blood pressure; *DBP*, diastolic blood pressure; *JNC*, Eighth Joint National Committee; *SBP*, systolic blood pressure.

[a]BP indicates blood pressure (based on an average of ≥2 careful readings obtained on ≥2 occasions).

Low Blood Pressure. Interpret relatively low levels of BP in the light of past readings and the patient's clinical state.

A pressure of 110/70 mm Hg would usually be normal but could also indicate significant hypotension if past pressures have been high.

Orthostatic Blood Pressure Measurements. If indicated, perform orthostatic BP measurements to assess *orthostatic* or *postural hypotension*, common in older adults. Measure BP in two positions—*supine* after the patient is resting from 3 to 10 minutes, and then within 3 minutes once the patient *stands up*. Normally, as the patient rises from the horizontal to the standing position, SBP drops slightly or remains unchanged, whereas DBP rises slightly.

Orthostatic hypotension is a sustained reduction in SBP of at least 20 mm Hg or in DBP of at least 10 mm Hg within 3 minutes of standing.

Causes of orthostatic hypotension include drugs, moderate or severe blood loss, prolonged bed rest, and diseases of the autonomic nervous system.

Special Patient-Related Situations

White Coat Hypertension. **White coat hypertension** *(isolated clinic hypertension)* is defined as BP ≥140/90 mm Hg in medical settings and mean awake ambulatory readings <135/85 mm Hg. This phenomenon, reported in up to 20% of patients with elevated office BP, is important to identify since it carries normal to slightly increased cardiovascular risk and does not require treatment. It is attributed to a conditioned anxiety response. Poor measurement technique, including rounding of measurements to zero, the presence of a physician or nurse, and even the prior diagnosis of hypertension can also substantially alter office readings. Replacing manual office measurements with an automated device that makes several readings with the patient seated alone in a quiet room has been shown to reduce the "white coat effect." White coat effect, however, is usually considered clinically significant when office SBP/DBPs are >20/10 mm Hg higher than home BP monitoring (HBPM) or ambulatory BP monitoring (ABPM) SBP/DBPs.

Masked Hypertension. **Masked hypertension**, defined as office BP <140/90 mm Hg, but an elevated daytime BP of >135/85 mm Hg on home or ambulatory testing, is more serious. Untreated adults with masked hypertension, an estimated 10% to 30% of the general population, have an increased risk of cardiovascular disease and end-organ damage. Consider HBPM or ABPM.

Concurrent Arrhythmias. Irregular rhythms produce variations in BP and therefore unreliable measurements. Ignore the effects of an occasional premature contraction. With frequent premature contractions or atrial fibrillation, determine the average of several observations and note that your measurements are approximate. Ambulatory monitoring for 2 to 24 hours is recommended.

Detection of an irregularly irregular rhythm suggests atrial fibrillation. For all irregular patterns, obtain an ECG to identify the type of rhythm.

Out-of-Office and Self-Monitoring of Blood Pressure. Self-monitoring of BP refers to the regular measurement of BP by a patient outside the clinic setting. When done at home, it is called **HBPM**. **ABPM**, on the other hand, is used to obtain out-of-office BP readings at preset intervals, usually programmed to obtain readings over a period of 24 hours while patients go about their normal daily activities. Although ABPM is generally accepted as the best out-of-office measurement method, HBPM is often a more practical approach in clinical practice (Box 8-23). Typically, a clinic BP of 140/90 mm Hg (hypertension) corresponds to:

- Home BP: 135/85 mm Hg
- Ambulatory BP:
  - 24-Hour average: 130/80 mm Hg
  - Daytime (awake) average: 135/85 mm Hg
  - Nighttime (asleep) average: 120/70 mm Hg

Both ABPM and HBPM typically provide BP estimates that can be helpful for confirmation and management of hypertension (Box 8-24). If you recommend out-of-office BP monitoring, advise patients about how to choose the best upper arm cuff for home use and have it recalibrated. Let them know that wrist and finger monitors are popular but less accurate. SBP increases in more distal arteries, whereas DBP falls, and hydrostatic effects introduce errors due to differences in position relative to the heart.

Box 8-23. Out-of-Office Methods for Measuring Blood Pressure

Method	Features
Home blood pressure monitoring (HBPM)	■ Accurate automated device applied by patient, easy to use, less expensive than ambulatory monitoring ■ Acceptable alternative if ambulatory monitoring not feasible; more predictive of cardiovascular risk than office measurements ■ Requires patient education for accurate technique, repeated measurements (two morning, two evening readings daily for 1 week); nighttime readings not recorded ■ Detects white coat hypertension—present in 20% of patients ■ Detects masked hypertension—present in 10% of patients ■ Sensitivity 85%, specificity 62% compared to ambulatory monitoring
Ambulatory blood pressure monitoring (ABPM)	■ Automated; clinical and research "gold standard" ■ Provides 24-hour average BPs and averages of daytime (awake), nighttime (asleep), systolic and diastolic BP ■ Shows whether nocturnal BP "dips" (normal) or stays elevated (a cardiovascular disease risk factor) ■ More expensive; may not be covered by insurance

BP, blood pressure.

Patient education about the correct use of home monitors is essential. Make sure that patients understand all the steps needed to ensure accurate readings at home, as detailed in this section.

Box 8-24. Corresponding Blood Pressure Values in mm Hg for Clinic, Home, Daytime, Nighttime, and 24-Hour Ambulatory Measurements

Clinic	HBPM	Daytime ABPM	Nighttime ABPM	24-Hour ABPM
120/80	120/80	120/80	100/65	115/75
130/80	130/80	130/80	110/65	125/75
140/90	135/85	135/85	120/70	130/80
160/100	145/90	145/90	140/85	145/90

ABPM, ambulatory blood pressure monitoring; *HBPM*, home blood pressure monitoring.

Source: Whelton PK, et al. Hypertension. 2018;71(6):1269–1324.

Pulse. Pulse is defined as rhythmic expansion of the arterial wall due to transmission of pressure waves along the walls of the arteries that are produced during each systole of the heart (Box 8-25). The ejection of blood from the aorta causes abrupt expansion of an artery and its transmission throughout the arterial system.

Box 8-25. Windkessel Effect

As the left ventricle ejects blood during systole, the elastic aorta expands to accommodate the stroke volume resulting in a rise in intra-aortic pressure from diastolic blood pressure to systolic blood pressure. The ejected blood has kinetic energy, whereas the stretched blood vessel possesses potential energy. During diastole, as the recoiling of the stretched blood vessel occurs, the stored potential energy gets converted into kinetic energy resulting in forward flow of the blood.

Examine the arterial pulses for rate, rhythm, volume, character, condition of the vessel wall, and equality. The radial pulse is commonly used to assess the rate and rhythm (Fig. 8-18). With the pads of your index, middle, and ring fingers, compress the radial artery until a maximal pulsation is detected. The index finger should be kept proximal to the heart and ring finger distally. The purpose of the distal finger is to obliterate the backflow coming from the ulnar artery. Light pressure is given by the ring finger to obliterate. Rest all parameters of the pulse are judged by the middle finger. For better feeling of the pulse, keep the forearm in semipronated position with the wrist slightly flexed.

If the rhythm is regular and the rate seems normal, count the rate for 30 seconds and multiply by 2. If the rate is unusually fast or slow, count for 60 seconds. The usual range of normal is 60 to 90 to 100 beats/min.

An elevated resting heart rate is associated with an increased risk of cardiovascular disease and mortality.

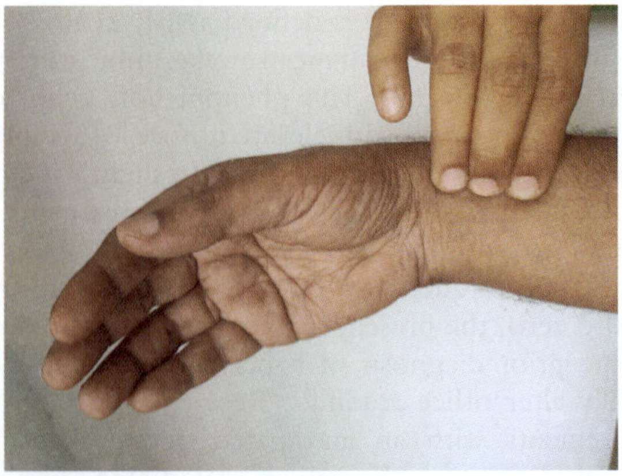

FIGURE 8-18. Palpating the radial pulse.

The normal range of the heart rates varies with age. A faster heart rate is seen in infants and children as compared to in adults. Factors affecting the heart rate are gender, activity, pain, stimulants, emotional state, medications, and disease state.

Tachycardia is a heart rate more than 100 beats/min in an adult. It is found in trauma, blood loss, anemia, infection, fear, fever, pain, hyperthyroidism, shock, and anxiety as a result of increased metabolic demands or low blood volume. In patients with cardiac disease, tachycardia may indicate congestive heart failure, myocardial ischemia, or dysrhythmia.

Bradycardia is a heart rate less than 60 beats/min in an adult. Drugs such as digoxin and β-blockers cause bradycardia. Bradycardia is also seen in myocardial infarction, hypothyroidism, increased intracranial pressure, and eye surgery.

Asystole is the absence of a pulse. Cardiac arrest, hypovolemia, pneumothorax, cardiac tamponade, and acidosis can cause asystole.

Assess for pulse deficit (Box 8-26) if the patient has irregular heart rate and signs and symptoms such as dyspnea, fatigue, chest pain, syncope, and palpitation.

Box 8-26. Pulse Deficit

- A pulse deficit provides an indirect evaluation of the ability of each heart contraction to eject enough blood into the peripheral circulation to create a pulse.
- To assess for a pulse deficit, the examiner and a colleague will assess the radial and the apical pulse rates at the same time and compare measurements. The pulse deficit is the difference between the apical and the radial pulse rate.
- Pulse deficits are frequently associated with arrhythmias. It is essential to recognize a pulse deficit because it indicates the heart's ability to perfuse the body adequately.

Rhythm. Begin by palpating the radial pulse. Is the rhythm regular or irregular? If there are any irregularities, assess the rhythm at the cardiac apex by listening with your stethoscope. If irregular, try to identify a pattern: (1) Do early beats appear in a basically regular rhythm? (2) Does the irregularity vary consistently with respiration? (3) Is the rhythm totally irregular?

The rhythm may vary with respirations, speeding up during inspiration and slowing with expiration. This is common in children and young adults and is called a sinus dysrhythmia or sinus arrhythmia.

Volume. Volume, or amplitude, indicates the volume of blood flowing through the vessel. It is the degree of expansion of the arterial walls during each pulse wave. The pulse volume gives an indication of the left ventricular stroke volume. It is described on a scale of 0 to 4+ (Box 8-27).

Box 8-27. Scale for Measuring Pulse Volume

Scale	Description
0	Nonpalpable or absent
1+	Weak, diminished, and barely palpable
2+	Normal, expected
3+	Full, increased
4+	Bounding

Usually in healthy individuals, the volume is normal and equal on both the sides. The normal pulse volume is 2+ (Box 8-28).

Box 8-28. Examination of Pulse Volume (Amplitude) and Contour

- The patient should be supine with the head of the bed elevated to about 30° angle. First, inspect the neck for carotid pulsations, often visible just medial to the sternocleidomastoid (SCM) muscles. Then place your index and middle fingers (Fig. 8-19) or left thumb (Fig. 8-20) on the right carotid artery in the lower third of the neck and palpate for pulsations.
- Press just inside the medial border of a relaxed SCM muscle, roughly at the level of the cricoid cartilage. Avoid pressing on the carotid sinus, which lies adjacent to the top of the thyroid cartilage. For the left carotid artery, use your right fingers or thumb. Slowly increase pressure until you feel a maximal pulsation, and then slowly decrease pressure until you best sense the arterial pressure and contour.

Low pulse volume is detected in heart failure, hypovolemia, shock, and arrhythmias. Bounding pulses are noted with early stages of septic shock, exercise, fever, and anxiety.

Pulsus alternans is a regular rhythm alternating with a strong and weak pulse; it indicates severe left ventricular failure.

Premature beats of low amplitude may not be transmitted to the peripheral pulses, leading to underestimates of the heart rate.

See Table 8-5, Selected Heart Rates and Rhythms, and Table 8-6, Selected Irregular Rhythms.

Always check an ECG to identify the type of rhythm.

Character. The character of the pulse is best appreciated by palpating the carotid artery in the neck (Figs 8-19 and 8-20). The normal carotid pulse has a smooth, rapid upstroke or ascending limb to a smooth, dome-shaped summit. The abnormalities in the pulse include the rate, rhythm, volume, and/or contour abnormalities. Depending on these changes, various types of abnormal pulses are described. The character of the pulse is described as "normal" if there is no abnormality detected.

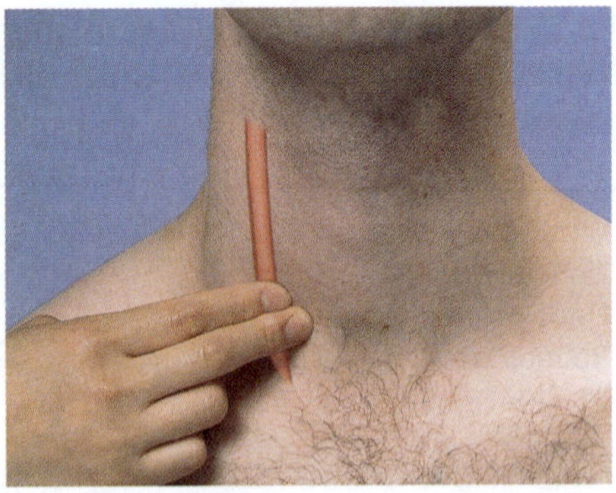

FIGURE 8-19. Palpating the carotid pulse with index and middle fingers.

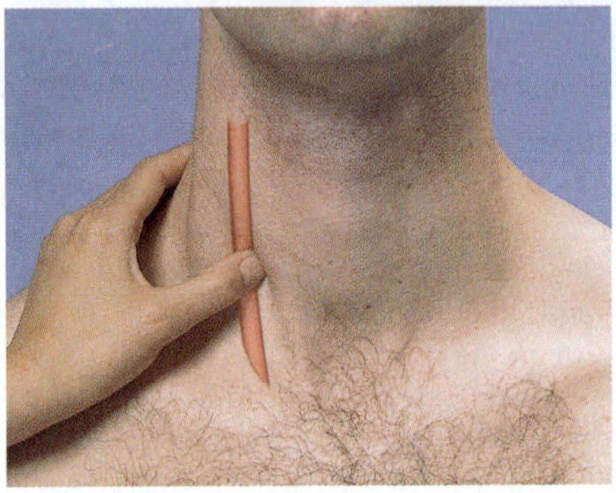

FIGURE 8-20. Palpating the carotid pulse with the thumb.

The contour of the pulses depends on the caliber of the blood vessel, stroke volume, ejection velocity, arterial compliance, and peripheral resistance. The arterial pulse upstroke increases with distance from the heart.

See Table 8-7, Abnormalities of the Arterial Pulse and Pressure Waves.

Equality. Pulse equality refers to simultaneous palpation of pulses at two sites for pulse volume and timings. For example, palpate the radial pulse on the right and left wrists at the same time and compare whether the pulse volume is equal. Similarly, palpate the right radial pulse and right femoral pulse at the same time. Assessment of pulse equality provides data about conditions such as arterial obstructions and aortic coarctation. However, never palpate the carotid pulses at the same time as this can decrease and/or compromise cerebral blood flow.

Inequality between the radial pulses may be due to anatomical variations, thoracic inlet syndromes, pre-subclavian coarctation, compression of the axillary artery, aortic arch syndrome, supravalvular aortic stenosis, and Volkmann's ischemic contracture.

If there is a palpable delay from the radial to the femoral pulse, it suggests coarctation of the aorta or at least an aortic obstruction below the origin of the left subclavian artery.

Difference of timing of the radial and dorsalis pedis pulses is 0.02 to 0.03 second. Inequality of the brachial pulse may be due to thrombosis, embolism, or atherosclerosis of the aorta.

Condition of the Vessel Wall. Examine the condition of the arterial wall for evidence of arterial thickening or undue mobility. The radial artery is generally palpated for this purpose.

Place three fingers over the radial artery. Press the proximal finger firmly to obliterate the blood flow so that loss of impulse is felt by the middle finger. Empty the artery with the distal finger, and roll the radial artery against the bone by the middle finger. Alternatively, apply sufficient pressure on the brachial artery to abolish pulsation in the radial artery. Now roll the radial artery over the bony surface and try to feel the arterial wall.

The normal vessel is soft and nonpalpable. The thickened vessel feels cord-like with consistency firm to hard.

Increase in vessel wall thickness occurs in atherosclerosis and Monckeberg medial calcific sclerosis.

Physiology OSCE Video:
Pulse

Respiration. Observe the rate, rhythm, depth, and effort of breathing. Count the number of respirations in 1 minute either by visual inspection or by subtly listening over the patient's trachea with your stethoscope during your examination of the head and neck or chest. Normally, adults take approximately 12 to 20 breaths/min in a quiet, regular pattern. An occasional sigh is normal. Check to see whether expiration is prolonged.

A respiration rate under 12 breaths/min or over 25 breaths/min while resting is considered abnormal.

Prolonged expiration is common in COPD.

Temperature. *Measure the core body temperature.* The core body temperature, measured internally, is approximately 37°C (98.6°F) and fluctuates approximately 1°C over the course of the day. It is lowest in the early morning and highest in the afternoon and evening. Women have a wider range of normal temperature than men.

Fever, or pyrexia, refers to an elevated body temperature. Hyperpyrexia refers to extreme elevation in temperature, above 41.1°C (106°F), whereas hypothermia refers to an abnormally low temperature, below 35°C (95°F) rectally.

Although the research gold standard for core body temperature is the blood temperature in the pulmonary artery, clinical practice relies on noninvasive oral, rectal, axillary, tympanic membrane, and temporal artery measurements. Tympanic membrane and temporal artery temperatures use infrared thermometry.

- *Oral and rectal temperature* measurements remain common. Oral temperatures are generally *lower* than the core body temperature. They are also *lower* than rectal temperatures by an average of 0.4 to 0.5°C (0.7 to 0.9°F), and *higher* than axillary temperatures by approximately 1°C (1.8°F).
- *Axillary temperatures* take 5 to 10 minutes to register and are considered less accurate than other measurements.
- *Tympanic membrane temperatures* can be more variable than oral or rectal temperatures.
- Studies vary in methodology, but suggest that in adults, *oral and temporal artery temperatures* correlate more closely with the pulmonary artery temperature but are about 0.5°C (0.9°F) lower.

Causes of fever include infection, trauma such as surgery or crush injuries, malignancy, drug reactions, and immune disorders such as collagen vascular disease.

The chief cause of hypothermia is exposure to cold. Other causes include reduced movement as in paralysis, interference with vasoconstriction from sepsis or excess alcohol, starvation, hypothyroidism, and hypoglycemia. Older adults are especially susceptible to hypothermia and also less likely to develop fever.

Oral Temperature. For *oral temperatures,* options include electronic or glass thermometers. Due to breakage and mercury exposure, glass thermometers have largely been replaced by electronic thermometers. If using an *electronic thermometer,* carefully place the disposable cover over the probe and insert the thermometer under the tongue. Position the tip of the thermometer as far back as possible on either side of the frenulum linguae. Ask the patient to close both lips, and then watch closely for the digital readout (Fig. 8-21). An accurate temperature recording usually takes about 10 seconds.

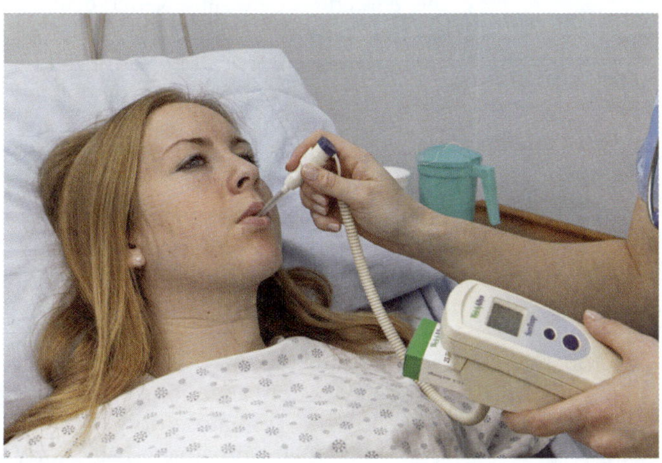

FIGURE 8-21. Taking the oral temperature using an electronic thermometer. (From Taylor C, et al. *Fundamentals of Nursing: The Art and Science of Person-Centered Nursing Care.* 8th ed. Wolters Kluwer; 2015:605, Fig. 24-1-2.)

For *glass thermometers,* shake the thermometer down to 35°C (96°F) or below, insert it under the tongue, instruct the patient to close both lips, and wait for 3 to 5 minutes. Then read the thermometer, reinsert it for a minute, and read it again. If the temperature is still rising, repeat this procedure until the reading remains stable. Note that hot or cold liquids, and even smoking, can alter the temperature reading. In these situations, delay taking the temperature for 10 to 15 minutes.

Rectal Temperature. For a *rectal temperature,* ask the patient to lie on one side with the hip flexed. Select a rectal thermometer with a stubby tip, lubricate it, and insert it about 3 to 4 cm (1.5 in) into the anal canal, in a direction pointing to the umbilicus. Remove it after 3 minutes, and then read. Alternatively, use an electronic thermometer after lubricating the probe cover. Wait about 10 seconds for the digital temperature recording to appear (Fig. 8-22).

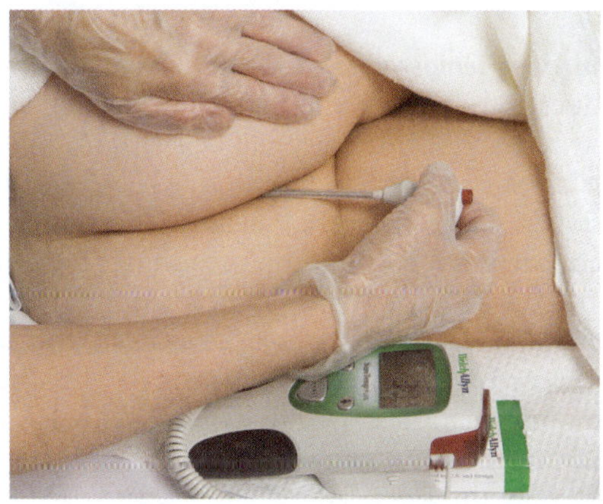

FIGURE 8-22. Taking the rectal temperature using an electronic thermometer. (From Craven RF, et al. *Fundamentals of Nursing: Human Health and Function.* 8th ed. Wolters Kluwer; 2017, Fig. 18-16.)

Rapid respiratory rates tend to increase the discrepancy between oral and rectal temperatures. In these situations, rectal temperatures are more reliable.

Tympanic Membrane Temperature. The tympanic membrane shares the same blood supply as the hypothalamus, where temperature regulation occurs in the brain. Accurate temperature readings require access to the tympanic membrane. Make sure that the external auditory canal is free of cerumen, which can lower temperature readings. Stabilize the patient's head; then gently pull the ear straight back (for children up to age 1) or up and back (for children age 1 and older to adults). Position the probe in the canal so that the infrared beam is aimed at the tympanic membrane, or otherwise the measurement will be invalid. Wait for 2 to 3 seconds until the digital temperature reading appears (Fig. 8-23).

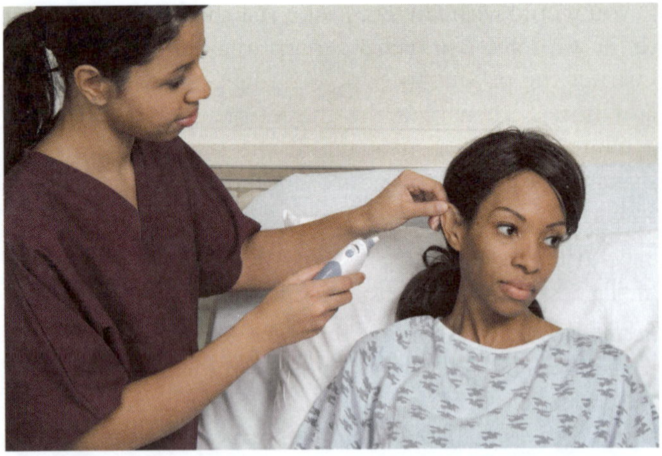

FIGURE 8-23. Taking the tympanic temperature using a tympanic thermometer. (From Springhouse. *Lippincott's Visual Encyclopedia of Clinical Skills*. Wolters Kluwer Health/Lippincott Williams & Wilkins; 2009:519.)

Temporal Artery Temperature. This method takes advantage of the location of the temporal artery, which branches off the external carotid artery and lies within a millimeter of the skin surface of the forehead, cheek, and behind the earlobes. Place the probe against the center of the forehead, depress the infrared scanning button, and brush the device across the forehead, down the cheek, and behind an earlobe (Fig. 8-24). Read the display, which records the highest measured temperature. Industry information suggests that combined forehead and behind-the-ear contact is more accurate than scanning only the forehead.

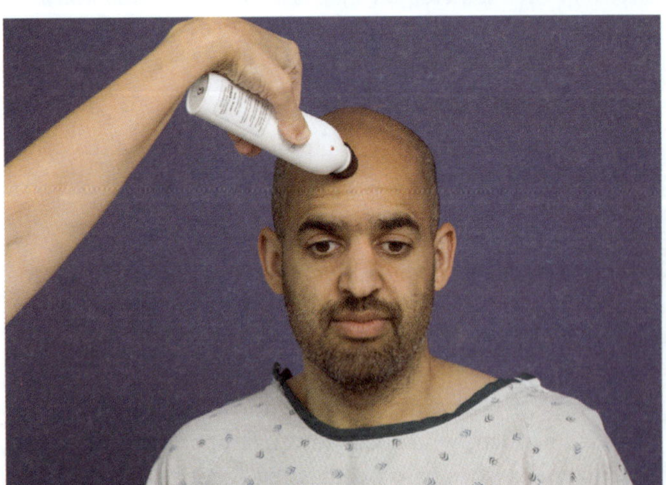

FIGURE 8-24. Taking the temporal temperature using a temporal thermometer. (From Lynn P. *Taylor's Clinical Nursing Skills: A Nursing Process Approach*. 5th ed. Wolters Kluwer; 2019:46, Fig. 2-9.)

ACUTE AND CHRONIC PAIN

The International Association for the Study of Pain defines **pain** as "an unpleasant sensory and emotional experience" associated with tissue damage. The experience of pain is complex and multifactorial. Pain involves sensory, emotional, and cognitive processing but may lack a specific physical etiology.

Acute pain is "the normal, predicted physiological response to an adverse chemical, thermal, or mechanical stimulus" that typically lasts less than 3 to 6 months and is commonly associated with surgery, trauma, and acute illness. It may also be a useful and life-sustaining function (protective function). Symptoms can last hours, days, or weeks but gradually resolve as the injured tissues heal.

Chronic pain is defined in several ways: pain not associated with cancer or other medical conditions that persists for more than 3 to 6 months, pain lasting more than 1 month beyond the course of an acute illness or injury, or pain recurring at intervals of months or years.

Types of Pain

Review the summary of types of pain to aid in your diagnosis and management (Box 8-29).

Box 8-29. Types of Pain	
Nociceptive (somatic) pain	■ **Nociceptive (somatic) pain** is linked to tissue damage to the skin, musculoskeletal system, or viscera (visceral pain), but the sensory nervous system is intact, as in arthritis or spinal stenosis. It can be acute or chronic. It is mediated by the afferent A-delta and C-nerve fibers of the sensory system. The involved afferent nociceptors can be sensitized by inflammatory mediators and modulated by both psychological processes and neurotransmitters like endorphins, histamines, acetylcholine, serotonin, norepinephrine, and dopamine. ■ It is usually described as *dull, pressing, pulling, throbbing, boring, spasmodic,* or *colicky*.
Neuropathic pain	■ **Neuropathic pain** is a direct consequence of a lesion or disease affecting the somatosensory system. Over time, neuropathic pain may become independent of the inciting injury. It may persist even after healing from the initial injury has occurred.

(continued)

Box 8-29. Types of Pain (*continued*)

Mechanisms postulated to evoke neuropathic pain include central nervous system—brain or spinal cord—injury from stroke or trauma; peripheral nervous system disorders causing entrapment or pressure on spinal nerves, plexuses, or peripheral nerves; and referred pain syndromes with increased or prolonged pain responses to inciting stimuli. These triggers appear to induce changes in pain signal processing through "neuronal plasticity," leading to pain that persists beyond healing from the initial injury.

- It is often described as *electric shock–like, stabbing, burning,* or *"pins and needles."*

Source: Institute of Medicine. *Relieving Pain in America: A Blueprint for Transforming Prevention, Care, Education, and Research (2011).* Available at https://www.nap.edu/catalog/13172/relieving-pain-in-america-a-blueprint-for-transforming-prevention-care. Accessed October 28, 2018.

Assessing Acute and Chronic Pain

Eliciting the Patient's History. Adopt a multidisciplinary, measurement-based approach to assessing pain, carefully listening to the patient's story, the many features of pain, and contributing factors. Elicit the full history of the patient's pain, tailoring your approach to each patient's unique experience. Ask the patient to describe the pain and how it started. Is it related to a site of injury, movement, or time of day? What is the quality of the pain—sharp, dull, burning? Ask whether the pain radiates or follows a particular pattern. What makes the pain better or worse? Pursue the seven features of pain, as you would with any symptom. Ask the patient to point to the pain because verbal descriptions can be imprecise.

Numerous validated brief screening tools are available for office use.

See Chapter 3, for discussion of the seven attributes of a symptom, p. 51.

Ask about treatments that the patient has tried, including medications, physical therapy, and alternative medicines. A comprehensive medication history identifies drugs that interact with analgesics and reduce their efficacy.

Explore any comorbid conditions such as arthritis, diabetes, HIV/AIDS, substance abuse, sickle cell disease, or psychiatric disorders. These can have significant effects on the patient's experience of pain.

Chronic pain is the leading cause of disability and impaired performance at work. Inquire about the effects of pain on the patient's daily activities, mood, sleep, work, and sexual activity.

Depressive, somatoform, and anxiety disorders affect the patient's coping strategies and have to be identified in order to effectively treat acute pain, in particular, chronic pain.

Assessing Severity of the Pain. Use a consistent method to assess pain severity. Three scales are common: the Visual Analog Scale (VAS), the Numeric Rating Scale (NRS), and the Wong–Baker FACES® Pain Rating Scale (Fig. 8-25). The VAS is usually a horizontal line with verbal descriptive anchors at each end to express the extremes of pain. Patients mark the point on the line that best corresponds to their symptom severity. In the NRS, there are numerical ratings from 0 to 10—zero indicates the absence of pain, while 10 represents the most intense pain possible. The patient indicates the number that corresponds to his or her pain intensity.

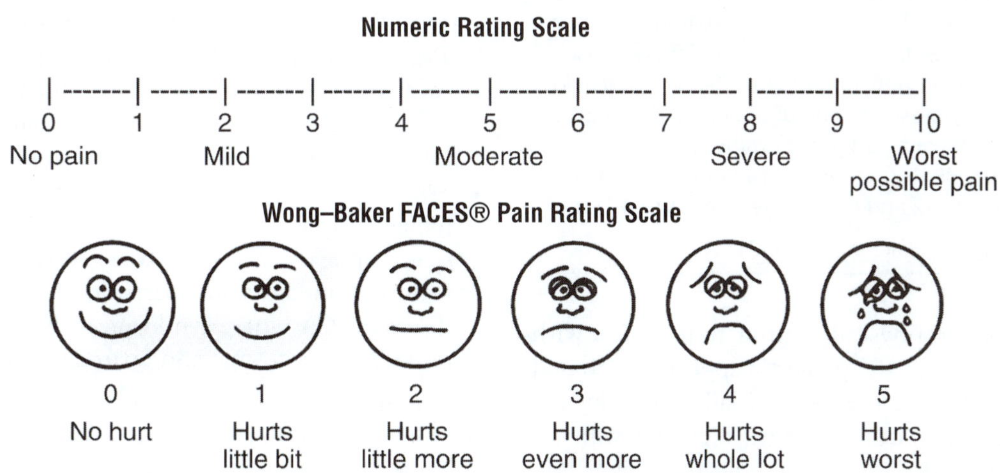

FIGURE 8-25. Numeric Rating Scale (NRS) and the Wong–Baker FACES® Pain Rating Scale. (From King MS, Lipsky MS. *Step-Up to Geriatrics.* Wolters Kluwer; 2017, Fig. 5-5.)

The Wong–Baker FACES® Pain Rating Scale can be used by children as well as patients with language barriers or cognitive impairment. Six faces depict different expressions, ranging from happy to extremely upset. Each is assigned a numerical rating between 0 (smiling) and 10 (crying). Patients can point to the picture that best represents the degree and intensity of their pain. The Faces Pain Scale—Revised (FPS-R) by the International Association for the Study of Pain is also commonly used. Numerous more detailed multidimensional tools like the Brief Pain Inventory and the McGill Pain Questionnaire are also available but take longer to administer.

The use of questionnaires, pain diaries, and analogue scales to complement history and physical examination is part of the essential documentation for every pain treatment plan.

RECORDING YOUR FINDINGS

Recording the General Examination

"Mrs. Pallavi is a young, healthy-appearing woman, well-groomed, fit, and cheerful. She is well hydrated and nourished. Skin is dry and intact without rashes or lesions. Nail beds pink with no pallor, cyanosis, and clubbing. Height is 5 ft 4 in; weight, 65 kg; BMI, 24; extremities are warm and without edema; BP, 120/80, right and left arms; pulse, 72 beats/min and regular; normal volume and character. All peripheral pulses are equal and symmetric. Arterial wall is not palpable; RR, 16; temperature, 37.5°C."

OR

"Mr. Anurag is an elderly man who looks pale and chronically ill. He is alert, with good eye contact but unable to speak more than two or three words at a time due to shortness of breath. He has intercostal muscle retraction when breathing and sits upright in bed. He is thin, with diffuse muscle wasting. He Is mildly dehydrated and fairly nourished. There is no pallor, cyanosis, clubbing, or lymphadenopathy. Height is 6 ft 2 in; weight, 82 kg; extremities are warm with dependent edema; BP, 160/95, right arm; pulse, 108 beats/min and irregular; RR, 32 and labored; temperature, 101.2°F."

These findings suggest exacerbation of COPD.

Your write-up of the physical examination begins with a general description of the patient's appearance, based on the general survey. Note that initially you may use sentences to describe your findings; later you will use phrases. Choose vivid and graphic adjectives, as if you are painting a picture in words. Avoid clichés such as "well developed," "well nourished," or "in no acute distress," because they are too general to convey the special features of the patient before you. Record the vital signs taken at the time of your examination rather than earlier in the day. (Common abbreviations for blood pressure, heart rate, and respiratory rate are self-explanatory.) The style below contains phrases appropriate for most write-ups.

HEALTH PROMOTION AND COUNSELING: EVIDENCE AND RECOMMENDATIONS

Important Topics for Health Promotion and Counseling

- Screening for hypertension
- Blood pressure and dietary sodium

Other related topics are addressed in more detail in the following sections:

- Optimal Weight (Chapter 6, p. 102)
- Nutrition and Diet (Chapter 6, p. 102)
- Exercise and Physical Activity (Chapter 6, pp. 102–103)

Screening for Hypertension

Epidemiology. Hypertension is an important public health problem in India. More than one-third of adults aged 20 years and older have *hypertension* (SBP ≥140 mm Hg or a DBP ≥90 mm Hg). Men and women have a similar prevalence of hypertension; however, prevalence markedly increases with age, ranging from 12% among adults aged 30 to 39, to 37% among adults aged 40 to 59 years, to more than 67% for adults ≥60 years of age. Uncontrolled hypertension is a major risk factor for ischemic heart disease, cerebrovascular disease, congestive heart failure, and chronic kidney disease.

- *Primary (essential) hypertension* is the most common cause of hypertension: risk factors include age, genetics, black race, obesity and weight gain, excessive salt intake, physical inactivity, and excessive alcohol use.
- *Secondary hypertension* accounts for <5% of hypertension cases. Causes include obstructive sleep apnea, chronic kidney disease, renal artery stenosis, medications, thyroid disease, parathyroid disease, Cushing syndrome, hyperaldosteronism, pheochromocytoma, and coarctation of the aorta.

Screening. Encourage annual BP screening of adults aged 40 years and older and those at an increased risk for high BP. Determinants of increased risk include having high-normal BPs (130 to 139/85 to 89 mm Hg) and being overweight or obese. Average-risk adults aged 18 to 39 can be screened every 3 to 5 years. The most important potential harm of screening is overdiagnosis, leading to unnecessary medication. However, the most recent guideline emphasized the importance of generally not beginning pharmacologic treatment until confirming elevated office readings with ABPM or HBPM. Immediate pharmacologic treatment is still recommended for patients with severe hypertension, particularly those with acute end-organ damage.

Blood Pressure and Dietary Sodium

A daily dietary intake of 2,300 mg of sodium is the acceptable upper intake level for adults.

Because more than 70% of consumed sodium comes from processed foods, patients should be advised to read the Nutrition Facts panel on food labels closely to help them adhere to the 2,300-mg/day guideline. Following eating plans such as the Dietary Approaches to Stop Hypertension (DASH Diet) or the American Heart Association Healthy Diet, which limit foods high in sodium, saturated fats, sugar, and dairy and encourage vegetable, fruit, and whole grain consumption, can reduce cardiovascular disease risk.

See Table 8-8, Patients With Hypertension: Recommended Changes in Diet.

TABLE 8-1. Causes of Anemia

Blood loss	Acute or chronic, overt or occult. Hematemesis, melena, hemoptysis, hematuria, menorrhagia, trauma, etc.
Impaired RBC Formation	■ Congenital: ■ Bone marrow aplasia ■ Pure red cell aplasia ■ Nutritional deficiencies: ■ Iron deficiency ■ Folate deficiency ■ Vitamin B_{12} deficiency ■ Bone marrow infiltration: ■ Leukemia ■ Fibrosis ■ Carcinoma ■ Infections: ■ Tuberculosis, HIV, Epstein–Barr virus ■ Endocrine disorders: ■ Hypothyroidism ■ Hypoadrenalism ■ Hypogonadism ■ Hypopituitarism ■ Drugs toxicity ■ Chloramphenicol ■ Sulfonamides ■ Phenytoin ■ Thalassemia ■ Sideroblastosis ■ Hepatic failure ■ Renal failure
Hemolysis	■ Intravascular hemolysis: ■ Microangiopathy (e.g., aortic stenosis, prosthetic valves) ■ Transfusion reactions (ABO incompatibility) ■ Paroxysmal nocturnal hemoglobinuria ■ Extravascular hemolysis: ■ Intrinsic RBC defects due to enzyme deficiencies, hemoglobinopathies, and membrane defects ■ Extrinsic RBC defects due to liver disease, hypersplenism, infections, autoimmune hemolytic anemia

TABLE 8-2. Causes of Cyanosis

Central cyanosis	High altitude due to decreased atmospheric pressure Impaired pulmonary function due to pneumonia, pulmonary edema, or COPD Shunting of systemic venous blood into the arterial circuit due to congenital heart diseases, pulmonary arteriovenous fistulae, and cardiac or pulmonary right-to-left shunts Methemoglobinemia, sulfhemoglobinemia
Peripheral cyanosis	Vasoconstriction due to cold exposure Decreased cardiac output Arterial obstruction, e.g., Raynaud phenomenon Venous obstruction, e.g., thrombophlebitis or deep venous thrombosis

COPD, chronic obstructive pulmonary disease.

TABLE 8-3. Types of Peripheral Edema

Approximately one third of total body water is extracellular fluid, which, in turn, is roughly 25% plasma; the remainder is interstitial fluid. Net plasma filtration appears to occur throughout the length of the capillary. Interstitial oncotic pressure is notably lower than plasma oncotic pressure, and lymphatic drainage plays a greater role in returning interstitial fluid to the circulation. Several clinical conditions disrupt these forces, resulting in *edema*, which is the clinically evident accumulation of interstitial fluid. Pitting characteristics reflect the viscosity of the edema fluid, based primarily on its protein concentration. When protein concentration is low, as in heart failure, pitting and recovery occur within a few seconds. In lymphedema, protein levels are higher and nonpitting is more typical. Not depicted below is *capillary leak syndrome*, in which protein leaks into the interstitial space, seen in burns, angioedema, snake bites, and allergic reactions.

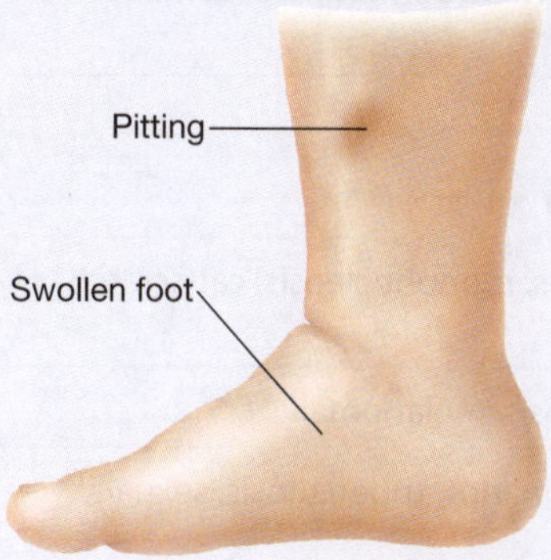

Pitting Edema

Edema is a soft, bilateral palpable swelling from increased interstitial fluid volume and retention of salt and water, demonstrated by pitting after 1 to 2 seconds of thumb pressure on the anterior tibiae and feet. Pitting edema occurs in several conditions: when legs are dependent from prolonged standing or sitting, which leads to increased hydrostatic pressure in the veins and capillaries; heart failure leading to decreased cardiac output; nephrotic syndrome, cirrhosis, or malnutrition leading to low albumin and decreased intravascular colloid oncotic pressure; and with selected medications.

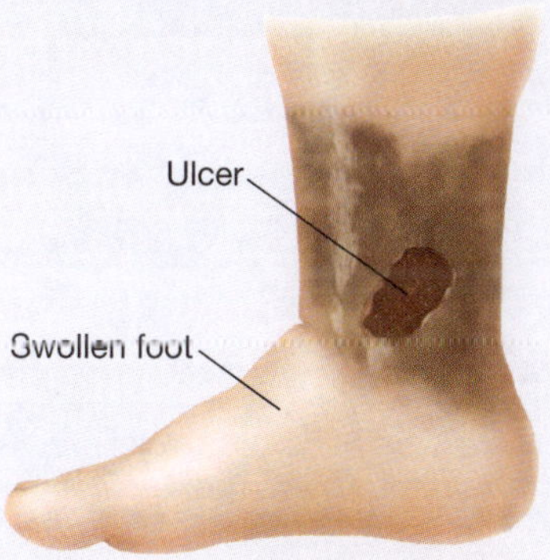

Chronic Venous Insufficiency

Edema is soft, with pitting on pressure, and occasionally bilateral. Look for brawny changes and skin thickening, especially near the ankle. Ulceration, brownish pigmentation, and edema in the feet are common. It arises from chronic obstruction and incompetent valves in the deep venous system.

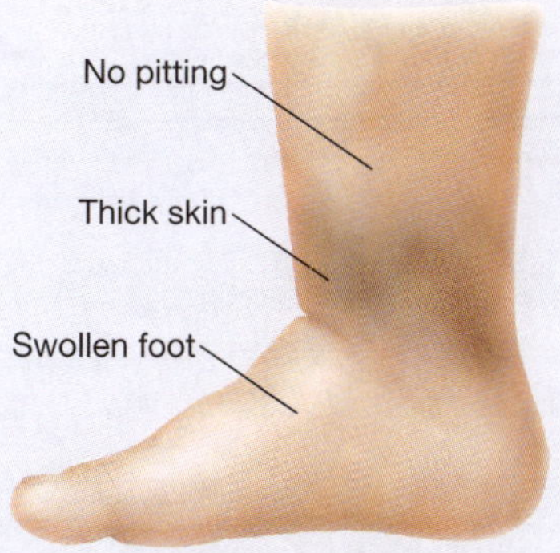

Lymphedema

Edema is initially soft and pitting, then becomes indurated, hard, and nonpitting. Skin is markedly thickened; ulceration is rare. There is no pigmentation. Edema often occurs bilaterally in the feet and toes. Lymphedema arises from interstitial accumulation of protein-rich fluid when lymph channels are infiltrated or obstructed by tumor, fibrosis, or inflammation, or disrupted by axillary node dissection and/or radiation.

TABLE 8-4. Causes of Lymphadenopathy

Site	Causes
Submental	Mononucleosis, cytomegalovirus, toxoplasmosis
Submandibular	Sinusitis, otitis media, conjunctivitis, pharyngitis
Posterior auricular	Otitis externa, tinea capitis, secondary syphilis, rubella
Tonsillar (Jugulodigastric)	Tuberculosis, pharyngitis, rubella
Occipital	Local infection, Tinea capitis, pediculosis capitis, seborrheic dermatitis, secondary syphilis, malignancies
Cervical	Tuberculosis, pharyngitis, rubella
Supraclavicular	Malignancies, tuberculosis, histoplasmosis, sarcoidosis
Epitrochlear	Staphylococcal skin infections, streptococcal infections, mononucleosis, cat-scratch disease, malignancies, sarcoidosis.
Axillary	Breast cancer, lymphoma, cat scratch disease, brucellosis, melanoma.
Inguinal	Infections of the leg and foot, lymphoma, pelvic malignancy, tuberculosis, sexually transmitted diseases.

TABLE 8-5. Selected Heart Rates and Rhythms

Cardiac rhythms may be classified as regular or irregular. When rhythms are irregular or rates are either fast or slow, obtain an ECG to identify the origin of the beats (sinus node, AV node, atrium, or ventricle) and the conduction pattern. The normal range for normal sinus rhythm is reported at 60 to 100 beats/min. Note that AV nodal rhythms, including AV block, may have a fast, normal, or slow ventricular rate.

Is the rhythm regular or irregular?		ECG Pattern	Usual Resting Rate (beats/min)
Regular → What is the rate?	Fast (>100)	Sinus tachycardia	100–180
		Supraventricular (atrial or nodal) tachycardia	150–250
		Atrial flutter with a regular ventricular response	100–175
		Ventricular tachycardia	110–250
	Or		
	Normal (60–90)	Normal sinus rhythm	60–90
		Second-degree AV block	60–100
		Atrial flutter with a regular ventricular response	75–100
	Or		
	Slow (<60)	Sinus bradycardia	<60
		Second-degree AV block	30–60
		Complete heart block	<40
Irregular → What is the pattern of irregularity?	Sporadic	Premature or extra beats at random intervals, but normal underlying rhythm: e.g., atrial or ventricular premature contractions, sinus arrhythmia	See Table 8-6
	Or		
	Regularly Irregular	Regular pattern of cadences: e.g., ventricular trigeminy	See Table 8-6
	Or		
	Irregularly Irregular	No discernible regularity: e.g., atrial fibrillation, atrial flutter	See Table 8-6

TABLE 8-6. Selected Irregular Rhythms

Type of Rhythm | **ECG Waves and Heart Sounds**

Sporadic sinus arrhythmia

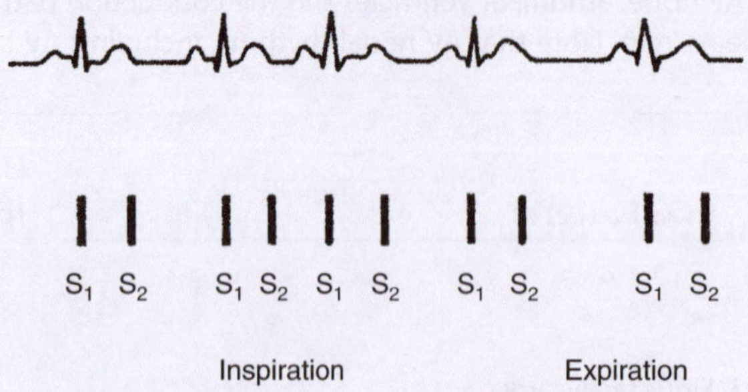

Rhythm. The heart varies cyclically, usually speeding up with inspiration and slowing down with expiration.

Heart sounds. Normal, although S_1 may vary with the heart rate.

Atrial or nodal premature contractions (*supraventricular*)

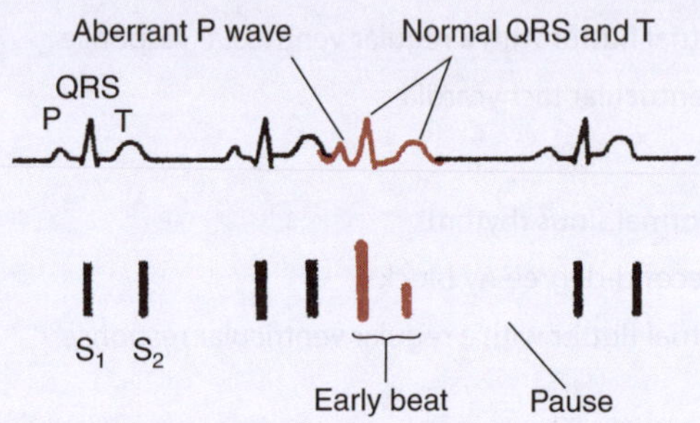

Rhythm. A beat of atrial or nodal origin comes earlier than the next expected normal beat. A pause follows, and then the rhythm resumes.

Heart sounds. S_1 may differ in intensity from the S_1 of normal beats, and S_2 may be decreased.

Sporadic ventricular premature contractions (*ventricular bigeminy or trigeminy*)

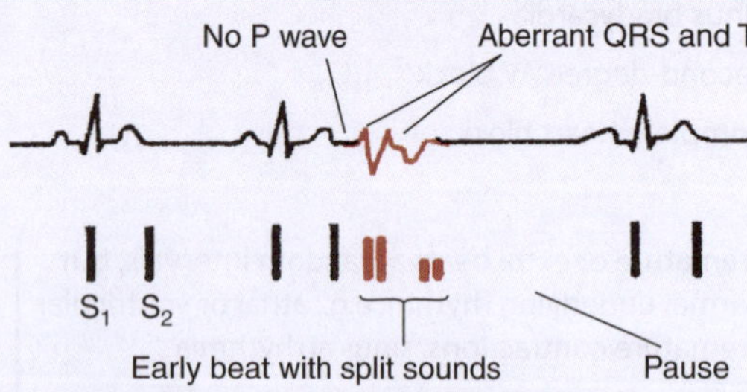

Rhythm. A beat of ventricular origin comes earlier than the next expected normal beat. A pause follows, and the rhythm resumes.

Heart sounds. S_1 may differ in intensity from the S_1 of the normal beats, and S_2 may be decreased. Both sounds are likely to be split.

Irregularly irregular atrial fibrillation and atrial flutter with varying Av block

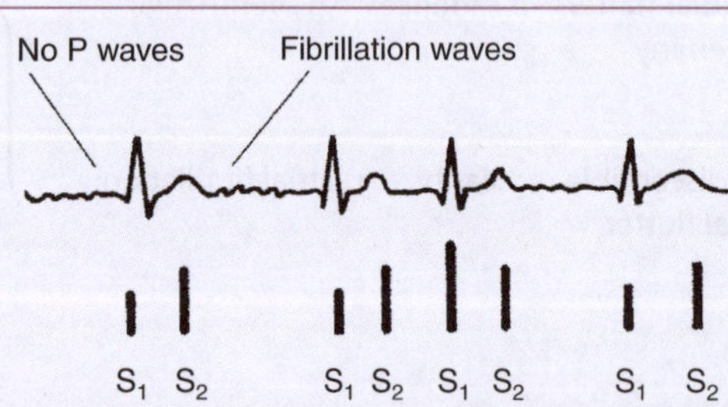

Rhythm. The ventricular rhythm is totally irregular, although short runs of the irregular ventricular rhythm may seem regular.

Heart sounds. S_1 varies in intensity.

TABLE 8-7. Abnormalities of the Arterial Pulse and Pressure Waves

Normal

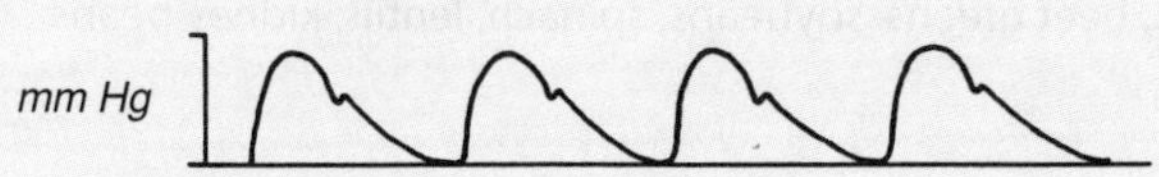

The pulse pressure is approximately 30 to 40 mm Hg. The pulse contour is smooth and rounded. (The notch on the descending slope of the pulse wave is not palpable.)

Small weak pulses

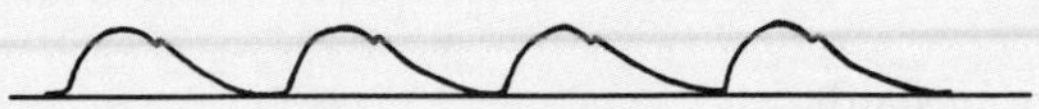

The pulse pressure is diminished, and the pulse feels weak and small. The upstroke may feel slowed, the peak prolonged. Causes include (1) decreased stroke volume, as in heart failure, hypovolemia, and severe aortic stenosis; and (2) increased peripheral resistance, as in exposure to cold and severe heart failure.

Large bounding pulses

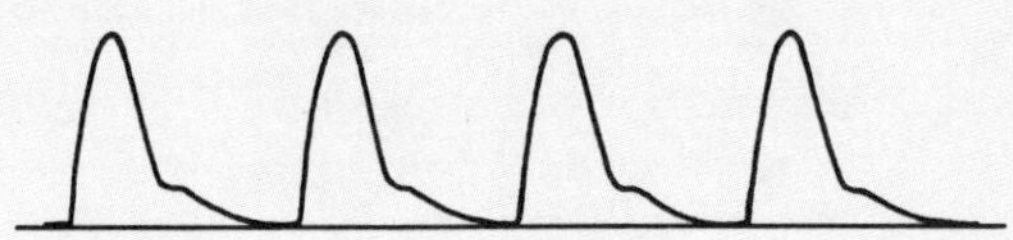

The pulse pressure is increased, and the pulse feels strong and bounding. The rise and fall may feel rapid, the peak brief. Causes include (1) increased stroke volume, decreased peripheral resistance, or both, as in fever, anemia, hyperthyroidism, aortic regurgitation, arteriovenous fistulas, and patent ductus arteriosus; (2) increased stroke volume because of slow heart rates, as in bradycardia and complete heart block; and (3) decreased compliance (increased stiffness) of the aortic walls, as in aging or atherosclerosis.

Bisferiens pulse

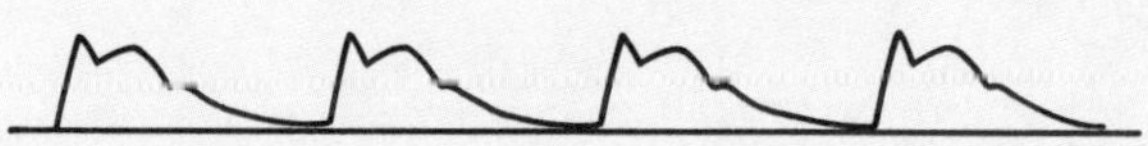

A bisferiens pulse is an increased arterial pulse with a double systolic peak, detected during moderate compression of the artery. Causes include pure aortic regurgitation, combined aortic stenosis and regurgitation, and hypertrophic cardiomyopathy.

Pulsus alternans

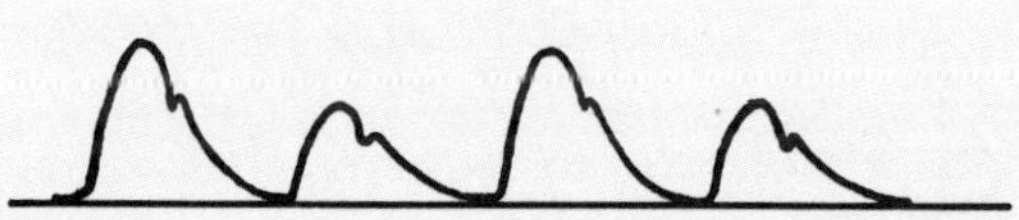

The pulse is completely regular but has alternating strong and weak beats. If there is only a slight difference between the strong and the weak beats, detection requires use of a blood pressure cuff (see p. 227). Pulsus alternans indicates severe left ventricular failure.

Bigeminal pulse

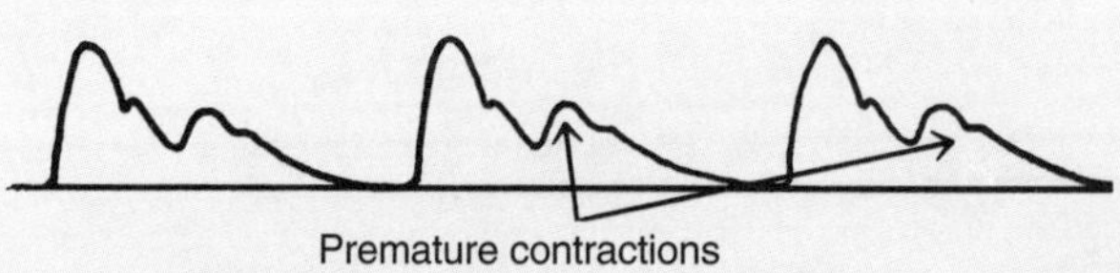

This disorder may mimic pulsus alternans. A bigeminal pulse is caused by a normal beat alternating with a premature contraction. The stroke volume of the premature beat is diminished in relation to that of the normal beats, and the pulse varies in amplitude accordingly.

Paradoxical pulse

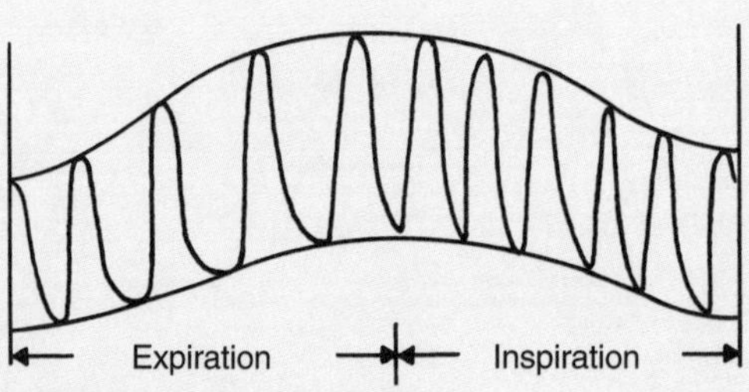

A paradoxical pulse may be detected by a palpable decrease in the pulse amplitude on quiet inspiration. If the sign is less pronounced, a blood pressure cuff is needed. Systolic pressure decreases by >10 to 12 mm Hg during inspiration. A paradoxical pulse occurs in pericardial tamponade, exacerbations of asthma and COPD, and constrictive pericarditis.

COPD, chronic obstructive pulmonary disease.

TABLE 8-8. Patients With Hypertension: Recommended Changes in Diet

Dietary Change	Food Source
Increase foods high in potassium	Baked white or sweet potatoes, white beans, beet greens, soybeans, spinach, lentils, kidney beans Yogurt Tomato paste, juice, puree, and sauce Bananas, plantains, many dried fruits, orange juice
Decrease foods high in sodium	Canned foods (soups, tuna fish) Pretzels, potato chips, pizza, pickles, olives Many processed foods (frozen dinners, ketchup, mustard) Batter-fried foods Table salt, including for cooking

CHAPTER

9

Cognition, Behavior, and Mental Status

ANATOMY AND PHYSIOLOGY

The anatomic and physiologic origin of psychiatric symptoms is less clearly defined than the origin of symptoms in other major systems in the body. For example, the conduction system of the heart or the process of digestion in the gastrointestinal tract generally has a fairly clear progression of cause and effect, whereas the complexity of the human brain makes narrowing down the source of mental disorder to any one component highly challenging. Through decades of neuroscience research, however, the roles certain brain regions play in mental disorders have been established.

The central nervous system (CNS) is made up of the *brain* and the *spinal cord*. The spinal cord, although crucial for motor and sensory functions, plays less of a role in mental disorder. The brain is further subdivided into: the *cerebrum* (cerebral hemispheres), which is the largest part of the brain and composed of *cortical structures* (frontal, temporal, parietal, and occipital lobes) and *subcortical structures* (fornix, cingulate cortex, basal ganglia, and basal forebrain), the *diencephalon* (made up of the thalamus, epithalamus, subthalamus, and the hypothalamus), the *cerebellum*, and the *brainstem*, which consists of the midbrain, pons, and the medulla.

See the anatomy of the nervous system in greater detail in Chapter 13, Nervous System.

Deep within the CNS, clusters of neurons, or *nuclei*, organized as *modulatory systems*, synthesize *neurotransmitters* that are crucial for higher-level CNS functions (Box 9-1).

- *Serotonergic* diffuse modulatory systems arise from the *raphe nuclei*. The raphe nuclei are clustered along the midline of the brainstem and project extensively to all levels of the CNS. The nuclei make *serotonin*, a neurotransmitter that helps regulate mood, arousal, and cognition (Fig. 9 1).
- *Norepinephrine* diffuse modulatory systems arise from the *locus coeruleus*. The small cluster of locus coeruleus neurons projects axons that innervate vast areas of the CNS, including the spinal cord, cerebellum, thalamus, and cerebral cortex. It makes *norepinephrine*, which regulates mood, arousal, attention, and cognition (Fig. 9-2).

Box 9-1. Key Neurotransmitters Involved in Mental Disorders

Neurotransmitter	Location of Synthesis	Regulatory Function
Serotonin	Brainstem: raphe nuclei	Helps regulate mood, arousal, and cognition
Norepinephrine	Brainstem: locus coeruleus	Regulates mood, arousal, attention, and cognition
Dopamine	Brainstem: substantia nigra	Regulates mood, arousal, cognition, and motor control
Acetylcholine	Basal forebrain: basal nucleus of Meynert	Regulate sleep, arousal, and attention

Low levels of serotonin, norepinephrine, and dopamine have been associated with depressive symptoms. Low concentrations of serotonin with high levels of norepinephrine have been associated with anxiety symptoms. Too much dopamine with low concentrations of serotonin in certain areas of the brain lead to symptoms of psychosis and mania. Dementia is notable for low concentration levels of acetylcholine.

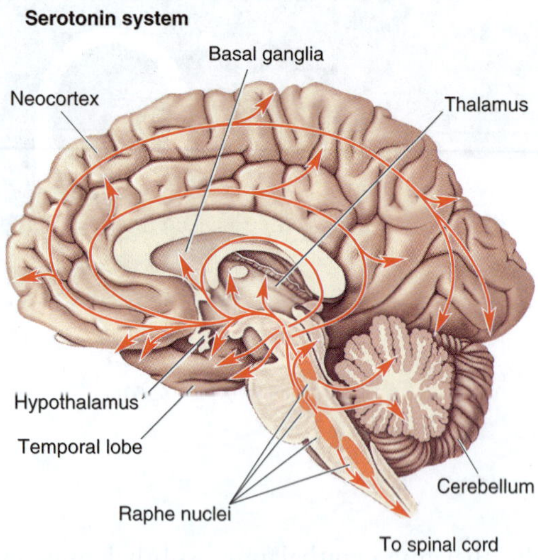

FIGURE 9-1. Serotonin system. (From Bear MF et al. *Neuroscience*. 4th ed. Wolters Kluwer; 2016, Fig. 15-13.)

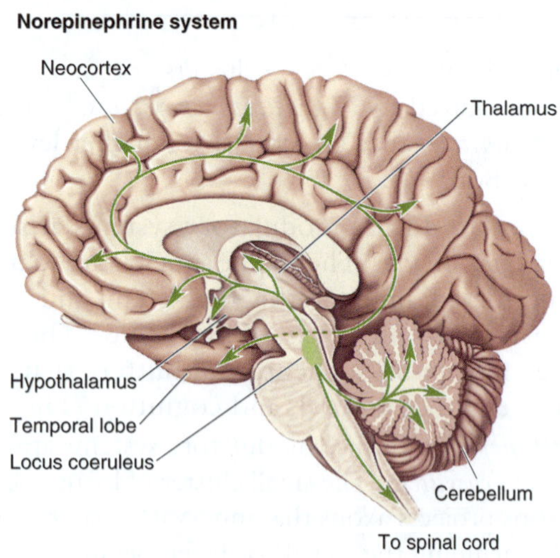

FIGURE 9-2. Norepinephrine system. (From Bear MF et al. *Neuroscience*. 4th ed. Wolters Kluwer; 2016, Fig. 15-12.)

- *Dopaminergic* diffuse modulatory systems arise from the *substantia nigra* and the *ventral tegmental area*, which make *dopamine*, a neurotransmitter that regulates mood, arousal, cognition, and motor control (Fig. 9-3). The substantia nigra and ventral tegmental area lie close together in the midbrain. They project to the striatum (caudate nucleus and putamen) and limbic and frontal cortical regions, respectively.
- *Cholinergic* diffuse modulatory systems arise from the *basal forebrain* and brainstem. The *medial septal nuclei* and *basal nucleus of Meynert* project widely upon the cerebral cortex, including the hippocampus. It is the major center for *acetylcholine* (ACh) production in the CNS. ACh helps regulate sleep, arousal, and attention (Fig. 9-4).

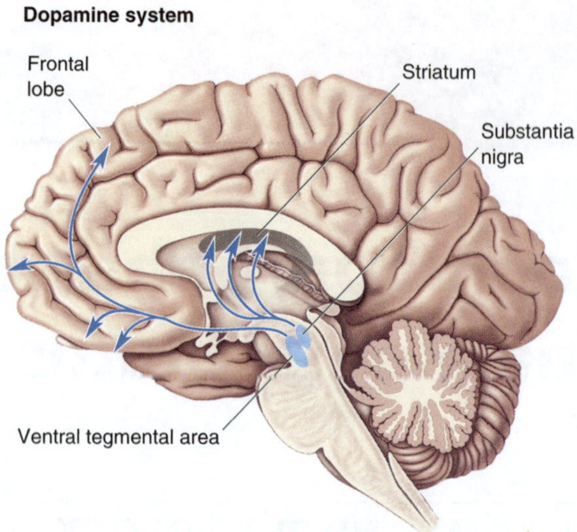

FIGURE 9-3. Dopamine system. (From Bear MF et al. *Neuroscience*. 4th ed. Wolters Kluwer; 2016, Fig. 15-14.)

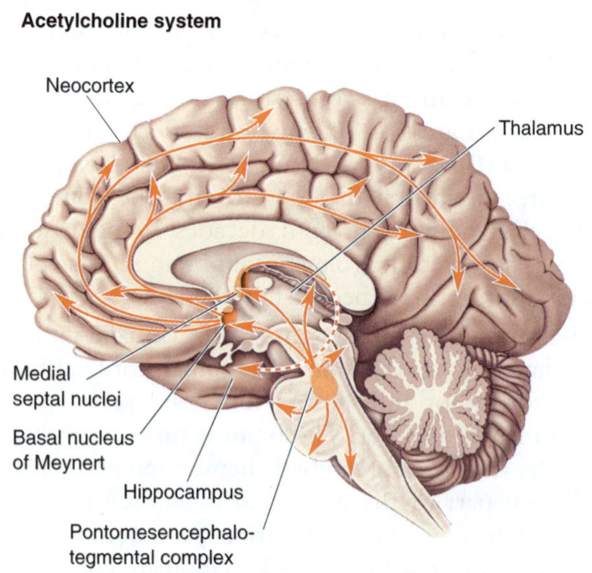

FIGURE 9-4. Acetylcholine system. (From Bear MF et al. *Neuroscience*. 4th ed. Wolters Kluwer; 2016, Fig. 15-1.)

These structures within the CNS are intricately connected to one another through a variety of complex pathways called *circuits* or *networks*. These networks process large amounts of information and carry out coordinated tasks in response. The complexity of these networks makes it difficult to attribute mental disorders and symptoms to any one particular area of the brain. Multiple deficits may occur within the network for illness to develop. The research on these networks is far from comprehensive and continues to evolve.

See discussion of structures, networks, their functions, and roles in psychiatric symptoms and disorders in Tables 9-1 and 9-2.

This chapter uses *mental disorder* to denote any condition or syndrome with clinical manifestations characterized by significant impairment in cognition, emotion regulation, or behavior, measured in terms of deviation from some normative concept and leading to significant distress and/or disability in social, occupational, or other important activities of daily life. This is also the term used in the current *Diagnostic and Statistical Manual of Mental Disorders*, Fifth Edition (*DSM-5*), the diagnostic manual used by psychiatrists and other mental health professionals. However, this nomenclature has inherent issues, and terms such as *mental illness* or *psychiatric illness* may be preferred. In fact, *DSM-5* acknowledges that the term may be misleading since it implies a distinction between mental disorders and physical disorders but continues using "mental disorder" because there is no appropriate substitute to date.

HEALTH HISTORY: GENERAL APPROACH

You are uniquely poised to detect clues to mental disorders and harmful behavior through empathic listening and close observation. Nonetheless, these clues are often missed. They may come as reports from family members of vague or changed behavior. Or, you may notice subtle behavioral changes, difficulty taking medications as prescribed, problems attending to household chores or paying bills, or loss of interest in their usual activities in patients as well as disorientation after surgery or during an acute illness.

Mental health disorders also are commonly masked by other clinical conditions, calling for sensitive and careful inquiry. Supplement your interview with questions in specific areas and pursue a formal mental status examination when indicated. Recognizing a mental disorder is especially important given its significant prevalence and morbidity, the high likelihood that it is treatable, the shortage of clinicians dealing with mental health issues, and the increasing importance of primary care clinicians as the first to encounter the patient's distress. Prompt identification of these problems is crucial because they impact family relationships and work status and may result in possible disability.

Patients with mental disorders also face significant stigma as a result of their diagnosis. They are often unfairly depicted as weak and responsible for their symptoms, and these prejudices often lead to discrimination at home, in the community, and in the workplace. When discussing a psychiatric diagnosis, it is important to elicit the patient's understanding of the diagnosis. The patient may hold internalized false beliefs about the disorder that are important to address. Reinforcing that psychiatric conditions, like cardiac conditions or pulmonary conditions, are real and treatable is crucial to mitigating damage from stigma.

Common or Concerning Symptoms

- Anxiety, excessive worrying
- Depressed mood
- Memory problems
- Medically unexplained symptoms

Anxiety, Excessive Worrying

Anxiety disorders include generalized anxiety disorder, social phobia, panic disorder, posttraumatic stress disorder (PTSD), and acute stress disorder. These are among the most common mental disorders, yet the chronic and disabling nature of these conditions is often seriously underestimated.

Common risk factors in patients with anxiety and related disorders include family history of anxiety, personal history of anxiety or mood disorder, childhood stressful life events or trauma, being female, chronic medical illness, and behavioral inhibition.

- In a patient with concerns of feeling nervous, uncontrollable worrying, being frightened or "on edge," try to explore with an open-ended question like, "Can you tell me how things have been going with you recently?" This provides an opportunity for patients to tell you in their own words what is happening (Box 9-2).

Box 9-2. High-Yield Screening Questions for Office Practice: Anxiety

- Over the past 2 weeks, have you been feeling nervous, anxious, or on edge?
- Over the past 2 weeks, have you been unable to stop or control worrying?
- Over the past 4 weeks, have you had an anxiety attack—suddenly feeling fear or panic?

- Ask about the *nature* of the anxiety. Is it worry, avoidance or obsession?

Worrying that predominates as the nature of the complaint may lead one to suspect a generalized anxiety disorder or panic disorder. Avoidance due to unreasonable fear of situations or activities that could lead to embarrassment (e.g., speaking to people) may point to a possible social anxiety disorder.

- Ask "What kinds of things do you worry about or make you feel anxious?" Common responses include family, finances, health, work, and relationships. Obsessions may include thoughts of hurting someone else, sexual thoughts, excessive concern about contamination/germs/disease, and mental rituals (e.g., counting, praying, repeating). Compulsions can manifest as repetitive acts of washing, cleaning, checking (e.g., doors, locks, appliances), arranging, and repeating (e.g., counting, touching, praying) as well as hoarding, collecting, and saving.

Obsessions which are repeated and unwanted thoughts that could lead to certain actions or habits (compulsions) could signify an obsessive–compulsive disorder.

- Ask about the *onset* and *duration* of the anxious feeling or worrying. "How long has this feeling of excessive worrying been going on?"

Excessive worry persisting over a 4-week period suggests a possible generalized anxiety disorder.

- Is this the *first occurrence* or has this been *recurrent*?

Panic disorder often presents with recurrent sudden episodes/spells/attacks of intense fear or discomfort that are unexpected or with intervening periods of living in fear or worrying of having another attack or facing the consequences of the attack.

- Is the worrying accompanied by *pervasive* thoughts and or behaviors that are *repetitive*? Difficulty sleeping? Feeling physically ill with headaches, stomach troubles, or fatigue?

Obsessive–compulsive disorder is characterized by intrusive thoughts and ritualistic behaviors.

- Explore associations with life events or trauma. Was there an inciting event that preceded this anxious feeling?

Consider posttraumatic stress disorder (PTSD) characterized by reexperiencing, avoidance, persistent negative alterations in cognition and mood, and alterations in arousal and reactivity. Also consider social anxiety disorder marked by anticipatory anxiety in social situations.

- It is important to identify other potential causes of the symptoms, including over-the-counter and prescribed medications, illicit substances, caffeine, alcohol, or other medical and psychiatric comorbidities.

Hyperthyroidism, cardiopulmonary disorders, and traumatic brain injury (TBI) are common comorbid conditions that accompany excessive or uncontrollable anxiety.

Anxiety is often comorbid with substance use and mood disorders.

- Always ask about the *impact* that the symptoms have had on the patient's current life and functioning.

Depressed Mood

Mood disorders with depressive symptoms include major depressive disorder (MDD), persistent depressive disorder (PDD), bipolar disorders, disruptive mood dysregulation disorder (DMDD), and premenstrual dysphoric disorder (PMDD).

There are numerous risk factors for depression, but the most common include a personal history of a depressive episode, a family history of first-degree family members with depression, personal history of recent stressful life events or significant childhood adversity, chronic and/or disabling medical illness, and female gender.

Assessing depression can sometimes be difficult as patients may be reluctant to share their symptoms with providers or may not recognize that they are struggling with depression. However, screening for depression is crucial since depression is a treatable risk factor for suicide. Several high-yield questions may help to clarify the presence of depressive symptoms and rule out other potential causes (Box 9-3).

Box 9-3. High-Yield Screening Questions for Office Practice: Depression

Over the past 2 weeks, have you felt down, depressed, or hopeless?

- Over the past 2 weeks, have you felt little interest or pleasure in doing things (anhedonia)?
- Over the past 2 weeks, have you had trouble falling or staying asleep, or have you been sleeping too much?
- Over the past 2 weeks, have you been feeling bad about yourself, or that you're a failure or have let your family down?
- Over the past 2 weeks, have you felt tired or had little energy?
- Over the past 2 weeks, have you had poor appetite or overeating?
- Over the past 2 weeks, have you had trouble concentrating on things, such as reading the newspaper or watching television?
- Over the past 2 weeks, have you been moving or speaking so slowly that other people could have noticed? Or have you been so fidgety or restless that you have been moving a lot more than usual?
- Over the past 2 weeks, have you had thoughts that you would be better off dead or thoughts of hurting yourself in some way?

- As with anxiety, it is important to start out with open-ended questions. "How have you been feeling?" or "How has your mood been?" can be helpful ways to start screening for depression. If the patient is struggling to answer these questions, you can take a more directive approach with, "Please describe your mood recently using three words."

People who are depressed may respond with moods other than "sad" or "depressed." Other common responses may include "guilty," "irritable," "angry," or "hopeless."

Sadness after a recent loss of a loved one is common and expected, and it may be part of normal bereavement rather than depression.

If patients describe their mood as any of the above, it is important to probe further. What do they think has been making them feel this way?

Feeling irritable or angry or sad after a recent stressor may actually be part of an adjustment disorder rather than a depressive disorder, especially in the absence of other depressive symptoms.

If depressive symptoms worsen in sync with a female patient's menstrual cycle, she may have premenstrual dysphoric disorder (PMDD).

- Next it is important to understand the *timeline* of their symptoms. How long have they been feeling this way? Do they feel like this most of the day on most days?

Major depressive disorder (MDD) is characterized by at least 2 weeks of depressed/irritable mood, with at least four of the following: anhedonia, insomnia or hypersomnia, decreased self-esteem, low energy, poor concentration or indecision, changes in appetite, feeling slowed or restless, and thoughts of death or suicide.

Persistent depressive disorder (PDD) is characterized by depressive/irritable mood lasting for at least 2 years with at least two of the aforementioned depressive symptoms.

- It is important to assess whether this is the patient's first presentation with mood symptoms or if such mood symptoms have occurred in the past. Someone with recurrent depressive episodes may have a worse prognosis than someone who is presenting with depressive symptoms for the first time. Ask, "Have you ever felt depressed like this before?" and "Have you ever had times when you felt excited, energetic, talkative, or restless for multiple days in a row and needed very little sleep during this time?"

Bipolar disorders present with both depressive episodes, such as in major depressive disorder (MDD), as well as manic or hypomanic episodes. Symptoms of manic episodes include euphoric/irritable mood, grandiosity, decreased need for sleep, talkativeness, racing thoughts, distractibility, increased goal-directed behavior or agitation, and an increase in reckless pleasure-seeking (having unprotected sex, spending excess money, foolish investments).

- Depressive symptoms can be mimicked by medical conditions and substance use. Screening for heart disease, stroke, diabetes, thyroid problems, and alcohol/drug use is crucial to clarifying the diagnosis.

Parkinson disease, traumatic brain injury (TBI), recent myocardial infarction (MI) or stroke, and hypothyroidism may mimic depressive symptoms. Additionally, alcohol use and recent substance use may present in a similar way to depressive symptoms.

Depression, particularly recurrent/chronic depression, is frequently comorbid with anxiety, personality disorders, and substance use.

- As with anxiety, assessing the *impact* of depressive symptoms on the patient's life is vital to the overall assessment.

Memory Problems

In the *DSM-5*, *delirium* and *dementia* fall under the new category of *neurocognitive disorders,* based on consultation with expert groups. Dementia is classified as a major cognitive disorder; a less severe level of cognitive impairment is now *mild neurocognitive disorder,* which applies to younger individuals with impairment from TBI or HIV infection. The *DSM-5* retains the term *dementia*, however, due to widespread clinical usage. Helpful tables in this chapter provide working definitions of each cognitive domain, with examples of symptoms related to everyday activities and related assessments.

See Table 9-3, Neurocognitive Disorders: Delirium and Dementia.

In assessing cognitive impairment, it is always helpful to obtain information from family members or loved ones who know the patient, as the patient may not always be aware of memory problems. Asking questions in a kind, compassionate, and curious way may help patients to discuss any memory problems they have of which they are aware.

- Starting out broadly with "Have you or anyone you know expressed concerns about your memory?"

Patients with milder forms of dementia may be able to acknowledge their forgetfulness. Patients with more severe forms of dementia may be more likely to remember other people worrying about their memory than episodes of forgetfulness.

- If patients or loved ones do confirm forgetfulness, ask about the *onset* and *duration*. "When did you first notice the forgetfulness?" "Did it happen over time, or was it sudden?"

Sudden-onset memory problems are concerning for major vascular neurocognitive disorders, wherein vascular occlusion damages structusres important for memory. Rapid-onset memory problems after a head injury should raise suspicion for a major neurocognitive disorder due to TBI.

Most other dementias have an insidious (or slowly progressing) onset.

- If patients or families report slow progression of forgetfulness, you should probe into other problems that may accompany the memory problems. "Have you noticed other concerning changes?" "Have you noticed unusual movements that you couldn't control?"

If the patient affirms one-sided hand tremor or difficulty starting movements, consider Parkinson disease. In a younger adult patient with unusual limb movements, you should assess the family history for Huntington disease.

"Have you noticed any changes in how you interact with other people?" "Have you noticed any changes in personality?" "Has the patient complained of seeing persons or things that are not there?"

If family members or caregivers have noticed personality changes in the patient, consider frontotemporal dementia. A patient starting to have visual hallucinations may be suffering from Lewy body dementia.

- Assessment of functional impairments due to memory issues should address activities of daily living affecting safety. Is the patient able to eat, bathe, and ambulate independently? If not, how much help is needed? Is the patient able to pay the bills, buy groceries, and clean the house? If not, what does the patient struggle with? Has the patient ever gotten lost or wandered away from home? Has the patient ever left the stove or the oven on? Has the patient ever made a mistake in taking medication?

This information is important because it may change the type of support that the family and the patient need to live their lives safely and comfortably.

Patients with Medically Unexplained Symptoms

Physical symptoms account for approximately 50% of clinic visits. Approximately 25% of these patients may present with persisting and recurrent symptoms that elude assessment and fail to improve. Overall, 30% of these symptoms are considered to be *medically unexplained*. Patients with medically unexplained symptoms fall into heterogeneous groupings ranging from selected impairment to behaviors meeting *DSM-5* criteria for mood and somatic symptom disorders. For example, many patients do not report symptoms of anxiety and depression, the most common mental health disorders in the general population, but focus on physical concerns instead. Roughly one-third of physical symptoms are unexplained. Two-thirds of patients with depression, for example, present with physical complaints, and half report multiple unexplained or somatic symptoms. Furthermore, functional syndromes have been shown to "frequently co-occur and share key symptoms and selected objective abnormalities."

See Table 9-4, Somatic Symptoms and Related Disorders.

Failure to recognize the admixture of physical symptoms, functional syndromes, and common mental disorders—anxiety, depression, unexplained and somatoform symptoms, and substance abuse—adds to the burden of patient undertreatment and poor quality of life.

PHYSICAL EXAMINATION: GENERAL APPROACH

The assessment of mental health is challenging and complex. Changes in mental health warrant careful evaluation for underlying pathologic and pharmacologic causes. The patient's personality, psychodynamics, family and life experiences, and cultural background all come into play. Amplify your findings from the history and physical examination as you select all or part of the formal mental status examination for further testing. The mental status examination is central to assessment of mental health. It is also a critical element in the assessment of the nervous system and the first segment of the nervous system write-up. Learn to describe the patient's mood, speech, behavior, and cognition and to relate these findings to your examination of the cranial nerves, motor and sensory systems, and reflexes.

The format that follows should help structure your observations but is not intended as a rigid step-by-step guide. Be flexible, but thorough. In some situations, however, sequence is important. If the patient's consciousness, attention, comprehension of words, and ability to speak are impaired, assess these deficits promptly. If the patient cannot give a reliable history, testing most of the other mental functions will be difficult and merits an evaluation for acute causes.

TECHNIQUES OF EXAMINATION

Key Components of the Mental Status Examination

- Assess *appearance* and *behavior*, including *level of consciousness* (alert, lethargy, obtundation, stupor, coma), *posture and motor behavior* (relaxed, slumped tense, restless, anxious, fidgeting, agitated, expansive), *dress, grooming, personal hygiene, facial expression* (e.g., anxiety, depression, apathy, anger, elation, immobility), *affect* (appropriate, flat, blunted, labile, inappropriate), and *manner* (e.g., anger, hostility, suspiciousness, evasiveness, apathy, detached, indifferent, anxious, depressed).
- Assess *speech* and *language*, including *quantity, rate* (fast, slow), *volume* (loud, soft), *articulation* (e.g., clear, nasal), and *fluency* (e.g., hesitancy, inflections, circumlocutions, paraphasia).
- Assess *mood* (e.g., sadness, melancholy, contentment, joy, euphoria, elation, anger, rage, anxiety, worry, detached, indifferent).
- Assess *thoughts* (logic, relevance, organization, coherence) and *perceptions* (illusions, hallucinations).
- Assess *insight* (aware, absent) and *judgment* (appropriate, poor).
- Assess *cognition*, including *orientation, attention* (digit span, serial 7s, spelling backward), *memory* (remote, recent, new learning), and *higher cognitive functions* (information and vocabulary, calculations, abstract thinking, constructional ability).

The mental status examination consists of six components: *appearance and behavior; speech and language; mood; thoughts and perceptions; insight and judgment*; and *cognitive function*. Each of these components will be discussed in the following sections.

Appearance and Behavior

Integrate the observations you have made throughout the history and physical examination, including the following aspects.

Level of Consciousness. Is the patient awake and alert? Does the patient understand your questions and respond appropriately and reasonably quickly, or tend to lose track of the topic, grow silent, or even fall asleep? If the patient does not respond to your questions, escalate the stimulus in steps (Box 9-4).

Box 9-4. Levels of Consciousness

Level	Patient Response
Alertness	The alert patient has eyes open, looks at you when spoken to in a *normal tone of voice*, and responds fully and appropriately to stimuli.
Lethargy	The lethargic patient appears drowsy but opens the eyes when spoken to in a *loud voice* and looks at you, responds to questions, and then falls asleep.
Obtundation	The obtunded patient opens the eyes when *tactile* stimulus is applied and looks at you but responds to you slowly and is somewhat confused.
Stupor	The stuporous patient arouses only after *painful* stimuli. Verbal responses are slow or even absent. The patient lapses into an unresponsive state when the stimulus ceases.
Coma	A comatose patient remains unarousable with eyes closed. There is no evident response to inner need or external stimuli.

Posture and Motor Behavior. Does the patient sit or lie quietly or prefer to walk around? Observe the patient's posture and ability to relax. Note the pace, range, and type of movement. Are movements voluntary and spontaneous? Are any limbs immobile? Are posture and motor activity affected by topics under discussion, type of activity, or who is in the room?

Look for tense posture, restlessness, and anxious fidgeting; the crying, pacing, and hand-wringing of agitated depression or anxiety; the hopeless slumped posture and slowed movements of depression; the poor eye contact and closed-off body posture of psychosis; the agitated and expansive movements of a manic episode.

Dress, Grooming, and Personal Hygiene. How is the patient dressed? Is the clothing clean and presentable? Is it appropriate for the patient's age and social group? Note the grooming of the patient's hair; nails; teeth; skin; and, if present, facial hair. How do the grooming and hygiene compare with that of peers of comparable age, lifestyle, and socioeconomic group? Compare one side of the body with the other.

Grooming and personal hygiene may deteriorate in depression, schizophrenia, and dementia. Excessive fastidiousness may be seen in obsessive–compulsive disorder (OCD). One-sided neglect may result from a lesion in the opposite parietal cortex, usually the nondominant side.

Facial Expression. Observe the face both at rest and during conversation. Watch for changes in expression. Are they appropriate for the topics being discussed? Or is the face relatively immobile throughout?

Note expressions of anxiety, depression, apathy, anger, or elation as well as facial immobility in parkinsonism.

Manner, Affect, and Relationship to People and Things. Assess the patient's **affect**, or the fluctuating pattern of observable behaviors that expresses subjective feelings or emotions through tone of voice, facial expression, and demeanor. It is the external expression of the inner emotional state. Is it appropriate to the topics being discussed? Or is the affect labile, blunted, or flat? Does it seem exaggerated at certain points? If so, how? Observe the patient's openness, approachability, and reactions to others and the surroundings. Does the patient hear or see things not present or converse with someone who is not there?

Watch for the anger, hostility, suspiciousness, or evasiveness of patients with paranoia; the elation and euphoria of mania; the flat affect and remoteness of schizophrenia; the *apathy* (dulled affect with detachment and indifference) of dementia; and anxiety or depression. Hallucinations occur in schizophrenia, alcohol withdrawal, and systemic toxicity.

Speech and Language

Language is the complex symbolic system for expressing, receiving, and comprehending words; as with consciousness, attention, and memory, language is essential for assessing other mental functions. Throughout the interview, note the following characteristics of the patient's speech.

Quantity. Is the patient talkative or unusually silent? Are comments spontaneous, or limited to direct questions?

Rate and Volume. Is speech fast or slow? Is speech loud or soft?

Note the slow speech of depression; the accelerated louder speech of mania.

Articulation of Words. Are the words clear and distinct? Does the speech have a nasal quality?

Dysarthria refers to defective articulation. **Aphasia** is a disorder of language. **Dysphonia** results from impaired volume, quality, or pitch of the voice.

Fluency. Fluency reflects the rate, flow, and melody of speech and the content and use of words. Watch for abnormalities of spontaneous speech such as:

- Hesitancies and gaps in the flow and rhythm of words
- Disturbed inflections, such as a monotone
- **Circumlocutions**, in which phrases or sentences are substituted for a word the person cannot think of, such as "what you write with" for "pen"
- **Paraphasias**, in which words are malformed ("I write with a den"), incorrect ("I write with a bar"), or invented ("I write with a dar").

If the patient's speech lacks meaning or fluency, proceed with further testing as outlined in Box 9-5. Check for deficits in vision, hearing, intelligence, and education that may affect responses. A person who can write a correct sentence does not have aphasia.

Box 9-5. Testing for Aphasia

Word Comprehension	Ask the patient to follow a one-stage command, such as "Point to your nose." Try a two-stage command: "Point to your mouth, then your knee."
Repetition	Ask the patient to repeat a phrase of one-syllable words (the most difficult repetition task): "No ifs, ands, or buts."
Naming	Ask the patient to name the parts of a watch.
Reading Comprehension	Ask the patient to read a paragraph aloud.
Writing	Ask the patient to write a sentence.

These questions help identify the type of aphasia. There are two common kinds of aphasia—*expressive*, or **Broca aphasia**, with preserved comprehension with slow, nonfluent speech and *receptive*, or **Wernicke aphasia**, with impaired comprehension with fluent speech. These are compared in Chapter 13, Nervous System, Table 13-5, Disorders of Speech.

Mood

Mood is the pervasive and sustained emotion that colors the person's perception of the world. This term is often confused with affect. Simply, affect is to mood as weather is to climate. Ask the patient to describe his or her mood, including usual mood level and fluctuations related to life events. "How did you feel about that?" for example, or, more generally, "How is your overall mood?" The reports from family and friends may be of value. For patients who struggle with naming emotions (*alexithymia*), it may be helpful to list some emotions for them to choose from. Moods range from sadness and melancholy; contentment, joy, euphoria, and elation; anger and rage; anxiety and worry; to detachment and indifference.

Has the mood been intense and unchanging, or labile? How long has it lasted? Is it appropriate to the patient's situation? With depression, have there been episodes of an elevated mood, suggesting a bipolar disorder?

For official diagnostic criteria of depressive and bipolar disorders, see the *DSM-5*.

If you suspect depression, assess its severity and any risk of suicide. Ask:

- Do you feel discouraged or depressed?
- How low do you feel?
- What do you see for yourself in the future?
- Have you had thoughts of death?
- Do you ever feel that life isn't worth living? Or that you want to be dead?
- Have you ever thought of killing yourself?
- Have you thought about how or when you would try to kill yourself? Do you have a plan?
- What do you expect is going to happen after you die?

It is your responsibility to ask directly about suicidal thoughts. This may be the only way to uncover suicidal ideation and plans that launch immediate intervention and treatment. Studies show that asking at-risk individuals if they are suicidal does not increase suicides or suicidal thoughts.

Thought

Thought Process. **Thought process** is the logic, organization, coherence, and relevance of the patient's thought as it leads to selected goals (*how* people think). Assess the the patient's thought processes throughout the interview.

Does speech progress logically toward a goal? Listen for patterns of speech that suggest disorders of thought processes, as outlined in Box 9-6.

Box 9-6. Variations and Abnormalities in Thought Processes

Blocking	Sudden interruption of speech in midsentence or before the idea is completed, attributed to "losing the thought." Blocking occurs in normal people.
Circumstantiality	The mildest thought disorder, consisting of speech with unnecessary detail, indirection, and delay in reaching the point. Some topics may have a meaningful connection. Many people without mental disorders have circumstantial speech.
Clanging	Speech with choice of words based on sound, rather than meaning, as in rhyming and punning. For example, "Look at my eyes and nose, wise eyes and rosy nose. Two to one, the ayes have it!"
Confabulation	Fabrication of facts or events in response to questions, to fill in the gaps from impaired memory.
Derailment (loosening of associations)	Tangential speech with shifting topics that are loosely connected or unrelated. The patient is unaware of the lack of association.
Echolalia	Repetition of the words and phrases of others.
Flight of ideas	An almost continuous flow of accelerated speech with abrupt changes from one topic to the next. Changes are based on understandable associations, plays on words, or distracting stimuli, but ideas are not well connected.
Incoherence	Speech that is incomprehensible and illogical, with lack of meaningful connections, abrupt changes in topic, or disordered grammar or word use. Flight of ideas, when severe, may produce incoherence.
Neologisms	Invented or distorted words, or words with new and highly idiosyncratic meanings.
Perseveration	Persistent repetition of words or ideas.

Blocking may be striking in schizophrenia.

Circumstantiality occurs in people with obsessions.

Clanging occurs in schizophrenia and manic episodes.

Confabulation is seen in Korsakoff syndrome from alcoholism.

Derailment is seen in schizophrenia, manic episodes, and other psychotic disorders.

Echolalia occurs in manic episodes and schizophrenia.

Flight of ideas is most frequently noted in manic episodes.

Incoherence is seen in severe psychotic disturbances (usually schizophrenia).

Neologisms are observed in schizophrenia, psychotic disorders, and aphasia.

Perseveration occurs in schizophrenia and other psychotic disorders.

Thought Content. **Thought content** is *what* the patient thinks about, including level of insight and judgment. To assess thought content, follow the patient's leads and cues rather than asking direct questions. For example, "You mentioned that a neighbor caused your entire illness. Can you tell me more about that?" Or, in another situation, "What do you think about at times like these?" For more focused inquiries, be tactful and accepting. "When people are upset like this, sometimes they can't keep certain thoughts out of their minds," or "... things seem unreal. Have you experienced anything like this?" In these ways, explore any of the patterns in Box 9-7.

Box 9-7. Abnormalities of Thought Content

Anxieties	Apprehensive anticipation of future danger or misfortune accompanied by feelings of worry, distress, and/or somatic symptoms of tension
Compulsions	Repetitive behaviors that the person feels driven to perform in response to an obsession, aimed at preventing or reducing anxiety or a dreaded event or situation; these behaviors are excessive and unrealistically connected to the provoking stimulus.

(continued)

Compulsions, obsessions, phobias, and anxieties often occur in anxiety disorders. See the *DSM-5*.

Box 9-7. Abnormalities of Thought Content (*continued*)

Delusions	False fixed personal beliefs that are not amenable to change in light of conflicting evidence; types of delusions include: ■ *persecutory* ■ *grandiose* ■ *jealous* ■ *erotomanic*—the belief that another person is in love with the individual ■ *somatic*—involves bodily functions or sensations ■ *unspecified*—includes delusions of reference without a prominent persecutory or grandiose component, or the belief that external events, objects, or people have a particular and unusual personal significance (e.g., commands from the radio or television)
Depersonalization	Sense that one's self or identity is different, changed, unreal; lost; or detached from one's mind or body
Derealization	Sense that the environment is strange, unreal, or remote
Obsessions	Recurrent persistent thoughts, images, or urges experienced as intrusive and unwanted that the person tries to ignore, suppress, or neutralize with other thoughts or actions (e.g., performing a compulsive behavior)
Phobias	Persistent irrational fears accompanied by a compelling desire to avoid the provoking stimulus

Delusions and feelings of unreality or depersonalization are often associated with psychotic disorders. For official diagnostic criteria of psychotic disorders, see the *DSM-5*.

Delusions may also occur in delirium, severe mood disorders, and dementia.

Perceptions

Perceptions are sensory awareness of objects in the environment and their interrelationships (external stimuli). They also refer to internal stimuli such as dreams or hallucinations (Box 9-8). Pursue false perceptions, for example, "When you heard the voice speaking to you, what did it say? How did it make you feel?" Or, "After you've been drinking a lot, do you ever see things that aren't really there?" Or, "Sometimes after major surgery like yours, people hear peculiar or frightening things. Has anything like this happened to you?" In these ways, find out about the following abnormal perceptions.

Box 9-8. Abnormalities of Perception

Hallucinations	Perception-like experiences that seem real but, unlike illusions, lack actual external stimulation. The person may or may not recognize the experiences as false. Hallucinations may be auditory, visual, olfactory, gustatory, tactile, or somatic. False perceptions associated with dreaming, falling asleep, and awakening are not classified as hallucinations. Hallucinations may occur in delirium, dementia (less commonly), posttraumatic stress disorder, schizophrenia, and substance use.
Illusions	Misinterpretations of real external stimuli, such as mistaking rustling leaves for the sound of voices. Illusions may occur in grief reactions, delirium, acute and posttraumatic stress disorders, and schizophrenia.

Insight. Insight is an awareness that symptoms or disturbed behaviors are normal or abnormal; for example, distinguishing between daydreams and hallucinations that seem real. Some of your first questions to the patient often yield important information about insight: "What brings you to the hospital?" "What seems to be the trouble?" "What do you think is wrong?" Note whether the patient is aware that a particular mood, thought, or perception is abnormal or part of an illness.

Patients with psychotic disorders often lack insight into their illness. Denial of impairment may accompany some neurologic disorders, particularly disorders affecting the parietal lobe.

Judgment. Judgment is the process of comparing and evaluating alternatives when deciding on a course of action; it reflects values that may or may not be based on reality and social conventions or norms. Assess judgment by noting the patient's responses to family situations, jobs, use of money, and interpersonal conflicts. "How do you plan to get help after leaving the hospital?" "How are you going to manage if you lose your job?" "If your husband starts to abuse you again, what will you do?" "Who will take care of your financial affairs while you are in the nursing home?"

Judgment may be poor in delirium, dementia, intellectual disability, and psychotic states.

Anxiety, mood disorders, intelligence, education, income, and cultural values also influence judgment.

Note whether decisions and actions are based on reality or impulse, wish fulfillment, or disordered thought content. What insights and values seem to underlie the patient's decisions and behavior? Allowing for cultural variations, how do these compare with a comparable mature adult? Because judgment reflects maturity, it may be variable and unpredictable during adolescence.

Cognitive Functions

Cognition refers to the mental processes involved in gaining knowledge and comprehension. Cognitive function includes *orientation, attention,* and *memory* (remote, recent, new learning) as well as *higher cognitive functions* such as information and vocabulary, calculations, abstract thinking, and constructional ability.

Orientation. Orientation is the awareness of personal identity, place, and time, which requires both memory and attention. You can usually assess orientation during the interview. For example, you can ask quite naturally for clarification about specific dates and times, the patient's address and telephone number, the names of family members, or the route to the hospital. At times, direct questions will be needed: "Can you tell me the time now...and what day it is?"

Disorientation is common when attention is impaired, as in delirium.

Attention. Attention is the ability to focus or concentrate over time on a particular stimulus or activity—an inattentive person is easily distractible and may have difficulty giving a history or responding to questions. The following tests of attention are commonly used.

Digit Span. Explain that you would like to test the patient's ability to concentrate, perhaps adding that this can be difficult if the patient is in pain or ill. Recite a series of digits, starting with two at a time and speaking each number clearly at a rate of about one per second. Ask the patient to repeat the numbers back to you. If this repetition is accurate, try a series of three numbers, then four, and so on as long as the patient responds correctly. Jot down the numbers as you say them to ensure your own accuracy. If the patient makes a mistake, try once more with another series of the same length. Stop after a second failure in a single series.

Causes of poor performance include delirium, dementia, intellectual disability, and performance anxiety.

When choosing digits, use street numbers, zip codes, telephone numbers, and other numerical sequences that are familiar to you, but avoid consecutive numbers, easily recognized dates, and sequences that are familiar to the patient.

Now, starting again with a series of two, ask the patient to repeat the numbers to you backward.

Normally, a person should be able to repeat correctly at least five digits forward and four backward.

Serial 7s. Instruct the patient, "Starting from 100, subtract 7, and keep subtracting 7...." Note the effort required and the speed and accuracy of the responses. Writing down the answers helps you keep up with the arithmetic. Normally, a person can complete serial 7s in 1½ minutes, with fewer than four errors. If the patient cannot do serial 7s, try 3s or counting backward.

Poor performance may result from delirium, the late stage of dementia, intellectual disability, anxiety, or depression. Also consider educational level.

Spelling Backward. This can substitute for serial 7s. Say a five-letter word, spell it, for example, W-O-R-L-D, and ask the patient to spell it backward.

Memory. Memory is the process of registering or recording information, tested by asking for immediate repetition of material, followed by storage or retention of information. *Recent* or *short-term* memory covers minutes, hours, or days; *remote* or *long-term* memory refers to intervals of years.

Remote (Long-Term) Memory. Inquire about important dates such as birthdays or anniversaries, names of schools attended, jobs held, or historical events relevant to the patient's past.

Remote memory is usually preserved in early stages of dementia but may be impaired in its later stages.

Recent (Short-Term) Memory. This can involve the events of the day. Ask questions with answers you can check against other sources to see if the patient is confabulating or making up facts to compensate for an impaired memory. These might include the day's weather or appointment time, current medications, or laboratory tests taken during the day.

Recent memory is impaired in dementia and delirium. Amnestic disorders impair memory or new learning ability and reduce social or occupational functioning but lack the global features of delirium or dementia. Anxiety, depression, and intellectual disability may also impair recent memory.

New Learning Ability. Give the patient three or four words such as "83, Water Street, and blue," or "table, flower, green, and hamburger." Ask the patient to repeat them so that you know that the information has been heard and registered. This step, like digit span, tests registration and immediate recall. Then proceed to other parts of the examination. After 3 to 5 minutes, ask the patient to repeat the words.

Note the accuracy of the response, awareness of whether it is correct, and any tendency to confabulate. Normally, a person should be able to remember the words.

Higher Cognitive Functions

Higher cognitive functions are assessed by vocabulary, fund of information, abstract thinking, calculations, and construction of objects that have two or three dimensions.

Information and Vocabulary. If observed clinically in the context of cultural and educational background, information and vocabulary provide a rough estimate of the patient's baseline abilities. Begin assessing fund of knowledge and vocabulary during the interview. Ask about work, hobbies, reading, favorite television programs, or current events. Start with simple questions, then move to more difficult questions. Note the person's grasp of information, complexity of the ideas, and choice of vocabulary.

Information and vocabulary are relatively unaffected by mental disorders except in severe cases. Testing helps distinguish adults with life-long intellectual impairment (whose information and vocabulary are limited) from those with mild or moderate dementia (whose information and vocabulary are fairly well preserved).

More directly, you can ask about specific facts such as:

- Name of the president, vice president, or governor
- Names of the last four or five presidents
- Names of five large cities in the country

Calculating Ability. Test the patient's ability to do arithmetical calculations, starting with simple addition ("What is 4 + 3?...8 + 7?") and multiplication ("What is 5 × 6?...9 × 7?"). Proceed to more difficult tasks using two-digit numbers ("15 + 12" or "25 × 6") or longer, written examples.

Poor performance suggests dementia or aphasia but should be measured against the patient's fund of knowledge and level of education.

Alternatively, pose practical functionally important questions, like: "If something costs 78 cents and you give the salesperson 1 dollar, how much change should you get back?"

Abstract Thinking. Test the capacity to think abstractly in two ways.

Proverbs. Ask the patient what the following proverbs mean:

- A stitch in time saves nine.
- Don't count your chickens before they're hatched.
- The proof of the pudding is in the eating.
- A rolling stone gathers no moss.
- The squeaky wheel gets the grease.

Note the relevance of the answers and their degree of concreteness or abstractness. For example, "You should sew a rip before it gets bigger" is concrete, whereas "Prompt attention to a problem prevents trouble" is abstract. Average patients should give abstract or semiabstract responses.

Concrete responses are common in people with intellectual disability, delirium, or dementia but may also reflect limited education. Patients with schizophrenia may respond concretely or with personal and bizarre interpretations.

Similarities. Ask the patient to tell you how the following are alike:

An orange and an apple	A church and a theater
A cat and a mouse	A piano and a violin
A child and a dwarf	Wood and coal

Note the accuracy and relevance of the answers and their degree of concreteness or abstractness. For example, "A cat and a mouse are both animals" is abstract, "They both have tails" is concrete, and "A cat chases a mouse" is not relevant.

Constructional Ability. The task here is to copy figures of increasing complexity onto a piece of blank unlined paper. Show each figure one at a time and ask the patient to copy it as well as possible (Figs. 9-5 and 9-6).

With intact vision and motor ability, poor constructional ability suggests dementia or parietal lobe damage. Intellectual disability can also impair performance.

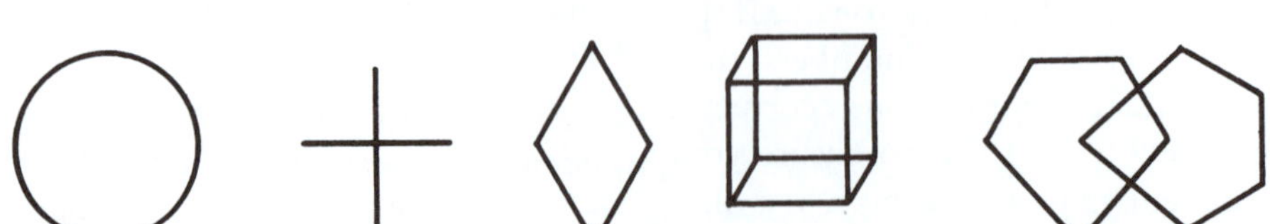

FIGURE 9-5. Ask the patient to copy these figures (starting from the left) on a piece of paper.

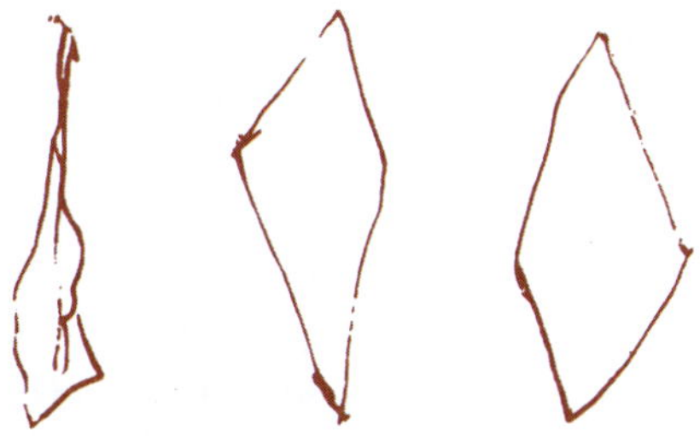

FIGURE 9-6. From left to right: poor, fair, and good attempts of drawn shapes.

In another approach, ask the patient to draw a clock face complete with numbers and hands (Figs. 9-7 and 9-8).

FIGURE 9-7. Patient-drawn clock face, with hands and numbers, rated as excellent.

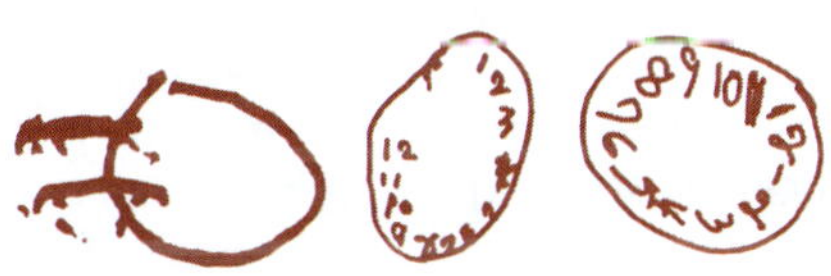

FIGURE 9-8. From left to right: poor, fair, and good attempts of clock face drawings.

RECORDING YOUR FINDINGS

Recording Behavior and Mental Status

"Mental Status: The patient is alert, well-groomed, and cheerful. Speech is fluent and words are clear. Thought processes are coherent, insight is good. The patient is oriented to person, place, and time. Serial 7s accurate; recent and remote memory intact. Calculations intact."

OR

"Mental Status: The patient appears sad and fatigued; clothes are wrinkled. Speech is slow and words are mumbled. Thought processes are coherent, but insight into current life reverses is limited. The patient is oriented to person, place, and time. Digit span, serial 7s, and calculations accurate, but responses delayed. Clock drawing is good."

These findings suggest depression.

HEALTH PROMOTION AND COUNSELING: EVIDENCE AND RECOMMENDATIONS

Important Topics for Health Promotion and Counseling

- Screening for depression
- Assessing for suicide risk
- Screening for neurocognitive disorders: dementia and delirium
- Screening for substance use disorders, including misuse of alcohol and prescription drugs

Mental health disorders impose a substantial burden of suffering. Depression and anxiety are a common cause of hospitalization in the United States, and mental illness is associated with increased risks for chronic medical conditions, decreased life expectancy, disability, substance abuse, and suicide.

Screening for Depression

Depression frequently accompanies chronic medical illness. High-risk patients may have subtle early signs of depression, including low self-esteem, loss of pleasure in daily activities (anhedonia), sleep disorders, and difficulty concentrating or making decisions. Look carefully for symptoms of depression in vulnerable patients, especially those who are young, female, single, divorced or separated, seriously or chronically ill, bereaved, or have other psychiatric disorders including substance abuse. A personal or family history of depression also places patients at risk.

- "Over the past 2 weeks, have you felt down, depressed, or hopeless?" screens for depressed mood.
- "Over the past 2 weeks, have you felt little interest or pleasure in doing things?" screens for anhedonia.

See Table 9-5, Screening for Depression: Geriatric Depression Scale, and Table 9-6, Screening for Depression: Patient Health Questionnaire (PHQ-9).

A single screening question, "Do you often feel sad or depressed?" has a sensitivity of 69% and specificity of 90%. All positive screening tests warrant full diagnostic interviews.

Assessing for Suicide Risk

Despite the public health burden of suicide, the current evidence is insufficient to assess the balance of benefits and harms of screening for suicide risk in a primary care setting (I statement), but clinicians should be aware of patient clues and risk factors.

Screening for Neurocognitive Disorders

Dementia. *Dementia* is "an acquired condition that is characterized by a decline in at least two cognitive domains (e.g., loss of memory, attention, language, or visuospatial or executive functioning) that is severe enough to affect social or occupational functioning." Affected patients may also exhibit behavioral and psychological symptoms. In the *DSM-5*, dementia is classified as a **major neurocognitive disorder.** The major dementia syndromes include Alzheimer disease (AD), vascular dementia, frontotemporal dementia, dementia with Lewy bodies, Parkinson disease with dementia, and dementia of mixed etiology. Risk factors include advancing age, family history, and the gene mutation apolipoprotein (APOE) ε4. Risk of AD more than doubles in first-degree relatives. Risk doubles in the presence of one APOE ε4 allele and increases fivefold or more in the presence of two alleles, although only 2% of the population carries these genes.

Box 9-9 highlights distinguishing features between age-related cognitive decline, mild cognitive impairment, and AD.

The *Mini-Mental State Examination* is the best-known screening test for dementia but is now copyrighted for commercial use, so is less accessible. Recommended screening tests now include the Mini-Cog and the Montreal Cognitive Assessment (MoCA) found in Tables 9-6 and 9-7. The *Mini-Cog* has a sensitivity and specificity in some studies as high as 91% and 86%, respectively, and is shorter to administer—about 3 minutes. The *MoCA* has comparable sensitivity and specificity, 91% and 81% in recent studies, and takes 10 minutes to administer.

See Table 9-3, Neurocognitive Disorders: Delirium and Dementia, Table 9-7, Screening for Dementia: The Mini-Cog, and Table 9-8, Screening for Dementia: Montreal Cognitive Assessment (MoCA).

Physiology OSCE Video:
Mini-Mental State Examination

Box 9-9. The Spectrum of Cognitive Decline

Age-related Cognitive Decline

- This diagnosis is suggested by mild forgetfulness, difficulty remembering names, and mildly reduced concentration.
- Such symptoms are sporadic and do not affect daily function.

Mild Cognitive Impairment (MCI)

- *Daily function is preserved,* but there is evidence of modest *cognitive decline in one or more cognitive domains* (complex attention, executive function, learning and memory, language, perceptual-motor, or social cognition) based on objective tasks, as reported by the patient, an informant, or the clinician or on clinical testing.
- *Alertness and attention are preserved* (unlike delirium).
- Other dementias are unlikely (see below).
- AD develops at a higher frequency in MCI patients, progressing to AD at a reported rate of 6% to 15% per year.

Alzheimer Disease

- *Probable AD,* based on *DSM-5* criteria, consists of evidence of a causative genetic mutation from family history or genetic testing, or the presence *of cognitive decline in two or more cognitive domains, with all three of the following features:* (1) clear evidence of a decline in memory and learning and at least one other cognitive domain (see above); (2) steady progressive decline in cognition without extended plateaus; and (3) no evidence of mixed etiology from other neurodegenerative, cerebrovascular, mental, or systemic disease.
- *Possible AD* is diagnosed when the patient meets all three criteria by evidence from genetic testing or when family history is absent.
- *Alertness and attention are preserved.*
- Other dementias are unlikely (see below).
- Memory difficulties may take the form of repeating questions, losing objects, or confusion when performing tasks such as shopping. Later stages include impaired judgment and disorientation progressing to aphasia, apraxia, left–right confusion, and ultimately, dependence of instrumental activities of daily living. Psychosis and agitation may also occur.
- The differentiation of dementia from MCI rests on the determination of whether or not there is significant interference in the ability to function at work or in usual daily activities.

Other Dementias

- *Vascular dementia* is suggested by vascular risk factors or cerebrovascular disease associated with cognitive impairment. Stepwise decline, especially in executive function, should correlate with the onset of a cerebrovascular event, but consider this dementia even if just risk factors are present. At times, there are gait changes and focal findings.
- *Lewy body disease* is suggested by evidence of parkinsonism. Visual hallucinations, delusions, and gait disorder may be early clues. At times, there are extrapyramidal symptoms, fluctuating mental status, and sensitivity to antipsychotic medications.
- *Frontotemporal dementia* is suggested by prominent behavioral or language disorders, at times with personality changes including impulsivity, aggression, and apathy. At times, there is excessive eating and drinking. There is relative preservation of memory and visual–spatial skills. Onset may occur before age 60 years.

See Table 9-7, Screening for Dementia: The Mini-Cog, and Table 9-8, Screening for Dementia: The Montreal Cognitive Assessment (MoCA).

Delirium. **Delirium**, a multifactorial syndrome, is an acute confusional state marked by sudden onset; fluctuating course; inattention; and, at times, changing levels of consciousness. Risk for developing delirium depends on both predisposing conditions that increase susceptibility and the immediate precipitating factors. Delirium is common in hospitalized general medical patients; rates are even higher following major elective surgeries. Intensive care unit admissions are associated with a high incidence of delirium regardless of age. Even though delirium is associated with poor patient outcomes, more than 50% of cases are undetected.

The Confusion Assessment Method (CAM) (Box 9-10) is recommended for screening at-risk patients. The CAM instrument can quickly and accurately detect delirium at the bedside.

Box 9-10. The Confusion Assessment Method (CAM) Diagnostic Algorithm

Diagnosing delirium requires features 1 and 2 and either 3 or 4.

1. Acute change in mental status and fluctuating course:
   Is there evidence of an acute change in cognition from baseline?
   Does the abnormal behavior fluctuate during the day?
2. Inattention:
   Does the patient have difficulty focusing attention?
3. Disorganized thinking:
   Does the patient have rambling or irrelevant conversations, unclear or illogical flow of ideas, or unpredictable switching from subject to subject?
4. Abnormal level of consciousness:
   Is the patient anything besides alert—hyperalert, lethargic, stuporous, or comatose?

Screening for Substance Use Disorders, Including Misuse of Alcohol and Prescription and Illicit Drugs

The harmful interactions between mental disorders and substance use disorders also present a major public health problem.

Every patient should be asked about alcohol use, substance abuse, and misuse of prescription drugs.

See discussion of screening tools in Chapter 6.

TABLE 9-1. Central Nervous System Structures and Mental Disorders

Structure	Roles	Clinical Manifestations of Dysfunction
Cortical Structures		
Parietal lobe	Involved in visuospatial sense, attention, and movement.	Deficits in parietal lobe function have been associated with attention-deficit/hyperactivity disorder (ADHD), obsessive–compulsive disorder (OCD), and schizophrenia.
Temporal lobe: primary auditory cortex	Responsible for auditory processing.	In schizophrenia, the primary auditory cortex activates even in the absence of sound, which often result in the experience of *auditory hallucinations*.
Temporal lobe: hippocampus	Critical to memory and learning. There is also high concentrations of cortisol receptors in the hippocampus.	Hippocampus dysfunction may contribute to cognitive impairment in Alzheimer disease (AD) and schizophrenia. Major depressive disorder (MDD) and posttraumatic stress disorder (PTSD) both cause significant increases of cortisol, which may cause memory and cognitive problems seen in these disorders. Hippocampus dysfunction is also thought to contribute to anxiety symptoms.
Temporal lobe: amygdala	Involved in the cortical processes that cause emotions. The fight-or-flight response, or fear response, is activated through the amygdala.	In people with posttraumatic stress disorder (PTSD), the amygdala is often hyperactivated and cannot be easily turned off. People with PTSD often startle easily and struggle with anxiety or panic. Excess amygdala activity is also seen in people with bipolar disorder, which is thought to contribute to irritability and labile mood.
Frontal lobe	Vital to executive function (which includes memory, cognition, behavioral control, and attention) and emotions.	Dysfunction has been associated with most mental disorders, including bipolar disorder, schizophrenia, attention-deficit/hyperactivity disorder, major depressive disorder (MDD), obsessive–compulsive disorder (OCD), posttraumatic stress disorder (PTSD), and AD.
Subcortical Structures		
Cingulate cortex	Manages attention, emotion, and memory.	Dysfunction in people with attention-deficit/hyperactivity disorder (ADHD), obsessive–compulsive disorder (OCD), generalized anxiety disorder (GAD), major depressive disorder (MDD), and schizophrenia.
Basal Forebrain		
Nucleus basalis of Meynert	Major center for acetylcholine production in the CNS which helps to regulate sleep, arousal, and attention.	Contributes to cognitive deficits in neurocognitive disorders
Nucleus accumbens	Vital to the functioning of the reward pathway.	Excess activation is commonly seen in addiction.

(*continued*)

TABLE 9-1. Central Nervous System Structures and Mental Disorders *(Continued)*

Structure	Roles	Clinical Manifestations of Dysfunction
Basal ganglia	Works with the nucleus accumbens to control reward.	Dysfunction seen in addiction, obsessive–compulsive disorder (OCD), major depressive disorder (MDD), attention-deficit/hyperactivity disorder (ADHD), schizophrenia, and bipolar disorder.
Epithalamus: pineal gland	Produces melatonin, which regulates sleep.	Contributes to sleep disturbances in major depressive disorder (MDD), obsessive–compulsive disorder (OCD), posttraumatic stress disorder (PTSD), and AD.
Epithalamus: habenula	Helps regulate reproductive behavior, pain, nutrition, sleep, stress, and learning.	Increased activity in the habenula can cause anhedonia in depression. Decreased habenula activity is associated with psychosis and addiction.
Hypothalamus	Periods of increased stress are associated with increased activity of the hypothalamic–pituitary–adrenal axis and increased release of corticotropin-releasing factor, which causes cortisol (a steroid hormone) release.	Increased cortisol can cause depressive symptoms.
Mammillary bodies	Crucial in memory	Damage to the mammillary bodies is seen in vitamin B_1 (thiamine) deficiency in people with alcohol use disorder. This may lead to Wernicke–Korsakoff syndrome, a condition characterized by severe memory impairment.
Cerebellum	Regulates motor coordination and motor learning	Alcohol use impairs cerebellar function, which can cause *ataxia*, or a loss of motor coordination.

Note: Based on current research, the occipital lobe does not significantly play a role in mental disorders as do other cortical and subcortical structures.

TABLE 9-2. Neurocircuitry of Mental Disorders

System/Network	CNS Structures Involved	Role When Activated	Mental Disorder
Limbic system	Hippocampus, amygdala, fornix, hypothalamus, thalamus, mammillary bodies, frontal lobes, temporal lobes, and cingulate gyrus	Responsible for experience of emotion as well as empathy	Dysfunction seen in the vast majority of mental disorders, including but not limited to schizophrenia, major depressive disorder (MDD), bipolar disorder, anxiety, and posttraumatic stress disorder (PTSD)
Fear network (subdivision of the limbic system)	Thalamus, frontal lobes, and amygdala		Dysfunction seen in anxiety, posttraumatic stress disorder (PTSD), and bipolar disorder
Attention network	Frontal lobes and parietal lobes	Responsible for controlling attention	Dysfunction seen in persons with attention-deficit/hyperactivity disorder (ADHD)
Salience network	Connections between the amygdala, basal ganglia, temporal lobes, and the cingulate cortex	Involved in monitoring internal states (homeostasis, emotion, pain) and external states (body position, environment); activity here has been associated with self-awareness, social behavior, and communication	Dysfunction associated with schizophrenia, mood disorder, anxiety, dementia, and substance use
Reward network	Composed of the amygdala, hippocampus, frontal lobes, cingulate cortex, brainstem, basal forebrain, and basal ganglia	Causes a pleasurable feeling of reward and contributes to the learning	Dysfunction occurs in addiction and attention-deficit/hyperactivity disorder (ADHD)
Default mode network	Frontal lobes, cingulate cortex, parietal lobes, and temporal lobes	Involved in rest and internal awareness	Dysfunction seen in schizophrenia and major depressive disorder (MDD), leading to delusions and negative thoughts, respectively
Executive network	Frontal lobes and cingulate cortex	Responsible for memory and planning	Dysfunction has been associated with numerous mental disorders, including posttraumatic stress disorder (PTSD), major depressive disorder (MDD), and schizophrenia

TABLE 9-3. Neurocognitive Disorders: Delirium and Dementia

Delirium and dementia are common and important disorders that affect multiple aspects of mental status. Both have many possible causes. Some clinical features of these two conditions and their effects on mental status are compared below. A delirium may be superimposed on dementia.

	Delirium	Dementia
Clinical Features		
Onset	Acute	Insidious
Course	Fluctuating, with lucid intervals; worse at night	Slowly progressive
Duration	Hours to weeks	Months to years
Sleep/Wake Cycle	Always disrupted	Sleep fragmented
General Clinical Illness or Drug Toxicity	Either or both present	Often absent, especially in Alzheimer disease
Mental Status		
Level of Consciousness	Disturbed. Person less alert to clearly aware of the environment and less able to focus, sustain, or shift attention	Usually normal until late in the course of the illness
Behavior	Activity often abnormally decreased (somnolence) or increased (agitation, hypervigilance)	Normal to slow; may become inappropriate
Speech	May be hesitant, slow or rapid, incoherent	Difficulty in finding words, aphasia
Mood	Fluctuating, labile, from fearful or irritable to normal or depressed	Often flat, depressed
Thought Processes	Disorganized, may be incoherent	Impoverished. Speech gives little information
Thought Content	Delusions common, often transient	Delusions may occur
Perceptions	Illusions, hallucinations, most often visual	Hallucinations may occur
Judgment	Impaired, often to a varying degree	Increasingly impaired over the course of the illness
Orientation	Usually disoriented, especially for time. A known place may seem unfamiliar.	Fairly well maintained, but becomes impaired in the later stages of illness
Attention	Fluctuates, with inattention. Person easily distracted, unable to concentrate on selected tasks	Usually unaffected until late in the illness
Memory	Immediate and recent memory impaired	Recent memory and new learning especially impaired
Examples of Cause	Delirium tremens (due to withdrawal from alcohol) Uremia Acute hepatic failure Acute cerebral vasculitis Atropine poisoning	*Reversible:* Vitamin B_{12} deficiency, thyroid disorders *Irreversible:* Alzheimer disease, vascular dementia (from multiple infarcts), dementia due to head trauma

TABLE 9-4. Somatic Symptom and Related Disorders

Type of Disorder	Diagnostic Features
Somatic symptom disorder	Somatic symptoms are either very distressing or result in significant disruption of functioning, as well as excessive and disproportionate thoughts, feelings, and behaviors related to those symptoms. Symptoms should be specific if with predominant pain.
Illness anxiety disorder	Preoccupation with having or acquiring a serious illness where somatic symptoms, if present, are only mild in intensity
Conversion disorder	Syndrome of symptoms of deficits mimicking neurologic or medical illness in which psychological factors are judged to be of etiologic importance
Psychological factors affecting other medical conditions	Presence of one or more clinically significant psychological or behavioral factors that adversely affect a medical condition by increasing the risk for suffering, death, or disability
Factitious disorder	Falsification of physical or psychological signs or symptoms, or induction of injury or disease, associated with identified deception. The individual presents himself or herself as ill, impaired, or injured even in the absence of external rewards.
Other Related Disorders or Behaviors	
Body dysmorphic disorder	Preoccupation with one or more perceived defects or flaws in physical appearance that are not observable or appear only slight to others.
Dissociative disorder	Disruption of and/or discontinuity in the normal integration of consciousness, memory, identity, emotion, perception, body representation, motor control, and behavior.

TABLE 9-5. Screening for Depression: The Geriatric Depression Scale (Short Form)

Administration

Ask the patient 15 questions for how he/she felt over the past week. Instruct the patient to respond either YES or NO. You may also ask the patient to complete the form using the self-rated form.

Scoring

Answers indicating depression are in bold; score 1 point for each one selected. Maximum score = 15; 0–4 = normal, depending on age, education, complaints; 5–8 = mild; 9–11 = moderate; 12–15 = severe

Choose the best answer for how you have felt over the past week:

1. Are you basically satisfied with your life? YES / **NO**
2. Have you dropped many of your activities and interests? **YES** / NO
3. Do you feel that your life is empty? **YES** / NO
4. Do you often get bored? **YES** / NO
5. Are you in good spirits most of the time? YES / **NO**
6. Are you afraid that something bad is going to happen to you? **YES** / NO
7. Do you feel happy most of the time? YES / **NO**
8. Do you often feel helpless? **YES** / NO
9. Do you prefer to stay at home, rather than going out and doing new things? **YES** / NO
10. Do you feel you have more problems with memory than most? **YES** / NO
11. Do you think it is wonderful to be alive now? YES / **NO**
12. Do you feel pretty worthless the way you are now? **YES** / NO
13. Do you feel full of energy? YES / **NO**
14. Do you feel that your situation is hopeless? **YES** / NO
15. Do you think that most people are better off than you are? **YES** / NO

TABLE 9-6. Screening for Depression: The Patient Health Questionnaire (PHQ-9)

Administration

The PHQ-9 should be completed by the patient and scored by a staff person or clinician.

Scoring

Count the number (#) of boxes checked in a column. Multiply that number by the value indicated below, then add the subtotal to produce a total score. The possible range is 0–27. Use the table below to interpret the PHQ-9 score.

- Not at all (#) _____ × 0 = _____
- Several days (#) _____ × 1 = _____
- More than half the days (#) _____ × 2 = _____
- Nearly every day (#) _____ × 3 = _____

Total score: _____

Total Score	Depression Severity	Proposed Treatment Action
0–4	None–Minimal	None
5–9	Mild	Watchful waiting; repeat PHQ-9 at follow-up
10–14	Moderate	Treatment plan, consider counseling, follow up and/or pharmacotherapy
15–19	Moderately severe	Active treatment with pharmacotherapy and/or psychotherapy
20–27	Severe	Immediate initiation of pharmacotherapy and, if severe impairment or poor response to therapy, expedited referral to a mental health specialist for psychotherapy and/or collaborative management

(continued)

TABLE 9-6. Screening for Depression: The Patient Health Questionnaire (PHQ-9) *(Continued)*

Patient Health Questionnaire (PHQ-9)

Nine Symptom Depression Checklist

Name: ______________________ **Date:** ______________

Over the *last 2 weeks*, how often have you been bothered by any of the following problems? (Please circle your answer.)

	Not at All	Several Days	More than Half the Days	Nearly Every Day
1. Little interest or pleasure in doing things	0	1	2	3
2. Feeling down, depressed, or hopeless	0	1	2	3
3. Trouble falling or staying asleep, or sleeping too much	0	1	2	3
4. Feeling tired or having little energy	0	1	2	3
5. Poor appetite or overeating	0	1	2	3
6. Feeling bad about yourself—or that you are a failure or have let yourself or your family down	0	1	2	3
7. Trouble concentrating on things, such as reading the newspaper or watching television	0	1	2	3
8. Moving or speaking so slowly that other people could have noticed. Or the opposite—being so fidgety or restless that you have been moving around a lot more than usual	0	1	2	3
9. Thoughts that you would be better off dead or of hurting yourself in some way	0	1	2	3

Add Columns, ______ + ______ + ______

Total Score*, ______ *Score is for healthcare provider incorporation

10. If you circled *any* problems, how *difficult* have these problems made it for you to do your work, take care of things at home, or get along with other people? (Please circle your answer.)	**Not Difficult at All**	**Somewhat Difficult**	**Very Difficult**	**Extremely Difficult**

A score of: 0–4 is considered non-depressed; 5–9 mild depression; 10–14 moderate depression; 15–19 moderately severe depression; and 20–27 severe depression.

Note: Perform suicide risk assessment in patients who respond positively to item 9 "Thoughts that you would be better off dead or of hurting yourself in some way." Additional information on administering the PHQ-2 and PHQ-9 can be found at: www.phqscreeners.com. (Copyright © 1999 Pfizer Inc. All rights reserved. Reproduced with permission. PRIME-MD© is a trademark of Pfizer Inc.)

TABLE 9-7. Screening for Dementia: The Mini-Cog

Administration

The test is administered as follows:

1. Instruct the patient to listen carefully to and remember three unrelated words and then to repeat the words.
2. Instruct the patient to draw the face of a clock, either on a blank sheet of paper or on a sheet with the clock circle already drawn on the page. After the patient puts the numbers on the clock face, ask him or her to draw the hands of the clock to read a specific time.
3. Ask the patient to repeat the three previously stated words.

Scoring

Give 1 point for each recalled word after the clock drawing test (CDT) distractor.

Patients recalling none of the three words are classified as demented (Score = 0).

Patients recalling all three words are classified as nondemented (Score = 3).

Patients with intermediate word recall of one to two words are classified based on the CDT (Abnormal = demented; Normal = nondemented).

Note: The CDT is considered normal if all numbers are present in the correct sequence and position, and the hands readably display the requested time.

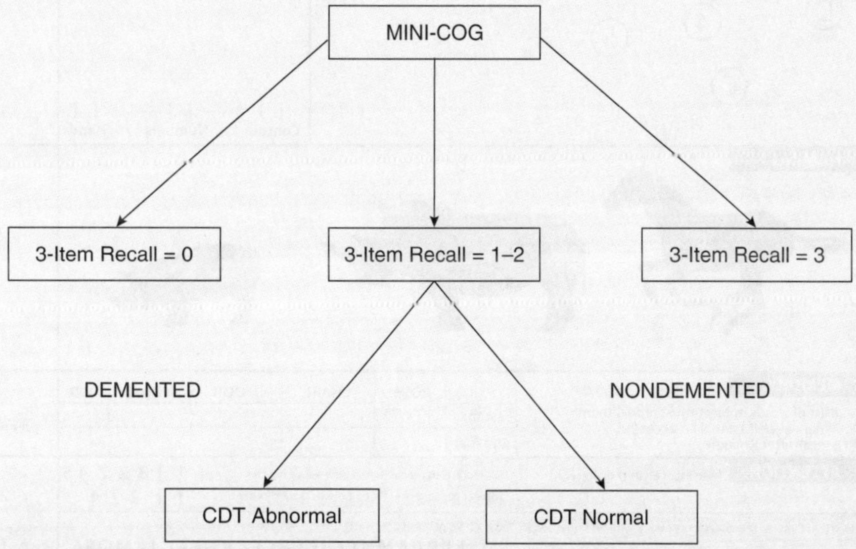

TABLE 9-8. Screening for Dementia: The Montreal Cognitive Assessment (MoCA)

Administration

The Montreal Cognitive Assessment (MoCA) was designed as a rapid screening instrument for mild cognitive dysfunction. It assesses different cognitive domains: attention and concentration, executive functions, memory, language, visuoconstructional skills, conceptual thinking, calculations, and orientation. Time to administer the MoCA is approximately 10 minutes.

Scoring

Sum all subscores listed on the right-hand side. Add one point for an individual who has 12 years or fewer of formal education, for a possible maximum of 30 points. A final total score of 26 and above is considered normal.

NAME:
Education: **Date of birth:**
Sex: **DATE:**

VISUOSPATIAL / EXECUTIVE

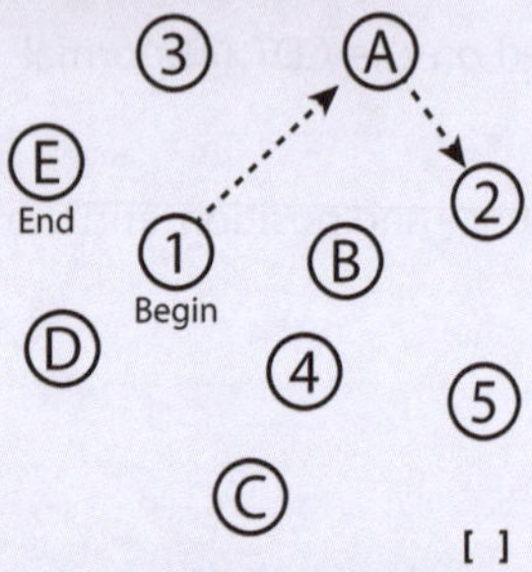

[ ]

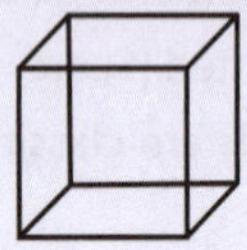

Copy cube [ ]

Draw Clock (Ten past eight) (3 points)

[ ] Contour [ ] Numbers [ ] Hands

SCORE ___/5

NAMING

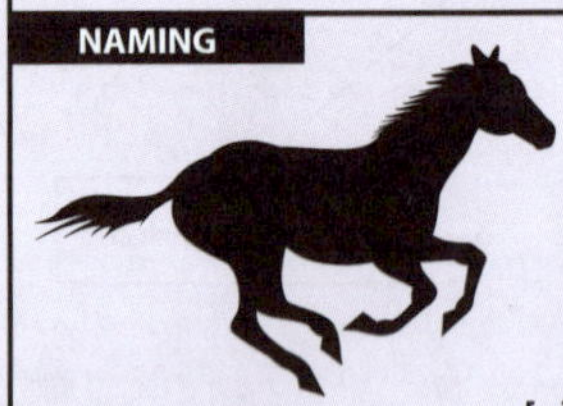

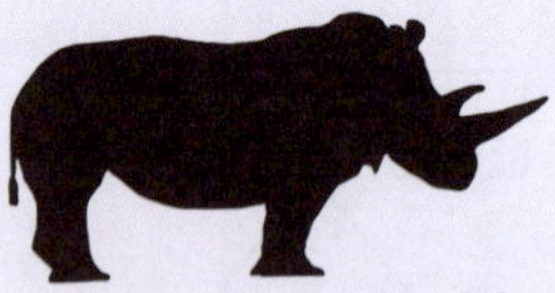

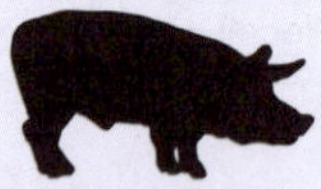

[ ] [ ] [ ] ___/3

MEMORY

Read list of words, subject must repeat them.
Do 2 trials, even if 1st trial is successful.
Do a recall after 5 minutes.

	ROSE	CHAIR	SPOON	HOUSE	RED
1st trial					
2nd trial					

No points

ATTENTION Read list of digits (1 digit /sec.).

Subject has to repeat them in the forward order [ ] 3 2 7 4 5
Subject has to repeat them inthe backward order [ ] 2 7 4 ___/2

Read list of letters. The subject must point with his finger at each letter C. No points if ≥ 2 errors.

[ ] FBCAMNCCJKLBCFCKDECCJAMOFA ___/1

Serial 7 subtraction starting at 100 [ ] 95 [ ] 86 [ ] 76 [ ] 65 [ ] 45
4 or 5 correct subtractions: **3 pts**, 2 or 3 correct: **2pts**, 1 correct: **1pt**, 0 correct: **0pt** ___/3

LANGUAGE Repeat : I only know that Judy is the one to help today. [ ]
The cat always hid under the couch when dogs were in the room. [ ] ___/2

Fluency / Name maximum number of words in one minute that begin with the letter F [ ]___ (N ≥ 11 words) ___/1

ABSTRACTION Similarity between e.g. banana - orange = fruit [ ] train - bicyle [ ] watch - ruler ___/2

DELAYED RECALL

		ROSE	CHAIR	SPOON	HOUSE	RED	
	Has to recall words **WITH NO CUE**	[ ]	[ ]	[ ]	[ ]	[ ]	Points for UNCUED recall only ___/5
Optional	Category cue						
	Multiple choice cue						

ORIENTATION [ ] Date [ ] Month [ ] Year [ ] Day [ ] Place [ ] City ___/6

Normal ≥ 26 / 30 TOTAL ___/30
Add 1 point if ≤ 12 yr edu

Administered by:______________

Copies are available at www.mocatest.org.

CHAPTER 10

Respiratory System

ANATOMY AND PHYSIOLOGY

The thorax is bounded anteriorly by the sternum and the ribs, laterally by the ribs, and posteriorly by the ribs and the thoracic spine. The superior boundary of the thorax comprises the clavicles and the neck tissues. Inferiorly, it is bounded by the diaphragm. The thorax encloses the major visceral organs—lungs and heart—and mechanically powers the work of breathing. Study the *anatomy of the chest wall*, identifying the structures illustrated (Fig. 10-1). Note that the number of the intercostal space between two ribs is the same number as the rib above it.

Locating Findings on the Chest

Describe chest findings in two dimensions: along the vertical axis and around the circumference of the chest.

Vertical Axis. To locate findings in the thorax, learn to count the ribs and intercostal spaces (Fig. 10-2). Place your finger in the hollow curve of the suprasternal notch, then move it down approximately 5 cm to the horizontal bony ridge where the manubrium joins the body of the sternum, called the *sternal angle* or the *angle of Louis.* Directly adjacent to the sternal angle is the 2nd rib and its costal cartilage. From here, using two fingers, "walk down" the interspaces *on an oblique line,* illustrated

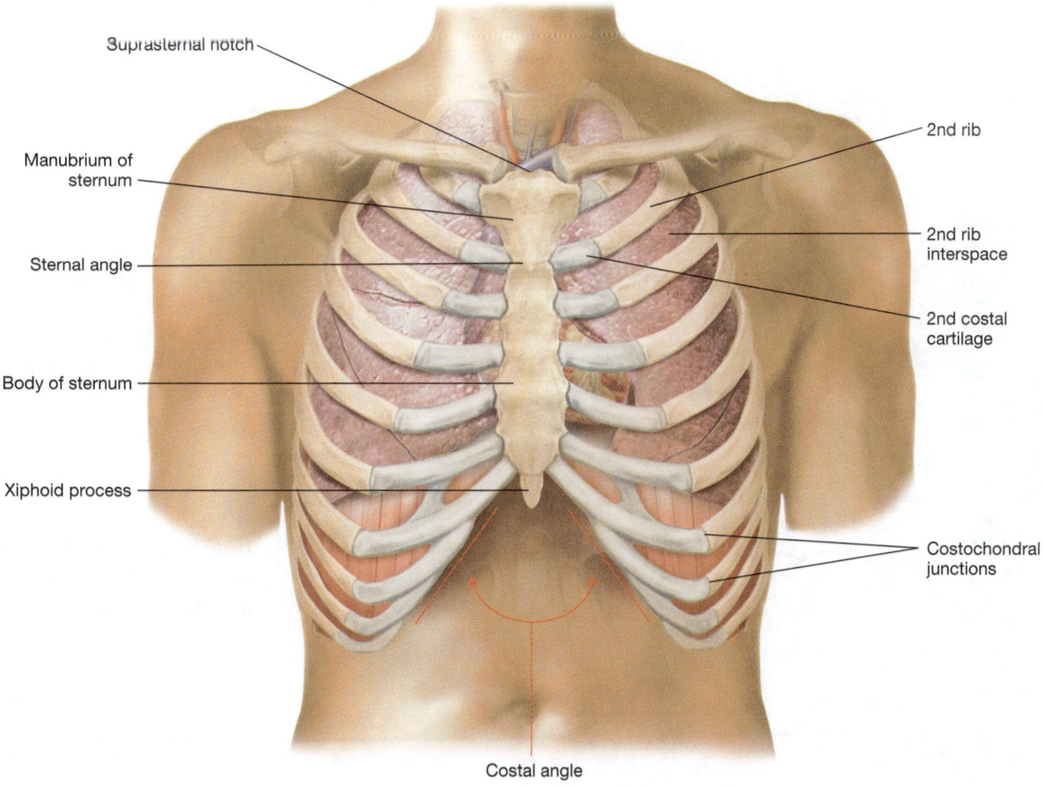

FIGURE 10-1. Chest wall anatomy.

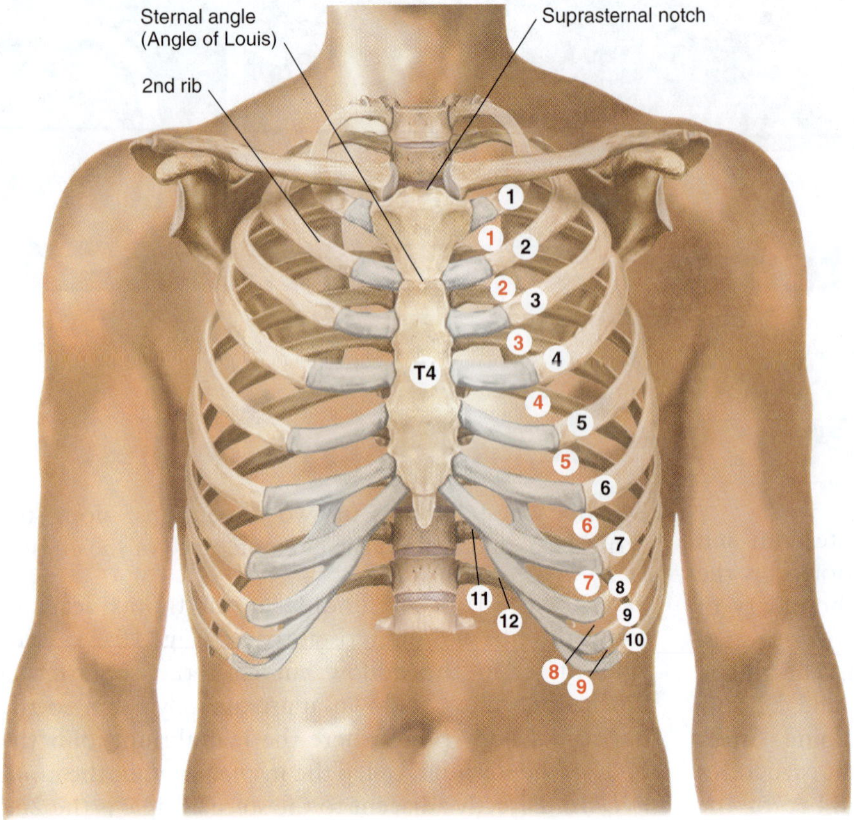

FIGURE 10-2. Anterior ribs (*black*) and intercostal spaces (*red*).

Note special landmarks:

- 2nd intercostal space for needle insertion for decompression of a tension pneumothorax.
- Intercostal space between the 4th and 5th ribs for chest tube insertion.
- Level of the 4th rib for the lower margin of a well-placed endotracheal tube on a chest x-ray.

Neurovascular structures run along the inferior margin of each rib, so needles and tubes should be placed just at the superior rib margins.

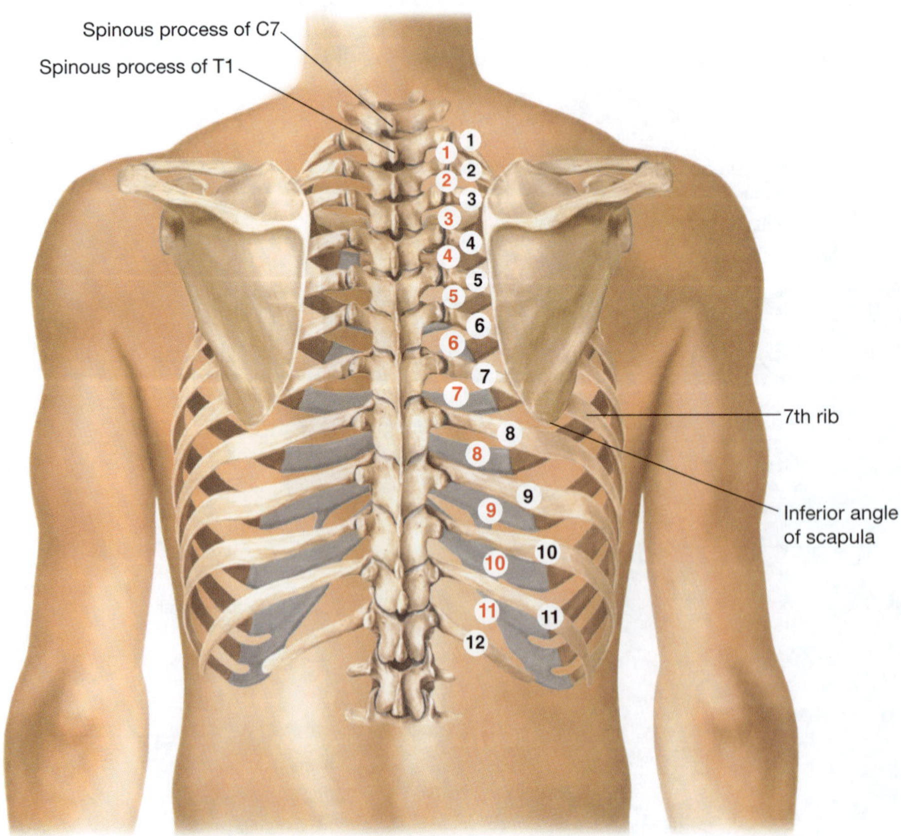

FIGURE 10-3. Posterior ribs (*black*) and intercostal spaces (*red*).

Note the intercostal space between the 7th and 8th ribs as a landmark for thoracentesis with needle insertion immediately superior to the 8th rib.

by the red numbers in Figure 10-2. (Note that the ribs at the lower edge of the sternum may be too close together to count correctly.) To count the intercostal spaces in a woman, displace the breast laterally by having the patient lie supine, or palpate more medially. Avoid pressing too hard on the tender breast tissue.

Note that the costal cartilages of the first seven ribs articulate with the sternum; the cartilages of the 8th, 9th, and 10th ribs articulate with the costal cartilages just above them. The 11th and 12th ribs, the "floating ribs," have no anterior attachments. The cartilaginous tip of the 11th rib usually can be felt laterally, and the 12th rib may be felt posteriorly. When palpated, costal cartilages and ribs feel identical.

Posteriorly, the 12th rib is a starting point for counting ribs and intercostal spaces and provides an alternative to the anterior approach (Fig. 10-3). With the fingers of one hand, press in and up against the lower border of the 12th rib; then "walk up" the intercostal spaces, numbered in red in Figure 10-3, or follow a more oblique line up and around to the front of the chest.

The inferior tip of the scapula is another useful bony landmark; it usually lies at the level of the 7th rib or intercostal space.

The spinous processes of the vertebrae are also useful landmarks. When the neck is flexed forward, the most protruding process is usually the vertebra of C7. If two processes are equally prominent, they are C7 and T1. You can often palpate and count the processes below them, especially when the spine is flexed.

Chest Circumference. Visualize a series of vertical lines as shown in Figures 10-4 through 10-6. The midsternal and vertebral lines are easily demarcated and reproducible; the others are visualized.

- *Midsternal line*—drops vertically along the sternum
- *Midclavicular line*—drops vertically from the midpoint of the clavicle
- *Anterior axillary line*—drops vertically from the anterior axillary fold

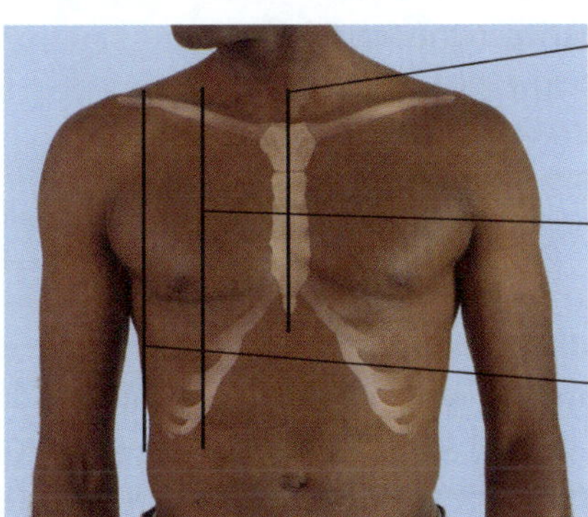

FIGURE 10-4. Midsternal and midclavicular lines.

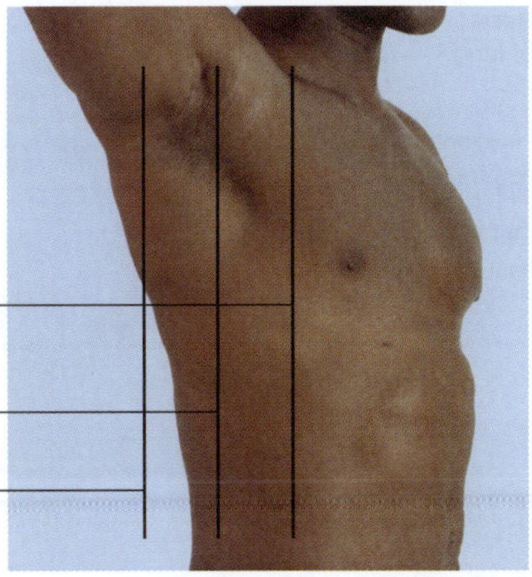

FIGURE 10-5. Anterior axillary, midaxillary, and posterior axillary lines.

The "triangle of safety" is an anatomical region in the midaxillary line formed by the lateral border of the pectoralis major muscle anteriorly, lateral border of the latissimus dorsi posteriorly, and the nipple line (4th or 5th intercostal space) inferiorly. This triangle represents a "safe position" for chest tube insertion.

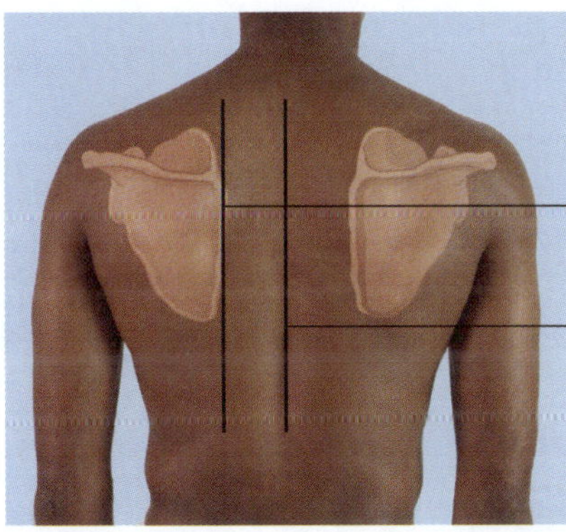

FIGURE 10-6. Vertebral and scapular lines.

- *Midaxillary line*—drops vertically from the apex of the axilla
- *Posterior axillary line*—drops vertically from the posterior axillary fold
- *Scapular line*—drops from the inferior angle of the scapula
- *Vertebral line*—overlies the thoracic spinous processes

Lungs, Fissures, and Lobes. Picture the lungs and their fissures and lobes on the chest wall. Anteriorly, the apex of each lung rises approximately 2 to 4 cm above the inner third of the clavicle (Fig. 10-7). The lower border of the lung crosses the 6th rib at the midclavicular line and the 8th rib at the midaxillary line. Posteriorly, the lower border of the lung lies at about the level of the T10 spinous process (Fig. 10-8). On inspiration, it descends in the chest cavity during contraction and descent of the diaphragm. Figure 10-9 identifies the right and left lungs on a chest radiograph.

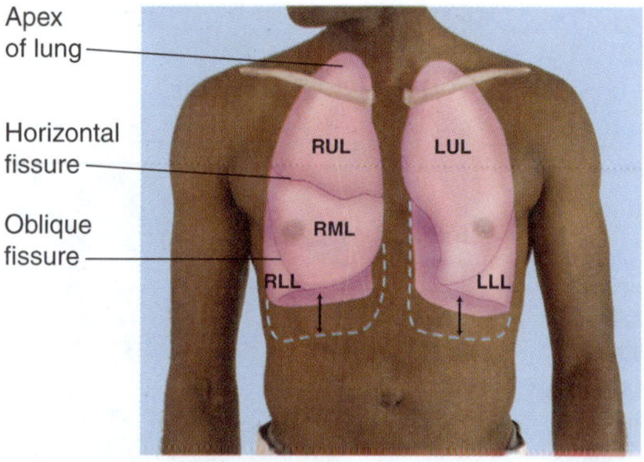

FIGURE 10-7. Anterior view of lung lobes.

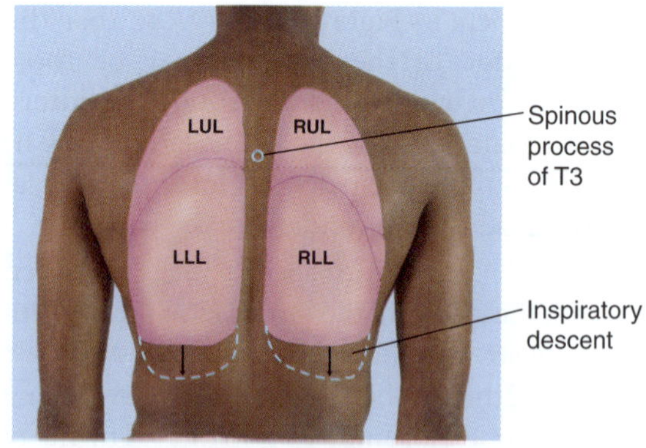

FIGURE 10-8. Posterior view of lung lobes.

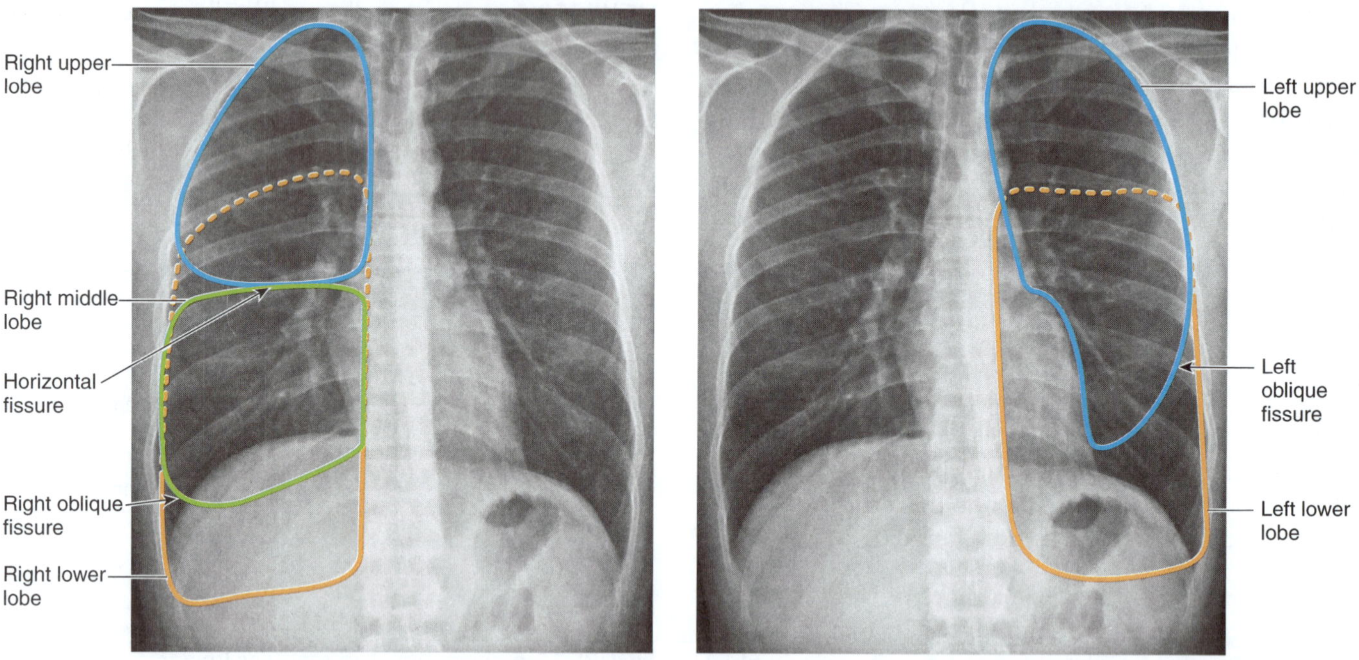

FIGURE 10-9. Right and left lungs in anterior view of a chest radiograph. (From Brant WE, Helms CA. *Brant and Helms Solution: Fundamentals of Diagnostic Radiology*. 3rd ed. Lippincott Williams & Wilkins; 2007, Fig. 1-5.)

Each lung is divided roughly in half by an *oblique (major) fissure*. This fissure may be approximated by a string that runs from the T3 spinous process obliquely down and around the chest to the 6th rib at the midclavicular line (Fig. 10-10). The *right lung* is further divided by the *horizontal (minor) fissure*. Anteriorly, this fissure runs close to the 4th rib and meets the oblique fissure in the midaxillary line near the 5th rib. The right lung is thus divided into *upper, middle*, and *lower lobes* (RUL, RML, and RLL). The left lung has only two lobes, *upper* and *lower* (LUL, LLL) as shown in Figure 10-11. Figures 10-12 and 10-13 identify the lobes of the right and left lungs on chest radiographs.

Learn the general anatomic terms used to locate chest findings as shown in Box 10-1.

Box 10-1. Anatomic Descriptors of the Chest

- *Supraclavicular*—above the clavicles
- *Infraclavicular*—below the clavicles
- *Interscapular*—between the scapulae
- *Infrascapular*—below the scapulae
- *Apices* of the lungs—the uppermost portions
- *Bases* of the lungs—the lowermost portions
- *Upper, middle,* and *lower lung fields*

Usually, physical examination findings correlate with the underlying lobes. Signs in the right upper lung field, for example, almost certainly originate in the right upper lobe. However, signs found laterally in the right middle lung field could come from any of the three different lobes.

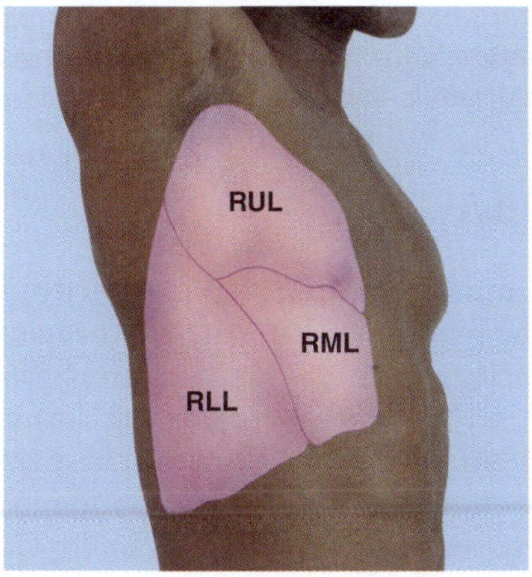

FIGURE 10-10. Right lung lobes and fissures.

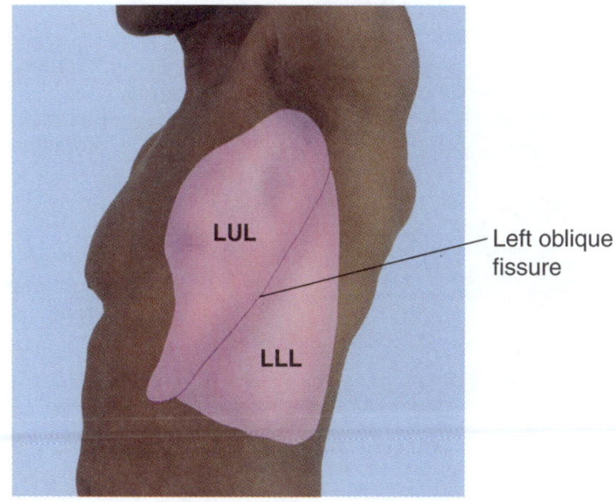

FIGURE 10-11. Left lung lobes and fissures.

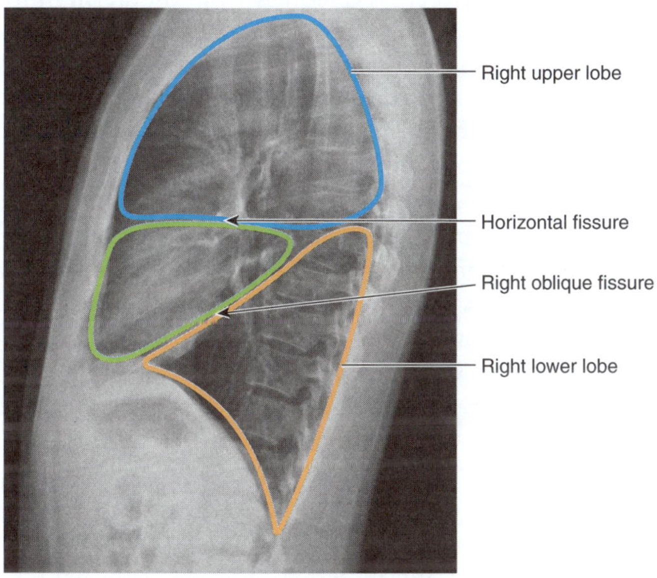

FIGURE 10-12. Lobes of the right lung in lateral view of a chest radiograph. (Modified from Brant WE, Helms CA. *Brant and Helms Solution: Fundamentals of Diagnostic Radiology.* 3rd ed. Lippincott Williams & Wilkins; 2007, Fig. 21-2.)

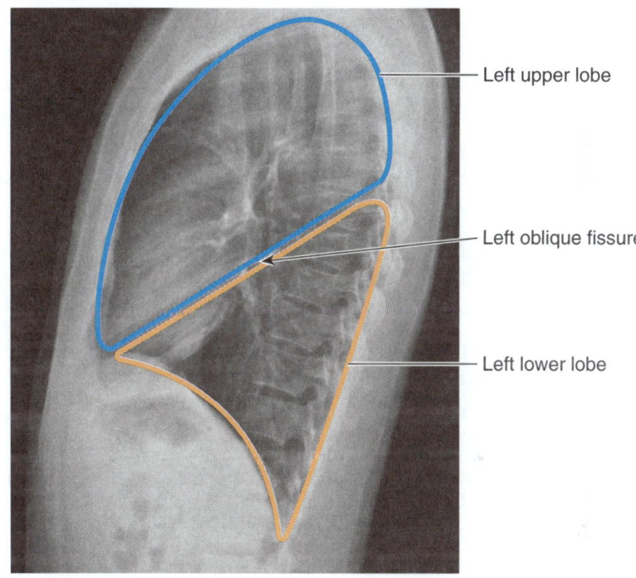

FIGURE 10-13. Lobes of the left lung in lateral view of a chest radiograph. (Modified from Brant WE, Helms CA. *Brant and Helms Solution: Fundamentals of Diagnostic Radiology.* 3rd ed. Lippincott Williams & Wilkins; 2007, Fig. 21-2.)

Trachea and Major Bronchi (Tracheobronchial Tree). Breath sounds over the trachea and bronchi have a harsher quality than those over the denser lung parenchyma. Learn the locations of these structures. The trachea bifurcates into its mainstem bronchi at the levels of the sternal angle anteriorly and the T4 spinous process posteriorly (Figs. 10-14 and 10-15). The *right main bronchus* is wider, shorter, and more vertical than the left main bronchus and directly enters the hilum of the lung. The *left main bronchus* extends inferolaterally from below the aortic arch and anterior to the esophagus and thoracic aorta and then enters the lung hilum. Each main bronchus then divides into *lobar* then into *segmental*

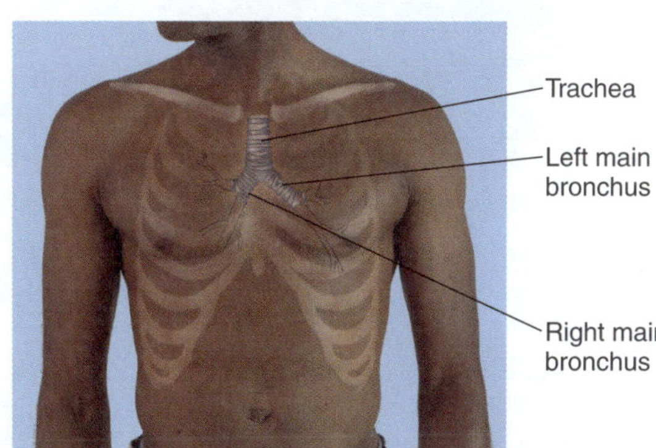

FIGURE 10-14. Trachea and mainstem bronchi, anterior view.

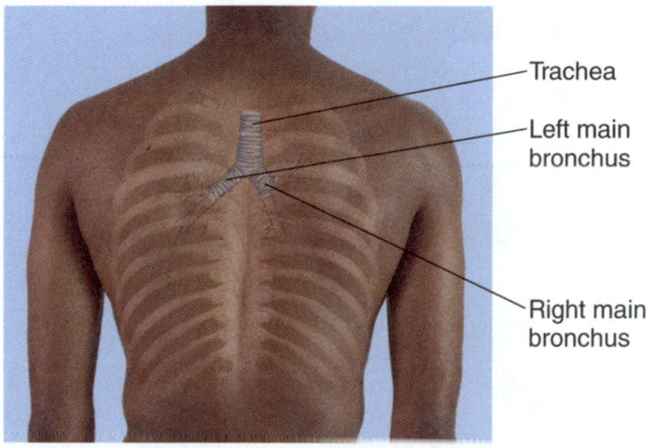

FIGURE 10-15. Trachea and mainstem bronchi, posterior view.

bronchi and *bronchioles*, terminating in the sac-like *alveoli*, where gas exchange occurs.

Aspiration pneumonia is more common in the right middle and lower lobes because the right main bronchus is more vertical. For this same reason, if an endotracheal tube is advanced too far during intubation, it will more likely enter the right mainstem bronchus.

Pleurae. Two continuous pleural surfaces, or serous membranes, separate the lungs from the chest wall. The *visceral pleura* covers the outer surface of the lungs. The *parietal pleura* lines the pleural cavity along the inner rib cage and the upper surface of the diaphragm. Between the visceral and parietal pleura is the *pleural space*, containing serous pleural fluid. The surface tension of the pleural fluid keeps the lung in contact with the thoracic wall, allowing the lung to expand and contract during respiration. The visceral pleura lacks sensory nerves, but the parietal pleura is richly innervated by the intercostal and phrenic nerves.

Accumulations of pleural fluid, or *pleural effusions*, may be *transudates*, seen in heart failure, cirrhosis, and nephrotic syndrome, or *exudates*, seen in numerous conditions including pneumonia, malignancy, pulmonary embolism, tuberculosis, and pancreatitis.

Irritation of the parietal pleura produces pleuritic pain with deep inspiration in viral pleurisy, pneumonia, pulmonary embolism, pericarditis, and collagen vascular diseases.

Breathing

Breathing is primarily automatic, controlled by respiratory centers in the brainstem that generate the neuronal drive for the muscles of respiration. The principal muscle of inspiration is the *diaphragm*. During inspiration, the diaphragm contracts, descends in the chest, and expands the thoracic cavity, compressing the abdominal contents and pushing out the abdominal wall. The muscles in the rib cage also expand the thorax, especially the *scalenes*, which run from the cervical vertebrae to the first two ribs, and the parasternal intercostal muscles, or *parasternals*, which cross obliquely from the sternum to the ribs. As the thorax expands, intrathoracic pressure decreases, drawing air through the tracheobronchial tree into the alveoli, or distal air sacs, filling the expanding lungs. Oxygen diffuses into the adjacent pulmonary capillaries as carbon dioxide exchanges from the blood into the alveoli.

During expiration, the chest wall and lungs recoil, and the diaphragm relaxes and rises passively. Abdominal muscles assist in expiration. As air flows outward, the chest and abdomen return to their resting positions.

Normal breathing is quiet and easy—barely audible near the open mouth as a faint whish. When a healthy person lies supine, the breathing movements of the thorax are relatively slight. By contrast, the abdominal movements are usually easy to see. In the sitting position, movements of the thorax become more prominent.

During exercise and in certain diseases, extra work is required to breathe, and accessory muscles are recruited; the sternocleidomastoid (SCM) muscles and the scalenes may become visible (Fig. 10-16).

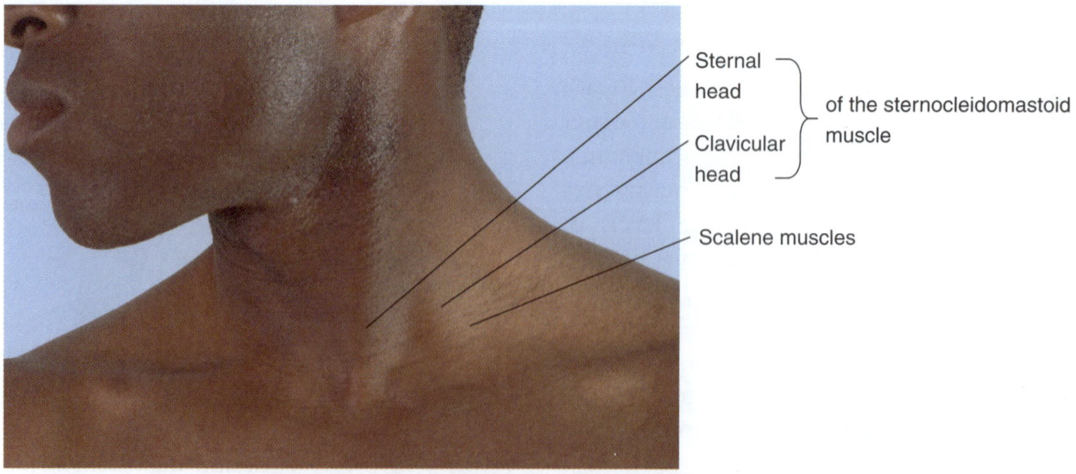

FIGURE 10-16. Accessory muscles in the neck.

HEALTH HISTORY: GENERAL APPROACH

Symptoms arising from disorders of the respiratory system are among the most common reasons for patients to see a healthcare provider, and, because these symptoms may result from life-threatening disorders, careful questioning is needed to establish their etiology and significance. Thus, it is important that you begin to learn how to identify signs and symptoms that warrant prompt medical intervention early in the clinical encounter (e.g., inability to speak in full sentences, use of accessory muscles, cyanosis, evidence of low oxygen saturation, and *pulsus paradoxus*). You should obtain a thorough account of the chief complaint or concern, allowing your patients to speak in their own words, with special attention to the effects of position and environmental exposures on their reported symptoms and the impact of these symptoms on their functional capacity. Many common respiratory symptoms may be a manifestation of other systemic disorders, particularly cardiovascular and hematologic diseases, so the examiner should integrate the health history for other systems as indicated by the chief complaint. A thorough past medical history and complete medication and allergy documentation are essential. Finally, because of its relevance and importance in the evaluation of patients with known or suspected pulmonary diseases, the social history should be thoroughly investigated, with special attention to tobacco and recreational drug use, occupational and environmental exposures, and travel history.

Common or Concerning Symptoms

- Shortness of breath (dyspnea) and wheezing
- Cough
- Blood-streaked sputum (hemoptysis)
- Chest pain (see also Chapter 16: Cardiovascular System)
- Daytime sleepiness, snoring and disordered sleep

Shortness of Breath (Dyspnea) and Wheezing

Shortness of breath, or *dyspnea*, is a painless but uncomfortable awareness of breathing that is inappropriate to the level of exertion. Thoroughly assess this telltale symptom of cardiac and pulmonary disease.

The degree of dyspnea, combined with spirometry, is a key component of important chronic obstructive pulmonary disease (COPD) classification systems that guide patient management.

Ask, "Have you had any difficulty breathing?" Find out if the symptom occurs at rest or with exertion, and how much exertion produces onset. Because of variations in age, body weight, and physical fitness, there is no absolute scale for quantifying shortness of breath. Instead, make every effort to determine its severity based on the patient's daily activities. How many steps or flights of stairs can the patient climb before pausing for breath? What about carrying bags of groceries, vacuuming, and making the bed? Has shortness of breath altered the patient's lifestyle and daily activities? How? Carefully elicit the timing and setting, any associated symptoms, and relieving or aggravating factors.

See Table 10-1, Dyspnea.

Most patients relate shortness of breath to their level of activity. Anxious patients present a different picture. They may describe difficulty taking a deep enough breath, a smothering sensation with inability to get enough air, and *paresthesias*, which are sensations of tingling or "pins and needles" around the lips or in the extremities.

Anxious patients may have episodic dyspnea during both rest and exercise and also hyperventilation, or rapid shallow breathing.

Wheezes are musical respiratory sounds that may be audible to the patient and to others.

Wheezing occurs in partial lower airway obstruction from secretions and tissue inflammation in asthma, or from a foreign body.

Medicine History Taking OSCE Video: **Shortness of Breath**

Cough

Cough is a common symptom that ranges in significance from trivial to ominous. Typically, cough is a reflex response to stimuli that irritate receptors in the larynx, trachea, or large bronchi. These stimuli include mucus, pus, and blood as well as external agents such as allergens, dust, foreign bodies, and even extremely hot or cold air. Other causes include inflammation of the respiratory mucosa, pneumonia, pulmonary edema, and compression of the bronchi or bronchioles from a tumor or enlarged peribronchial lymph nodes. Cough may also be cardiovascular in origin.

See Table 10-2, Cough and Hemoptysis.

Cough can signal left-sided heart failure.

For complaints of cough, pursue a thorough assessment. Establish the duration. Is the cough *acute*, lasting less than 3 weeks; *subacute*, lasting 3 to 8 weeks; or *chronic*, more than 8 weeks?

The most common cause of acute cough is viral upper respiratory infections. Also consider acute bronchitis, pneumonia, left-sided heart failure, asthma, foreign body, smoking, and ACE-inhibitor therapy. Postinfectious cough, pertussis, acid reflux, bacterial sinusitis, and asthma can cause subacute cough. Chronic cough is seen in postnasal drip, asthma, gastroesophageal reflux, chronic bronchitis, and bronchiectasis.

Ask whether the cough is *dry* or *productive* of sputum, or phlegm.

Mucoid sputum is translucent, white, or gray and seen in viral infections and cystic fibrosis; purulent sputum—yellow or green—often accompanies bacterial pneumonia.

Ask the patient to describe the *volume* of any sputum and its *color*, *odor*, and *consistency*.

Foul-smelling sputum is present in anaerobic lung abscess, thick tenacious sputum in cystic fibrosis.

To help patients quantify volume, try a multiple-choice question. "How much do you think you cough up in 24 hours: a teaspoon, tablespoon, quarter cup, half cup, cupful?" If possible, ask the patient to cough into a tissue; inspect the phlegm, and note its characteristics. The symptoms associated with a cough often lead to its cause.

Large volumes of purulent sputum are present in bronchiectasis and lung abscess.

Diagnostically helpful symptoms include fever and productive cough in pneumonia; wheezing in asthma; and chest pain, dyspnea, and orthopnea in acute coronary syndromes.

Medicine History Taking OSCE Video: **Cough**

Hemoptysis

Hemoptysis refers to blood coughed up from the lower respiratory tract; it may vary from blood-streaked sputum to frank blood. For patients reporting hemoptysis, quantify the volume of blood produced, the setting and activity, and any associated symptoms. Hemoptysis is rare in infants, children, and adolescents.

See Table 10-2, Cough and Hemoptysis. Causes include bronchitis; malignancy; cystic fibrosis; and, less commonly, bronchiectasis, mitral stenosis, Goodpasture syndrome, and granulomatosis with polyangiitis (formerly Wegener granulomatosis). *Massive hemoptysis* (>500 mL over a 24-hour period or ≥100 mL/hr) may be life-threatening.

Before using the term "hemoptysis," try to confirm the source of the bleeding. Blood or blood-streaked material may originate in the nose, mouth, pharynx, or gastrointestinal (GI) tract and is easily mislabeled. If vomited, it probably originates in the GI tract. Occasionally, however, blood from the nasopharynx or the GI tract is aspirated and then coughed out.

Blood originating in the stomach is usually darker than blood from the respiratory tract and may be mixed with food particles.

Medicine History Taking OSCE Video: **Hemoptysis**

Chest Pain

Complaints of chest pain or chest discomfort raise concerns about the heart but often arise from other structures in the thorax and lungs. To assess this symptom, you must pursue a dual investigation of both thoracic and cardiac causes. Sources of chest pain are listed in Box 10-2. For this important symptom, keep all of these possibilities in mind.

See Table 10-3, Chest Pain.

Box 10-2. Sources of Chest Pain and Related Causes

Source	Possible Causes
Myocardium	Angina pectoris, myocardial infarction, myocarditis
Pericardium	Pericarditis
Aorta	Aortic dissection
Trachea and large bronchi	Bronchitis
Parietal pleura	Pericarditis, pneumonia, pneumothorax, pleural effusion, pulmonary embolus, connective tissue disease
Chest wall, including the skin, musculoskeletal and neurologic systems	Costochondritis, herpes zoster
Esophagus	Gastroesophageal reflux disease, esophageal spasm, esophageal tear
Extrathoracic structures such as the neck, gallbladder, and stomach	Cervical arthritis, biliary colic, gastritis

Chest pain is reported in one in four patients with panic and anxiety disorders.

This section focuses on *pulmonary complaints*. For symptoms of exertional chest pain, palpitations, shortness of breath when supine (*orthopnea*) or at night relieved by sitting upright (*paroxysmal nocturnal dyspnea*), and edema, see Chapter 11, Cardiovascular System.

Always start your interview with an open-ended question. "Do you have any discomfort or unpleasant feelings in your chest?" Ask the patient to point to the location of the pain in the chest. Watch for any gestures as the patient describes the pain. Elicit all seven attributes of chest pain to distinguish among its various causes.

A clenched fist over the sternum (*Levine sign*) suggests angina pectoris; a finger pointing to a tender spot on the chest wall suggests musculoskeletal pain; a hand moving from the neck to the epigastrium may suggest heartburn.

Lung tissue has no pain fibers. The pericardium also has few pain fibers.

Pain in conditions such as pneumonia and pulmonary infarction usually arises from inflammation of the adjacent parietal pleura. Muscle strain from prolonged recurrent coughing or costochondral inflammation may also be responsible. The pain of pericarditis stems from inflammation of the adjacent parietal pleura.

Extrapulmonary sources of chest pain include gastroesophageal reflux disease and anxiety, but the mechanism remains obscure.

Medicine History Taking OSCE Video:
Chest Pain

Daytime Sleepiness, Snoring and Disordered Sleep

Patients may report excessive daytime sleepiness and fatigue. Ask about problems with snoring, witnessed *apneas* (defined as breathing cessation for >10 seconds), awakening with a choking sensation, or morning headache.

These symptoms, especially daytime sleepiness and snoring, are hallmarks of obstructive sleep apnea (OSA), commonly seen in patients with obesity, posterior malocclusion of the jaw (*retrognathia*), treatment-resistant hypertension, heart failure, atrial fibrillation, stroke, and type 2 diabetes. Mechanisms include instability of the brainstem respiratory center, disordered sleep arousal, disordered contraction of upper airway muscles (*genioglossus malfunction*), and anatomic changes contributing to airway collapse such as obesity, among others.

PHYSICAL EXAMINATION: GENERAL APPROACH

The physical examination of the thorax and lungs employs the four classic techniques of inspection, palpation, percussion, and auscultation discussed in this chapter; however, the physical examination of the respiratory system should begin during the interview of the patient. You can elicit a large amount of information just from observing the patient speak. The inability to speak in full sentences before stopping to take a breath suggests increased respiratory drive or impairment of ventilation with reduced vital capacity. Likewise, evidence of increased work of breathing (supraclavicular retractions, use of accessory muscles of ventilation, and the *tripod position*, characterized by sitting with hands braced on the knees) is indicative of increased airways resistance or stiff lungs and/or chest wall.

When measuring vital signs, you should accurately assess the respiratory rate by carefully observing the rate of rise of the chest wall. In addition, you should ask patients with exertional dyspnea to walk under observation in order to reproduce the symptoms while closely monitoring their oximetry to note any desaturation at rest or with activity. During the general examination, look for signs of hypoxemia (cyanosis), anemia (pale conjunctivae), and extrapulmonary manifestations of lung disease (clubbing). Examination of the chest should focus on symmetry of movement; percussion (dullness indicative of pleural effusion or atelectasis, hyperresonance a sign of emphysema); and auscultation (wheezes, crackles, rhonchi, prolonged expiratory phase, and/or diminished breath are clues to disorders of the airways or lung parenchyma). A careful cardiac examination is necessary to identify signs of elevated right-sided heart pressures (jugular venous distention, peripheral edema, accentuated pulmonic component of the second heart sound), left ventricular dysfunction (S_3 and S_4 gallops), and valvular disease (murmurs). Finally, it is also important to examine the abdomen with the patient in the supine position to identify whether there is paradoxical movement of the abdomen (inward motion during inspiration), a sign of diaphragmatic weakness. For best results, examine the posterior chest while the patient is sitting, and the anterior chest with the patient supine. Be considerate when draping the patient, allowing for maximal exposure of the area to be examined yet mindful of the patient's sense of comfort with the examination.

TECHNIQUES OF EXAMINATION

Key Components of the Thorax and Lung Examination

- Survey respiration (rate, rhythm, depth, effort of breathing, signs of respiratory distress).
- Examine the anterior and posterior chest:
  - Inspect the chest (deformities, muscle retraction, lag).
  - Palpate the chest (tenderness, bruising, sinus tracts, respiratory expansion, fremitus).
  - Percuss the chest (flat, dull, resonant, hyperresonant or tympanitic).
  - Auscultate the chest (breath sounds, adventitious, transmitted voice sounds).

Initial Survey

Carefully observe the *rate, rhythm, depth*, and *effort of breathing*. A healthy resting adult breathes quietly and regularly about 20 times a minute. Note whether expiration lasts longer than usual.

See Table 10-4, Abnormalities in Rate and Rhythm of Breathing, including bradypnea, tachypnea, hyperventilation, Cheyne–Stokes breathing, and ataxic breathing. Delayed expiration occurs in COPD.

Signs of Respiratory Distress. Begin by observing the patient for signs of respiratory distress.

- Assess the respiratory rate for *tachypnea* (>25 breaths/min).
- Inspect the patient's color for *cyanosis* or *pallor*. Recall earlier relevant findings, such as the shape and color of the fingernails.

  Cyanosis in the lips, tongue, and oral mucosa signals hypoxia. Pallor and sweating (*diaphoresis*) are common in acute coronary syndromes and heart failure. Clubbing of the nails occurs in bronchiectasis, congenital heart disease, pulmonary fibrosis, cystic fibrosis, lung abscess, and malignancy.

- Listen for *audible sounds of breathing*. Is there audible whistling during inspiration over the neck or lungs?

  Audible high-pitched inspiratory whistling, or **stridor**, is an ominous sign of upper airway obstruction in the larynx or trachea that requires urgent airway evaluation.

- Inspect the neck. During inspiration, is there contraction of the accessory muscles, namely the SCM and scalene muscles, or supraclavicular retraction? During expiration, is there contraction of the intercostal or abdominal oblique muscles? Is the trachea midline?

  Accessory muscle use can signal increased ventilatory requirements due to airways and/or parenchymal lung disease or respiratory muscle fatigue. Lateral displacement of the trachea occurs in pneumothorax, pleural effusion, and atelectasis.

- Also observe the shape of the chest, which is normally wider than it is deep. The ratio of the anteroposterior (AP) diameter to the lateral chest diameter is usually 0.7 to 0.75 up to 0.9 and increases with aging.

  The AP ratio may exceed 0.9 in COPD, producing a barrel-chest appearance, although evidence of this correlation is conflicting.

Posterior Chest

With the patient sitting, examine the posterior chest. The patient's arms should be folded across the chest with hands resting, if possible, on the opposite shoulders. This position swings the scapulae laterally and increases access to the lung fields. Then ask the patient to lie down.

For patients who cannot sit up, ask for assistance so that you can examine the posterior chest in the sitting position. If this is not possible, roll the patient to one side and then to the other. Percuss and auscultate both lungs in each position. Because ventilation is relatively greater in the dependent lung, you are more likely to hear abnormal wheezes or crackles on the dependent side.

Inspection. Standing in a midline position behind the patient, try to visualize the underlying lobes and compare the right lung field with the left, carefully noting any asymmetries. Note the shape of the chest such as a **barrel chest** or and how the chest moves, including the following:

See Table 10-5, Deformities of the Thorax.

- Deformities or asymmetry in chest expansion

  Asymmetric expansion occurs in large pleural effusions.

- Abnormal muscle retraction of the intercostal spaces during inspiration, most visible in the lower intercostal spaces

  Retraction occurs in severe asthma, COPD, or upper airway obstruction.

- Impaired respiratory movement on one or both sides or a unilateral *lag* (or delay) in movement

  Unilateral impairment or *lagging* suggests pleural disease from asbestosis or silicosis; it is also seen in phrenic nerve damage or trauma.

Palpation. As you palpate the chest, focus on areas of tenderness or bruising, respiratory expansion, and fremitus.

Intercostal tenderness can develop over inflamed pleurae, costal cartilage tenderness in costochondritis.

- Identify tender areas. Carefully palpate any area where the patient reports pain or has visible lesions or bruises. Note any palpable *crepitus*, defined as a crackling or grinding sound over bones, joints, or skin, with or without pain, due to air in the subcutaneous tissue.

  Tenderness, bruising, and bony "step-offs" are common over a fractured rib. Crepitus may be palpable in overt fractures and arthritic joints; crepitus and chest wall edema are seen in mediastinitis.

- Assess any skin abnormalities such as masses or *sinus tracts* (blind, inflammatory, tube-like structures opening onto the skin).

  Although rare, sinus tracts suggest infection of the underlying pleura and lung (as in tuberculosis or actinomycosis).

- Test *chest expansion*. Place your thumbs at about the level of the 10th ribs, with your fingers loosely grasping and parallel to the lateral rib cage (Fig. 10-17). As you position your hands, slide them medially just enough to raise a loose fold of skin between your thumbs over the spine. Ask the patient to inhale deeply. Watch the distance between your thumbs as they move apart during inspiration and feel for the range and symmetry of the rib cage as it expands and contracts. This movement is sometimes called *lung excursion*.

Unilateral decrease or delay in chest expansion occurs in chronic fibrosis of the underlying lung or pleura, pleural effusion, lobar pneumonia, pleural pain with associated splinting, unilateral bronchial obstruction, and paralysis of the hemidiaphragm.

Physiology OSCE Video:
Chest Movements

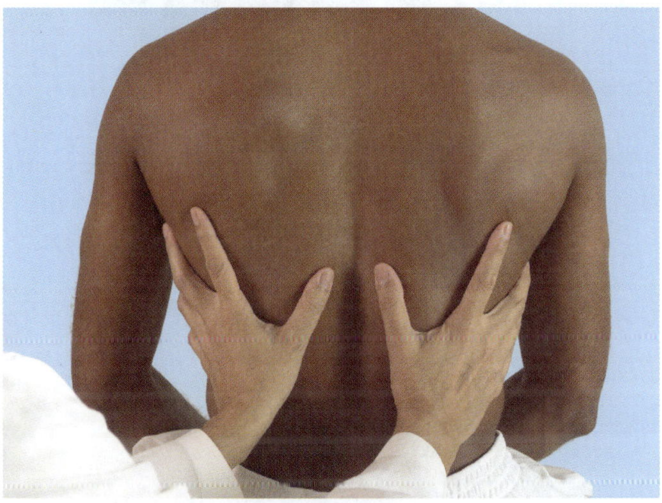

FIGURE 10-17. Assessing chest expansion.

- Palpate both lungs for symmetric *tactile fremitus* (Fig. 10-18). *Fremitus* refers to the palpable vibrations that are transmitted through the bronchopulmonary tree to the chest wall as the patient is speaking and is normally symmetric. Fremitus is typically more prominent in the interscapular area than in the lower lung fields and easier to detect over the right lung than the left. It disappears below the diaphragm.

Tactile fremitus is decreased or absent when the voice is higher pitched or soft or when the transmission of vibrations from the larynx to the surface of the chest is impeded by a thick chest wall, an obstructed bronchus, COPD, pleural effusion, fibrosis, air (*pneumothorax*), or an infiltrating tumor.

Physiology OSCE Video:
Tactile Vocal Fremitus

To detect fremitus, use either the ball (the bony part of the palm at the base of the fingers) or the ulnar surface of your hand to optimize the vibratory sensitivity of the

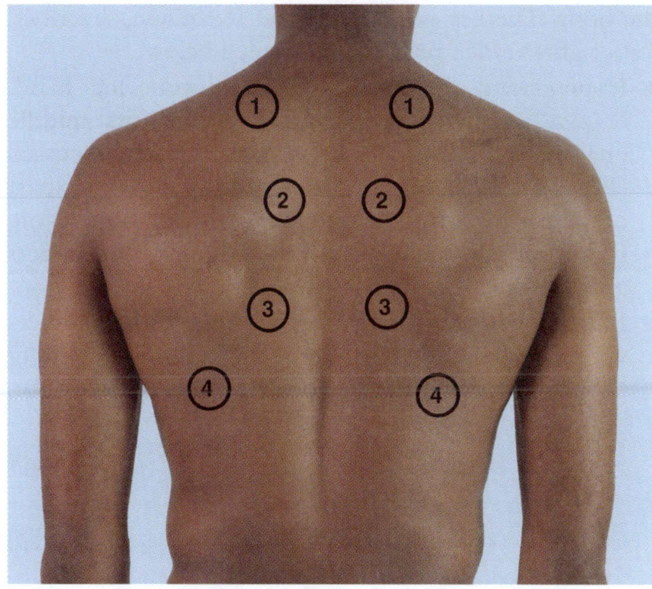

FIGURE 10-18. Locations for palpating fremitus.

bones in your hand. Ask the patient to repeat the words "*ninety-nine*" or "*one-one-one.*" Initially practice with one hand until you feel the transmitted vibrations. Use both hands to palpate and *compare symmetric areas of the lungs* in the pattern shown in Figure 10-18. Identify and locate any areas of *increased*, *decreased*, or *absent* fremitus. If fremitus is faint, ask the patient to speak more loudly or in a deeper voice.

Asymmetric decreased fremitus raises the likelihood of unilateral pleural effusion, pneumothorax, or neoplasm, which decreases transmission of low-frequency sounds; asymmetric increased fremitus occurs in unilateral pneumonia which increases transmission through consolidated tissue.

Tactile fremitus is a somewhat imprecise assessment technique but does direct your attention to possible asymmetries. Confirm any disparities by listening for underlying breath sounds, voice sounds, and whispered voice sounds. All these attributes should increase or decrease together.

Percussion. Percussion is one of the most important techniques of physical examination of the chest. Percussion sets the chest wall and underlying tissues in motion, producing audible sound and palpable vibrations. Percussion helps you establish whether the underlying tissues are air-filled, fluid-filled, or consolidated. The percussion blow penetrates only 5 to 7 cm into the chest, however, and will not aid in detection of deep-seated lesions. The technique of percussion can be practiced on any surface. As you practice, listen for changes in percussion notes over different types of materials or different parts of the body. The key points for good technique, described for a right-handed person, are detailed below:

- Hyperextend the middle finger of your left hand, known as the *pleximeter finger*. Press its middle phalanx firmly on the lung surface to be percussed (Fig. 10-19). Avoid surface contact by any other part of the hand because this dampens out vibrations. Note that the thumb and second, fourth, and fifth fingers are not touching the chest wall.
- Position your right forearm quite close to the surface, with the hand cocked upward. The middle finger should be partially flexed, relaxed, and poised to strike.

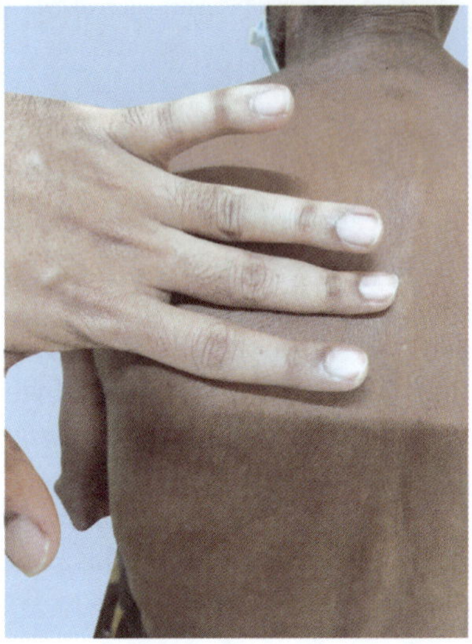

FIGURE 10-19. The pleximeter finger is placed firmly on the chest wall.

- With a quick, sharp but relaxed wrist motion, strike the pleximeter finger with the right middle finger, called the *plexor finger* (Fig. 10-20). Aim at your middle phalanx of pleximeter finger. Your goal is to transmit vibrations through the bones of this joint to the underlying chest wall. Use the same force for each percussion strike and the same pleximeter pressure to avoid changes in the percussion note due to your technique rather than underlying findings.

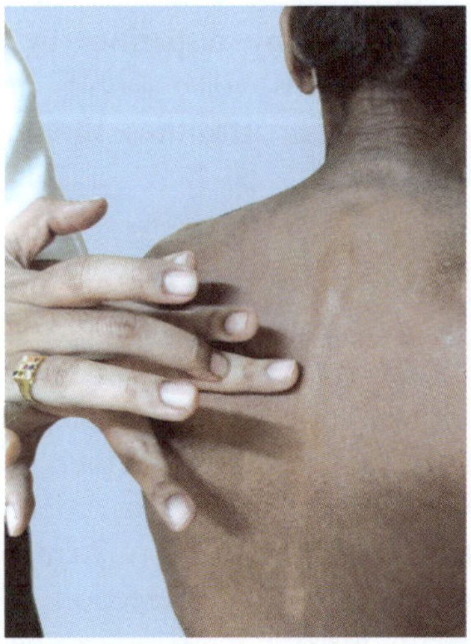

FIGURE 10-20. Striking the pleximeter finger with the right middle finger.

- Strike using the tip of the plexor finger, not the finger pad. The striking finger should be almost at right angles to the pleximeter. A short fingernail is recommended to avoid injuring your knuckle.
- Withdraw your striking finger quickly to avoid damping the vibrations you have created (Fig. 10-21).

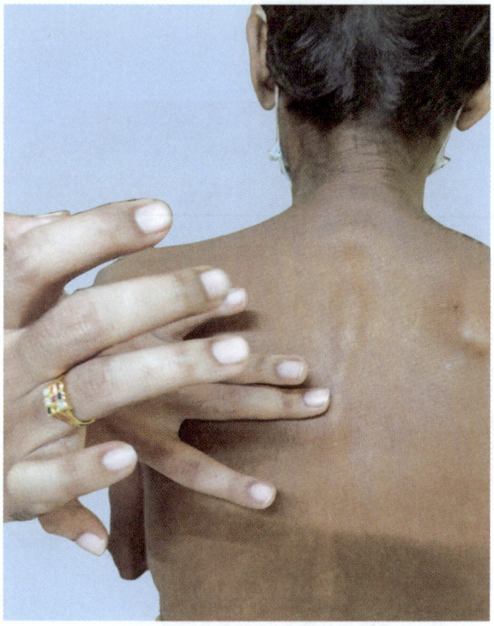

FIGURE 10-21. Withdraw the striking finger quickly.

In summary, the movement is at the wrist. It is directed, brisk, yet relaxed and slightly bouncy.

Percussion Notes. With your plexor or striking finger, use the lightest percussion that produces a clear note. A thick chest wall requires a more forceful percussion blow than a thin one. However, if a louder note is needed, apply more pressure with the pleximeter finger.

When percussing the lower posterior chest, stand somewhat to the side rather than directly behind the patient. In this position it is easier to place your pleximeter finger more firmly on the chest, making your plexor strike more effective by creating a better percussion note.

- When comparing two areas, use the same percussion technique in both areas. Percuss or strike twice in each location and listen for differences in the percussion notes at the two locations.
- Learn to identify five percussion notes—*flat, dull, resonant, hyperresonant,* and *tympanitic* (Box 10-3).

Box 10-3. Percussion Notes and Their Characteristics

	Relative Intensity	Relative Pitch	Relative Duration	Example of Location	Pathologic Examples
Flat	Soft	High	Short	Thigh	Large pleural effusion
Dull	Medium	Medium	Medium	Liver	Lobar pneumonia
Resonant	Loud	Low	Long	Healthy lung	Simple chronic bronchitis
Hyperresonant	Very loud	Lower	Longer	Usually none	COPD, pneumothorax
Tympanitic	Loud	High[a]	Longer	Gastric air bubble or puffed-out cheek	Large pneumothorax

[a]Distinguished mainly by its musical timbre.

You can practice four of them on yourself. These notes differ in their basic qualities of sound, intensity, pitch, and duration. Train your ear by concentrating on one quality at a time as you percuss first in one location, then in another. Review the description of percussion notes on p. 190. Healthy lungs are resonant.

While the patient keeps both arms crossed in front of the chest, percuss the thorax in symmetric locations on each side from the apex to the base.

- Percuss one side of the chest and then the other at each level in a *ladder-like pattern*, as shown in Figure 10-22. Omit the areas over the scapulae—the thickness of muscle and bone alters the percussion notes over the lungs. Identify and locate the area and quality of any abnormal percussion note.

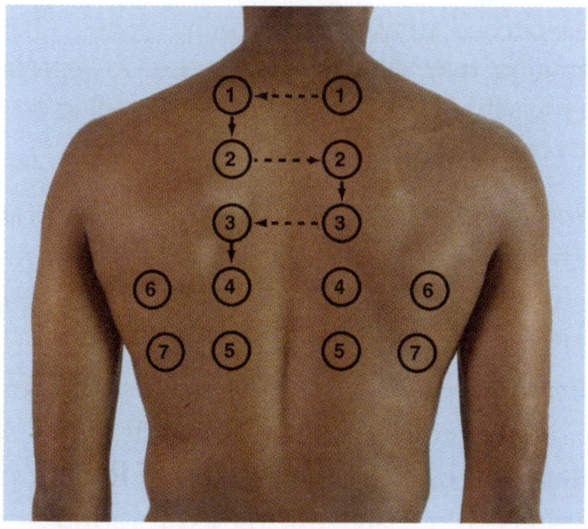

FIGURE 10-22. "Ladder" pattern for percussion and auscultation.

Dullness replaces *resonance* when fluid or solid tissue replaces air-containing lung or occupies the pleural space beneath your percussing fingers. Examples include: lobar pneumonia, in which the alveoli are filled with fluid and blood cells, and pleural accumulations of serous fluid (pleural effusion), blood (*hemothorax*), pus (*empyema*), fibrous tissue, or tumor. Dullness makes pneumonia and pleural effusion three to four times more likely, respectively.

Generalized hyperresonance is common over the hyperinflated lungs of COPD or asthma. Unilateral hyperresonance suggests a large pneumothorax or an air-filled bulla.

- Identify the descent of the diaphragm, or *diaphragmatic excursion*. First, determine the level of diaphragmatic dullness during quiet respiration. Holding the pleximeter finger above and parallel to the expected level of dullness, percuss downward in progressive steps until dullness clearly replaces resonance. Confirm this level of change by percussing downward from adjacent areas both medially and laterally (Fig. 10-23).

This technique tends to overestimate actual movements of the diaphragm.

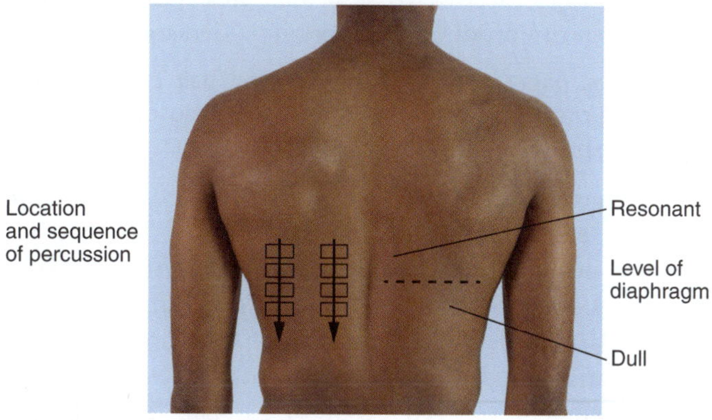

FIGURE 10-23. Identifying the extent of diaphragmatic excursion.

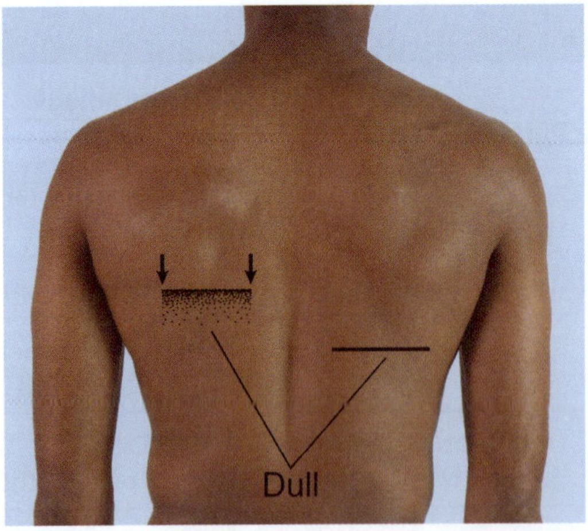

FIGURE 10-24. Absent descent of the diaphragm can indicate pleural effusion.

An abnormally high level suggests a pleural effusion or an elevated hemidiaphragm from atelectasis or phrenic nerve paralysis (Fig. 10-24).

Note that with this technique, you are identifying the boundary between the resonant lung tissue and the duller structures below the diaphragm. You are not percussing the diaphragm itself. You can infer the probable location of the diaphragm from the level of dullness.

Now, estimate the extent of diaphragmatic excursion by determining the distance between the level of dullness on full expiration and the level of dullness on full inspiration, normally about 3 to 5.5 cm.

Auscultation. Auscultation is the most important examination technique for assessing air flow through the tracheobronchial tree. Auscultation involves (1) listening to the sounds generated by breathing; (2) listening for any *adventitious* (added) sounds; and (3), if abnormalities are suspected, listening to the sounds of the patient's spoken or whispered voice as they are transmitted through the chest wall. Before beginning auscultation, ask the patient to cough once or twice to clear mild atelectasis or airway mucus that can produce unimportant added sounds.

Bedclothes, paper gowns, and even chest hair can generate confusing crackling sounds that interfere with auscultation. For chest hair, press harder or moisten the hair.

Listen to the breath sounds with the *diaphragm* of your stethoscope after instructing the patient to breathe deeply through an open mouth. Always place the stethoscope directly on the skin. Clothing alters the characteristics of the breath sounds and can introduce friction and added sounds.

Like auscultating over clothing, air movement through a partially obstructed nose or nasopharynx can also introduce abnormal sounds.

Use the *ladder pattern* suggested for percussion, moving from one side to the other and comparing symmetric areas of the lungs. Listen to at least one full breath—both inspiration and expiration—in each location. If you hear or suspect abnormal sounds, auscultate adjacent areas to assess the extent of any abnormality. If the patient becomes lightheaded from hyperventilation, allow the patient to take a few normal breaths.

Note the *intensity* of the breath sounds, which reflects the air flow rate at the mouth, and may vary from one area to another. Breath sounds are usually louder in the lower posterior lung fields. If the breath sounds seem faint, ask the patient to breathe more deeply. Both shallow breathing and a thick chest wall can alter breath sound intensity.

Breath sounds may be decreased when air flow is decreased (as in obstructive lung disease or respiratory muscle weakness) or when the transmission of sound is poor (as in pleural effusion, pneumothorax, or COPD).

Is there a *silent gap* between the inspiratory and expiratory sounds?

A gap suggests **bronchial breath sounds**.

Listen for the *pitch, intensity*, and *duration* of the *inspiratory and expiratory sounds.* Are **vesicular breath sounds** distributed normally over the chest wall? Are breath sounds diminished, or are there bronchovesicular or bronchial breath sounds in unexpected places? If so, in what distribution?

Breath Sounds (Lung Sounds). Learn to identify breath sounds by their intensity, their pitch, and the relative duration of their inspiratory and expiratory phases (Box 10-4). Normal breath sounds are:

In cold or tense patients, watch for muscle contraction sounds—muffled, low-pitched rumbling, or roaring noises. Changing the patient's position may eliminate this noise. To reproduce these sounds on yourself, do a *Valsalva maneuver* (straining down) as you listen to your own chest.

- *Vesicular* are soft and low pitched. They are heard throughout inspiration, continue without pause through expiration, and then fade away about one third of the way through expiration.
- *Bronchovesicular*, with inspiratory and expiratory sounds about equal in length, are at times separated by a silent interval. Detecting differences in pitch and intensity is often easier during expiration.
- *Bronchial* are louder, harsher and higher in pitch, with a short silence between inspiratory and expiratory sounds. Expiratory sounds last longer than inspiratory sounds.
- *Tracheal* are loud harsh sounds heard over the trachea in the neck.

Box 10-4. Characteristics of Breath Sounds

	Duration of Sounds	Intensity of Expiratory Sound	Pitch of Expiratory Sound	Locations Where Heard Normally
Vesicular*	Inspiratory sounds last longer than expiratory sounds.	Soft	Relatively low	Over most of both lungs
Bronchovesicular	Inspiratory and expiratory sounds are almost equal.	Intermediate	Intermediate	Often in the first and second interspaces anteriorly and between the scapulae
Bronchial	Expiratory sounds last longer than inspiratory ones.	Loud	Relatively high	Over the manubrium (larger proximal airways)
Tracheal	Inspiratory and expiratory sounds are almost equal.	Very loud	Relatively high	Over the trachea in the neck

*The thickness of the bars indicates intensity; the steeper their incline, the higher the pitch.

Sources: Loudon R, Murphy LH. *Am Rev Respir Dis.* 1994;130:663; Bohadana A et al. *N Engl J Med.* 2014;370:744; Wilkins RL et al. *Chest.* 1990;98:886; Schreur HJW et al. *Thorax.* 1992;47:674; Bettancourt PE et al. *Am J Resp Crit Care Med.* 1994;150:1921.

If bronchovesicular or bronchial breath sounds are heard in locations distant from those listed, suspect replacement of air-filled lung by fluid-filled or consolidated lung tissue.

See Table 10-6, Normal and Altered Breath and Voice Sounds.

Adventitious (Added) Sounds. Listen for any added, or *adventitious,* sounds that are superimposed on the usual breath sounds (Box 10-5). Detection of adventitious sounds—**crackles** (sometimes called *rales*), **wheezes**, and **rhonchi**—is an important focus of your examination, often leading to diagnosis of cardiac and pulmonary conditions.

Box 10-5. Adventitious or Added Breath Sounds

Crackles (or Rales)	Wheezes and Rhonchi
Discontinuous	**Continuous**
■ Intermittent, nonmusical, and brief	■ Sinusoidal, musical, prolonged (but not necessarily persisting throughout the respiratory cycle)
■ Like dots in time	■ Like dashes in time
■ *Fine crackles:* soft, high-pitched (~650 Hz), very brief (5–10 ms)	■ *Wheezes:* relatively high-pitched (≥400 Hz) with hissing or shrill quality (>80 ms)
■ *Coarse crackles:* somewhat louder, lower in pitch (~350 Hz), brief (15–30 ms)	■ *Rhonchi:* relatively low-pitched (150–200 Hz) with snoring quality (>80 ms)

Sources: Loudon R, Murphy LH. *Am Rev Respir Dis.* 1994;130:663; Bohadana A et al. *N Engl J Med.* 2014;370:744.

Crackles can arise from abnormalities of the lung parenchyma (pneumonia, interstitial lung disease, pulmonary fibrosis, atelectasis, heart failure) or of the airways (bronchitis, bronchiectasis).

Wheezes arise in the narrowed airways of asthma, COPD, and bronchitis.

Many clinicians use the term "rhonchi" to describe sounds from secretions in large airways that may change with coughing.

For further discussion and other added sounds, see Table 10-7, Adventitious (Added) Lung Sounds: Causes and Qualities.

If you hear crackles, especially those that do not clear after coughing, listen carefully for the following characteristics. These are clues to the underlying condition:

- *Loudness, pitch,* and *duration,* summarized as *fine* or *coarse* crackles

  Fine late inspiratory crackles that persist from breath to breath suggest abnormal lung tissue.

- *Number,* few to many
- *Timing* in the respiratory cycle—inspiratory or expiratory?
- *Location* on the chest wall

  The crackles of heart failure are usually best heard in the posterior inferior lung fields.

- *Persistence* of their pattern from breath to breath
- Any *change* after a cough or change in the patient's position

  Clearing of crackles, wheezes, or rhonchi after coughing or position change suggests inspissated secretions, seen in bronchitis or atelectasis.

In some normal people, crackles may be heard at the anterior lung bases after maximal expiration. Crackles in dependent portions of the lungs may also occur after prolonged recumbency.

If you hear wheezes or rhonchi, note their timing and location. Do they change with deep breathing or coughing? Beware of the silent chest, in which air movement is minimal.

In the advanced airway obstruction of severe asthma, wheezes and breath sounds may be absent due to low respiratory airflow ("silent chest"), a clinical emergency.

Note that tracheal sounds originating in the neck such as stridor and vocal cord dysfunction can be transmitted to the chest and mistaken for wheezing, leading to inappropriate or delayed treatment.

Stridor and laryngeal sounds are loudest over the neck, whereas true wheezes and rhonchi are faint or absent over the neck.

Note any *pleural friction rubs,* which are coarse, grating biphasic sounds heard primarily during expiration.

Pleural friction rubs may be heard in pleurisy, pneumonia, and pulmonary embolism.

Transmitted Voice Sounds. If you hear abnormally located bronchovesicular or bronchial breath sounds, assess transmitted voice sounds using the three techniques below. With the diaphragm of your stethoscope, listen in symmetric areas over the chest wall for abnormal vocal resonances suspicious for pneumonia or pleural effusion.

Increased **transmitted voice sounds** suggest that embedded airways are blocked by inflammation or secretions. See Table 10-6, Normal and Altered Breath and Voice Sounds.

- *Egophony.* Ask the patient to say "ee." You will normally hear a muffled long E sound.

  If "ee" sounds like "A" and has a nasal bleating quality, an E-to-A change, or **egophony**, is present.

- *Bronchophony.* Ask the patient to say "ninety-nine." Normally the sounds transmitted through the chest wall are muffled and indistinct. Louder voice sounds are called bronchophony.

  Localized **bronchophony** and egophony are seen in lobar consolidation from pneumonia. In patients with fever and cough, the presence of bronchial breath sounds and egophony more than triples the likelihood of pneumonia.

Physiology OSCE Video: **Vocal Resonance**

- *Pectoriloquy.* Ask the patient to whisper "ninety-nine" or "one-two-three." The whispered voice is normally heard faintly and indistinctly, if at all.

  Louder, clearer whispered sounds are called **whispered pectoriloquy**.

Anterior Chest

With the patient supine, examine the anterior chest. For women, this position allows the breasts to be gently displaced. When examined in the supine position, the patient should lie comfortably with the arms somewhat abducted. If the patient is having difficulty breathing, raise the head of the examining table or the bed to increase respiratory excursion and ease of breathing.

Persons with severe COPD may prefer to sit leaning forward, with lips pursed during exhalation and arms supported on their knees or a table.

Inspection. Observe the shape of the patient's chest and the movement of the chest wall. Note:

- *Deformities* or *asymmetry* of the thorax

  See Table 10-5, Deformities of the Thorax.

- Abnormal *retraction* of the lower intercostal spaces during inspiration, or any supraclavicular retraction

  Abnormal retraction occurs in severe asthma, COPD, or upper airway obstruction.

- Local *lag* or *impairment* in respiratory movement

  Lag occurs in underlying diseases of the lung or pleura.

Palpation. Palpate the anterior chest wall and perform the following techniques.

Assess the *position of trachea*. Try to identify the thyroid and cricoid cartilages and the trachea below them. Feel the tracheal rings by the index finger. Look for any deviation of the trachea from its usual midline position. Place your finger along one side of the trachea and note the space between it and the SCM muscle (Fig. 10-25). Compare it with the other side. The spaces should be symmetric.

Trachea is displayed by neck masses, such as goiters and enlarged lymph nodes, gross deformity of the spine and skeletal system, pleural diseases such as pleural effusion, pneumothorax and hydropneumothorax or lung diseases such as collapse or fibrosis of the lung.

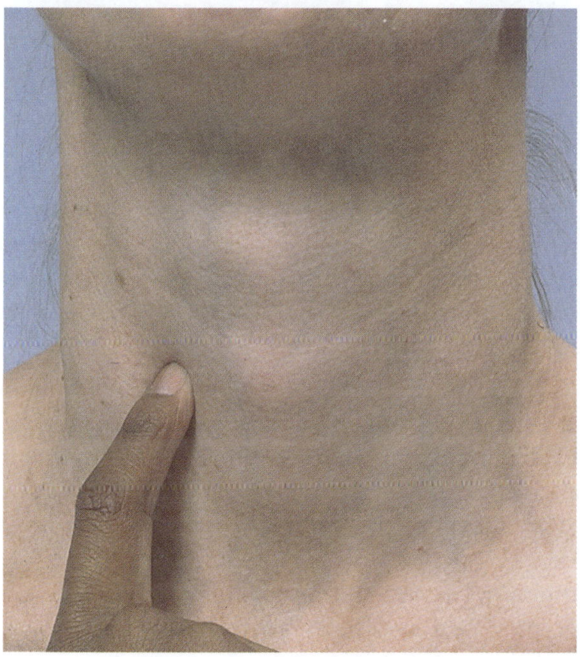

FIGURE 10-25. Palpating the trachea.

Physiology OSCE Video:
Palpation of Trachea

- Identify any *tender areas.*

  Tender pectoral muscles or costal cartilages suggest, but do not prove, that chest pain has a localized musculoskeletal origin.

- Assess for the presence of *bruising, sinus tracts*, or other *skin changes.*
- Assess *chest expansion.* Place your thumbs along each costal margin, your hands along the lateral rib cage (Fig. 10-26). As you position your hands, slide them medially a bit to raise loose skin folds between your thumbs. Ask the patient to inhale deeply. Observe how far your thumbs diverge as the thorax expands and feel for the extent and symmetry of respiratory movement.

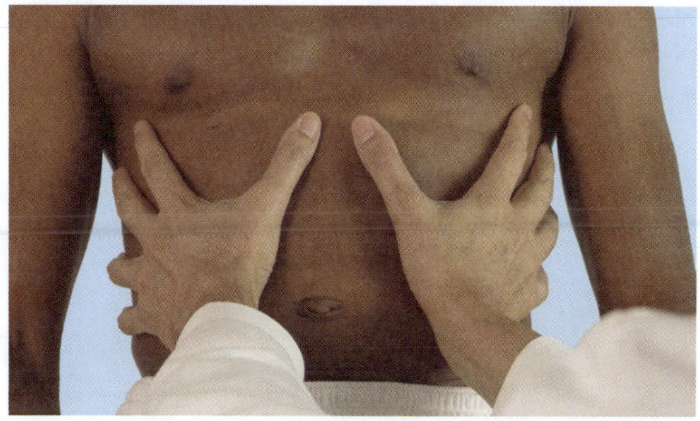

FIGURE 10-26. Assessing chest expansion anteriorly.

Physiology OSCE Video:
Chest Movements

- Assess *tactile fremitus.* If needed, compare both sides of the chest, using the ball or ulnar surface of your hand. Fremitus is usually decreased or absent over the precordium. When examining a woman, gently displace the breasts as necessary (Fig. 10-27).

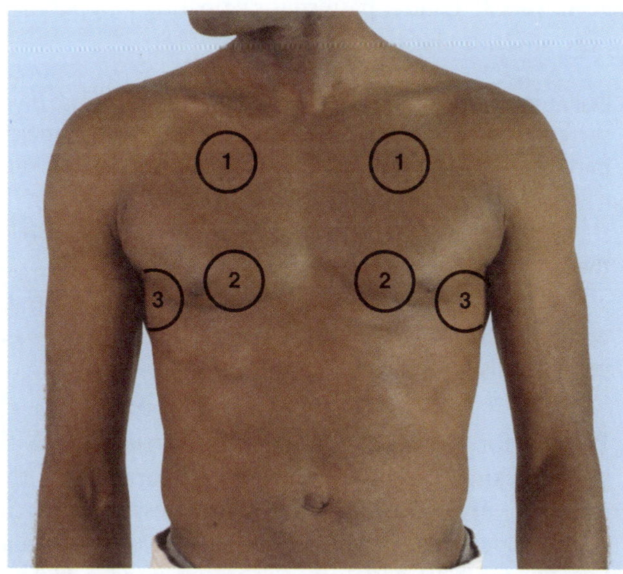

FIGURE 10-27. Locations for palpating tactile fremitus in the anterior chest.

Physiology OSCE Video:
Tactile Vocal Fremitus

Percussion. If clinically indicated, percuss the anterior and lateral chest, again comparing both sides (Fig. 10-28). The heart normally produces an area of dullness to the left of the sternum from the third to the fifth interspaces. In a woman, to enhance percussion, gently displace the breast with your left hand while percussing with the right or ask the patient to move the breast for you.

- Identify and locate any area with an *abnormal percussion note.*

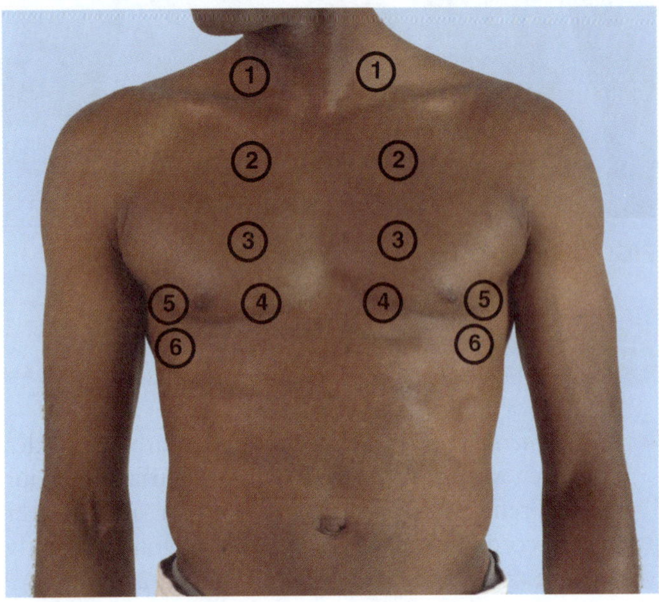

FIGURE 10-28. Ladder pattern for palpating and percussing the anterior chest.

Dullness represents airway obstruction from inflammation or secretions. Because pleural fluid usually sinks to the lowest part of the pleural space (posteriorly in a supine patient), only a very large effusion can be detected anteriorly.

The hyperresonance of COPD may obscure dullness over the heart.

The dullness of right middle lobe pneumonia typically occurs behind the right breast. Unless you displace the breast, you may miss the abnormal percussion note.

- Percuss for *liver dullness* and *gastric tympany.* With your pleximeter finger above and parallel to the expected upper border of liver dullness, percuss in progressive steps downward in the right midclavicular line (Fig. 10-29). Identify the upper border of liver dullness. This is the method you will use to estimate the size of the liver. As you percuss down the chest on the left, the *resonance of normal lung* usually changes to the *tympany of the gastric air bubble.*

The hyperinflated lung of COPD often displaces the upper border of the liver downward and lowers the level of diaphragmatic dullness posteriorly.

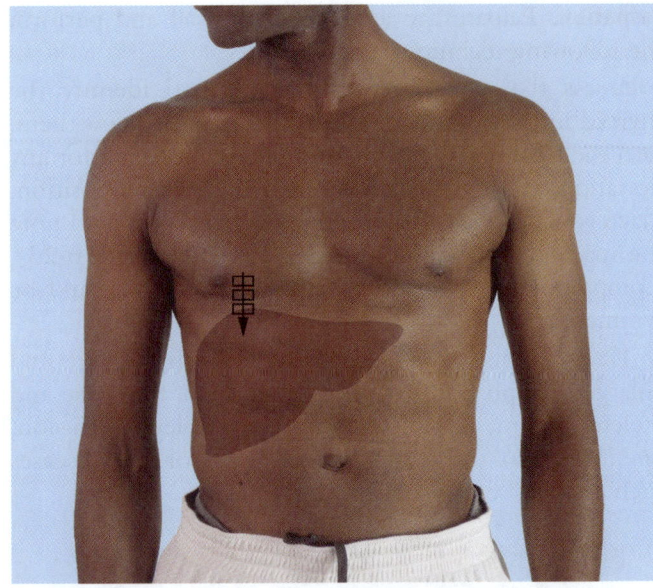

FIGURE 10-29. Percussing for liver dullness and gastric tympany.

Auscultation. Listen to the chest anteriorly and laterally as the patient breathes with mouth open, and somewhat more deeply than normal. Compare symmetric areas of the lungs, using the pattern suggested for percussion and extending it to adjacent areas, if indicated.

- Listen to the *breath sounds,* noting their intensity and identifying any variations from normal vesicular breathing. Breath sounds are usually louder in the upper anterior lung fields. Bronchovesicular breath sounds may be heard over the large airways, especially on the right.
- Identify any *adventitious sounds,* time them in the respiratory cycle, and locate them on the chest wall. Do they clear with deep breathing?

See Table 10-7, Adventitious (Added) Lung Sounds: Causes and Qualities, and Table 10-8, Physical Findings in Selected Chest Disorders.

- If clinically indicated, listen for *transmitted voice sounds.*

SPECIAL TECHNIQUES

Clinical Assessment of Pulmonary Function

Walk tests are practical, simple ways to assess cardiopulmonary function commonly used in rehabilitation and pre- and postoperative settings. The 2002 American Thoracic Society guidelines that standardize the 6-minute walk test continue to predict clinical outcomes in most patients with COPD. The test is easy to administer and requires only a 100-foot hallway. It measures "the distance that a patient can quickly walk on a flat, hard surface in a period of 6 minutes" and provides a global evaluation of the pulmonary and cardiovascular systems, neuromuscular units, and muscle metabolism.

Forced Expiratory Time

This test assesses the expiratory phase of breathing, which is typically slowed in obstructive pulmonary disease. Ask the patient to take a deep breath in and then breathe out as quickly and completely as possible with mouth open. Listen over the trachea with the diaphragm of a stethoscope and time the audible expiration. Try to get three consistent readings, allowing a short rest between efforts, if necessary. Forced expiratory time of 6 seconds or more is regarded as abnormal.

Patients ≥age 60 years with a forced expiratory time of ≥9 seconds are four times more likely to have COPD.

Identification of a Fractured Rib

Local pain and tenderness of one or more ribs raise the question of fracture. By compression of the chest in the AP plane, you can help to distinguish a fracture from a soft-tissue injury. With one hand on the sternum and the other on the thoracic spine, squeeze the chest. Ask "Is this painful, and where?"

An increase in the local pain (distant from your hands) suggests rib fracture rather than just soft-tissue injury.

RECORDING YOUR FINDINGS

Note that initially you may use sentences to describe your findings; later you will use phrases.

Recording the Respiratory System Examination

"Chest is symmetric with good expansion. Lungs resonant. Breath sounds vesicular; no crackles, wheezes, or rhonchi. Diaphragms descend 4 cm bilaterally."

OR

"Chest symmetric with moderate kyphosis and increased AP diameter, decreased expansion. Lungs are hyperresonant. Breath sounds distant with delayed expiratory phase and scattered expiratory wheezes. Fremitus decreased; no bronchophony, egophony, or whispered pectoriloquy. Diaphragms descend 2 cm bilaterally."

These findings suggest COPD.

HEALTH PROMOTION AND COUNSELING: EVIDENCE AND RECOMMENDATIONS

Important Topics for Health Promotion and Counseling

- Lung cancer screening
- Latent tuberculosis
- Screening for obstructive sleep apnea (OSA)
- Tobacco cessation (See Chapter 6)
- Immunizations—influenza and streptococcal pneumonia vaccines (See Chapter 6)

Lung Cancer

Epidemiology. Lung cancer is the frequently diagnosed cancer in both men and women. More people die of lung cancer than of colon, breast, and prostate cancer combined. More than 230,000 new cases and nearly 155,000 deaths (accounting for about 25% of all cancer deaths) were expected in 2018. However, incidence rates and death rates have been decreasing over the past few decades concurrent with a decline in smoking rates. Cigarette smoking is far and away the leading risk factor for lung cancer, accounting for about 85% of lung cancer cases. Radon, an invisible, odorless, radioactive gas released from soil and rocks in the ground, is the second leading cause of lung cancer in the United States. Other environmental and occupational exposures include second-hand smoke, asbestos, diesel exhaust, heavy metals, organic chemicals, ionizing radiation, and air pollution. Lung cancer also has a familial risk, especially if the relative was diagnosed at a younger age.

Prevention. Longer smoking histories and greater number of cigarettes smoked are associated with higher lung cancer risk. Tobacco cessation and prevention (see Chapter 6) will have the greatest effect on reducing the burden of lung cancer.

Screening. Screening for lung cancer is an appealing strategy because cancers diagnosed at an early stage (confined to the lung) have a 56% 5-year relative survival compared to a dismal 4.5% relative survival for cancers diagnosed at a distant stage (metastatic). Unfortunately, only 16% of lung cancers are diagnosed at an early stage.

Annual LDCT screening is recommended for current smokers (or those who have quit within the last 15 years) if they have smoked an average of one pack of cigarettes for 30 years and are aged 55 to 80. The American Cancer Society also recommends annual screening, though only until age 74. Both organizations agree that all current smokers should be counseled about smoking cessation and offered smoking cessation interventions.

Latent Tuberculosis

Epidemiology. One fourth of the world's population is infected with tuberculosis, and there are about 1.7 million tuberculosis-related deaths worldwide. As opposed to persons with active tuberculosis, persons with latent tuberculosis have no symptoms and are not contagious. However, they may develop active tuberculosis if they do not receive treatment for their latent tuberculosis infection. Immunocompetent patients with latent tuberculosis have a 5% to 10% lifetime risk of developing active tuberculosis. Risk for latent tuberculosis is increased for those born in or previously residing in countries with high tuberculosis prevalence and those living in high-risk settings such as homeless shelters or correctional facilities.

Screening. Screening tests include the TST and interferon-gamma release assay (IGRA) blood tests. The TST requires intradermal placement of purified protein derivative and interpretation of response 48 to 72 hours later. The skin test reaction is measured in millimeters of *induration* (a palpable, raised, hardened area or swelling). The presence of induration indicates a positive result. IGRA requires a single venous blood sample and laboratory processing within 8 to 30 hours after collection.

Obstructive Sleep Apnea

Epidemiology. Obstructive sleep apnea (OSA) is a disorder characterized by repeated episodes of upper airway collapse, particularly during rapid eye movement (REM) sleep, leading to hypoxemia and disrupted sleep. OSA can cause excessive daytime sleepiness, which increases risk for motor vehicle and occupational accidents, and is associated with higher risks for cognitive impairment, diabetes, cardiovascular morbidity, and all-cause mortality. The estimated prevalence of OSA in adults ages 30 to 70 is about 15% for men and 5% for women, though OSA is often undiagnosed. Risk factors for OSA include obesity, male sex, older age, craniofacial and upper airway abnormalities, and being postmenopausal. Symptoms suggesting OSA include excessive daytime sleepiness (which can be assessed with the Epworth sleepiness scale shown in Box 10-6), loud snoring, or choking or gasping during sleep.

Box 10-6. Epworth Sleepiness Scale

Consider how you have felt over the past week or two. How likely are you to doze off or fall asleep in the following situations?

0 = Never

1 = Slight chance

2 = Moderate chance

3 = High chance

Situation	Score
Sitting and reading	
Watching television	
Sitting inactive in a public space (e.g., theater or meeting)	
As a passenger in a car for an hour without a break	
Lying down in the afternoon when able	
Sitting quietly after lunch without alcohol	
In a car while stopped for a few minutes in traffic	
	Total:

Scores >10 are consistent with excessive daytime sleepiness.

Source: Adapted from Johns MW. *Sleep*. 1991;14(6):540–545. Reproduced by permission from American Sleep Disorders Association and Sleep Research Society.

Asymptomatic patients with morbid obesity or refractory hypertension may also have OSA. The definitive diagnosis is made by polysomnography performed in a sleep lab that measures brain waves, airflow, respiratory effort, oxygenation, and heart rhythms. Severity of OSA is based on the hourly number of episodes of apnea (breathing cessation for ≥10 seconds) and hypopnea (breathing flow reduction for ≥10 seconds accompanied by oxygen desaturation or sleep arousal). Home sleep apnea testing devices, measuring at least airflow, respiratory effort, and oxygenation, are increasingly being used to diagnose OSA.

Screening. The American College of Physicians offered weak recommendations for ordering sleep studies in patients with unexplained daytime somnolence or in patients suspected to have OSA. The American Academy of Sleep Medicine recommends obtaining sleep histories and evaluating clinical risk factors, including obesity, upper airway narrowing, and comorbidities highly co-prevalent with OSA, during routine health maintenance examinations. Patients at high risk for OSA should undergo a sleep evaluation. A number of screening questionnaires and clinical prediction tools have been developed to assess whether patients are likely to have OSA, including the STOP-Bang Questionnaire (Box 10-7).

Box 10-7. STOP-Bang

STOP

S: Do you *snore* loudly (louder than talking or loud enough to be heard through closed doors)?

T: Do you often feel *tired*, fatigued, or sleepy during the day?

O: Has anyone *observed* you stop breathing during the day?

P: Do you have or are you being treated for high blood *pressure*?

Bang

B: *Body* mass index >35 kg/m^2

A: *Age* >50 years?

N: *Neck* circumference >40 cm (16 in)?

G: *Gender* male?

Source: Reprinted from Chung F et al. *Br J Anaesth*. 2012;108(5):768–775.

TABLE 10-1. Dyspnea

Problem	Process	Timing	Factors That Aggravate
Left-Sided Heart Failure (Left Ventricular Failure or Mitral Stenosis)	Elevated pressure in pulmonary capillary bed with transudation of fluid into interstitial spaces and alveoli, decreased compliance (increased stiffness) of the lungs, increased work of breathing	Dyspnea may progress slowly, or suddenly as in acute pulmonary edema	Exertion, lying down
Chronic Bronchitis	Excessive mucus production in bronchi, followed by chronic obstruction of airways	Chronic productive cough followed by slowly progressive dyspnea	Exertion, inhaled irritants, respiratory infections
Chronic Obstructive Pulmonary Disease (COPD)	Overdistention of air spaces distal to terminal bronchioles, with destruction of alveolar septa, alveolar enlargement, and limitation of expiratory air flow	Slowly progressive dyspnea; relatively mild cough later	Exertion
Asthma	Reversible bronchial hyperresponsiveness involving release of inflammatory mediators, increased airway secretions, and bronchoconstriction	Acute episodes, separated by symptom-free periods. Nocturnal episodes common	Variable, including allergens, irritants, respiratory infections, exercise, cold, and emotion
Diffuse Interstitial Lung Diseases (e.g., Sarcoidosis, Widespread Neoplasms, Idiopathic Pulmonary Fibrosis, and Asbestosis)	Abnormal and widespread infiltration of cells, fluid, and collagen into interstitial spaces between alveoli; many causes	Progressive dyspnea, which varies in its rate of development with the cause	Exertion
Pneumonia	Infection of lung parenchyma from the respiratory bronchioles to the alveoli	An acute illness, timing varies with the causative agent	Exertion, smoking
Spontaneous Pneumothorax	Leakage of air into pleural space through blebs on visceral pleura, with resulting partial or complete collapse of the lung	Sudden onset of dyspnea	
Acute Pulmonary Embolism	Sudden occlusion of part of pulmonary arterial tree by a blood clot that usually originates in deep veins of legs or pelvis	Sudden onset of tachypnea, dyspnea	Exertion
Anxiety with Hyperventilation	Overbreathing, with resultant respiratory alkalosis and fall in arterial partial pressure of carbon dioxide (pCO_2)	Episodic, often recurrent	Often occurs at rest; an upsetting event may not be evident

Sources: Parshall MB et al. Am J Respir Crit Care Med. 2012;185:435; Wenzel RP, Fowler AA. N Engl J Med. 2006;355:2125; Badgett RG et al. Am J Med. 1993;94:188; Holleman DR, Simel DL. JAMA. 1995;273:63; Straus SE et al. JAMA. 2000;283:1853; Panettieri RA. Ann Intern Med. 2007;146:ITC6–1; Littner M. Ann Intern Med. 2011;154:ITC4–1; Neiwoehner DR. N Engl J Med. 2010;362:1407; Global Strategy for the Diagnosis. Management and prevention of COPD, Global Initiative for Chronic Obstructive Lung Disease (GOLD) 2017. Available from: http://goldcopd.org. Accessed April 28, 2018; Neiderman M. Ann Intern Med. 2009;151:ITC4–1–ITC4–16; Agnelli G, Becattini C. N Engl J Med. 2010;363:266; Katerndahl DA. Prim Care Companion J Clin Psychiatry. 2008;10:376.

Factors That Relieve	Associated Symptoms	Setting
Rest, sitting up, though dyspnea may become persistent	Often cough, orthopnea, paroxysmal nocturnal dyspnea; sometimes wheezing	History of heart disease or its predisposing factors
Expectoration; rest, though dyspnea may become persistent	Chronic productive cough, recurrent respiratory infections; wheezing may develop	History of smoking, air pollutants, recurrent respiratory infections; often present with COPD
Rest, though dyspnea may become persistent	Cough, with scant mucoid sputum	History of smoking, air pollutants, sometimes a familial deficiency in α_1-antitrypsin
Separation from aggravating factors	Wheezing, cough, tightness in chest	Environmental conditions
Rest, though dyspnea may become persistent	Often weakness, fatigue; cough less common than in other lung diseases	Varied; exposure to trigger substances
Rest, though dyspnea may become persistent	Pleuritic pain, cough, sputum, fever, though not necessarily present	Varied
	Pleuritic pain, cough	Often a previously healthy young adult or adult with emphysema
Rest, though dyspnea may become persistent	Often none; retrosternal oppressive pain if massive occlusion; pleuritic pain, cough, syncope, hemoptysis, and/or unilateral leg swelling and pain from instigating deep vein thrombosis; anxiety (see below)	Postpartum or postoperative periods; prolonged bed rest; heart failure, chronic lung disease, and fractures of hip or leg; deep venous thrombosis (often not clinically apparent); also hypercoagulability, hereditary (i.e., protein C, S, factor V Leiden deficiency) or acquired (e.g., cancer, hormonal therapy)
Breathing in and out of a paper or plastic bag may help	Sighing, lightheadedness, numbness or tingling of the hands and feet, palpitations, chest pain	Other manifestations of anxiety may be present, such as chest pain diaphoresis, palpitations

TABLE 10-2. Cough and Hemoptysis

Problem	Cough and Sputum	Associated Symptoms and Setting
Acute Inflammation		
Laryngitis	Dry cough, may become productive of variable amounts of sputum	Acute fairly minor illness with hoarseness. Often associated with viral rhinosinusitis.
Acute Bronchitis	Cough, may be dry or productive	Acute, often viral, illness generally without fever or dyspnea; at times with burning retrosternal discomfort.
Mycoplasma and Viral Pneumonias	Dry hacking cough, may become productive of mucoid sputum	Acute febrile illness, often with malaise, headache, and possibly dyspnea.
Bacterial Pneumonias	Sputum is mucoid or purulent; may be **blood-streaked, diffusely pinkish, or rusty**	Acute illness with chills, often high fever, dyspnea, and chest pain. Commonly from *Streptococcus pneumoniae*; *Haemophilus influenzae*; *Moraxella catarrhalis*; *Klebsiella pneumoniae* in alcoholism, especially if underlying smoking, chronic bronchitis, and COPD; cardiovascular disease; diabetes.
Chronic Inflammation		
Postnasal Drip	Chronic cough; sputum mucoid or mucopurulent	Postnasal discharge may be seen in posterior pharynx. Associated with allergic rhinitis, with or without sinusitis.
Chronic Bronchitis	Chronic cough; sputum mucoid to purulent, may be **blood-streaked or even bloody**	Often with recurrent wheezing and dyspnea, and prolonged history of tobacco abuse.
Bronchiectasis	Chronic cough; sputum purulent, often copious and foul-smelling; may be **blood-streaked or bloody**	Recurrent bronchopulmonary infections common; sinusitis may coexist.
Pulmonary Tuberculosis	Cough, dry or with mucoid or purulent sputum; may be **blood-streaked or bloody**	Early, no symptoms. Later, anorexia, weight loss, fatigue, fever, and night sweats.
Lung Abscess	Sputum purulent and foul-smelling; may be **bloody**	Usually from aspiration pneumonia with fever and infection from oral anaerobes and poor dental hygiene; often with dysphagia or episode of impaired consciousness.
Asthma	Cough, at times with thick mucoid sputum, especially near end of an attack	Episodic wheezing and dyspnea, but cough may occur alone. Often with a history of allergies.
Gastroesophageal Reflux	Chronic cough, especially at night or early in the morning	Wheezing, especially at night (often mistaken for asthma), early morning hoarseness, and repeated attempts to clear the throat. Often with heartburn and regurgitation.

(continued)

TABLE 10-2. Cough and Hemoptysis *(Continued)*

Problem	Cough and Sputum	Associated Symptoms and Setting
Neoplasm		
Lung Cancer	Cough, dry to productive; sputum may be **blood-streaked or bloody**	Commonly with dyspnea, weight loss, and history of tobacco abuse.
Cardiovascular Disorders		
Left Ventricular Failure or Mitral Stenosis	Often dry, especially on exertion or at night; may progress to the **pink frothy sputum** of pulmonary edema or to frank hemoptysis	Dyspnea, orthopnea, paroxysmal nocturnal dyspnea.
Pulmonary Embolism	Dry cough, at times with hemoptysis	Tachypnea, chest or pleuritic pain, dyspnea, fever, syncope, anxiety; factors that predispose to deep venous thrombosis.
Irritating Particles, Chemicals, or Gases	Variable. There may be a latent period between exposure and symptoms.	Exposure to irritants. Eyes, nose, and throat may be affected.

Sources: Irwin RS, Madison JM. N Engl J Med. 2000;343:1715; Metlay JP et al. JAMA. 1997;378:1440; Neiderman M. Ann Intern Med. 2009;151:ITC4–1; Barker A. N Engl J Med. 2002;346:1383; Wenzel RP, Fowler AA. N Engl J Med. 2006;355:2125; Kerlin MP. Ann Intern Med. 2014;160:ITC3–1; Escalante P. Ann Intern Med. 2009;150:ITC6–1; Agnelli G, Becattini C. N Engl J Med. 2010;363:266.

TABLE 10-3. Chest Pain

Problem	Process	Location	Quality	Severity
Cardiovascular				
Angina Pectoris	Temporary myocardial ischemia, usually secondary to coronary atherosclerosis	Retrosternal or across the anterior chest, often radiates to the shoulders, arms, neck, lower jaw, or upper abdomen	Pressing, squeezing, tight, heavy, occasionally burning	Mild to moderate, sometimes perceived as discomfort rather than pain
Myocardial Infarction	Prolonged myocardial ischemia, resulting in irreversible muscle damage or necrosis	Same as in angina	Same as in angina	Often, but not always, a severe pain
Pericarditis	Irritation of parietal pleura adjacent to the pericardium	Retrosternal or left precordial, may radiate to the tip of left shoulder	Sharp, knifelike	Often severe
Aortic Dissection	A splitting within the layers of the aortic wall, allowing passage of blood to dissect a channel	Anterior or posterior chest, radiating to the neck, back, or abdomen	Ripping, tearing	Very severe
Pulmonary				
Pleuritic Pain	Inflammation of the parietal pleura, as in pleurisy, pneumonia, pulmonary infarction, or neoplasm; rarely, subdiaphragmatic abscess	Chest wall overlying the process	Sharp, knifelike	Often severe
Gastrointestinal and Other				
Gastrointestinal Reflux Disease	Irritation or inflammation of the esophageal mucosa due to reflux of gastric acid from lowered esophageal sphincter tone	Retrosternal, may radiate to the back	Burning, may be squeezing	Mild to severe
Diffuse Esophageal Spasm	Motor dysfunction of the esophageal muscle	Retrosternal, may radiate to the back, arms, and jaw	Usually squeezing	Mild to severe
Chest Wall Pain, Costochondritis	Variable, including trauma, inflammation of costal cartilage	Often below the left breast or along the costal cartilages	Stabbing, sticking, or dull, aching	Variable
Anxiety, Panic Disorder	Unclear	Precordial, below the left breast, or across the anterior chest	Stabbing, sticking, or dull, aching	Variable

Note: Chest pain may be referred from extrathoracic structures in the neck (arthritis) and abdomen (biliary colic, acute cholecystitis).

Problem	Timing	Factors That Aggravate	Factors That Relieve	Associated Symptoms
Cardiovascular				
Angina Pectoris	Usually 1–3 min but up to 10 min. Prolonged episodes up to 20 min	Often exertion, especially in the cold; meals; emotional stress. May occur at rest	Often, but not always, rest, nitroglycerin	Sometimes dyspnea, nausea, sweating
Myocardial Infarction	20 min to several hours	Not always triggered by exertion	Not relieved by rest	Dyspnea, nausea, vomiting, sweating, weakness
Pericarditis	Persistent	Breathing, changing position, coughing, lying down, sometimes swallowing	Sitting forward may relieve it	Seen in autoimmune disorders, postmyocardial infarction, viral infection, chest irradiation
Aortic Dissection	Abrupt onset, early peak, persistent for hours or more	Hypertension		If thoracic, hoarseness, dysphagia; also syncope, hemiplegia, paraplegia
Pulmonary				
Pleuritic Pain	Persistent	Deep inspiration, coughing, movements of the trunk		Of the underlying illness
Gastrointestinal and Other				
Gastrointestinal Reflux Disease	Variable	Large meal; bending over, lying down	Antacids, sometimes belching	Sometimes regurgitation, dysphagia; also cough, laryngitis, asthma
Diffuse Esophageal Spasm	Variable	Swallowing of food or cold liquid; emotional stress	Sometimes nitroglycerin	Dysphagia
Chest Wall Pain, Costochondritis	Fleeting to hours or days	Coughing; movement of chest, trunk, arms		Often local tenderness
Anxiety, Panic Disorder	Fleeting to hours or days	May follow effort, emotional stress		Breathlessness, palpitations, weakness, anxiety

TABLE 10-4. Abnormalities in Rate and Rhythm of Breathing

When observing respiratory patterns, note the rate, depth, and regularity of the patient's breathing.

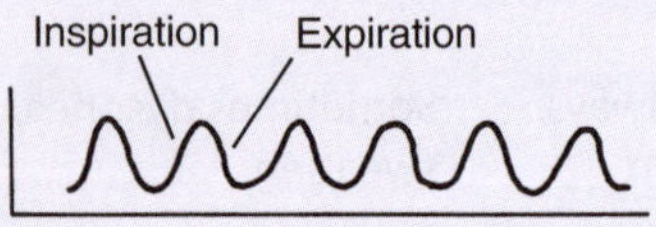

Normal

The respiratory rate is about 14–20 per min in normal adults and up to 44 per min in infants.

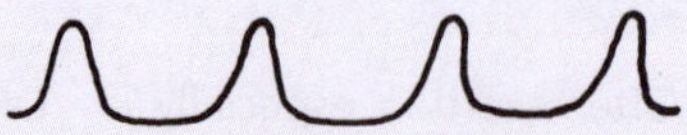

Slow Breathing (*Bradypnea*)

Slow breathing with or without an increase in tidal volume that maintains alveolar ventilation. Abnormal alveolar hypoventilation without increased tidal volume can arise from uremia, drug-induced respiratory depression, and increased intracranial pressure.

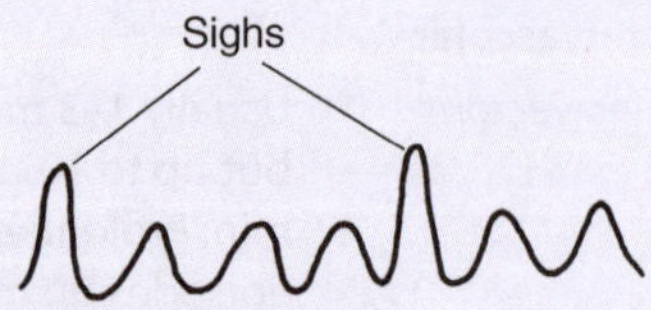

Sighing Respiration

Breathing punctuated by frequent sighs suggests *hyperventilation syndrome*—a common cause of dyspnea and dizziness. Occasional sighs are normal.

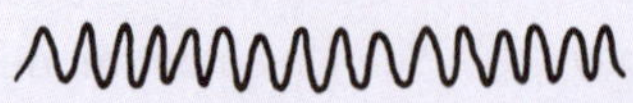

Rapid Shallow Breathing (*Tachypnea*)

Rapid shallow breathing has numerous causes, including salicylate intoxication, restrictive lung disease, pleuritic chest pain, and an elevated diaphragm.

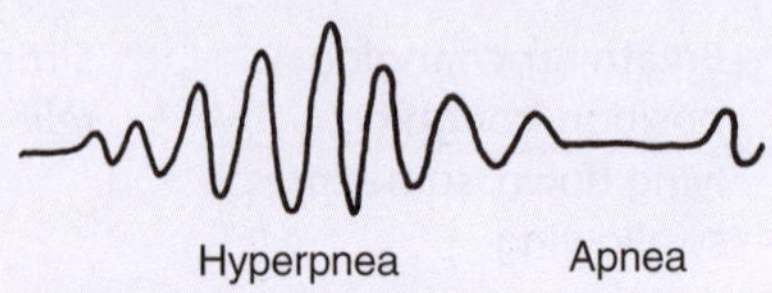

Cheyne–Stokes Breathing

Periods of deep breathing alternate with periods of *apnea* (no breathing). This pattern is normal in children and older adults during sleep. Causes include heart failure, uremia, drug-induced respiratory depression, and brain injury (typically bihemispheric).

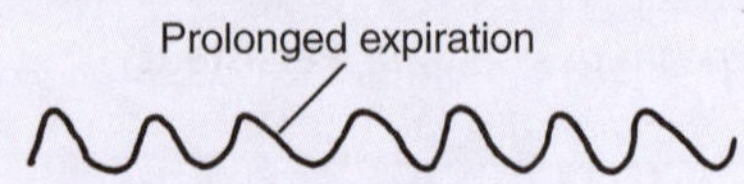

Obstructive Breathing

In obstructive lung disease, expiration is prolonged due to narrowed airways increase the resistance to air flow. Causes include asthma, chronic bronchitis, and COPD.

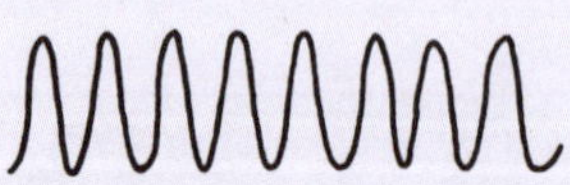

Rapid Deep Breathing (*Hyperpnea, Hyperventilation*)

In *hyperpnea,* rapid deep breathing occurs in response to metabolic demand from causes such as exercise, high altitude, sepsis, and anemia. In *hyperventilation,* this pattern is independent of metabolic demand, except in respiratory acidosis. Lightheadedness and tingling may arise from decreased CO_2 concentration. In the comatose patient, consider hypoxia, or hypoglycemia affecting the midbrain or pons. *Kussmaul breathing* is compensatory overbreathing due to systemic acidosis. The breathing rate may be fast, normal, or slow.

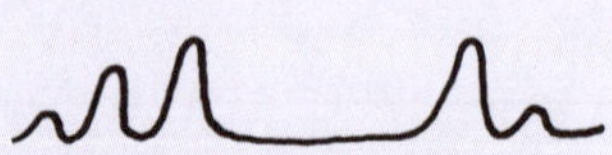

Ataxic Breathing (*Biot Breathing*)

Breathing is irregular—periods of apnea alternate with regular deep breaths which stop suddenly for short intervals. Causes include meningitis, respiratory depression, and brain injury, typically at the medullary level.

TABLE 10-5. Deformities of the Thorax

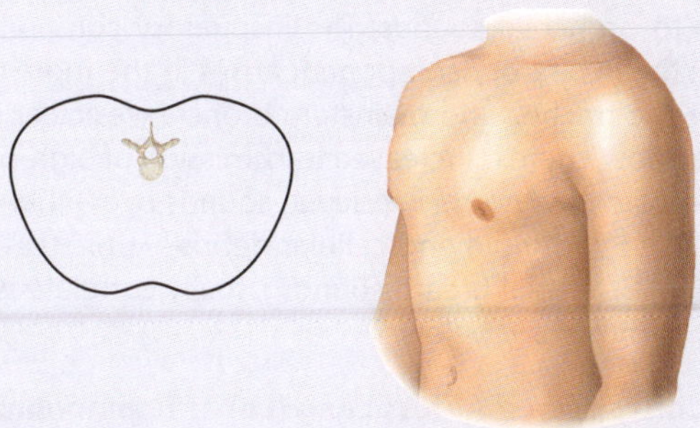

Normal Adult

The lateral diameter of the thorax in the normal adult is greater than its AP diameter. The ratio of its AP diameter to the lateral diameter is normally ~0.7 up to 0.9 and increases with aging.

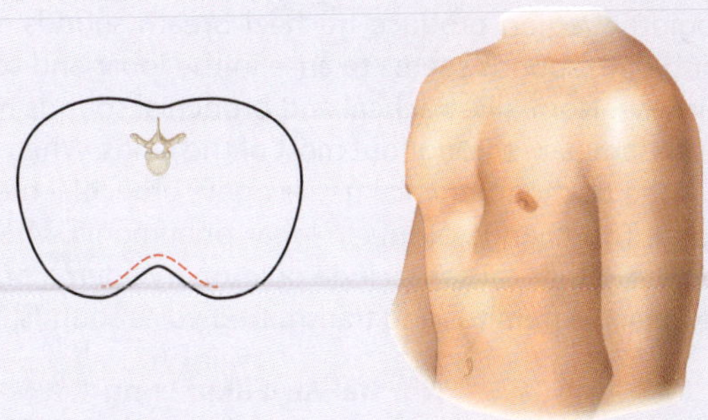

Funnel Chest (*Pectus Excavatum*)

Note depression in the lower portion of the sternum. Compression of the heart and great vessels may cause murmurs.

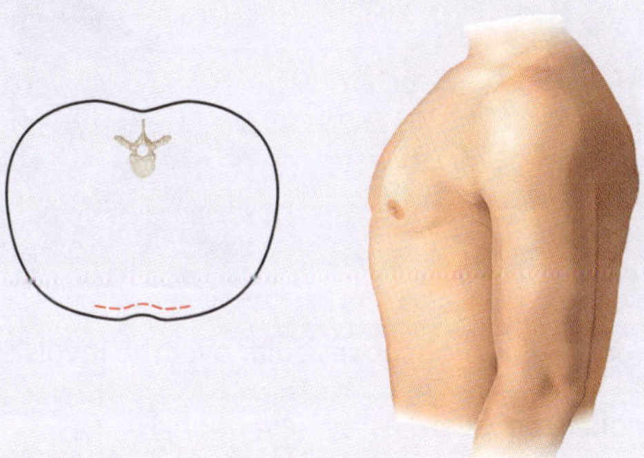

Barrel Chest

There is an increased AP diameter. This shape is normal during infancy, and often accompanies aging and chronic obstructive pulmonary disease.

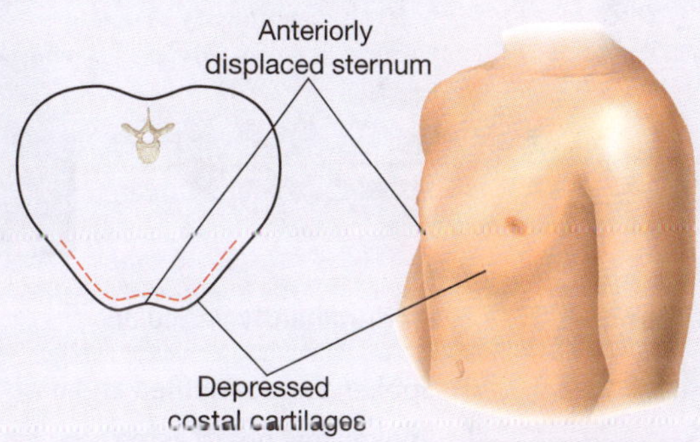

Pigeon Chest (*Pectus Carinatum*)

The sternum is displaced anteriorly, increasing the AP diameter. The costal cartilages adjacent to the protruding sternum are depressed.

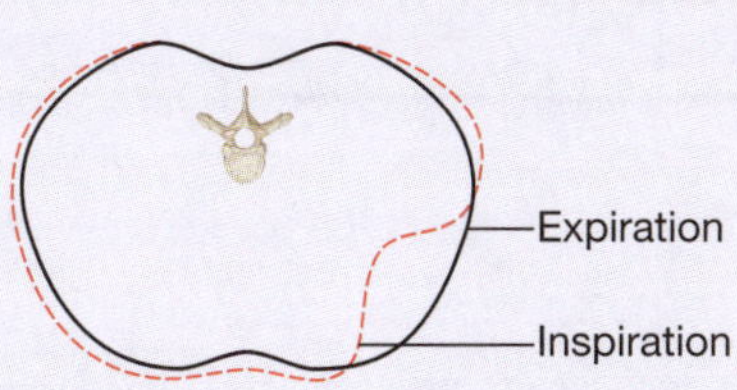

Traumatic Flail Chest

Multiple rib fractures may result in paradoxical movements of the thorax. As descent of the diaphragm decreases intrathoracic pressure, on inspiration, the injured area caves inward; on expiration, it moves outward.

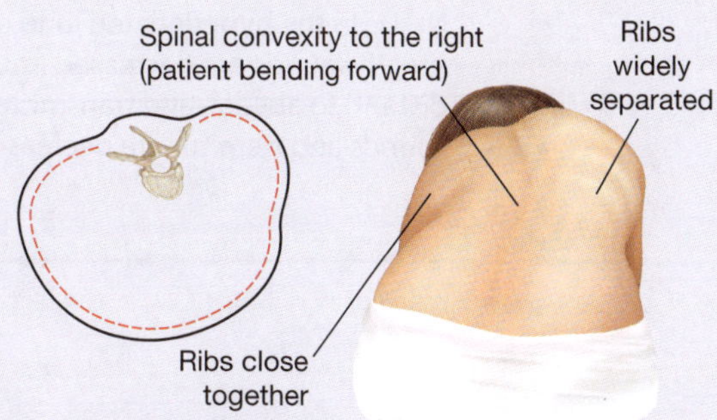

Posterior view of patient in forward flexion.

Thoracic Kyphoscoliosis

Abnormal spinal curvatures and vertebral rotation deform the chest. Distortion of the underlying lungs may make interpretation of lung findings very difficult.

TABLE 10-6. Normal and Altered Breath and Voice Sounds

The origins of breath sounds continue to be investigated. Acoustic studies indicate that turbulent air flow in the pharynx, glottis, and subglottic region produce tracheal breath sounds, which are similar to bronchial sounds. The inspiratory component of vesicular breath sounds seems to arise in the lobar and segmental airways; the expiratory component arises in the more central larger airways. Normally, tracheal and bronchial sounds may be heard over the trachea and mainstem bronchi; vesicular breath sounds predominate throughout most of the lungs. When lung tissue loses airflow, there is increased transmission of high-pitched sounds. If the tracheobronchial tree is open, bronchial breath sounds may replace the normal vesicular sounds over airless areas of the lung. This change occurs in lobar pneumonia when the alveoli get filled with fluid and cellular debris—a process called *consolidation*. Other causes include pulmonary edema or, rarely, hemorrhage. Bronchial breath sounds usually correlate with an increase in tactile fremitus and transmitted voice sounds. These findings are summarized below.

	Normal Air-Filled Lung	Consolidated Airless Lung (Lobar Pneumonia)
	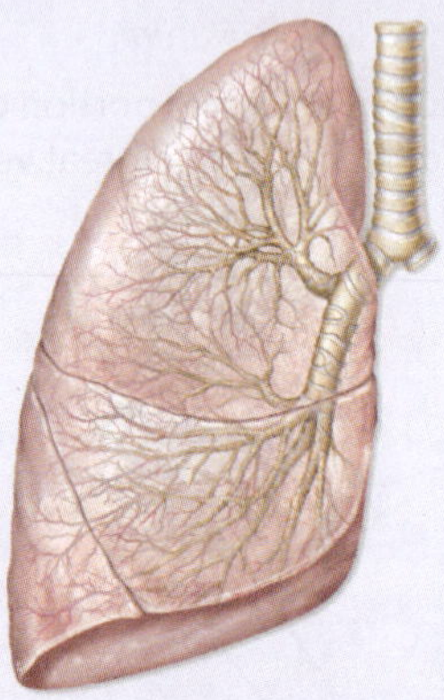 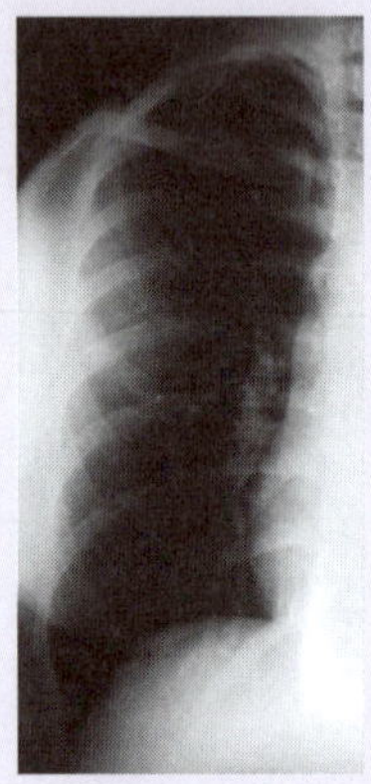	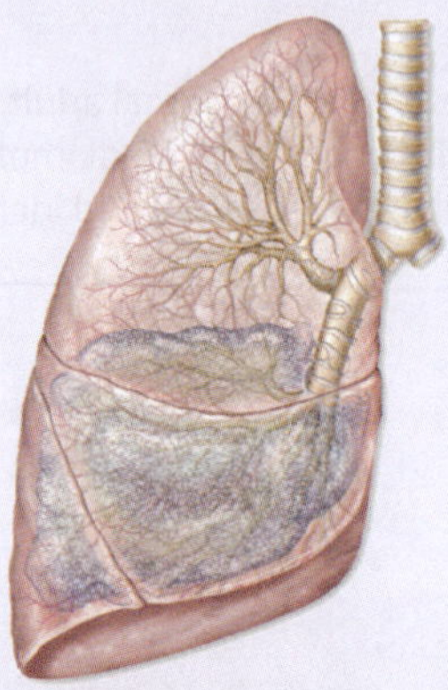 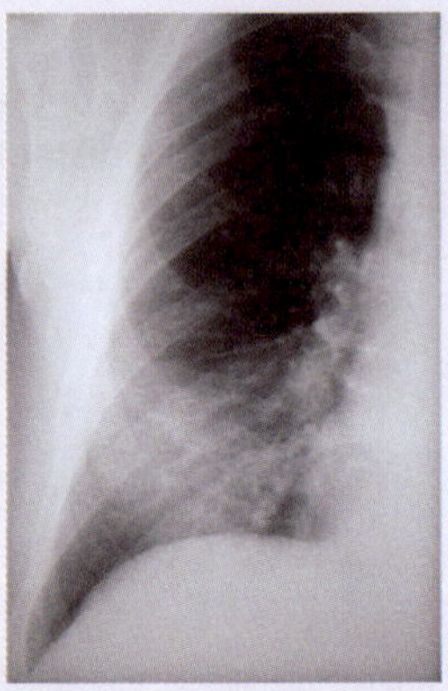
Breath Sounds	Predominantly vesicular	Bronchial or bronchovesicular over the involved area
Transmitted Voice Sounds	Spoken words muffled and indistinct Spoken "ee" heard as "ee" Whispered words faint and indistinct, if heard at all	Spoken "ee" heard as "ay" (*egophony*) Spoken words louder (*bronchophony*) Whispered words louder, clearer (*whispered pectoriloquy*)
Tactile Fremitus	Normal	Increased
	NOTE: In the hyperinflated lung of COPD, breath sounds are decreased (muffled to distant) to absent, and transmitted voice sounds and fremitus are decreased.	NOTE: In the dull lung of pleural effusion, breath sounds are decreased to absent (bronchial sounds possible at upper margin of effusion). Transmitted voice sounds are decreased to absent (but may be increased at upper margin of effusion). Fremitus is decreased.

TABLE 10-7. Adventitious (Added) Lung Sounds: Causes and Qualities

Sound	Causes and Qualities
Crackles	Crackles are discontinuous nonmusical sounds that can be early inspiratory (as in *COPD*), late inspiratory (as in *pulmonary fibrosis*), or biphasic (as in *pneumonia*). They are currently considered to result from a series of tiny explosions when small distal airways, deflated during expiration, pop open during inspiration. With few exceptions, recent acoustic studies indicate that the role of secretions as a cause of crackles is less likely.
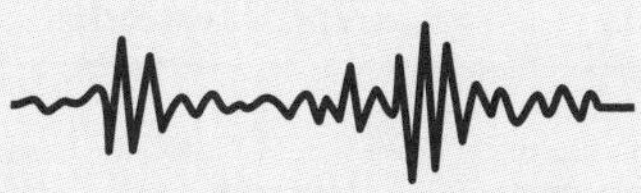	***Fine crackles*** are softer, higher pitched, and more frequent per breath than coarse crackles. They are heard from *mid to late inspiration*, especially in the dependent areas of the lung, and change according to body position. They have a shorter duration and higher frequency than coarse crackles. Fine crackles appear to be generated by the "sudden inspiratory opening of small airways held closed by surface forces during the previous expiration." Examples include *pulmonary fibrosis* (known for "Velcro rales") and interstitial lung diseases such as *interstitial fibrosis* and *interstitial pneumonitis*.
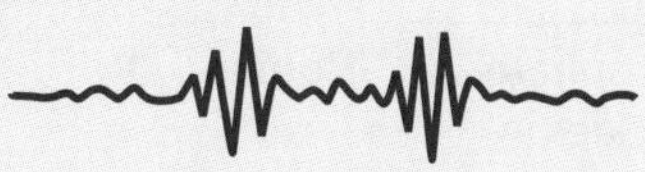	***Coarse crackles*** appear in early inspiration and last throughout expiration (*biphasic*), have a popping sound, are heard over any lung region, and do not vary with body position. They have a longer duration and lower frequency than fine crackles, change or disappear with coughing, and are transmitted to the mouth. Coarse crackles appear to result from "boluses of gas passing through airways as they open and close intermittently." Examples include *COPD, asthma, bronchiectasis, pneumonia* (crackles may become finer and change from mid to late inspiratory during recovery), and *heart failure*.
Wheezes and Rhonchi 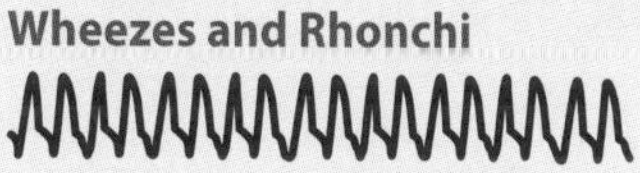	***Wheezes*** are continuous musical sounds that occur during rapid airflow when bronchial airways are narrowed almost to the point of closure. Wheezes can be inspiratory, expiratory, or biphasic. They may be localized, due to a foreign body, mucous plug, or tumor, or heard throughout the lung. Although wheezes are typical of asthma, they can occur in a number of pulmonary diseases. Recent studies suggest that as the airways become more narrowed, wheezes become less audible, culminating finally in "the silent chest" of severe asthma requiring immediate intervention.
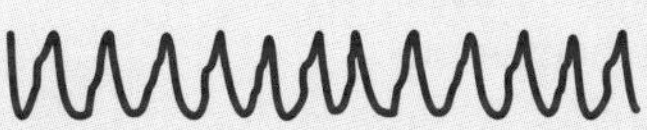	***Rhonchi*** are considered by some to be a variant of wheezes, arising from the same mechanism, but lower in pitch. Unlike wheezes, rhonchi may disappear with coughing, so secretions may be involved.
Stridor 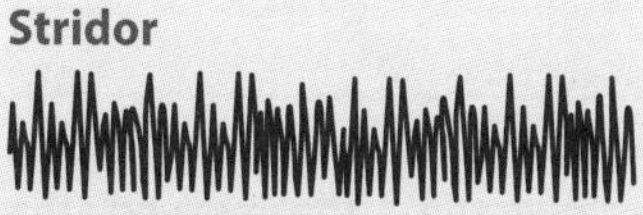	***Stridor*** is a continuous, high-frequency, high-pitched musical sound produced during airflow through a narrowing in the upper respiratory tract. Stridor is best heard over the neck during inspiration but can be biphasic. Causes of the underlying airway obstruction include tracheal stenosis from intubation, airway edema after device removal, epiglottitis, foreign body, and anaphylaxis. Immediate intervention is warranted.
Pleural Rub 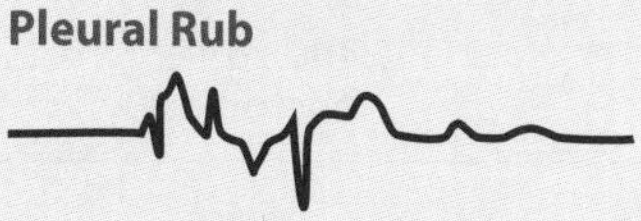	A ***pleural rub*** is a discontinuous, low-frequency, grating sound that arises from inflammation and roughening of the visceral pleura as it slides against the parietal pleura. This nonmusical sound is biphasic, heard during inspiration and expiration, and often best heard in the axilla and base of the lungs.
Mediastinal Crunch (*Hamman Sign*)	A ***mediastinal crunch*** is a series of precordial crackles synchronous with the heartbeat, not with respiration. Best heard in the left lateral position, it arises from air entry into the mediastinum causing mediastinal emphysema (*pneumomediastinum*). It usually produces severe central chest pain and may be spontaneous. It has been reported in cases of tracheobronchial injury, blunt trauma, pulmonary disease, use of recreational drugs, childbirth, and rapid ascent from scuba diving.

Sources: Bohadana A et al. N Engl J Med. 2014;370:744; McGee S. Evidence-Based Physical Diagnosis. 3rd ed. Saunders; 2012; Loudon R, Murphy LH. Am Rev Respir Dis. 1994;130:663.

TABLE 10-8. Physical Findings in Selected Chest Disorders

The red boxes in this table provide a framework for the clinical assessment of common chest disorders. Start with the three boxes under percussion. Note resonant, dull, and hyperresonant. Then move from each of these to other boxes that emphasize some of the key differences among various conditions. The changes described vary with the extent and severity of the disorder. Abnormalities deep in the chest usually produce fewer signs than superficial ones and may cause no signs at all. Use the table for the direction of typical changes, not for absolute distinctions.

Condition	Percussion Note	Trachea	Breath Sounds	Adventitious Sounds	Tactile Fremitus and Transmitted Voice Sounds
Normal The tracheobronchial tree and alveoli are open; pleurae are thin and close together; mobility of the chest wall is unimpaired.	**Resonant**	Midline	Vesicular, except perhaps bronchovesicular and bronchial sounds over the large bronchi and trachea, respectively	None, except a few transient inspiratory crackles at the bases of the lungs	Normal
Left-Sided Heart Failure Increased pressure in the pulmonary veins causes congestion and interstitial edema (around the alveoli); bronchial mucosa may become edematous.	**Resonant**	Midline	Vesicular (normal)	Late inspiratory crackles in the dependent portions of the lungs; possibly wheezes	Normal
Chronic Bronchitis The bronchi are chronically inflamed, and a productive cough is present. Airway obstruction may develop.	**Resonant**	Midline	Vesicular (normal)	None; possible scattered coarse crackles in early inspiration and expiration; possible wheezes or rhonchi	Normal
Lobar Pneumonia (*Consolidation*) Alveoli fill with fluid, as in pneumonia	**Dull** over the airless area	Midline	Bronchial over the involved area	Late inspiratory crackles over the involved area	Increased over the involved area, with egophony, bronchophony, and whispered pectoriloquy
Partial Lobar Obstruction (*Atelectasis*) When a plug (from mucus or a foreign object) obstructs bronchial air flow, affected alveoli collapse and become airless.	**Dull** over the airless area	May be shifted toward involved side	Usually absent when bronchial plug persists. Exceptions include right upper lobe atelectasis, where adjacent tracheal sounds may be transmitted.	None	Usually absent when the bronchial plug persists. In right upper lobe atelectasis may be increased.

(continued)

TABLE 10-8. Physical Findings in Selected Chest Disorders *(Continued)*

Condition	Percussion Note	Trachea	Breath Sounds	Adventitious Sounds	Tactile Fremitus and Transmitted Voice Sounds
Pleural Effusion Fluid accumulates in the pleural space and separates air-filled lung from the chest wall, blocking the transmission of breath sounds.	**Dull** to flat over the fluid	Shifted toward the unaffected side in a large effusion	Decreased to absent, but bronchial breath sounds may be heard near top of large effusion.	None, except a possible pleural rub	Decreased to absent, but may be increased toward the top of a large effusion
Pneumothorax When air leaks into the pleural space, usually unilaterally, the lung recoils away from the chest wall. Pleural air blocks transmission of sound.	**Hyperresonant** or tympanitic over the pleural air	Shifted toward the unaffected side if tension pneumothorax	Decreased to absent over the pleural air	None, except a possible pleural rub	Decreased to absent over the pleural air
Chronic Obstructive Pulmonary Disease (COPD) Slowly progressive disorder in which the distal air spaces enlarge and lungs become hyperinflated. Chronic bronchitis may precede or follow the development of COPD.	Diffusely **hyperresonant**	Midline	Decreased to absent, with delayed expiration	None, or the crackles, wheezes, and rhonchi of associated chronic bronchitis	Decreased
Asthma Widespread, usually reversible, airflow obstruction with bronchial hyperresponsiveness and underlying inflammation. During attacks, as air flow decreases lungs hyperinflate.	**Resonant** to diffusely **hyperresonant**	Midline	Often obscured by wheezes	Wheezes, possibly crackles	Decreased

CHAPTER 11

Cardiovascular System

ANATOMY AND PHYSIOLOGY

Combining your knowledge of anatomy and physiology with hands-on practice of inspection, palpation, and auscultation brings rewards of proven diagnostic value.

Surface Projections of the Heart and Great Vessels

The *mediastinum* is a connective tissue–lined compartment located centrally in the thoracic cavity. It is bordered by the lungs on either side, the sternum anteriorly, and the thoracic vertebral bodies posteriorly. The mediastinum houses the heart and its great vessels—the *aorta, pulmonary artery,* and *superior* and *inferior vena cavae*—as well the esophagus, trachea, thoracic duct, and thoracic lymph nodes.

Visualize the underlying structures of the heart and other mediastinal structures as you inspect the anterior chest. Note that the *right ventricle* (RV) is the most anterior structure of the heart. This chamber and the pulmonary artery form a wedge-like structure behind and to the left of the sternum, outlined in Figure 11-1.

The inferior border of the RV lies below the junction of the sternum and the xiphoid process. The RV narrows superiorly and joins the pulmonary artery at the level of the sternal angle, or "base of the heart," a clinical term that refers to the superior aspect of the heart at the valve plane, which is near the right and left second intercostal spaces adjacent to the sternum. This should be distinguished from the "apex of the heart," which is located inferolaterally.

The *left ventricle* (LV), behind the RV and to the left, forms the left lateral margin of the heart (see Fig. 11-1). Its tapered inferior tip is often termed the *cardiac apex.* It is clinically important because it produces the apical impulse, identified during palpation of the precordium as the **point of maximal impulse** (**PMI**). This impulse

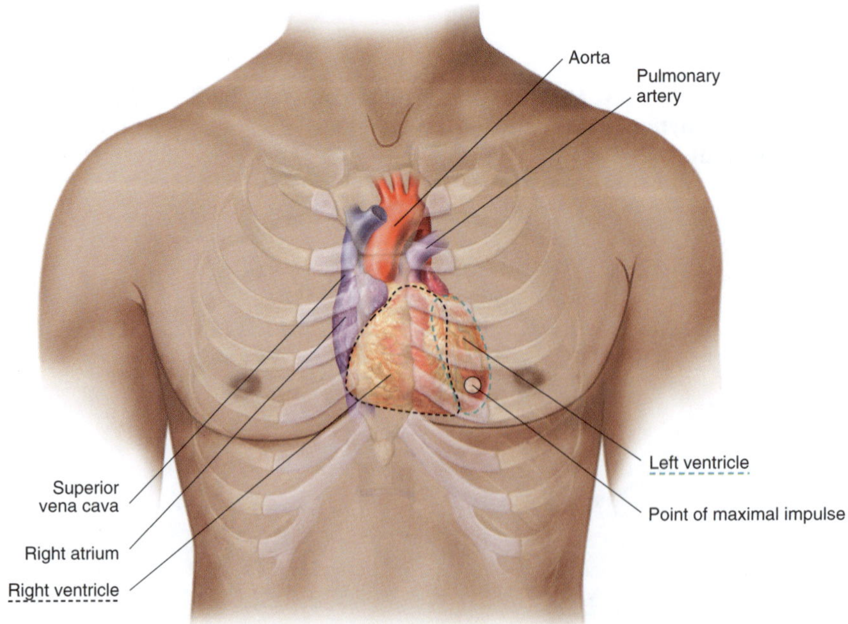

FIGURE 11-1. Major cardiac structures as visualized through the chest wall.

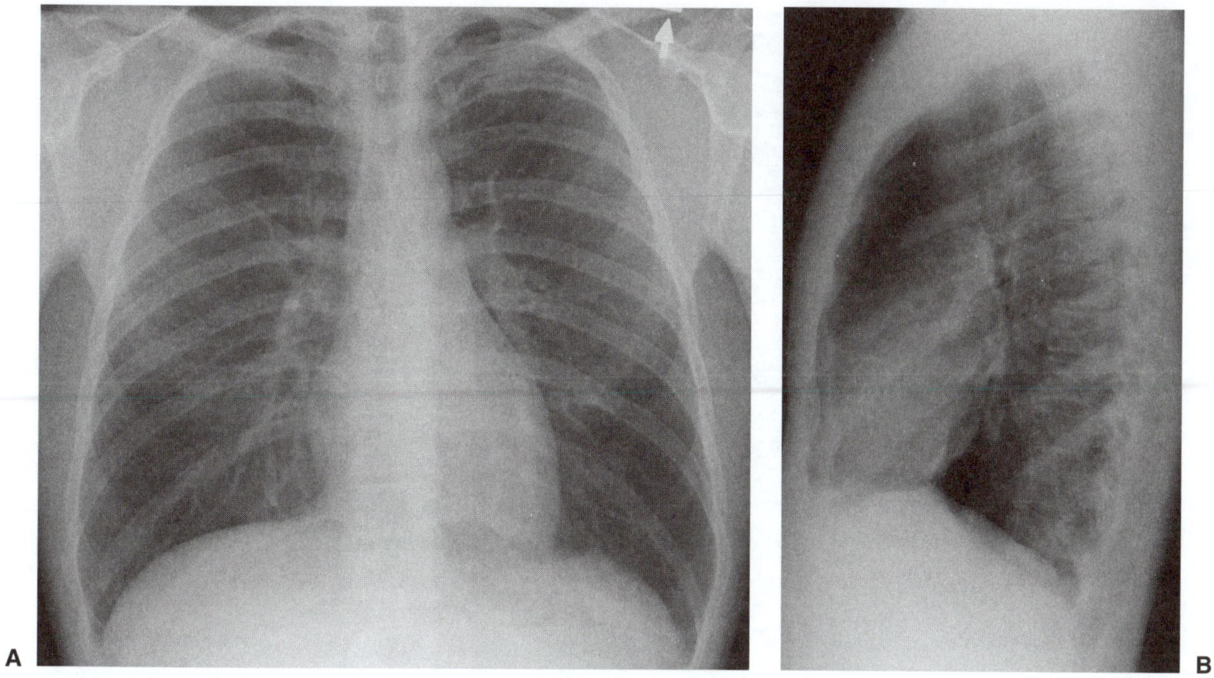

FIGURE 11-2. Normal posteroanterior (**A**) and lateral (**B**) chest radiographs. (From Collins J, Stern EJ. *Chest Radiology: The Essentials.* 3rd ed. Wolters Kluwer; 2015, Fig. 1-2ab.)

locates the left border of the heart and is normally found in the fifth intercostal space at or just medial to the left midclavicular line (or 7 to 9 cm lateral to the midsternal line). In supine patients, the diameter of the PMI is approximately 1 to 2.5 cm. The PMI is not always palpable, even in a healthy patient with a normal heart. Detection is affected by both the patient's body habitus and position during the examination.

Rarely, in **dextrocardia**, the PMI is located on the right side of the chest.

A PMI >2.5 cm is evidence of left ventricular hypertrophy (LVH), often seen in hypertension or dilated cardiomyopathy.

In some patients, the most prominent precordial impulse may not be at the apex of the left ventricle. For example, in patients with chronic obstructive pulmonary disease (COPD), the most prominent palpable impulse or PMI may be in the xiphoid or epigastric area due to right ventricular hypertrophy.

Displacement of the PMI lateral to the midclavicular line or >10 cm lateral to the midsternal line occurs in LVH and also in ventricular dilatation from myocardial infarction (MI) or heart failure.

Above the heart lie the great vessels. The *pulmonary artery* bifurcates quickly into its left and right branches. The *aorta* curves upward from the left ventricle to the level of the sternal angle, where it arches posteriorly to the left and then downward. On the medial border, the *superior* and *inferior venae cavae* channel venous blood from the upper and lower portions of the body into the right atrium.

Also familiarize yourself with the appearance of the heart and great vessels in a chest radiograph (Figs. 11-2 and 11-3). Understanding the contours of these structures can help in describing the location of pathologic processes.

Cardiac Chambers, Valves, and Circulation

Circulation through the heart is diagrammed below. Identify the cardiac chambers, valves, and direction of blood flow. Because of their location, the *mitral* and *tricuspid* valves are often called *atrioventricular (AV) valves.* The *aortic* and *pulmonic* valves are called *semilunar valves* because the valve leaflets are shaped like half-moons.

In most adults, the diastolic sounds of S_3 and S_4 are pathologic, and are correlated with systolic and diastolic heart failure, respectively.

As the heart valves close, the heart sounds of S_1 and S_2 arise from vibrations emanating from the leaflets, the adjacent cardiac structures, and the flow of blood. Study carefully the opening and closing of the AV and semilunar valves in relation to events in the cardiac cycle to improve your diagnostic accuracy as you auscultate the heart. In Figure 11-4, note that the aortic and pulmonic valves are closed, and the mitral and tricuspid valves are open, as seen in diastole.

An S_3 corresponds to an abrupt deceleration of inflow across the mitral valve.

An S_4 corresponds to increased left ventricular end diastolic stiffness which decreases compliance.

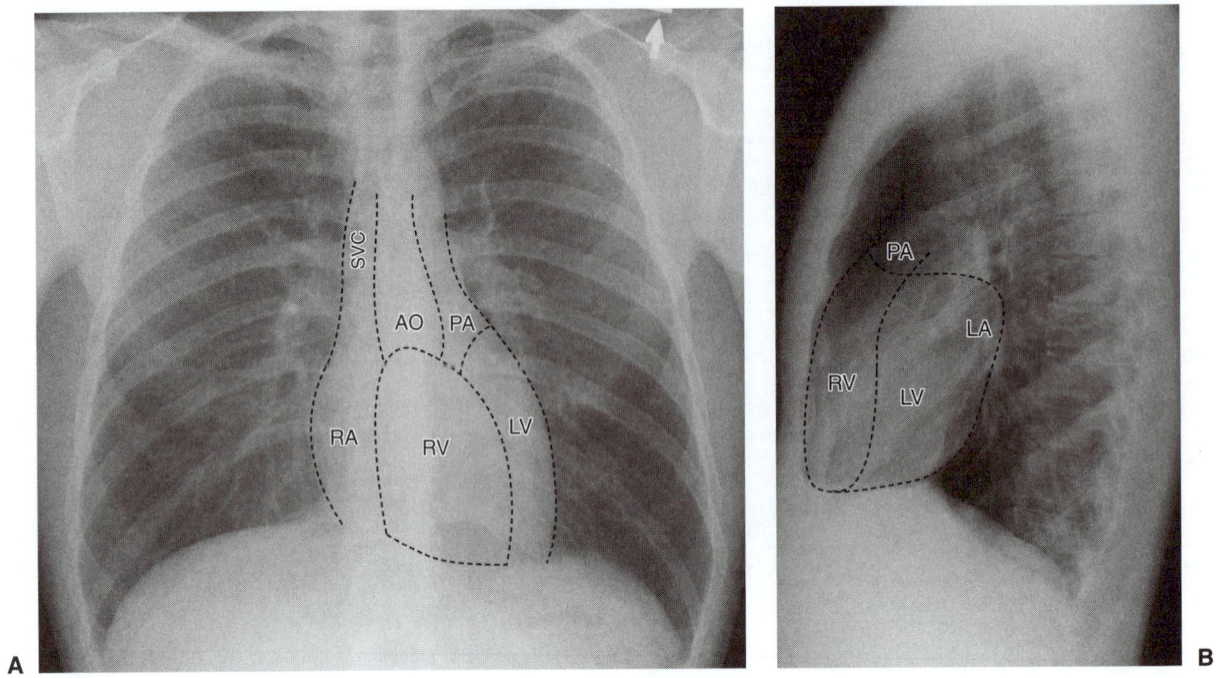

FIGURE 11-3. Normal posteroanterior **(A)** and lateral **(B)** chest radiographs with cardiac chambers and great vessels outlined. AO, aorta; LA, left atrium; LV, left ventricle; PA, pulmonary artery; RA, right atrium; RV, right ventricle; SVC, superior vena cava. (Modified from Collins J, Stern EJ. *Chest Radiology: The Essentials.* 3rd ed. Wolters Kluwer; 2015, Fig. 1-2ab.)

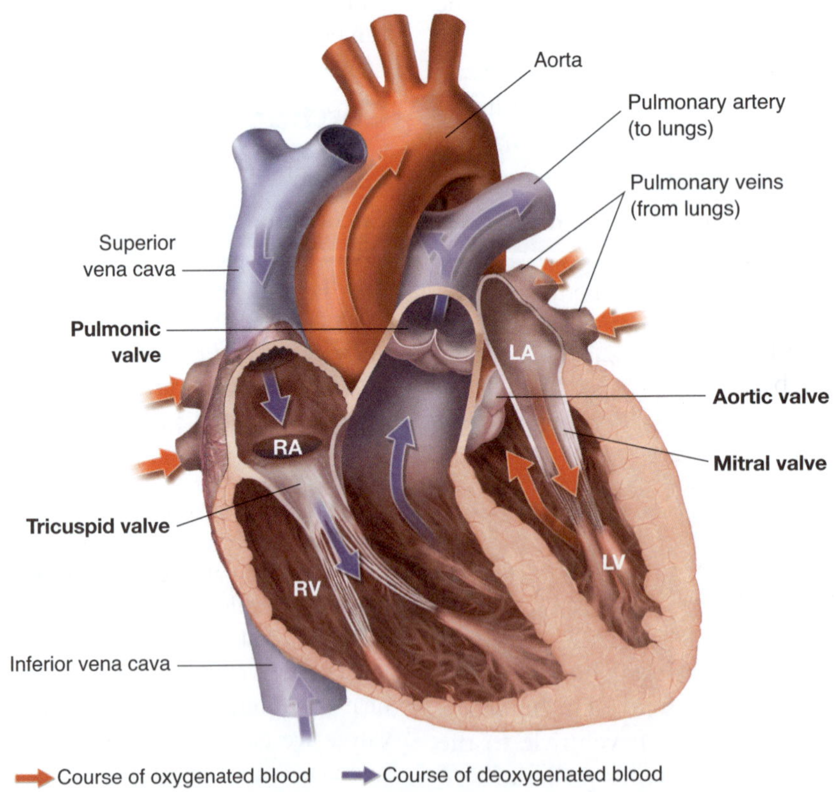

FIGURE 11-4. Cardiac chambers, valves, and circulation. RA, right atrium; LA, left atrium; RV, right ventricle; LV, left ventricle.

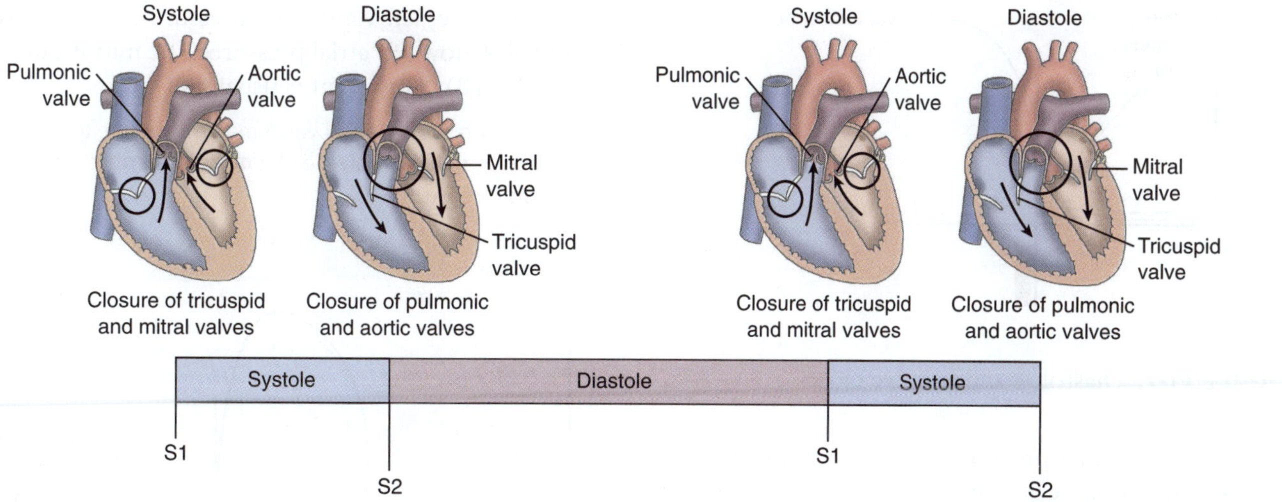

FIGURE 11-5. Cardiac cycle, direction of blood flow. (Modified from Jensen S. *Nursing Health Assessment: A Best Practice Approach.* 3rd ed. Wolters Kluwer; 2019, Fig. 17-8.)

Events in the Cardiac Cycle

The *cardiac cycle* describes the complete movement of the heart and includes the period from the beginning of one heartbeat to the beginning of the next one. The heart serves as a pump that generates varying pressures as its chambers contract and relax throughout the cycle phases of systole and diastole (Fig. 11-5). *Systole* is the period of ventricular contraction when the left ventricle ejects blood into the aorta. After the ventricle ejects much of its blood into the aorta, the pressure levels off and starts to fall. Ventricular pressure falls further, and blood flows from atrium to ventricle. This period of ventricular relaxation is called *diastole*. Late in diastole, ventricular pressure rises slightly during inflow of blood from atrial contraction.

Note that during *systole* the aortic valve is open, allowing ejection of blood from the LV into the aorta. The mitral valve is closed, preventing blood from regurgitating back into the left atrium. In contrast, during *diastole* the aortic valve is closed, preventing regurgitation of blood from the aorta back into the LV. The mitral valve is open, allowing blood to flow from the left atrium into the relaxed LV. At the same time, during systole, the pulmonic valve opens, and the tricuspid valve closes as blood is ejected from the RV into the pulmonary artery. During diastole, the pulmonic valve closes, and the tricuspid valve opens as blood flows into the relaxed right ventricle.

Understanding the interrelationships of the pressure gradients in the left heart (the left atrium, left ventricle, and aorta), together with the position and movement of the four heart valves, is fundamental to understanding heart sounds. An extensive literature explores how heart sounds are generated. Possible explanations include closure of the valve leaflets; tensing of related structures, leaflet positions, and pressure gradients at the time of atrial and ventricular systole; and the acoustic effects of moving columns of blood.

Trace the changing left ventricular pressures and sounds through one cardiac cycle. Note that S_1 and S_2 define the duration of systole and diastole. The explanations given here are oversimplified and focused on left-sided cardiac pressures but retain clinical usefulness to understanding the cycle.

During diastole, pressure in the blood-filled left atrium slightly exceeds that in the relaxed LV, and blood flows from left atrium to left ventricle across the open mitral valve (Fig. 11-6). Just before the onset of systole, atrial contraction produces a slight pressure rise in both chambers.

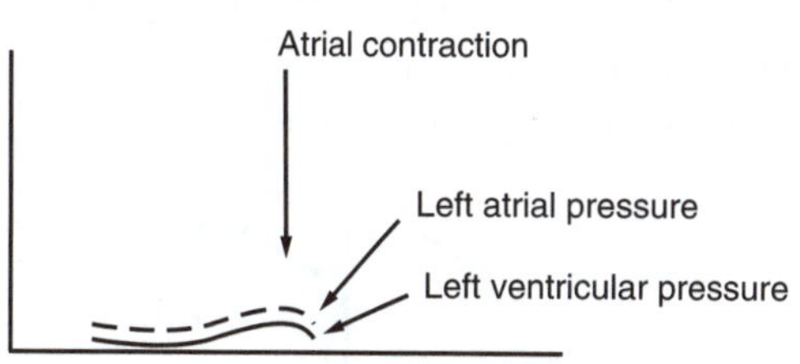

FIGURE 11-6. Diastole—atrial contraction.

During systole, the LV starts to contract, and ventricular pressure rapidly exceeds left atrial pressure, closing the mitral valve (Fig. 11-7). Closure of the mitral valve and the tricuspid valve in the right side of the heart produce the first heart sound, S_1.

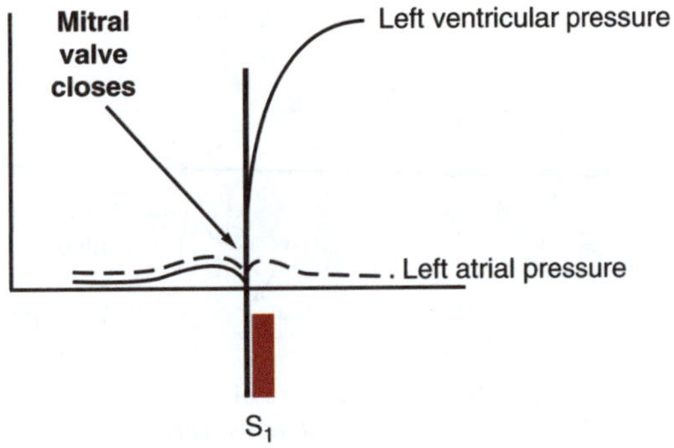

FIGURE 11-7. Diastole—mitral valve closes.

As left ventricular pressure continues to rise, it quickly exceeds the pressure in the aorta and forces the aortic valve open (Fig. 11-8).

In some pathologic conditions, an early systolic ejection sound (E_j) accompanies the opening of the aortic valves (see Fig. 11-8).

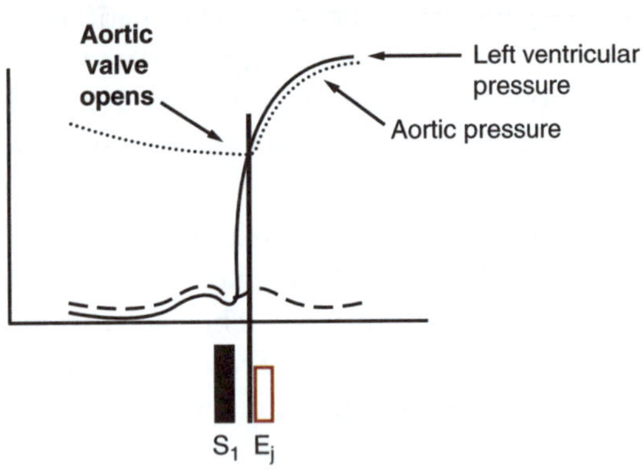

FIGURE 11-8. Systole—aortic valve opens.

Normally, maximal left ventricular pressure corresponds to systolic blood pressure. As the LV ejects most of its blood, ventricular pressure begins to fall. When left ventricular pressure drops below aortic pressure, the aortic valve closes (Fig. 11-9). Aortic valve closure, as well as the closure of the pulmonic valves, produces the second heart sound, S_2, and another diastole begins.

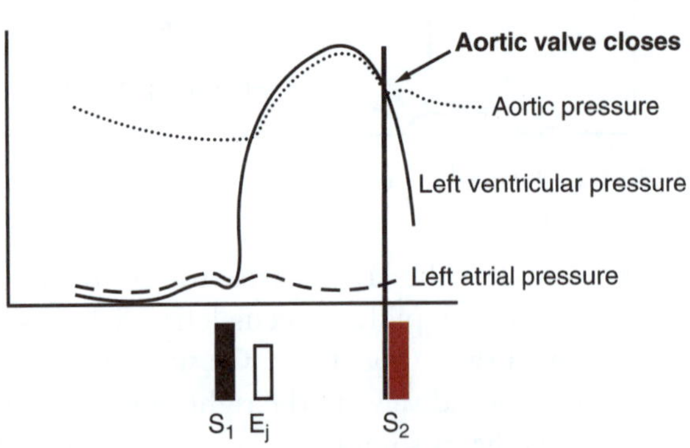

FIGURE 11-9. Systole—aortic valve closes.

In diastole, left ventricular pressure continues to drop and falls below left atrial pressure. The mitral valve opens (Fig. 11-10). This event is usually silent.

The opening of the mitral valve may be audible as a pathologic opening snap (OS) if valve leaflet motion is restricted, as in mitral stenosis (see Fig. 11-10).

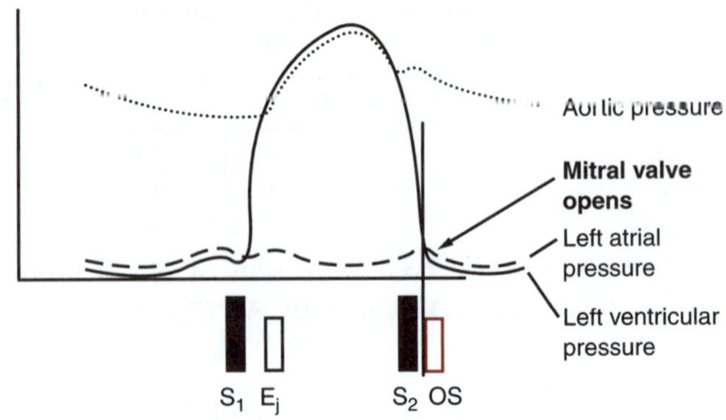

FIGURE 11-10. Diastole—mitral valve opens.

After the mitral valve opens, there is a period of rapid ventricular filling as blood flows early in diastole from left atrium to LV (Fig. 11-11).

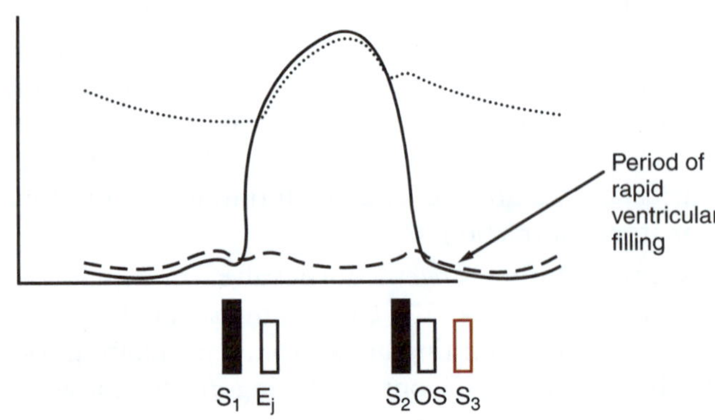

FIGURE 11-11. Diastole—rapid ventricular filling; S_3.

In children and young adults, a third heart sound, S_3, may arise from rapid deceleration of the column of blood against the ventricular wall (see Fig. 11-11).

In older adults, an S_3, sometimes termed "an S_3 gallop," usually indicates pathology.

Although not often heard in normal adults, a fourth heart sound, S_4, marks atrial contraction (Fig. 11-12). It immediately precedes S_1 of the next beat and can also reflect a pathologic ventricular stiffness, as seen in hypertension or an acute myocardial infarction.

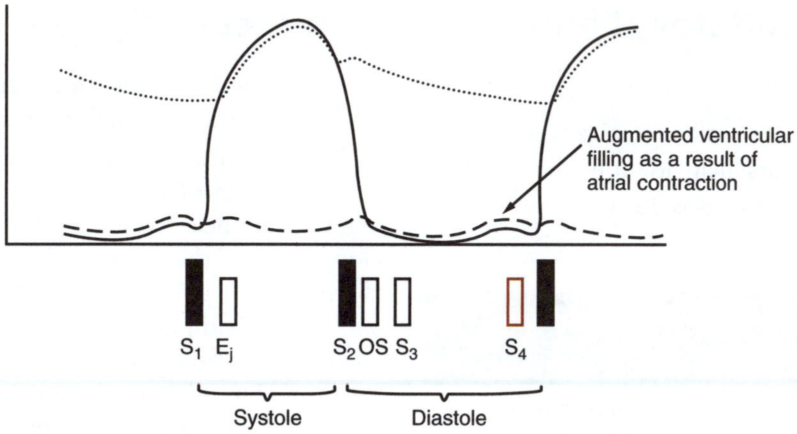

FIGURE 11-12. Diastole—atrial contraction; S_4.

Splitting of Heart Sounds

While these events are occurring on the left side of the heart, similar changes are occurring on the right side, which involves the right atrium, tricuspid valve, RV, pulmonic valve, and pulmonary arteries. Right ventricular and pulmonary arterial pressures are significantly lower than corresponding pressures on the left side. Note that right-sided cardiac events usually occur slightly later than those on the left.

The second heart sound, S_2, and its two components, A_2 and P_2, are caused primarily by closure of the aortic and pulmonic valves, respectively. During inspiration, the right heart filling time is increased, which increases right ventricular stroke volume and the duration of right ventricular ejection compared with the neighboring LV. This delays the closure of the pulmonic valve, P_2, splitting S_2 into its two audible components. During expiration, the right ventricular ejection period is faster, and A_2 and P_2 fuse into a single sound, S_2 (Fig. 11-13). Note that because the walls of veins contain less smooth muscle, the venous system has more capacitance than the arterial system and lower systemic pressure. Distensibility and impedance in the pulmonary vascular bed contribute to the "hangout time" that delays P_2.

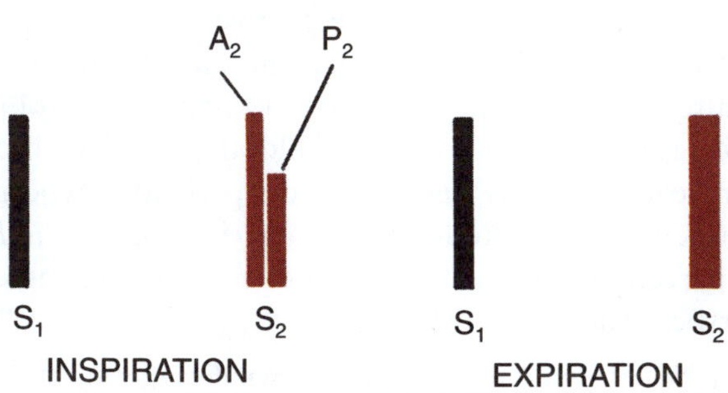

FIGURE 11-13. Splitting of S_2 during inspiration.

Of the two components of the S_2, A_2 is normally louder, reflecting the high pressure in the aorta. It is heard throughout the precordium. In contrast, P_2 is relatively soft, reflecting the lower pressure in the pulmonary artery and as such is best auscultated near its anatomic location, the second and third left intercostal spaces close to the sternum. It is here that you should search for the splitting of S_2.

S_1 also has two components, an earlier mitral and a later tricuspid sound. The mitral sound can be heard throughout the precordium and is loudest at the cardiac apex. The softer tricuspid component is heard best at the lower left sternal border; it is here that you may hear a split S_1, which is a normal finding. The earlier louder mitral component may mask the tricuspid sound, however, and splitting is not always detectable. Splitting of S_1 does not vary with respiration.

Heart Murmurs

Heart murmurs are distinct heart sounds distinguished by their pitch and their longer duration. They are attributed to turbulent blood flow and usually indicate valvular heart disease. At times, they may also represent "innocent" flow murmurs, especially in young adults. A *stenotic* valve has an abnormally narrowed orifice that obstructs blood flow, as in aortic stenosis, and causes a characteristic murmur. Valves can also close abnormally, resulting in *regurgitation.* Such a valve allows blood to leak backward in a retrograde direction and produces a regurgitant murmur.

To identify murmurs accurately, you must learn where they are best heard on the chest wall, their timing in systole or diastole, and their descriptive qualities. In the Techniques of Examination section, you will learn to integrate location and timing with the murmur's shape, maximal intensity, direction of radiation, grade of intensity, pitch, and quality (see p. 232).

Relation of Auscultatory Findings to the Chest Wall

The locations on the chest wall where you auscultate heart sounds and murmurs help identify the valve or chamber where they originate (Box 11-1).

Box 11-1. Chest Wall Location and Origin of Valve Sounds and Murmurs

Chest Wall Location	Typical Origin of Sounds and Murmurs
Right second intercostal space or cardiac apex	Aortic valve
Left second and third intercostal spaces close to the sternum, but also at higher or lower levels	Pulmonic valve
At or near the lower left sternal border	Tricuspid valve
At and around the cardiac apex	Mitral valve

These areas overlap, as illustrated in Figure 11-14. Integrating the auscultatory location with the timing of the sound or murmur, either systole or diastole, is an important first step in identifying sounds and murmurs correctly, and often leads to accurate bedside diagnosis when integrated with other cardiac findings.

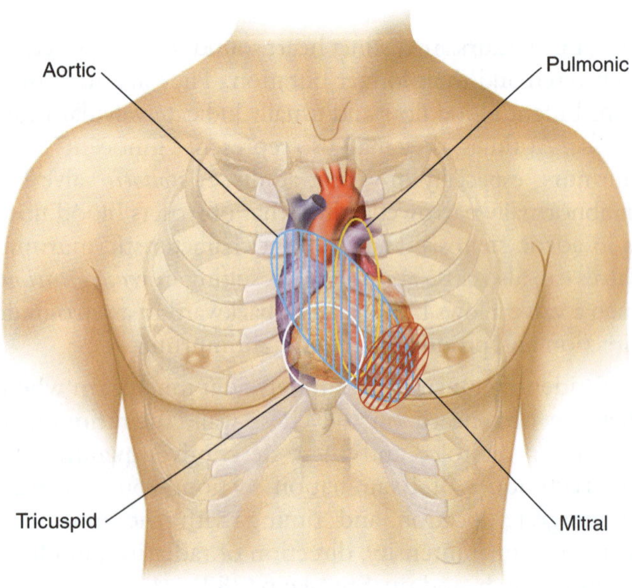

FIGURE 11-14. Precordial areas of cardiac auscultation.

Conduction System

An electrical conduction system stimulates and coordinates the contraction of cardiac muscle.

Normally, each electrical impulse originates in the *sinus node*, a group of specialized cardiac cells located in the right atrium near the junction of the vena cava. The sinus node acts as the cardiac pacemaker and automatically discharges an impulse anywhere from *60 to 100 times a minute*. This impulse travels through both atria to the *AV node*, a specialized group of cells located low in the atrial septum. Here, the impulse is delayed before passing down the *bundle of His* and its branches to the ventricular myocardium. Muscular contraction follows: first the atria, then the ventricles. The normal conduction system is diagrammed in Figure 11-15 in simplified form. The *electrocardiogram*, or *ECG*, records these events. Contraction of cardiac smooth muscle produces electrical activity, resulting in a series of waves on the ECG. You will need further instruction and considerable practice to interpret recordings from patients.

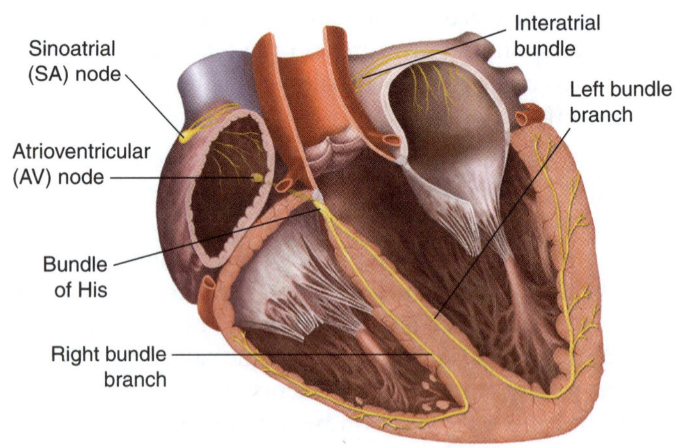

FIGURE 11-15. Cardiac conduction system.

The Heart as a Pump

The left and right ventricles pump blood into the systemic and pulmonary arterial trees, respectively. *Cardiac output*, the volume of blood ejected from each ventricle in 1 minute, is the product of heart rate and stroke volume. *Stroke volume* is the volume of blood ejected with each heartbeat, and it is dependent on preload, myocardial contractility, and afterload. The *ejection fraction (EF)* is the percentage of ventricular volume ejected during each heartbeat and is normally 60%.

Heart failure has two common manifestations, and the classification is determined by the EF. The terms *heart failure with preserved EF* and *heart failure with reduced EF* are two distinct clinical entities with different treatment algorithms.

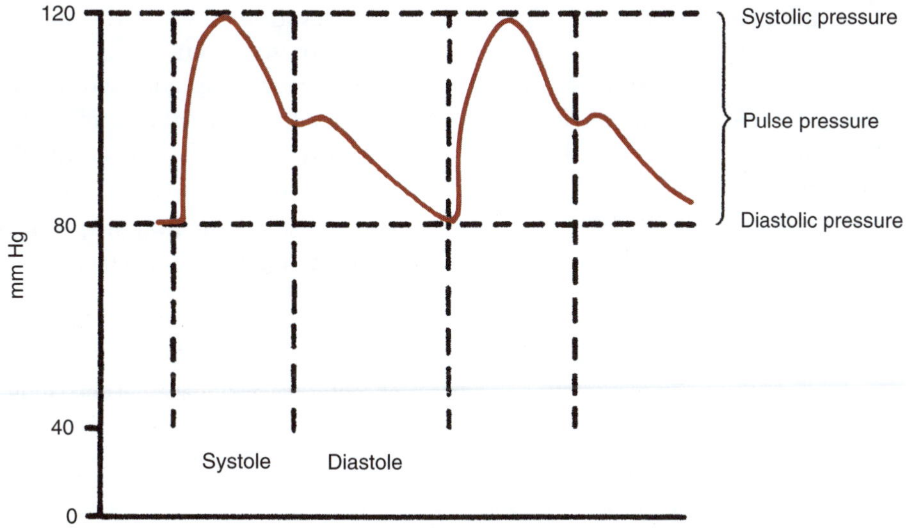

FIGURE 11-16. Blood pressure and pulse pressure in the cardiac cycle.

- *Preload* refers to the load that stretches the cardiac muscle before contraction. The volume of blood in the RV at the end of diastole constitutes its preload for the next beat. Right ventricular preload is increased by increasing venous return to the right heart. Physiologic causes include inspiration and the increased volume of blood flow from exercising muscles. The increased blood volume of a dilated RV in heart failure also increases preload.

  Causes of decreased right ventricular preload include exhalation, dehydration, and pooling of blood in the capillary bed or the venous system.

- *Myocardial contractility* refers to the ability of the cardiac muscle, when given a load, to shorten. Contractility increases when stimulated by action of the sympathetic nervous system and decreases when blood flow or oxygen delivery to the myocardium is impaired, as occurs in MI.
- *Afterload* refers to the degree of vascular resistance to ventricular contraction. Sources of resistance to contraction include the tone in the walls of the aorta, the large arteries, and the peripheral vascular tree (primarily the small arteries and arterioles), as well as the volume of blood already in the aorta.

  Pathologic increases in preload and afterload, called *volume overload* and *pressure overload*, respectively, produce changes in ventricular function that may result in clinical heart failure, when the heart becomes ineffective as a pump.

Arterial Pulses and Blood Pressure

With each contraction, the LV ejects a volume of blood into the aorta that then perfuses the arterial tree. As the ensuing pressure wave moves rapidly through the arterial system, it generates the arterial pulse. Although the pressure wave travels quickly, many times faster than the blood itself, a palpable delay between ventricular contraction and peripheral pulses makes the pulses in the arms and legs unsuitable for timing events in the cardiac cycle.

Blood pressure in the arterial system varies during the cardiac cycle, peaking in systole and falling to its lowest trough in diastole (Fig. 11-16). These are the levels that are measured with the blood pressure cuff, or *sphygmomanometer*. Box 11-2 lists factors that can affect blood pressure. The difference between systolic and diastolic pressures is known as the *pulse pressure*.

Box 11-2. Factors Affecting Blood Pressure

- Left ventricular stroke volume
- Distensibility of the aorta and the large arteries
- Peripheral vascular resistance, particularly at the arteriolar level
- Volume of blood in the arterial system

Changes in any of these four factors alter systolic pressure, diastolic pressure, or both. Blood pressure levels fluctuate strikingly throughout any 24-hour period, varying with physical activity; emotional state; pain; noise; environmental temperature; use of coffee, tobacco, and other drugs; and even time of day.

Jugular Venous Pressure and Pulsations

The jugular veins provide an important index of right heart pressures and cardiac function. Jugular venous pressure (JVP) reflects right atrial pressure, which, in turn, equals central venous pressure and right ventricular end-diastolic pressure. The JVP is best estimated from the right internal jugular vein, which has the most direct channel into the right atrium. Some affirm that the right external jugular vein can also be used. Because the jugular veins lie deep to the sternocleidomastoid (SCM) muscles, learn to identify the pulsations they transmit to the surface of the neck, briefly described below, and measure their highest point of oscillation.

See p. 224 for more detailed discussion of the JVP and techniques for its examination.

Changing pressures in the right atrium during diastole and systole produce oscillations of filling and emptying in the jugular veins, or *jugular venous pulsations* (Fig. 11-17). Atrial contraction produces an *a wave* in the jugular veins just before S_1 and systole caused by retrograde blood flow into the neck veins, followed by the *x descent* of continued atrial relaxation. As right atrial pressure begins to rise with inflow from the vena cava during right ventricular systole, there is a second elevation, the *v wave*, followed by the *y descent* as blood passively empties from the right atrium into the RV during early and middiastole. A simplified way to remember the three peaks is: *a* for *a*trial contraction, *c* for *c*arotid transmission (although this may represent closure of the tricuspid valve), and *v* for *v*enous filling.

Abnormally prominent **cannon a waves** occur in increased resistance to right atrial contraction, as in tricuspid stenosis; also in severe first-, second-, and third-degree AV block, supraventricular tachycardia, junctional tachycardia, pulmonary hypertension, and pulmonic stenosis.

Absent *a* waves signal atrial fibrillation.

Increased *v* waves occur in tricuspid regurgitation, atrial septal defects, and constrictive pericarditis.

Changes Over the Life Span

Aging may affect the location of the apical impulse, the pitch of heart sounds and murmurs, the stiffness of the arteries, and blood pressure. For example, the PMI is usually easily palpated in children and young adults; as the chest deepens

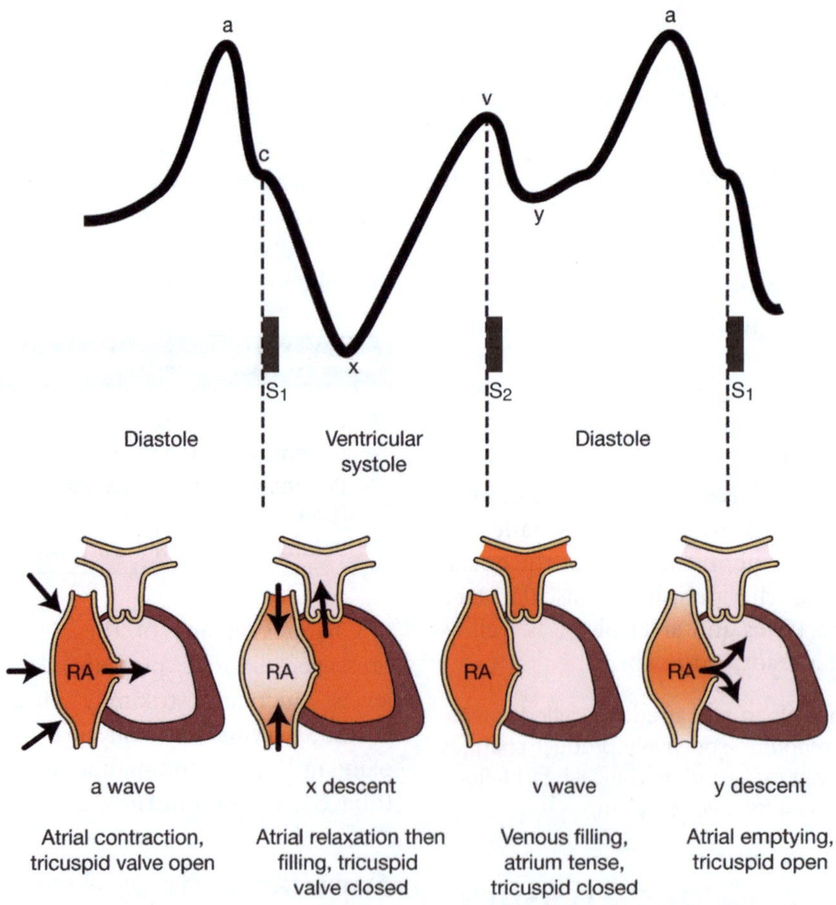

FIGURE 11-17. Jugular venous pulsations and corresponding wave patterns caused by changing pressures in the right atrium during diastole and systole.

in its anteroposterior (AP) diameter, the impulse gets harder to find. For the same reason, splitting of S_2 may be harder to hear in older people as its pulmonic component becomes less audible. Furthermore, at some time during the life span, almost everyone has a heart murmur. Most murmurs occur without other evidence of cardiovascular abnormality and are considered normal variants. These common murmurs vary with age, and knowing their patterns helps you to distinguish normal from abnormal.

Murmurs may originate in large blood vessels as well as in the heart. The jugular venous hum, which is common in children, may still be heard through young adulthood. A second more important example is the cervical systolic murmur, or bruit, which may be innocent in children but suspicious for atherosclerotic disease in adults.

HEALTH HISTORY: GENERAL APPROACH

In approaching the patient, you should seek answers to the three questions below that relate to the most common manifestations of cardiac disease:

- Is the blood supply to the heart adequate?
- Is the electrical system of the heart functioning normally?
- Is the heart adequately moving blood through the circulation and supplying the organs?

Determine if the patient is experiencing a chest pain syndrome and whether that syndrome worsens when the heart requires more oxygen such as when the patient is exercising. If the patient is experiencing palpitations, or the sensation of abnormal, irregular, or extra heart beats, consider disease of the conduction system of the heart. Finally, you must ensure that the heart is fulfilling its role as a pump. If the LV is not moving blood adequately, fluid will be retained in the lungs (*pulmonary edema*), and the patient will experience shortness of breath, especially with exertion or with lying flat (**orthopnea**). Additionally, the patient can experience lightheadedness or loss of consciousness if the blood supply to the brain is inadequate. If the RV is not moving blood adequately, fluid can build up in the legs, a condition known as *peripheral edema*.

It is important for you to remember that the end result of all heart disease is pump malfunction. The patient with an abnormal heart rhythm may present with loss of consciousness, as the abnormal rhythm prevents adequate LV function and cerebral perfusion. If the blood supply to the heart is compromised, patients can experience shortness of breath in addition to chest pain.

The final category of heart disease is valvular heart disease. Valvular heart disease usually presents without symptoms, but if symptoms are present, they are usually symptoms related to a failing heart.

Common or Concerning Symptoms

- Chest pain
- Palpitations
- Shortness of breath: dyspnea, orthopnea, or paroxysmal nocturnal dyspnea
- Swelling (*edema*)
- Fainting (*syncope*)

For chest symptoms, be systematic as you think through the range of possible cardiac and pulmonary etiologies as well as those outside the thoracic cavity. This section approaches chest symptoms from a cardiac standpoint, and includes the important symptoms of chest pain, palpitations, shortness of breath from orthopnea or paroxysmal nocturnal dyspnea (PND), swelling from edema, and fainting.

Chest Pain

Chest pain is one of the most serious of all patient complaints and accounts for 1% of primary care outpatient visits. Classic exertional pain; pressure; or discomfort in the chest, shoulder, back, neck, or arm in angina pectoris is seen in 18% of patients with acute MI; atypical descriptors also are common, such as cramping; grinding; pricking; or, rarely, tooth or jaw pain.

Medicine History Taking OSCE Videos: **Chest Pain**

Begin with open-ended questions . . . "Please tell me about any symptoms you might be having in your chest." Then elicit more specific details. Ask the patient to point to the pain and describe all features of the symptom. Clarify:

- "Is the pain related to exertion?"
- "What kinds of activities bring on the pain?"
- "How intense is the pain, on a scale of 1 to 10?"
- "Does it radiate into the neck, shoulder, back, or down your arm?"

Anterior chest pain, often tearing or ripping and radiating into the back or neck, occurs in acute aortic dissection.

- "Are there any associated symptoms like shortness of breath, sweating, palpitations, or nausea?"
- "Does it ever wake you up at night?"
- "What do you do to make it better?"

It is important to quantify the patient's baseline level of activity. Does the pain occur with climbing stairs? How many flights? How many steps? How about with walking—50 feet, one block, more? What about carrying heavy items, or such day-to-day activities as putting on clothes? How does this compare with these activities in the past? When did the symptoms appear or change? Quantifying the baseline level of activity helps establish both the *severity* of the patient's symptoms and their *significance* as you consider the next steps for management.

Both men and women with acute coronary syndrome usually present with the classic symptoms of exertional angina; however, women, particularly those over age 65, are more likely to report atypical symptoms that may go unrecognized, such as upper back, neck, or jaw pain; shortness of breath; paroxysmal nocturnal dyspnea; nausea or vomiting; and fatigue, making careful history-taking especially important. Failure to identify cardiac causes of chest pain can have dire consequences. Inappropriate discharge from the emergency room results in a 25% mortality rate.

Causes of chest pain in the absence of obstructive coronary artery disease on angiogram include microvascular coronary dysfunction and abnormal cardiac nocioception, which require specialized testing. Roughly half of women with chest pain and normal angiograms have microvascular coronary dysfunction.

Acute coronary syndrome is increasingly used to describe the clinical syndromes caused by acute myocardial ischemia, which include unstable angina, non–ST elevation MI, and ST elevation infarction.

As you evaluate your patient's history of chest pain, always consider life-threatening diagnoses such as angina pectoris, MI, dissecting aortic aneurysm, and pulmonary embolus. Learn to distinguish cardiovascular causes from disorders of the pericardium, trachea and bronchi, parietal pleura, esophagus, and chest wall as well as from extrathoracic causes in the neck, shoulder, gallbladder, and stomach.

Palpitations

Palpitations involve an unpleasant awareness of the heartbeat. Patients use various terms to describe palpitations such as skipping, racing, fluttering, pounding, or stopping of the heart. Palpitations may be irregular, rapidly slow down or accelerate, or arise from the increased forcefulness of cardiac contraction. Palpitations do not necessarily mean heart disease.

Anxious and hyperthyroid patients may report palpitations.

The most serious dysrhythmias, such as ventricular tachycardia, often do not produce palpitations.

If there are symptoms or signs of irregular heart action, obtain an ECG. This includes atrial fibrillation, which causes an "irregularly irregular" pulse often identified at the bedside.

Reword your questions if needed—"Are you ever aware of your heartbeat? What is it like?" Ask the patient to tap out the rhythm with a hand or finger. Was it fast or slow? Regular or irregular? How long did it last? If there was an episode of rapid heartbeats, did they start and stop suddenly or gradually? For this group of symptoms, an ECG is indicated.

Clues in the history include transient skips and flip-flops (possible premature contractions); rapid regular beating of sudden onset and offset (possible paroxysmal supraventricular tachycardia); and a rapid regular rate of $<$120 beats/min, especially if gradually starting and stopping (possible sinus tachycardia).

Teach selected patients how to take serial measurements of their pulse rates in case they have further episodes.

Medicine History Taking OSCE Videos:
Palpitation

Shortness of Breath

Shortness of breath is a common patient concern that can represent *dyspnea*, *orthopnea*, or *paroxysmal nocturnal dyspnea* (*PND*). *Dyspnea* is an uncomfortable awareness of breathing that is inappropriate to a given level of exertion. This complaint is common in patients with cardiac or pulmonary problems.

As with chest pain, it is important to quantify how the current shortness of breath started and how it has changed or not, over time. Does this occur at rest, during exercise, or after exertion? Sudden shortness of breath has different implications in an athlete compared to a person who only walks from one room to another.

Medicine History Taking OSCE Videos:
Shortness of Breath

Sudden dyspnea occurs in pulmonary embolus, spontaneous pneumothorax, and anxiety.

Ask if the patient can lie down flat without getting short of breath. *Orthopnea* is dyspnea that occurs when the patient is supine and improves when the patient sits up. Classically, it is quantified by the number of pillows the patient uses for sleeping, or by the fact that the patient needs to sleep sitting up. Make sure that the patient is using extra pillows or sleeping upright due to shortness of breath and not due to other causes.

Orthopnea and PND occur in left ventricular heart failure and mitral stenosis and also in obstructive lung disease.

Ask, "Do you experience any nighttime episodes of sudden dyspnea that awakens you usually 1 or 2 hours after falling sleep, prompting you to sit up and stand up?" This is called *paroxysmal nocturnal dyspnea (PND)*. Ask also about any associated wheezing and coughing. The episode usually subsides but may recur at about the same time on subsequent nights.

PND may be mimicked by nocturnal asthma attacks.

Swelling (Edema)

See Chapter 8, Edema in General Examination.

Medicine History Taking OSCE Videos:
Edema

Fainting (Syncope)

Fainting, blacking out, or **syncope**, is a transient loss of consciousness followed by recovery. This is usually caused by vasovagal syncope, which is further discussed in Chapter 13 and see Table 11-1, Syncope and Similar Disorders, for discussion of the symptoms and causes of syncope.

The more concerning causes of syncope involve the heart not providing adequate blood flow to the brain, as occurs in end-stage heart failure and arrhythmias.

PHYSICAL EXAMINATION: GENERAL APPROACH

Listening to the heart has come to epitomize the art of bedside diagnosis. Mastering the skills of cardiac examination requires patience, practice, and repetition.

Although the main focus of your cardiovascular examination will be on auscultation, other parts of the physical examination will yield even more important information that answers the question: Is the heart adequately providing blood to the remainder of the body? In addition, knowing how well these findings, by themselves or in concert with others, predict the presence or absence of cardiac disease is vitally important.

In the physical examination of the cardiovascular system, remember to answer the following questions to assess the integrity of the pump:

- Is the forward pump function normal?
  - Is the blood pressure in normal range?
  - Are the extremities well perfused?
  - Are the pulses brisk and easily palpable?
  - Is the JVP normal?
  - Is there edema in the lower extremities?
- Is the heart normal in size?
  - Is the point of maximal impulse displaced, or over the right ventricle?
- Is there evidence of valvular heart disease?
  - Are there any systolic or diastolic murmurs?
- Is there pulmonary edema?

TECHNIQUES OF EXAMINATION

Key Components of the Cardiovascular Examination

- Note general appearance and measure blood pressure and heart rate.
- Estimate the level of jugular venous pressure.
- Auscultate the carotids (bruit) one at a time.
- Palpate the carotid pulse including carotid upstroke (amplitude, contour, timing) and presence of a thrill.
- Inspect the anterior chest wall (apical impulse, precordial movements).
- Palpate the precordium for any heaves, thrills, or palpable heart sounds.
- Palpate and locate the PMI or apical impulse.
- Palpate for a systolic impulse of the right ventricle, pulmonary artery, and aortic outflow tract areas on the chest wall.
- Auscultate S_1 and S_2 in six positions from the base to the apex.
- Identify physiologic and paradoxical splitting of S_2.
- Auscultate and recognize abnormal sounds in early diastole, including an S_3 and OS of mitral stenosis and an S_4 later in diastole.
- Distinguish systolic and diastolic murmurs, using maneuvers when needed. If present, identify their timing, shape, grade, location, radiation, pitch, and quality.

Blood Pressure and Heart Rate

Note the patient's general appearance and vital signs. The patient's general appearance provides many clues to cardiac illness, so pay special attention to the patient's color, respiratory rate, and level of anxiety, in addition to blood pressure and heart rate. Since auscultation is so important for detecting subtle findings, examine the patient in a quiet comfortable room where distractions and noise are at a minimum.

As you begin, *review the blood pressure and pulse* recorded at the start of the visit. If you need to repeat these measurements, or if they have not already been done, measure the blood pressure and pulse using optimal technique.

In brief review, after letting the patient rest for at least 5 minutes in a quiet setting with feet on the floor, choose a correctly sized cuff and position the patient's unclothed arm at heart level, either resting on a table if the patient is seated, or supported at midchest level if supine or standing. Heart level is usually at the fourth intercostal space at the sternum. Make sure the bladder of the cuff is centered over the brachial artery. Inflate the cuff approximately 30 mm Hg above the pressure at which the brachial or radial pulse disappears. As you deflate the cuff, listen first for the *Korotkoff sounds* of at least two consecutive heartbeats; these mark the *systolic* pressure. Then listen for the disappearance point of the heartbeats, which marks the *diastolic* pressure. For *heart rate,* palpate the radial pulse using the pads of your index and middle fingers, or auscultate the apical pulse with your stethoscope. At higher arm levels, the blood pressure recordings will be lower; at lower levels, the blood pressure recordings will be higher.

Physiology OSCE Videos:
Blood Pressure and Pulse

A growing literature documents the poor reliability of clinic blood pressure measurements. Multiple averaged measurements improve precision, especially when using automated home and ambulatory blood pressure readings, which are more reliable, accurate, and better correlated with cardiovascular outcomes than clinic readings. See Box 8-23, Out-of-Office Methods for Measuring Blood Pressure.

Jugular Venous Pressure

Identify and estimate the jugular venous pressure (JVP). Estimating the JVP is one of the most important and frequently used skills of physical examination. The JVP closely parallels pressure in the right atrium, or central venous pressure, related primarily to volume in the venous system.

Identifying the Jugular Venous Pressure. The JVP is best assessed from pulsations in the right internal jugular vein, which is directly in line with the superior vena cava and right atrium. The internal jugular veins lie deep to the SCM muscles in the neck and are not directly visible, so you must learn to identify the pulsations of the internal jugular vein that are transmitted to the surface of the neck (Fig. 11-18). Pulsations in the *right external jugular vein* can also be used, but the route from the vena cava is more tortuous, and examination can be impaired by kinking and obstruction at the base of the neck and by obesity. Note that the jugular veins and pulsations are difficult to see in children under 12 years of age, so inspection is not useful in this age group.

See discussion of the double peak of the *a* and *v* waves and of the *x* and *y* descent on p. 220.

Although the JVP accurately predicts elevations in fluid volume in heart failure, its prognostic value for heart failure outcomes and mortality is unclear.

Pressure changes from right atrial filling, contraction, and emptying cause fluctuations in the JVP and its

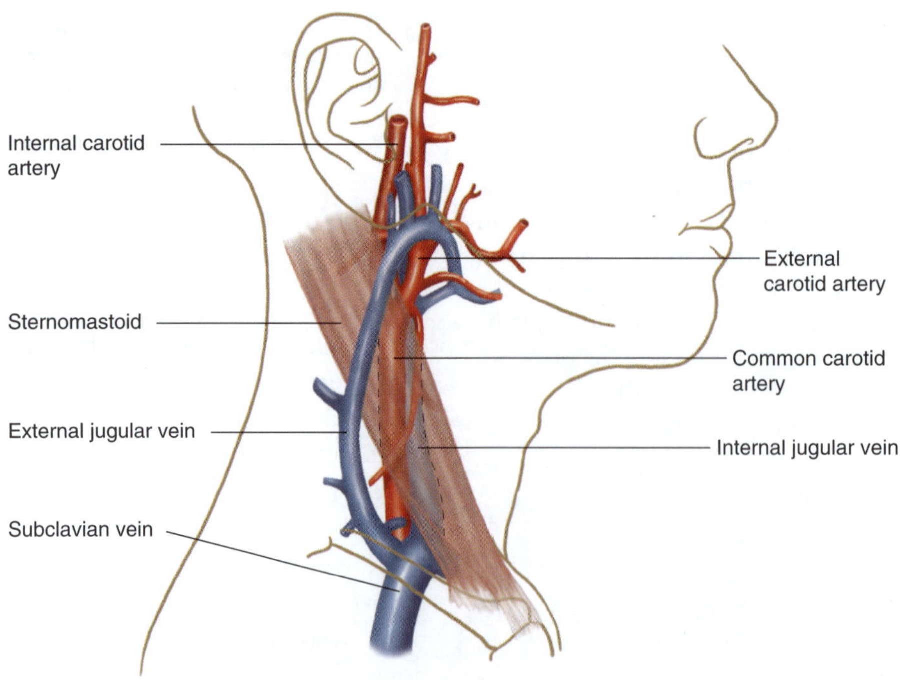

FIGURE 11-18. Internal and external jugular veins.

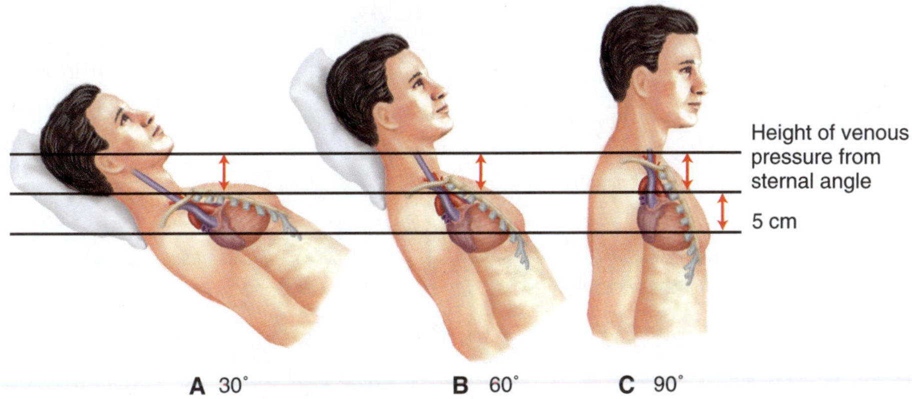

FIGURE 11-19. JVP height remains relatively constant in three positions. Sometimes, the JVP can only be detected while the patient is recumbent or upright.

waveforms that are visible to the examiner. The dominant movement of the JVP is inward, coinciding with the *x descent*. In contrast, the dominant movement of the carotid pulse, often confused with the JVP, is outward. Careful observation of the fluctuations of the JVP yields clues about volume status, right and left ventricular function, patency of the tricuspid and pulmonary valves, pressures in the pericardium, and arrhythmias caused by junctional rhythms and AV blocks.

JVP falls with loss of blood or decreased venous vascular tone and increases with right or left heart failure, pulmonary hypertension, tricuspid stenosis, AV dissociation, increased venous vascular tone, and pericardial compression or tamponade.

Measuring the Jugular Venous Pressure. To estimate the level of the JVP, learn to find the *highest point of oscillation in the internal jugular vein* or, alternatively, the point above which the external jugular vein appears collapsed. The JVP is usually measured in vertical distance above the *sternal angle* (also called the *angle of Louis*), the bony ridge located around T4 adjacent to the second rib where the manubrium joins the body of the sternum.

Study carefully the illustrations in Figure 11-19. Note that in the three positions, the sternal angle remains roughly 5 cm above the right mid-atrium. In this patient, the pressure in the internal jugular vein is somewhat elevated.

- In *Position A*, the head of the bed is raised to the usual level, approximately 30°, but the JVP cannot be measured because the *level of oscillation*, or *meniscus*, is above the jaw and, therefore, not visible.
- In *Position B*, the head of the bed is raised to 60°. The "top" of the internal jugular vein is now easily visible, so the vertical distance from the sternal angle or right atrium can now be measured.
- In *Position C*, the patient is upright, and the veins are barely discernible above the clavicle, making measurement untenable.

Note that the height of the venous pressure as measured from the sternal angle is *similar* in all three positions, but your ability to *measure* the height of the column of venous blood, or JVP, differs according to how you position the patient.

To help you learn the techniques for this challenging portion of the cardiac examination, steps for assessing the JVP are outlined in Box 11-3.

Box 11-3. Steps for Measuring the Jugular Venous Pressure

1. Make the patient comfortable. Raise the head slightly on a pillow to relax the SCM muscles.
2. Raise the head of the bed or examining table to about 30°. Turn the patient's head slightly away from the side you are inspecting.
3. Use tangential lighting and examine both sides of the neck. Identify the external jugular vein on each side, then find the internal jugular venous pulsations.
4. If necessary, raise or lower the head of the bed until you can see the oscillation point or meniscus of the internal jugular venous pulsations in the lower half of the neck.
5. Focus on the right internal jugular vein. Look for pulsations in the suprasternal notch, between the attachments of the SCM muscle on the sternum and clavicle, or just posterior to the SCM. Distinguish the pulsations of the internal jugular vein from those of the carotid artery (see Box 11-4).
6. Identify the highest point of pulsation in the right jugular vein. Extend a long rectangular object or card horizontally from this point and a centimeter ruler vertically from the sternal angle, making an exact right angle. Measure the vertical distance in centimeters above the sternal angle where the horizontal object crosses the ruler and add to this distance 5 cm, the distance from the sternal angle to the center of the right atrium (Fig. 11-20). The sum is the JVP.

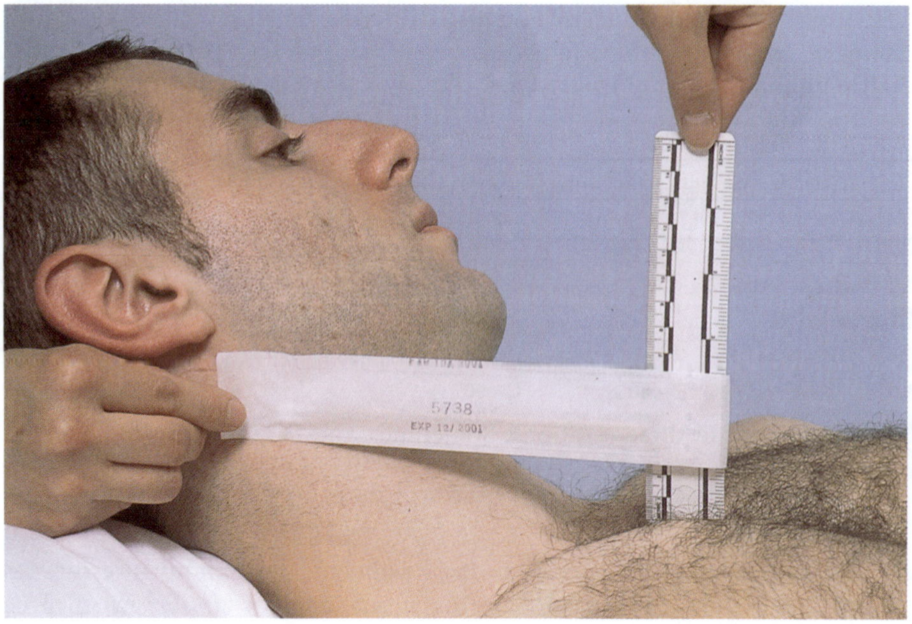

FIGURE 11-20. Measuring the JVP with a horizontal card and vertical ruler.

An elevated JVP is highly correlated with both acute and chronic heart failure. It is also seen in tricuspid stenosis, chronic pulmonary hypertension, superior vena cava obstruction, cardiac tamponade, and constrictive pericarditis.

An elevated JVP is >95% specific for an increased left ventricular end-diastolic pressure and low left ventricular EF, although its role as a predictor of hospitalization and death from heart failure is less clear.

In patients with obstructive lung disease, the JVP can appear elevated on expiration, but the veins collapse on inspiration. This finding does not indicate heart failure.

Distinguishing Jugular Venous Pulsations from Carotid Pulsations. The features listed in Box 11-4 help to distinguish jugular from carotid artery pulsations.

Box 11-4. Distinguishing Internal Jugular and Carotid Pulsations

Internal Jugular Pulsations	Carotid Pulsations
■ Rarely palpable	■ Palpable
■ Soft biphasic undulating quality, usually with two elevations and *characteristic inward deflection* (x descent)	■ A more vigorous thrust with a *single outward component*
■ Pulsations eliminated by light pressure on the vein(s) just above the sternal end of the clavicle	■ Pulsations not eliminated by pressure on veins at sternal end of clavicle
■ Height of pulsations changes with position, normally dropping as the patient becomes more upright	■ Height of pulsations unchanged by position
■ Height of pulsations usually falls with inspiration	■ Height of pulsations not affected by inspiration

Jugular Venous Pressure and Volume Status. As you begin your assessment, consider the patient's volume status and whether you need to alter the elevation of the head of the bed or examining table. The usual starting position for the head of the bed or examining table when assessing the JVP is 30°. Turn the patient's head lightly to the left, then the right, and identify the external jugular vein on each side. Then focus on the internal jugular venous pulsations on the right, transmitted from deep in the neck to the overlying soft tissues. The JVP is the highest oscillation point, or meniscus, of the jugular venous pulsations that is usually evident in euvolemic patients.

Some authors report that at 30° to 45°, the estimated JVP may be 3 cm lower than catheter measurements from the right mid-atrium.

In conditions wherein you anticipate that *the JVP will be low,* you may have to *lower the head of the bed,* sometimes even to 0°, to see the point of oscillation best. Likewise, if you suspect that *the JVP will be high,* you may have to *raise the head of the bed.* In some patients, the JVP will only be measurable when the patient is upright.

JVP measured at >3 cm above the sternal angle, or more than 8 cm in total distance above the right atrium, is considered *elevated above normal.*

Carotid Arteries

Auscultation. Next, *auscultate both the carotid arteries to listen for a bruit.* As the presence of carotid atherosclerosis could potentially narrow the carotid arteries, it is important to auscultate the carotid arteries prior to palpating the carotid pulse.

The most feared complication of carotid artery palpation is the dislodgment of an atherosclerotic plaque, which could result in stroke.

A **bruit** is a murmur-like sound arising from turbulent arterial blood flow. Ask the patient to stop breathing for ~10 seconds, then listen with the diaphragm of the stethoscope, which generally detects the higher-frequency sounds of arterial bruits better than the bell.

Note that higher-grade stenoses may have lower-frequency or even absent sounds, more amenable to detection with the bell.

Place the diaphragm near the upper end of the thyroid cartilage below the angle of the jaw, which overlies the bifurcation of the common carotid artery into the external and internal carotid arteries. A bruit in this location is less likely to be confused with a transmitted murmur from the heart or subclavian or vertebral artery bruits. In some patients, carotid bruits may only be detected by auscultation over the mastoid process, posterior to the ear.

Although usually caused by atherosclerotic luminal stenosis, bruits are also caused by a tortuous carotid artery, external carotid arterial disease, aortic stenosis, the hypervascularity of hyperthyroidism, and external compression from thoracic outlet syndrome. Bruits do not correlate with clinically significant underlying disease.

Listen for bruits in older patients and patients with suspected cerebrovascular disease.

Carotid artery stenosis causes ~10% of ischemic strokes and doubles the risk of coronary heart disease.

Palpation. Next, *palpate the carotid pulse, including the carotid upstroke*, its amplitude and contour, and the presence or absence of *thrills*. The carotid pulse provides valuable information about cardiac function, especially aortic valve stenosis and regurgitation.

For the assessment of *amplitude and contour*, see Chapter 8, Pulse in General Examination, p. 141.

A tortuous and kinked carotid artery may produce a unilateral pulsatile bulge.

Causes of decreased pulsations include decreased stroke volume from shock or MI and local atherosclerotic narrowing or occlusion.

Thrills. As you palpate the carotid artery, you may detect vibrations, or **thrills**, like the throat vibrations of a cat when it purrs.

Thrills in aortic stenosis are transmitted to the carotid arteries from the suprasternal notch or second right intercostal space.

Pulsus Alternans. In **pulsus alternans**, the rhythm of the pulse remains *regular*, but the *force* of the arterial pulse alternates because of alternating strong and weak ventricular contractions. Pulsus alternans almost always indicates severe left ventricular dysfunction. It is usually best felt by applying light pressure on the radial or femoral arteries. Use a blood pressure cuff to confirm your finding. After raising the cuff pressure, lower it slowly to just below the systolic level. The initial Korotkoff sounds are the strong beats. As you lower the cuff, you will hear the softer sounds of the alternating weak beats, which will eventually disappear, causing the remaining Korotkoff sounds to double.

Alternately loud and soft Korotkoff sounds or a sudden doubling of the apparent heart rate as the cuff pressure declines signals pulsus alternans.

Placing the patient in the upright position may accentuate this finding.

Paradoxical Pulse. *Paradoxical pulse* or **pulsus paradoxus** is a greater-than-normal drop in systolic blood pressure during inspiration. If the pulse varies in amplitude with respiration or you suspect cardiac tamponade (because of jugular venous distention, dyspnea, tachycardia, muffled heart tones, or hypotension), use a blood pressure cuff to check for a *paradoxical pulse*. As the patient breathes quietly, lower the cuff pressure to the systolic level. Note the pressure level at which the first sounds can be heard. Then drop the pressure very slowly until sounds can be heard throughout the respiratory cycle. Again, note the pressure level. The difference between these two levels is normally no greater than 3 or 4 mm Hg.

The pressure when Korotkoff sounds are first heard is the highest systolic pressure during the respiratory cycle. The pressure when sounds are heard throughout the cycle is the lowest systolic pressure. A difference between these levels of ≥10 mm Hq to 12 mm Hg constitutes a *paradoxical pulse*.

Paradoxical pulse is found in pericardial tamponade, a life-threatening condition. It is also (more commonly) found in acute asthma and obstructive pulmonary disease. It also occurs in constrictive pericarditis and acute pulmonary embolism.

Pulsus alternans and a bigeminal pulse vary beat to beat; a paradoxical pulse varies with respiration.

In patients with carotid obstruction, kinking, or thrills, assess the pulse in the *brachial artery*, applying the techniques described previously for determining amplitude and contour.

Heart

Positioning the Patient. For the precordial examination, stand at the patient's right side. The patient should be supine, with the upper body and head of the bed or examining table raised to about 30°. To assess the PMI and extra heart sounds such as S_3 or S_4, ask the patient to turn to the left side—the *left lateral decubitus position*, which brings the ventricular apex closer to the chest wall. To bring the left ventricular outflow tract closer to the chest wall and improve detection of aortic regurgitation,

Box 11-5. Sequence of Patient Positions in the Cardiac Examination

Patient Position	Examination	Accentuated Abnormal Findings
Supine, with the head elevated 30°	After examining the JVP and carotid pulse, inspect and palpate the precordium: the second right and left intercostal spaces; the RV; and the LV, including the apical impulse (diameter, location).	
Left lateral decubitus	Palpate the apical impulse to assess its diameter. Listen at the apex with the *bell* of the stethoscope.	Left lateral decubitus: low-pitched extra sounds such as an S_3, opening snap, diastolic rumble of *mitral stenosis*
Supine, with the head elevated 30°	Listen at the second right and left intercostal spaces, down the left sternal border to the fourth and fifth intercostal spaces, and across to the apex the six listening areas with the *diaphragm*, then the *bell*. As indicated, listen at the lower right sternal border for right-sided murmurs and sounds, often accentuated with inspiration, with the *diaphragm* and *bell.*	
Sitting, leaning forward, after full exhalation	Listen down the left sternal border and at the apex with the *diaphragm.*	Sitting, leaning forward: Soft decrescendo higher-pitched diastolic murmur of *aortic regurgitation*

have the patient sit up, lean forward, and exhale. See Box 11-5 for the patient positions and a suggested sequence for the examination.

Location and Timing of Cardiac Findings. Identify both the anatomical location of impulses, heart sounds, and murmurs and where they fall in the cardiac cycle. Remember to integrate your findings with the characteristics of the patient's JVP and carotid upstroke.

- Identify the *anatomical location* of cardiac findings in terms of intercostal spaces and the distance of the PMI from the midclavicular line. The midclavicular line correlates with left ventricular pathology, as long as the midpoint between the acromioclavicular and sternoclavicular joints is carefully identified.
- Identify the *timing of impulses, sounds,* and *murmurs* in relation to the cardiac cycle. Timing of sounds is often possible through auscultation alone but aided by inspection and palpation as well. In most patients with normal or slow heart rates, it is easy to identify the paired heart sounds of S_1 and S_2 that mark the onset of systole and diastole. The relatively long diastolic interval after S_2 separates one pair from the next (Fig. 11-21).

The relative intensity of S_1 and S_2 is also helpful. S_1 is usually louder than S_2 at the apex; S_2 is usually louder than S_1 at the base.

"*Inching*" your stethoscope also helps clarify the timing of S_1 and S_2. Return to a place on the chest, typically the base, where it is easy to identify S_1 and S_2. Get their rhythm clearly in mind. Then inch your stethoscope down the left sternal border in steps until you hear changes in the sounds.

At times, the intensities of S_1 and S_2 may be abnormal, or, at rapid heart rates, the duration of diastole may shorten, making it difficult to distinguish systole from diastole. Palpation of the carotid artery during auscultation is an invaluable aid to the timing of sounds and murmurs. Since the carotid upstroke always occurs in systole immediately after S_1, sounds or murmurs coinciding with the upstroke are systolic; sounds or murmurs following the carotid upstroke are diastolic.

S_1 is diminished in first-degree heart block; S_2 is diminished in aortic stenosis.

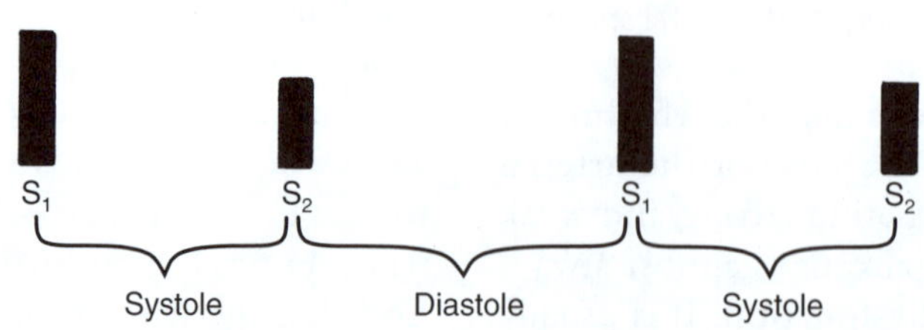

FIGURE 11-21. Diastole (S_2 to S_1) lasts longer than systole (S_1 to S_2).

Inspection. *Carefully inspect the anterior chest,* which may reveal the location of the *apical impulse* or *PMI,* or less commonly, the ventricular movements of a left-sided S_3 or S_4. Shine a tangential light across the chest wall over the cardiac apex to make these movements more visible. Plan to further characterize these movements as you proceed to palpation. Keep in mind the anatomic locations diagrammed in Figure 11-22.

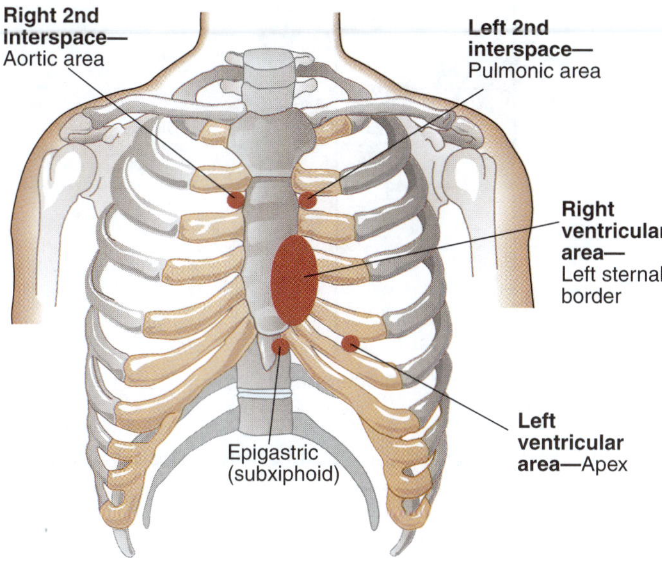

FIGURE 11-22. Palpation areas on the chest wall.

Palpation. Next, palpate the chest wall for:

- Heave
- Thrill
- Palpable S_1 and S_2
- Palpable S_3 or S_4
- Apical impulse and PMI
- Systolic impulse of the RV
- Pulmonary artery area
- Aortic outflow area

Palpation is less useful in patients with a thickened chest wall (obesity) or increased AP diameter (obstructive lung disease).

Palpation of the chest wall provides considerable information to the examiner and should not be neglected. Begin with general palpation of the chest wall. In women, keeping the right chest draped, gently lift the breast with your left hand or ask the woman to do this to assist you. Then using the techniques below, palpate in the second right intercostal space, the second left intercostal space, along the sternal border, and at the apex for heaves, lifts, thrills, impulses from the RV, and the four heart sounds.

Heaves and Thrills. To palpate **heaves**, use your palm and/or hold your fingerpads flat or obliquely against the chest. Heaves are sustained impulses that rhythmically lift your fingers, usually produced by an enlarged right or left ventricle (depending on the location of the heave) and occasionally by ventricular aneurysms.

For *thrills,* press the ball of your hand (the padded area of your palm near the wrist) firmly on the chest to check for a buzzing or vibratory sensation caused by underlying turbulent flow. If present, auscultate the same area for murmurs. Conversely, once a murmur is detected, it is easier to palpate a thrill in the position that accentuates the murmur, such as the leaning forward position after detecting aortic regurgitation.

The presence of a thrill changes the grading of the murmur, as described on p. 236.

Palpate impulses from the *RV* in the right ventricular area, normally at the lower left sternal border and in the subxiphoid area (see p. 231).

Palpating S_1, S_2, S_3, and S_4. To palpate *S_1 and S_2*, using firm pressure, place your right hand on the chest wall. With your left index and middle fingers, palpate the carotid upstroke to identify S_1 and S_2 just before and just after the upstroke. S_1 and S_2 are usually not palpable.

For *S_3 and S_4*, position the patient in the left lateral decubitus position, then palpate the cardiac apex gently with one finger as the patient exhales and briefly stops breathing. By marking an X on the apex, you may be able to palpate these brief early and late diastolic ventricular movements that are synchronous with pathologic third and fourth heart sounds.

A brief early to middiastolic impulse represents a palpable S_3; an outward movement just before S_1 signifies a palpable S_4.

Apical Impulse and Point of Maximal Impulse. Next, *identify the apical impulse and the* **point of maximal impulse (PMI)**. The apical impulse represents the brief early pulsation of the LV as it moves anteriorly during systole and contacts the chest wall. In most examinations, the apical impulse is the PMI. If you cannot find the apical impulse, ask the patient to exhale fully and stop breathing for a few seconds. When examining a woman, it may be helpful to displace the left breast upward or laterally as necessary, or ask her to do this for you.

Physiology OSCE Videos:
Palpation of Apex

Pathologic conditions such as right ventricular hypertrophy, a dilated pulmonary artery, or an aortic aneurysm may produce a different pulsation that is more prominent than the apex beat.

In *dextrocardia with situs inversus,* a rare congenital transposition of the heart, the heart is situated in the right chest cavity and generates a right-sided apical impulse. Use percussion to help locate the heart border, the liver, and stomach. In full *situs inversus totalis,* the heart, trilobed lung, stomach, and spleen are on the right, and the liver and gallbladder are on the left.

If you cannot identify the apical impulse with the patient supine, ask the patient to roll partly onto the left side into the *left lateral decubitus* position. Palpate again, using the palmar surfaces of several fingers (Fig. 11-23). The apex beat is palpable in 25% to 40% of adults in the supine position and in 50% to 73% of adults in the left lateral decubitus position, especially those who are thin.

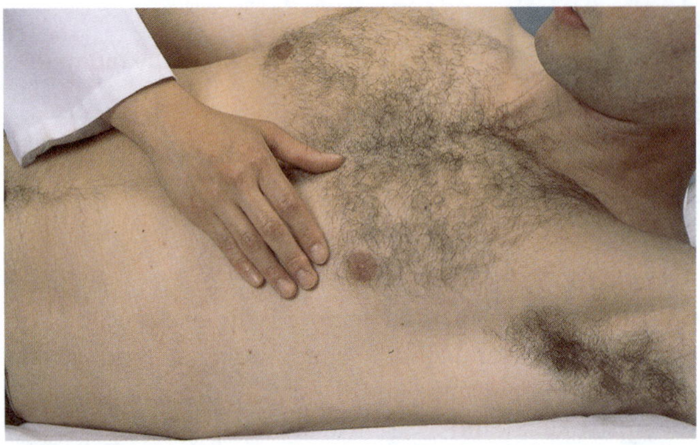

FIGURE 11-23. Palpating the apical impulse in the left lateral decubitus position.

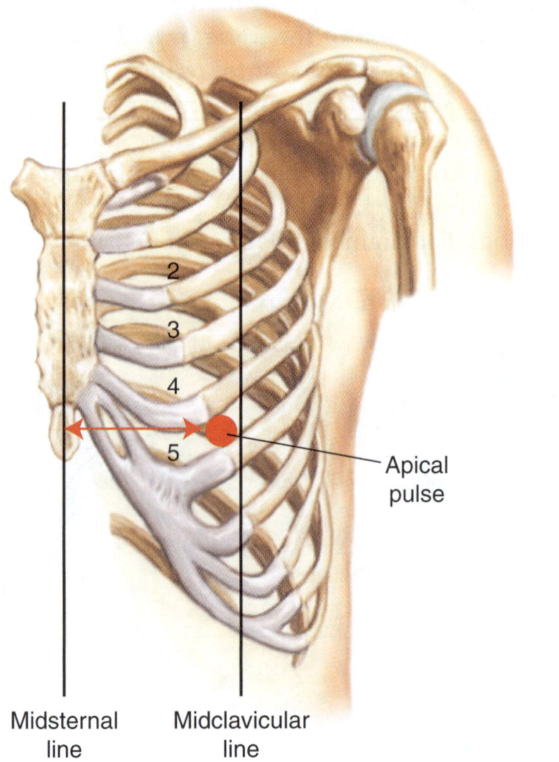

FIGURE 11-24. Describing the location of the PMI in relation to the midsternal or midclavicular lines.

Locate two points: the intercostal spaces, usually the fifth or possibly the fourth, which give the vertical location, and the distance in centimeters from the *midclavicular line* (or *midsternal line*), which gives the horizontal location (Fig. 11-24). It is always best to describe the apical impulse in relation to the midsternal or midclavicular line, or the anterior axillary line if the apical impulse is displaced.

Obesity, a very muscular chest wall, or an increased AP diameter of the chest may obscure detection of the apical impulse.

Once you have found the apical impulse, make finer assessments with your fingertips, and then with one finger (Fig. 11-25). With experience, you will learn to palpate the apical impulse in most patients.

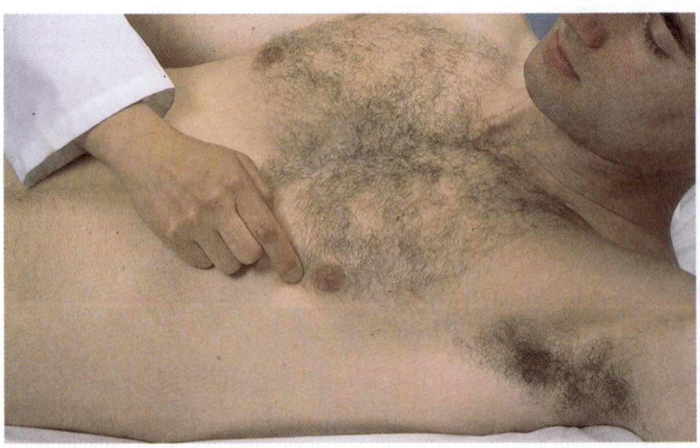

FIGURE 11-25. Palpating the apical impulse with one finger.

See Table 11-2, Variations and Abnormalities of the Ventricular Impulses.

Pregnancy or a high left diaphragm may shift the apical impulse upward and to the left.

Lateral displacement toward the anterior axillary line from ventricular dilatation is seen in heart failure, cardiomyopathy, and ischemic heart disease as well as in thoracic deformities and mediastinal shift.

A markedly dilated failing heart may have a hypokinetic apical impulse displaced far to the left.

A large pericardial effusion may make the impulse undetectable.

One descriptive feature of the apical impulse that may be helpful clinically is its *diameter* or *area.* In the supine patient, it usually measures less than 2.5 cm, about the size of a quarter, and occupies only one interspace. It may feel larger in the left lateral decubitus position.

A *diffuse* PMI (usually >3 cm) may indicate left ventricular enlargement.

Other characteristics that may be clinically useful are its *amplitude* and *duration*. Normally, its amplitude feels brisk and nonsustained (a tap).

If the PMI is forceful and terminates quickly (does not extend through systole), it is *hyperkinetic* and may occur in hypermetabolic states such as severe anemia, hyperthyroidism and also may occur in volume overload of the left ventricle from aortic regurgitation.

Right Ventricular Area. *Now, palpate for the systolic impulse of the RV.* With the patient supine and the head elevated to 30°, ask the patient to exhale and briefly stop breathing, then place the tips of your curved fingers in the left third, fourth, and fifth intercostal spaces (Fig. 11-26). If there is a palpable impulse, assess its location, amplitude, and duration. In thin individuals, you may detect a brief systolic tap, especially when stroke volume is increased by conditions such as anxiety.

A sustained left parasternal movement beginning at S_1 points to pressure overload from pulmonary hypertension and pulmonic stenosis or the chronic ventricular volume overload of an atrial septal defect. A sustained movement later in systole can be seen in mitral regurgitation.

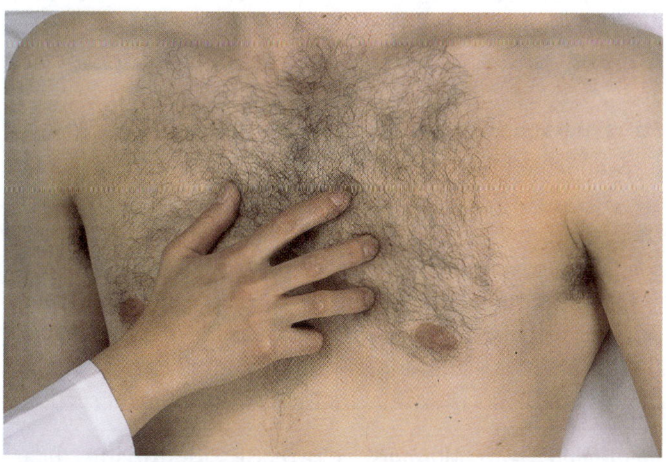

FIGURE 11-26. Palpating the right ventricular systolic impulse.

Occasionally, the diastolic movements of *right-sided S_3 and S_4* are palpable in the left fourth and fifth intercostal spaces. Time them by auscultation or palpation of the carotid upstroke.

In patients with an increased AP diameter, ask the patient to inhale and briefly stop breathing and palpate for the RV in the *epigastric* or *subxiphoid area*.

In obstructive pulmonary disease, hyperinflation of the lungs may prevent palpation of the hypertrophied RV in the left parasternal area. The RV impulse is readily palpated high in the epigastrium where heart sounds are also more audible.

Pulmonary Artery Area. This intercostal space overlies the *pulmonary artery*. As the patient holds expiration, inspect and palpate for pulmonary artery pulsations and transmitted heart sounds, especially if patients are excited or examined after exercise.

A prominent pulsation here often accompanies dilatation or increased flow in the pulmonary artery. A *palpable S_2*, also known as a "*pulmonary artery tap*," points to increased pulmonary artery pressure from pulmonary hypertension.

Aortic Outflow Tract Area. This intercostal space overlies the aortic outflow tract. Search for pulsations and palpable heart sounds.

A pulsation in this area suggests a dilated or aneurysmal aorta.

Auscultation. Auscultation of heart sounds and murmurs is a preeminent skill that leads directly to important clinical diagnoses (Box 11-6). Cardiac auscultation is the most widely used method of screening for valvular heart disease. Review the six auscultatory areas in Figure 11-27, with the following caveats: (1) many authorities discourage designations such as "aortic area," because murmurs may be loudest in other areas, and (2) these areas do not apply to patients with cardiac dilatation or hypertrophy, anomalies of the great vessels, or dextrocardia.

Box 11-6. Appropriate Use of the Stethoscope for the Cardiac Examination

It is important to understand the uses of both the diaphragm and the bell.

- *The diaphragm.* The diaphragm is better for picking up the relatively high-pitched sounds of S_1 and S_2, the murmurs of aortic and mitral regurgitation, and pericardial friction rubs. *Listen throughout the precordium* with the diaphragm, pressing it firmly against the chest.
- *The bell.* The bell is more sensitive to the low-pitched sounds of S_3 and S_4 and the murmur of mitral stenosis. Apply the bell lightly, with just enough pressure to produce an air seal with its full rim. *Use the bell at the apex, then move medially along the lower sternal border.* Resting the heel of your hand on the chest like a fulcrum may help you to maintain light pressure.

  Firm pressure on the bell can stretch the underlying skin and make it function more like the diaphragm. Low-pitched sounds like S_3 and S_4 may then disappear—an observation that can help identify them. In contrast, high-pitched sounds such as a midsystolic click, an ejection sound, or an OS will persist or get louder.

See Tools of the Trade, p. 70, in Chapter 4, Physical Examination.

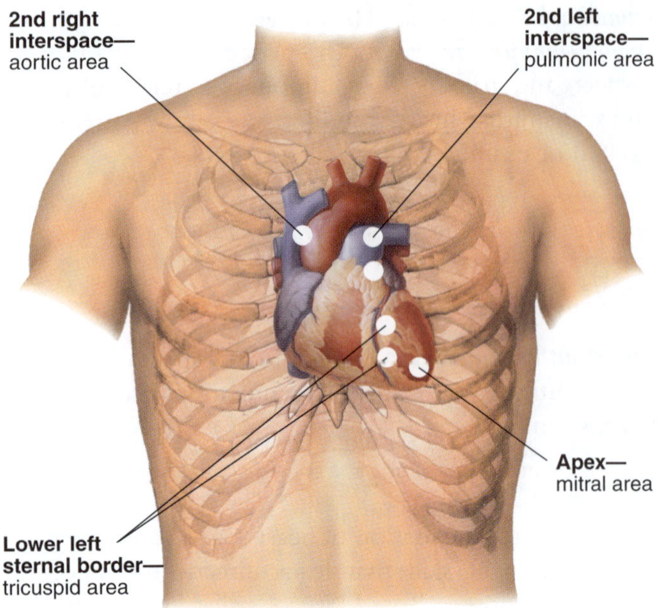

FIGURE 11-27. Auscultatory areas on the chest wall.

Heart sounds and murmurs that originate in the four valves radiate widely, as illustrated in Figure 11-28. Use anatomical location rather than valve area to describe your findings.

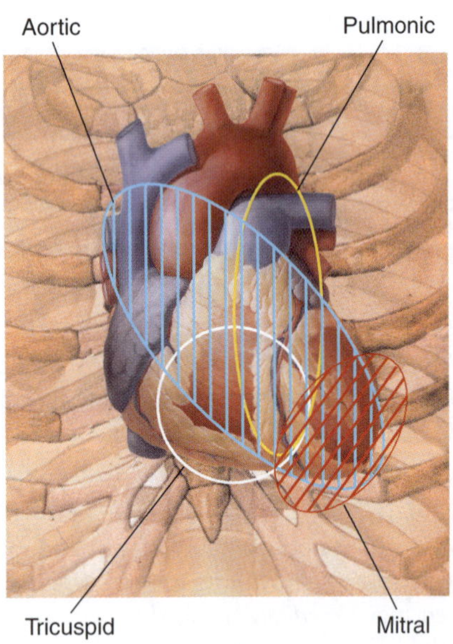

FIGURE 11-28. Radiation of heart sounds and murmurs.

Throughout your examination, take your time at each of the six auscultatory areas. Concentrate on each of the events in the cardiac cycle, listening carefully to S_1, then S_2, then other sounds and murmurs occurring in systole and diastole. Techniques for assessing these events are described in the pages that follow.

Identifying Systole and Diastole. *Auscultate and identify S_1 and S_2.* By carefully noting the intensities of S_1 and S_2, you will confirm each of these sounds and thereby correctly identify *systole,* the interval between S_1 and S_2, and *diastole,* the interval between S_2 and S_1. The correct timing of systole and diastole is the fundamental prerequisite for identifying events in the cardiac cycle.

To facilitate the correct identification of systole and diastole, as you auscultate the chest, palpate the right carotid artery in the lower third of the neck with your index and middle fingers—S_1 falls just before the carotid upstroke and S_2 follows the carotid upstroke. Be sure to compare the intensities of S_1 and S_2 as you move your stethoscope through the listening areas. At the *base*, you will note that S_2 is louder than S_1 and may split with respiration. At the *apex*, S_1 is usually louder than S_2 unless the PR interval is prolonged..

Pattern of Auscultation. In a quiet room, auscultate the heart with your stethoscope with the patient's head and upper chest elevated to 30°. Start at either the base or apex, listening first with the diaphragm, then with the bell.

The examination *starts at the base. Following the base, "inch" your stethoscope to the apex:* with your stethoscope in the right second intercostal space close to the sternum, move along the left sternal border in each intercostal space from the second through the fifth, and then toward the apex, making sure to auscultate in each of the six anatomic areas marked by the white circles in Figure 11-27.

Some recommend *starting at the apex and moving to the base:* Move the stethoscope from the PMI medially to the left sternal border, superiorly to the second intercostal space, then across the sternum to the second intercostal space at the right sternal border. To clarify findings, "inch" the stethoscope in smaller increments as needed. Review the guides to auscultation in Box 11-7 and learn the tips for identifying heart murmurs that follow in the next section.

Identifying Heart Murmurs. Correctly identifying heart murmurs is a diagnostic challenge. A systematic approach; thorough understanding of cardiac anatomy and physiology; and, above all, your dedication to the practice and mastery of techniques of examination, will lead to your success. Whenever possible, compare your findings with those of an experienced clinician to improve your clinical acumen. Review the tips for identifying heart murmurs in Box 11-8, then carefully study the subsequent sections on the timing, shape, location, radiation, intensity, pitch, and quality of heart murmurs for more details. Study the tables at the end of the chapter to further expand your skills. Reinforce your learning by listening to heart sound recordings, which can increase accurate identification of heart murmurs (and generally transfers to actual patients).

Box 11-7. Auscultatory Sounds

Heart Sounds	Guides to Auscultation	
S_1	■ Note its intensity and any apparent splitting. ■ S_1 splitting is a normal finding detectable along the lower left sternal border.	See Table 11-3, Variations in the First Heart Sound—S_1. Note that S_1 is louder at more rapid heart rates, and PR intervals are shorter.
S_2	■ Note its intensity.	
Split S_2	■ Listen for splitting of this sound in the second and third left intercostal spaces. Ask the patient to breathe quietly and then slightly more deeply than normal.	See Table 11-4, Variations in the Second Heart Sound—S_2.
	■ Does S_2 split into its two components, as it normally does? If not, ask the patient to (1) breathe a little more deeply, or (2) sit up. Listen again. ■ A thick chest wall may make the pulmonic component of S_2 inaudible.	When either A_2 or P_2 is absent, as in aortic or pulmonic valve disease, S_2 is persistently single.
	■ *Width of split*. How wide is the split? It is normally quite narrow. ■ *Timing of split*. When in the respiratory cycle do you hear the split? It is normally heard late in inspiration.	Expiratory splitting suggests a valvular abnormality.
	■ Does the split disappear as it should, during exhalation? If not, listen again with the patient sitting up.	Persistent splitting results from delayed closure of the pulmonic valve or early closure of the aortic valve.
	■ *Intensity of A_2 and P_2*. Compare the intensity of the two components, A_2 and P_2; A_2 is usually louder.	A loud P_2 points to pulmonary hypertension.
Extra Sounds in Systole	■ These may include ejection sounds or systolic clicks. ■ Note their location, timing, intensity, and pitch, and variations with respiration.	The systolic click of mitral valve prolapse is the most common extra sound. See Table 11-5, Extra Heart Sounds in Systole.
Extra Sounds in Diastole	■ Such as S_3, S_4, or an opening snap ■ Note the location, timing, intensity, and pitch and variations with respiration. ■ An S_3 or S_4 in athletes is a normal finding.	See Table 11-6, Extra Heart Sounds in Diastole.
Systolic and Diastolic Murmurs	■ Murmurs are differentiated from S_1, S_2, and extra sounds by their longer duration.	See Table 11-7, Midsystolic Murmurs; Table 11-8, Pansystolic (Holosystolic) Murmurs; and Table 11-9, Diastolic Murmurs.

Box 11-8. Tips for Identifying Heart Murmurs

- Time the murmur—is it in systole or diastole? What is its duration?
- Locate where on the precordium the murmur is loudest—at the base, along the sternal border, at the apex? Does it radiate?
- Conduct any necessary maneuvers, such as having the patient lean forward and exhale or turn to the left lateral decubitus position to accentuate the murmurs.
  - Ask the patient to roll into the left lateral decubitus position, which brings the LV closer to the chest wall. Place the bell of your stethoscope lightly on the apical impulse (Fig. 11-29).
  - Ask the patient to *sit up, lean forward, exhale completely, and briefly stop breathing after expiration.* Pressing the diaphragm of your stethoscope on the chest, listen along the left sternal border and at the apex, pausing periodically so the patient may breathe (Fig. 11-30).
- Determine the shape of the murmur—for example, is it crescendo or decrescendo, is it holosystolic?
- Grade the intensity of the murmur from 1 to 6 (systolic) or 1 to 4 (diastolic) and determine its pitch (high, medium, or low) and quality (blowing, harsh, rumbling, or musical).
- Identify associated features such as the quality of S_1 and S_2; the presence of extra sounds such as S_3, S_4, or an OS; or the presence of additional murmurs.
- Be sure you are listening in a quiet room!

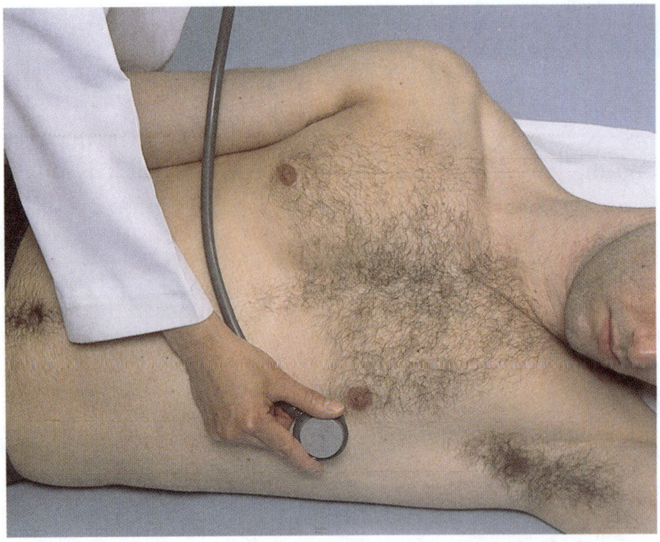

FIGURE 11-29. Auscultating for mitral stenosis in the left lateral decubitus position.

This position accentuates a left-sided S_3 and S_4 and mitral murmurs, especially mitral stenosis. Otherwise, you may miss these important findings.

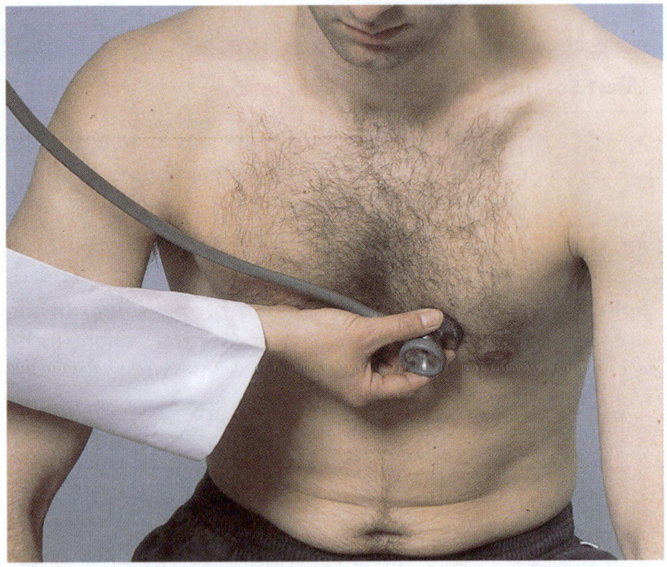

FIGURE 11-30. Auscultating for aortic regurgitation with the patient leaning forward.

You may easily miss the soft diastolic decrescendo murmur of aortic regurgitation unless you listen at this position.

Timing of Murmur. First decide if you are hearing a *systolic murmur,* falling between S_1 and S_2 (Box 11-9), or a *diastolic murmur,* falling between S_2 and S_1 (Box 11-10). Box 11-11 shows continuous murmurs, and Box 11-12 shows murmur shapes. Palpating the carotid pulse as you listen can help you with timing. Murmurs that coincide with the carotid upstroke are systolic.

Diastolic murmurs usually represent valvular heart disease. Systolic murmurs point to valvular disease but can be physiologic flow murmurs arising from normal heart valves.

Box 11-9. Systolic Murmurs

Systolic murmurs are typically *midsystolic* or *pansystolic.* Midsystolic murmurs can be *functional murmurs;* these are typically short midsystolic murmurs that decrease in intensity with maneuvers that reduce left ventricular volume, such as standing, sitting up, and straining during the Valsalva maneuver. These murmurs are often heard in healthy patients and are not pathologic. Early systolic murmurs are uncommon and are not depicted below.

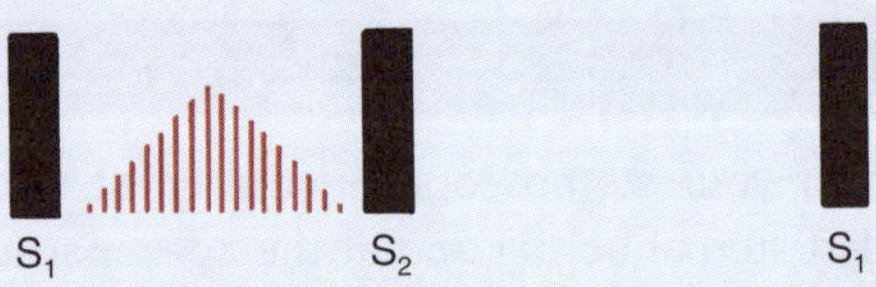

Midsystolic murmur: Begins after S_1 and stops before S_2. Brief gaps are audible between the murmur and the heart sounds. Listen carefully for the gap just before S_2, which is more readily detected and, if present, usually confirms the murmur as midsystolic, not pansystolic.

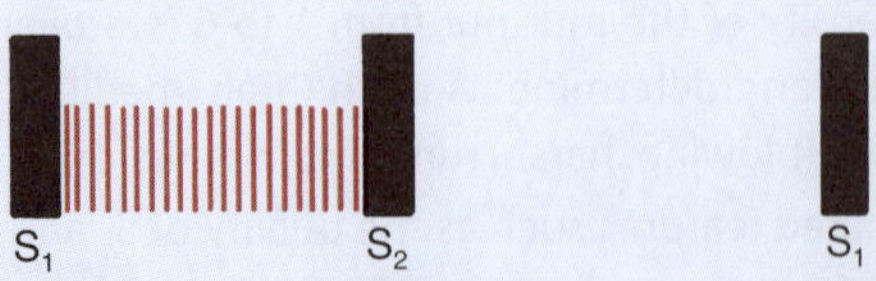

Pansystolic (holosystolic) murmur: Starts with S_1 and stops at S_2, without a gap between murmur and heart sounds.

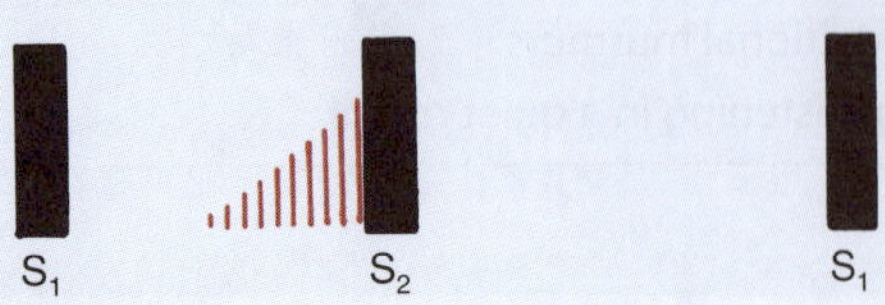

Late systolic murmur: Usually starts in mid- or late systole and persists up to S_2.

Murmurs detected during pregnancy should be promptly evaluated for possible risk to the mother and fetus, especially those of aortic stenosis or pulmonary hypertension.

Midsystolic murmurs typically arise from blood flow across the semilunar (aortic and pulmonic) valves. See Table 11-7, Midsystolic Murmurs.

Pansystolic murmurs often occur with regurgitant (backward) flow across the AV valves. See Table 11-8, Pansystolic (Holosystolic) Murmurs.

This is the murmur of mitral valve prolapse and is often, but not always, preceded by a systolic click; the murmur of mitral regurgitation may also be late systolic.

Box 11-10. Diastolic Murmurs

Diastolic murmurs may be early diastolic, middiastolic, or late diastolic.

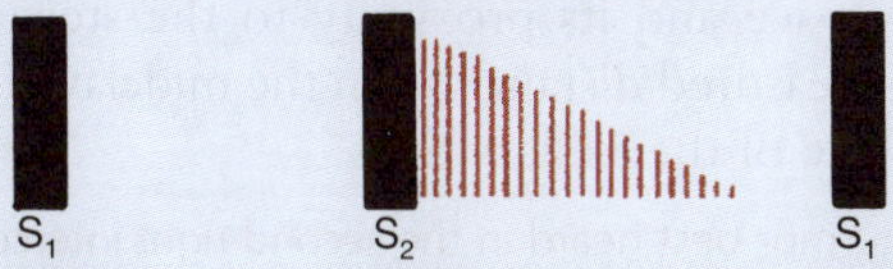

Early diastolic murmur: Starts immediately after S_2, without a discernible gap, then usually fades into silence before the next S_1.

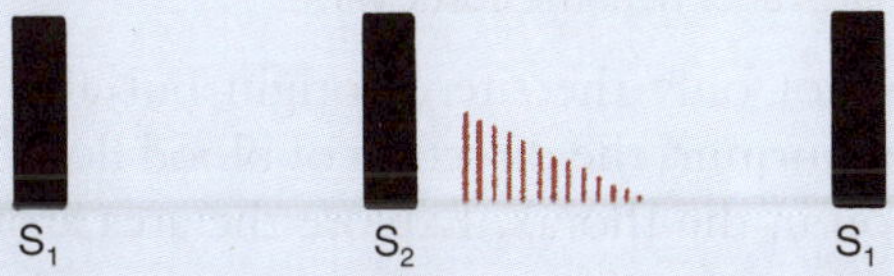

Middiastolic murmur: Starts a short time after S_2. It may fade away, as illustrated, or merge into a late diastolic murmur.

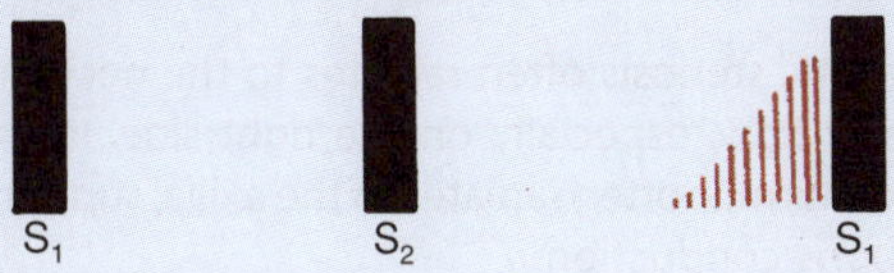

Late diastolic (presystolic) murmur: Starts late in diastole and typically continues up to S_1.

Early diastolic murmurs typically reflect regurgitant flow across incompetent semilunar valves.

Middiastolic and presystolic murmurs reflect turbulent flow across the AV valves. See Table 11-9, Diastolic Murmurs.

Box 11-11. Continuous Murmurs

Some congenital and clinical conditions produce continuous murmurs.

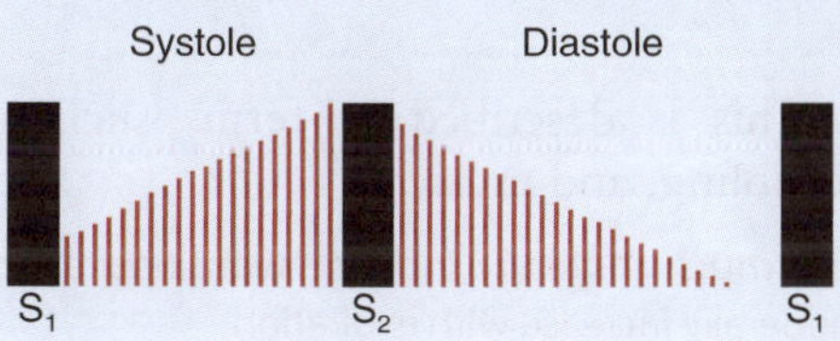

Continuous murmur: Begins in systole and extends into all or part of diastole (but is not necessarily uniform throughout).

Congenital patent ductus arteriosus and AV fistulas, common in dialysis patients, produce continuous murmurs that are nonvalvular in origin. Venous hums and pericardial friction rubs also have both systolic and diastolic components. See Table 11-10, Cardiovascular Sounds with Both Systolic and Diastolic Components.

Box 11-12. Murmur Shapes

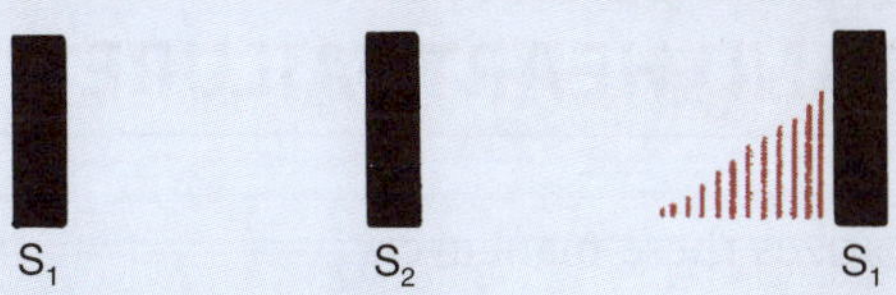

Crescendo murmur: Grows louder.

Note the presystolic murmur of mitral stenosis in normal sinus rhythm.

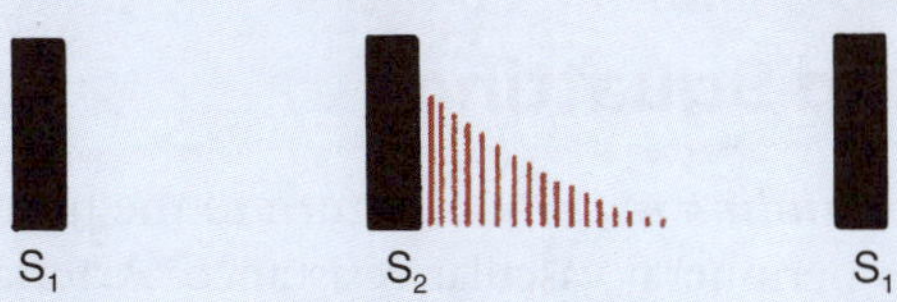

Decrescendo murmur: Grows softer.

Note the early diastolic murmur of aortic regurgitation.

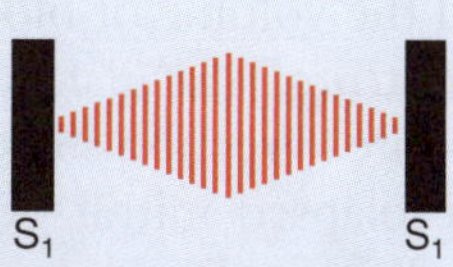

Crescendo–decrescendo murmur: First rises in intensity, then falls.

Listen for the midsystolic murmur of aortic stenosis and innocent flow murmurs.

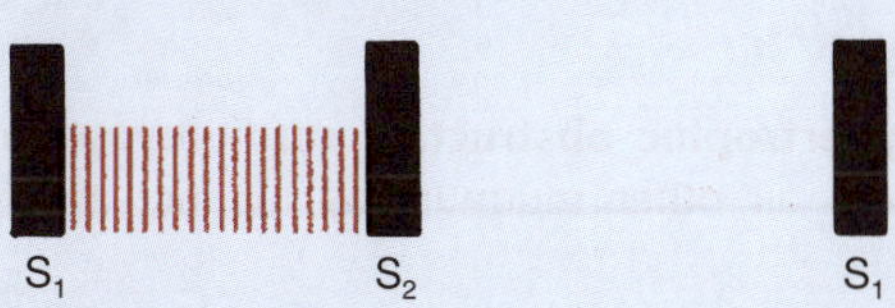

Plateau murmur: Has the same intensity throughout.

Note the pansystolic murmur of mitral regurgitation.

Shape of Murmur. The shape or configuration of a murmur is determined by its intensity over time.

Intensity and Grade. Intensity is usually graded on an objective scale and expressed as a fraction. The *numerator* describes the intensity of the murmur wherever it is loudest; the *denominator* indicates the scale you are using. Intensity is influenced by the thickness of the chest wall and the presence of intervening tissue.

An identical degree of turbulence would cause a louder murmur in a thin person than in a very muscular or obese person. Emphysematous lungs may diminish the intensity of murmurs.

Grade systolic murmurs using the six-point scale in Box 11-13 (the Levine grading system). Note that grades 4 through 6 require the added presence of a palpable thrill. Grade diastolic murmurs using the four-point scale in Box 11-14. A different scale is used by convention for diastolic murmurs as they are not commonly associated with a palpable thrill.

For maneuvers, see Special Techniques, p. 237.

Box 11-13. Gradations of Systolic Murmurs

Grade	Description
Grade 1/6	Softer in volume than S_1 and S_2, very faint
Grade 2/6	Equal in volume to S_1 and S_2, quiet, but heard immediately
Grade 3/6	Louder in volume than S_1 and S_2, moderately loud
Grade 4/6	Louder in volume than S_1 and S_2, with *palpable thrill*
Grade 5/6	Louder in volume than S_1 and S_2, with *thrill*; may be heard when the stethoscope is partly off the chest
Grade 6/6	Louder in volume than S_1 and S_2, with *thrill*; may be heard with stethoscope entirely off the chest

Box 11-14. Gradations of Diastolic Murmurs

Grade	Description
Grade 1/4	Barely audible
Grade 2/4	Faint but immediately audible
Grade 3/4	Easily heard
Grade 4/4	Very loud

Location of Maximal Intensity and Its Radiation/Transmission. This is determined by the site where the murmur originates. Find the location by exploring the area where you hear the murmur. Describe where you hear it best in terms of the intercostal space and its proximity to the sternum, the apex, or its measured distance from the midclavicular, midsternal, or one of the axillary lines.

For example, a murmur best heard in the second right intercostal space often originates at or near the aortic valve.

This reflects not only the site of origin but also the intensity of the murmur, the direction of blood flow, and bone conduction in the thorax. Explore the area around a murmur and determine where else you can hear it.

The murmur of aortic stenosis often radiates to the neck in the direction of arterial flow, especially on the right side. In mitral regurgitation, the murmur often radiates to the axilla, supporting transmission by bone conduction.

Pitch of Murmur. This is categorized as high, medium, or low.

A fully described murmur might be: a "medium-pitched, grade 2/4, blowing decrescendo diastolic murmur, best heard in the fourth left intercostal space, with radiation to the apex" (aortic regurgitation).

Quality of Murmur. This is described in terms such as blowing, harsh, rumbling, and musical.

Right-sided heart murmurs generally increase with inspiration; left-sided murmurs generally increase with expiration.

SPECIAL TECHNIQUES: BEDSIDE MANEUVERS TO IDENTIFY MURMURS AND HEART FAILURE

Box 11-15 summarizes these maneuvers.

Standing and Squatting

When a person is *standing up*, venous return to the heart decreases, as does peripheral vascular resistance. Arterial blood pressure, stroke volume, and the volume of blood in the LV all decline. With *squatting*, vascular and volume changes occur in the opposite direction. These maneuvers help (1) to identify a prolapsed mitral valve and (2) to distinguish hypertrophic cardiomyopathy from aortic stenosis.

The murmur of **hypertrophic obstructive cardiomyopathy** is distinguished from all other murmurs by an increase in

Box 11-15. Bedside Maneuvers to Identify Systolic Murmurs

Maneuver	Cardiovascular Effect	Effect on Systolic Sounds and Murmurs: Mitral Valve Prolapse	Hypertrophic Cardiomyopathy	Aortic Stenosis
Squatting; Valsalva: Release Phase	**Increased left ventricular volume** from ↑ venous return to heart	↓ prolapse of mitral valve	↓ outflow obstruction	↑ blood volume ejected into aorta
	Increased vascular tone: ↑ arterial blood pressure; ↑ peripheral vascular resistance	*Delay of click and murmur shortens*	↓ **intensity of murmur**	↑ **intensity of murmur**
Standing; Valsalva: Strain Phase	**Decreased left ventricular volume** from ↓ venous return to heart	↑ prolapse of mitral valve	↑ outflow obstruction	↓ blood volume ejected into aorta
	Decreased vascular tone: ↓ arterial blood pressure	*Click moves earlier in systole and murmur lengthens*	↑ **intensity of murmur**	↓ **intensity of murmur**

intensity during squatting-to-standing action (95% sensitivity, 84% specificity) and by a decrease in intensity during standing-to-squatting action (95% sensitivity, 85% specificity).

Secure the patient's gown so that it will not interfere with your examination and prepare for prompt auscultation. Instruct the patient to squat next to the examining table and hold on to it for balance. Listen to the heart with the patient in the squatting position and again in the standing position.

Valsalva Maneuver

The **Valsalva maneuver** involves forcible exhalation against a closed glottis after full inspiration, causing increased intrathoracic pressure. The normal systolic blood pressure response follows four phases: (1) transient increase during onset of the "strain" phase when the patient bears down, due to increased intrathoracic pressure; (2) sharp decrease to below baseline as the "strain" phase is maintained, due to decreased venous return; (3) further acute drop of both blood pressure and left ventricular volume during the "release" phase, due to decreased intrathoracic pressure; and (4) "overshoot" increased blood pressure, due to reflex sympathetic activation and increased stroke volume. This maneuver has several uses at the bedside.

To distinguish the murmur of *hypertrophic cardiomyopathy,* ask the supine patient to "bear down, like straining during a bowel movement." Alternatively, place one hand on the patient's midabdomen and ask the patient to push against it. With your other hand, place your stethoscope on the patient's chest and listen at the lower left sternal border.

The murmur of hypertrophic cardiomyopathy is the only systolic murmur that increases during the "strain phase" of the Valsalva maneuver due to increased outflow tract obstruction (65% sensitivity, 96% specificity).

The Valsalva maneuver can also identify *heart failure* and *pulmonary hypertension.* Inflate the blood pressure cuff to 15 mm Hg greater than the systolic blood pressure and ask the patient to perform the Valsalva maneuver for 10 seconds, then resume normal respiration. Keep the cuff pressure locked at 15 mm Hg above the baseline systolic pressure during the entire maneuver and for 30 seconds afterward. Listen for Korotkoff sounds over the brachial artery throughout. Typically, only phases 2 and 4 are significant, since phases 1 and 3 are too short for clinical detection. *In healthy patients, phase 2, the "strain" phase, is silent; Korotkoff sounds are heard after straining is released during phase 4.*

In patients with severe heart failure, blood pressure remains elevated and there are Korotkoff sounds during the phase 2 strain phase, but not during phase 4 release, termed *"the square wave" response.* This response is highly correlated with volume overload and elevated left ventricular end-diastolic pressure and pulmonary capillary wedge pressure, in some studies outperforming brain natriuretic peptide.

Isometric Handgrip

Isometric handgrip increases the systolic murmurs of mitral regurgitation, pulmonic stenosis, and ventricular septal defect as well as the diastolic murmurs of aortic regurgitation and mitral stenosis.

Transient Arterial Occlusion

Transient compression of both arms by bilateral blood pressure cuff inflation to 20 mm Hg greater than peak systolic blood pressure augments the murmurs of mitral regurgitation, aortic regurgitation, and ventricular septal defect.

The murmurs of mitral regurgitation and ventricular septal defect could be differentiated from other systolic murmurs by augmentation of their intensity with handgrip (68% sensitivity, 92% specificity) and during transient arterial occlusion (78% sensitivity, 100% specificity).

RECORDING YOUR FINDINGS

Note that initially you may use sentences to describe your findings; later you will use phrases. The style below contains phrases appropriate for most write-ups.

Recording the Cardiovascular Examination

"The JVP is 3 cm above the sternal angle with the head of bed elevated to 30°. Carotid upstrokes are brisk, without bruits. The PMI is tapping, 1 cm lateral to the midclavicular line in the left fifth intercostal space. Crisp S_1 and S_2. At the base, S_2 is louder than S_1 with physiologic split of $A_2 > P_2$. At the apex, S_1 is louder than S_2. There are no murmurs or extra sounds."

OR

"The JVP is 5 cm above the sternal angle with the head of bed elevated to 50°. Carotid upstrokes are brisk; a bruit is heard over the left carotid artery. The PMI is diffuse, 3 cm in diameter, palpated at the anterior axillary line in the left fifth and sixth intercostal spaces. S_1 and S_2 are soft. S_3 is present at the apex. High-pitched harsh 2/6 holosystolic murmur best heard at the apex, radiating to the axilla."

These findings suggest heart failure with volume overload with possible left carotid occlusion and mitral regurgitation.

HEALTH PROMOTION AND COUNSELING: EVIDENCE AND RECOMMENDATIONS

Important Topics for Health Promotion and Counseling

- Challenges of cardiovascular disease prevention
- Health disparities in cardiovascular disease
- Assessing cardiovascular disease risk factors
  - *Step 1:* Screen for individual cardiovascular disease risk factors
  - *Step 2:* Calculate 10-year and lifetime global cardiovascular disease risk using a web-based calculator
  - *Step 3:* Address individual risk factors—hypertension, diabetes, dyslipidemias, metabolic syndrome, smoking, family history, and obesity
- Promoting lifestyle changes and risk factor modification.

Cardiovascular disease (CVD), including hypertension (which accounts for the vast majority of diagnoses), CHD, heart failure, and stroke, is the leading global cause of death and is expected to account for >23.6 million deaths by 2030.

Health promotion to prevent CVD includes screening for and addressing important risk factors, knowledge of evidence-based guidelines and interventions, and acquisition of interviewing and counseling skills that nurture healthier lifestyles and behaviors. As emerging clinicians, your task is threefold:

1. To understand the epidemiology of CVD
2. To identify modifiable CVD risk factors
3. To help patients reduce CVD risk by adopting lifestyle changes and by taking appropriate pharmacologic treatments

See discussion of Promoting Lifestyle Modification, p. 97 in Chapter 6, Health Maintenance and Screening, and Chapter 2, Interviewing, Communication, and Interpersonal Skills, p. 35, for discussion of motivational interviewing.

Challenges of Cardiovascular Disease Prevention

New studies continually refine our understanding of the epidemiology of CVD and provide evidence-based guidance for preventive interventions. Many CVDs share common risk factors, and major professional societies of related disciplines are now issuing joint guidelines. As a result, screening guidelines are becoming more complex as approaches to specific risk groups become more customized. For example, recommendations for prescribing statins for primary prevention are based on gender, age, cholesterol levels, blood pressure, and the presence of risk factors such as smoking and diabetes. Increasingly, clinicians are urged to engage patients in shared decision making, helping them make informed personalized decisions about preventive interventions that can have both benefits and harms. As an aid to decision making, online calculators are available for rapidly assessing risk for CHD and stroke.

Challenge of Risk Factor Reduction. The American Heart Association (AHA) promotes the concept of "*ideal cardiovascular health*," defined as the absence of clinically manifest CVD and the simultaneous presence of optimal levels of seven health metrics.

- Health behaviors
  - Body mass index <25 kg/m^2
  - Not smoking
  - Being physically active
  - Following a healthy diet
- Health factors
  - Untreated total cholesterol <200 mg/dL
  - Blood pressure <120/<80 mm Hg
  - Fasting blood glucose <100 mg/dL

Health Disparities in Cardiovascular Disease

CVD manifests differently in certain population groups. This may be due to biologic differences, but also because management of CVD risk factors and disease may differ across populations due to socioeconomic, environmental, behavioral, and cultural factors.

Sex and Gender Disparities. Women have become increasingly aware that CVD is their leading cause of death. Improved CVD prevention and treatment efforts for women have led to dramatic decreases in the age-adjusted mortality rates for CHD—a decrease of nearly two-thirds between 1980 and 2000. The statistics in Box 11-16 illuminate concerning issues for cardiovascular health in women.

Racial and Ethnic Disparities. CHD death rates show marked ethnic disparities. In 2015, the CHD death rate among black women was 21% higher than in white women and 55% higher than in Hispanic women. The CHD death rate among black men was 7% higher than in white men and 49% higher than in Hispanic men. Selected racial disparities in disease prevalence and risk factors are shown in Box 11-17.

Box 11-16. Screening for Major Cardiovascular Risk Factors

Risk Factor	Screening Recommendation	Goal
Family history of premature CVD	Ask about family history	Estimate CVD risk
Cigarette smoking	Ask about tobacco use	Cessation or continued abstinence
Unhealthy diet	Ask about diet	Improved overall eating pattern
Physical inactivity	Ask about physical activity	30 minutes moderate intensity exercise five times weekly
Obesity	Estimate BMI and/or measure waist circumference	BMI ≤25 kg/m^2; waist circumference: ≤40 in for men, ≤35 in for women
Hypertension	Measure blood pressure	<130/80 mm Hg for adults
Dyslipidemias	Obtain baseline fasting lipids at age 21. Measure fasting lipids in average risk adults every 5 years from ages 40 to 75	Initiate statin therapy if meeting ACC/AHA guidelines
Diabetes	Check hemoglobin A1c or fasting glucose every 3 years (if normal) beginning at age 45 years; more frequently at any age if with risk factors	Prevent/delay diabetes for those with HbA1c of 5.7%–6.4%
Atrial fibrillation	Assess heart rhythm	Identify and treat atrial fibrillation

Box 11-17. Selected Web-Based Global CVD Risk Calculators

American College of Cardiology/ American Heart Association	http://www.cvriskcalculator.com
American College of Cardiology	http://tools.acc.org/ASCVD-Risk-Estimator-Plus/#!/calculate/estimate

Screening for Cardiovascular Risk Factors

Heart disease has "a long asymptomatic latent period," and about half of all coronary deaths occur without previous warning signs or cardiac diagnoses. Consequently, clinicians are encouraged to assess *lifetime risk* in asymptomatic patients, possibly beginning as early as age 20 years. Earlier risk assessment may lead to more timely interventions to lower the burden of CVD.

Step 1: Screen for Individual CV Risk Factors. Begin routine screening at 20 years for individual risk factors and for any family history of premature heart disease (age <55 years in first-degree male relatives and age <65 years in first-degree female relatives). Recommended screenings are listed in Box 11-16.

Step 2: Calculate 10-Year and Lifetime Global CVD Risk Using a Web-Based Calculator. Use the global CVD risk calculators shown in Box 11-17 to establish 10-year and lifetime risk for patients ages 40 to 79 years. Unfortunately, there is insufficient data to reliably predict risk for those <40 or >79 years of age. The risk estimates, which incorporate age, sex, smoking history, total cholesterol level, high-density lipoprotein (HDL) cholesterol level, systolic blood pressure, antihypertensive therapy, and diabetes, are based on pooled data from population-based studies. The primary use of these risk estimates is to support and facilitate important clinician–patient discussions regarding risk reduction.

The new calculators provide sex and race/ethnicity (white and black)–specific risk estimates for a first MI, CHD death, or fatal or nonfatal stroke. A revised calculator, which used more recent data and newer statistical methods, improved on the accuracy of the ACC/AHA CVD risk calculator. Regardless, the risk prediction information should be integrated in the context of other considerations, including recommended lifestyle interventions, patient preferences for taking medications, potential adverse drug reactions or interactions, and the likelihood of successfully intervening for a particular patient.

Step 3: Address Individual Risk Factors—Hypertension, Diabetes, Dyslipidemias, Metabolic Syndrome, Smoking, Family History, and Obesity. Approximately 80% of CVDs can be prevented through not smoking, eating a healthy diet, engaging in regular physical activity, maintaining a healthy weight, and controlling high blood pressure, diabetes, and elevated lipid levels.

Hypertension.

- *Primary (essential) hypertension* is the most common cause of hypertension: risk factors include age, genetics, black race, obesity and weight gain, excessive salt intake, physical inactivity, and excessive alcohol use.
- *Secondary hypertension* accounts for less than 5% of hypertension cases. Causes include obstructive sleep apnea, chronic kidney disease, renal artery stenosis, medications, thyroid disease, parathyroid disease, Cushing syndrome, hyperaldosteronism, pheochromocytoma, and coarctation of the aorta.

Diabetes. Although diabetes unequivocally increases the risk of CVD, early detection and intensive glycemic control has not been firmly established to improve cardiovascular outcomes. Dyslipidemia has been hypothesized to play a significant role in the accelerated atherosclerosis found in patients with diabetes. The fact that treatment of hyperlipidemia has consistently been shown to reduce CVD events in patients with diabetes supports this view. Guidelines recommend treating adults with diabetes with at least a moderate dose of statin therapy (Fig. 11-31).

Dyslipidemias. Start low-to-moderate dose statins for primary CVD prevention in adults aged 40 to 75 years who have one or more CVD risk factors (dyslipidemia, diabetes, hypertension, or smoking) and a 10-year calculated CVD event risk ≥10%. Measure periodically (every 5 years is considered a reasonable interval) lipid levels in all adults aged 40 to 75 years without existing CVD.

In 2018, the ACC/AHA published "a guideline on the treatment of blood cholesterol to reduce atherosclerotic cardiovascular risk in adults." This guideline, summarized in Figure 11-31, offers evidence-based recommendations for initiating statin therapy based on risk level as estimated by CVD risk calculator (see Box 11-17). The guideline notes that high-intensity therapy lowers low-density lipoprotein (LDL) cholesterol by about 50% and moderate-intensity therapy lowers LDL cholesterol by 30% to 50%. The guideline also states that clinicians and patients should engage in shared decision making, addressing the potential benefits and harms of prescribing statins and eliciting patient preferences before initiating therapy. The guideline firmly emphasizes the importance of encouraging all patients to adhere to a healthy lifestyle.

Metabolic Syndrome. *Metabolic syndrome* consists of a cluster of risk factors that increase risk of both CVD and diabetes. Metabolic syndrome is diagnosed when any three of the following five risk factors are present (1) an elevated

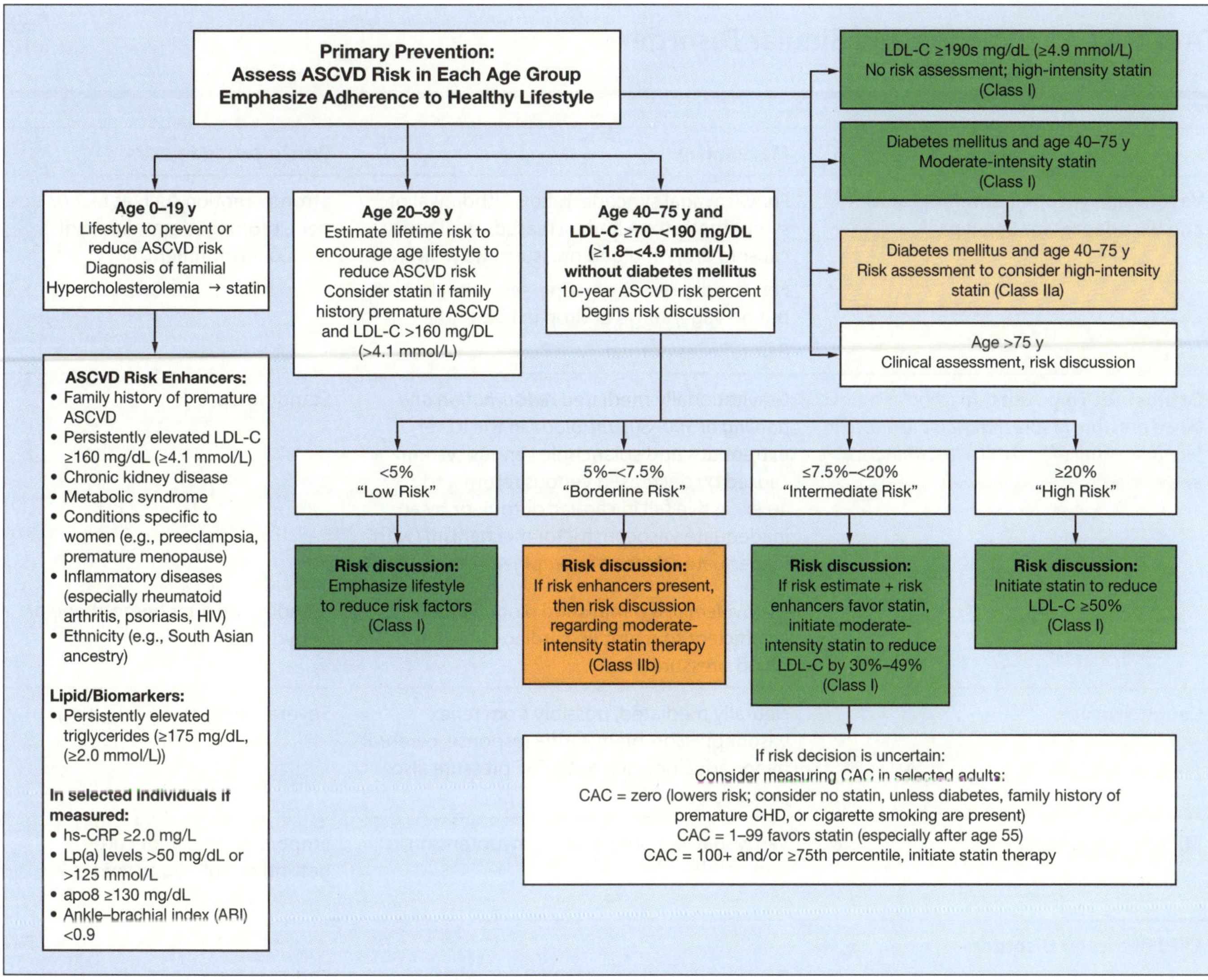

FIGURE 11-31. American College of Cardiology/American Heart Association cholesterol guideline, 2018. ASCVD, atherosclerotic cardiovascular disease; CAC, coronary artery calcium; CHD, coronary heart disease; HIV, human immunodeficiency syndrome; hs-CRP, high-sensitivity C-reactive protein; LDL-C, low-density lipoprotein cholesterol. (Reprinted with permission from Grundy SM et al. *Circulation*. 2018;139(25):e1082–e1143. Copyright © 2018 American Heart Association, Inc.)

waist circumference (population- and country-specific), (2) elevated triglycerides, (3) reduced HDL cholesterol, (4) elevated blood pressure, and (5) elevated fasting plasma glucose. When a patient presents with comorbid conditions, the risk for future CVD is greater than with any one factor presenting alone. Metabolic syndrome should be considered largely a "disease of unhealthy lifestyle."

Other Risk Factors: Smoking, Family History, and Obesity. Risk factors such as smoking, family history, and obesity contribute substantially to the population burden of CVD. *Smoking* increases a person's risk of CHD and stroke by two- to fourfold compared to nonsmokers or past smokers who quit >10 years previously. Among adults, 12% report a *family history* of heart attack or angina before age 50 years. Along with a family history of premature revascularization, this risk factor is associated with about a 50% increased lifetime risk for CHD and for CVD mortality. *Obesity*, or BMI over 30 kg/m^2, is significantly associated with increased overall mortality and death from CVD.

Promoting Lifestyle Change and Risk Factor Modification

Motivating behavior change is challenging, but it is an essential clinical skill for risk factor reduction.

The ACC/AHA recommendations on lifestyle management address diet, physical activity, body weight, and tobacco avoidance, as well as controlling hypertension and diabetes.

TABLE 11-1. Syncope and Similar Disorders

	Mechanism	Precipitating Factors
Vasovagal Syncope (Common Faint) and Vasodepressor Syncope	For vasovagal syncope: reflex withdrawal of sympathetic tone and increased vagal tone causing drop in blood pressure and heart rate For vasodepressor syncope: same mechanism but no vagal surge or drop in heart rate Baroreflexes normal	Strong emotion such as fear or pain, prolonged standing, hot humid environment
Orthostatic Hypotension *(drop in systolic blood pressure of ≥20 mm Hg or in diastolic blood pressure of ≥10 mm Hg within 3 min of standing)*	Gravitationally mediated *redistribution and pooling of 300–800 mL blood* in the lower extremities and splanchnic venous system, caused by decreased venous return and an excessive fall in cardiac output, or by an inadequate vasoconstrictor mechanism (with inadequate release of norepinephrine)	Standing up
	Hypovolemia, a diminished blood volume insufficient to maintain cardiac output and blood pressure	Standing up after hemorrhage or dehydration
Cough Syncope	Neurally mediated, possibly from reflex vasodepressor–bradycardia response; cerebral hypoperfusion, increased CSF pressure also proposed	Severe paroxysm of coughing
Micturition Syncope	Vasovagal response, sudden hypotension proposed	Emptying the bladder after getting out of bed to void
Cardiovascular Disorders		
Arrhythmias	Decreased cardiac output from cardiac ischemia, ventricular arrhythmias, prolonged QT syndrome, persistent bradycardia, infrafascicular block causing cerebral hypoperfusion; often sudden onset, sudden offset	Sudden change in rhythm to bradycardia or tachyarrhythmia
Aortic Stenosis and Hypertrophic Cardiomyopathy	Vascular resistance falls with exercise, but cardiac output does not rise due to outflow obstruction	Exercise
Myocardial Infarction	Sudden arrhythmia or decreased cardiac output	Variable, often exertion
Massive Pulmonary Embolism	Sudden hypoxia or decreased cardiac output	Variable, including prolonged bed rest, major surgery, clotting disorders, pregnancy

Predisposing Factors	Prodromal Manifestations	Postural Associations	Recovery
Fatigue, hunger, preload reduction from dehydration, diuretics, vasodilators	Usually >10 s; palpitations, nausea, blurred vision, warmth, pallor, diaphoresis, lightheadedness	Usually occurs when standing, at times when sitting	Prompt return of consciousness after lying down, but pallor, weakness, nausea, and slight confusion may persist for a time; most common type of syncope
Aging; antihypertensive vasodilator drugs; prolonged bed rest central disorders: Parkinson disease, multiple system atrophy; dementia with Lewy bodies; peripheral neuropathy: diabetes, amyloidosis	Lightheadedness, dizziness, cognitive slowing, fatigue; often none	Occurs soon after standing Supine hypertension is common	Prompt return to normal when lying down
Bleeding from the GI tract or trauma, potent diuretics, vomiting, diarrhea, polyuria	Lightheadedness and palpitations (tachycardia) on standing up	Occurs soon after standing up	Improves with volume repletion
COPD, asthma, pulmonary hypertension; typically occurs in overweight middle-aged patients	Often none except for cough; blurred vision, lightheadedness may occur	May occur in any position	Prompt return to normal after a few seconds
Nocturia, usually in elderly or adult men	Often none	Commonly just after (or during) voiding after standing up	Prompt return to normal
Ischemic or valvular heart disease, conduction abnormalities, pericardial disease, cardiomyopathy; aging decreases tolerance of abnormal rhythms	Palpitations, usually lasting <5 s; often none	May occur in any position	Prompt return to normal when arrhythmia resolves; most common cause of cardiac syncope; cardiogenic syncope has a 6-mo mortality >10%
Cardiac disorders	Chest pain, often none; onset is sudden	Occurs with or after exercise	Usually a prompt return to normal
Coronary artery disease, coronary ischemia or vasospasm	Ischemic chest pain; may be silent	May occur in any position	Variable; related to time to diagnosis and treatment
Deep vein thrombosis, bed rest, hypercoagulable states (systemic lupus erythematosus, cancer), protein S or C deficiency antithrombin III deficiency; estrogen therapy	Tachypnea, chest or pleuritic pain, dyspnea, anxiety, cough	May occur in any position	Related to time to diagnosis and treatment

(*continued*)

TABLE 11-1. Syncope and Similar Disorders *(Continued)*

	Mechanism	Precipitating Factors
Disorders Resembling Syncope		
Hypocapnia due to Hyperventilation	Constriction of cerebral blood vessels from hypocapnia induced by hyperventilation	Anxiety, panic disorder
Hypoglycemia	Insufficient glucose to maintain cerebral metabolism; epinephrine release contributes to symptoms; true syncope is uncommon	Variable, including fasting
Fainting from Conversion Disorder (Termed "Functional Neurologic Symptom Disorder" in DSM-5)	Unknown mechanism Skin color, vital signs may be normal; sometimes with bizarre purposeful movements; usually occurs when other people present	Stress or trauma, psychological or physical Sometimes no precipitant identified

Predisposing Factors	Prodromal Manifestations	Postural Associations	Recovery
Anxiety	Dyspnea, palpitations, chest discomfort, numbness, and tingling in hands and around the mouth lasting several minutes; consciousness is often maintained	May occur in any position	Slow improvement as hyperventilation ceases
Insulin therapy and a variety of metabolic disorders	Sweating, tremors, palpitations, hunger, headache, confusion, abnormal behavior, coma	May occur in any position	Variable, depending on severity and treatment
History of multiple somatic symptoms Often dissociative symptoms such as depersonalization, derealization, dissociative amnesia, or maladaptive personality traits; associated with past child abuse or neglect	Variable	A slump to the floor, often from a standing position, without injury	Variable; may be prolonged, often with fluctuating responsiveness and inconsistent neurologic findings

TABLE 11-2. Variations and Abnormalities of the Ventricular Impulses

In the healthy heart, the *left ventricular impulse* is usually the PMI. This brief impulse is generated by the movement of the ventricular apex against the chest wall during contraction. The *right ventricular impulse* is normally not palpable beyond infancy, and its characteristics are indeterminate. Learn the classical descriptors of the normal left ventricular PMI:

- *Location:* in the fourth or fifth left intercostal space, at the midclavicular line
- *Diameter:* discrete, or ≤2 cm
- *Amplitude: brisk* and *tapping*
- *Duration:* ≤2/3 of systole

The characteristics of the ventricular impulse change as the left and right ventricles adapt to high-output states (anxiety, hyperthyroidism, and severe anemia) and to the more pathologic conditions of chronic pressure or volume overload. In addition to the normal *brisk tapping* PMI, learn to recognize three additional types of ventricular impulses and their distinguishing features in the table below:

- *Hyperkinetic:* The *hyperkinetic ventricular impulse* from transiently increased stroke volume—this change does not necessarily indicate heart disease.
- *Sustained:* The *sustained* ventricular impulse of ventricular hypertrophy from chronic pressure load, known as increased afterload.
- *Diffuse:* The *diffuse* ventricular impulse of ventricular dilation from chronic volume overload, or *increased preload*.

	Left Ventricular Impulse			**Right Ventricular Impulse**		
	Hyperkinetic	**Pressure Overload**	**Volume Overload**	**Hyperkinetic**	**Pressure Overload**	**Volume Overload**
Examples of Causes	Anxiety, hyperthyroidism, severe anemia	Aortic stenosis, hypertension	Aortic or mitral regurgitation; cardiomyopathy	Anxiety, hyperthyroidism, severe anemia	Pulmonic stenosis, pulmonary hypertension	Atrial septal defect
Location	Normal	Normal	Displaced to the left and possibly downward	Third, fourth, or fifth left intercostal spaces	Third, fourth, or fifth left intercostal spaces, subxiphoid area	Left sternal border, extending toward the left cardiac border, subxiphoid area
Diameter	~2 cm, though increased amplitude may make diameter feel larger	>2 cm	>2 cm	Not useful	Not useful	Not useful
Amplitude	More forceful tapping	More forceful tapping	*Diffuse*	Slightly more forceful	More forceful	Slightly to markedly more forceful
Duration	<2/3 systole	*Sustained* (up to S_2)	Often slightly sustained	Normal	*Sustained*	Normal to slightly sustained

TABLE 11-3. Variations in the First Heart Sound—S_1

Variation	Diagram	Description
Normal Variations	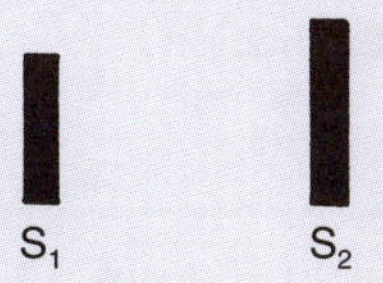	S_1 is softer than S_2 at the *base* (right and left second intercostal spaces).
		S_1 is often but not always louder than S_2 at the apex.
Accentuated S_1	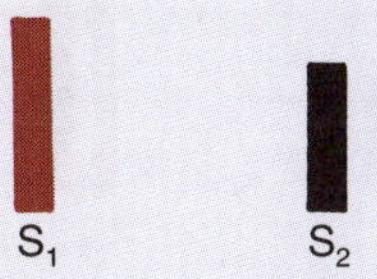	S_1 is accentuated in (1) tachycardia, rhythms with a short PR interval, and high cardiac output states (e.g., exercise, anemia, hyperthyroidism) and (2) mitral stenosis.
Diminished S_1	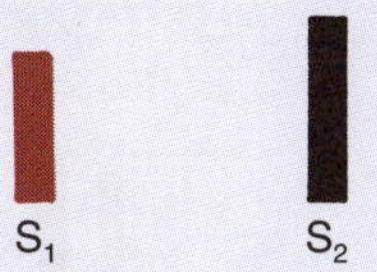	S_1 is diminished in first-degree heart block, left bundle branch block, and myocardial infarction. Early mitral valve closure occurring before ventricular contraction also causes a soft S_1, seen in severe aortic regurgitation.
Varying S_1	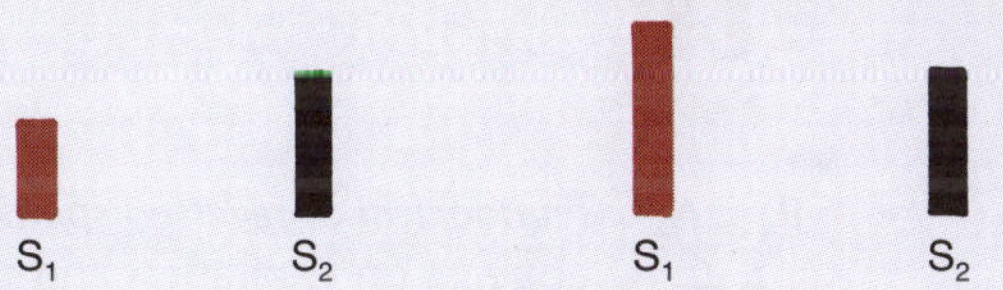	S_1 varies in intensity (1) in complete heart block, when atria and ventricles are beating independently of each other and (2) in any totally irregular rhythm (e.g., atrial fibrillation). In these situations, the mitral valve is in varying positions before being shut by ventricular contraction. Its closure sound, therefore, varies in loudness.
Split S_1	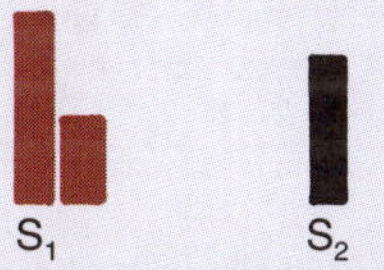	Delayed closure of the tricuspid valve increases splitting of S_1, best heard along the lower left sternal border where the tricuspid component, often too faint to be heard, becomes audible. A more prominent split S_1 than normal occurs in right bundle branch block. This split may rarely be heard at the apex, but must be distinguished from an S_4, an aortic ejection sound, and an early systolic click.

TABLE 11-4. Variations in the Second Heart Sound—S_2

	Inspiration	Expiration	
Physiologic Splitting	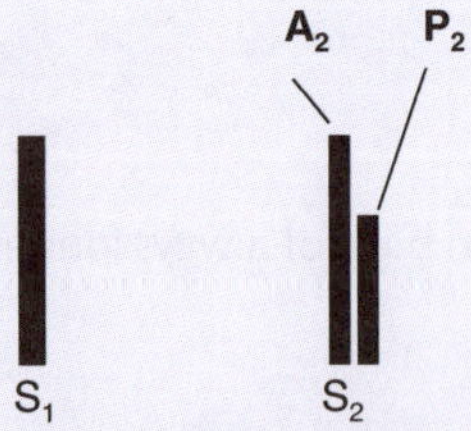	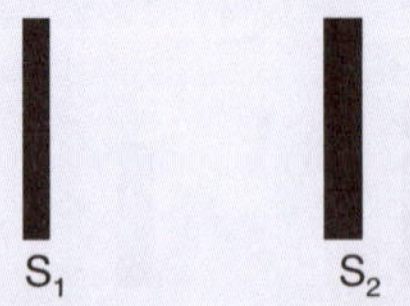	Listen for *splitting* of S_2 in the *second or third left intercostal space*. The pulmonic component of S_2 is usually too faint to be heard at the apex or aortic area, where S_2 is a single sound derived only from aortic valve closure. Normal splitting is *accentuated by inspiration*, which increases the interval between A_2 and P_2, and *disappears on expiration.*
Pathologic Splitting (*Audible splitting occurs during expiration and suggests heart disease.*)	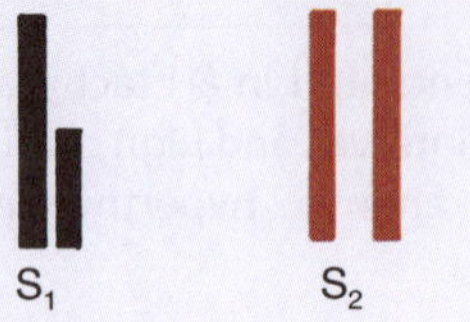	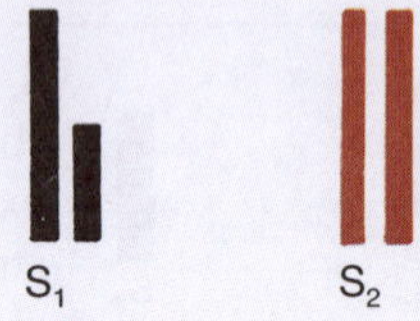	*Wide physiologic splitting* of S_2 refers to an increase in the usual splitting of S_2 during inspiration that persists throughout the respiratory cycle. Wide splitting is caused by delayed closure of the pulmonic valve (as in pulmonic stenosis or right bundle branch block) or early closure of the aortic valve (mitral regurgitation). Right bundle branch block is illustrated here.
	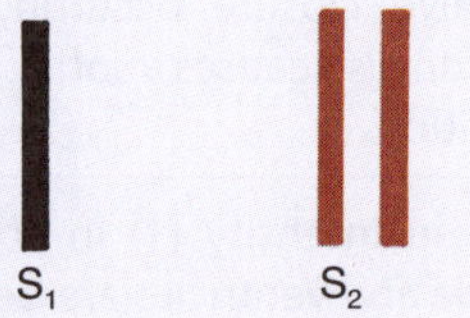	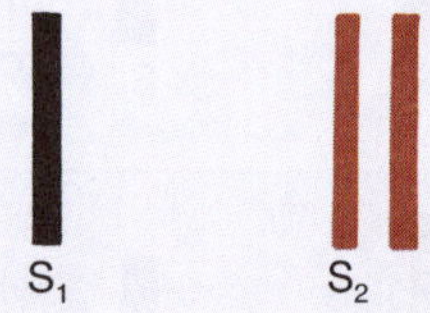	*Fixed splitting* refers to wide splitting that does not vary with respiration, often due to prolonged right ventricular systole, seen in atrial septal defect.
	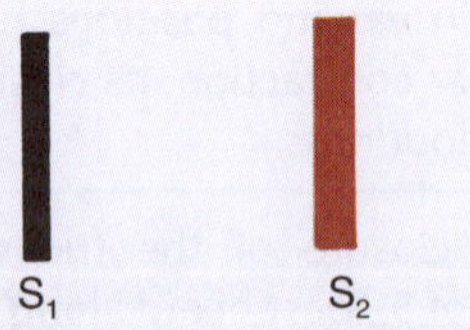	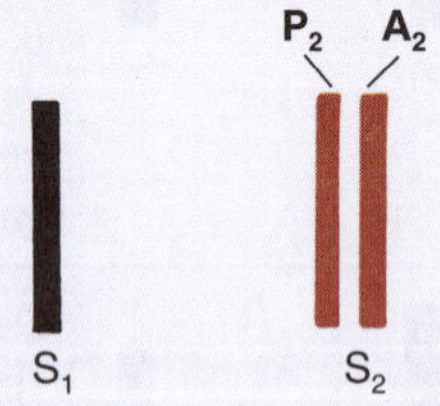	*Paradoxical or reversed splitting* refers to splitting that appears on expiration and disappears on inspiration. Closure of the aortic valve is abnormally delayed so that A_2 follows P_2 in expiration. Normal inspiratory delay of P_2 makes the split disappear. The most common cause is left bundle branch block.

A_2 and P_2: Second Right Intercostal Space

A_2 with Increased Intensity (A_2 can usually be heard only in right second intercostal space): occurs in systemic hypertension because of the increased pressure load. Increased intensity also occurs when the aortic root is dilated, attributed to the increased proximity of the aortic valve to the chest wall.

P_2 with Increased Intensity: When P_2 is equal to or louder than A_2, suspect pulmonary hypertension. Other causes include a dilated pulmonary artery and an atrial septal defect. When a split S_2 is heard widely, extending to the apex and the right base, P_2 is accentuated.

A_2 Decreased or Absent: occurs in calcific aortic stenosis due to valve immobility. If A_2 is inaudible, no splitting is heard.

P_2 Decreased or Absent: This usually occurs from the increased AP diameter of the chest associated with aging. It can also result from pulmonic stenosis. If P_2 is inaudible, no splitting is heard.

TABLE 11-5. Extra Heart Sounds in Systole

There are two kinds of extra heart sounds in systole: (1) early ejection sounds and (2) clicks, commonly heard in mid- and late systole.

Early Systolic Ejection Sounds

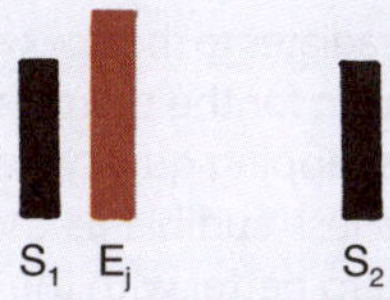

Early systolic ejection sounds occur shortly after S_1, coincident with sudden pathologic halting of the aortic and pulmonic valves as they open in early systole. They are relatively high in pitch, have a sharp clicking quality, and are best heard with the diaphragm. An ejection sound indicates CVD.

Listen for an *aortic ejection sound* at both the base and apex. It may be louder at the apex and usually does not vary with respiration. An aortic ejection sound may accompany a dilated aorta, or aortic valve disease from congenital stenosis or a bicuspid aortic valve.

A *pulmonic ejection sound* is heard best in the second and third left intercostal spaces. When S_1, usually relatively soft in this area, appears to be loud, consider a possible pulmonic ejection sound. Its intensity often *decreases with inspiration*. Causes include dilatation of the pulmonary artery, pulmonary hypertension, and pulmonic stenosis.

Systolic Clicks

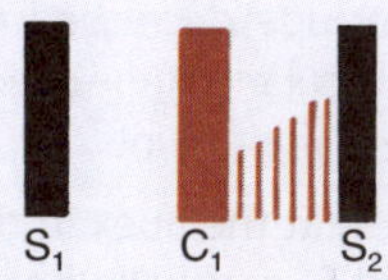

Systolic clicks are usually caused by *mitral valve prolapse*—an abnormal systolic ballooning of part of the mitral valve into the left atrium related to leaflet redundancy and elongation of the chordae tendineae. The clicks are usually mid- or late systolic. Systolic clicks may also be of extracardiac or mediastinal origin.

Squatting

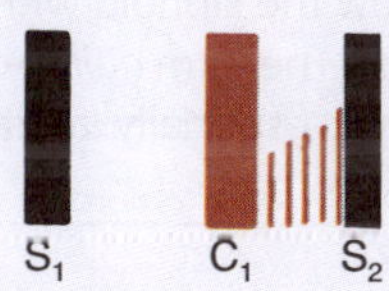

The click is usually single, but there may be more than one, usually at or medial to the apex, but also at the lower left sternal border. The click is high pitched, so best heard with the diaphragm. It is often followed by a late systolic murmur from mitral regurgitation that crescendos up to S_2. Auscultatory findings are notably variable. Most patients have only a click, some have only a murmur, and some have both.

Standing

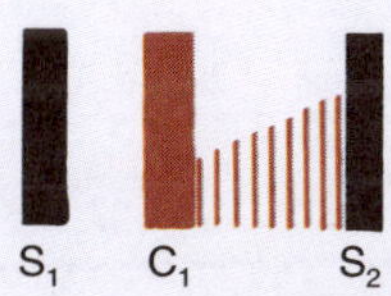

In *mitral valve prolapse,* findings vary from one examination to the next and often change with body position. Several positions are recommended to identify the syndrome: supine, seated, squatting, and standing. *Squatting (and the Valsalva release phase) delays the click and murmur due to increased venous return; standing (and the Valsalva strain phase) moves them closer to S_1.*

TABLE 11-6. Extra Heart Sounds in Diastole

Opening Snap

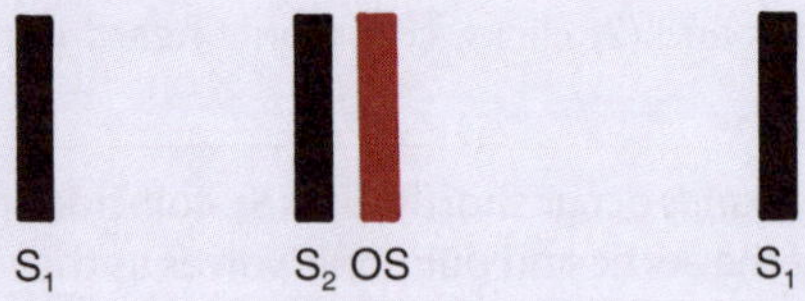

The opening snap (OS) is a very early diastolic sound caused by abrupt deceleration during the opening of a *stenotic mitral valve*. It is best heard just medial to the apex and along the lower left sternal border. If loud, an OS radiates to the apex and to the pulmonic area, where it may be mistaken for the pulmonic component of a split S_2. Its high pitch and snapping quality help to distinguish it from an S_2, but it becomes less audible as the valve leaflets become more calcified. It is heard better with the *diaphragm*.

S_3

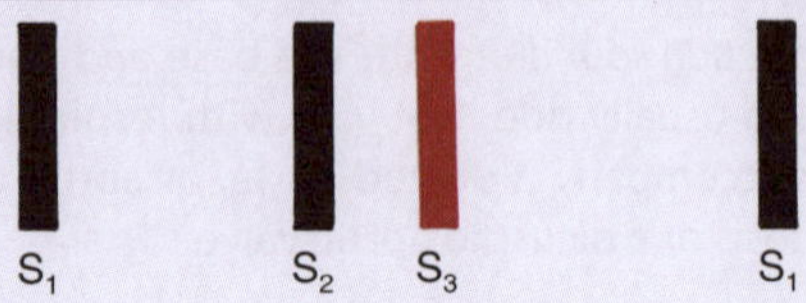

You will detect *physiologic* S_3 frequently in children and young adults to the age of 35 or 40 years, and often during the last trimester of pregnancy. Occurring early in diastole during rapid ventricular filling, it is later than an OS, dull and low in pitch, and heard best at the apex in the left lateral decubitus position. The bell of the stethoscope should be used with very light pressure.

A *pathologic S_3* or *ventricular gallop* sounds like a physiologic S_3. An S_3 in adults over age 40 years is usually pathologic, arising from high left ventricular filling pressures and abrupt deceleration of inflow across the mitral valve at the end of the rapid filling phase of diastole. Causes include decreased myocardial contractility, heart failure, and ventricular volume overload from aortic or mitral regurgitation, and left-to-right shunts.

Listen for a *left-sided S_3* at the apex in the left lateral decubitus position. A *right-sided S_3* is usually heard along the lower left sternal border or below the xiphoid with the patient supine and is louder on inspiration. The term *gallop* comes from the cadence of three heart sounds, especially at rapid heart rates, which sounds like "Kentucky."

(*continued*)

TABLE 11-6. Extra Heart Sounds in Diastole *(Continued)*

S_4

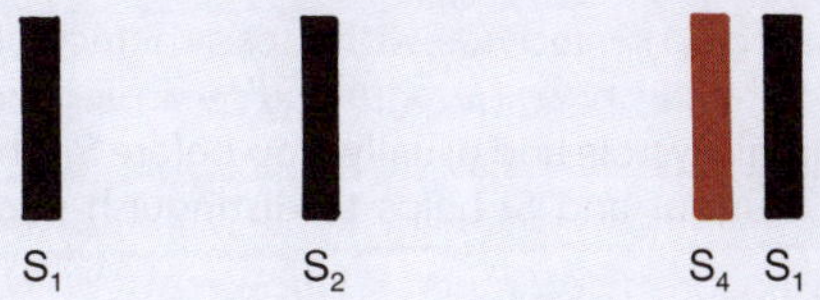

An S_4 (*atrial sound* or *atrial gallop*) occurs just before S_1. It is dull, low in pitch, and best heard at the apex with the bell. Listen at the lower left sternal border for a right ventricular S_4 (or in the subxiphoid area if obstructive lung disease). An S_4 is occasionally normal, especially in trained athletes and older age groups. More commonly, it is due to ventricular hypertrophy or fibrosis causing stiffness and increased resistance (or decreased compliance) during ventricular filling following atrial contraction.

Causes of a left-sided S_4 include hypertensive heart disease, aortic stenosis, and ischemic and hypertrophic cardiomyopathy.

A *left-sided S_4* is heard best at the apex in the left lateral decubitus position, with a cadence like "Tennessee." The less common *right-sided S_4* is heard along the lower left sternal border or below the xiphoid. It often gets louder with inspiration. Causes include pulmonary hypertension and pulmonic stenosis.

An S_4 is also associated with delayed conduction between the atria and ventricles. This delay separates the normally faint atrial sound from the louder S_1 and makes it audible. An S_4 is never heard when there are no atrial contractions (absent during atrial fibrillation).

Occasionally, a patient has both an S_3 and an S_4, producing a *quadruple rhythm* of four heart sounds. At rapid heart rates, the S_3 and S_4 may merge into one loud extra heart sound, called a *summation gallop*.

TABLE 11-7. Midsystolic Murmurs

Midsystolic ejection murmurs are the most common kind of heart murmur. They may be (1) *innocent*—without any detectable physiologic or structural abnormality; (2) *physiologic*—from physiologic changes in body metabolism; or (3) *pathologic*—arising from structural abnormalities in the heart or great vessels. Midsystolic murmurs tend to peak near midsystole and usually stop before S_2. The crescendo–decrescendo or "diamond" shape is not always audible. The gap between the murmur and S_2 helps to distinguish midsystolic from pansystolic murmurs.

	Innocent Murmurs	**Physiologic Murmurs**
	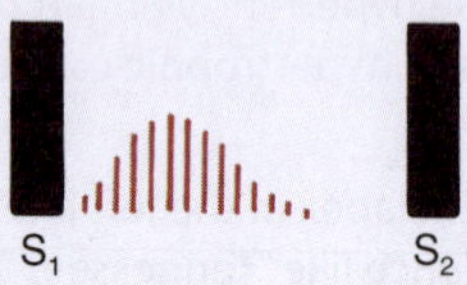	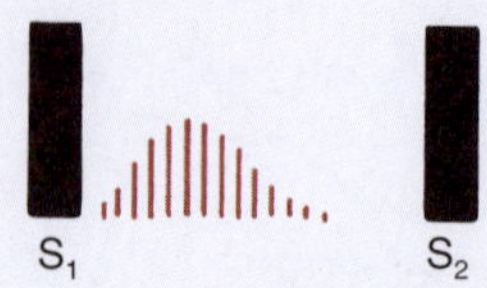
Murmur	*Location.* Left second to fourth intercostal spaces between the left sternal border and the apex *Radiation.* Minimal *Intensity.* Grades 1 to 2, possibly 3 *Pitch.* Soft to medium *Quality.* Variable *Maneuvers.* Usually decreases or disappears on sitting	Similar to innocent murmurs
Associated Findings	None: normal splitting, no ejection sounds, no diastolic murmurs, and no palpable evidence of ventricular enlargement. Occasionally, both an innocent murmur and pathologic murmur are present.	Signs of physiologic causes (see mechanisms below)
Mechanism	Turbulent blood flow, probably generated by ventricular ejection of blood into the aorta from the left and occasionally the right ventricle. Very common in children and young adults but may also be present in older adults. There is no underlying CVD.	Turbulence due to a temporary increase in blood flow in predisposing conditions such as anemia, pregnancy, fever, and hyperthyroidism.

Pathologic Murmurs

Aortic Stenosis	Hypertrophic Cardiomyopathy	Pulmonic Stenosis
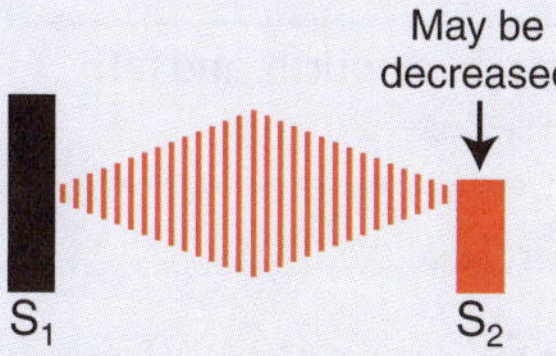	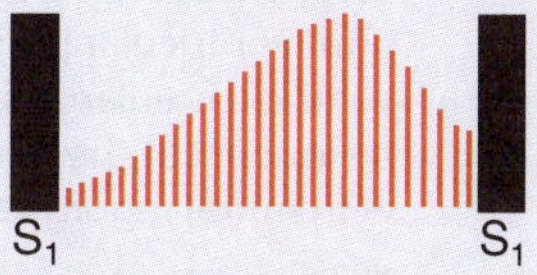	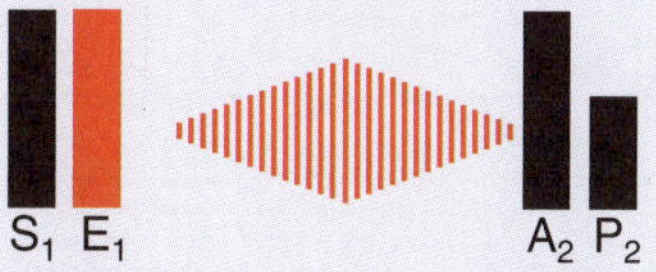
Location. Right second and third intercostal spaces	*Location.* Left third and fourth intercostal spaces	*Location.* Left second and third intercostal spaces
Radiation. Often to the carotids, down the left sternal border, even to the apex. If severe, may radiate to left second and third intercostal spaces	*Radiation.* Down the left sternal border to the apex, possibly to the base, but not to the neck	*Radiation.* If loud, toward the left shoulder and neck
Intensity. Sometimes soft, but often loud, with a thrill	*Intensity.* Variable. See Maneuvers.	*Intensity.* Soft to loud; if loud, associated with a thrill
Pitch. Medium, harsh; crescendo–decrescendo may be higher at the apex	*Pitch.* Medium	*Pitch.* Medium; crescendo–decrescendo
Quality. Often harsh; may be more musical at the apex	*Quality.* Harsh	*Quality.* Often harsh
Maneuvers. Heard best with the patient sitting and leaning forward	*Maneuvers.* Intensity decreases with squatting and Valsalva release phase (increases venous return), *increases with standing and Valsalva strain phase* (decreases left ventricular volume) (see p. 528)	
As aortic stenosis worsens, the murmur peaks later in systole, and A_2 decreases in intensity. A_2 may be delayed and merged with $P_2 \rightarrow$ single S_2 on expiration or a paradoxical S_2 split. Carotid upstroke may be delayed, with a slow rise, small amplitude, and decreased volume. The hypertrophied left ventricle may produce a sustained apical impulse and an S_4 due to decreased compliance. After age 40 years there may be a dilated aorta and murmur of aortic regurgitation. Subendocardial ischemia due to poor coronary perfusion distal to the valve causes angina and syncope.	The carotid upstroke rises quickly, unlike aortic stenosis. The apical impulse is sustained. S_2 may be single. An S_4 is usually present at the apex (unlike mitral regurgitation). Usually benign, but progresses in 25% to syncope, ischemia, atrial fibrillation, dilated cardiomyopathy and heart failure, and stroke, with increased risk of sudden death.	The JVP is usually normal but may have prominent a wave. The right ventricular impulse is often sustained. An early pulmonic ejection sound is present in mild to moderate stenosis. In severe stenosis, S_2 is widely split and P_2 softens. May hear a right-sided S_4 over the left sternal border.
Significant stenosis causes turbulent blood flow across the valve and increases left ventricular afterload. The most common cause is valve calcification in older adults, at times progressing from nonobstructing sclerosis (present in 25%) to stenosis. The second most common cause is a congenital bicuspid aortic valve, often not recognized until adulthood.	Unexplained diffuse or focal ventricular hypertrophy with myocyte disarray and fibrosis associated with unusually rapid ejection of blood from the left ventricle during systole. Outflow tract obstruction of flow may coexist. Associated distortion of the mitral valve may cause mitral regurgitation.	Primarily a congenital disorder with valvular, supravalvular, or subvalvular stenosis. Stenosis impairs flow across the valve, increasing right ventricular afterload. In an atrial septal defect, increased flow across the pulmonic valve may mimic pulmonic stenosis.

TABLE 11-8. Pansystolic (Holosystolic) Murmurs

Pansystolic (holosystolic) murmurs are pathologic, arising from blood flow from a chamber with high pressure to one of lower pressure, through a valve or other structure that should be closed. The murmur begins immediately with S_1 and continues up to S_2.

	Mitral Regurgitation	Tricuspid Regurgitation	Ventricular Septal Defect
	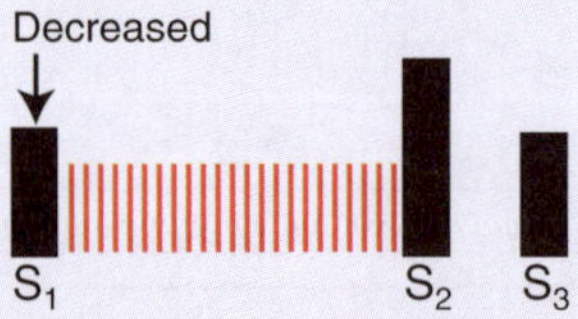	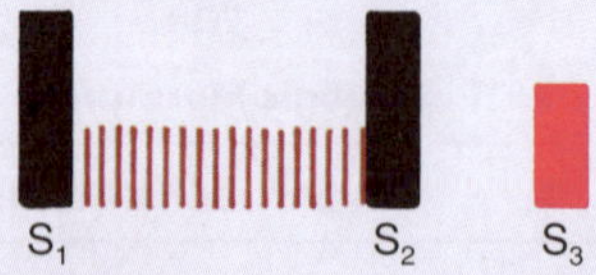	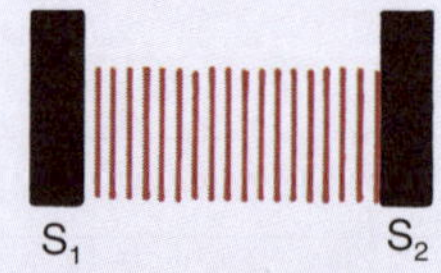
Murmur	*Location.* Apex *Radiation.* To the left axilla, less often to the left sternal border *Intensity.* Soft to loud; if loud, associated with an apical thrill *Pitch.* Medium to high *Quality.* Blowing, holosystolic *Maneuvers.* Unlike tricuspid regurgitation, the intensity of the murmur does not change with inspiration.	*Location.* Lower left sternal border. If right ventricular pressure is high and the ventricle is enlarged, the murmur may be loudest at the apex and confused with mitral regurgitation. *Radiation.* To the right of the sternum, to the xiphoid area, and at times to the left midclavicular line, but not into the axilla. *Intensity.* Variable *Pitch.* Medium *Quality.* Blowing, holosystolic *Maneuvers.* Unlike mitral regurgitation, the intensity increases with inspiration.	*Location.* Left third, fourth, and fifth intercostal spaces *Radiation.* Often wide, depending on the size of the defect. *Intensity.* Often very loud, with a thrill. Smaller defects have louder murmurs. *Pitch.* High, holosystolic. Smaller defects have murmurs with a higher pitch. *Quality.* Often harsh
Associated Findings	S_1 normal (75%), loud (12%), soft (12%) An apical S_3 reflects volume overload of the left ventricle. The apical impulse may be *diffuse* and laterally displaced. There may be a sustained lower left parasternal impulse from a dilated left atrium.	The right ventricular impulse is increased in amplitude and may be sustained. The JVP is often elevated in severe tricuspid regurgitation, with large *v* waves in the jugular veins, a pulsatile liver, ascites, and edema.	S_2 may be obscured by the loud murmur. Findings and associated findings vary with the size of the defect. Larger defects cause left-to-right shunts, pulmonary hypertension, and right ventricular overload.
Mechanism	When the *mitral valve fails to close fully in systole,* blood regurgitates from left ventricle to left atrium, causing the murmur and increasing left ventricular preload, ultimately leading to left ventricular dilatation. Causes are structural, from mitral valve prolapse, infectious endocarditis, rheumatic heart disease, and collagen vascular disease; and functional, from ventricular dilatation and dilatation of the mitral valve annulus and from leaflet, papillary muscle, or chordae tendineae dysfunction.	When the *tricuspid valve fails to close fully in systole,* blood regurgitates from RV to right atrium, producing a murmur. The most common causes are: right ventricular failure and dilatation, with resulting enlargement of the tricuspid orifice, often induced by pulmonary hypertension or left ventricular failure; and endocarditis—the RV and pulmonary artery pressures are low, so the murmur is early systolic.	A ventricular septal defect is a congenital abnormality classified according to one of four locations in the ventricular septum. The defect is a conduit for *blood flow from the relatively high-pressure left ventricle into the low-pressure right ventricle.* The defect may be accompanied by aortic regurgitation, tricuspid regurgitation, and aneurysms of the ventricular septum; an uncomplicated lesion is described here.

TABLE 11-9. Diastolic Murmurs

Diastolic murmurs are always pathologic. There are two basic types in adults. Early decrescendo diastolic murmurs signify regurgitant flow through an incompetent semilunar valve, usually the aortic. Rumbling diastolic murmurs in mid- or late diastole point to stenosis of an AV valve, usually the mitral. Diastolic murmurs are less common than systolic murmurs and more difficult to hear, requiring more meticulous examination.

	Aortic Regurgitation	**Mitral Stenosis**
	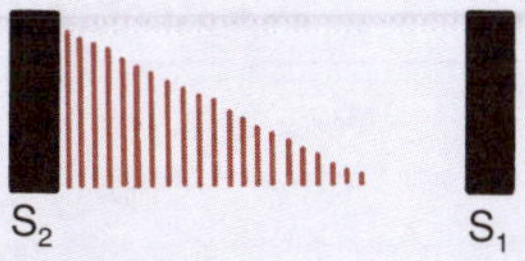	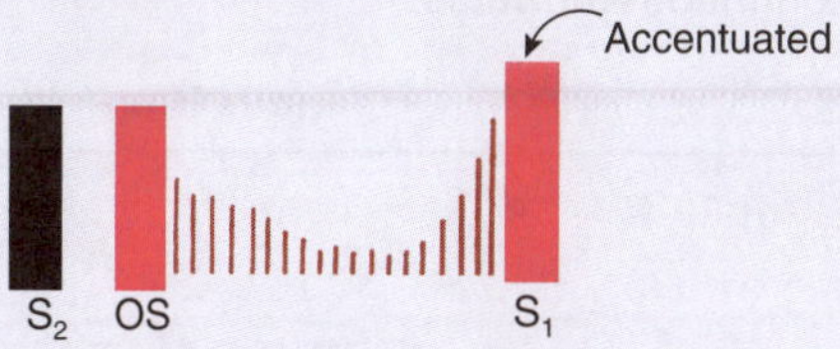
Murmur	*Location.* Left second to fourth intercostal spaces *Radiation.* If loud, to the apex, perhaps to the right sternal border *Intensity.* Grades 1 to 4 *Pitch.* High. *Use the diaphragm.* *Quality.* Blowing decrescendo; may be mistaken for breath sounds *Maneuvers.* The murmur is heard best with the *patient sitting, leaning forward,* with breath held after exhalation.	*Location.* Usually limited to the apex *Radiation.* Little or none *Intensity.* Grades 1 to 4 *Pitch.* Decrescendo low-pitched rumble with presystolic accentuation. *Use the bell.* *Maneuvers.* Placing the bell exactly on the apical impulse, turning the patient into *a left lateral position,* and mild exercise like handgrips make the murmur audible. It is heard better in exhalation.
Associated Findings	With advancing severity, the diastolic pressure drops to as low as 50 mm Hg; the pulse pressure can widen by >80 mm Hg. The apical impulse becomes *diffuse,* displaced laterally and downward, and increased in diameter, amplitude, and duration. A systolic ejection sound may be present; S_2 is increased in aortic root dilatation and decreased if leaflets are thickened and calcified; and an S_3 often reflects ventricular dysfunction from both volume and pressure overload. A midsystolic flow murmur or a mitral diastolic (*Austin Flint*) murmur, usually with middiastolic and presystolic components, reflect increased regurgitant flow. The arterial pulse wave collapses suddenly creating bounding arterial pulses with *pistol shot sounds* on light pressure of the diaphragm, especially with arm elevation (*Corrigan pulse*), a *to–fro murmur* over the brachial or femoral artery with firm pressure (*Duroziez sign*), and capillary pulsations with nail blanching (*Quincke pulses*).	S_1 is loud and may be palpable at the apex. An OS often follows S_2 and initiates the murmur. If pulmonary hypertension develops, P_2 is accentuated, the right ventricular parasternal impulse becomes palpable, and the *a* wave of the JVP is more prominent. The apical impulse is small and tapping. Atrial fibrillation occurs in about a third of symptomatic patients, with ensuing risks of thromboembolism.
Mechanism	The aortic valve leaflets fail to close completely during diastole, causing regurgitation from the aorta back into the left ventricle and left ventricular overload. The associated midsystolic flow murmur results from the ejection of this increased stroke volume across the aortic valve. The mitral diastolic (*Austin Flint*) murmur is seen in moderate to severe disease and attributed to diastolic impingement of the regurgitant flow on the anterior leaflet of the mitral valve. Causes include leaflet abnormalities, aortic pathology (Marfan syndrome), and subvalvular abnormalities such as subaortic stenosis or an atrial septal defect.	The stiffened mitral valve leaflets move into the left atrium in midsystole and narrow the valve opening, causing turbulence. The resulting murmur has two components: (1) middiastolic (during rapid ventricular filling) and (2) presystolic accentuation, possibly related to ventricular contraction. The most common cause worldwide is rheumatic fever, which causes fibrosis, calcification, and thickening of the leaflets and commissures, and chordal fusion.

TABLE 11-10. Cardiovascular Sounds with Both Systolic and Diastolic Components

Some cardiovascular sounds extend beyond one phase of the cardiac cycle. Three examples, all nonvalvular in origin, are: (1) a *venous hum,* a benign sound produced by turbulence of blood in the jugular veins—common in children; (2) a *pericardial friction rub,* produced by inflammation of the pericardial sac; and (3) *patent ductus arteriosus,* a congenital anomaly that persists after birth causing a left-to-right shunt from the aorta to the pulmonary artery. *Continuous murmurs* begin in systole and extend through S_2 into all or part of diastole, as in *patent ductus arteriosus.* Arteriovenous fistulas, common in patients on hemodialysis, also produce continuous murmurs.

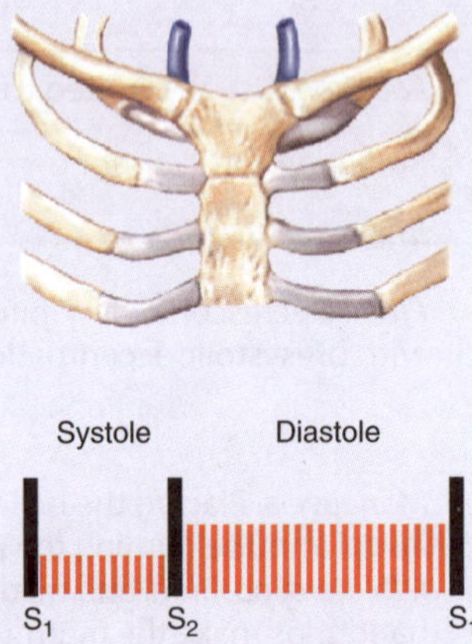

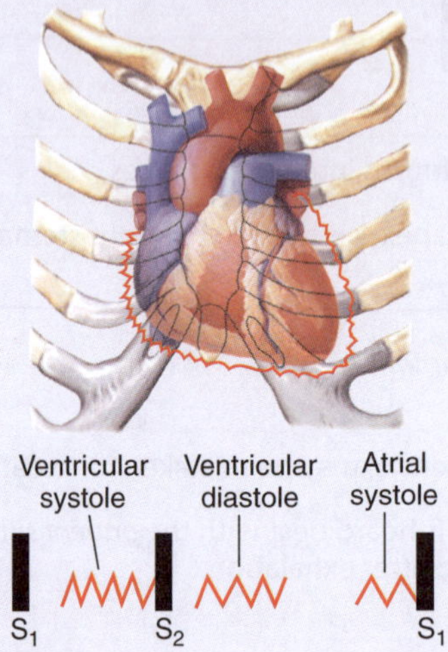

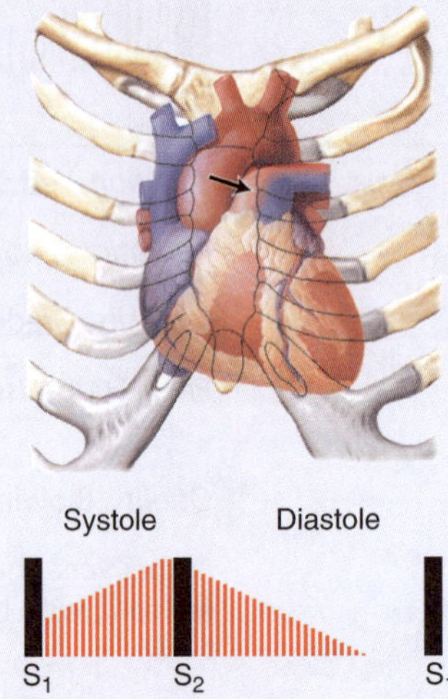

	Venous Hum	**Pericardial Friction Rub**	**Patent Ductus Arteriosus**
Timing	Continuous murmur without a silent interval. Loudest in diastole.	Inflammation of the visceral and parietal pericardium from pericarditis produces a coarse grating sound with one, two, or three components (ventricular systole; ventricular filling and atrial contraction during diastole). Rubs are heard with and without pericardial effusions.	Continuous murmur in both systole and diastole, often with a silent interval late in diastole. Loudest in late systole, obscures S_2, and fades in diastole.
Location	Above the medial third of the clavicles, especially on the right, often when the head is turned in the opposite direction. Best heard when patient in sitting position; disappears when patient supine.	Usually best heard in the left third intercostal space next to the sternum with the patient sitting and leaning forward with breath held after forced expiration. (In contrast, a pleural rub is heard only during inspiration.) May come and go spontaneously and require auscultation in several positions. Causes include myocardial infarction, uremia, connective tissue disease.	Left second intercostal space
Radiation	Right or left first and second intercostal spaces	Minimal.	Toward the left clavicle
Intensity	Soft to moderate. The hum is obliterated by pressure on the internal jugular vein.	Superficial sound of varying intensity that seems "close to the stethoscope."	Usually loud, sometimes associated with a thrill
Quality	Humming, roaring	Scratchy, scraping, grating	Harsh, machinery-like
Pitch	Low (heard better with the *bell*)	High (heard better with the *diaphragm*)	Medium

CHAPTER

12

Gastrointestinal System

ANATOMY AND PHYSIOLOGY

The gastrointestinal (GI) system extends from the mouth to the anus and includes the mouth, pharynx, esophagus, stomach, small intestine, large intestine, liver, biliary system, pancreas, rectum, and anus. It is responsible for ingestion of food, absorption of nutrients, and elimination of waste products. GI system examination is essentially an examination of the patient's abdomen.

The *abdomen* lies between the thorax and pelvis and is bordered superiorly by the inferior surface of the dome of the diaphragm (at about the fifth anterior intercostal space); posteriorly by the *lumbar vertebrae*, anterolaterally by flexible multilayered wall of muscles and sheet-like tendons (*rectus abdominis*, *transversus abdominis*, *internal* and *external oblique*); and inferiorly by the pelvic brim, which consists of the *iliac crest*, *anterior superior iliac spine*, *inguinal ligament pubic tubercle*, and *symphysis pubis*. Try to visualize these anatomic landmarks as shown in Figure 12-1.

The *abdominopelvic cavity* lies between the thoracic diaphragm and the pelvic diaphragm and contains two continuous cavities, the *abdominal cavity* and the *pelvic cavity*. This extended cavity houses most of the digestive organs, the spleen, and parts of the urogenital system

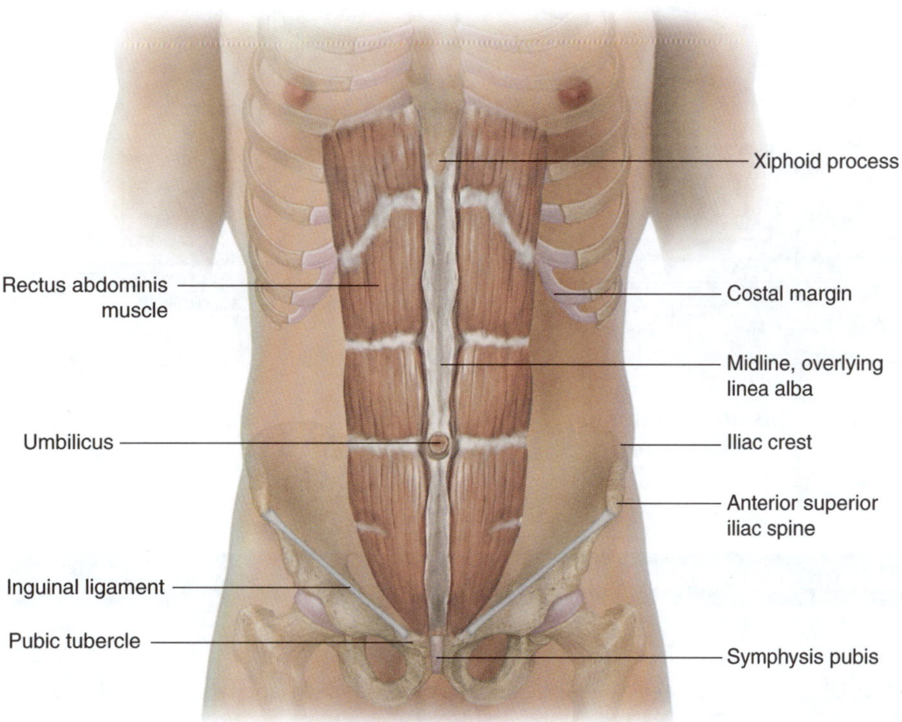

FIGURE 12-1. Landmarks of the abdomen.

(Fig. 12-2). Several organs are often palpable except for the stomach and much of the liver and spleen, which lie high in the abdominal cavity close to the diaphragm, where they are protected by the thoracic ribs beyond the reach of the palpating hand. Lining this cavity and folding over viscera are the *parietal* and *visceral* peritoneum.

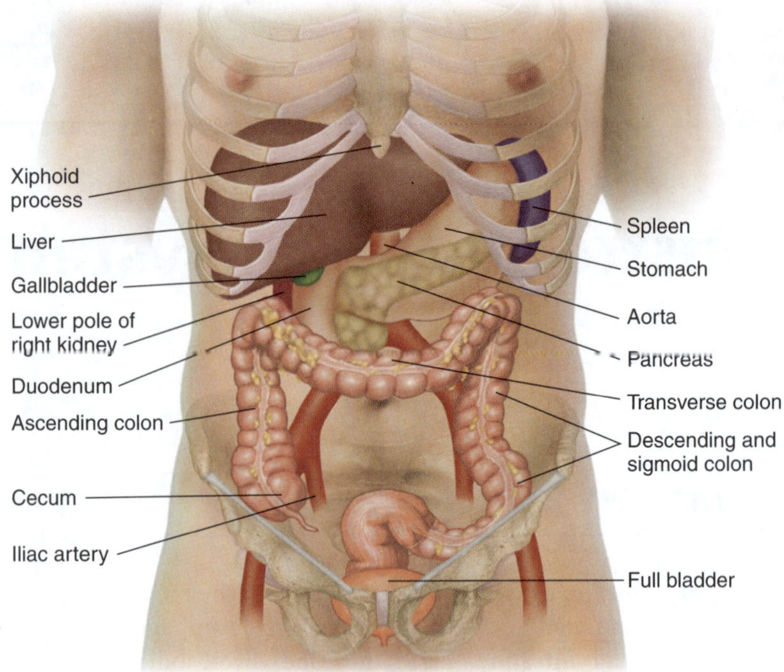

FIGURE 12-2. Abdominal viscera in situ.

Abdominal Cavity and Contents

For descriptive purposes, the abdomen is often divided by imaginary horizontal and vertical lines crossing at the umbilicus, forming the right upper, right lower, left upper, and left lower quadrants (Fig. 12-3). Box 12-1 provides the anatomic structures located within each quadrant. Another system divides the abdomen into nine regions. Terms for three of them are commonly used: *epigastric*, *umbilical*, and *hypogastric* or *suprapubic* (Fig. 12-4).

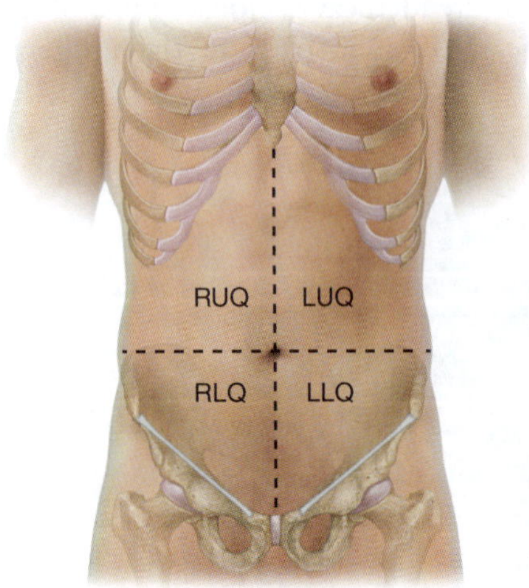

FIGURE 12-3. Quadrants of the abdomen.

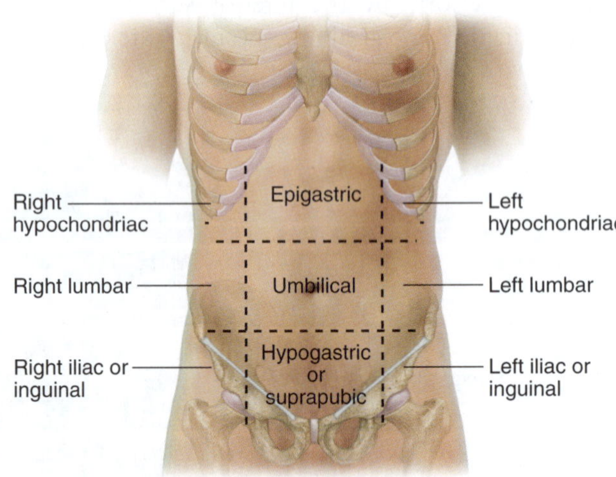

FIGURE 12-4. Regions of the abdomen.

Box 12-1. Abdominal Structures by Quadrant	
Right upper quadrant (RUQ)	Liver, gallbladder, pylorus, duodenum, hepatic flexure of colon, and head of pancreas
Left upper quadrant (LUQ)	Spleen, splenic flexure of colon, stomach, and body and tail of pancreas
Left lower quadrant (LLQ)	Sigmoid colon, descending colon, and left ovary
Right lower quadrant (RLQ)	Cecum, appendix, ascending colon, terminal ileum, and right ovary

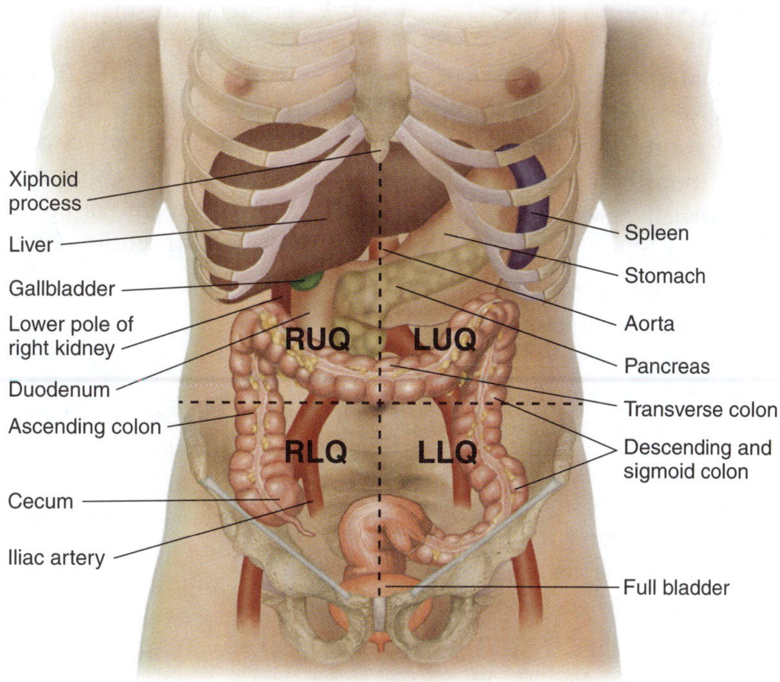

FIGURE 12-5. Abdominal quadrants and underlying structures.

In the *right upper quadrant (RUQ)*, the soft consistency of the *liver* makes it difficult to palpate through the abdominal wall. The lower margin of the liver, the liver edge, can be palpable at the right costal margin. The *gallbladder*, which rests against the inferior surface of the liver, and the more deeply lying *duodenum* are generally not palpable unless pathologic. Moving medially, the examiner encounters the rib cage with its *xiphoid process*, which protects the *stomach*. The *abdominal aorta* can have visible pulsations and may be palpable in the upper abdomen, or epigastrium in thin patients. At a deeper level, the lower pole of the right kidney and the tip of the 12th floating rib may be palpable, especially in children and thin individuals with relaxed abdominal muscles.

In the *left upper quadrant (LUQ)*, the *spleen* is lateral to and behind the stomach, just above the left kidney in the left midaxillary line. Its upper margin rests against the dome of the diaphragm. The 9th, 10th, and 11th ribs protect most of the spleen. The tip of the spleen may be palpable below the left costal margin in a small percentage of adults (in contrast to readily palpable splenic enlargement, or *splenomegaly*). In healthy people the *pancreas* cannot be detected.

The *left lower quadrant (LLQ)* contains the *sigmoid colon*. Portions of the distal colon (descending and sigmoid) may be palpable, especially if stool is present. In the lower midline are the *urinary bladder*, which can often be palpated when distended and in women, the *uterus* and *ovaries*.

The *appendix* is located in the right lower quadrant (RLQ) at the base of the *cecum*, the first part of the large intestine where the *terminal ileum* enters the large intestine at the *ileocecal valve*. In healthy people, these are not palpable (Fig. 12-5).

The *kidneys* lie posteriorly in the abdominal cavity behind the peritoneum (*retroperitoneal*). The ribs protect their upper poles (Fig. 12-6). The *costovertebral angle (CVA)*, formed by the lower border of the 12th rib and the transverse processes of the upper lumbar vertebrae, defines where to elicit for kidney tenderness, called *costovertebral angle tenderness*.

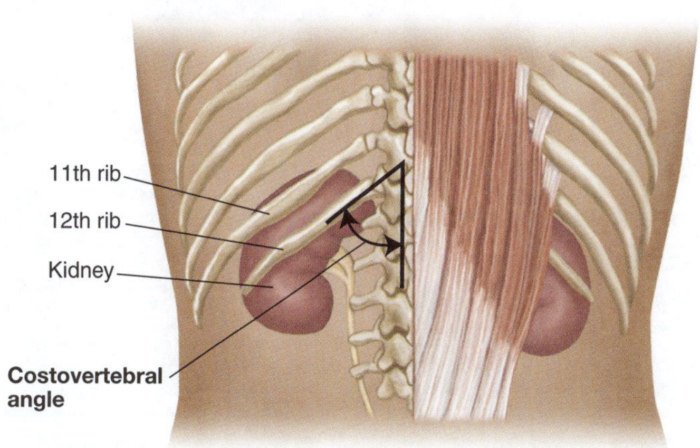

FIGURE 12-6. Kidneys and the costovertebral angle.

Pelvic Cavity and Contents

Continuous with the abdominal cavity, but angulated posteriorly, lies the funnel-shaped *pelvic cavity*, which contains the terminal ureters; bladder; pelvic genital organs; and, at times, loops of small and large intestine. These organs are partially protected by the surrounding pelvis.

The *sigmoid colon* terminates at the *rectum*, the most distal part of the lower GI tract, which extends from the *rectosigmoid junction* at the *sacral promontory*, anterior to the S3 vertebra, to the *anorectal junction*. The rectum then merges into the short segment of the *anal canal* (Fig. 12-7).

The *anus* extends proximally from the anorectal ring distally to the anal verge. The **anal verge** is the junction of hair-bearing and hairless skin at the external anus. Beyond the verge extending externally is the *perianal skin*, which is also referred to as the *anal margin*. The *external anal sphincter* is composed of skeletal muscle that is under voluntary control. The *internal anal sphincter* is an extension of the outer smooth muscle layer of the rectum and is under involuntary control. The *anorectal ring* can be palpated superior to the external anal sphincter.

Carefully note the angle of the anal canal, on a line roughly between the anus and the umbilicus. Unlike the rectum, the canal is liberally supplied by somatic sensory nerves, and a poorly directed finger or instrument will produce pain.

A serrated line marking the change from skin to mucous membrane demarcates the anal canal from the rectum (Fig. 12-8). This *anorectal junction*, often called the *pectinate or dentate line*, is also the boundary between somatic and visceral nerve supplies and is where transitional columnar epithelium is adjacent to the distal squamous epithelium. It is easily visible on anoscopic or endoscopic examination but is not palpable.

Groin

The *groin* or the *inguinal area* lies in the junctional area between the lower part of the abdomen and the thigh on either side of the pubic bone. The basic landmarks in the groin are the *anterior superior iliac spine* in the iliac bone, the *pubic tubercle* of the superior ramus of the pubic bone, and the *inguinal ligament* that runs between them, which are readily identified (Fig. 12-9).

The *inguinal canal*, which lies medial to and roughly parallel to the *inguinal ligament*, forms a tunnel for the vas deferens as it passes through the abdominal muscles. The internal opening of the canal, the *internal inguinal ring*, is approximately 1 cm above the midpoint of the inguinal ligament. Neither the canal nor the internal ring is palpable through the abdominal wall. The exterior opening of the tunnel, the *external inguinal ring*, is a triangular slit-like structure palpable just above and lateral to the pubic tubercle.

The *femoral canal* lies below the inguinal ligament. Although this canal is not visible, you can estimate its

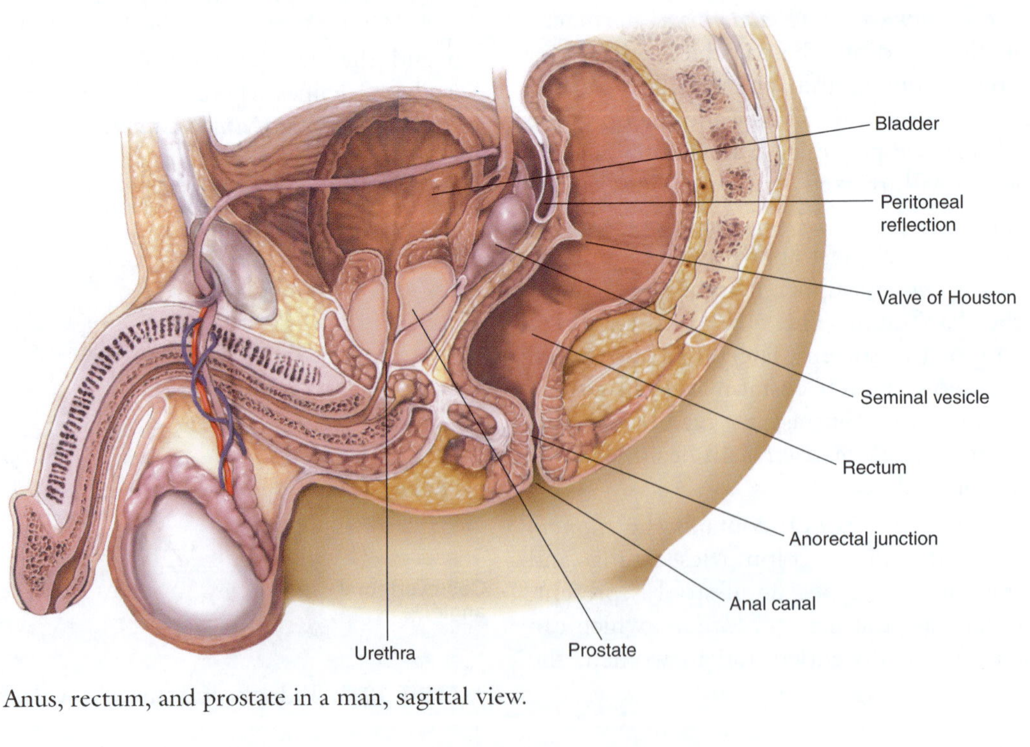

FIGURE 12-7. Anus, rectum, and prostate in a man, sagittal view.

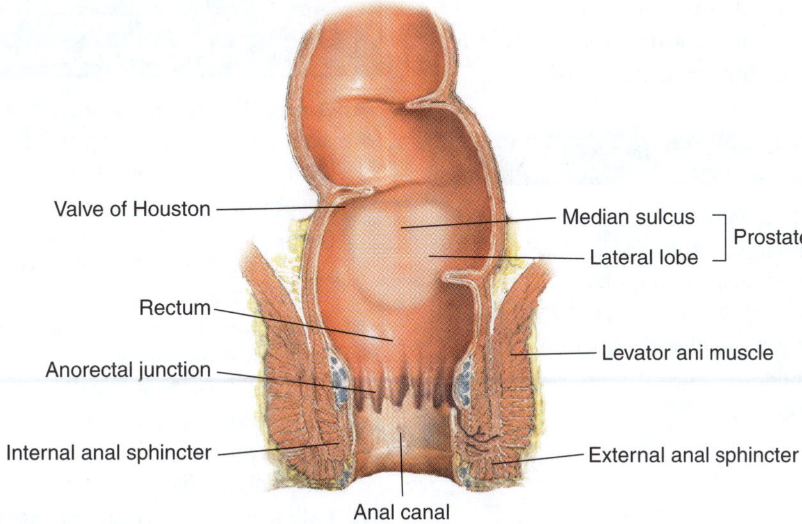

FIGURE 12-8. Anus and rectum, coronal view showing the anterior wall.

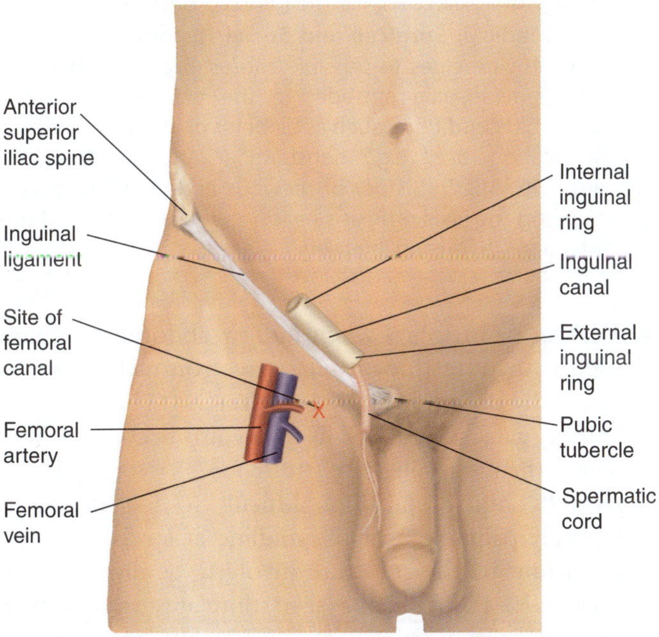

FIGURE 12-9. Anatomic landmarks of the right groin.

location by placing your right index finger, from below, on the right femoral artery. Your middle finger will then overlie the femoral vein and your ring finger, the femoral canal.

Femoral hernias protrude at this location and are more likely to present as emergencies with bowel incarceration or strangulation.

The *femoral artery* enters the thigh from behind the inguinal ligament as the common femoral artery. The *femoral vein*, which drains blood from the lower extremity, ends at the inferior margin of the inguinal ligament where it becomes the external iliac vein. The femoral vein accompanies and lies medial to the femoral artery in the *femoral sheath* right behind the inguinal ligament.

When loops of bowel force their way through the *inguinal canal*, they produce inguinal hernias. Indirect inguinal hernias develop at the internal inguinal ring, where the spermatic cord exits the abdomen. **Direct inguinal hernias** arise more medially due to weakness in the floor of the inguinal canal and are associated with straining and heavy lifting. See Table 12-1, Course, Presentation, and Differentiation of Hernias in the Groin.

HEALTH HISTORY: GENERAL APPROACH

The interview of patients presenting with symptoms concerning the abdomen requires a systematic approach. It is often advisable to align your history taking in parallel with the structures within the abdominopelvic cavity as well as its layers. Keep the anatomical placement of the structures in the abdomen in mind to guide your questions. Ask clarifying questions to exactly know what is meant by each symptom. For example, the term "heartburn" may mean pain from reflux but may also mean angina. "Spitting up blood" may mean blood arising from the GI tract but may also mean blood coming from the upper airways. Qualify each symptom by learning about the acuity of onset, triggering events, quality, progression, and exacerbating and relieving factors. Over time, you will be able to modify this structure-based approach and ask fewer but more focused questions that are relevant to the given presenting complaint. Remember that it takes time to become competent at this. Your skills in history taking and examination, and clustering your findings, are important determinants of sound clinical reasoning and an astute differential diagnosis.

Common or Concerning Symptoms

- Abdominal pain, acute and chronic
- Associated gastrointestinal symptoms including indigestion, nausea, vomiting including blood (hematemesis), loss of appetite (anorexia), early satiety
- Difficulty swallowing (dysphagia) and/or painful swallowing (odynophagia)
- Change in bowel function
- Diarrhea
- Constipation
- Jaundice
- Pain with defecation; rectal bleeding or tenderness
- Anal warts or fissures

GI complaints rank high among reasons for office and emergency room visits. You will encounter a wide variety of upper GI symptoms, including abdominal pain, reflux, nausea and vomiting with or without blood, difficulty or pain with swallowing, loss of appetite, and jaundice. Lower GI complaints are also common: pain; diarrhea; constipation; change in bowel habits; and blood in the stool, which can be further classified as bright red blood or dark and tarry (*melena*).

Numerous symptoms also originate in the genitourinary (GU) tract: difficulty initiating urination, urgency and frequency, hesitancy and decreased stream in men, high urine volume, frequent urination at night (*nocturia*), incontinence, blood in the urine (*hematuria*), and flank pain and colic from renal stones or infection. These are often accompanied by GI symptoms such as abdominal pain, nausea, and vomiting.

Abdominal Pain

The history of present illness is arguably the most important part of the interview for the patient presenting with abdominal pain. Attempt to clarify the presenting symptoms carefully and obtain clues from accompanying symptoms as described in Box 12-2. A careful history alone can lead to the correct diagnosis in most cases.

Medicine History Taking OSCE Videos: **Abdominal Pain**

Before exploring common symptoms, review the mechanisms and clinical patterns of abdominal pain. There are three broad categories of abdominal pain:

See Table 12-2, Abdominal Pain.

Box 12-2. Key Information to Obtain in the Medical Interview of a Patient with Abdominal Pain

- **Onset:** The timing as to when the patient's symptoms occurred and its progression can help determine the likelihood of an emergent cause.
- **Location:** The knowledge of where the viscera are positioned in the abdominal cavity is a key part in narrowing the differential diagnosis to the potential affected organs. (See Fig. 12-5.)
- **Character:** Determining the underlying pathophysiologic process of the patent's pain (*visceral* or *somatic*) may help in elucidating the cause. (See Table 12-2.)
- **Radiation:** Presence or absence of pain migration can help determine the cause, especially in disease processes involving the liver, biliary tract, and appendix.
- **Palliative, Provoking, or Associated Factors:** These may provide insight into the differential diagnosis. Examples include relief of pain by vomiting, increased pain with eating, anorexia, fever, diarrhea, and constipation.
- **Past Medical, Surgical, and Social History:** These can help provide clues to possible causes. Examples include prior similar pain episodes in the past; presence of comorbid conditions, such as diabetes or atrial fibrillation; medication use (e.g., nonsteroidal anti-inflammatory drugs [NSAIDs]), history of previous abdominal surgery; smoking and illicit drug use; history of sexually transmitted infections (STIs); and infertility.

- *Visceral* pain occurs when hollow abdominal organs such as the intestine or biliary tree contract unusually forcefully or are distended or stretched (Fig. 12-10). Solid organs such as the liver can also become painful when their capsules are stretched. Visceral pain is typically nonspecific and difficult to localize. It is typically palpable near the midline at levels that vary according to the structure involved, as illustrated in Figure 12-10. Ischemia also stimulates visceral pain fibers. Visceral pain varies in quality and may be gnawing, cramping, or aching. As the pain progresses, systemic symptoms such as sweating, pallor, nausea, vomiting, and restlessness may follow.

Visceral pain in the RUQ suggests liver distention against its capsule from the various causes of hepatitis, including alcoholic hepatitis or biliary pathology.

Visceral periumbilical pain can be suggestive of early acute appendicitis from distention of an inflamed appendix. It gradually changes to parietal pain in the RLQ from inflammation of the adjacent parietal peritoneum.

For pain disproportionate to physical findings, suspect intestinal mesenteric ischemia.

- *Somatic or parietal* pain originates from inflammation of the parietal peritoneum, called *peritonitis*, which can be localized or diffuse. It is a steady, aching pain

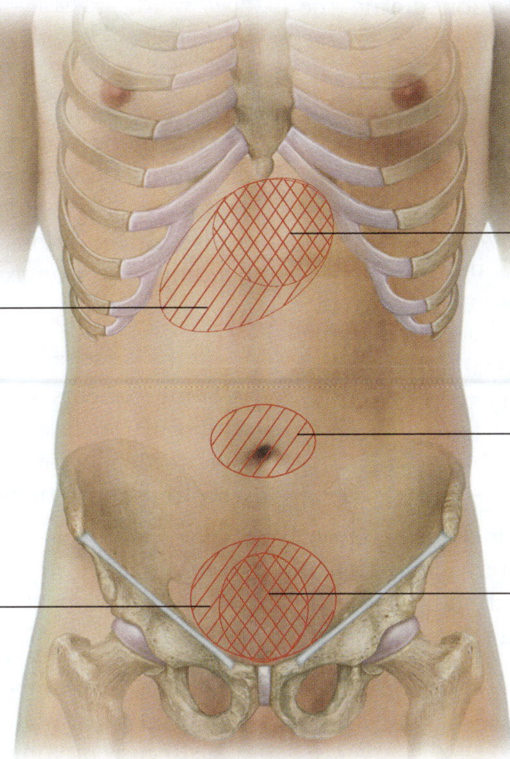

FIGURE 12-10. Areas of manifestation of visceral pain from abdominal viscera.

that is usually more severe than visceral pain and more precisely localized over the involved structure. It is typically aggravated by movement or coughing. Patients with parietal pain usually prefer to lie still.

In contrast to peritonitis, patients with colicky pain from a renal stone move around frequently trying to find a comfortable position.

- *Referred* pain is felt in more distant sites that are innervated at approximately the same spinal levels as the disordered structures. Referred pain often develops as the initial pain becomes more intense and seems to radiate or travel from the initial site. Palpation at the site of referred pain often does not result in tenderness.

Pain of duodenal or pancreatic origin may be referred to the back, pain from the biliary tree, to the right scapular region or the right posterior thorax.

Pain from pleurisy or inferior wall myocardial infarction may be referred to the epigastric area.

Pain may also be referred to the abdomen from the chest, spine, or pelvis, further complicating the assessment of abdominal pain.

Upper Abdominal Pain, Discomfort, and Heartburn. Understanding carefully defined terminology will help you identify the patient's underlying condition. *Discomfort* is defined as a subjective negative feeling that is nonpainful. It can include various symptoms such as bloating, nausea, upper abdominal fullness, and heartburn.

Studies suggest that neuropeptides such as 5 hydroxytryptophan and substance P mediate interconnected symptoms of pain, bowel dysfunction, and stress.

Acute Upper Abdominal Pain or Discomfort. For patients with abdominal pain, causes range from benign to life threatening, so take the time to conduct a careful history.

- First determine how the pain started. Was there an inciting event? Then establish the timing of the pain. Is it acute or chronic? Acute abdominal pain has many patterns. Did the pain start suddenly or gradually? When did it begin? How long does it last? What is its pattern over a 24-hour period? Over weeks or months? Is the illness acute, or chronic and recurring?

In emergency rooms, 40% to 45% of patients have nonspecific pain, but 15% to 30% need surgery, usually for appendicitis, intestinal obstruction, or cholecystitis.

- Ask patients to *describe the pain in their own words.* Pursue important details: "Where does the pain start?" "Does it radiate or travel anywhere?" "What is the pain like?" Only if the patient has trouble describing the pain, you should try offering several choices: "Is it sharp or dull, constant or intermittent?" "Has the pain traveled or changed in nature since the onset?"
- Then ask the patient to *point to the pain.* Patients cannot always clearly describe the location of pain in words. The quadrant where the pain is located helps identify the underlying organs that may be involved.

If clothes interfere, repeat the question during the physical examination.

Epigastric pain can occur with gastroesophageal reflex disease (GERD), pancreatitis, and perforated duodenal ulcers. RUQ pain is associated with pathology with the biliary tree and the liver.

- Ask the patient to rank the *severity of the pain* on a scale of 1 to 10. Note that severity does not always help identify the cause. Sensitivity to abdominal pain varies widely and tends to diminish in older adults, masking acute abdominal conditions. Individual differences in pain thresholds and accommodation to pain during daily activities also affect ratings of severity.
- As you explore *factors that aggravate or relieve the pain*, pay special attention to body position, association with meals, alcohol, medications (including aspirin, NSAIDs, and any over-the-counter medications), stress, and use of antacids. Ask if indigestion or discomfort is related to exertion and relieved by rest.

Note that angina from inferior wall coronary artery disease may present as "indigestion," but is precipitated by exertion and relieved by rest.

Chronic Upper Abdominal Discomfort or Pain. *Dyspepsia* is defined as chronic or recurrent discomfort or pain centered in the upper abdomen, characterized by epigastric pain or burning (or both) and postprandial fullness or early satiety (or both). Note that bloating, nausea, or belching can occur alone but also can accompany other disorders. If these conditions occur alone, they do not meet the criteria for dyspepsia.

Bloating may occur with a spectrum of disorders ranging from benign to more concerning, such as lactose intolerance, irritable bowel syndrome (IBS), inflammatory bowel disease (IBD), and GERD, to early presentation of malignancies.

Many patients with upper abdominal discomfort or pain will have *functional*, or *non-ulcer, dyspepsia*, defined as a 3-month history of nonspecific upper abdominal discomfort or nausea not attributable to structural abnormalities or peptic ulcer disease (PUD). Symptoms are usually recurring and present for more than 6 months.

Multifactorial causes include delayed gastric emptying (20% to 40%), PUD with or without *Helicobacter pylori* (20% to 60%), PUD (up to 15% if *H. pylori* is present), IBS, and psychosocial factors.

Many patients with chronic upper abdominal discomfort or pain complain of heartburn, dysphagia, or effortless regurgitation.

If patients report heartburn and effortless regurgitation together more than once a week, the accuracy of diagnosing GERD is over 90%.

These symptoms or mucosal damage on endoscopy are the diagnostic criteria for GERD. Risk factors include reduced salivary flow, which increases mucosal acid exposure by dampening the actions of the bicarbonate buffer; obesity; delayed gastric emptying; selected medications; hiatal hernia and increased intraabdominal pressure.

Heartburn is a rising retrosternal burning pain or discomfort occurring weekly or more often. It is typically aggravated by foods such as alcohol; chocolate; citrus fruits; coffee; onions; and peppermint; or positions like bending over, exercising, lifting, or lying supine.

Angina from inferior wall coronary ischemia along the diaphragm may also present as heartburn.

Some patients with GERD have atypical respiratory symptoms such as chest pain, cough, wheezing, and aspiration pneumonia. Others complain of pharyngeal symptoms, such as hoarseness chronic sore throat, and laryngitis.

A total of 30% to 90% of patients with asthma and 10% with specialty referral for throat conditions have GERD-like symptoms.

- Some patients may have "alarm symptoms," such as
  - Difficulty swallowing (*dysphagia*)
  - Pain with swallowing (*odynophagia*)
  - Recurrent vomiting
  - Evidence of GI bleeding
  - Early satiety
  - Weight loss
  - Anemia
  - Risk factors for gastric cancer
  - Palpable mass
  - Painless jaundice

Patients who have uncomplicated GERD who fail empiric therapy, age >55 years, and "alarm symptoms" warrant endoscopy to evaluate possible esophagitis, peptic strictures, Barrett esophagus, or esophageal cancer.

Of those with suspected GERD, ~50% to 85% have no disease on endoscopy.

Approximately 10% of patients with chronic longstanding heartburn have *Barrett esophagus*, a metaplastic change in the esophageal lining from normal squamous to columnar epithelium. In those affected, dysplasia on endoscopy increases the risk of esophageal cancer from 0.1% to 0.5% (no dysplasia) to 6% to 19% per patient year (high-grade dysplasia).

Lower Abdominal Pain and Discomfort. Lower abdominal pain and discomfort may be acute or chronic. Asking the patient to point to the pain and characterize all its features, combined with findings on the physical examination, is key to identifying possible causes. Some acute pain, especially in the suprapubic area or radiating from the flank, may originate in the GU tract.

Acute Lower Abdominal Pain. Patients may complain of acute pain localized to the RLQ. Find out if it is sharp and continuous, or intermittent and cramping, causing them to double over.

RLQ pain or pain that migrates from the periumbilical region, combined with nausea, vomiting, and loss of appetite is suspicious for *appendicitis*. In women, consider pelvic inflammatory disease (PID), ruptured ovarian follicle, and ectopic pregnancy.

Combining clinical examination findings with laboratory inflammatory markers and imaging (CT scan, ultrasound) markedly reduces misdiagnosis and unnecessary surgery.

Cramping pain radiating to the flank or groin accompanied by urinary symptoms may be suggestive of *nephrolithiasis* (renal stone).

When patients report acute pain in the LLQ or diffuse abdominal pain, investigate associated symptoms such as fever and loss of appetite.

Pain in the LLQ accompanied by diarrhea in a patient with a history of constipation is suggestive of *diverticulitis*. Nonspecific diffuse abdominal pain with abdominal distention, nausea, emesis, and lack of flatus and/or bowel movements is symptomatic of a *bowel obstruction*.

Patients who have peritonitis require surgical evaluation urgently. *Peritonitis* is marked by severe diffuse abdominal pain with guarding and rigidity on examination. Patients may or may not have accompanying abdominal **distention**.

Chronic Lower Abdominal Pain. If there is *chronic pain* in the quadrants of the lower abdomen, ask about change in bowel habits and alternating diarrhea and constipation.

Change in bowel habits with a palpable mass warns of late-stage colon cancer.

Diagnostic criteria for IBS is a diagnosis of exclusion and requires intermittent pain for 12 weeks of the preceding 12 months with relief from defecation, change in frequency of bowel movements, or change in form of stool (loose, watery, pellet-like), linked to luminal and mucosal irritants that alter motility, secretion, and pain sensitivity.

Abdominal Pain and Associated Gastrointestinal Symptoms

Patients often experience abdominal pain in conjunction with other symptoms. Begin by asking "How is your appetite?" then pursue symptoms such as *indigestion*, *nausea*, *vomiting*, and *anorexia*.

Indigestion. *Indigestion* is a general term for distress associated with eating that can have many meanings. Urge your patient to be more specific.

Anorexia, nausea, and vomiting accompany many disorders ranging from benign to more insidious, including pregnancy, diabetic ketoacidosis, adrenal insufficiency, hypercalcemia, uremia, liver disease, emotional states, and adverse drug reactions. Induced vomiting without nausea is more indicative of bulimia.

Nausea and Vomiting. *Nausea*, often described as "feeling sick to my stomach," may progress to retching and vomiting. *Retching* describes involuntary spasm of the stomach, diaphragm, and esophagus that precedes and culminates in *vomiting*, the forceful expulsion of gastric contents out of the mouth.

Medicine History Taking OSCE Videos: **Vomiting**

Some patients may not actually vomit but raise esophageal or gastric contents without nausea or retching, called *regurgitation*.

Regurgitation is a common symptom of GERD; however, it can also be a presenting symptom of esophageal stricture, Zenker diverticulum, or esophageal or gastric malignancy.

Ask about any vomitus or regurgitated material and inspect it if possible, noting the color, odor, and quantity. Help the patient to specify the amount: a teaspoon? Two teaspoons? A cupful?

Vomiting and nausea with constipation or **obstipation** (severe constipation with inability to pass both stool and gas) is indicative of a bowel obstruction and warrants further imaging workup.

Patients with symptoms and abdominal pain and tenderness may have ischemia, which requires urgent cross-sectional imaging and surgical consultation.

Hematemesis. Ask specifically if the vomitus contains any blood and quantify the amount. Gastric juice is clear and mucoid. Small amounts of yellowish or greenish bile are common and have no special significance. Brownish or blackish vomitus with a "coffee grounds" appearance suggests blood altered by gastric acid. Bloody emesis is called *hematemesis*.

Hematemesis may accompany esophageal or gastric varices, Mallory–Weiss tears, or PUD.

Is there any dehydration from prolonged vomiting or significant blood loss? Do the patient's symptoms suggest any complications of vomiting, such as aspiration into the lungs, seen in debilitated, obtunded, or elderly patients?

Symptoms of blood loss such as lightheadedness or syncope depend on the rate and volume of bleeding and are rare until blood loss exceeds 500 mL.

Anorexia. *Anorexia* is loss or lack of appetite. Find out if it arises from intolerance to certain foods, fear of abdominal discomfort (or "*food fear*"), or distortions in self-image. Check for associated nausea and vomiting.

Early Satiety. Patients may complain of unpleasant abdominal fullness after light or moderate meals, or early satiety, the inability to eat a full meal. A dietary assessment or recall may be warranted.

If fullness or early satiety, consider diabetic gastroparesis, anticholinergic medications, gastric outlet obstruction, and gastric cancer.

Difficulty Swallowing (Dysphagia) and/or Painful Swallowing (Odynophagia)

Less commonly, patients may report difficulty swallowing from impaired passage of solid foods or liquids from the mouth to the stomach, or **dysphagia**. Food seems to stick or "not go down right," suggesting motility disorders or structural anomalies. The sensation of a lump or foreign body in the throat at rest that improves or disappears with swallowing, called a *globus sensation*, is not true dysphagia.

Xerostomia (insufficient saliva) commonly present in older adult men and women ≥70 years can give rise to the sensation of difficulty swallowing food. For types of dysphagia, see Table 12-3.

Indicators of oropharyngeal dysphagia include delay in initiating swallowing, postnasal regurgitation or coughing from aspiration, and repetitive swallowing to achieve clearance. Causes may be *neurologic* like stroke, Parkinson disease, or amyotrophic lateral sclerosis; *muscular* like muscular dystrophy or myasthenia gravis; or *structural* as seen in esophageal stricture and hypopharyngeal diverticuli (Zenker diverticulum). Causes are generally structural in younger adults and neurologic/muscular in older adults.

Ask the patient to point to where the dysphagia occurs.

Pointing to below the sternoclavicular notch suggests esophageal dysphagia.

Pursue which types of foods provoke symptoms: solids, or solids and liquids? Establish the timing. When does the dysphagia start? Is it intermittent or persistent? Is it progressing? If so, over what time period? Are there associated symptoms and clinical conditions?

If solid foods, consider structural causes like esophageal stricture, webbing or narrowing (*Schatzki ring*), and neoplasm; if solids and liquids, a motility disorder like *achalasia* is more likely.

Is there **odynophagia**, or pain on swallowing?

Consider esophageal ulceration from ingestion of aspirin or NSAIDs; caustic ingestion; radiation; or infection with *Candida*, cytomegalovirus, herpes simplex, or HIV.

Change in Bowel Function

To assess bowel function, start with open-ended questions: "How are your bowel movements?" "How often do they occur in a week?" "Do you have any difficulties?" "Have you noticed any change in stool pattern or appearance?" The range of normal frequency is broad and can be as low as three bowel movements per week.

Some patients may complain of passing excessive gas, or *flatus*.

Causes include excessive and repetitive air swallowing (*aerophagia*), ingestion of legumes or other gas-producing foods, intestinal lactase deficiency, and IBS.

Diarrhea

Diarrhea is defined as painless loose or watery stools during ≥75% of defecations for the prior 3 months, with symptom onset at least 6 months prior to diagnosis. Stool volume may increase to >200 g in 24 hours.

See Table 12-4, Diarrhea.

- Ask about the *duration*. **Acute diarrhea** is defined as diarrhea that lasts less than 14 days, **persistent diarrhea** as lasting 14 to 30 days, and **chronic diarrhea** as more than 30 days.

  Acute diarrhea, especially foodborne, is usually caused by infection. *Chronic diarrhea* is typically noninfectious in origin, as in IBS (Crohn disease and ulcerative colitis) or food allergy.

  Nosocomial diarrhea is a subset of acute diarrhea that starts in the hospital, generally after 72 hours, and is less than 2 weeks in duration. The most common is *Clostridium difficile infection*.

- Ask about the *characteristics of the diarrhea*, including volume, frequency, and consistency.

  High-volume frequent watery stools are usually from the small intestine; small-volume stools with tenesmus or diarrhea with mucus, pus, or blood occur in rectal inflammatory conditions.

- Is there mucus, pus, or blood? Is there associated *tenesmus*, a constant urge to defecate, accompanied by pain, cramping, and involuntary straining?
- Does diarrhea occur at night?

  Nocturnal diarrhea is usually pathologic.

- Are the stools greasy or oily? Frothy? Foul-smelling? Floating on the surface because of excessive gas?

  Oily residue, sometimes frothy or floating, occurs with *steatorrhea* (fatty diarrheal stools) from malabsorption in celiac sprue, pancreatic insufficiency, and small bowel bacterial overgrowth.

- Explore associated features that are important in identifying possible causes. These include current and alternative medications, especially antibiotics, recent travel, diet patterns, baseline bowel habits, and risk factors for immunocompromise.

Diarrhea is common with use of penicillin and macrolides, magnesium-based antacids, metformin, and herbal and alternative medicines.

In patients with recent hospitalizations or antibiotic use or those that are immunocompromised, it is important to consider *C. difficile* infection.

Constipation

Ask about stool characteristics identified by the Rome IV criteria, which stipulate that **constipation** should be present for the last 3 months with symptom onset at least 6 months prior to diagnosis and should have at least two of the following conditions: less than three bowel movements per week, ≥25% or more defecations with either straining or sensation of incomplete evacuation, lumpy or hard stools, or manual facilitation.

See Table 12-5, Constipation.

In *primary* or *functional constipation*, the cause cannot be identified from the history and physical examination. Types include normal transit, slow transit, impaired expulsion (from pelvic floor dysfunction), and combined causes. *Secondary* or *organic constipation* has an identified underlying cause, which may include medications, amyloidosis, diabetes, and central nervous system disorders.

- Check if the patient actually looks at the stool and can describe its color and bulk.

Thin, pencil-like stool occurs in an obstructing "apple-core" lesion of the distal colon.

- What remedies has the patient tried? Do medications or stress play a role? Are there associated systemic disorders?

Anticholinergic agents, antidepressants, calcium-channel blockers, calcium and iron supplements, and opioids can cause medication-induced constipation. Constipation also occurs with diabetes, hypothyroidism, hypercalcemia, hypomagnesemia, multiple sclerosis, Parkinson disease, and systemic sclerosis.

- Occasionally, there is no passage of either stool or gas (*obstipation*).

Obstipation signifies intestinal obstruction.

- Inquire about the color of stools. Is there *melena*, or black tarry stools, or *hematochezia*, stools that are red or maroon-colored? Determine the quantity and frequency of any blood.

See Table 12-6, Black and Bloody Stool.

Melena may appear with as little as 60 mL of blood from upper GI bleeding; hematochezia, if more than 1,000 mL of blood, is usually from lower GI bleeding, but if massive can have an upper GI source.

- Is the blood mixed in with stool or on the surface? Does the blood appear as streaks on the toilet paper or is it more copious?

Blood on the surface or toilet paper may point to the presence of hemorrhoids.

Jaundice

See Chapter 8 for jaundice.

Pain on Defecation

Is there any pain on defecation? Any itching? Any extreme tenderness in the anus or rectum? Is there mucopurulent discharge or bleeding? Any ulcerations? Does the patient have receptive anal intercourse?

Anorectal pain, tenesmus, or discharge and/or bleeding suggest *proctitis*. Causes include IBD; sexually transmitted infections (STIs), such as gonorrhea, chlamydia, lymphogranuloma venereum, herpes simplex, or chancres of primary syphilis (see Table 14-6, Sexually Transmitted Infections of Male Genitalia); trauma from receptive anal intercourse; bacterial infections; and radiation therapy.

Anal Warts and Fissures

Is there any history of anal warts or anal fissures?

Genital warts may arise from human papillomavirus (HPV) or condylomata lata in secondary syphilis. Anal fissures are seen in proctitis and Crohn disease.

PHYSICAL EXAMINATION: GENERAL APPROACH

Once you have carefully interviewed the patient, gathering more information through the physical examination helps narrow the possible causes to specific areas and/or organ systems. A complete physical examination includes a review of patients' vital signs and an inspection of other body areas outside of the GI system, particularly the GU system, cardiopulmonary system, and skin. To begin, explain the steps for examining the abdomen to the patient and ensure you have good lighting. The patient should have an empty bladder. Pay special attention when draping to expose the abdomen, as pictured throughout and detailed in Box 12-3.

Atypical presentations of abdominal pain can be seen in elderly patients who might not mount an adequate response.

Box 12-3. Tips for Examining the Abdomen

- Make the patient comfortable in the supine position, with a pillow under the head and perhaps under the knees.
- Ask the patient to keep the arms at the sides. When the arms are above the head, the abdominal wall stretches and tightens, which hinders palpation.
- *Draping the patient.* Place the drape or sheet at the level of the symphysis pubis, then expose the abdomen by raising the patient's gown to just below the nipple line above the xiphoid process. The groin should be visible, but the genitalia should remain covered. The abdominal muscles should be relaxed to enhance all aspects of the examination, especially palpation.
- Before you begin, ask the patient to point to any areas of pain so that you can examine these areas last.
- Warm your hands by rubbing them together or placing them under lukewarm water.
- Approach the patient calmly and avoid quick, unexpected movements. Avoid having long fingernails that can scratch or scrape the patient's skin.
- Position yourself at the patient's *right side* and proceed in a systematic fashion with inspection, percussion, and palpation. Mentally visualize each organ in the region you are examining. *Watch the patient's face for any signs of pain or discomfort.*
- If necessary, distract the patient with conversation or questions. If the patient is frightened or ticklish, begin palpation with the patient's hand under yours. After a few moments, slip your hand underneath to palpate directly.

TECHNIQUES OF EXAMINATION

Key Components of the Abdominal Examination

Abdomen

- Note the patient's general appearance (demeanor, distress, color, mental status).
- Inspect the surface, contours, and movements of the abdomen including skin temperature, color, and presence of scars or striae.
- Prior to palpation or percussion, place the diaphragm of your stethoscope in one abdominal region and listen for bowel sounds (presence, characteristics, bruits).
- Percuss the abdomen lightly in all four quadrants (tympany, dullness, area of change).
- Palpate lightly with one hand in all four quadrants (masses, tenderness, guarding).
- Palpate deeply with two hands in all four quadrants (liver edge, masses, tenderness, pulsations).

(continued)

- Check for signs of peritonitis (guarding, rigidity, rebound tenderness).

Liver

- Estimate the liver size along right midclavicular line by percussion.
- Palpate and characterize the liver edge (surface, consistency, tenderness).

Spleen

- Percuss for splenic enlargement along Traube space.
- Palpate for the splenic edge with the patient supine and in the right lateral decubitus position.

Kidneys

- Check for costovertebral angle (CVA) tenderness using fist percussion.

Urinary Bladder

- Percuss the urinary bladder (distention, tenderness).

Special Techniques

- Perform special techniques if indicated (ascites, appendicitis, cholecystitis, ventral hernia, abdominal wall mass).
- Evaluate for groin hernias.

Abdomen

Inspection. First, observe the general appearance of the patient. A patient who is pale or confused or writhing with discomfort may pinpoint to an illness of higher acuity compared to someone who is lying quietly.

From the right side of the bed, *inspect the surface, contours, and movements of the abdomen*. Watch for bulges or peristalsis. Try to also lower your viewing plane by bending over or stooping down so that you can observe the abdomen tangentially (Fig. 12-11).

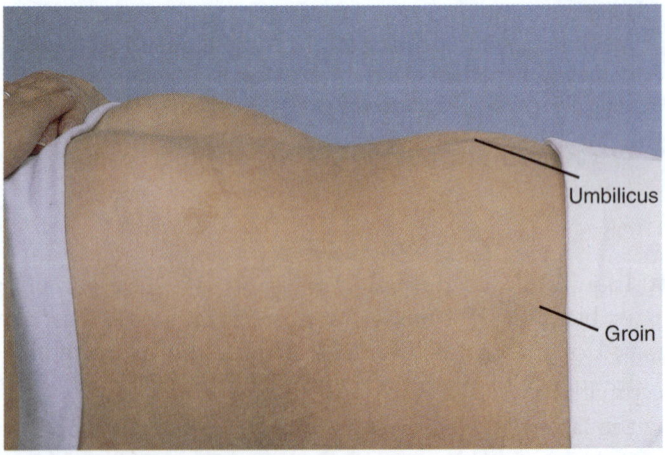

FIGURE 12-11. Inspecting the contours of the abdomen.

Note especially:

- *Skin*, including:
  - *Temperature*. Check if the skin is warm or cool and clammy.
  - *Color*. Note any bruises, erythema, or jaundice.
  - *Scars*. Describe or diagram their location.
  - *Striae*. Old silver striae or stretch marks are normal.

  Pink–purple striae are a hallmark of Cushing syndrome.

  - *Dilated veins*. A few small veins may be visible normally.

  Dilated veins suggest portal hypertension from cirrhosis (caput medusae) or inferior vena cava obstruction.

  - *Rashes* or *ecchymoses*

  Ecchymosis of the abdominal wall is seen in intraperitoneal or retroperitoneal hemorrhage.

  - *Umbilicus*. Observe its contour and location and any inflammation or bulges suggesting a hernia.

  See Table 12-7, Localized Bulges in the Abdominal Wall.

- *Contour of the abdomen*
  - Is it flat, rounded, protuberant, or scaphoid (markedly concave or hollowed)?

  See Table 12-8, Protuberant Abdomens.

  - Do the flanks bulge, or are there any local bulges? Also survey the inguinal and femoral areas.

  Observe for the bulging flanks of ascites, the suprapubic bulge of a distended bladder or pregnant uterus and ventral, femoral, or inguinal hernias.

  - Is the abdomen symmetric?

  Asymmetry suggests a hernia, an enlarged organ, or a mass.

  - Are there visible organs or masses? An enlarged liver or spleen may descend below the rib cage.

  Inspect for lower abdominal masses or hernias.

- *Pulsations*. The normal aortic pulsation is frequently visible in the epigastrium in thin patients.

Inspect for the increased pulsations of an abdominal aortic aneurysm (AAA) or increased pulse pressure.

Auscultation. Auscultate the abdomen before performing percussion or palpation, maneuvers that may alter the characteristics of the bowel sounds. Place the diaphragm of your stethoscope gently on the abdomen for a maximum of 5 minutes. Listen for bowel sounds, which may consist of clicks and gurgles, occurring at an estimated frequency of 5 to 34 per minute. Frequency within this range is considered to be *normoactive* bowel sounds. Occasionally you may hear the prolonged gurgles or rumbling of hyperperistalsis from "stomach growling," called *borborygmi*.

Frequency <5 per minute is considered to arise from *hypoactive* bowel sounds and of >34 per minute from *hyperactive* bowel sounds.

Because bowel sounds are widely transmitted through the abdomen, listening in one area, such as the RLQ, is usually sufficient. Although auscultation of the abdomen is common, it might be of limited use. Changes in bowel sounds heard on auscultation are typically nonspecific and nondiagnostic.

If an abdominal pulsatile mass is seen on physical examination suggestive of an AAA, *auscultation over the mass* may identify the presence of turbulent flow (*bruits*) within the aorta (Fig. 12-12).

A total of 4% to 20% of healthy individuals have abdominal bruits. See Table 12-9, Sounds in the Abdomen.

Friction rubs are infrequently found on abdominal examination but can occur over the liver, spleen, or an abdominal mass.

Friction rubs are present in hepatoma, gonococcal infection around the liver, splenic infarction, and pancreatic carcinoma.

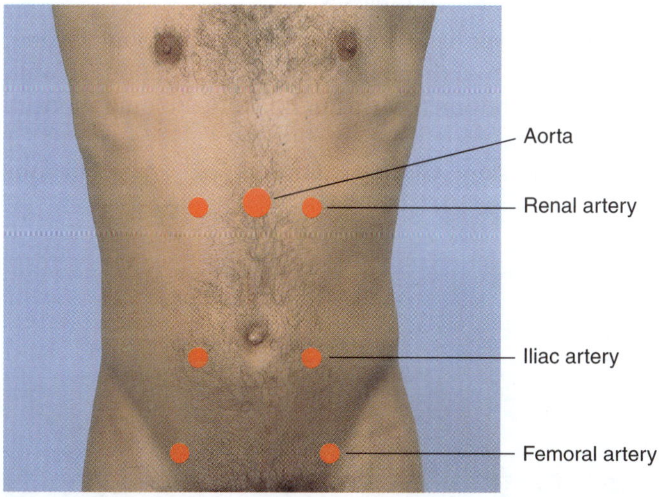

FIGURE 12-12. Abdominal auscultatory areas for bruits.

Percussion. Percussion helps you assess the amount and distribution of gas in the abdomen, viscera and masses that are solid or fluid-filled, and the size of the liver and spleen.

Percuss the abdomen lightly in all four quadrants to determine the distribution of *tympany* and *dullness*. Tympany usually predominates because of gas in the GI tract, but scattered areas of dullness from fluid and feces are also common.

A protuberant abdomen that is tympanitic throughout suggests intestinal obstruction or paralytic ileus. See Table 12-8, Protuberant Abdomens.

- Note any dull areas suggesting an underlying mass or enlarged organ. This observation will guide subsequent palpation.

Dull areas characterize an intrauterine pregnancy, an ovarian tumor, a distended bladder, large volume ascites, or a large liver or spleen.

- On each side of a protuberant abdomen, note where abdominal tympany changes to the dullness of solid posterior structures.

Dullness in both flanks prompts further assessment for ascites.

- Briefly percuss the lower anterior chest above the costal margins. On the right, you will usually find the dullness of the liver; on the left, the tympany that overlies the gastric air bubble and the splenic flexure of the colon.

In the rare condition of *situs inversus,* organs are reversed—air bubble on the right, liver dullness on the left.

Palpation

Light Palpation. Gentle palpation aids detection of abdominal tenderness, muscular resistance, and some superficial organs and masses.

Keeping your hand and forearm on a horizontal plane, with fingers together and flat on the abdominal wall, palpate the abdomen with a light gentle dipping motion. As you move your hand to different quadrants, raise it just off the skin. Gliding smoothly, palpate in all four quadrants (Fig. 12-13).

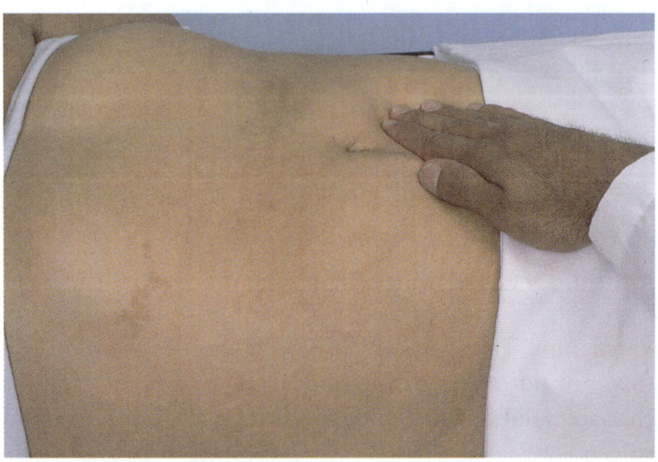

FIGURE 12-13. Using one hand to lightly palpate the abdomen in all four quadrants.

Identify any superficial organs, masses or hernias and any area of tenderness or increased resistance to palpation. If resistance is present, try to distinguish voluntary guarding from **involuntary guarding** or rigidity. *Voluntary guarding* usually decreases with the techniques listed below.

Involuntary guarding or rigidity typically persists despite these maneuvers, suggesting **peritonitis**.

- Ask the patient to bend the lower extremities at the hip to make the abdominal muscles less tense.
- Ask the patient to mouth-breathe with the jaws wide open.
- Palpate after asking the patient to exhale, which usually relaxes the abdominal muscles.

Deep Palpation. Deep palpation is usually required to delineate the liver edge, the kidneys, and abdominal masses. Use one hand over the other to perform this technique. Again, using the palmar surfaces of your fingers, press down in all four quadrants (Fig. 12-14). Identify any masses; note their location, size, shape, consistency, tenderness, pulsations, and any mobility with respiration or pressure from the examining hand. Correlate your findings from palpation with their percussion notes.

Abdominal masses may be categorized in several ways: physiologic (pregnant uterus), inflammatory (diverticulitis), vascular (an AAA), neoplastic (colon cancer), or obstructive (a distended bladder or dilated loop of bowel).

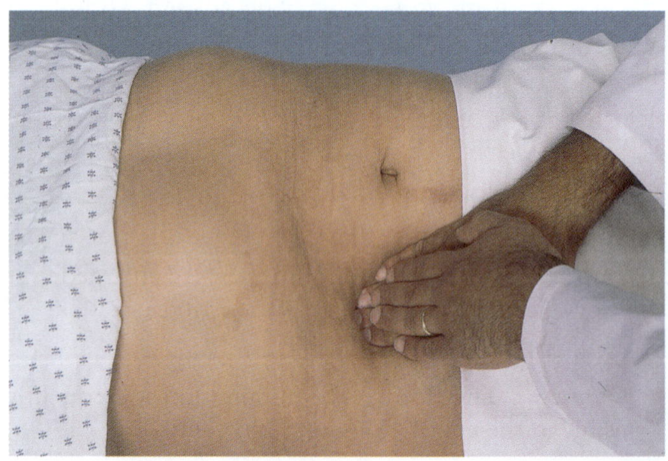

FIGURE 12-14. Using two hands to deeply palpate the abdomen in all four quadrants.

Assessing Possible Peritonitis. Inflammation of the parietal peritoneum, or peritonitis, signals an acute intraabdominal inflammatory process requiring further urgent evaluation and workup. Signs of peritonitis include a *positive cough test, involuntary guarding, rigidity,* ***rebound tenderness,*** *and percussion tenderness.*

When positive, these signs roughly double the likelihood of peritonitis; rigidity makes peritonitis almost four times more likely. Causes include any inflammatory, infectious or ischemic intraabdominal process, such as appendicitis, diverticulitis, cholecystitis, bowel ischemia or perforation.

Even before palpation, ask the patient to cough and identify where the cough produces pain. Then palpate gently, starting with one finger then with your hand, to localize the area of pain. As you palpate, check for the peritoneal signs of guarding, rigidity, and rebound tenderness (Box 12-4).

Box 12-4. Signs of Peritonitis

- *Guarding* is a voluntary contraction of the abdominal wall, often accompanied by a grimace that may diminish when the patient is distracted.
- *Rigidity* is an involuntary reflex contraction of the abdominal wall from peritoneal inflammation that persists over several examinations.
- *Rebound tenderness* refers to pain expressed by the patient after the examiner presses down on an area of tenderness and suddenly removes the hand. To assess rebound tenderness, ask the patient, "Which hurts more, when I press or let go?" Press down with your fingers firmly and slowly, then withdraw your hand quickly. *The maneuver is positive if withdrawal produces pain.* Percuss gently to check for percussion tenderness.

See also Table 12-10, Tender Abdomens.

Liver

Because the rib cage shelters most of the liver, direct assessment is limited. Liver size and shape can be estimated by palpation and percussion. Pressure from your palpating hand helps you to evaluate the surface, consistency, and tenderness of the liver. Percussion helps you approximate the liver size.

In chronic liver disease, finding an enlarged palpable liver edge below the ribs is suggestive of an enlarged liver and cirrhosis.

Percussion. *Estimate the size of the liver by percussion.* Measure the vertical span of liver dullness in the right midclavicular line after carefully locating the midclavicular line to improve accurate measurement (Fig. 12-15). Use a light to moderate percussion strike, because a heavier strike can lead to underestimates of liver size. Starting at a level well below the umbilicus in the RLQ (in an area of tympany, not dullness), percuss upward toward the liver. Identify the lower border of dullness in the midclavicular line (Fig. 12-16).

Estimates of liver span by percussion have a 60% to 70% correlation with actual span.

Next, identify the upper border of liver dullness. Starting at the nipple line, percuss downward in the midclavicular line until lung resonance shifts to liver dullness, as shown in Figure 12-16. Gently displace a woman's breast as necessary to be sure that you start in a resonant area. Now, measure the distance between your two points in centimeters—this is the vertical span of liver dullness. If the liver seems enlarged, outline the lower edge by percussing medially and laterally.

Palpation. *Palpate for the liver edge* below the right costal margin. Place your right hand on the patient's right abdomen lateral to the rectus muscle, with your fingertips (Fig. 12-17). This is done to prevent mistaking the rectus muscle for the underlying and adjacent liver. Also place your hand *well below where you would expect the lower border of the liver, which you previously percussed.* Starting palpation too close to the right costal margin risks missing the lower edge of an enlarged liver that extends into the RLQ. Some examiners point their fingers up toward the patient's head, whereas others prefer a somewhat more oblique position. In either case, press gently in and up.

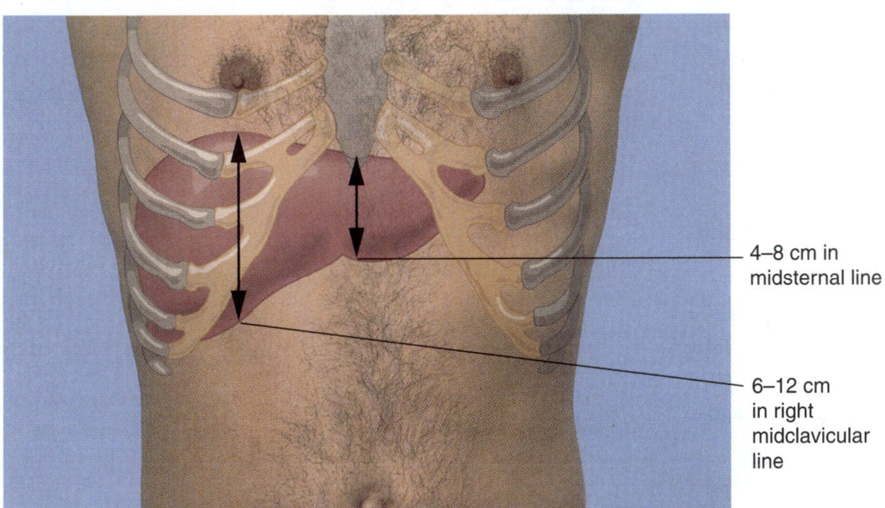

FIGURE 12-15. Area of percussion for estimating liver size along the right midclavicular line.

The span of liver dullness is increased when the liver is enlarged. The span of liver dullness is decreased when the liver is small or when there is free air below the diaphragm, as from a perforated bowel or hollow viscus.

Liver dullness may be displaced downward by the low diaphragm of chronic obstructive pulmonary disease. Span, however, remains normal.

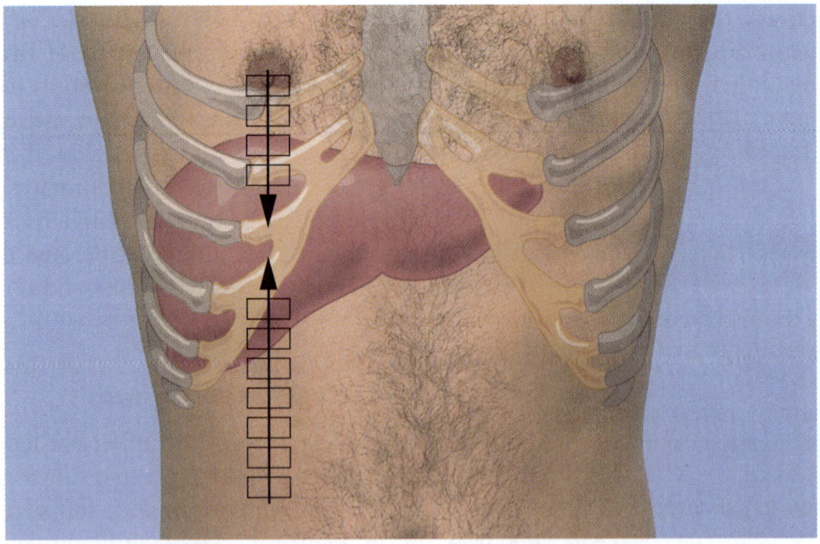

FIGURE 12-16. Percussing for liver dullness.

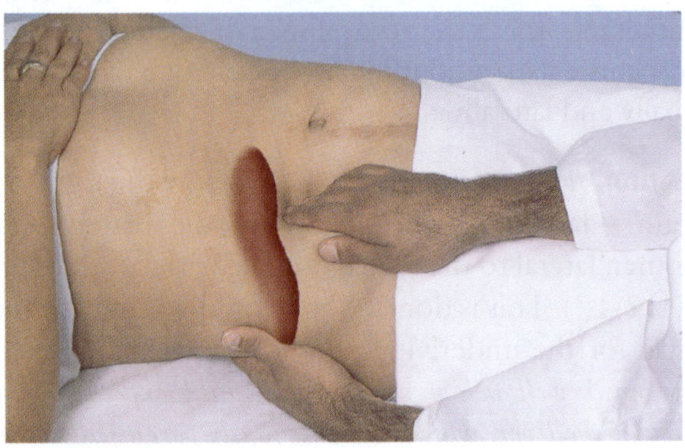

FIGURE 12-17. Palpating for the liver edge.

Ask the patient to take a deep breath. Try to feel the liver edge as the air-filled lungs and the diaphragm push the liver down to meet your fingertips. When palpable, the normal liver edge is soft, distinct in outline, and with a smooth surface. If you feel the edge, slightly lighten the pressure of your palpating hand so that the liver can slip under your fingerpads and you can feel its anterior surface. Note any tenderness (the normal liver may be slightly tender).

Firmness or hardness of the liver, bluntness or rounding of its edge, and surface irregularity are suspicious for liver disease.

On inspiration, the liver is palpable about 3 cm below the right costal margin in the midclavicular line. Some patients breathe more with the chest than with the diaphragm. It may be helpful to ask such patients to "breathe with the abdomen," which brings the liver, as well as the spleen and kidneys, into a palpable position during inspiration.

An obstructed distended gallbladder may merge with the liver, forming a firm oval mass below the liver edge and an area that is dull to percussion.

To palpate the liver edge, you may have to adapt your examining pressure to the thickness and resistance of the abdominal wall. If you cannot feel the edge, move your palpating hand closer to the costal margin and try again. A palpable liver edge *does not* reliably indicate hepatomegaly.

See Table 12-11, Liver Enlargement: Apparent and Real.

Physiology OSCE Video:
Palpation of Liver

Trace the liver edge both laterally and medially. Palpation through the rectus muscles is especially difficult. Describe the liver edge and measure its distance from the right costal margin in the midclavicular line.

Hooking Technique. The "hooking technique" may be helpful, especially when the patient is obese. Stand to the right of the patient's chest. Place both hands, side by side, on the right abdomen below the border of liver dullness. Press in with your fingers and up toward the costal margin (Fig. 12-18). Ask the patient to take a deep breath. The liver edge shown in Figure 12-19 is palpable with the fingerpads of both hands.

Spleen

When a spleen enlarges, it expands anteriorly, downward, and medially, often replacing the tympany of stomach and colon with the dullness of a solid organ. It then becomes palpable below the costal margin. Dullness to percussion suggests splenic enlargement but may be absent when enlarged spleens lie above the costal margin. Continue to examine the patient from the patient's right side.

Physiology OSCE Videos:
Palpation of Spleen

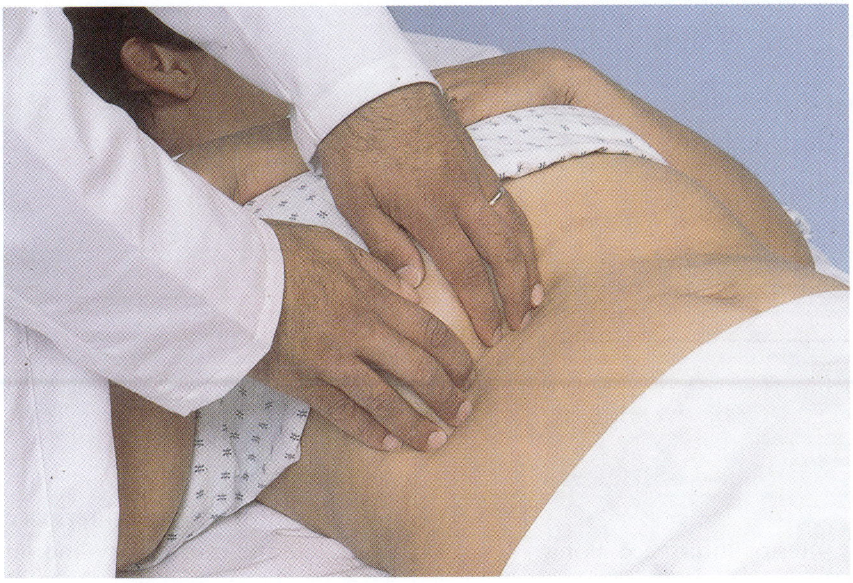

FIGURE 12-18. Hooking technique for palpating the liver edge.

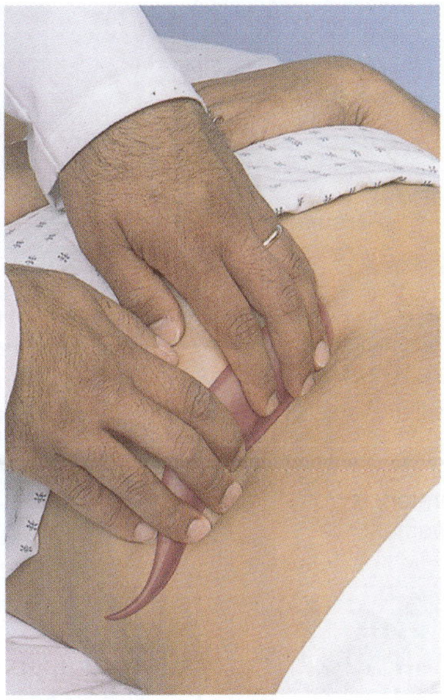

FIGURE 12-19. Applying the "hooking" technique to palpate the liver edge.

Percussion. Two techniques may help you to detect *splenomegaly,* an enlarged spleen:

Percussion is moderately accurate in detecting splenomegaly (sensitivity, 60% to 80%; specificity, 72% to 94%).

- *Percuss the left lower anterior chest wall* roughly from the border of cardiac dullness at the sixth rib to the anterior axillary line and down to the costal margin, an area termed *Traube (semilunar) space.* As you percuss along the routes marked by the arrows in the Figures 12-20 and 12-21, you should note tympany. If tympany is prominent, especially laterally, splenomegaly is unlikely.

If percussion dullness is present, palpation correctly detects splenomegaly more than 80% of the time.

Fluid or solids in the stomach or colon may also cause dullness in Traube space.

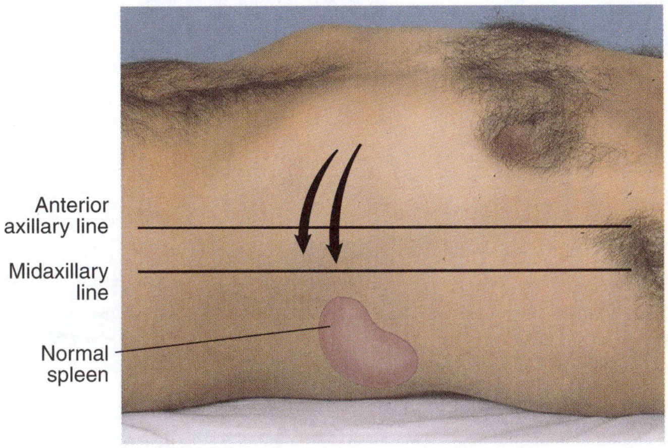

FIGURE 12-20. Area of percussion to detect splenic enlargement along Traube space.

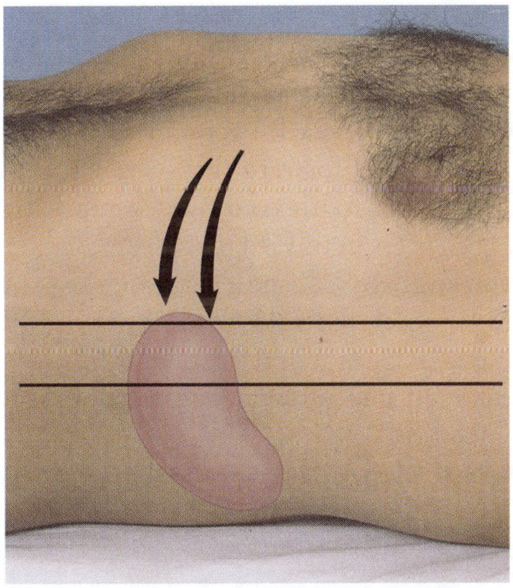

FIGURE 12-21. Area of percussion dullness in splenic enlargement.

- *Check for a splenic percussion sign (Castell sign).* Percuss the lowest interspace in the left anterior axillary line (Fig. 12-22). This area is usually tympanitic. Then ask the patient to take a deep breath to let the air-filled lungs and diaphragm push the spleen and percuss again. When spleen size is normal, the percussion note usually remains tympanitic despite this downward displacement by the diaphragm.

A change in percussion note from tympany to dullness on inspiration is a *positive splenic percussion sign,* but this sign is only moderately useful for detecting splenomegaly (Fig. 12-23).

If either or both of these tests are positive, pay extra attention to palpation of the spleen.

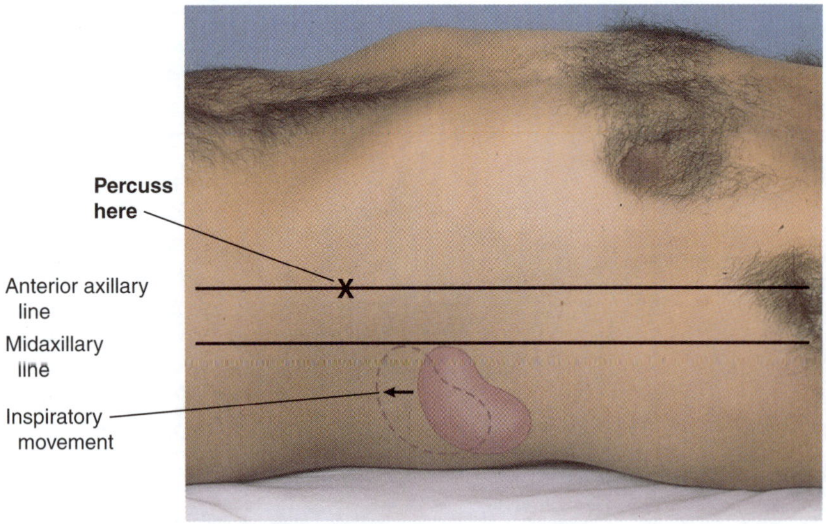

FIGURE 12-22. Percussion tympany on most inferior interspace along left anterior axillary line on deep inspiration (negative splenic percussion sign).

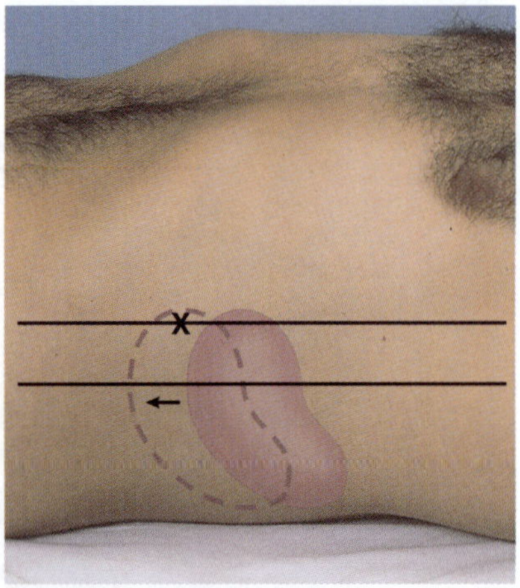

FIGURE 12-23. Percussion dullness on most inferior interspace along left anterior axillary line on deep inspiration (positive splenic percussion sign).

Palpation. *Palpate for the splenic edge.* To enhance relaxation of the abdominal wall, the patient should keep arms at the sides and, if needed, flex the hips and legs. With your left hand, reach over and around the patient to support and press forward the lower left rib cage and adjacent soft tissue. With your right hand below the left costal margin, press in toward the spleen. Begin palpation low enough so that you can detect an enlarged spleen. If your hand is too close to the costal margin, you will not be able to reach up under the rib cage. The examiner may miss an enlarged spleen by starting palpation too high in the abdomen.

Splenomegaly is eight times more likely when the spleen is palpable. Causes include portal hypertension, hematologic malignancies, HIV infection, infiltrative diseases like amyloidosis, and splenic infarct or hematoma.

- Ask the patient to take a deep breath. Try to feel the tip or edge of the spleen as it comes down to meet your fingertips (Fig. 12-24). Note any tenderness, assess the splenic contour, and measure the distance between the spleen's lowest point and the left costal margin. Approximately 5% of normal adults have a palpable spleen tip.

The spleen tip, illustrated in Figure 12-25, is just palpable deep to the left costal margin.

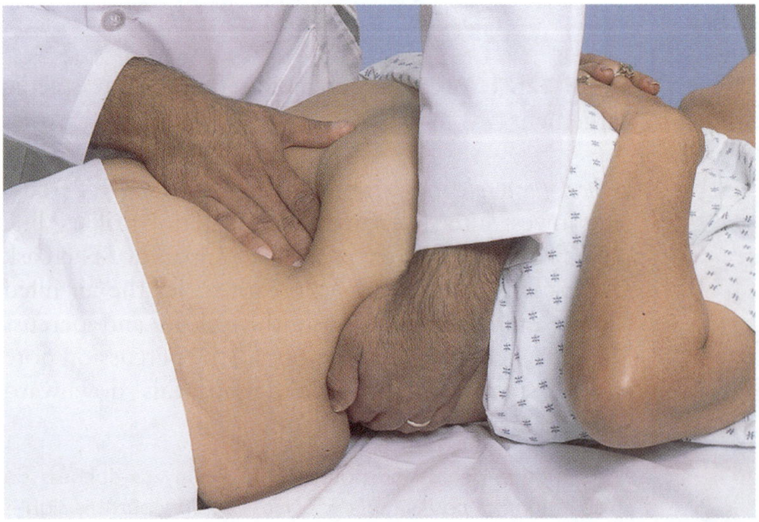

FIGURE 12-24. Palpating for the splenic edge.

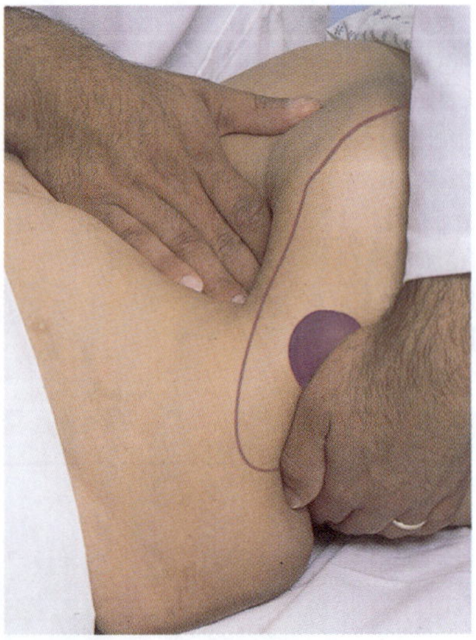

FIGURE 12-25. Spleen tip (purple) palpable below costal margin.

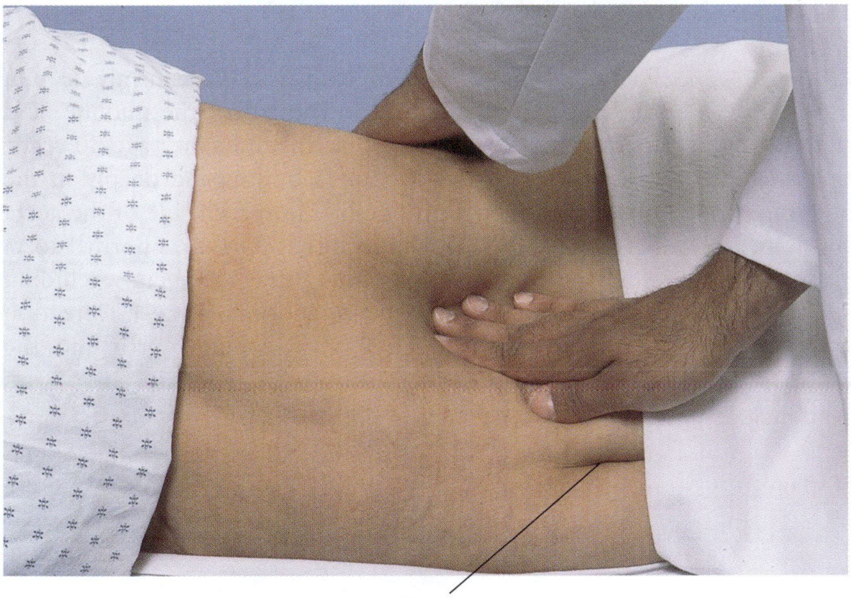

FIGURE 12-26. Palpating the splenic edge with patient lying on right side.

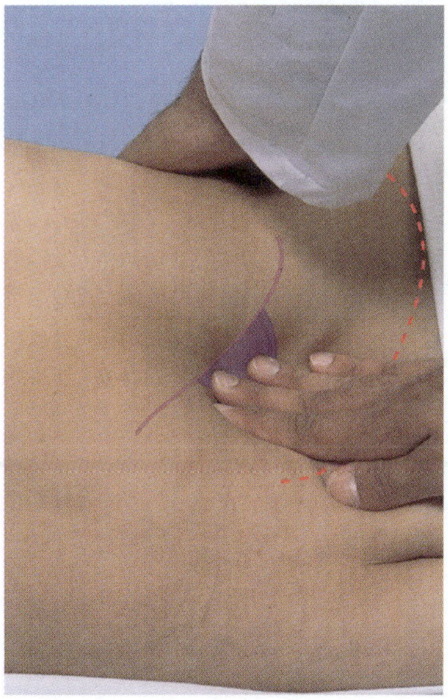

FIGURE 12-27. Edge of enlarged spleen palpable about 2 cm below the right costal margin on deep inspiration.

- Repeat with the patient lying on the right side with the hips and knees partially flexed (Fig. 12-26). In this position, gravity may bring the spleen forward and to the right into a palpable location (Fig. 12-27).

Kidneys

The kidneys are retroperitoneal and usually not palpable unless markedly enlarged.

Percussion. *Assess percussion tenderness over the CVA.* In patients suspected to have renal colic or pyelonephritis, *CVA tenderness* can be elicited due to inflammation of the renal capsule. Start by explaining the maneuver to the patient. Place the palm of one hand along the CVA area. Then make a fist with the other hand and strike the hand already on the CVA with the ulnar surface of your fist (Fig. 12-28). Use enough force to cause a perceptible but painless jar or thud on the area.

Physiology OSCE Videos:
Palpation of Kidneys

Pain with pressure or fist percussion supports pyelonephritis if associated with fever and dysuria but may also be musculoskeletal.

To save the patient from repositioning, integrate this assessment into your examination of the posterior thorax, lungs, or back.

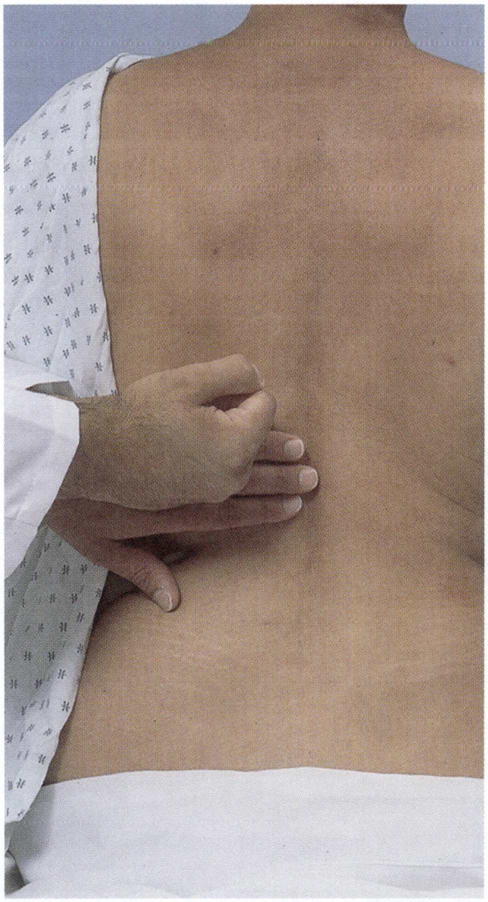

FIGURE 12-28. Fist percussion to detect costovertebral angle (CVA) tenderness.

Urinary Bladder

Normally, the urinary bladder is not palpable unless it is distended above the symphysis pubis.

Percussion. *Percuss for dullness and the height of the urinary bladder* above the symphysis pubis. Bladder volume must be 400 to 600 mL before dullness appears. On palpation, the dome of the distended bladder feels smooth and round. Check for tenderness.

Causes of bladder distention are outlet obstruction from a urethral stricture or prostatic hyperplasia; medication side effects; and neurologic disorders, such as stroke and multiple sclerosis.

Suprapubic tenderness is common in bladder infection.

Aorta

Palpation. *Identify aortic pulsations.* Press firmly deep in the epigastrium, slightly to the left of the midline, and identify the aortic pulsations. In adults over age 50 years, assess the width of the aorta by pressing deeply in the upper abdomen with one hand on each side of the aorta (Figs. 12-29 to 12-31). In this age group, a normal aorta is not more than 3 cm wide (average, 2.5 cm, excluding the thickness of the skin and abdominal wall). Detection of pulsations is affected by abdominal girth and the diameter of the aorta.

Risk factors for AAA are age ≥65 years, history of smoking, male gender, and a first-degree relative with a history of AAA repair.

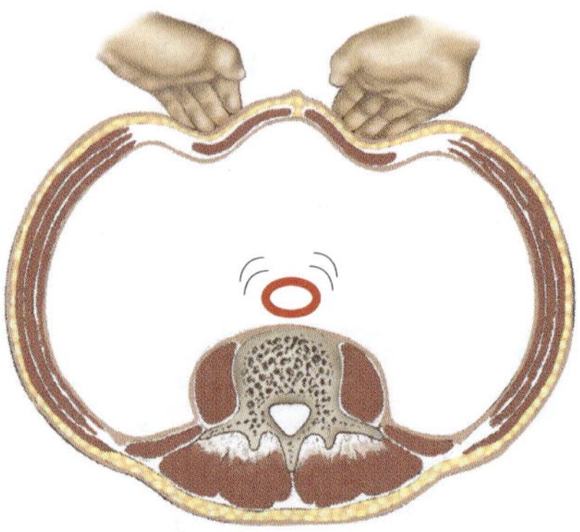

FIGURE 12-29. Detecting aortic pulsations by applying firm pressure on epigastrium, cross section.

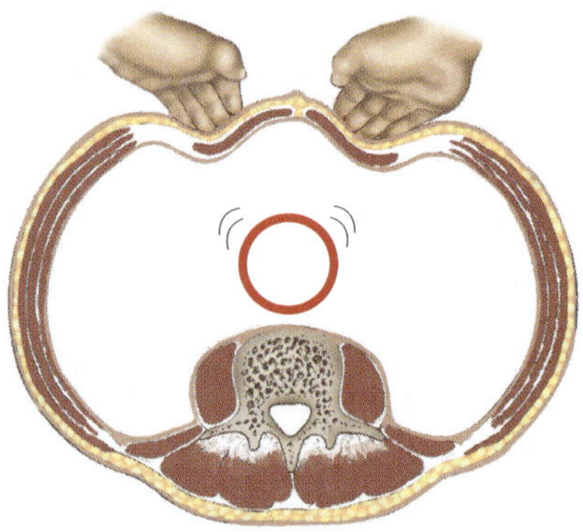

FIGURE 12-30. Identifying expanded aortic width on pressure on firm application of pressure on epigastrium, cross section.

A periumbilical or upper abdominal mass with expansile pulsations that is ≥3 cm in diameter suggests an AAA. Sensitivity of palpation increases as AAAs enlarge: for widths of 3 to 3.9 cm, 29%; 4 to 4.9 cm, 50%; ≥5 cm, 76%, but caution is warranted for palpating a large pulsatile mass. Consider assessment by ultrasound or radiology.

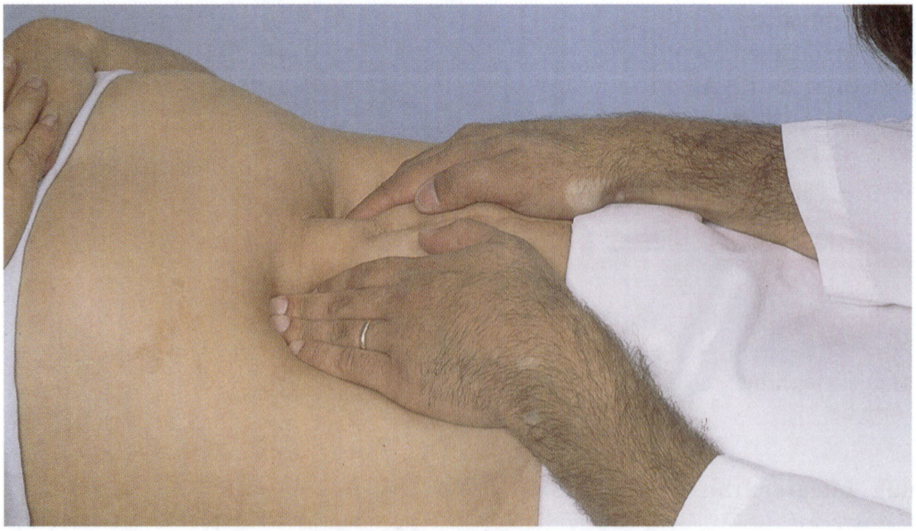

FIGURE 12-31. Palpating the epigastrium on both sides of the aorta.

Pain may signal rupture. Rupture is 15 times more likely in AAAs >4 cm than in smaller aneurysms and carries an 85% to 90% mortality rate.

SPECIAL TECHNIQUES

Assessment techniques exist for ascites, appendicitis, acute cholecystitis, ventral hernia, and abdominal wall mass.

Assessing Possible Ascites

A protuberant abdomen with bulging flanks is suspicious for *ascites,* the most common complication of cirrhosis. Because ascitic fluid characteristically sinks with gravity, whereas gas-filled loops of bowel rise, dullness appears in the dependent areas of the abdomen. There are two techniques for comparative percussion for detecting ascites:

- *Percuss from area of central tympany to area of dullness on supine patient.* Start with the patient supine then percuss for dullness outward in several directions from the central area of tympany in the abdomen. Map the border between tympany and dullness (Fig. 12-32).

Ascites reflects the increased hydrostatic pressure in cirrhosis (the most common cause of ascites), heart failure, constrictive pericarditis, or inferior vena cava or hepatic vein obstruction. It may signal decreased osmotic pressure in nephrotic syndrome, malnutrition, or ovarian cancer.

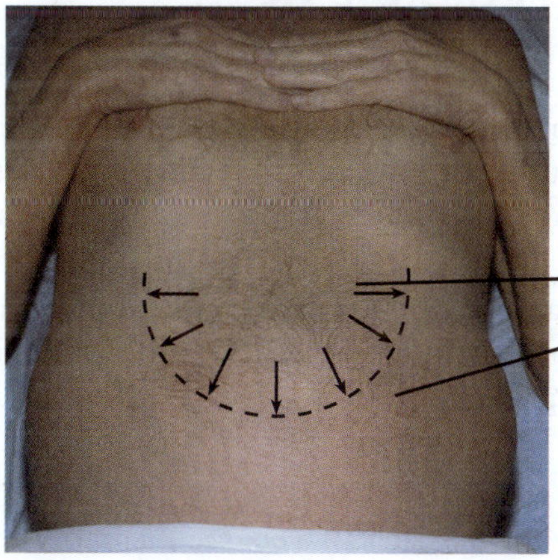

FIGURE 12-32. Area and direction outward to map percussion dullness from ascites.

- *Test for shifting dullness.* Percuss the border of tympany and dullness with the patient supine, then ask the patient to roll onto one side. Percuss and mark the borders again. In a person without ascites, the border between tympany and dullness usually stays relatively constant (Fig. 12-33).

Physiology OSCE Videos:
Ascites

In ascites, dullness shifts to the more dependent side, whereas tympany shifts to the top. Sensitivity of this test is 83% with a specificity of 56%.

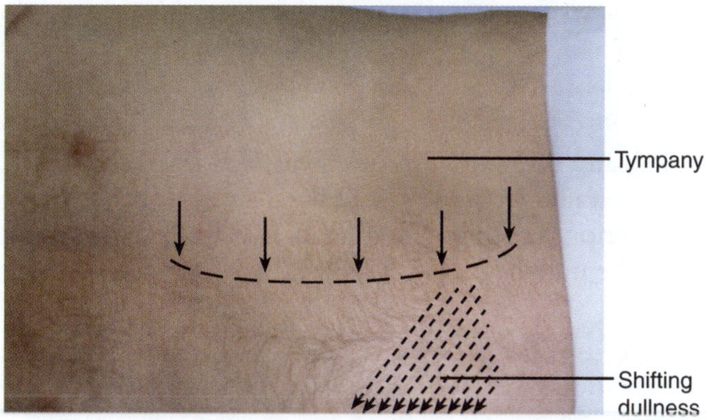

FIGURE 12-33. Area of percussion for shifting dullness with the patient turned to right side.

A previously utilized test to detect an impulse transmitted through ascitic fluid from one flank to the opposite side (test for a *fluid wave*) is often negative until ascites is quite obvious, and the test is sometimes positive even in people without ascites.

Identifying an Organ or a Mass in an Abdomen with Ascites. Try to *ballotte* the organ or mass, exemplified here by an enlarged liver (Fig. 12-34). Straighten and stiffen the fingers of one hand together, place them on the abdominal surface, and make a brief jabbing movement directly toward the anticipated structure. This quick movement often displaces the fluid so that your fingertips can briefly touch the surface of the structure through the abdominal wall (Fig. 12-35).

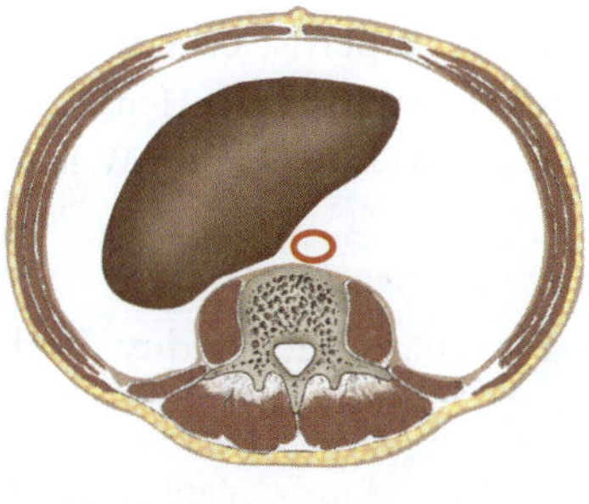

FIGURE 12-34. Note enlarged liver surrounded by ascitic fluid.

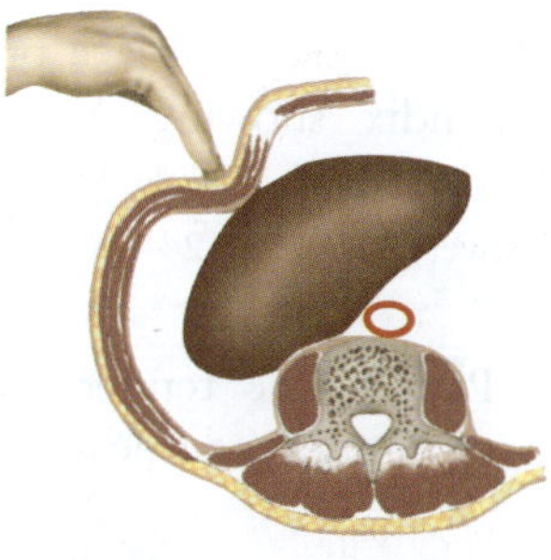

FIGURE 12-35. Displacement of ascitic fluid by ballottement allowing palpation of liver.

Assessing Possible Appendicitis

Appendicitis is a common cause of acute abdominal pain especially in the RLQ. Assess for signs of McBurney point tenderness, Rovsing sign (indirect tenderness), the psoas sign, and the obturator sign.

Appendicitis is twice as likely in the presence of RLQ tenderness, Rovsing sign (indirect tenderness), and the psoas sign; it is three times more likely if there is McBurney point tenderness (**McBurney sign**).

- Palpate carefully for an area of local tenderness. Classically, *McBurney point* lies 2 in from the anterior superior iliac spine on a line drawn from that process to the umbilicus (Fig. 12-36).

Localized tenderness anywhere in the RLQ, even in the right flank, suggests *appendicitis*.

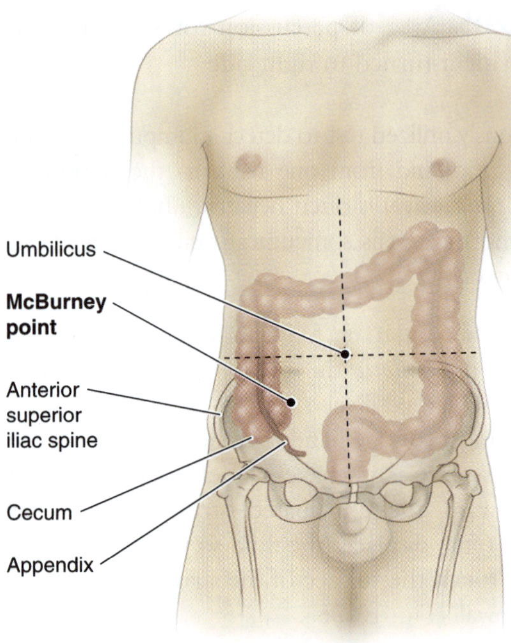

FIGURE 12-36. Surface projection of pelvis, cecum, and appendix showing McBurney point. (From Honan L. *Focus on Adult Health: Medical-Surgical Nursing*. 2nd ed. Wolters Kluwer; 2019, Fig. 24-2.)

- Palpate the tender area for guarding, rigidity, and rebound tenderness.

Early voluntary guarding may be replaced by involuntary muscular rigidity and signs of peritoneal inflammation. There may also be RLQ pain on quick withdrawal or deferred rebound tenderness.

- Palpate for **Rovsing sign** *(indirect tenderness)* and referred rebound tenderness. With the patient supine, press deeply and evenly in the *LLQ*. Then quickly withdraw your fingers.

Pain in the RLQ during *left*-sided pressure is a *positive Rovsing sign*.

- Assess the *psoas sign*. With the patient supine, place your hand just above the patient's right knee and ask the patient to raise that thigh against your hand. Alternatively, ask the patient to turn onto the left side. Then extend the patient's right thigh at the hip. Flexion of the thigh at the hip makes the psoas muscle contract; extension stretches it.

Increased abdominal pain on either technique is a *positive psoas sign*, suggesting irritation of the right psoas muscle by an inflamed retrocecal appendix.

- Though less helpful, assess the *obturator sign*. Flex the patient's right thigh at the hip, with the knee bent, and rotate the leg internally at the hip. This maneuver stretches the internal obturator muscle. Internal rotation of the hip is described on p. 449.

Right hypogastric pain is a *positive obturator sign*, from irritation of the right obturator internus muscle by an inflamed appendix located in the pelvis. This sign has very low sensitivity.

- *Perform a rectal examination and, in women, a pelvic examination*. These maneuvers have low sensitivity and specificity, but they may identify an inflamed appendix atypically located within the pelvic cavity or other causes of the abdominal pain.

Right-sided rectal tenderness suggests appendicitis but may also be caused by an inflamed adnexa or seminal vesicle.

Assessing Possible Acute Cholecystitis

When a patient present with RUQ pain suspicious for acute cholecystitis but does not have any tenderness on palpation in the RUQ, the test for Murphy sign can be performed.

Deeply palpate the RUQ at the location of the patient's pain. Ask the patient to take a deep breath, which forces the liver and gallbladder down toward the examining fingers.

A sharp halting in inspiratory effort due to pain from palpation of the gallbladder on examination is a *positive Murphy sign*. When positive, Murphy sign triples the likelihood of acute cholecystitis. Of note, this finding is only useful in a patient who does not have tenderness in the RUQ with regular palpation.

Assessing Ventral Hernias

Ventral hernias are hernias in the abdominal wall exclusive of groin hernias. If you suspect but do not see an umbilical or incisional hernia, ask the patient to raise both legs off the table or perform a Valsalva maneuver to increase intraabdominal pressure.

The bulge of a hernia will usually appear with this action, but should not be confused with *diastasis recti*, which is a benign 2- to 3-cm gap in the rectus muscles often seen in obese and postpartum patients.

Abdominal Wall Mass

Occasionally, there are masses in the abdominal wall rather than inside the abdominal cavity. Ask the patient either to raise the head and shoulders or to strain down, thus tightening the abdominal muscles. Feel for the mass again.

A mass in the abdominal wall remains palpable; an intraabdominal mass is obscured by muscular contraction.

Evaluating Groin Hernias

The lifetime risk of developing a *groin hernia (inguinal* or *femoral hernia)* is approximately 25% in men but <5% in women. Approximately 96% of groin hernias are inguinal and 4% are femoral. However, femoral hernias, which occur more often in older women (median age of presentation is 60 to 79 years), lead to a higher proportion of emergency operations due to the higher risk of the hernia contents being trapped within the hernia sac (*incarceration*) and causing ischemia and necrosis (*strangulation*).

Examination for groin hernias is best performed with the patient standing but can also be performed with the patient in the supine position. The techniques for examination and examiner hand placement are the same for both positions. The techniques that follow apply to the standing position, but can be replicated for the supine position depending on examiner preference.

Inspection

Sitting comfortably in front of the patient, with the patient standing and an assistant present, if indicated, inspect the inguinal regions and genitalia for bulging areas and asymmetry.

A bulge suggests a groin hernia. Groin hernias in women often do not have a visible bulge.

Femoral hernias most commonly present inferior to the inguinal ligament and medial to the femoral artery.

Palpation

Palpate for an inguinal hernia, using the techniques given next. Continue to face the patient, who should still be standing.

See Table 12-1, Course, Presentation, and Differentiation of Hernias in the Groin.

- To examine for an inguinal hernia on either side (Fig. 12-37) place the tip of your dominant index finger at the anterior inferior margin of the scrotum, staying superficial to the testes, and then move your finger and hand upward toward the external inguinal ring, invaginating the redundant scrotal skin beneath the peripubic fat pad next to the base of the penis.

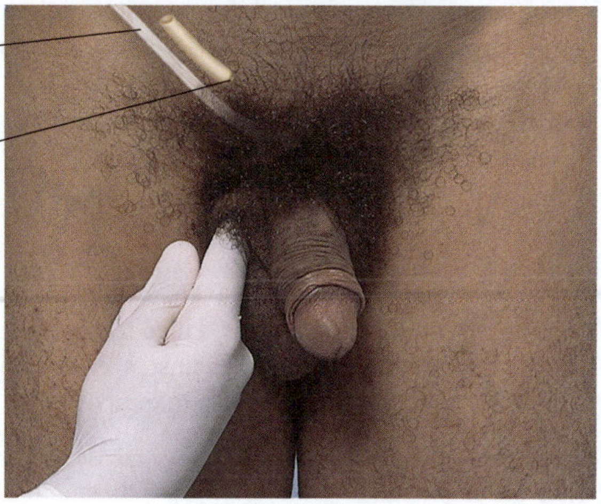

FIGURE 12-37. Invaginating redundant scrotal skin toward external inguinal ring to detect a right inguinal hernia.

- Follow the spermatic cord upward to the inguinal ligament. Find the triangular slit-like opening of the external inguinal ring just above and lateral to the pubic tubercle. Palpate the external inguinal ring and its floor. Ask the patient to cough. Palpate for a distinct bulge or mass that moves against your stationary finger during the cough.

A bulge near the external inguinal ring suggests a direct inguinal hernia. A bulge near the internal inguinal ring suggests an indirect inguinal hernia.

Experts note that distinguishing the type of hernia is difficult, with sensitivity and specificity of 74% and 96%, respectively. Ultrasonography of the groin may be particularly useful in clinically doubtful cases.

- The external ring may be large enough for you to gently palpate obliquely along the inguinal canal toward the internal inguinal ring. Again, ask the patient to cough. Check for a bulge that slides down the inguinal canal and taps against the fingertip.

Hernias warrant surgical evaluation, especially when symptomatic or incarcerated. Chance of incarceration is low, estimated at 0.3% to 3% per year, and is 10 times more common with indirect hernias.

- Use the same techniques with the same dominant finger to examine both sides.

If your findings suggest an inguinal hernia, but it does not spontaneously return to the abdomen on lying down, gently try to reduce it by sustained pressure with your fingers. Do not attempt this maneuver if the mass is tender or the patient reports nausea and vomiting.

A hernia is *incarcerated* when its contents cannot be returned to the abdominal cavity. A hernia is *strangulated* when the blood supply to the entrapped contents is compromised. Suspect strangulation in the presence of tenderness, nausea, and vomiting, and consider surgical intervention.

- Can you get your fingers above the mass in the scrotum?

If you can place your fingers above the mass, it is probably not a hernia, and you should suspect the presence of a hydrocele.

- With the patient standing, palpate the spermatic cord about 2 cm above the testis. Have the patient hold his breath and "bear down" against a closed glottis for about 4 seconds (the Valsalva maneuver).

During this maneuver, a temporary increase in the diameter of the spermatic cord indicates filling of abnormally dilated spermatic veins draining the testis, suggesting a varicocele.

- Swelling in the scrotum can also be evaluated by *transillumination*. After darkening the room, hold a strong light source behind the scrotum, which will demonstrate whether the mass is cystic (light shines through as a red glow) or solid (light blocked by the mass).

Transillumination of the scrotal mass may help distinguish a *hydrocele* from an intestine-containing hernia. Those containing blood or tissue, such as a normal testis, a tumor, or most hernias, do not transilluminate.

Palpate for a femoral hernia by placing your fingers on the anterior thigh in the region medial to the femoral canal. Start by locating the femoral pulse in the upper portion of the thigh and moving medially toward the pubic tubercle. Ask the patient to strain down again or cough. Note any swelling or tenderness.

Evaluating a Possible Scrotal Mass. To assess a possible groin hernia presenting as a mass in the scrotum, ask the patient to lie down. If the mass disappears by returning to the abdomen by itself (*reducible*), it is likely to be an indirect inguinal hernia. The patient can often tell you what happens to his swelling when lying down and may be able to demonstrate how he reduces it himself.

RECORDING YOUR FINDINGS

Note that initially you may use sentences to describe your findings; later you will use phrases. The style below contains phrases appropriate for most write-ups.

Recording the Abdominal Examination

"Abdomen is protuberant, soft and nontender; no palpable masses or hepatosplenomegaly. Liver span is 7 cm in the right midclavicular line; edge is smooth and palpable 1 cm below the right costal margin. Spleen and kidneys not felt. No costovertebral angle (CVA) tenderness."

"No perirectal lesions or fissures. External sphincter tone intact. Rectal vault without masses. Prostate smooth, symmetric, and nontender with palpable median sulcus. (Or, in a female, uterine cervix nontender.) Stool brown; no fecal blood."

OR

"Abdomen is flat. No bowel sounds heard. It is firm and boardlike, with increased tenderness, guarding, and rebound in the right lower quadrant. Liver percusses to 7 cm in the midclavicular line; edge not felt. Spleen and kidneys not felt. No palpable masses. No CVA tenderness. Psoas sign positive."

"No perirectal lesions or fissures; no ulcerations, warts, or discharge. Rectal vault tenderness on the right side. Prostate smooth, symmetric, and nontender with palpable median sulcus. (Or, in a female, uterine cervix nontender.) Stool brown; no fecal blood."

These findings suggest peritonitis from possible appendicitis.

HEALTH PROMOTION AND COUNSELING: EVIDENCE AND RECOMMENDATIONS

Important Topics for Health Promotion and Counseling

- Viral hepatitis
- Colon cancer

Viral Hepatitis

Hepatitis A. HAV infection is rarely fatal; it does not cause a chronic hepatitis, and deaths usually occur only in those with other liver diseases. Viral transmission is primarily person to person through the fecal–oral route and can be reduced by handwashing with soap and water after using the bathroom or changing diapers and before preparing or eating food.

The Advisory Committee on Immunization Practices (ACIP) recommends hepatitis A vaccination for all children at age 1 year, for persons with chronic liver disease, and for groups at increased risk of acquiring HAV—persons traveling to or working in countries with high endemic rates of infection, men who have sex with men, injection and illicit drug users, persons with occupational risk for infection, and persons who have clotting-factor disorders.

Postexposure prophylaxis among previously unvaccinated individuals is a single dose of immune globulin administered as soon as possible, ideally within 2 weeks. Recommendations for immune globulin apply to close personal contacts of persons with confirmed HAV; co-workers of infected food handlers; and staff and attendees (and their household members) of child care centers where HAV has been diagnosed in children, staff, or households of attendees. Hepatitis A vaccine is additionally recommended if the person also has an indication for vaccination. The vaccine alone may be administered at any time before traveling to endemic areas.

Hepatitis B. Hepatitis B virus (HBV) infection is a more serious health threat than hepatitis A; the fatality rate for acute infection can be up to 1.5%, and HBV infection can become chronic. HBV is spread by the blood, semen, or other bodily fluids of an infected person; sexual contact, injection drug use, and perinatal transmission are the most common pathways. Most infections in healthy adults are self-limited, with elimination of the virus and development of immunity. Risk of chronic HBV infection is highest when the immune system is immature; chronic infection occurs in up to 90% of infected infants and 30% of children infected before age 6 years. Chronic HBV infection also develops more often in persons who are immunosuppressed or have diabetes. Most persons with chronic infection are asymptomatic until the onset of advanced liver disease.

HBV infection is preventable. The ACIP recommends universal vaccination for all infants beginning at birth as well as for previously unvaccinated children younger than 19 years. For adults, vaccine recommendations target high-risk groups (Box 12-5). HBV infection is also treatable.

Box 12-5. Recommendations for Hepatitis B Vaccination: High-Risk Groups and Settings

- *Sexual contacts*, including sex partners of hepatitis B surface antigen–positive persons, people with more than one sex partner in the prior 6 months, people seeking evaluation and treatment for sexually transmitted infections, and men who have sex with men
- *Persons with percutaneous or mucosal exposure to blood*, including injection drug users, household contacts of antigen-positive persons, residents and staff of facilities for the developmentally disabled, health care workers, persons with diabetes, and dialysis patients
- *Others*, including travelers to endemic areas, people with chronic liver disease and HIV infection, and people seeking protection from hepatitis B infection who do not acknowledge a specific risk factor
- *All adults in high-risk settings*, such as sexually transmitted infection clinics, HIV testing and treatment programs, drug-abuse treatment programs and programs for injection drug users, correctional facilities, programs for men having sex with men, chronic hemodialysis facilities and end-stage renal disease programs, and facilities for people with developmental disabilities

Source: Schillie S et al. *MMWR Morb Mortal Wkly Rep.* 2018;67(15):455–458.

Hepatitis C. Hepatitis C virus (HCV) is mainly transmitted by percutaneous exposures, particularly injection drug use, health care workers with needlestick injury or mucosal exposure to HCV-positive blood, blood transfusion or organ transplantation before 1992, and transfusion with clotting factors before 1987. Other causes include long-term hemodialysis, getting an unregulated tattoo, and birth from an HCV-positive mother; sexual transmission is uncommon, although it occurs among HIV-positive persons, particularly among men who have sex with men. Hepatitis C becomes a chronic illness in more than 75% of those who are infected and is a major risk factor for subsequently developing cirrhosis and hepatocellular carcinoma and for undergoing transplantation for end-stage liver disease. However, the majority of persons with chronic HCV are unaware of being infected.

Screening tests for HCV are very sensitive. Antiviral treatment regimens can achieve high rates of sustained virologic response (aviremia 24 weeks or more after completing treatment) and improve clinical outcomes.

Colorectal Cancer

Epidemiology. Overall, about 80% of new cases and nearly 90% of deaths occur after age 55; the median age at diagnosis is 67 years and the median age at death is 73 years. The lifetime risk for being diagnosed with colorectal cancer is about 4%, while the lifetime risk for dying from colorectal cancer is just under 2%.

Risk Factors. The strongest risk factors for colorectal cancer are increasing age; personal history of colorectal cancer, adenomatous polyps, or longstanding inflammatory bowel disease (IBD); and family history of colorectal neoplasia—particularly with diagnoses in multiple first-degree relatives, a single first-degree relative diagnosed before age 60, or a hereditary colorectal cancer syndrome. While the lifetime risk of colorectal cancer is extremely high in patients with hereditary syndromes, about 75% of colorectal cancers arise in people without any obvious hereditary risk or family history.

Prevention. The most effective prevention strategy is to screen for and remove precancerous adenomatous polyps. Screening programs using fecal blood testing or flexible sigmoidoscopy have been shown in randomized trials to reduce the risk of developing colorectal cancer by about 5% to 25%. Physical activity, aspirin, and other NSAIDs, and postmenopausal combined hormone replacement therapy (estrogen and progestin) also protect against colorectal cancer.

Screening. Screening tests include stool tests that detect occult fecal blood, such as fecal immunochemical tests and high-sensitivity guaiac-based tests, and those that detect abnormal DNA in the stool. Endoscopic tests are also used for screening, including colonoscopy, which visualizes the entire colon and can remove polyps, and flexible sigmoidoscopy, which visualizes the distal 60 cm of the bowel. CT colonography is used to image the colon. Any abnormal finding on a stool test, imaging study, or flexible sigmoidoscopy warrants further evaluation with colonoscopy. Screening programs using fecal blood testing or flexible sigmoidoscopy have been shown in randomized trials to reduce the risk of colorectal cancer death by about 15% to 30% (Box 12-6).

Although colonoscopy is the gold standard diagnostic test for screening, there is no direct evidence from randomized trials that screening with colonoscopy reduces colorectal cancer incidence or mortality. Additionally, no randomized trials have evaluated the efficacy of screening with CT colonography or fecal DNA tests (which are now combined with fecal immunochemical tests).

Box 12-6. Screening for Colorectal Cancer

Screen all adults aged 45 to 75 years

A variety of factors are considered in deciding the test: frequencies of screening, location of screening (home or office), methods of screening (stool-based or direct visualization), pre-procedure bowel preparation, anesthesia or sedation during the test, and follow-up procedures for abnormal findings.

Recommended screening strategies include:

- High-sensitivity guaiac fecal occult blood test (HSgFOBT) or fecal immunochemical test (FIT) every year
- Stool DNA-FIT every 1 to 3 years
- Computed tomography colonography every 5 years
- Flexible sigmoidoscopy every 5 years
- Flexible sigmoidoscopy every 10 years + annual FIT
- Colonoscopy screening every 10 years

Selectively screen adults aged 76 to 85 years: individualized decision making

Decisions should take into consideration patient's overall health status (life expectancy, comorbid conditions), prior screening history, and preferences.

Do not screen adults older than age 85

Because "competing causes of mortality preclude a mortality benefit that would outweigh the harms"

TABLE 12-1. Course, Presentation, and Differentiation of Hernias in the Groin

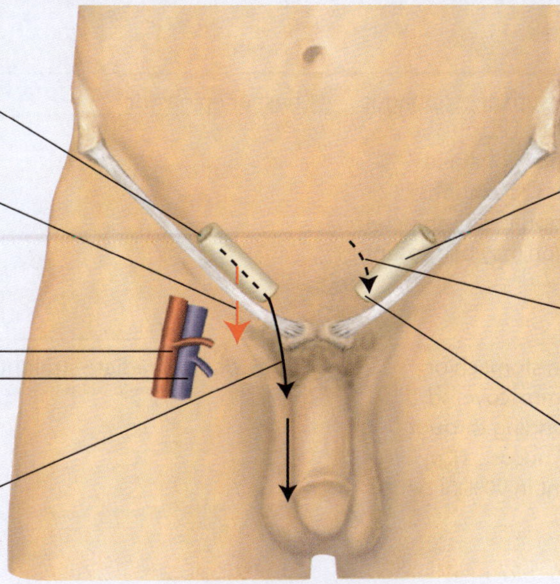

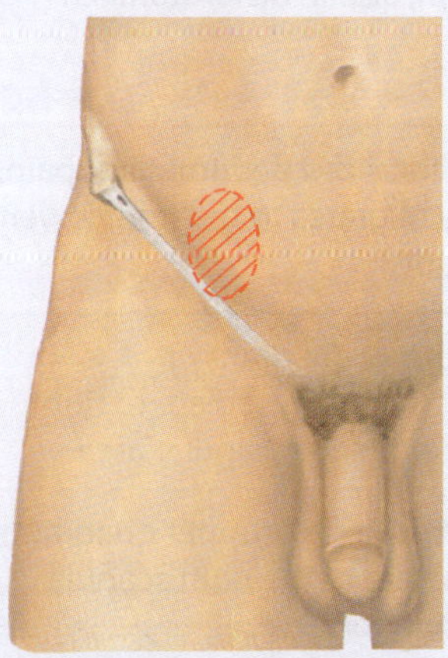

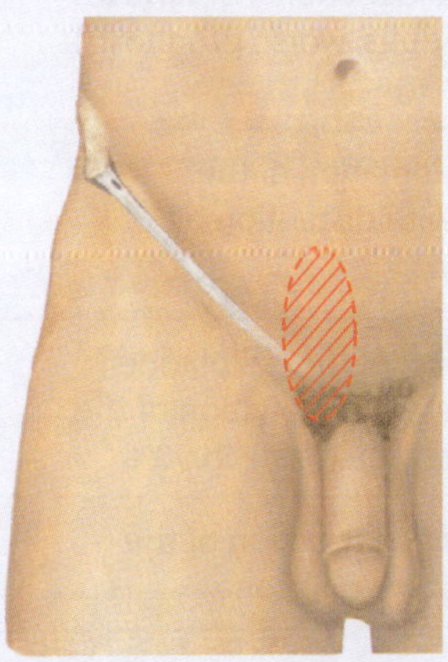

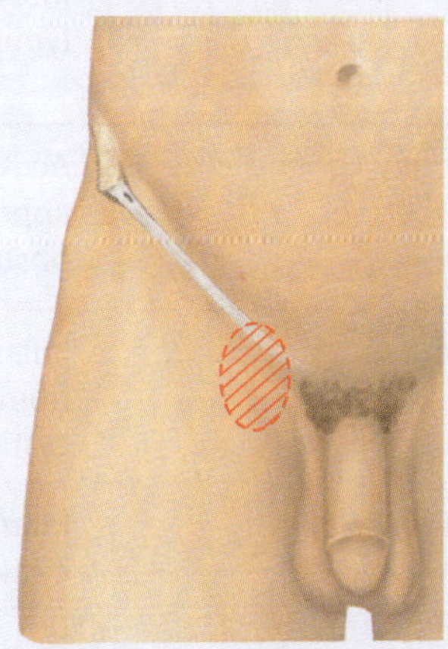

	Inguinal Hernias: Indirect	Inguinal Hernias: Direct	Femoral Hernias
Frequency, Age, and Sex	Most common, all ages and sexes. Often in children; may occur in adults.	Less common. Usually in men older than 40 yrs; rare in women.	Least common. More common in women than in men.
Point of Origin	Above inguinal ligament, near its midpoint (the internal inguinal ring).	Above inguinal ligament, close to the pubic tubercle (near the external inguinal ring).	Below the inguinal ligament; appears more lateral than an inguinal hernia. Can be hard to differentiate from lymph nodes.
Course *(Examining finger in inguinal canal during coughing or straining)*	Often into the scrotum. The hernia comes down the inguinal canal and touches the fingertip.	Rarely into the scrotum. The hernia bulges anteriorly and pushes the side of the finger forward.	Never into the scrotum. The inguinal canal is empty.

TABLE 12-2. Abdominal Pain

Problem	Process	Location	Quality
Gastroesophageal Reflux Disease (GERD)	Prolonged exposure of esophagus to gastric acid due to impaired esophageal motility or excess relaxations of the lower esophageal sphincter; *Helicobacter pylori* may be present	Chest or epigastric	Heartburn, regurgitation
Peptic Ulcer and Dyspepsia	Mucosal ulcer in stomach or duodenum >5 mm, covered with fibrin, extending through the muscularis mucosa; *H. pylori* infection present in 90% of peptic ulcers	Epigastric, may radiate straight to the back	Variable: epigastric gnawing or burning (dyspepsia); may also be boring, aching, or hungerlike No symptoms in up to 20%
Gastric Cancer	Adenocarcinoma in 90–95%, either intestinal (older adults) or diffuse (younger adults, worse prognosis)	Increasingly in "cardia" and GE junction; also in distal stomach	Variable
Acute Appendicitis	Acute inflammation of the appendix with distention or obstruction	Poorly localized periumbilical pain, usually migrates to the right lower quadrant	Mild but increasing, possibly cramping Steady and more severe
Acute Cholecystitis	Inflammation of the gallbladder, from persistent obstruction of the cystic duct by gallstone in 90%	Right upper quadrant or epigastrium; may radiate to right shoulder or interscapular area	Steady, persistent, aching
Biliary Colic	Intermittent obstruction of the cystic duct by a gallstone	Epigastric or right upper quadrant; may radiate to the right scapula and shoulder	Intermittent pain that resolves
Acute Pancreatitis	Intrapancreatic trypsinogen activation to trypsin and other enzymes, resulting in autodigestion and inflammation of the pancreas	Epigastric, may radiate straight to the back or other areas of the abdomen; 20% with severe sequelae of organ failure	Usually steady, progressive, severe
Chronic Pancreatitis	Irreversible destruction of the pancreatic parenchyma from recurrent inflammation	Epigastric, radiating to the back	Longstanding persistent pain
Pancreatic Cancer	Predominantly adenocarcinoma (95%); 5% 5-yr survival	If cancer in body or tail, epigastric, in either upper quadrant, often radiates to the back	Steady, deep, nonspecific

Timing	Aggravating Factors	Relieving Factors	Associated Symptoms and Setting
After meals, especially spicy foods	Lying down, bending over; physical activity; diseases such as scleroderma, gastroparesis; drugs like nicotine that relax the lower esophageal sphincter	Antacids, proton pump inhibitors; avoiding alcohol, smoking, fatty meals, chocolate, selected drugs such as theophylline, calcium channel blockers	Wheezing, chronic cough, shortness of breath, hoarseness, choking sensation, dysphagia, regurgitation, halitosis, sore throat; increases risk of Barrett esophagus and esophageal cancer
Intermittent; duodenal ulcer is more likely than gastric ulcer or dyspepsia to cause pain that (1) wakes the patient at night, and (2) occurs intermittently over a few wks, disappears for months, then recurs	Variable	Food and antacids may bring relief (less likely in gastric ulcers)	Nausea, vomiting, belching, bloating; heartburn (more common in duodenal ulcer); weight loss (more common in gastric ulcer); dyspepsia is more common in the young (20–29 yrs), gastric ulcer in those over 50 yrs, and duodenal ulcer in those 30–60 yrs
Pain is persistent, slowly progressive; duration of pain is typically shorter than in peptic ulcer	Often food; *H. pylori* infection	Not relieved by food or antacids	Anorexia, nausea, early satiety, weight loss, and sometimes bleeding; most common in ages 50–70 yrs
Continues to worsen until intervention/treatment	Movement or cough	If it subsides temporarily, suspect perforation of the appendix.	Anorexia, nausea, possibly vomiting, which typically follow the onset of pain; low fever
Gradual onset; course longer than in biliary colic	Prior history of biliary colic symptoms		Anorexia, nausea, vomiting, fever; no jaundice
Rapid onset over a few min, lasts one to several hrs and subsides gradually; often recurrent	Large fatty meals		Anorexia, nausea, vomiting,
Acute onset, persistent pain	Movement	Hydration, bowel rest	Nausea, vomiting, abdominal distention, 80% with history of alcohol abuse or gallstones
Chronic or recurrent course	Alcohol, medication, frequent attacks of acute pancreatitis	None	Pancreatic enzyme insufficiency, diarrhea with fatty stools (*steatorrhea*) and diabetes mellitus
Persistent pain; relentlessly progressive illness	Smoking, chronic pancreatitis	Often intractable	Painless jaundice, anorexia, weight loss; glucose intolerance, depression

(*continued*)

TABLE 12-2. Abdominal Pain *(Continued)*

Problem	Process	Location	Quality
Acute Diverticulitis	Acute inflammation of colonic diverticula, outpouchings, usually in sigmoid or descending colon	Left lower quadrant, pelvic	May be cramping at first, then steady
Acute Bowel Obstruction	Obstruction of the bowel lumen, most commonly caused by (1) adhesions or hernias (small bowel), or (2) cancer or strictures (colon)	Generalized abdominal pain, nonspecific, result of distention	Cramping, colicky
Mesenteric Ischemia	Occlusion of blood flow to small bowel, from arterial or venous thrombosis, cardiac embolus, or hypoperfusion	Vague nonspecific	Pain out of proportion to examination is hallmark of mesenteric ischemia

Timing	Aggravating Factors	Relieving Factors	Associated Symptoms and Setting
Often gradual onset		Analgesia, bowel rest, antibiotics	Fever, diarrhea, urinary symptoms, anorexia
Progressive, intermittent	Ingestion of food or liquids	Bowel rest, hydration	No passage of flatus or bowel movement, nausea, vomiting, progressive abdominal distention
Usually abrupt in onset, then persistent	Underlying thromboembolic disease, low flow states, hypercoagulable conditions	Volume resuscitation	Vomiting, bloody stool, soft distended abdomen, systemic shock

TABLE 12-3. Dysphagia

Process and Problem	Timing	Factors That Aggravate	Factors That Relieve	Associated Symptoms and Conditions
Oropharyngeal Dysphagia	Acute or gradual onset and a variable course, depending on the underlying disorder	Attempts to start the swallowing process		Aspiration into the lungs or regurgitation into the nose with attempts to swallow; from motor disorders affecting the pharyngeal muscles such as stroke, bulbar palsy, or other neuromuscular conditions
Esophageal Dysphagia				
Mechanical Narrowing				
Mucosal rings and webs	Intermittent	Solid foods	Regurgitation of the bolus of food	Usually none
Esophageal stricture	Intermittent; may become slowly progressive	Solid foods	Regurgitation of the bolus of food	A long history of heartburn and regurgitation
Esophageal cancer	May be intermittent at first; progressive over months	Solid foods, with progression to liquids	Regurgitation of the bolus of food	Pain in the chest and back and weight loss, especially late in the course of illness
Motor Disorders				
Diffuse esophageal spasm	Intermittent	Solids or liquids	Maneuvers described below; sometimes nitroglycerin	Chest pain that mimics angina pectoris or myocardial infarction and lasts minutes to hours; possibly heartburn
Scleroderma	Intermittent; may progress slowly	Solids or liquids	Repeated swallowing; movements such as straightening the back, raising the arms, or a Valsalva maneuver (straining down against a closed glottis)	Heartburn; other manifestations of scleroderma
Achalasia	Intermittent; may progress	Solids or liquids		Regurgitation, often at night when lying down, with nocturnal cough; possibly chest pain precipitated by eating

TABLE 12-4. Diarrhea

Problem	Process	Characteristics of Stool	Timing	Associated Symptoms	Setting, Persons at Risk
Acute Diarrhea (≤14 days)					
Secretory Infection (Noninflammatory)	Infection by viruses, preformed bacterial toxins (such as *Staphylococcus aureus, Bacillus cereus, Clostridium perfringens,* toxigenic *Escherichia coli, Vibrio cholerae*), cryptosporidium, *Giardia lamblia*, rotavirus	Watery, without blood, pus, or mucus	Duration of a few days, possibly longer; lactase deficiency may lead to a longer course	Nausea, vomiting, periumbilical cramping pain; temperature normal or slightly elevated	Often travel, a common food source, or an epidemic
Inflammatory Infection	Colonization or invasion of intestinal mucosa (nontyphoid *Salmonella, Shigella, Yersinia, Campylobacter*, enteropathic *E. coli, Entamoeba histolytica, C. difficile*)	Loose to watery, often with blood, pus, or mucus	An acute illness of varying duration	Lower abdominal cramping pain and often rectal urgency, tenesmus; fever	Travel, contaminated food or water; frequent anal intercourse
Drug-Induced Diarrhea	Action of many drugs, such as magnesium-containing antacids, antibiotics, antineoplastic agents, and laxatives	Loose to watery	Acute, recurrent, or chronic	Possibly nausea; usually little if any pain	Prescribed or over-the-counter medications
Chronic Diarrhea (≥30 days)					
Diarrheal Syndrome					
Irritable bowel syndrome	Altered motility or secretion from luminal and mucosal irritants that change mucosal permeability, immune activation, and colonic transit, including maldigested carbohydrates, fats, excess bile acids, gluten intolerance, enteroendocrine signaling, and changes in microbiomes	Loose; ~50% with mucus; small to moderate volume. Small, hard stools with constipation. May be mixed pattern.	Worse in the morning; rarely at night.	Crampy lower abdominal pain, abdominal distention, flatulence, nausea; urgency, pain relieved with defecation	Young and middle-aged adults, especially women
Fecal impaction/motility disorders	Partial obstruction by impacted stool only allowing passage of loose feces	Loose, small volume	Variable	Crampy abdominal pain, incomplete evacuation	Older adults immobilized and institutionalized patients; ensues from selected medications

(continued)

TABLE 12-4. Diarrhea *(Continued)*

Problem	Process	Characteristics of Stool	Timing	Associated Symptoms	Setting, Persons at Risk
Cancer of the sigmoid colon	Partial obstruction by a malignant neoplasm	May be blood-streaked	Variable	Change in usual bowel habits, crampy lower abdominal pain, constipation	Middle-aged and older adults, especially older than 55 yrs
Inflammatory Bowel Disease					
Ulcerative colitis	Mucosal inflammation typically extending proximally from the rectum (*proctitis*) to varying lengths of the colon (*colitis to pancolitis*), with microulcerations and, if chronic, inflammatory polyps	Frequent, watery, bloody	Onset typically abrupt; often recurrent, persisting, and may awaken at night	Cramping, with urgency, tenesmus; fever, fatigue, weakness; abdominal pain if complicated by toxic megacolon; may include episcleritis, uveitis, arthritis, erythema nodosum	Often young adults, Ashkenazi Jewish descendants; linked to altered CD4+ T-cell Th2 response; increases risk of colon cancer
Crohn disease of the small bowel (*regional enteritis*) or colon (*granulomatous colitis*)	Chronic transmural inflammation of the bowel wall, with skip pattern involving the terminal ileum and/or proximal colon (and rectal sparing); may cause strictures	Small, soft to loose or watery, with bleeding if colitis, obstructive symptoms, if enteritis	More insidious onset; chronic or recurrent	Crampy periumbilical, right lower quadrant (*enteritis*) or diffuse (*colitis*) pain, with anorexia, fever, and/or weight loss; perianal or perirectal abscesses and fistulas; may cause small or large bowel obstruction	Often teens or young adults, but also adults of middle age; more common in Ashkenazi Jewish descendants; linked to altered CD4+ T-cell helper Th1 and 17 response; increases risk of colon cancer

(continued)

TABLE 12-4. Diarrhea *(Continued)*

Problem	Process	Characteristics of Stool	Timing	Associated Symptoms	Setting, Persons at Risk
Voluminous Diarrhea					
Malabsorption syndrome	Defective membrane transport or absorption of intestinal epithelium (Crohn, celiac disease, surgical resection); impaired luminal digestion (pancreatic insufficiency); epithelial defects at brush border (lactose intolerance)	Typically, bulky, soft, light yellow to gray, mushy, greasy or oily, and sometimes frothy; particularly foul-smelling; usually floats in toilet (*steatorrhea*)	Onset of illness typically insidious	Anorexia, weight loss, fatigue, abdominal distention, often crampy lower abdominal pain. Symptoms of nutritional deficiencies such as bleeding (vitamin K), bone pain and fractures (vitamin D), glossitis (vitamin B), and edema (protein)	Variable, depending on cause
Osmotic diarrhea					
■ Lactose intolerance	Intestinal lactase deficiency	Watery diarrhea of large volume	Follows the ingestion of milk and milk products; relieved by fasting	Crampy abdominal pain, abdominal distention, flatulence	In >50% of African Americans, Asians, Native Americans, Hispanics; in 5–20% of Caucasians
■ Abuse of osmotic purgatives	Laxative habit, often surreptitious	Watery diarrhea of large volume	Variable	Often none	Persons with anorexia nervosa or bulimia nervosa
Secretory diarrhea	Variable: bacterial infection, secreting villous adenoma, fat or bile salt malabsorption, hormone-mediated conditions (gastrin in *Zollinger–Ellison syndrome*, vasoactive intestinal peptide)	Watery diarrhea of large volume	Variable	Weight loss, dehydration, nausea, vomiting, and cramping abdominal pain	Variable depending on cause

TABLE 12-5. Constipation

Problem	Process	Associated Symptoms and Setting
Life Activities and Habits		
Inadequate Time or Setting for the Defecation Reflex	Ignoring the sensation of a full rectum inhibits the defecation reflex	Hectic schedules, unfamiliar surroundings, bed rest
False Expectations of Bowel Habits	Expectations of "regularity" or more frequent stools than a person's norm	Beliefs, treatments, and advertisements that promote the use of laxatives
Diet Deficient in Fiber	Decreased fecal bulk	Other factors such as debilitation and constipating drugs may contribute
Irritable Bowel Syndrome	Functional change in frequency or form of bowel movement without known pathology; possibly from change in intestinal bacteria.	Three patterns: diarrhea—predominant, constipation—predominant, or mixed. Symptoms present ≥6 mo and abdominal pain for ≥3 mo plus at least 2 of 3 features (improvement with defecation; onset with change in stool frequency; onset with change in stool form and appearance)
Mechanical Obstruction		
Cancer of the Rectum or Sigmoid Colon	Progressive narrowing of the bowel lumen from adenocarcinoma	Change in bowel habits; often diarrhea, abdominal pain, bleeding, occult blood in stool; in rectal cancer, tenesmus and pencil-shaped stools; weight loss
Fecal Impaction	A large, firm, immovable fecal mass, most often in the rectum	Rectal fullness, abdominal pain, and diarrhea around the impaction; common in debilitated, bedridden, and often older adults and institutionalized patients
Other Obstructing Lesions (such as diverticulitis, volvulus, intussusception, or hernia)	Narrowing or complete obstruction of the bowel	Colicky abdominal pain, abdominal distention, and in intussusception, often "currant jelly" stools (red blood and mucus)
Painful Anal Lesions	Pain may cause spasm of the external sphincter and voluntary inhibition of the defecation reflex.	Anal fissures, painful hemorrhoids, perirectal abscesses
Drugs	A variety of mechanisms	Opiates, anticholinergics, antacids containing calcium or aluminum, and many others
Depression	A disorder of mood	Fatigue, anhedonia, sleep disturbance, weight loss
Neurologic Disorders	Interference with the autonomic innervation of the bowel	Spinal cord injuries, multiple sclerosis, Hirschsprung disease, and other conditions
Metabolic Conditions	Interference with bowel motility	Pregnancy, hypothyroidism, hypercalcemia

TABLE 12-6. Black and Bloody Stool

Problem	Selected Causes	Associated Symptoms and Setting
Melena		
Refers to passage of black tarry stool Fecal blood tests are positive Involves loss ≥60 mL of blood into the gastrointestinal tract (less in children), usually from the esophagus, stomach, or duodenum with transit time of 7–14 hrs Less commonly, if slow transit, blood loss originates in the jejunum, ileum, or ascending colon In infants, melena may result from swallowing blood during the birth	Gastritis, gastroesophageal reflux disease, peptic ulcer (gastric or duodenal) Gastritis or stress ulcers Esophageal or gastric varices Reflux esophagitis, Mallory–Weiss tear in esophageal mucosa due to retching and vomiting	Usually epigastric discomfort from heartburn, dysmotility; if peptic ulcer, pain after meals (delay of 2–3 hrs if duodenal ulcer; may be asymptomatic) Recent ingestion of alcohol, aspirin, or other anti-inflammatory drugs; recent bodily trauma, severe burns, surgery, or increased intracranial pressure Cirrhosis of the liver or other causes of portal hypertension Retching, vomiting, often recent ingestion of alcohol
Black Stool		
Black stool from other causes with negative fecal blood tests; stool change has no pathologic significance	Ingestion of iron, bismuth salts, licorice, or even chocolate cookies	Asymptomatic
Stool with Red Blood (*Hematochezia*)		
Usually originates in the colon, rectum, or anus; much less frequently from the jejunum or ileum	Colon cancer	Often a change in bowel habits, weight loss
	Hyperplasia or adenomatous polyps	Often no other symptoms
Upper gastrointestinal hemorrhage may also cause red stool, usually with large blood loss ≥1 L	Diverticula of the colon	Often no symptoms unless inflammation causes diverticulitis
Rapid transit leaves insufficient time for the blood to turn black from oxidation of iron in hemoglobin	Inflammatory conditions of the colon and rectum Ulcerative colitis, Crohn disease Infectious diarrhea	See Table 12-4, Diarrhea
	Proctitis (various causes including anal intercourse)	Rectal urgency, tenesmus (see Table 12-4)
	Ischemic colitis	Lower abdominal pain sometimes fever or shock in older adults; abdomen typically soft to palpation
	Hemorrhoids	Blood on the toilet paper, on the surface of the stool, or dripping into the toilet, typically painless
	Anal fissure	Blood on the toilet paper or on the surface of the stool; anal pain with defecation
Reddish but Nonbloody Stool	Ingestion of beets	Pink urine, which usually precedes the reddish stool; from poor metabolism of betacyanin

TABLE 12-7. Localized Bulges in the Abdominal Wall

Localized bulges in the abdominal wall include *ventral hernias* (defects in the wall through which tissue protrudes) and subcutaneous tumors such as *lipomas*. The more common ventral hernias are umbilical, incisional, and epigastric. Hernias and diastasis recti usually become more evident when the patient is supine and raises the head and shoulders.

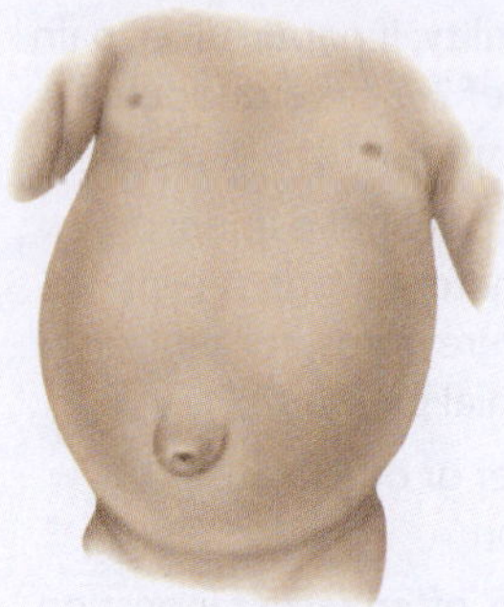

Umbilical Hernia

A protrusion through a defective umbilical ring. When present in infants, it usually closes spontaneously within 1–2 yrs.

Diastasis Recti

Separation of the two rectus abdominis muscles, through which abdominal contents form a midline ridge typically extending from the xiphoid to the umbilicus and seen only when the patient raises the head and shoulders. Often present in patients with repeated pregnancies, obesity, and chronic lung disease. It is clinically benign.

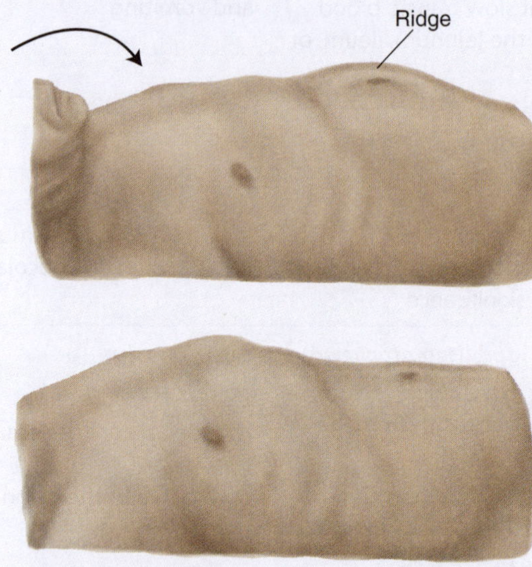

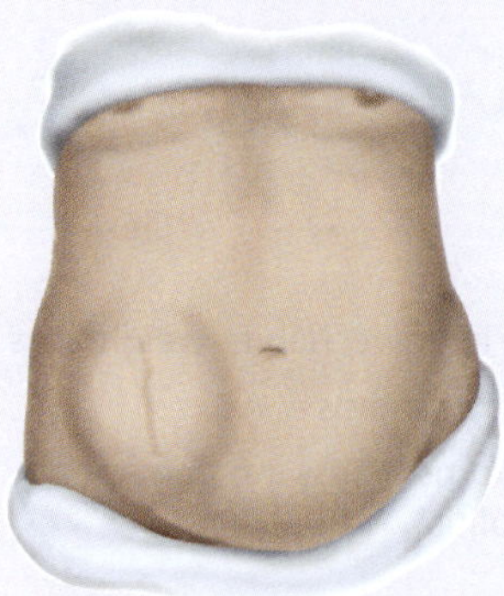

Incisional Hernia

This is a protrusion through an operative scar. Palpate to detect the length and width of the defect in the abdominal wall. A small defect, through which a large hernia has passed, has a greater risk for complications than a large defect.

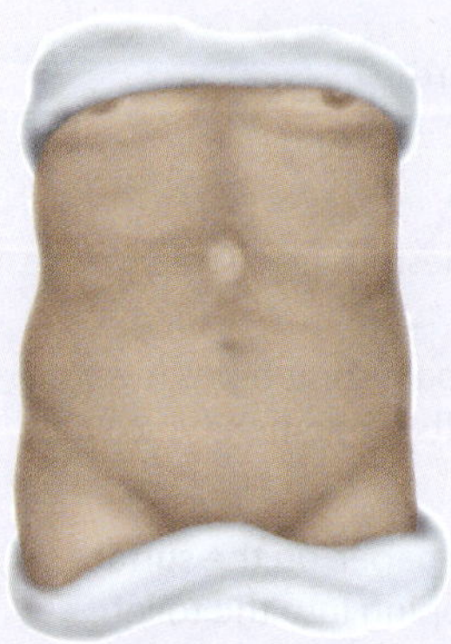

Epigastric Hernia

A small midline protrusion through a defect in the linea alba occurs between the xiphoid process and the umbilicus. With the patient coughing or performing a Valsalva maneuver, palpate by running your fingerpad down the linea alba.

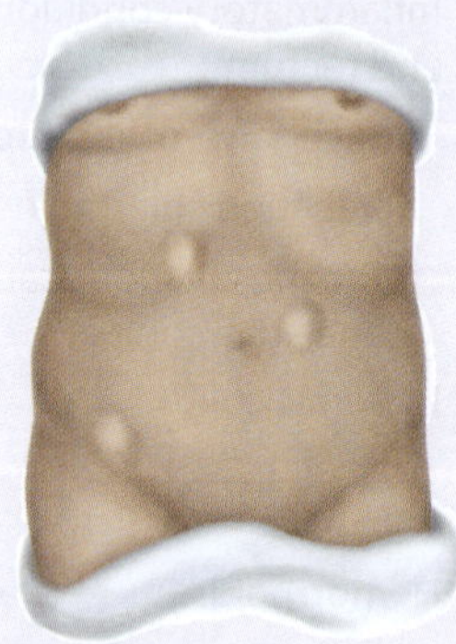

Lipoma

Common, benign, fatty tumors usually in the subcutaneous tissues almost anywhere in the body, including the abdominal wall. Small or large, they are usually soft and often lobulated. Press your finger down on the edge of a lipoma. The tumor typically slips out from under your finger and is well demarcated, nonreducible, and usually nontender.

TABLE 12-8. Protuberant Abdomens

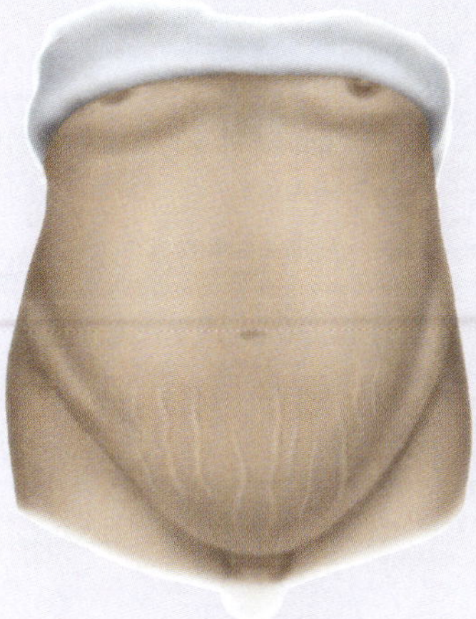

Fat

Fat is the most common cause of a protuberant abdomen. Fat thickens the abdominal wall, the mesentery, and omentum. The umbilicus may appear sunken. A *pannus,* or apron of fatty tissue, may extend below the inguinal ligaments. Lift it to look for inflammation in the skin folds or even for a hidden hernia.

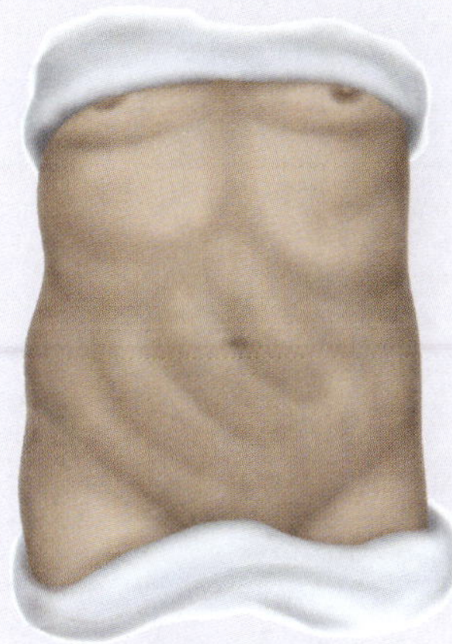

Gas

Gaseous distention may be localized or generalized. It causes a tympanitic percussion note. Selected foods may cause mild distention from increased intestinal gas production. More serious causes are intestinal obstruction and adynamic (paralytic) ileus. Note the location of the distention. Distention is more marked in obstruction in the colon than in the small bowel.

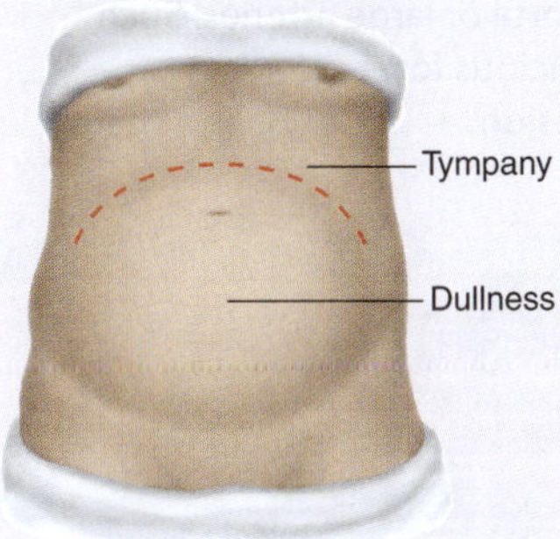

Tumor

A large solid tumor, usually rising out of the pelvis, is dull to percussion. Air-filled bowel is displaced to the periphery. Causes include ovarian tumors and uterine fibroids. Occasionally, a markedly distended bladder is mistaken for such a tumor.

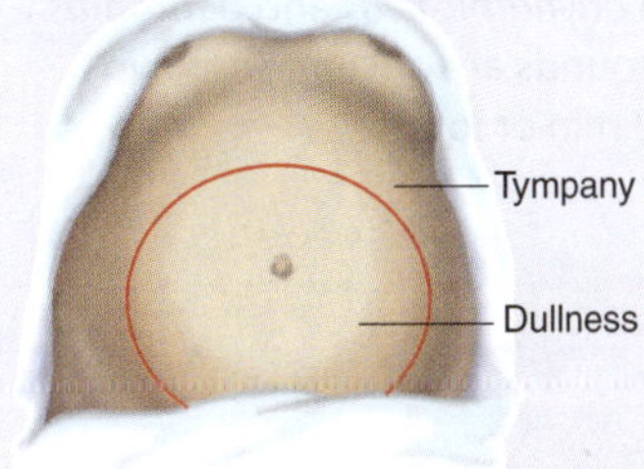

Pregnancy

Pregnancy is a common pelvic "mass." Listen for the fetal heart (see p. 1093).

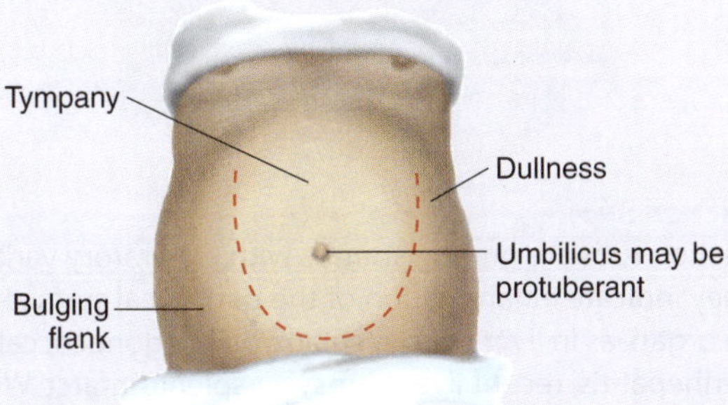

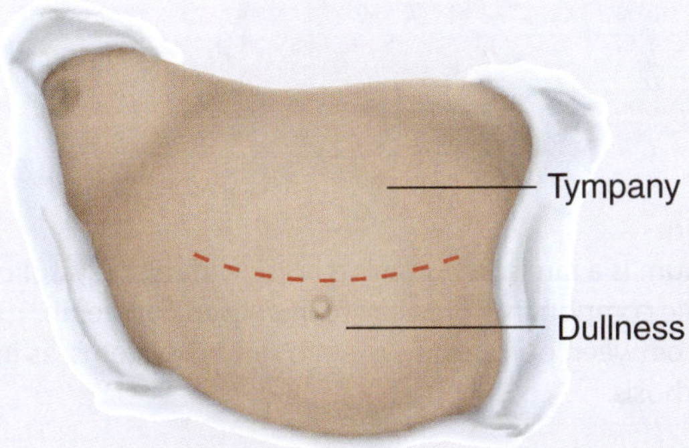

Ascitic Fluid

Ascitic fluid seeks the lowest point in the abdomen, producing bulging flanks that are dull to percussion. The umbilicus may protrude. Turn the patient onto one side to detect the shift in position of the fluid level (shifting dullness). (See p. 277 for the assessment of ascites.)

TABLE 12-9. Sounds in the Abdomen

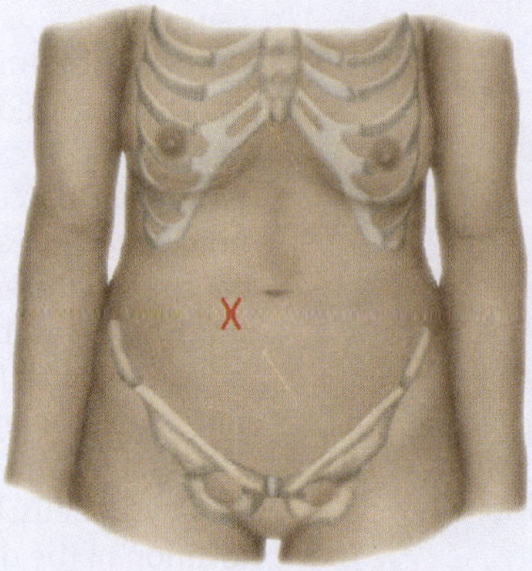

Bowel Sounds

Bowel sounds may be:

- *Increased,* as in diarrhea or early intestinal obstruction
- *Decreased,* then absent, as in *adynamic ileus* and *peritonitis.* Before deciding that bowel sounds are absent, sit down and listen where shown for 2 min or longer.

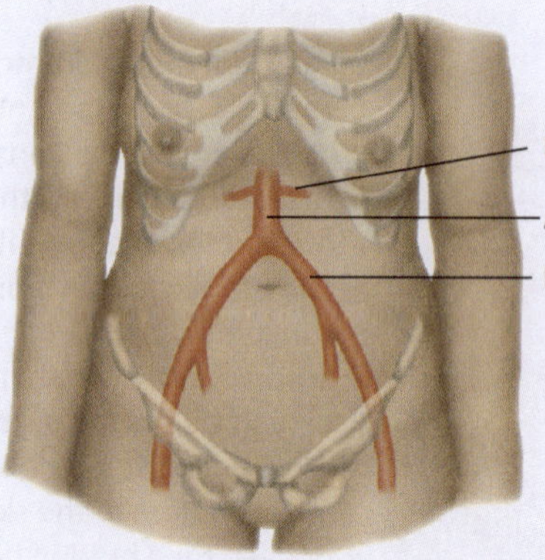

Bruits

A *hepatic bruit* suggests carcinoma of the liver or cirrhosis. *Arterial bruits* with both systolic and diastolic components suggest partial occlusion of the aorta or large arteries. Such bruits in the epigastrium are suspicious for renal artery stenosis or renovascular hypertension.

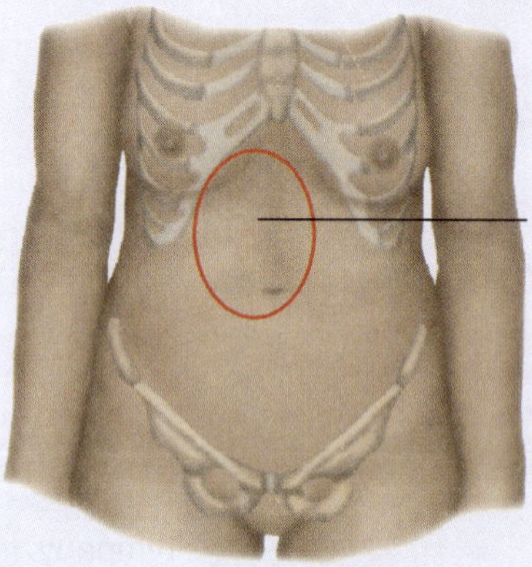

Venous Hum

A venous hum is a rare soft humming noise with both systolic and diastolic components. It points to increased collateral circulation between portal and systemic venous systems, as in hepatic cirrhosis.

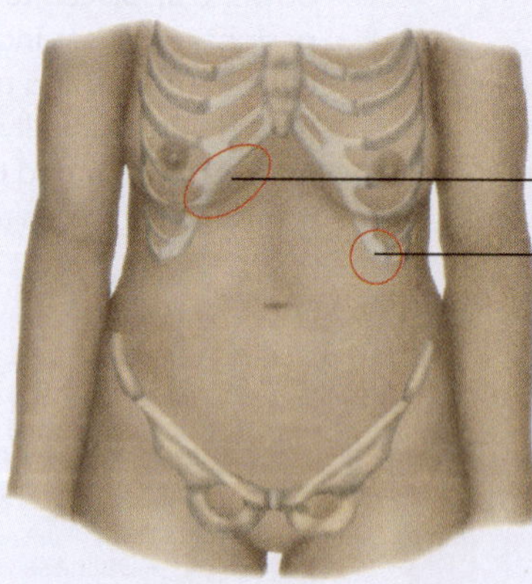

Friction Rubs

Friction rubs are grating sounds with respiratory variation. They indicate inflammation of the peritoneal surface of an organ, as in liver cancer, chlamydial or gonococcal perihepatitis, recent liver biopsy, or splenic infarct. When a systolic bruit accompanies a hepatic friction rub, suspect carcinoma of the liver.

TABLE 12-10. Tender Abdomens

Abdominal Wall Tenderness

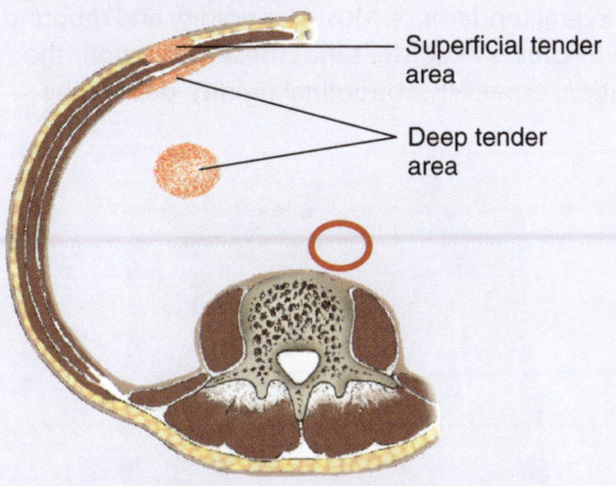

Tenderness may originate in the abdominal wall. When the patient raises the head and shoulders, this tenderness persists, whereas tenderness from a deeper lesion (protected by the tightened muscles) decreases.

Visceral Tenderness

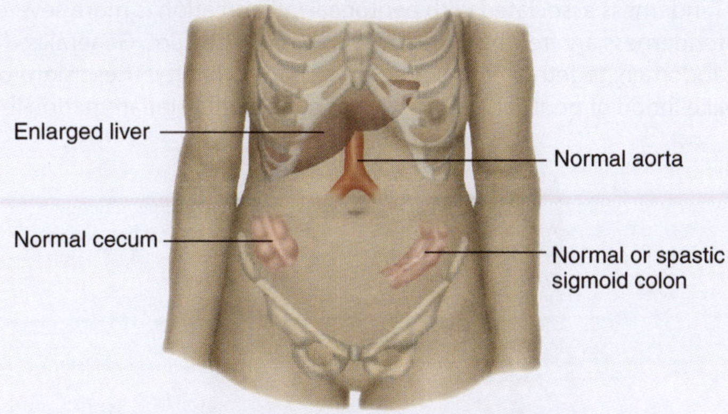

The structures shown may be tender to deep palpation. Usually the discomfort is dull with no muscular rigidity or rebound tenderness. A reassuring explanation to the patient may prove helpful.

Tenderness from Disease in the Chest and Pelvis

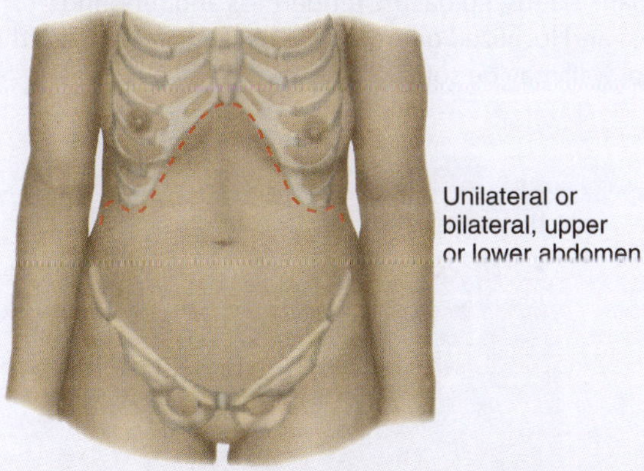

Acute Pleurisy

Abdominal pain and tenderness may result from acute pleural inflammation. When unilateral, it can mimic acute cholecystitis or appendicitis. Rebound tenderness and rigidity are less common; chest signs are usually present.

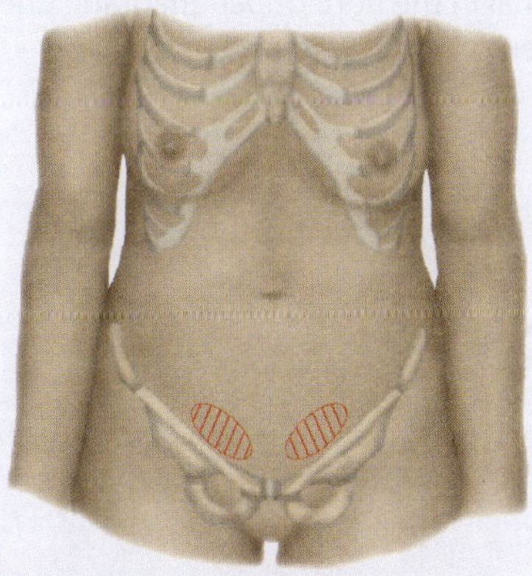

Acute Salpingitis

Frequently bilateral, the tenderness of acute salpingitis (inflammation of the fallopian tubes) is usually maximal just above the inguinal ligaments. Rebound tenderness and rigidity may be present. On pelvic examination, motion of the cervix and uterus causes pain.

(continued)

TABLE 12-10. Tender Abdomens *(Continued)*

Tenderness of Peritoneal Inflammation

Tenderness associated with peritoneal inflammation is more severe than visceral tenderness. Muscular rigidity and rebound tenderness are frequently but not necessarily present. Generalized peritonitis causes exquisite tenderness throughout the abdomen, together with board-like muscular rigidity. These signs on palpation, especially abdominal rigidity, double the likelihood of peritonitis. Local causes of peritoneal inflammation include:

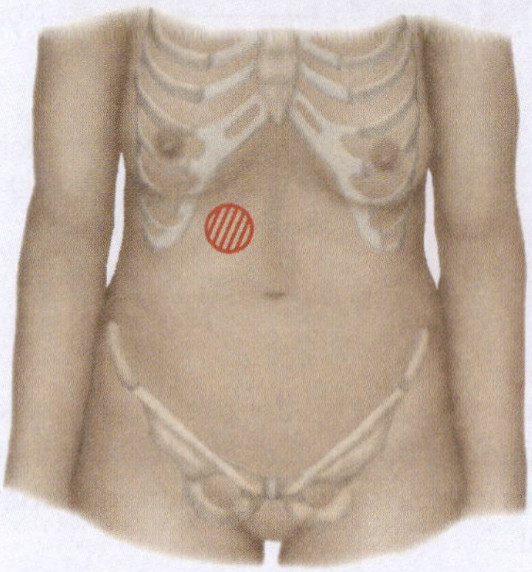

Acute Cholecystitis

Signs are maximal in the right upper quadrant. Check for Murphy sign (see p. 278).

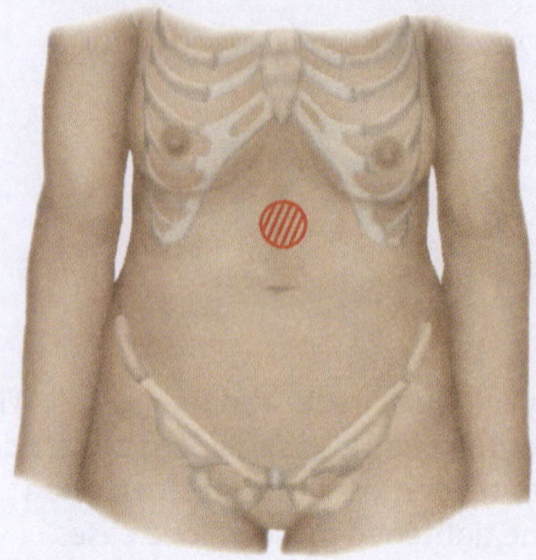

Acute Pancreatitis

In acute pancreatitis, epigastric tenderness and rebound tenderness and localized guarding are usually present, but the abdominal wall may be soft.

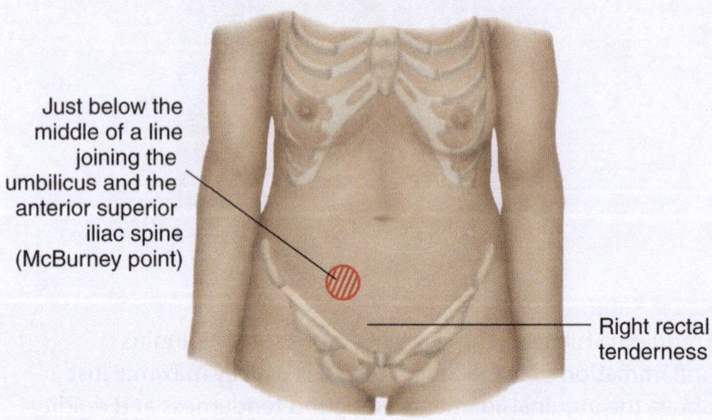

Acute Appendicitis

Right lower quadrant signs are typical of acute appendicitis but may be absent early in the course. The typical area of tenderness, McBurney point, is illustrated. Examine other areas of the right lower quadrant as well as the right flank.

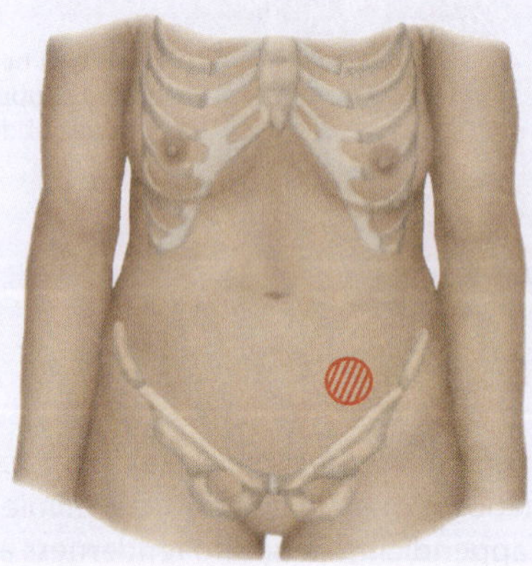

Acute Diverticulitis

Acute diverticulitis is a confined inflammatory process, usually in the left lower quadrant, that involves the sigmoid colon. If the sigmoid colon is redundant there may be suprapubic or right-sided pain. Look for localized peritoneal signs and a tender underlying mass. Microperforation, abscess, and obstruction may ensue.

TABLE 12-11. Liver Enlargement: Apparent and Real

A palpable liver does not necessarily indicate hepatomegaly (an enlarged liver), but more often results from a change in consistency—from the normal softness to an abnormal firmness or hardness, as in cirrhosis. Clinical estimates of liver size should be based on both percussion and palpation, although even these techniques are imperfect compared to ultrasound.

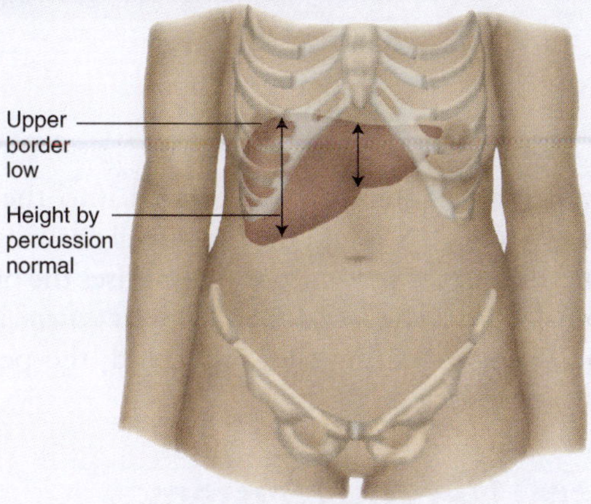

Downward Displacement of the Liver by a Low Diaphragm
This finding is common when the diaphragm is flattened and low, as in COPD. The liver edge may be palpable well below the costal margin. Percussion, however, reveals a low upper edge, and the vertical span of the liver is normal.

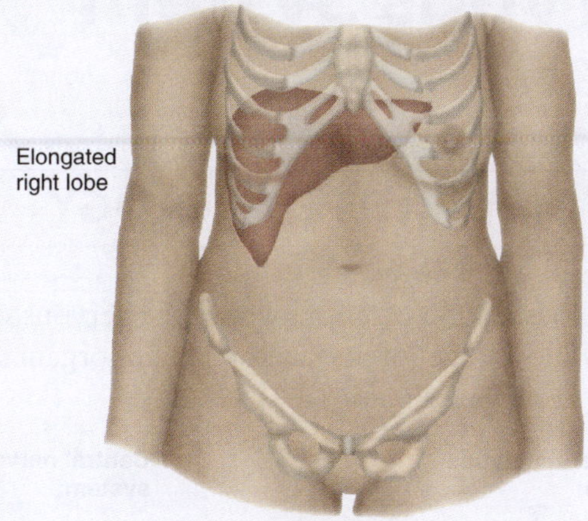

Normal Variations in Liver Shape
In some individuals the right lobe of the liver may be elongated and easily palpable as it projects downward toward the iliac crest. Such an elongation, sometimes called *Riedel lobe*, represents a variation in shape, not an increase in liver volume or size.

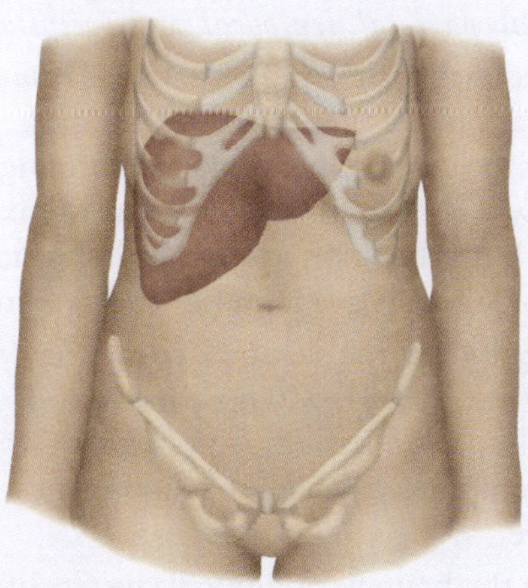

Smooth Large Liver
Cirrhosis may produce an enlarged liver with a firm, *nontender* edge. The cirrhotic liver may also be scarred and contracted. Many other diseases may produce similar findings such as hemochromatosis, amyloidosis, and lymphoma. An enlarged liver with a smooth, *tender* edge suggests inflammation, as in hepatitis, or venous congestion, seen in right-sided heart failure.

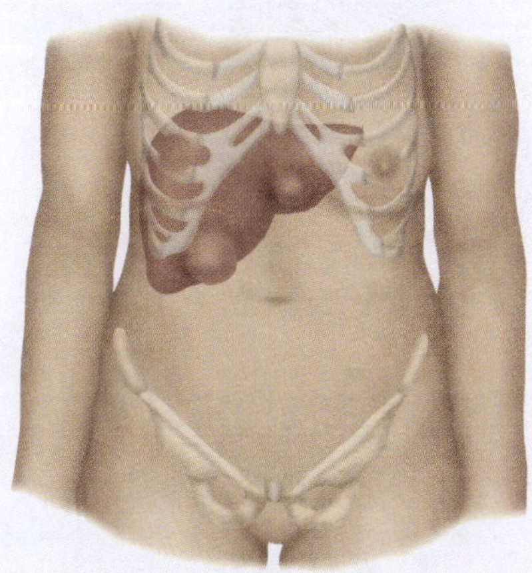

Irregular Large Liver
An enlarged liver that is firm or hard with an irregular edge or surface suggests hepatocellular carcinoma. There may be one or more nodules. The liver may or may not be tender.

CHAPTER 13

Nervous System

ANATOMY AND PHYSIOLOGY

Accurate localization of lesions within the nervous system requires knowledge of its anatomy and organization. Begin by reviewing Figure 13-1.

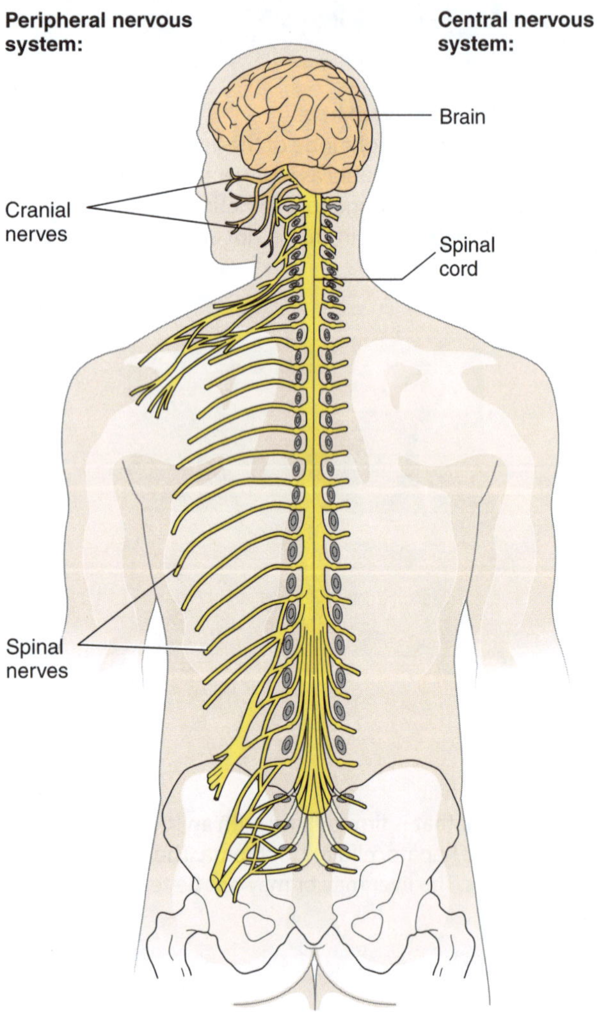

FIGURE 13-1. Central nervous system (CNS) and peripheral nervous system (PNS), coronal section. (Modified from Cohen BJ, Hull KL. *Memmler's The Human Body in Health and Disease*. 14th ed. Jones & Bartlett Learning; 2019, Fig. 9-1.)

The nervous system can be divided into the central nervous system (CNS) and the peripheral nervous system (PNS). The *central nervous system* comprises the brain and the spinal cord. The *peripheral nervous system* includes the spinal nerves exiting the spinal cord, the peripheral nerves, and muscles.

Central Nervous System

Brain. The brain is a vast network of nerve cells, called *neurons*, interconnected through *axons*—single long fibers that conduct impulses from one neuron to another (Fig. 13-2). The largest part of the brain is called the *cerebrum* and is divided into two halves called *cerebral hemispheres*. Each cerebral hemisphere is subdivided into *frontal, parietal, temporal,* and *occipital lobes.*

Brain tissue may be gray or white. *Gray matter* consists of aggregations of neuronal cell bodies. It rims the surfaces of the cerebral hemispheres, forming the *cerebral cortex. White matter* consists of neuronal axons that are coated with myelin. The *myelin sheaths*, which create the white color, allow nerve impulses to travel more rapidly.

Each region of the cerebral cortex has a specialized function (Fig. 13-3). Comprehension of speech, for example, is controlled by a portion of the posterior, superior temporal lobe in the dominant (usually left) hemisphere.

Deep in the brain lie additional clusters of gray matter. These include the *basal ganglia*, which affect movement, and the inferior surface of the frontal lobes (*diencephalon*), which includes the thalamus and the hypothalamus. The *thalamus* processes sensory impulses and relays them to the cerebral cortex. The *hypothalamus* maintains homeostasis and regulates temperature, heart rate, and blood pressure. It also affects the endocrine system and governs emotional behaviors such as anger and sexual drive. Hormones secreted in the hypothalamus act directly on the pituitary gland. The *internal capsule* is a white-matter structure where myelinated fibers converge from the cerebral cortex and descend into the brainstem.

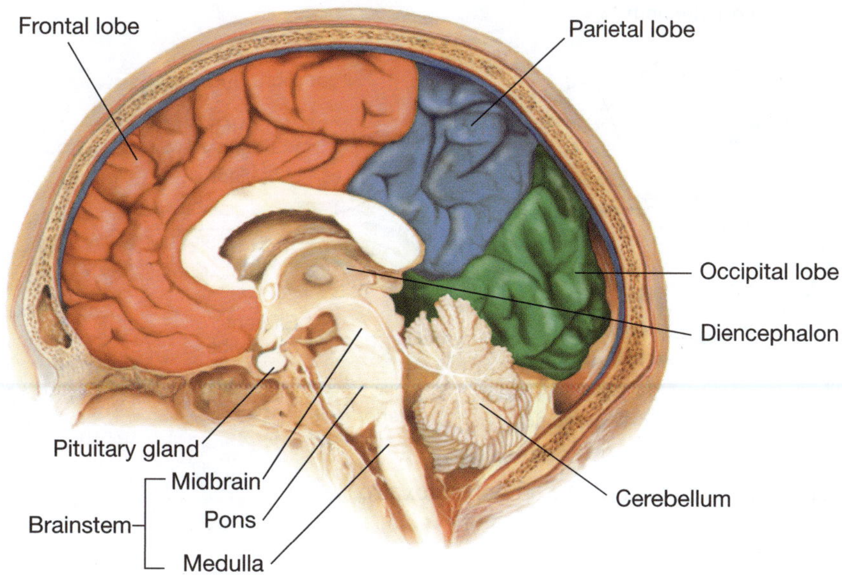

FIGURE 13-2. Right half of the brain, medial view.

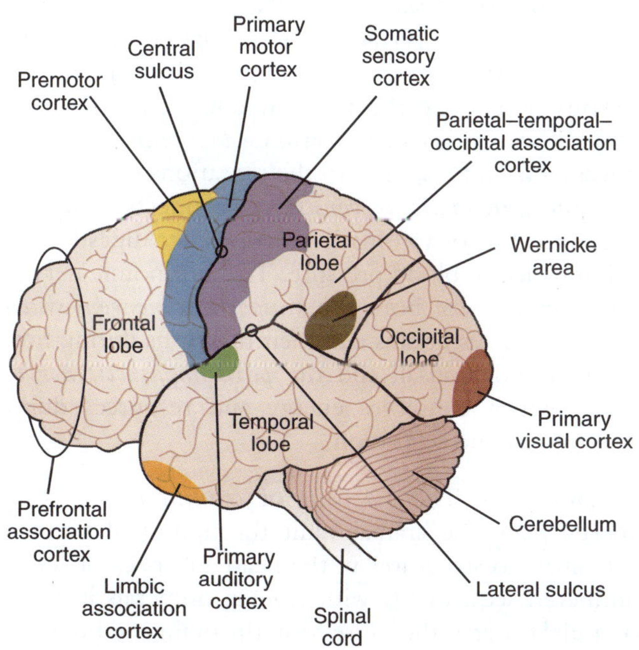

FIGURE 13-3. Regions of the cerebral cortex and selected functions. (From Rhoades RA, Bell DR. *Medical Physiology: Principles for Clinical Medicine*. 5th ed. Wolters Kluwer; 2018, Fig. 7-12.)

The major descending motor pathway, the *corticospinal tract*, runs through the internal capsule.

The *brainstem* connects the upper part of the brain with the spinal cord and has three sections: the *midbrain*, the *pons*, and the *medulla* (see Fig. 13-2). Consciousness relies on the interaction between intact cerebral hemispheres and a structure in the inferior surface of the frontal lobes (*diencephalon*) and upper brainstem, the *reticular activating (arousal) system*. The *cerebellum*, which lies at the base of the brain, coordinates all movement and helps maintain the body upright in space (see Fig. 13-3).

Spinal Cord. The lower brainstem (*medulla*) connects directly to the *spinal cord*. Like the brain, the spinal cord contains both gray matter and white matter. The gray matter consists of aggregations of neuronal cell bodies; note the butterfly appearance of the gray matter nuclei and their *anterior* and *posterior horns* (Fig. 13-4). The outer portions are made up of white matter tracts relaying signals between the brain and PNS.

As shown in Figure 13-5, the *spinal cord* is encased within the bony *vertebral column* and terminates at the first or second lumbar vertebra (L1, L2). The cord provides a series of segmental relays with the periphery, serving as a conduit for information flow to and from the brain. Motor signals exit the cord through *anterior nerve roots* and sensory signals are relayed in via *posterior nerve roots*. The nerve roots join to form *spinal nerves* which in turn form *peripheral nerves*.

The spinal cord is divided into segments related to pairs of exiting spinal nerves: *cervical*, from C1 to C8; *thoracic*, from T1 to T12; *lumbar*, from L1 to L5; *sacral*, from S1 to S5; and *coccygeal*. The spinal cord is thickest in the cervical segment, which contains nerve tracts to and from both the upper and lower extremities. Note that the spinal cord is not as long as the vertebral canal. The lumbar and sacral roots travel the longest intraspinal distance and fan out like a horse's tail after the spinal cord ends at L1–L2, giving rise to the term *cauda equina*.

To avoid injury to the spinal cord, most lumbar punctures are performed at the L3–L4 or L4–L5 vertebral interspaces.

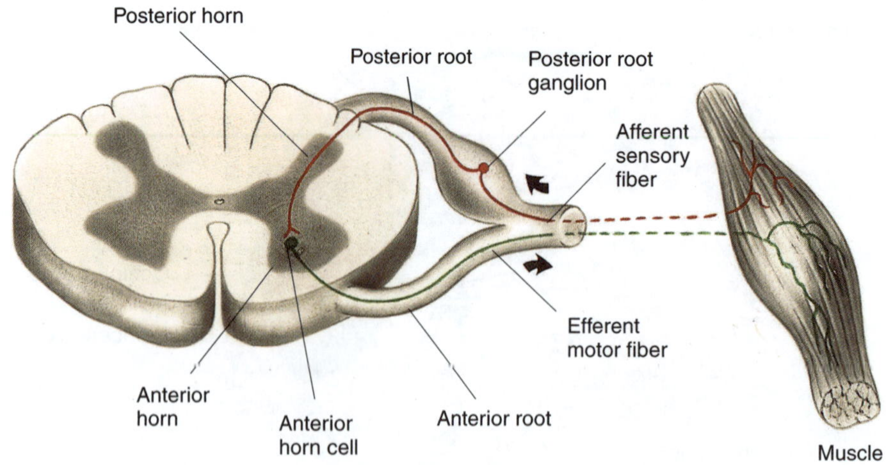

FIGURE 13-4. Spinal cord, cross section and the spinal reflex arc.

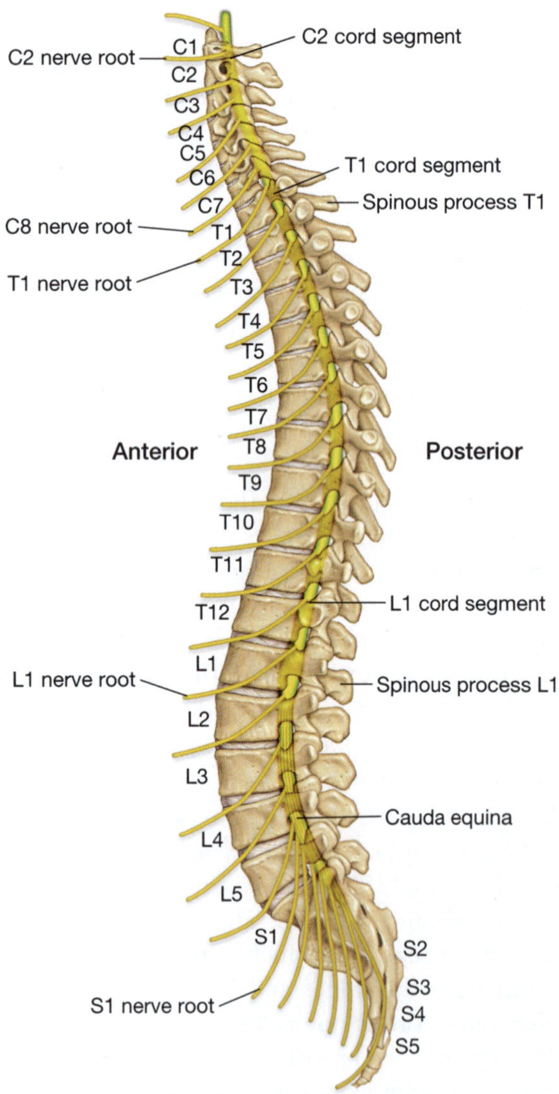

FIGURE 13-5. Spinal cord, lateral view.

Peripheral Nervous System

The *peripheral nervous system* (PNS) includes the *cranial nerves* (CNs) and *peripheral nerves* that project to the heart, visceral organs, skin, and limbs. Both the somatic nervous system and the autonomic nervous system rely on the PNS. The *somatic nervous system* regulates muscle movements and response to the sensations of touch and pain; the *autonomic nervous system* connects to internal organs to control automatic functions like digestion and maintenance of blood pressure. The autonomic nervous system consists of both the *sympathetic nervous system*, which mobilizes organs and their functions during times of stress and arousal, and the *parasympathetic nervous system*, which conserves energy and resources during times of rest and relaxation.

Cranial Nerves. The 12 pairs of *cranial nerves (CNs)* emerge from the cranial vault through skull foramina and canals to structures in the head and neck. They are numbered sequentially with Roman numerals in rostral to caudal order as they arise from the brain and brainstem (Box 13-1). CNs III through XII arise from the brainstem analogous to other peripheral nerves, as illustrated in Figure 13-6. CNs I and II are actually white matter tracts emerging as direct extensions from the brain. Some CNs are limited to general motor and/or sensory functions, whereas others are specialized, serving smell (I), vision (II), or hearing (VIII).

Peripheral Nerves. Spinal and peripheral nerves carry impulses to and from the spinal cord. A total of 31 pairs of spinal nerves attach to the spinal cord: *8 cervical, 12 thoracic, 5 lumbar, 5 sacral, and 1 coccygeal.* Each nerve has an *anterior (ventral) root* containing motor fibers,

Box 13-1. Cranial Nerves

No.	Name	Function
I	Olfactory	Sense of smell
II	Optic	Vision
III	Oculomotor	Pupillary constriction, opening the eye (lid elevation), and most extraocular movements 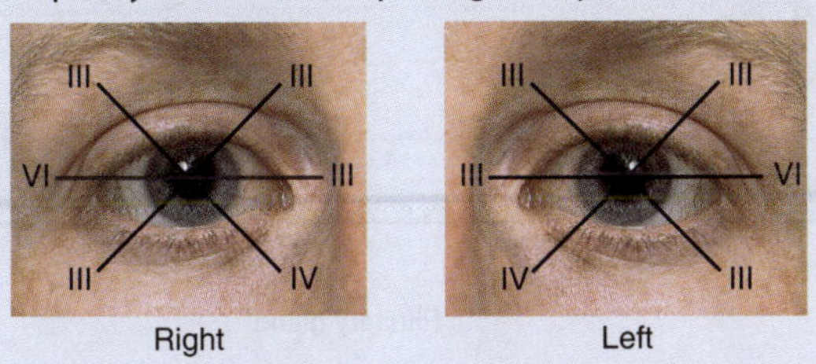
IV	Trochlear	Downward, internal rotation of the eye
V	Trigeminal	*Motor*—temporal and masseter muscles (jaw clenching), lateral pterygoids (lateral jaw movement) 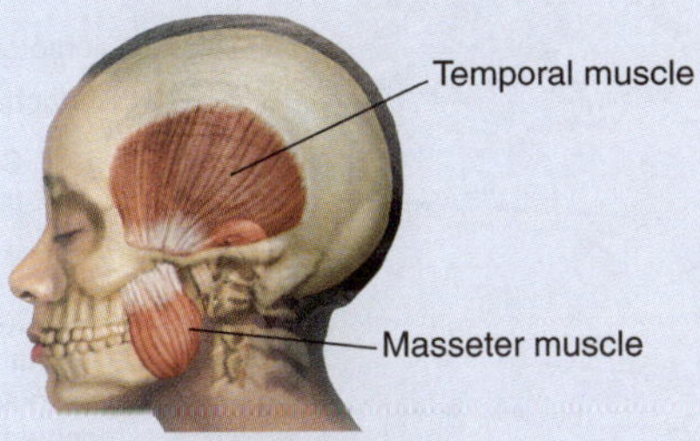 C2 = cervical spine 2. *Sensory*—facial. The nerve has three divisions: (1) ophthalmic, (2) maxillary, and (3) mandibular. 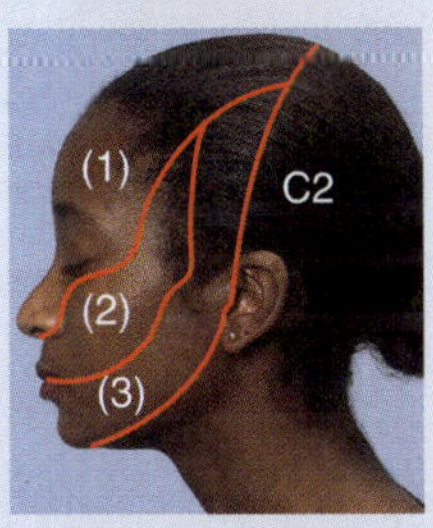
VI	Abducens	Lateral deviation of the eye
VII	Facial	*Motor*—facial movements, including those of facial expression, closing the eye, and closing the mouth *Sensory*—taste for salty, sweet, sour, and bitter substances on the anterior two-thirds of the tongue and sensation from the ear
VIII	Vestibulocochlear	Hearing (cochlear division) and balance (vestibular division)
IX	Glossopharyngeal	*Motor*—pharynx sensory—posterior portions of the eardrum and ear canal, the pharynx, and the posterior tongue, including taste (salty, sweet, sour, bitter)
X	Vagus	*Motor*—palate, pharynx, and larynx *Sensory*—pharynx and larynx

(continued)

Box 13-1. Cranial Nerves (*continued*)

No.	Name	Function
XI	Spinal accessory	*Motor*—the sternocleidomastoid and trapezius 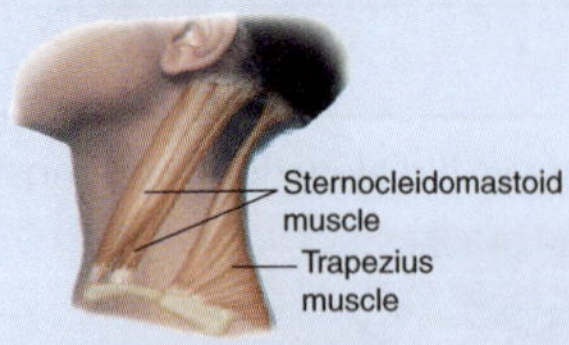
XII	Hypoglossal	*Motor*—tongue

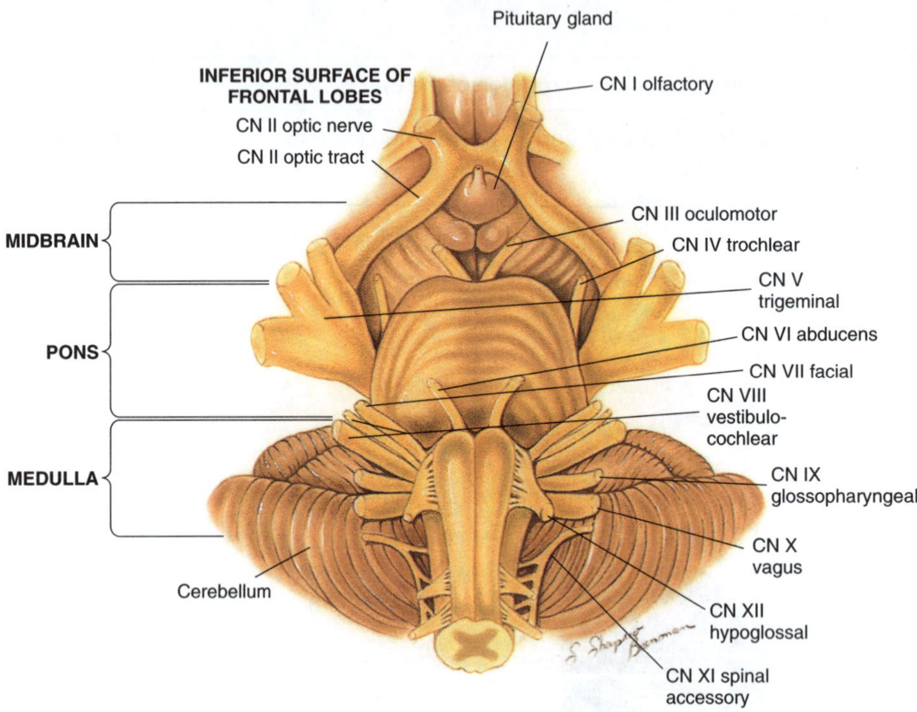

FIGURE 13-6. Cranial nerves, inferior surface of the brain.

and a *posterior (dorsal) root* containing sensory fibers. The anterior and posterior roots merge to form a short *spinal nerve*, <5 mm long. Spinal nerve fibers commingle with each other in plexuses outside the cord, from which peripheral nerves emerge. Most peripheral nerves contain both sensory (*afferent*) and motor (*efferent*) fibers.

Motor Pathways

The primary motor system controlling voluntary movement is called the *corticospinal* or *pyramidal* system. It is best thought of as a two-part system, consisting of *upper motor neurons* and *lower motor neurons.* The cell bodies of upper motor neurons lie in the motor strip of the cerebral cortex (see Fig. 13-7). Their axons project to lower motor neurons through a white matter bundle called the *corticospinal tract.* Motor fibers travel to the brainstem through the internal capsule deep in the brain. In the lower medulla, the corticospinal tracts form an anatomical structure resembling a pyramid—hence the alternative name, the *pyramidal tracts.* At the junction of the medulla and the cervical spinal cord, most of these fibers *decussate,* or cross to the opposite side of the medulla. Because of this crossing, the right side of the brain controls movement on the left side of the body, and vice/versa.

After crossing, corticospinal tract fibers continue downward through the spinal cord to synapse with lower motor neurons. The cell bodies of lower motor neurons reside in the anterior horns of the spinal cord, so they are also called *anterior horn cells.* Some lower motor neurons controlling the motor function of cranial nerves reside

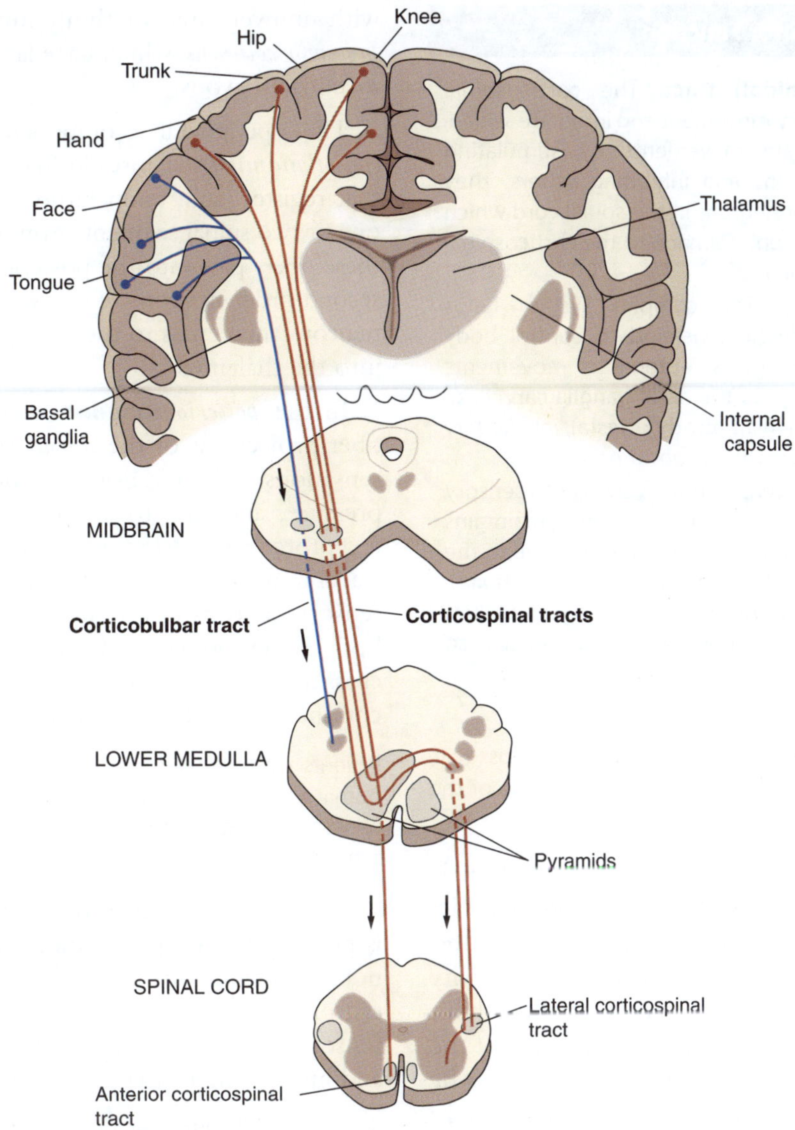

FIGURE 13-7. Motor pathways: corticospinal and corticobulbar tracts.

in the brainstem, however. The *corticobulbar tract* refers to those upper motor neuron axons that project to these lower motor neurons. Axons from lower motor neurons transmit impulses either through cranial nerves, or through the anterior roots of the spinal cord and spinal nerves into peripheral nerves. These impulses terminate at the *neuromuscular junction*, which mediates muscle contraction.

Box 13-2 describes three systems that control motor function. The corticospinal tracts have an inhibitory effect on lower motor neurons; upper motor neuron or corticospinal tract damage leads to *increased muscle tone* and *hyperreflexia* because the lower motor neurons are disinhibited. By contrast, lower motor neuron damage causes *decreased muscle tone* and *hyporeflexia*; *atrophy* and *fasciculations* can also be seen. Characteristic upper motor neuron signs (increased muscle tone, hyperreflexia) and lower motor neuron signs (decreased muscle tone, hyporeflexia, fasciculations and atrophy) can be demonstrated on neurologic examination to help distinguish between the two possibilities.

Weakness can be caused by damage to upper motor neurons or their projections (the corticospinal tract) or by damage to lower motor neurons or their projections (the cranial nerves, spinal nerve roots, or peripheral nerves).

Higher motor pathways depend on intact lower motor neurons to affect movement. Damage to lower motor neurons leads to paralysis or weakness of the affected segment(s) even if the higher motor pathways are intact. When the corticospinal tract is damaged or destroyed, its functions are reduced or lost below the level of injury. The affected limb becomes weak or paralyzed, and skilled, complicated, or delicate movements are performed poorly when compared with gross movements.

When upper motor neuron systems are damaged above their crossover in the medulla, motor impairment develops on the

Box 13-2. Control of Motor Function

- **Corticospinal (pyramidal) tract.** The corticospinal tracts mediate voluntary movement and integrate skilled, complicated, or delicate movements by stimulating selected muscular actions and inhibiting others. They synapse on lower motor neurons in the spinal cord which directly mediate movement. Damage to the corticospinal tract system causes *weakness.*
- **Basal ganglia system.** This complex system helps to maintain normal muscle tone and to control body movements, especially gross automatic movements such as walking. Damage to the basal ganglia can cause *rigidity, slowness of movement* (**bradykinesia**), *involuntary movements, and/or disturbances in posture and gait.*
- **Cerebellar system.** The cerebellum receives both sensory and motor input and coordinates motor activity, maintains equilibrium, and helps to control posture. Damage to the cerebellar system can *impair coordination* (called **ataxia**), *gait, equilibrium,* and *decrease muscle tone.* The cerebellum also helps coordinate eye movements and speech, so other signs like *nystagmus* or *dysarthria* may be seen.

opposite or contralateral side. In damage below the crossover, motor impairment occurs on the *same or ipsilateral* side of the body.

Two other systems do not control movement directly but help modulate the effects of the corticospinal tract system. The *basal ganglia* are collections of gray matter deep within the cerebral hemispheres. Their activity helps facilitate desired voluntary movement and inhibit unwanted movements. The *cerebellum* at the base of the brain helps coordinate movement and control posture by integrating visual, proprioceptive, and vestibular sensory inputs together with the desired motor plan.

Disease of the basal ganglia system or cerebellar system does not cause paralysis but can be disabling.

Sensory Pathways

Sensory impulses give rise to conscious sensation, locate body position in space, and help regulate internal autonomic functions such as blood pressure, heart rate, and respiration.

A complex system of sensory receptors relays impulses from skin, mucous membranes, muscles, tendons, and viscera that travel through peripheral projections into the dorsal (posterior) root ganglia, where a second projection of the ganglia directs impulses centrally into the spinal cord (Fig. 13-8). Sensory impulses then travel to the sensory cortex of the brain via one of two pathways: the *spinothalamic tract*, consisting of smaller sensory neurons with unmyelinated or thinly myelinated axons, and the *posterior columns*, which have larger neurons with heavily myelinated axons.

The peripheral component of the small-fiber *spinothalamic tract* arises in free nerve endings in the skin that register pain, temperature, and crude touch. Within one or two spinal segments from their entry into the cord, these fibers pass into the posterior horn and synapse with second-order neurons. The axons of these second-order neurons then cross to the opposite side and pass upward into the thalamus.

In the *posterior column system*, the peripheral large-fiber projections of the *dorsal root ganglia* transmit the sensations of vibration, proprioception, kinesthesia, pressure, and fine touch from skin and joint position receptors to the dorsal root ganglia. Central projections travel upwards in the posterior columns to second-order sensory neurons in the medulla on the same side of the body. Axons projecting from these second-order neurons cross to the opposite side at the medullary level and continue on to the thalamus.

Patients with diabetes with small-fiber neuropathy report sharp, burning, or shooting foot pain, whereas those with large-fiber neuropathy experience numbness and tingling or even no sensation at all.

At the thalamic level, the general quality of sensation is perceived (e.g., pain, cold, pleasant, unpleasant), but not fine distinctions. For full perception, a third group of sensory neurons sends impulses from the thalamus to the sensory cortex of the brain. Here, stimuli are localized, and higher-order discriminations are made.

See Table 13-1, Disorders of the Central and Peripheral Nervous Systems.

Dermatomes. A *dermatome* is the band of skin innervated by the sensory root of a single spinal nerve. Knowledge and testing of dermatomes are valuable when localizing a lesion to a specific spinal cord segment. See the dermatome maps on pp. 328–329.

Lesions at different points in the sensory pathways produce different kinds of sensory loss. A lesion in the sensory cortex may not impair the perception of pain, touch, and position, for example, but does impair finer discrimination. A patient with this lesion cannot appreciate the size, shape, or texture of an object by feeling it and therefore cannot identify it. Loss of position and vibration sense, with preservation of other sensations, points to disease of the posterior columns. Loss of all sensations from the waist down, together with paralysis and hyperactive reflexes in the legs, indicates severe transverse damage to the spinal cord. Crude and light touch are often preserved despite partial damage to the cord because impulses originating on one side of the body travel up both sides of the cord.

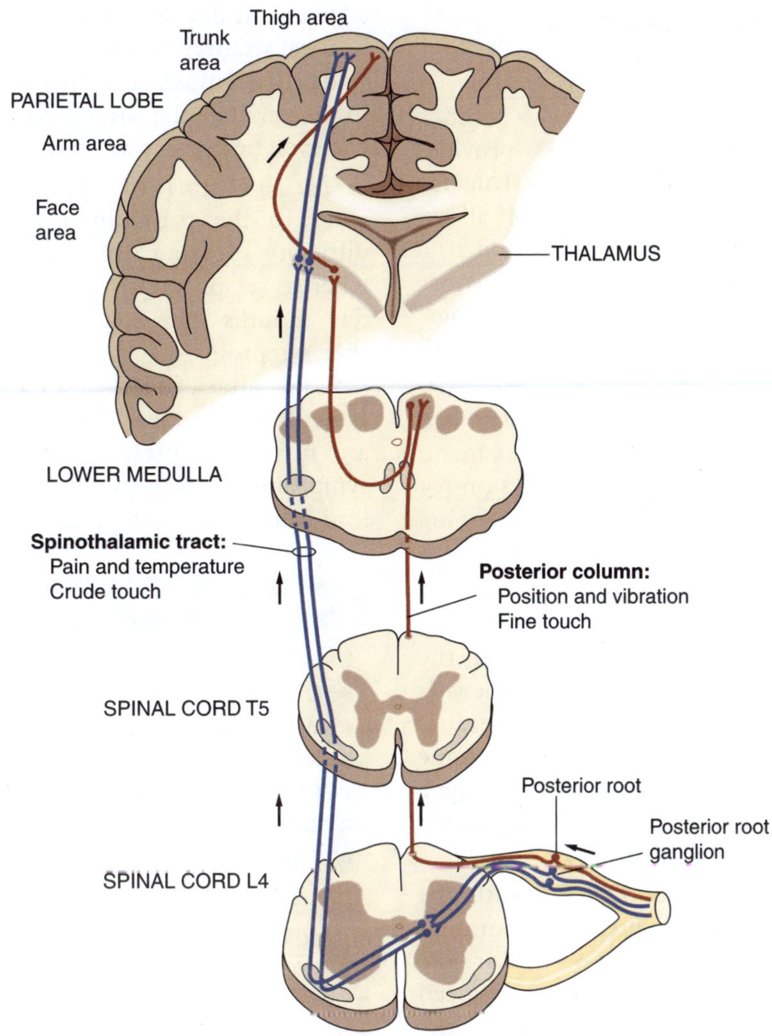

FIGURE 13-8. Sensory pathways: spinothalamic tract and posterior columns.

Spinal Reflexes: Muscle Stretch Response

The *muscle stretch reflexes* are relayed over structures of both the CNS and PNS. Since the tendons are not the primary structures involved, the term muscle stretch reflexes is more precise than the commonly used *deep tendon reflexes.* A *reflex* is an involuntary stereotypical response that may involve as few as two neurons, one afferent (sensory) and one efferent (motor), across a single synapse. The muscle stretch reflexes in the arms and legs are such *monosynaptic reflexes.* They illustrate the simplest unit of sensory and motor function. Other reflexes are *polysynaptic*, involving interneurons interposed between sensory and motor neurons.

For the reflex to occur, all components of the reflex arc must be intact: sensory nerve fibers, spinal cord synapse, motor nerve fibers, neuromuscular junction, and muscle fibers. Tapping the tendon activates special sensory fibers in the partially stretched muscle, triggering a sensory impulse that travels to the spinal cord via a peripheral nerve. The stimulated sensory fiber synapses directly with the anterior horn cell innervating the same muscle. When the impulse crosses the neuromuscular junction, the muscle suddenly contracts, completing the reflex arc.

Because each muscle stretch reflex involves specific spinal segments, together with their sensory and motor fibers, an abnormal reflex helps you locate a pathologic lesion. Learn the segmental levels of the muscle stretch reflexes, which are listed in Box 13-3 in descending order from C6–C7 through S1.

Box 13-3. Muscle Stretch Reflexes

Reflex	Level
Triceps reflex	Cervical 6, 7
Brachioradialis (supinator) reflex	Cervical 5, 6
Biceps reflex	Cervical 5, 6
Knee reflex	Lumbar 2, 3, 4
Ankle reflex	Sacral 1

HEALTH HISTORY: GENERAL APPROACH

For many of the body systems, the history provides the essential clues to diagnosis. While this is true for the nervous system, the neurologic examination allows you to assess all levels of nervous system function to a unique degree. With practice, you can obtain a history and perform a thorough yet efficient neurologic examination that enables you to detect the wide breadth of neurologic illness.

When neurologic disease is suspected, two complimentary questions should guide your assessment: (1) What is the localization of the responsible lesion (or lesions) in the nervous system? (2) What is the underlying pathophysiology that explains the patient's symptoms and neurologic findings?

These questions are not answered separately, but iteratively as you learn about the patient from the patient's spontaneous responses during the interview. It is important to consider both of these questions because different pathophysiologic processes may affect the same structures and produce similar symptoms. Reaching a neurologic diagnosis through this process is considered difficult by many and requires practice.

Assessment of the nervous system begins with the first moments of the patient encounter and continues throughout the interview. If you suspect that the patient's mental status is abnormal, you may need to proceed directly to formal mental status testing, described in Chapter 9, Cognition, Behavior, and Mental Status. If there is significant impairment, for example, disorientation to person or place, the history may be unreliable, so you will need other observers to obtain critical information.

See Chapter 9, techniques to conduct the formal mental status examination.

The *pattern of symptoms* often aids with localization. If the patient complains of weakness, for example, identify whether one side of the body is affected or both. Identify if proximal muscles, distal muscles, or both are weak. Always ask about other neurologic symptoms even if they are not volunteered by the patient. A patient complaining of trouble walking and falls may not realize that numbness in the feet could be related, for example.

Remember that lesions at different levels of the nervous system can cause the same symptoms. For example, distal leg weakness can be caused by lesions in the brain, brainstem, spinal cord, spinal nerve root, peripheral nerve, and muscles. In addition, neurologic disease can have positive or negative effects, or both. There may be *irritative phenomena*, for example, such as a "pins-and-needles" sensation (*paresthesia*), **myoclonus**, or focal seizures with jerking of a limb on one side of the body. In contrast, some parts of the nervous system, as in the parietal lobe, are *relatively silent*—extensive lesions can even be present without causing any symptoms at all.

The time course of a patient's symptoms can provide clues to the pathophysiology. The sudden onset of difficulty speaking, for example, may suggest a stroke whereas a progressive worsening of speech over a few months may suggest a brain tumor. Remember that symptoms may be transient, such as in a transient ischemic attack (TIA) or an attack of multiple sclerosis. Patients may be less likely to volunteer symptoms that are no longer present; specifically asking about past symptoms can help better elucidate the time course and lead to more accurate diagnosis.

Common or Concerning Symptoms

- Headache
- Dizziness or lightheadedness
- Weakness (generalized, proximal, or distal)
- Numbness or abnormal or absent sensation
- Fainting and blacking out (near-syncope and syncope)
- Seizures
- Tremors or involuntary movements

Other common symptoms that may involve the nervous system are addressed in more detail in the following sections:

- Confusion (see Chapter 9)
- Memory loss (see Chapter 9)
- Trouble speaking (see Table 13-2)
- Vision loss or double vision (see Chapter 20)
- Difficulty walking (see Table 13-3)

Headache

Headache is one of the most common symptoms in clinical practice, with a lifetime prevalence of 30% in the general population. Among types of headaches, tension headache predominates, affecting half of all individuals during their lifetime. Neurologic causes such as subarachnoid hemorrhage, meningitis, or mass lesions are especially ominous. Headaches are generally classified as *primary* (without an identified underlying disease) or *secondary* (with an identified underlying disease). However, every headache warrants careful evaluation for life-threatening secondary causes such as meningitis, subarachnoid hemorrhage, or mass lesion.

Medicine History Taking OSCE Videos: **Headache**

Primary headaches include migraine, tension, cluster, trigeminal autonomic cephalalgias and chronic daily headaches; *secondary headaches* arise from underlying structural, systemic, or infectious causes such as meningitis or subarachnoid hemorrhage and may be life threatening.

Obtaining a thorough history is critical because the physical examination will often be normal in patients with headache. In fact, the presence of any abnormal findings on examination raises concern for a secondary headache and should always prompt additional work-up.

See Tables 13-4 and 13-5 on Primary Headaches and Secondary Headaches and Cranial Neuralgias.

The approach to headache is similar to your approach to assessing pain elsewhere in the body—ask about the location, character, severity, onset, and time course of the headache. Is it unilateral or bilateral? Severe with sudden onset, like a thunderclap? Steady or throbbing? Continuous or intermittent? Is there an aura? Is the headache "typical" or is there something different?

Subarachnoid hemorrhage classically presents as "the worst headache of my life" with instantaneous onset. Severe headache and stiff neck accompany meningitis. Dull headache increased by coughing and sneezing, especially when recurring in the same location, occurs in mass lesions from brain tumors or abscess.

An atypical presentation of the patient's usual migraine may be suspicious for stroke, especially in women using hormonal contraceptives.

Migraine headache is often preceded by an aura or prodrome, and is highly likely if three of the five "POUND" features are present: **P**ulsatile or throbbing; **O**ne-day duration, or lasts 4 to 72 hours if untreated; **U**nilateral; **N**ausea or vomiting; **D**isabling or intensity causing interruption of daily activity.

Exacerbating or Alleviating Symptoms. Identify any exacerbating or alleviating factors; for example, does the headache get worse with coughing, sneezing, or sudden head movements, which can alter intracranial pressure dynamics?

Presenting and Associated Symptoms. The three most important attributes of headache are its *severity*, its *chronologic pattern*, and its *associated symptoms*. Is the headache severe and of sudden onset? Does it intensify over several hours? Is it episodic? Or is it chronic or recurring? Is there a recent change in its pattern? Does the headache recur at the same time every day? What other symptoms, especially weakness or numbness in an arm or leg?

If headache is severe and of sudden onset, consider subarachnoid hemorrhage or meningitis.

Migraine and tension headaches are episodic and tend to peak over several hours. New and persisting, progressively severe headaches raise concerns of tumor, abscess, or mass lesion.

Look for important signs (red flags) that warn of headaches needing prompt investigation such as sudden onset "like a thunderclap," onset after age 50 years, and associated symptoms such as fever and stiff neck (Box 13-4). Examine for papilledema and focal neurologic signs.

Box 13-4. Headache Warning Signs

- Progressively frequent or severe over a 3-month period
- Sudden onset like a "thunderclap" or "the worst headache of my life"
- New onset after age 50 years
- Aggravated or relieved by change in position
- Precipitated by Valsalva maneuver or exertion
- Associated symptoms of fever, night sweats, or weight loss
- Presence of cancer, HIV infection, or pregnancy
- Recent head trauma
- Change in pattern from past headaches
- Lack of a similar headache in the past
- Associated papilledema, neck stiffness, or focal neurologic deficits

Thunderclap headaches reaching maximal intensity over several minutes occur in 70% of patients with subarachnoid hemorrhage and are often preceded by a sentinel leak headache from a vascular leak into the subarachnoid space.

Ask about any associated symptoms such as double vision, visual changes, weakness, or loss of sensation. Is there fever, stiff neck, or a parameningeal focus like ear, sinus, or throat infection that may signal meningitis?

Ask about nausea and vomiting.

Nausea and vomiting are common with migraine, but also occur with brain tumors and subarachnoid hemorrhage.

Is there a prodrome of unusual feelings such as euphoria, craving for food, fatigue, or dizziness?

Approximately 60% to 70% of patients with migraine have a symptom prodrome prior to onset. About a third experience a visual aura, such as spark photopsias (flashes of light), fortifications (zig-zag arcs of light), and scotomas (areas of visual loss with surrounding normal vision).

Does the patient report an aura with neurologic symptoms, such as change in vision, numbness, or weakness?

Note that, due to increased risk of ischemic stroke and cardiovascular disease, the World Health Organization advises women with migraines over age 35 years and women with migraines with aura avoid use of estrogen–progestin contraceptives.

Ask if coughing, sneezing, or changing the position of the head affects the headache. If head position affects the headache, ask if leaning forward or lying down increases the headache, or if lying down increases the headache.

Valsalva maneuvers and leaning forward may increase pain from acute sinusitis. Valsalva and lying down may increase pain from mass lesions due to changing intracranial pressure.

Is there any overuse of analgesics, ergotamines, or triptans?

Medication for overuse headache may cause headache if present ≥15 days a month for 3 months and reverts to <15 days a month when the medication is discontinued.

Ask about family history.

Genetic inheritance is present in 30% to 50% of patients with migraine.

After your usual open-ended assessment, ask the patient to point to the area of pain or discomfort.

Unilateral headache occurs in migraine and cluster headaches. Tension headaches often arise in the temporal areas; cluster headaches may be retro-orbital.

Dizziness or Lightheadedness

Dizziness and *lightheadedness* are common, somewhat vague, complaints that prompt a more specific history and neurologic examination, with emphasis on detection of nystagmus and focal neurologic signs. Especially in older patients, ask about medications.

Feeling lightheaded, weak in the legs, or about to faint point to presyncope from vasovagal stimulation, orthostatic hypotension, arrhythmia, or side effects from blood pressure and other medications.

See Table 11-1, Syncope and Similar Disorders.

Does the patient feel faint or about to fall or pass out (*presyncope*)? Or unsteady and off balance (*dysequilibrium* or *ataxia*)? Or is there *vertigo,* a spinning sensation within the patient or of the surroundings? If there is true vertigo, establish the time course of symptoms, which helps distinguish among the different types of peripheral vestibular disorders. Although these distinctions are helpful, note that patients may have difficulty describing their symptoms and distinguishing between these categories of dizziness.

Vertigo often reflects vestibular disease, usually from peripheral causes in the inner ear such as benign positional vertigo, labyrinthitis, or Ménière disease.

See Table 21-1, Dizziness and Vertigo, for distinguishing symptoms and time course.

If there are localizing symptoms or signs like double vision (*diplopia*), difficulty forming words (*dysarthria*), or problems with gait or balance (*ataxia*), investigate the central causes of vertigo.

Ataxia, diplopia, and dysarthria are suspicious for *vertebrobasilar* TIA or stroke. Also consider posterior fossa tumor and migraine with brainstem aura.

See Table 13-6, Types of Stroke.

Weakness

Complaints of weakness may have different meanings, including fatigue, apathy, drowsiness, or actual loss of strength. True motor weakness can arise from lesions affecting the CNS, a peripheral nerve, the neuromuscular junction, or a muscle. Time course and location are especially relevant. Is the onset sudden, gradual or subacute, or chronic, over a long period of time?

Medicine History Taking OSCE Videos: **Weakness of the Limbs**

Abrupt onset of motor and sensory deficits occurs in *TIA* and *stroke.* Progressive but rapid development of lower extremity weakness followed by upper extremity weakness suggests Guillain–Barré syndrome. Chronic, more gradual, progression of weakness may be seen from expanding tumors or amyotrophic lateral sclerosis (ALS).

What areas of the body are involved? Is the weakness generalized, or focal to the face or a limb? Does it involve one side of the body or both sides? What movements are affected? As you listen to the patient's story, identify the patterns below:

- *Proximal*—in the shoulder and/or hip girdle, for example
- *Distal*—in the hands and/or feet
- *Symmetric*—in the same areas on both sides of the body
- *Asymmetric*—types of weakness include *focal,* in a portion of the face or extremity; *monoparesis,* in an extremity; *paraparesis,* in both lower extremities; and *hemiparesis,* in one side of the body

Focal or asymmetric weakness has both central (ischemic, thrombotic, or mass lesions) and peripheral causes ranging from nerve injury to the neuromuscular junction disorders to myopathies.

To identify *proximal weakness,* ask about difficulty with movements such as combing hair, reaching up to a shelf, getting up out of a chair, or climbing stairs. Does the weakness get worse with repetition and improve after rest (suggesting myasthenia gravis)? Are there associated sensory or other symptoms?

Proximal limb weakness, when symmetric with intact sensation, occurs in myopathies from alcohol, drugs like glucocorticoids, and inflammatory muscle disorders like polymyositis and dermatomyositis. In the neuromuscular junction disorder myasthenia gravis, there is proximal weakness that gets worse with effort (fatigability), often with associated *bulbar symptoms* such as diplopia, ptosis, dysarthria, and dysphagia.

To identify *distal weakness,* ask about hand strength when opening a jar or using scissors or buttoning buttons, or problems tripping when walking.

Bilateral predominantly distal weakness, often with sensory loss, suggests a polyneuropathy, as in diabetes.

Numbness or Abnormal or Absent Sensation

In a patient who reports numbness, ask the patient to be more precise. Is there tingling like "pins and needles," called *paresthesia*, distorted sensations (*dysesthesias*), or is sensation reduced or completely absent?

Sensory changes can arise at several levels: local nerve compression, or *"entrapment,"* can cause hand numbness in distributions specific to the median, ulnar, or radial nerve; nerve root compression can cause dermatomal sensory loss from vertebral bone spurs or herniated discs; or central lesions from stroke or multiple sclerosis can cause hemianesthesia.

With dysesthesias, light touch or pinprick, for example, may cause a burning or irritating sensation. Burning pain occurs in painful sensory neuropathies from conditions like diabetes.

Establish the pattern of sensory loss. Is there a stocking-glove distribution? Are sensory deficits patchy, nondermatomal, and occurring in more than one limb?

A pattern of stocking, then glove, sensory loss occurs in polyneuropathies, especially from diabetes; multiple patchy areas of sensory loss in different limbs suggest mononeuritis multiplex, seen in vasculitis and rheumatoid arthritis.

Fainting and Blacking Out (Near-Syncope and Syncope)

Patient reports of fainting or "passing out" are common and warrant a meticulous history to guide management and possible hospital admission.

Begin by finding out whether the patient has actually lost consciousness. Did the patient hear external noise or voices throughout the episode, feel light-headed or weak, but fail to actually lose consciousness, consistent with *near syncope* or *presyncope*? Or did the patient actually experience complete loss of consciousness, a more serious symptom representing true *syncope*, defined as a sudden but temporary loss of consciousness and postural tone from transient global hypoperfusion of the brain? Seizures may be confused with syncope, but impairment of consciousness in seizure results from disordered neuronal firing rather than hypoperfusion of brain tissue.

Causes include "neurocardiogenic" conditions such as vasovagal syncope, postural tachycardia syndrome, carotid sinus syncope, and orthostatic hypotension, and cardiac disease causing arrhythmias, especially ventricular tachycardia and bradyarrhythmias. Stroke or TIA are unlikely causes of syncope, though strokes affecting the reticular activating system can impair consciousness.

Elicit a complete description of the event. What was the patient doing when the episode occurred? Was the patient standing, sitting, or lying down? Were there any triggers or warning symptoms? How long did the episode last? Could voices still be heard? Importantly, were onset and offset slow or fast? Were there any palpitations? Is there a history of heart disease?

The presence of a history of heart disease has a sensitivity for a cardiac cause of more than 95% (with a specificity of ~45%).

In vasovagal syncope, the most common cause of syncope, look for the prodrome of nausea, diaphoresis, and pallor triggered by a fearful or unpleasant event, then vagally mediated hypotension, often with slow onset and offset. In syncope from arrhythmias, onset and offset are often sudden, reflecting loss and recovery of cerebral perfusion.

Try to interview any witnesses. Consider the possibility of a seizure based on the features described in the following section, especially if the onset was abrupt and without warning.

Seizures

Patients may report "spells" or episodes of losing consciousness that raise suspicion of *seizure*, a sudden excessive electrical discharge from cortical neurons. Seizures may be related to a genetic disorder, symptomatic, with an identifiable cause, or idiopathic. A careful history is important to rule out other causes of loss of consciousness and acute symptomatic seizures that have discernible explanations.

See Table 13-7, Seizure Disorders.

If there is more than one seizure, consider *epilepsy*, defined as two or more seizures that are not provoked by other illnesses or circumstances. There are many genetic forms of epilepsy, which are more common in infants and children; the neurologic examination may be normal. In older adults, epilepsy may have a structural cause, for example a brain tumor. In more than 60% to 70% of affected patients, no cause is identified. Epilepsy does not always involve loss of consciousness, depending on the type.

Common causes of acute symptomatic seizures include head trauma; alcohol, cocaine, and other drugs; withdrawal from alcohol, benzodiazepines, and barbiturates; metabolic insults from low or high glucose or low calcium or sodium; acute stroke; and meningitis or encephalitis.

Seizures are usually classified as focal or generalized, based on the location in the cortex of the initial seizure focus. If available, ask a witness how the patient looked before, during, and after the episode. Was there any seizure-like movement of the arms or legs? Any incontinence of the bladder or bowel? What about any drowsiness or impaired memory after the event suggestive of a postictal state?

Tonic–clonic motor activity, bladder or bowel incontinence, and an altered level of consciousness after a seizure episode (*postictal state*) characterize generalized seizures. Unlike syncope, tongue biting or bruising of limbs may occur.

Ask about age at onset, frequency, change in frequency or symptom pattern, and use of medications, alcohol, or illicit drugs. Check for any history of head injury.

Generalized epilepsy syndromes usually begin in childhood or adolescence; adult-onset seizures are usually partial.

Tremors or Involuntary Movements

Tremor, "a rhythmic oscillatory movement of a body part resulting from the contraction of opposing muscle groups," is the most common movement disorder. It may be an isolated finding or part of a neurologic disorder. Ask about any tremor, shaking, or body movements that the patient seems unable to control. Does the tremor occur at rest? Does it get worse with voluntary intentional movement or with sustained postures?

See Table 13-8, Tremors and Involuntary Movements.

Low-frequency unilateral resting tremor, rigidity, bradykinesia, and postural instability typify Parkinson disease. *Essential tremor* is a high-frequency, bilateral, upper extremity tremor that occur with both limb movement and sustained posture and subsides when the limb is relaxed; head, voice, and leg tremor may also be present.

Distinct from these symptoms is restless legs syndrome, described as an unpleasant sensation in the legs, especially at night, that gets worse with rest and improves with movement of the symptomatic limb(s).

Reversible causes of restless legs syndrome include pregnancy, renal disease, and iron deficiency.

PHYSICAL EXAMINATION: GENERAL APPROACH

As you interview the patient, remember the dual goals of your assessment: localizing the lesion(s) and identifying the underlying pathophysiology causing the patient's symptoms. Once again, these questions are answered iteratively as you learn about the patient from your neurologic findings. As you acquire the skills of nervous system examination, it is important to test your findings against those of your teachers and neurologists to refine your clinical expertise. When you conduct the neurologic examination, it is advisable to adopt a fixed routine or examination sequence to minimize omission of one of its important components. Whether you perform a comprehensive or screening examination, organize your thinking into five categories: (1) mental status, speech, and language; (2) cranial nerves (CNs); (3) motor system; (4) sensory system; and (5) reflexes.

The neurologic examination begins as soon as the patient enters the room. An abnormal gait, for example, may provide an important clue to the neurologic diagnosis even before you begin taking a history. While talking, you may detect aphasia—difficulty producing or understanding language. By observing the patient's natural behavior, you may notice weakness on one side of the face while speaking or an intermittent tremor in the hands while they rest in the patient's lap.

The pattern of deficits identified on examination can be especially helpful for localizing the lesion. If there is weakness, for example, is it symmetric or affecting only one side of the body? Is the weakness restricted to the distribution of a single peripheral nerve, or instead only to a spinal nerve root? Start by grouping your findings into patterns of central or peripheral disorders. Remember that accompanying upper motor neuron or lower motor neuron signs may help. For example, look for fasciculations or atrophy alongside weakness to suggest a peripheral disorder, or hyperreflexia to suggest a central disorder.

In many neurologic conditions the neurologic examination may be normal, as when a patient recovers from attacks of epilepsy or a TIA. In some neurologic diseases such as migraine, normal findings are expected—abnormal findings would trigger alarm and further evaluation. In some instances, symptoms in the absence of findings would raise concern, as with a TIA.

The amount of detail in an appropriate neurologic examination varies widely. In healthy patients, your examination will be relatively brief, as outlined in the Screening Neurologic Examination recommended by the American Academy of Neurology (Box 13-5). If the patient complains of neurologic symptoms or if you detect abnormal findings, your examination should be more comprehensive. Recognize that neurologists use many additional techniques in specific situations.

As you become more skilled at performing the neurologic examination, you will integrate the neurologic examination with other parts of the examination for efficiency. Survey the patient's mental status and speech during the interview even if you do more detailed testing later during the neurologic examination. Assess the CNs as you examine the head and neck, and any neurologic abnormalities in the arms and legs as you evaluate the peripheral vascular and musculoskeletal systems. Chapter 4 provides an outline for this kind of integrated approach. Think about, describe, and record your findings, however, in terms of the nervous system as a whole.

Box 13-5. American Academy of Neurology: Guidelines for a Screening Neurologic Examination

A screening neurologic examination that is sufficient for detection of significant neurologic disease should be performed in all patients, even those without neurologic complaints. Although the screening examination sequence may vary, it should cover the major components of the full examination—mental status, cranial nerves (CNs), motor system (strength, gait, and coordination), sensation, and reflexes. One example of a screening examination is given here.

Mental Status (level of alertness, appropriateness of responses, orientation to date and place)

Cranial Nerves

- Visual acuity
- Pupillary light reflex
- Eye movements
- Hearing
- Facial strength (smile, eye closure)
- Speech

Motor Function

- Strength (shoulder abduction, elbow flexion/extension, wrist extension, finger abduction, hip flexion, knee flexion/extension, ankle dorsiflexion)

Reflexes

- Deep tendon reflexes (biceps, patellar, Achilles)
- Plantar responses

Sensation (one modality at toes—can be light touch, pain, temperature, vibration, or proprioception)

Coordination (fine finger movements, finger-to-nose or finger-to-chin)

Gait (casual and tandem)

Note: If there is reason to suspect neurologic disease based on the patient's history or the results of any components of the screening examination, a more complete neurologic examination may be necessary.

Source: Safdieh JE et al. *Neurology.* 2019;92(13):619–626.

TECHNIQUES OF EXAMINATION

Key Components of the Examination of the Nervous System

- Assess mental status: level of alertness, language function (fluency, comprehension, repetition, and naming), memory (short-term and long-term), calculation, visuospatial processing, abstract reasoning.
- Test cranial nerves:
  - Test sense of smell (I)

(continued)

  - Test visual acuity in each eye (II)
  - Inspect optic fundi with an ophthalmoscope (disc bulging, blurred margins, pallor, cup enlargement) (II)
  - Test visual fields by confrontation (visual field defects) (II)
  - Inspect size and shape of pupils (size, asymmetry) (II, III)
  - Test pupillary reactions to light (II, III)
  - Check pupillary constriction, convergence, and lens accommodation (II, III)
  - Test extraocular movements (asymmetry, weakness, palsy, nystagmus) (III, IV, VI)
  - Palpate temporal and masseter muscles (motor weakness) (V)
  - Test sensation in face (sensory loss) (V)
  - Inspect face (asymmetry, lower lid droop, abnormal movements) (VII)
  - Test muscles of facial expression: raise eyebrows, frown, close eyes tightly against resistance, show teeth, smile, puff cheeks (asymmetry) (VII)
  - Assess gross hearing with whispered voice test (VIII)
  - Determine hearing loss with tuning fork tests (Rinne and Weber if indicated) (VIII)
  - Assess swallowing and palate/uvula movement (IX, X)
  - Assess speech (articulation, voice quality) (V, VII, IX, X, XII)
  - Test trapezii or sternocleidomastoid strength against resistance (weakness, asymmetry) (XI)
  - Inspect and test tongue movement (deviation, atrophy, fasciculations) (XII)
- Assess the motor system for involuntary movements, muscle bulk, muscle tone (resistance to passive manipulation, pronator drift).
  - Test muscle strength:
    - Shoulder abduction (C5, C6—deltoid)
    - Elbow flexion (C5, C6—biceps and brachioradialis)/extension (C6, C7, C8—triceps)
    - Wrist flexion/extension (C6, C7, C8, radial nerve—extensor carpi radialis longus and brevis, extensor carpi ulnaris)
    - Finger extension (C7, C8, radial nerve—extensor digitorum)/abduction (C8, T1, ulnar nerve—first dorsal interosseous and abductor digiti minimi)
    - Thumb abduction (C8, T1, median nerve—abductor pollicis brevis)
    - Hip flexion (L2, L3, L4—iliopsoas)/extension (S1—gluteus maximus)
    - Knee flexion (L5, S1, S2—hamstrings)/extension (L2, L3, L4—quadriceps)
    - Ankle dorsiflexion (L4, L5—tibialis anterior)/plantar flexion (S1—gastrocnemius, soleus)
  - Assess coordination:
    - Rapid alternating movements
      - Rapid alternating arm movements
      - Rapid finger tapping

(continued)

Key Components of the Examination of the Nervous System (*continued*)

- Point-to-point movements
  - Finger-to-nose test
  - Heel-to-shin test
- Gait
  - Casual walk
  - Walk on toes and on heels
  - Walk heel to toe in a straight line (tandem)
- Assess position sense (Romberg test)
- Assess the sensory system for light touch, pain, temperature, proprioception, vibration, and discriminative sensation (stereognosis).
- Elicit muscle stretch reflexes:
  - Biceps reflex (C5, C6)
  - Triceps reflex (C6, C7)
  - Brachioradialis reflex (C5, C6)
  - Quadriceps (patellar) reflex (L2, L3, L4)
  - Achilles (ankle) reflex (primarily S1)
- Elicit cutaneous or superficial stimulation reflexes (abdominal reflex, plantar response, anal reflex).

Cranial Nerves

The examination of the CNs can be summarized as follows (Box 13-6).

Cranial Nerve I—Olfactory. *Test the sense of smell* by presenting the patient with familiar nonirritating odors. First, make sure that each nasal passage is patent by compressing one side of the nose and asking the patient to sniff through the other. Then ask the patient to close both eyes. Occlude one nostril and test smell in the other with substances like coffee, soap, or vanilla. Avoid noxious odors like ammonia that might stimulate CN V.

Box 13-6. Summary: Cranial Nerves I–XII

I	Smell
II	Visual acuity, visual fields, and ocular fundi
II, III	Pupillary light reflex
III, IV, VI	Extraocular movements
V	Facial sensation (sensory) and jaw movements (motor)
V, VII	Corneal reflex
VII	Facial movements and strength
VIII	Hearing
IX, X	Swallowing and palatal movement, gag reflex
V, VII, X, XII	Voice and speech
XI	Shoulder and neck movements (head rotation, shoulder elevation)
XII	Tongue symmetry, position, and movement

Ask the patient to identify each odor. Test smell on the other side. Normally the patient perceives odors on each side and identifies them correctly.

Loss of smell occurs in sinus conditions, head trauma, smoking, aging, use of cocaine, and *Parkinson disease.*

Cranial Nerve II—Optic. Test visual acuity in each eye.

See Chapter 20, Eyes, for more detailed discussion of the techniques for examining Visual Acuity and Visual Fields, p. 575; pupils, p. 578; and the optic fundi using an ophthalmoscope, p. 580.

Inspect the optic fundi with your ophthalmoscope, paying special attention to the optic discs.

Inspect each disc carefully for bulging and blurred margins (papilledema); pallor (optic atrophy); and cup enlargement (glaucoma).

Test the visual fields by confrontation. Test each eye separately. When complaining of partial loss of vision, patients may not be able to distinguish between vision loss affecting a single eye and a *visual field defect* affecting both eyes. In stroke patients, for example, testing of both eyes may reveal a visual field defect such as *homonymous hemianopsia.* Testing only one eye would miss this finding. At least once, present stimuli on both the left and right sides of the face simultaneously to look for **extinction**.

Physiology OSCE Videos:
Assessment of Vision and Visual Fields

See Table 20-2, Visual Field Defects. Look for prechiasmal, or anterior, defects seen in glaucoma, retinal emboli, optic neuritis (visual acuity poor); bitemporal hemianopsias from defects at the optic chiasm, usually from pituitary tumor; and homonymous hemianopsias or quadrantanopsias in postchiasmal lesions, usually in the occipital, temporal, or parietal lobe, with associated findings of stroke (visual acuity normal).

Cranial Nerves II and III—Optic and Oculomotor. *Inspect the size and shape of the pupils and* compare one side with the other. **Anisocoria**, or a difference of >0.4 mm in the diameter of one pupil compared to the other, is seen in up to 38% of healthy individuals. Test the *pupillary reactions to light.*

See Table 20-6, Pupillary Abnormalities. If the large pupil reacts poorly to light or anisocoria worsens in light, the large pupil has abnormal pupillary constriction, seen in CN III palsy. Consider intracranial aneurysm if the patient is awake and transtentorial herniation if the patient is comatose.

Also check the *near response* (p. 579), which tests pupillary constriction (pupillary constrictor muscle), convergence (medial rectus muscles), and accommodation of the lens (ciliary muscle).

If anisocoria worsens in darkness, with normal pupillary reaction to light but abnormal pupillary dilation in one eye, this suggests *Horner syndrome* affecting sympathetic innervation.

Cranial Nerves III, IV, and VI—Oculomotor, Trochlear, and Abducens. Test the *extraocular movements* in the six cardinal directions of gaze and look for loss of conjugate movements in any of the six directions. Check convergence of the eyes. Ask patients if they experience **diplopia** when testing. Ask which direction of gaze makes the diplopia worse and inspect the eyes closely for asymmetric deviation of movement. Determine if the diplopia is *monocular* or *binocular* by asking the patient to cover one eye, then the other.

See Chapter 20, Eyes, p. 579, for a more detailed discussion of testing extraocular movements.

See Table 20-7, Dysconjugate Gaze. Monocular diplopia is seen in problems with glasses or contact lenses, or ocular problems such as cataracts or astigmatism. Binocular diplopia occurs in CN III, IV, and/or VI neuropathy (40% of patients), internuclear ophthalmoplegia, myasthenia gravis, and eye muscle disorders including trauma and thyroid ophthalmopathy.

Identify any **nystagmus**, an involuntary jerking movement of the eyes with quick and slow components. Note the direction of gaze in which it appears, the plane of the nystagmus (*horizontal, vertical, rotary*, or *mixed*), and the direction of the *fast* and *slow components*. Nystagmus is named for the direction of the fast component (e.g., left-beating nystagmus). Ask the patient to fix vision on a distant object and observe if the nystagmus increases or decreases.

See Table 13-9, Nystagmus. Nystagmus is seen in cerebellar disease (increases with retinal fixation, may be accompanied by ataxia and dysarthria), vestibular disorders (decreases with retinal fixation), and internuclear ophthalmoplegia.

Look for **ptosis** (drooping of the upper eyelids) by observing where on the eye the eyelid falls in relationship to the iris and pupil (Fig. 13-9). A slight difference in the width of the palpebral fissures is a normal variant in approximately one-third of patients.

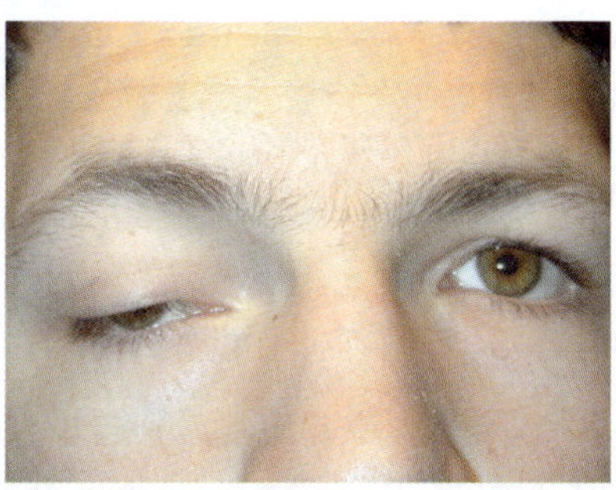

FIGURE 13-9. Right upper eyelid ptosis from CN III palsy. (From Savino PJ, Danesh-Meyer HV. *Neuro-Ophthalmology*. 3rd ed. Wolters Kluwer; 2019, Fig. 10-1a.)

Ptosis is seen in third nerve palsy (CN III), Horner syndrome (ptosis, miosis, forehead anhidrosis), or myasthenia gravis.

Cranial Nerve V—Trigeminal

Motor. While palpating the temporal and masseter muscles in turn, *ask the patient to firmly clench the teeth* (Figs. 13-10 and 13-11). Note the strength of muscle contraction. Ask the patient to open and move the jaw from side to side.

Difficulty clenching the jaw or moving it to the opposite side suggests masseter and lateral pterygoid weakness, respectively. Jaw deviation during opening points to weakness on the deviating side.

Look for unilateral weakness in CN V pontine lesions; bilateral weakness in bilateral hemispheric disease.

CNS patterns from stroke include ipsilateral facial and body sensory loss from contralateral cortical or thalamic lesions; ipsilateral face, but contralateral body sensory loss in brainstem lesions.

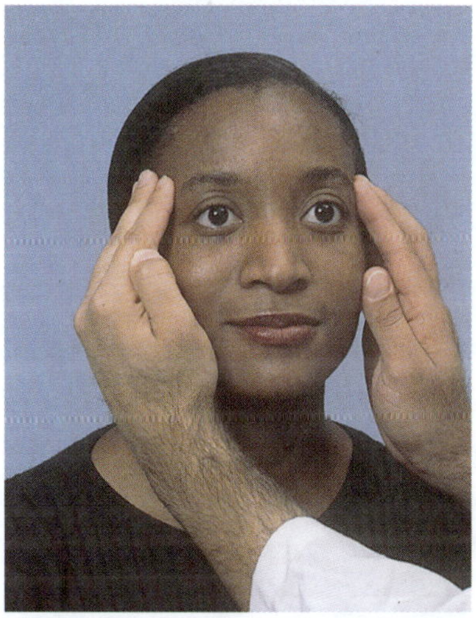

FIGURE 13-10. Palpating the temporal muscles.

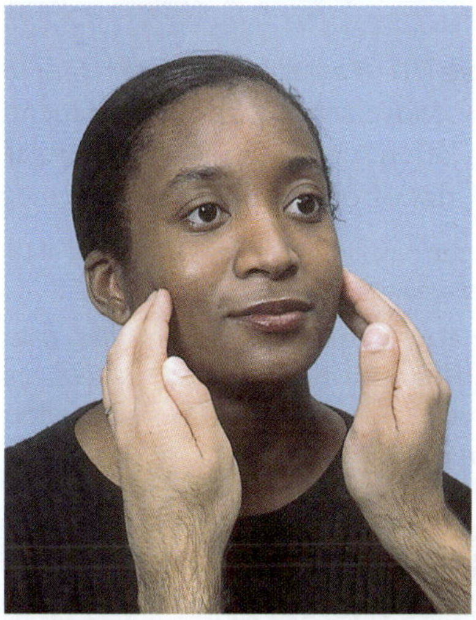

FIGURE 13-11. Palpating the masseter muscles.

Sensory. After explaining what you plan to do, test sensation for each of the three divisions of CN V on each side using the circled areas in Figure 13-12. The patient's eyes should be closed. Test for *light touch* by using a fine wisp of cotton. Ask the patient to respond whenever you touch the skin. Test for *pain* sensation using a suitable sharp object such as a pin. You can create a sharp wood splinter by breaking or twisting a cotton swab. To avoid transmitting infection, use a new object for each patient. While testing, occasionally substitute the blunt end for the point as a contrasting stimulus. Ask the patient to report whether each stimulus is "sharp" or "dull" and to compare sides. If you detect sensory loss, confirm it by testing *temperature sensation*. Two test tubes, filled with hot and ice-cold water, are the traditional stimuli. You can also use a tuning fork, which usually feels cool, and make it warm or cool with running water. Dry it, then touch the skin and ask the patient to identify "hot" or "cold."

Isolated sensory loss occurs in peripheral nerve disorders, including lesions of the trigeminal nerve (CN V).

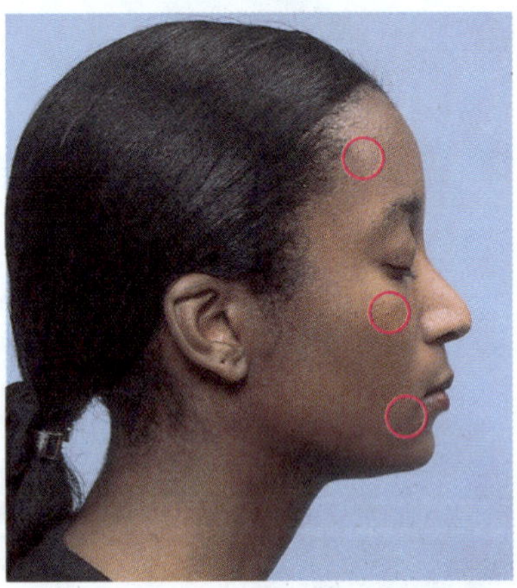

FIGURE 13-12. Areas for testing sensation of the three divisions of CN V.

Cranial Nerve VII—Facial. *Inspect the face* both at rest and during conversation with the patient. Note any asymmetry, often visible in the nasolabial folds, and observe any tics or other abnormal movements.

Flattening of the nasolabial fold and drooping of the lower eyelid suggest facial weakness.

A peripheral injury to CN VII, as seen in Bell palsy, affects both the upper and lower face; a central lesion affects mainly the lower face. Loss of taste, hyperacusis, and increased or decreased tearing can also occur in Bell palsy.

See Table 13-10, Types of Facial Paralysis.

Ask the patient to:

1. Raise both eyebrows
2. Frown

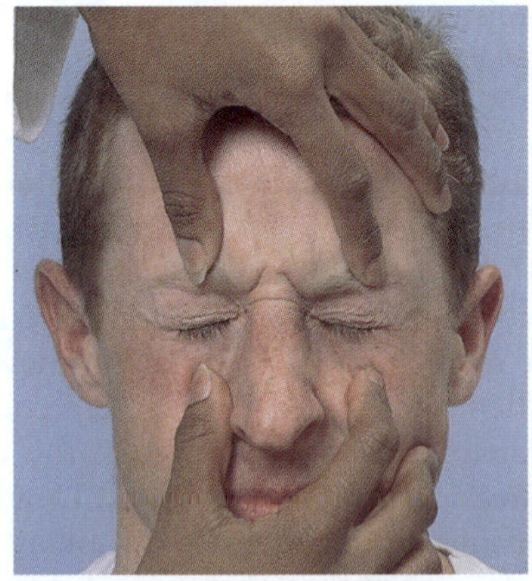

FIGURE 13-13. Testing the eye muscle strength.

3. Close both eyes tightly so that you cannot open them. Test muscular strength by trying to open them, as illustrated in Figure 13-13.
4. Show both upper and lower teeth
5. Smile
6. Puff out both cheeks

In unilateral facial paralysis, the mouth droops on the paralyzed side when the patient smiles or grimaces.

Cranial Nerve VIII—Vestibulocochlear. *Assess gross hearing with the whispered voice test.* Ask the patient to repeat numbers whispered into one ear while blocking or rubbing your fingers next to the contralateral ear.

Physiology OSCE Videos:
Tests for Hearing

See Whispered Voice Test for Auditory Acuity in Chapter 21, Ears and Nose, p. 607.

The whispered voice test is both sensitive (>90%) and specific (>80%) when assessing presence or absence of hearing loss.

If hearing loss is present, determine if the loss is *conductive*, from impaired "air through ear" transmission, or *sensorineural*, from damage to the cochlear branch of CN VIII. Test for *air and bone conduction*, using the Rinne test, and *lateralization*, using the Weber test.

See techniques for Weber and Rinne tests in Chapter 21, Ears and Nose, pp. 607–608, and Table 21-4, Patterns of Hearing Loss.

Excess cerumen, otosclerosis, and *otitis media* cause conductive hearing loss; *presbyacusis* from aging is usually from sensorineural hearing loss.

Disorders that affect the vestibular function of CN VIII may produce nystagmus. For caloric stimulation testing of comatose patients, see p. 338. Specific tests of the vestibular function of CN VIII are otherwise rarely included in the typical neurologic examination.

Vertigo with hearing loss and nystagmus typifies Ménière disease.

See Table 21-1, Dizziness and Vertigo in Chapter 21, Ears and Nose, and Table 13-9, Nystagmus.

Cranial Nerves IX and X—Glossopharyngeal and Vagus. *Listen to the patient's voice.* Is it hoarse, or does it have a nasal quality?

Hoarseness occurs in vocal cord paralysis; nasal voice in paralysis of the palate.

Is there difficulty in swallowing?

Difficulty swallowing suggests pharyngeal or palatal weakness.

Ask the patient to say "ah" or to yawn as you watch the *movements of the soft palate and the pharynx.* The soft palate normally rises symmetrically, the uvula remains in the midline, and each side of the posterior pharynx moves medially, like a curtain. The slightly curved uvula seen occasionally as a normal variation should not be mistaken for a uvula deviated by a lesion of CN IX or X.

The palate fails to rise with a bilateral lesion of CN X. In unilateral paralysis, one side of the palate fails to rise and, together with the uvula, is pulled toward the normal side (Fig. 13-14). For testing the gag reflex, see p. 339.

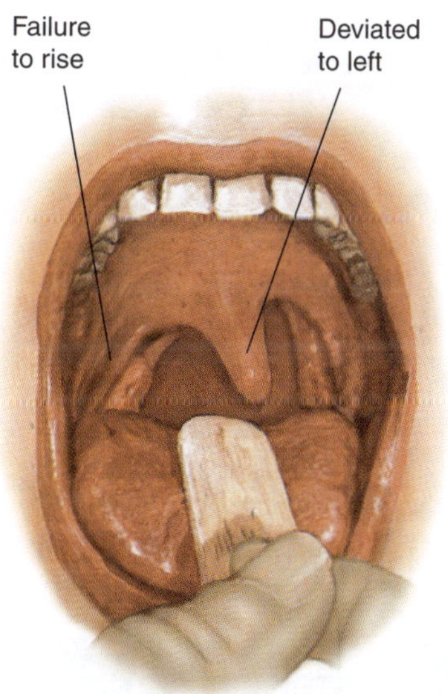

FIGURE 13-14. Weakness of the right palate leads to a deviation of the uvula to the left (unaffected side).

Cranial Nerve XI—Spinal Accessory. Standing behind the patient, look for atrophy or fasciculations in the trapezius muscles, and compare one side with the other. **Fasciculations** are small irregular twitching movements affecting small groups of muscle fibers. *Ask the patient to shrug both shoulders upward against your hands* (Fig. 13-15). Note the strength and contraction of the trapezii.

In trapezius muscle paralysis, the shoulder droops, and the scapula is displaced downward and laterally.

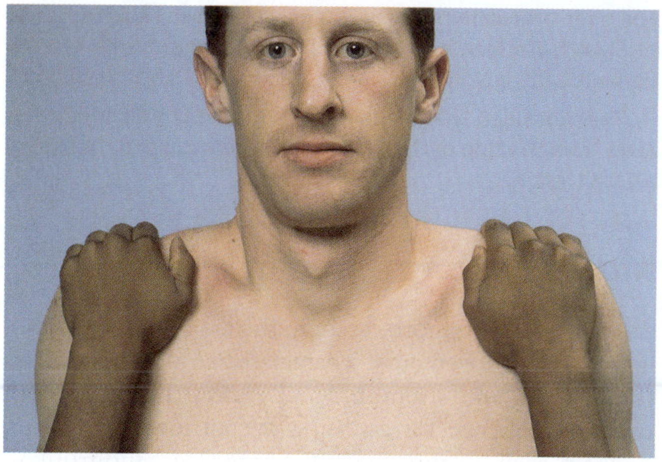

FIGURE 13-15. Testing trapezius strength.

Ask the patient to turn the head to each side against your hand (Fig. 13-16).

A supine patient with bilateral weakness of the SCM muscles has difficulty raising the head off the pillow.

Observe the contraction of the opposite sternocleidomastoid (SCM) muscle and note the force of the movement against your hand.

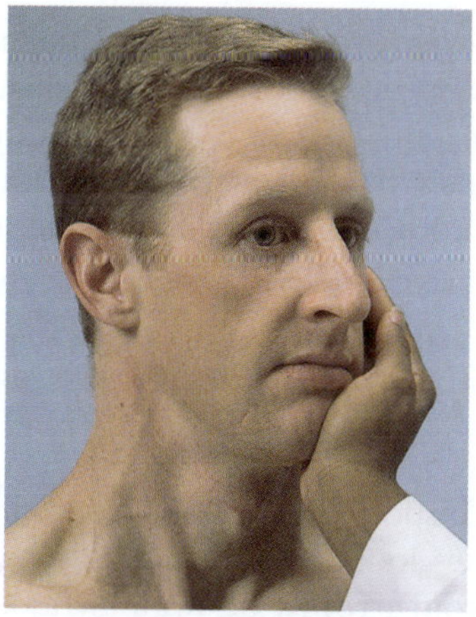

FIGURE 13-16. Testing sternocleidomastoid strength.

Cranial Nerve XII—Hypoglossal. Listen to the articulation of the patient's words. This relies on CNs V, VII, IX, and X, as well as XII. Inspect the patient's tongue as it lies resting on the floor of the mouth. Look for any atrophy or fasciculations. Some coarse, restless movements are normal. Then, with the patient's tongue protruded, look for asymmetry, atrophy, or deviation from the midline. Ask the patient to move the tongue from side to side and note the symmetry of the movement. In ambiguous cases, ask the patient to push the tongue against the inside of each cheek in turn as you palpate externally for strength.

For poor articulation, or *dysarthria*, see Table 13-2, Disorders of Speech. Tongue atrophy and fasciculations can be seen in patients with amyotrophic lateral sclerosis and a history of polio.

The protruded tongue deviates to the weak side. It deviates away from the side of the cortical lesion, and toward the side of a CN XII lesion.

Motor System

As you assess the motor system, focus on body position, involuntary movements, characteristics of the muscles (bulk, tone, and strength), and coordination. You can use this sequence for assessing overall motor function, or check each component in the arms, legs, and trunk in turn. If you detect an abnormality, identify the muscle(s) involved and determine if it is central or peripheral in origin. Learn which nerves innervate the major muscle groups.

Body Position. Observe the patient's body position during movement and at rest.

Abnormal positions alert you to conditions such as mono- or hemiparesis from stroke. See Table 13-11, Abnormal Body Postures.

Involuntary Movements. Watch for involuntary movements such as tremors, tics, chorea, or fasciculations. Noting their location, quality, rate, rhythm, and amplitude can help characterize the type of movement. Observe their relation to posture, activity, fatigue, emotion, and distraction.

Patients with Parkinson disease may have a slow, "pill-rolling" resting tremor. See Table 13-8, Tremors and Involuntary Movements.

Muscle Bulk. Inspect the size and contours of muscles. Do the muscles look flat or concave, suggesting loss of muscle bulk from **atrophy** or wasting? If so, is the process unilateral or bilateral? proximal or distal?

Atrophy is a sign of lower motor neuron pathology and can be seen in motor neuron disease, diseases affecting the nerve roots exiting the spinal cord (radiculopathy), or peripheral neuropathy.

When inspecting for atrophy, pay particular attention to the hands, shoulders, thighs, and calves. The spaces between the metacarpals, where the dorsal interosseous muscles lie, should be full or only slightly depressed (Fig. 13-17). The thenar and hypothenar eminences of the hands should be full and convex (Fig. 13-18). Mild atrophy of the hand muscles occurs in normal aging (Figs. 13-19 and 13-20).

Furrowing between the metacarpals and flattening of the thenar and hypothenar eminences (seen in median and ulnar nerve damage, respectively), suggest atrophy.

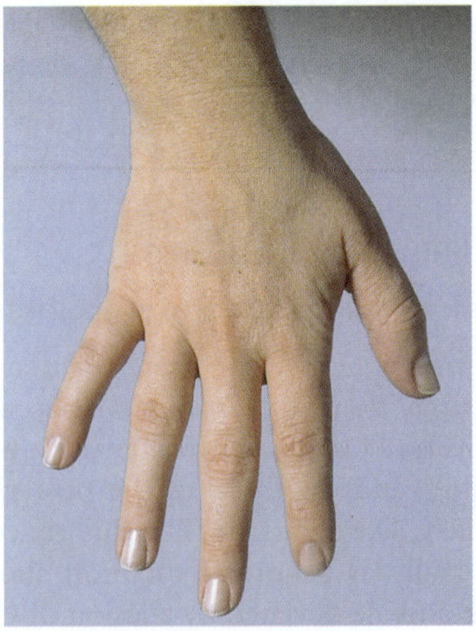

FIGURE 13-17. No interosseous atrophy—44-year-old woman.

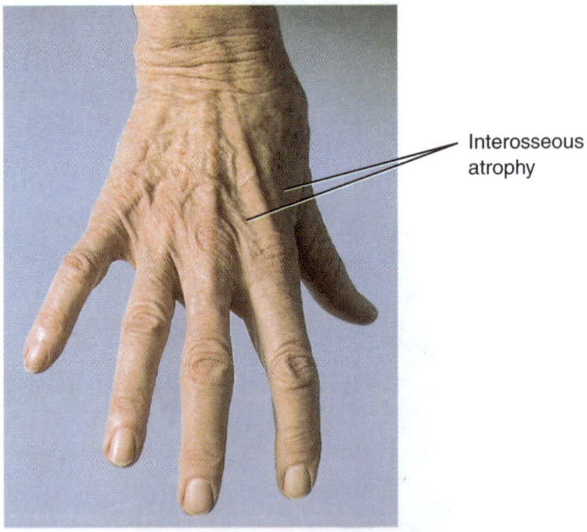

FIGURE 13-18. Interosseous atrophy—84-year-old woman.

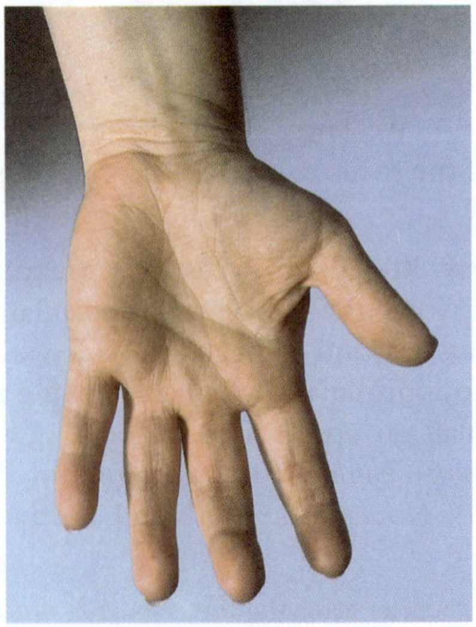

FIGURE 13-19. No hypothenar atrophy—44-year-old woman.

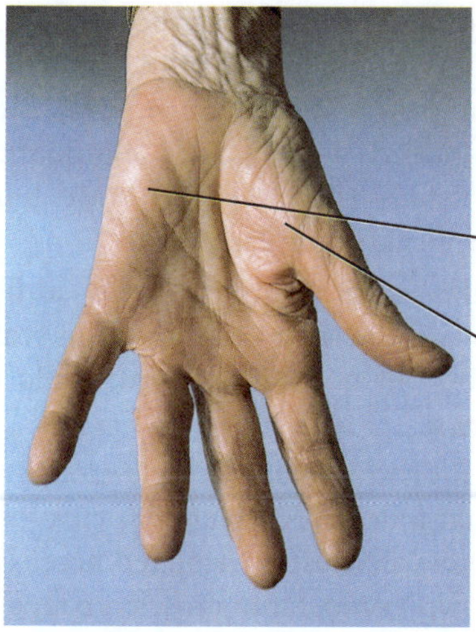

FIGURE 13-20. Hypothenar atrophy—84-year-old woman.

Hypertrophy is an increase in muscle bulk with normal or increased strength. In the Duchenne form of muscular dystrophy, weak muscles may exhibit pseudohypertrophy, an apparent increase in muscle bulk caused by increased fat and connective tissue replacing muscle.

Inspect for fasciculations, another sign of lower motor neuron pathology, in atrophic muscles. Tapping on the muscles with a reflex hammer can stimulate fasciculations if they are not seen at rest.

Fasciculations with atrophy and muscle weakness suggest peripheral motor neuron disease. Diseases of the muscles themselves (*myopathy*) can also cause atrophy but do not cause fasciculations. Corticospinal tract injury can sometimes cause mild atrophy due to decreased muscle use.

Muscle Tone. When a normal muscle with an intact nerve supply is relaxed voluntarily, it maintains a slight residual tension known as *muscle tone*. This is best assessed by feeling the muscle's resistance to passive stretch. Encourage the patient to relax. Hold one hand with yours and, while supporting the elbow, flex and extend the patient's fingers, wrist, and elbow, and put the shoulder through a moderate range of motion. With practice, you can combine these actions into a single smooth movement. On each side, note muscle tone—the resistance offered to your movements. Patients who are tense may show increased resistance. With repeated practice, you will learn the feel of normal resistance.

Decreased resistance suggests disease of the PNS or cerebellum, or the acute stages of spinal cord injury. See Table 13-12, Disorders of Muscle Tone.

If you suspect decreased resistance, hold the forearm and shake the hand loosely back and forth. Normally the hand moves back and forth freely but is not completely floppy.

Marked floppiness indicates muscle hypotonia or flaccidity, usually from a peripheral motor system disorder.

If resistance is increased, determine if it varies as you move the limb or persists throughout the range of movement and if it persists in both directions, for example, during both flexion and extension. Vary the speed at which you move the limb. Feel for any jerkiness in the resistance.

Spasticity is increased tone that is velocity-dependent and worsens at the extremes of range of motion. Resistance increases with more rapid movement. Spasticity is seen in central diseases affecting the corticospinal tract.

Rigidity is increased tone that remains the same throughout the range of motion; it is not velocity dependent.

Rigidity is seen in central disorders affecting the basal ganglia, such as *Parkinson disease*.

To assess muscle tone in the legs, support the patient's thigh with one hand, grasp the foot with the other, and flex and extend the patient's knee and ankle on each side. Note the resistance to moving the limb. (See also Figures 13-31 and 13-32.)

Test for Pronator Drift. Have the patient hold both arms straight forward with palms up (Fig. 13-21). Normally patients hold this arm position well.

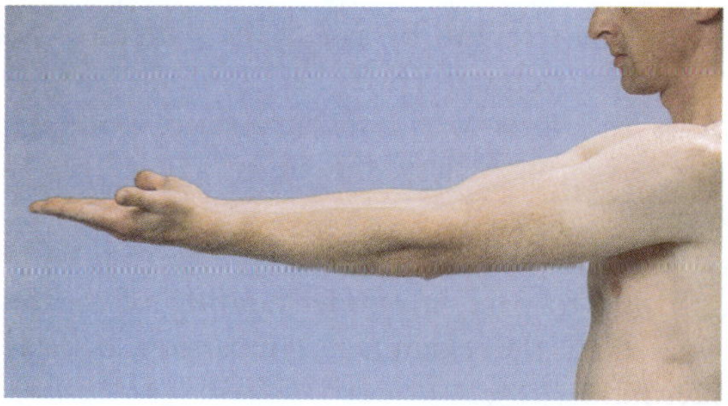

FIGURE 13-21. Testing for pronator drift.

Pronator drift occurs when one forearm and palm turn inward and down (Fig. 13-22) and is both sensitive and specific for a corticospinal tract lesion in the contralateral hemisphere.

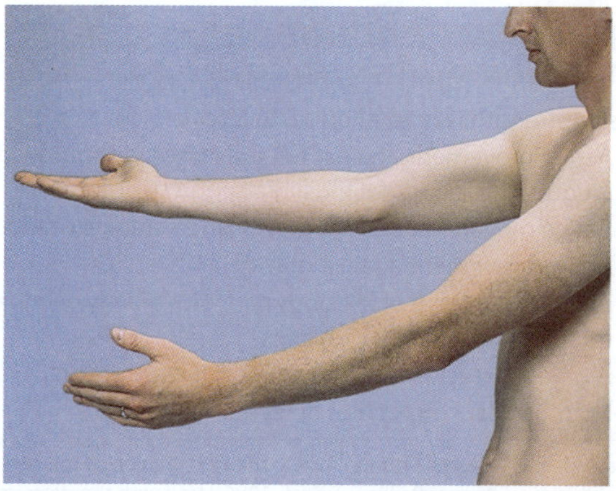

FIGURE 13-22. Positive test for pronator drift of left side.

Downward drift of the arm with flexion of fingers and elbow is also seen. In loss of position sense the arms drift sideward or upward, sometimes with writhing movements of the hands; the patient may not recognize the displacement and when asked, corrects it poorly.

Next, instruct the patient to keep the arms out and eyes shut and *tap the arms briskly downward*. The arms normally return smoothly to the horizontal position. This response requires muscular strength, coordination, and good position sense.

In cerebellar incoordination, the arm overshoots its original position and bounces.

Muscle Strength. Normal strength varies widely, so your standard of normal should allow for factors like age, sex, and muscular training. The patient's dominant side is usually slightly stronger than the nondominant side, though differences can be hard to detect. Keep this difference in mind as you compare sides.

Impaired strength or weakness is called *paresis*. Absent strength is *paralysis*, or *plegia*. **Hemiparesis** refers to weakness of one side of the body; *hemiplegia* refers to paralysis of one side of the body. *Paraplegia* means paralysis of the legs; *quadriplegia* means paralysis of all four limbs.

Test muscle strength by asking the patient to actively resist your movement (Box 13-7). Remember that a muscle is strongest when shortest, and weakest when longest. Give the patient the advantage as you try to overcome the resistance and judge true the muscle's true strength. Some patients give way during tests of muscle strength due to pain, misunderstanding of the test, an effort to help the examiner, conversion disorder, or malingering.

See Table 13-1, Disorders of the Central and Peripheral Nervous Systems.

If the muscles are too weak to overcome resistance, test them against gravity alone or with gravity eliminated. When the forearm rests in a pronated position, for example, dorsiflexion at the wrist can be tested against gravity alone. When the forearm is midway between pronation and supination, extension at the wrist can be tested with gravity eliminated. Finally, if the patient fails to move the body part, observe or palpate for weak muscular contraction.

Box 13-7. Scale for Grading Muscle Strength

Muscle strength is graded on a 0 to 5 scale:

- 5—Active movement against full resistance without evident fatigue. This is normal muscle strength.
- 4—Active movement against gravity and some resistance
- 3—Active movement against gravity
- 2—Active movement of the body part with gravity eliminated (planar motion)
- 1—A barely detectable flicker or trace of contraction
- 0—No muscular contraction detected

Source: Medical Research Council. Aids to the examination of the peripheral nervous system. London: Bailliere Tindall, 1986. Used with the permission of the Medical Research Council.

Many clinicians make further distinctions by adding plus or minus signs toward the stronger end of this scale. Thus, 4+ indicates good but not full strength, while 5− means a trace of weakness.

Methods for testing individual major muscle groups are described in the text that follows. A screening neurologic examination need not test all muscles depicted here. For all muscles, use your own comparable muscle groups to ensure you are accurately and fairly judging strength.

Also, be sure to isolate only the muscle group you intend to test. For example, when testing elbow flexion and extension you should support the patient's upper arm so that the shoulder muscles do not need to do any work.

The spinal root innervations and the muscles affected are shown in parentheses. To localize lesions in the spinal cord or the PNS more precisely, consult texts of neurology for specialized additional testing.

Test abduction at the shoulder (C5, C6—deltoid). Ask the patient to raise the arm from the side to shoulder level. Then press down firmly on the patient's upper arm with shoulder abducted (Fig. 13-23). Both arms can be tested simultaneously to aid in side-to-side comparison.

Test elbow flexion (C5, C6—biceps and brachioradialis) *and extension* (C6, C7, C8—triceps) by having the patient pull (Fig. 13-24) and push (Fig. 13-25) against your hand.

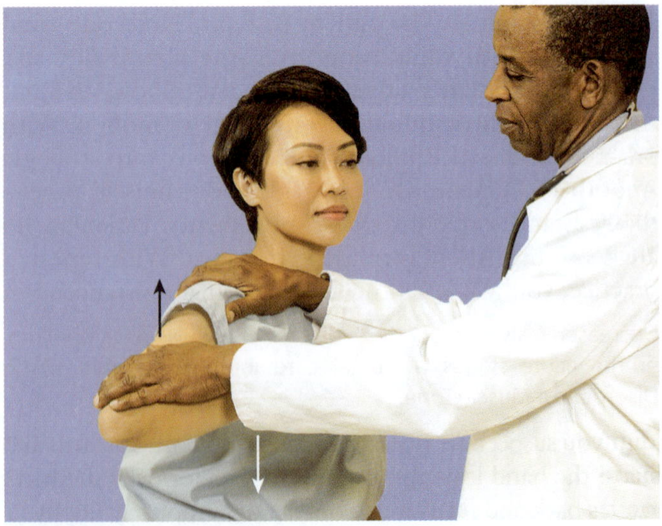

FIGURE 13-23. Testing shoulder abduction (C5, C6—deltoid).

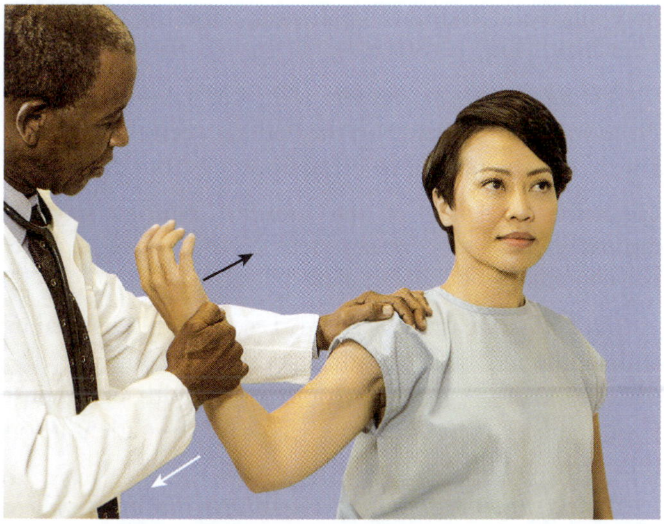

FIGURE 13-24. Testing elbow flexion (C5, C6—biceps, brachioradialis).

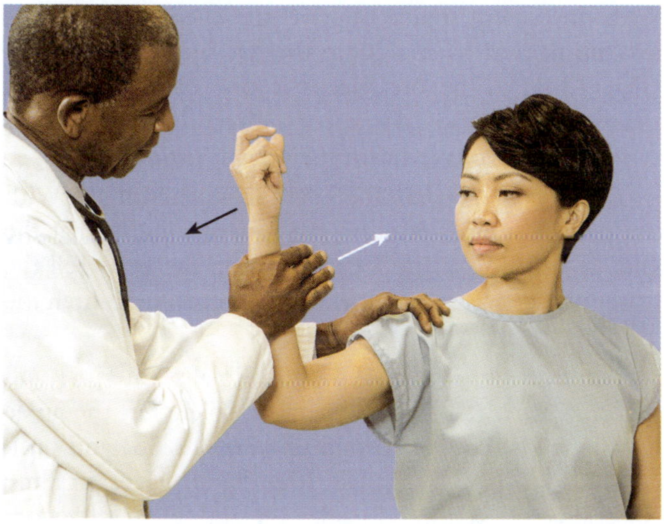

FIGURE 13-25. Testing elbow extension (C6, C7, C8—triceps).

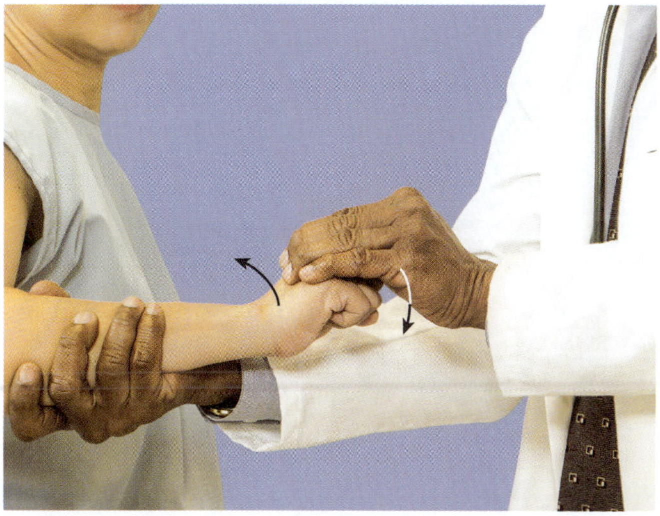

FIGURE 13-26. Testing wrist extension (C6, C7, C8, radial nerve—extensor carpi radialis longus and brevis, extensor carpi ulnaris).

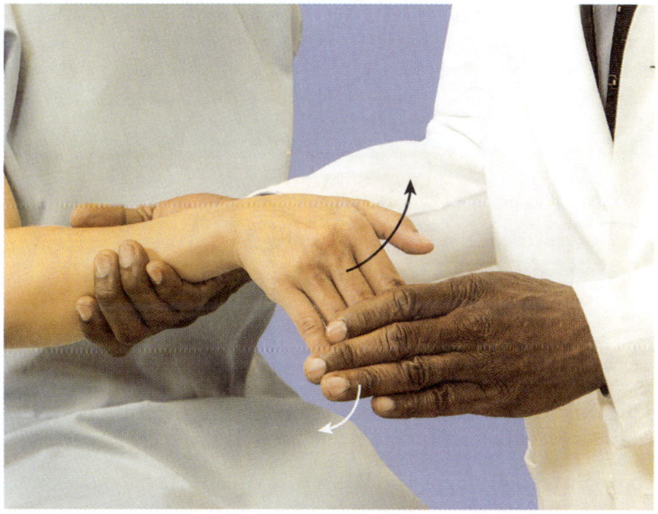

FIGURE 13-27. Testing finger extension (C7, C8, radial nerve—extensor digitorum).

Test extension at the wrist (C6, C7, C8, radial nerve—extensor carpi radialis longus and brevis, extensor carpi ulnaris) by asking the patient to make a fist and resist as you press down (Fig. 13-26). Or ask the patient to extend the forearms with fingers straight and palms up, then press the palms downward.

Wrist and finger extensor weakness is seen in peripheral radial nerve damage, and in the hemiplegia of CNS disease seen in stroke or multiple sclerosis.

Test finger extension (C7, C8, radial nerve—extensor digitorum). Grasp the patient's forearm or palm with one hand. Use the fingers of your other hand to press down on the patient's outstretched fingers (Fig. 13-27).

Test finger abduction (C8, T1, ulnar nerve—first dorsal interosseous and abductor digiti minimi). Position the patient's hand with palm down or on its side and with fingers spread. Instruct the patient to prevent you from moving any fingers as you try to force them together (Fig. 13-28).

Weak finger abduction occurs in ulnar nerve disorders.

Test abduction of the thumb (C8, T1, median nerve—abductor pollicis brevis). Place the forearm in a fully supinated position. Ask the patient to point the thumb straight upwards toward the ceiling. Try to push the thumb straight down into the palm (Fig. 13-29).

Inspect for weak abduction of the thumb in median nerve disorders such as carpal tunnel syndrome (see Chapter 15, Musculoskeletal System, p. 437).

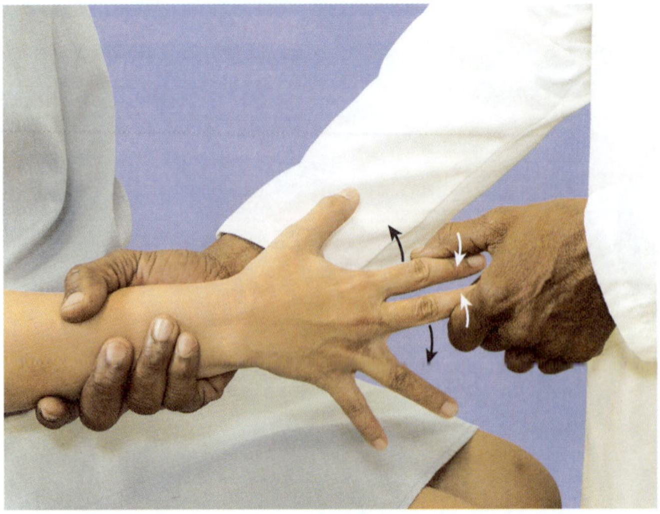

FIGURE 13-28. Testing finger abduction (C8, T1, ulnar nerve—first dorsal interosseous and abductor digiti minimi).

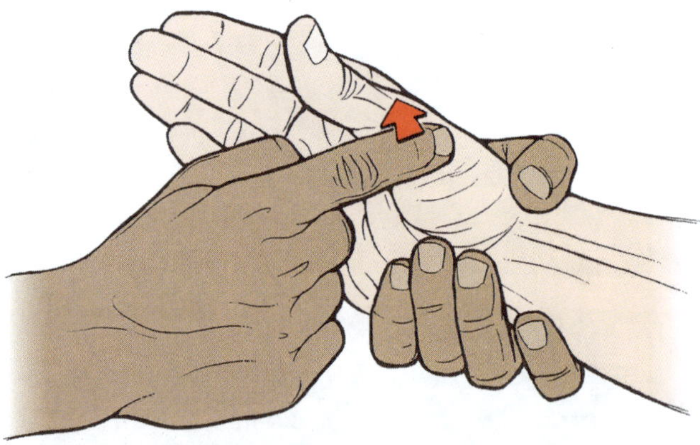

FIGURE 13-29. Testing abduction of the thumb (C8, T1, median nerve—abductor pollicis brevis).

Test flexion at the hip (L2, L3, L4—iliopsoas). With the patient sitting or supine, place your hand on the patient's mid-thigh and asking the patient to raise the leg against your hand (Fig. 13-30).

Test adduction at the hips (L2, L3, L4—adductors). Place your hands firmly on the bed between the patient's knees. Ask the patient to bring both legs together.

Symmetric weakness of the proximal muscles suggests myopathy; symmetric weakness of distal muscles suggests polyneuropathy, or disorders of peripheral nerves.

Test abduction at the hips (L4, L5, S1—gluteus medius and minimus). Place your hands firmly outside the patient's knees. Ask the patient to spread both legs against your hands. To test against gravity, have the patient lie on their side and lift their top leg upward.

Test extension at the hips (S1—gluteus maximus). Have the patient lie on the stomach and lift the leg off the bed. Push down on the posterior thigh.

Test extension at the knee (L2, L3, L4—quadriceps). With the patient supine, support the knee in flexion and ask the patient to straighten the leg against your hand (Fig. 13-31). The quadriceps is one of the strongest muscles in the body, so expect a forceful response. This can also be performed with the patient sitting.

Test flexion at the knee (L5, S1, S2—hamstrings). With the patient supine, position the patient's leg so that the knee is flexed with the foot resting on the bed. Tell the patient to keep the foot down as you try to straighten the leg (Fig. 13-32).

Test foot dorsiflexion (L4, L5—tibialis anterior) and *plantarflexion* (S1—gastrocnemius, soleus) at the ankle by asking the patient to pull up (Fig. 13-33) and push down (Fig. 13-34) against your hand. Heel and toe walk also assess foot dorsiflexion and plantar flexion, respectively.

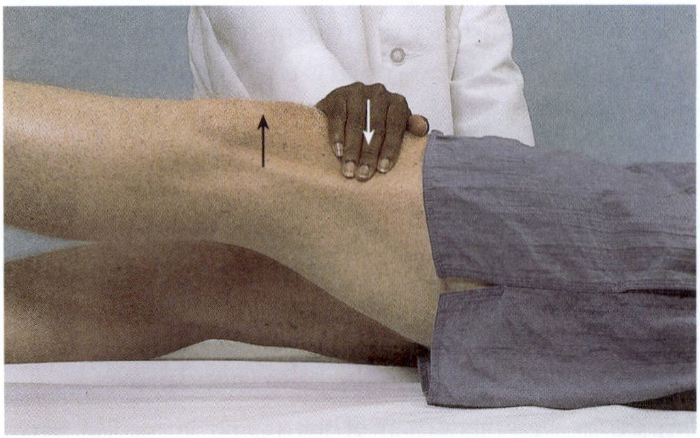

FIGURE 13-30. Testing hip flexion (L2, L3, L4—iliopsoas).

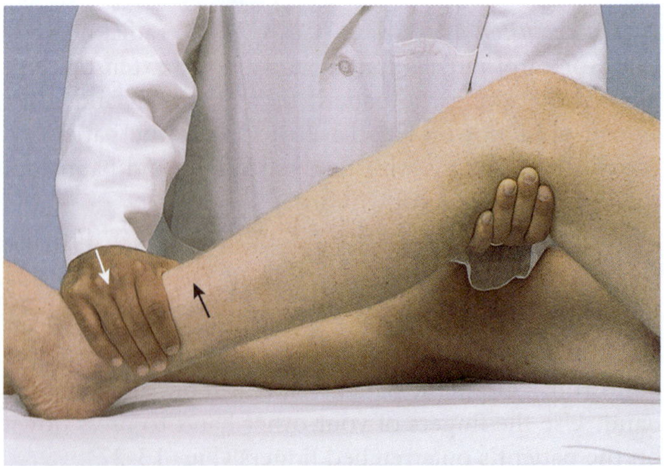

FIGURE 13-31. Testing knee extension (L2, L3, L4—quadriceps).

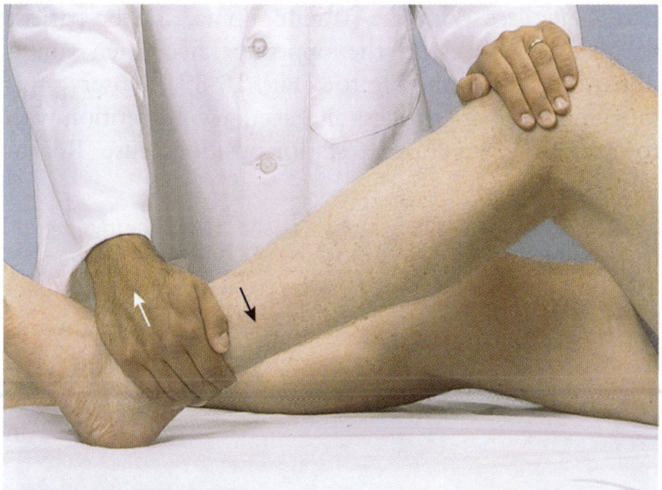

FIGURE 13-32. Testing knee flexion (L5, S1, S2—hamstrings).

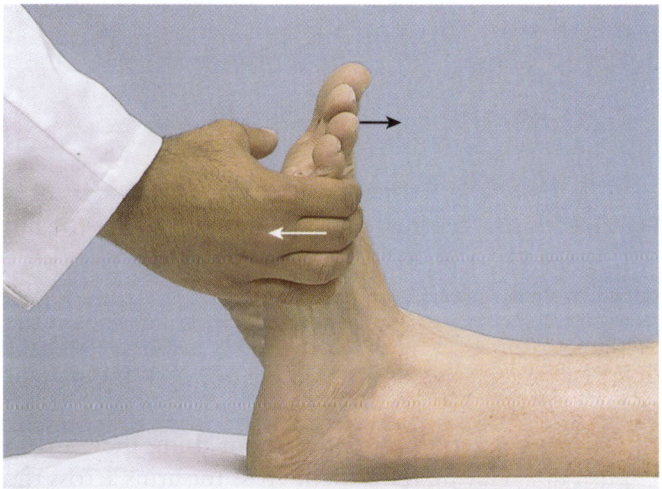

FIGURE 13-33. Testing foot dorsiflexion (L4, L5—tibialis anterior).

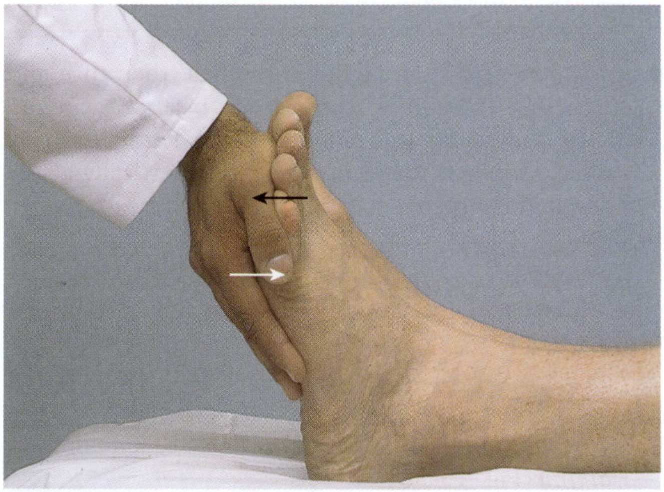

FIGURE 13-34. Testing plantar flexion (S1—gastrocnemius, soleus).

Coordination. Coordination of muscle movement requires four areas of the nervous system to function in an integrated way:

- Motor system, for muscle strength
- Vestibular system, for balance and for coordinating eye, head, and body movements

In cerebellar disease, look for nystagmus, dysarthria, hypotonia, and ataxia.

- Sensory system, for position sense

Ataxia refers to a loss of control of coordinated voluntary movements.

- Cerebellar system for integrating the above information to produce normal rhythmic movement and steady posture

To assess coordination, observe the patient performing:

- Rapid alternating movements
- Point-to-point movements
- Gait and stance

Rapid Alternating Movements

Arms. Show the patient how to strike one hand on the thigh, raise the hand, turn it over, and then strike the back of the hand down on the same place. Urge the patient to repeat these alternating movements as rapidly as possible (Fig. 13-35).

In cerebellar disease, instead of alternating quickly, these movements are slow, irregular, and clumsy, an abnormality called **dysdiadochokinesis**.

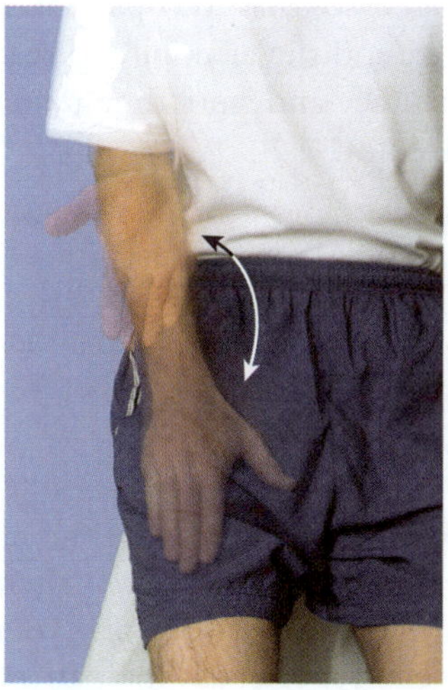

FIGURE 13-35. Testing coordination with rapid alternating arm movement.

Observe the speed, rhythm, and smoothness of the movements. Repeat with the other hand. The nondominant hand may perform less well.

Show the patient how to tap the distal joint of the thumb with the tip of the index finger, again as rapidly as possible (Fig. 13-36). Again, observe the speed, rhythm, and smoothness of the movements. The nondominant side often performs less well.

Cerebellar disease causes finger tapping to be imprecise, with an irregular rhythm. Upper motor neuron weakness and basal ganglia disease can also impair these movements, but not in the same manner. Movements will be slow and low amplitude.

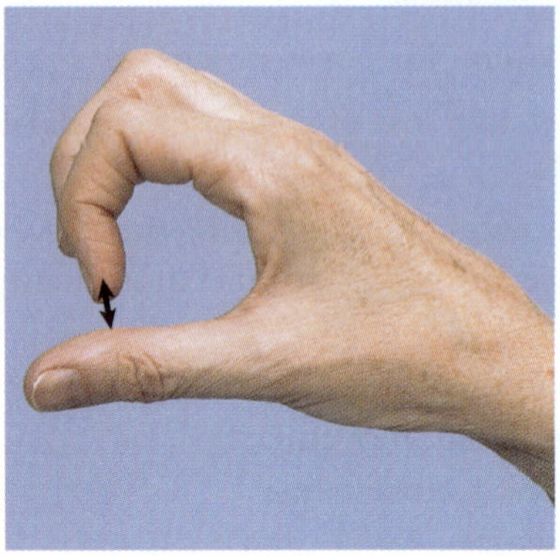

FIGURE 13-36. Testing coordination with rapid finger tapping.

Legs. Ask the patient to tap the ball of each foot in turn as quickly as possible on your hand or the floor. Note any slowness or awkwardness. Normally the feet do not perform as well as the hands.

Point-to-Point Movements

Finger-to-Nose Test. Ask the patient to touch your index finger and then his or her nose alternately several times. Move your finger so that the patient has to change directions and extend the arm fully to reach your finger. Observe the accuracy and smoothness of movement and watch for any tremor.

In cerebellar disease, movements are clumsy, unsteady, and inappropriately variable in their speed, force, and direction. If the patient's finger over- or undershoots your finger, this is called **dysmetria**. An intention tremor may appear toward the end of the movement. See Table 13-8, Tremors and Involuntary Movements.

Now hold your finger in one place so that the patient can touch it with one finger with the arm completely outstretched. Ask the patient to alternate between touching his or her nose and touching your finger several times. After several repeats, ask the patient to close both eyes and try several more times. Repeat on the other side. Normally the patient touches the examiner's finger successfully with eyes open or closed. With eyes closed, the patient must rely on position sense and the function of both the labyrinth of the inner ear and the cerebellum to accurately direct movement.

If the accuracy of movement significantly worsens with eyes closed, this indicates a loss of position sense, also called *sensory ataxia.*

Heel-to-Shin Test. With the patient supine, ask the patient to place one heel on the opposite knee, then run it down the shin to the big toe (Fig. 13-37). Observe this movement for smoothness and accuracy. Repetition with the patient's eyes closed tests for position sense. Repeat on the other side.

In cerebellar disease, the heel may overshoot the knee (*dysmetria*), then oscillate from side to side down the shin (*intention tremor*). If position sense is absent, the heel lifts too high and the patient tries to look. With eyes closed, performance is poor.

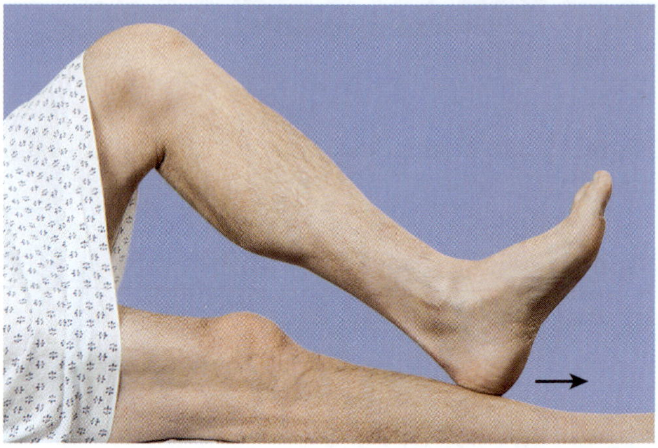

FIGURE 13-37. Testing coordination with heel-to-shin test. (From Weber JR, Kelley JH. *Health Assessment in Nursing.* 6th ed. Wolters Kluwer; 2018, Fig. 25-22.)

Gait. Gait abnormalities increase risk of falls. Ask the patient to:

- *Rise from a sitting position* without using the arms to push up. (Having the patient cross the arms across the chest will guarantee this.)

  Difficulty rising from a chair suggests proximal weakness (extensors of the hip), weakness of the quadriceps (extensor of the knee), or both. See Box 25-7, Timed Get Up and Go Test in Chapter 25, Older Adult.

- *Walk across the room* or down the hall, then turn and come back. Observe posture, stance, balance, swinging of the arms, and movements of the legs. Normally balance is intact, the arms swing symmetrically at the sides, and turns are smooth.

  A wide-based, uncoordinated gait with reeling and instability is *ataxic.* Ataxia is seen in cerebellar disease, loss of position sense, and intoxication. Patients with Parkinson disease walk slowly with a stooped posture, shuffling short steps, and minimal arm-swing, See Table 13-3, Abnormalities of Gait and Posture.

- *Walk heel-to-toe* in a straight line—called *tandem walking* (Fig. 13-38).

  Tandem walking may reveal ataxia that is not otherwise obvious.

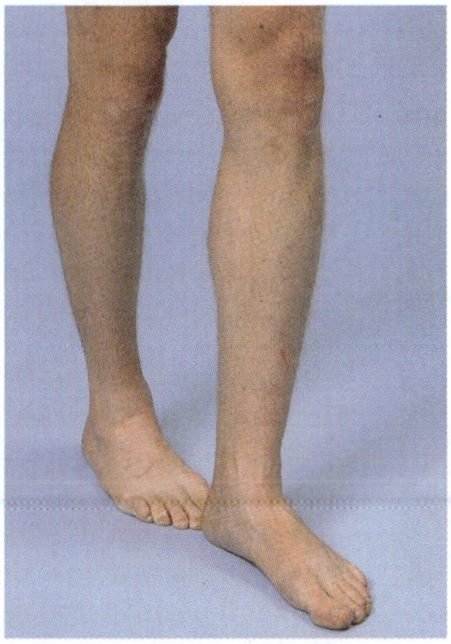

FIGURE 13-38. Testing tandem gait (heel-to-toe).

- *Walk on the toes, then on the heels*—these test plantarflexion and dorsiflexion of the ankles as well as balance.

Walking on toes and heels may reveal distal leg weakness. Inability to heel-walk is a sensitive test for corticospinal tract damage.

Physiology OSCE Videos:
Gait

Romberg Test. This is mainly a test of *position sense*. The patient should first stand with feet together and eyes open and then close both eyes for about 30 seconds without support. Note the patient's ability to maintain an upright posture. Normally any swaying is minimal.

In *sensory ataxia* from loss of position sense, vision compensates for the sensory loss. The patient stands fairly well with eyes open but loses balance when they are closed, a positive Romberg sign. In *cerebellar ataxia,* the patient has difficulty standing with feet together whether the eyes are open or closed.

Physiology OSCE Videos:
Test for Co-ordination

Sensory System

To evaluate the sensory system, you will test several kinds of sensation:

- Pain and temperature (spinothalamic tracts)
- Position and vibration (posterior columns)
- Light touch (both of these pathways)
- Discriminative sensations, which rely on some of the above sensations but also involve processing by the sensory cortex

Assess the patient carefully to establish the pattern of any sensory loss, which can help determine whether the underlying lesion is central or peripheral. Is the sensory loss bilateral or unilateral? Is it symmetric? Which modalities are involved? The pattern you find may suggest a dermatomal distribution, a polyneuropathy, or a spinal cord syndrome.

See Table 13-1, Disorders of the Central and Peripheral Nervous Systems.

Correlate any abnormal findings with motor and reflex activity to establish the location of the causative lesion. Accurate physical diagnosis of the many conditions with impaired sensation requires time and practice.

Certain spinal cord syndromes produce crossed sensory findings, both ipsilateral and contralateral to the spinal cord injury. Refer to specialty textbooks for further discussion.

Physiology OSCE Videos:
Sensory System

Patterns of Testing. Because sensory testing is tiring for many patients and can produce unreliable results, conduct the examination as efficiently as possible. You need not test all modalities in all patients. Focus on areas that have numbness or pain, motor or reflex abnormalities suggesting a lesion of the spinal cord or PNS, and trophic changes such as absent or excessive sweating, atrophic skin, or cutaneous ulceration.

Meticulous sensory mapping helps establish the level of a spinal cord lesion, or if a peripheral lesion is localized to a nerve root, a major peripheral nerve, or one of its branches. You may need to retest at another time to confirm abnormalities.

The following patterns of testing help you to identify sensory deficits accurately and efficiently (Box 13-8).

Before each of the following tests, show the patient what you plan to do and explain how you would like the patient to respond. The patient's eyes should be closed during actual testing.

Pain. Use the stick portion of a broken cotton swab, or other suitable tool. Occasionally, substitute the blunt end for the point. Ask the patient, "Is this sharp or dull?" or, when making comparisons, "Does this feel the same as this?" Apply the lightest pressure needed for the stimulus to feel sharp; avoid heavy pricks that draw blood. To prevent transmitting any infection, safely discard the device after use. Do not reuse it on another person.

Analgesia refers to absence of pain sensation, *hypalgesia* refers to decreased sensitivity to pain, and *hyperalgesia* refers to increased pain sensitivity.

Temperature. Testing skin temperature is often omitted if pain sensation is normal. If there are sensory deficits, use a tuning fork warmed or cooled by running water. Touch the skin and ask the patient to identify "hot" or "cold."

Box 13-8. Tips for Detecting Sensory Deficits

- *Compare symmetric areas* on the two sides of the body, including the arms, legs, and trunk.
- *Vary the pace of your testing* so that the patient does not merely respond to your repetitive rhythm.
- When you detect an area of sensory loss or hypersensitivity, *map out its boundaries* in detail. Stimulate first at a point of reduced sensation, then in progressive steps until the patient reports a change to normal sensation.

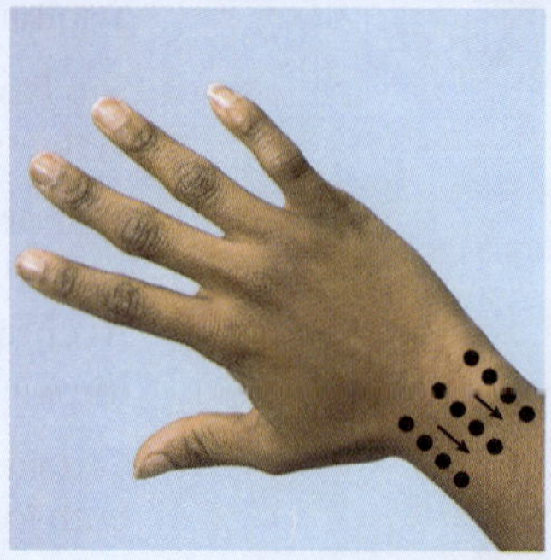

A hemisensory loss pattern suggests a lesion in the contralateral cerebral hemisphere; a sensory level (when one or more sensory modalities are reduced below a dermatome on one or both sides) suggests a spinal cord lesion.

Here, all sensation in the hand is lost. Testing in a progressively more proximal direction reveals a gradual return to normal sensation at the wrist. This pattern does not fit either a peripheral nerve or dermatomal distribution (see p. 328). If bilateral, it suggests the "glove" of the "stocking-glove" sensory loss of polyneuropathy, often seen in diabetes.

- For *pain*, *temperature*, and *touch* sensation, *compare distal to proximal areas* of the extremities. Scatter the stimuli to sample most of the dermatomes and major peripheral nerves (see Figs. 13-42 to 13-45). One suggested pattern is to include:
  - both shoulders (C5)
  - inner and outer aspects of the forearms (C6 and T1)
  - thumbs and little fingers (C6 and C8)
  - fronts of both thighs (L3)
  - ankle at the medial malleolus (L4)
  - dorsum of the foot (L5)
  - fifth toes (S1)
  - medial aspect of each buttock (S3)
- For *vibration* and *position* sensation, test the fingers and toes first. If these are normal, you may safely assume that more proximal areas are also be normal.

Symmetric distal sensory loss suggests a *polyneuropathy*. You may miss this finding unless you compare distal and proximal sensation.

Light Touch. With a fine wisp of cotton, touch the skin lightly, avoiding pressure. Ask the patient to respond whenever a touch is felt, and to compare one area with another. Avoid testing calloused skin, which is normally relatively insensitive.

Anesthesia is absence of touch sensation, *hypesthesia* is decreased sensitivity to touch, and *hyperesthesia* is increased sensitivity.

Vibration. Use a relatively low-pitched tuning fork of 128 Hz. Tap the prongs on the heel of your hand and place the base firmly over a distal interphalangeal joint of the patient's finger, then over the interphalangeal joint of the big toe (Fig. 13-39). Ask what the patient feels. If you are not sure whether the patient is feeling pressure or vibration, ask the patient to tell you when the vibration stops. Then touch the tuning fork to stop it from vibrating and confirm this change with the patient. If vibration sense is impaired, proceed to more proximal bony prominences (e.g., wrist, elbow; medial malleolus, shin, patella, anterior superior iliac spine, spinous processes, clavicles).

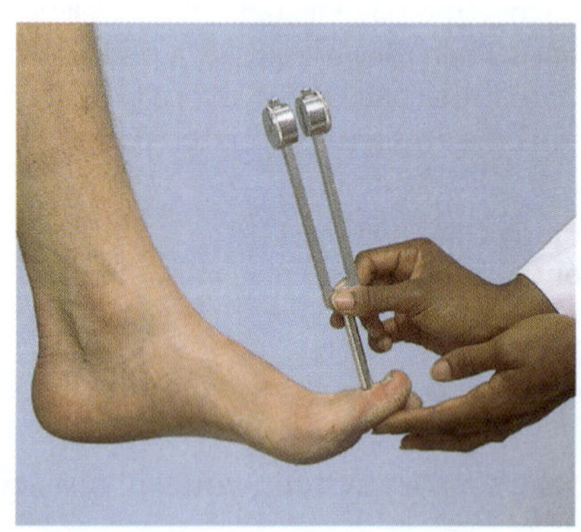

FIGURE 13-39. Testing vibration sense.

Vibration sense is often the first sensation lost in a peripheral neuropathy and increases the likelihood of peripheral neuropathy 16-fold. Causes include diabetes, alcoholism, and certain medications. Posterior column disease, seen in tertiary syphilis or vitamin B_{12} deficiency, also causes loss of vibration sense.

Testing vibration sense in the trunk is useful when identifying the level of a cord lesion.

Proprioception (Joint Position Sense). Grasp the patient's big toe, *holding it by its sides* between your thumb and index finger, then pull it away from the other toes (Fig. 13-40). This prevents extraneous tactile stimuli from affecting testing. Demonstrate "up" and "down" as you move the patient's toe clearly upward and downward. Then, with the patient's eyes closed, ask the patient to say "up" or "down" when moving the large toe in a small arc.

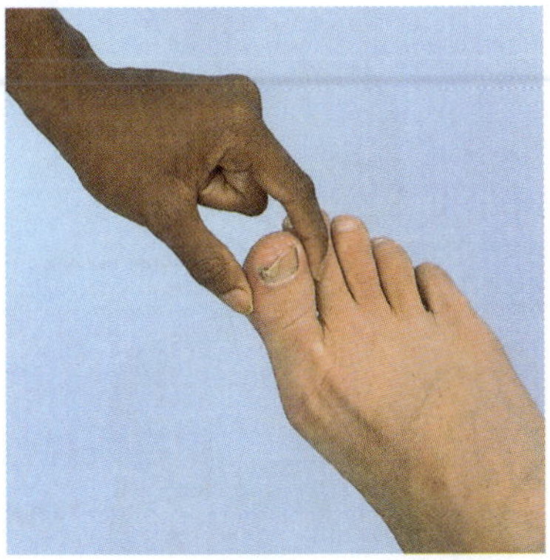

FIGURE 13-40. Testing joint position sense (proprioception).

Loss of position sense, like loss of vibration sense, is seen in tertiary syphilis, multiple sclerosis, or B_{12} deficiency from posterior column damage, and in diabetic neuropathy.

Move the toe several times on each side. If position sense is impaired, move proximally to test the ankle joint. In a similar fashion, test position in the fingers, moving proximally, if indicated, to the metacarpophalangeal joints, wrist, and elbow.

Discriminative Sensations. Several additional techniques test the ability of the sensory cortex to correlate, analyze, and interpret sensations. Because discriminative sensations depend on touch and position sense, they are useful only when these sensations are either intact or only slightly impaired.

If touch and position sense are normal, decreased or absent, discriminative sensation indicates a lesion in the sensory cortex. Stereognosis, number identification, and two-point discrimination are also impaired in posterior column disease.

Screen a patient with *stereognosis,* and proceed to other methods, if indicated. The patient's eyes should be closed during all these tests.

- *Stereognosis.* Stereognosis refers to the ability to identify an object by feeling.it. Place a familiar object such as a coin, paper clip, key, pencil, or cotton ball, in the patient's hand and ask the patient to tell you what it is. Normally a patient will manipulate it skillfully and identify it correctly within 5 seconds. Asking the patient to distinguish "heads" from "tails" on a coin is a sensitive test of stereognosis.

  Astereognosis refers to the inability to recognize objects placed in the hand.

- *Number identification (graphesthesia).* If arthritis or other conditions prevent the patient from manipulating an object well enough to identify it, test the ability to identify numbers. With the blunt end of a pen or pencil, draw a large number in the patient's palm (Fig. 13-41). Normally, a person can identify most such numbers.

  The inability to recognize numbers, or *graphesthesia,* indicates a lesion in the sensory cortex.

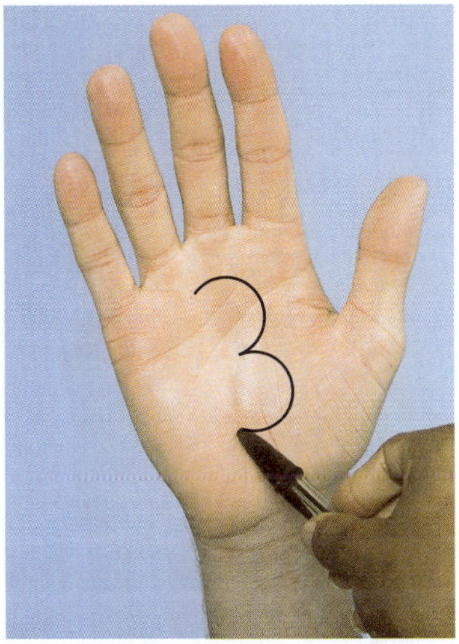

FIGURE 13-41. Testing discriminative sensation using number identification (graphesthesia).

- *Point localization.* Briefly touch a point on the patient's skin. Then ask the patient to open both eyes and point to the place touched. Normally a person can do so accurately.

  Lesions of the sensory cortex impair the ability to localize points accurately.

- *Extinction.* Touch each arm individually, then simultaneously touch corresponding areas on both arms. Ask where the patient feels your touch with each stimulus. Normally both stimuli are felt. The face and legs can also be tested in the same manner.

  In sensory neglect, stimuli on one side of the body are ignored despite intact primary sensory modalities. With extinction to double simultaneous stimulation, patients will correctly identify a tactile stimulus if the affected side is touched individually but will report touch only on the unaffected side if both sides are touched simultaneously.

  Lesions in the cerebral hemisphere cause extinction of the contralateral side, especially lesions in the right parietal lobe or right basal ganglia.

Dermatomes. A *dermatome* is the band of skin innervated by the sensory root of a single spinal nerve. Knowledge of dermatomes helps you localize neurologic lesions to a specific level of the spinal cord, particularly in spinal cord injury. Dermatome and peripheral nerve patterns are illustrated in Figures 13-42 to 13-45, which reflect the international standard recommended by the American Spinal Injury Association. Dermatome levels are more variable between individuals than these diagrams suggest. They overlap at their upper and lower margins and also slightly across the midline. Do not try to memorize all the dermatomes. Instead, focus on learning the dermatomes shaded in green.

In spinal cord injury, all dermatomes below the level of injury can be affected. The sensory level may be several segments *lower* than the spinal lesion, for reasons that are not well understood.

Percussing for the level of vertebral pain may be helpful. In radiculopathy, damage to a spinal nerve root causes sensory loss limited to that dermatome.

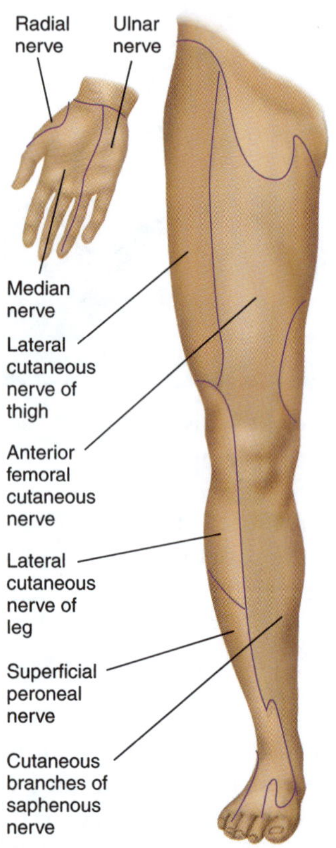

FIGURE 13-42. Areas innervated by peripheral nerves (anterior surface of right lower extremity).

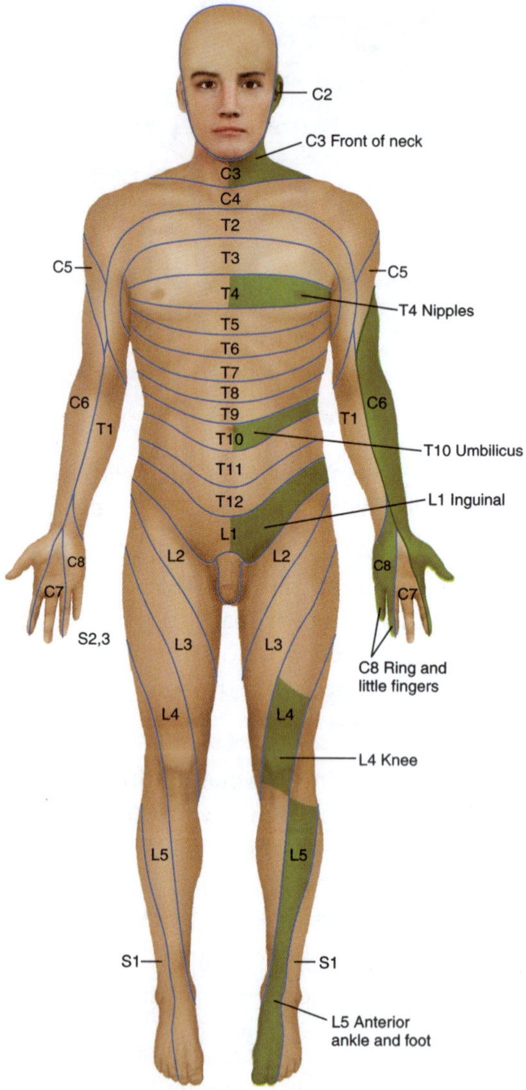

FIGURE 13-43. Dermatomes innervated by posterior roots.

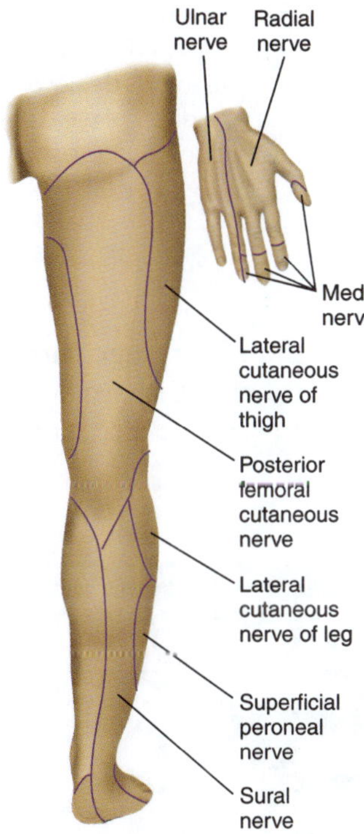

FIGURE 13-44. Areas innervated by peripheral nerves (posterior surface of right lower extremity).

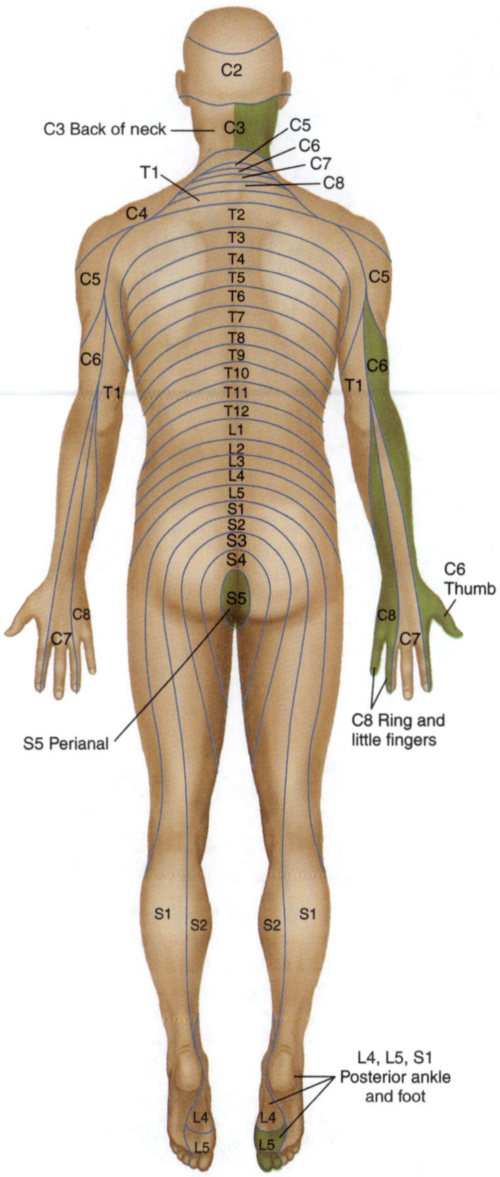

FIGURE 13-45. Dermatomes innervated by posterior roots.

Muscle Stretch Reflexes

Eliciting the *muscle stretch reflexes* requires special handling of the reflex hammer. Select a properly weighted reflex hammer and learn the different uses of the pointed end and the flat end. For example, the pointed end is useful for striking small areas, such as your finger as it overlies the biceps tendon.

Test the reflexes as follows:

- Encourage the patient to relax, then position the limbs properly and symmetrically.

  Hold the reflex hammer *loosely* between your thumb and index finger so that it swings freely in an arc within the limits set by your palm and other fingers (Fig. 13-46).

- With your wrist relaxed, strike the tendon briskly using a rapid wrist movement. Allow the hammer to do the work. Your strike should be *quick and direct*, not glancing.

Note the speed, force, and amplitude of the reflex response and grade the response using the scale in Box 13-9. Always compare the response of one side with the other. Reflexes are usually graded on a 0 to 4 scale.

Physiology OSCE Videos:
Deep Tendon Reflexes

Reflex response depends partly on the force of your strike on the tendon. Only use enough force to provoke a definite response. Symmetrically increased, diminished, or even absent reflexes can be normal. Differences between sides are more definitive for disease

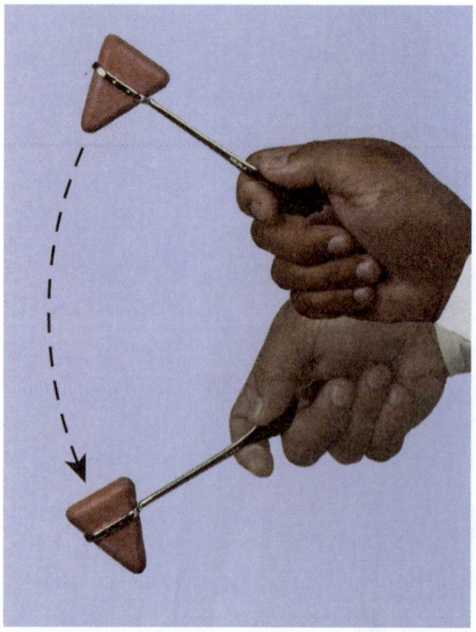

FIGURE 13-46. Proper use of a reflex hammer: Striking with a brisk relaxed swing.

Box 13-9. Scale for Grading Reflexes

4	Very brisk, with *clonus* (rhythmic oscillations between flexion and extension)
3	Brisker than average; possibly but not necessarily indicative of disease
2	Average; normal
1	Somewhat diminished, or requires reinforcement
0	Reflex absent

Hyperactive reflexes (hyperreflexia) occur in CNS lesions affecting the descending corticospinal tract. Look for associated upper motor neuron findings of weakness, spasticity, and/or a positive Babinski sign.

Hypoactive or *absent reflexes (hyporeflexia)* occur in PNS lesions affecting the spinal nerve roots, brachial or lumbosacral plexus, or peripheral nerves. Look for associated lower motor neuron findings of weakness, atrophy, and/or fasciculations.

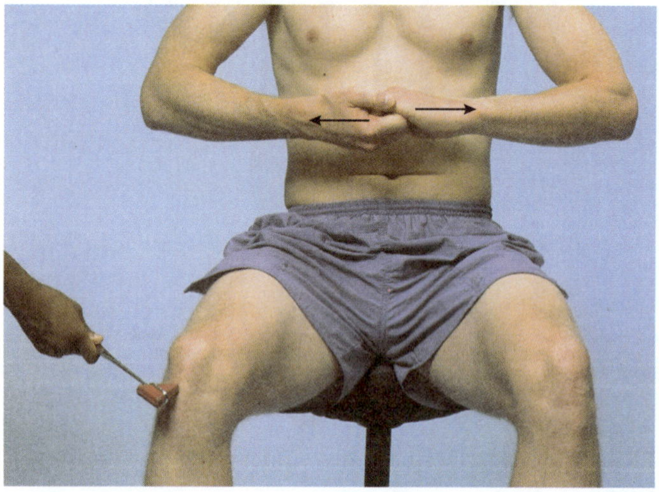

FIGURE 13-47. Reinforcing the quadriceps (patellar) reflex.

and are usually easier to detect than symmetric changes on both sides.

If a reflex seems diminished or absent, use *reinforcement*, a technique involving isometric contraction of other muscles for up to 10 seconds that may increase reflex activity. If reinforcement is required to obtain a reflex, grade the response a "1." To reinforce the arm reflexes, ask the patient to clench the teeth or to squeeze both knees together. If leg reflexes are diminished or absent, ask the patient to lock fingers and pull one hand against the other. Tell the patient to pull just before you strike the patellar or Achilles tendon (Fig. 13-47).

Biceps Reflex (C5, C6). The patient's elbow should be partially flexed, and the forearm pronated with palm down. Place your thumb or finger firmly on the biceps tendon. Aim the strike with the reflex hammer directly through your digit toward the biceps tendon (Figs. 13-48 and 13-49).

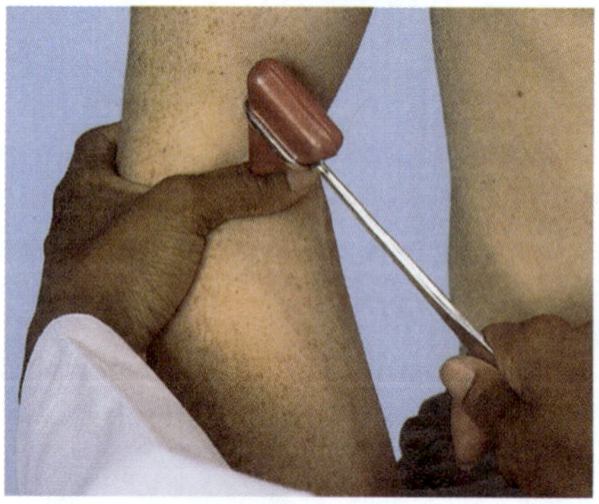

FIGURE 13-48. Biceps reflex (C5, C6)—patient sitting.

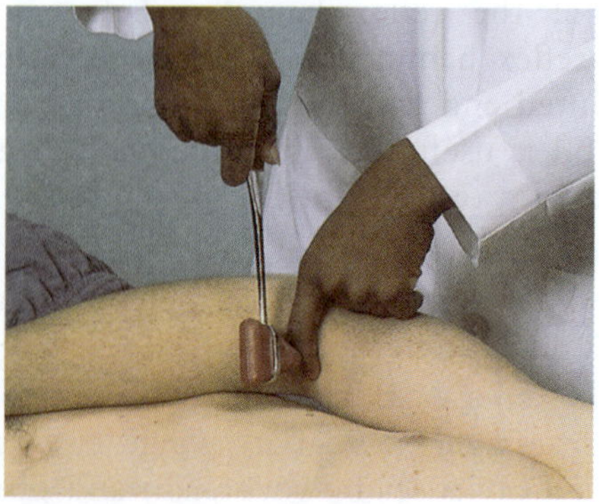

FIGURE 13-49. Biceps reflex (C5, C6)—patient supine.

Observe flexion at the elbow and watch for and feel the contraction of the biceps muscle.

Triceps Reflex (C6, C7). The patient may be sitting or supine. Flex the patient's arm at the elbow, with palm toward the body, and pull it slightly across the chest. Strike the triceps tendon with a direct blow directly behind and just above the elbow (Figs. 13-50 and 13-51). Watch for contraction of the triceps muscle and extension at the elbow.

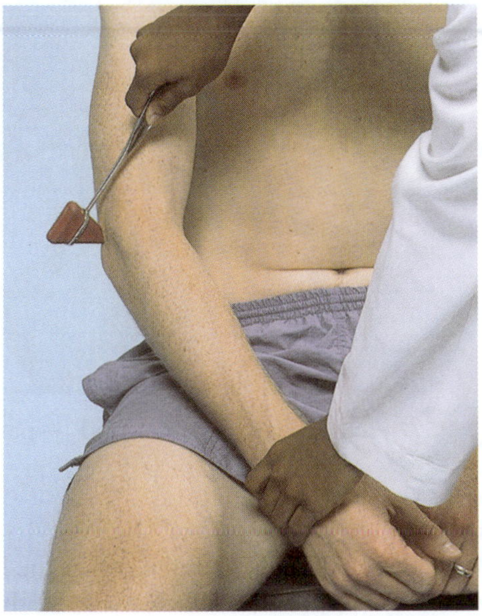

FIGURE 13-50. Triceps reflex (C6, C7)—patient sitting.

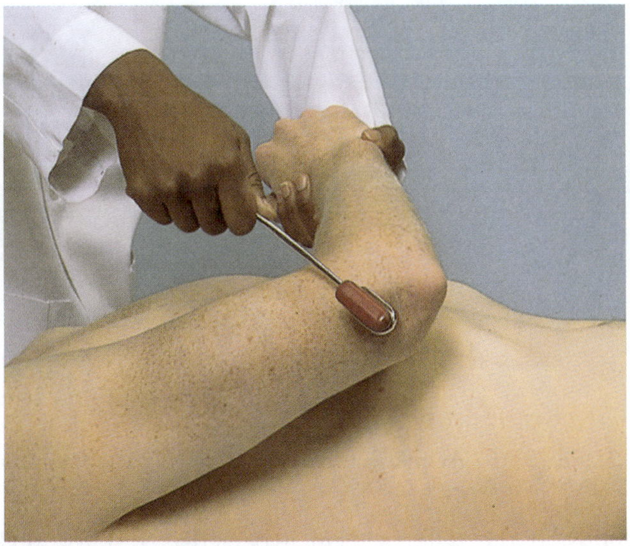

FIGURE 13-51. Triceps reflex (C6, C7)—patient supine.

If you have difficulty getting the patient to relax, try supporting the upper arm. Ask the patient to let the arm go limp, as if it were "hung up to dry." Then strike the triceps tendon (Fig. 13-52).

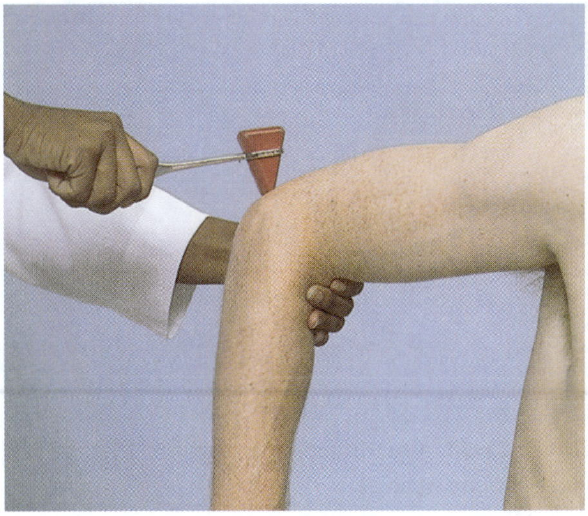

FIGURE 13-52. Triceps reflex (C6, C7)—patient sitting, and elbow supported.

Brachioradialis Reflex (C5, C6). The patient's hand should rest on the abdomen or the lap, with the forearm partly pronated. Strike the radius with the point or flat edge of the reflex hammer, about 2 to 4 inches above the wrist (Fig. 13-53). Watch for flexion at the elbow and supination of the forearm.

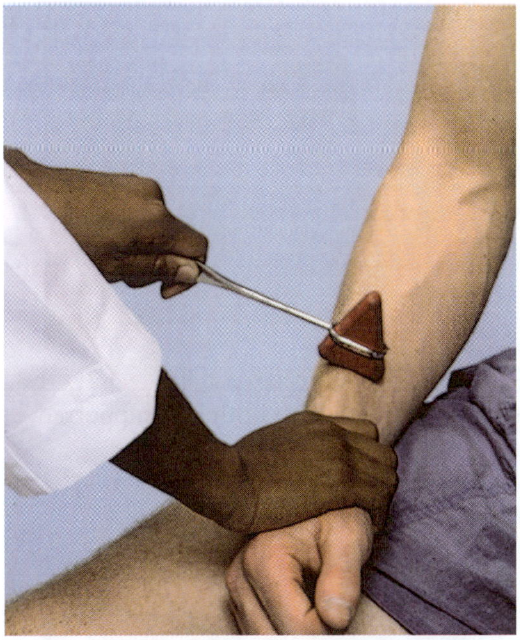

FIGURE 13-53. Brachioradialis reflex (C5, C6).

Quadriceps (Patellar) Reflex (L2, L3, L4). The patient may be either sitting or lying down as long as the knee is flexed. Briskly tap the patellar tendon just below the patella (Fig. 13-54). Note contraction of the quadriceps with extension at the knee. Placing your hand on the patient's anterior thigh lets you feel this reflex.

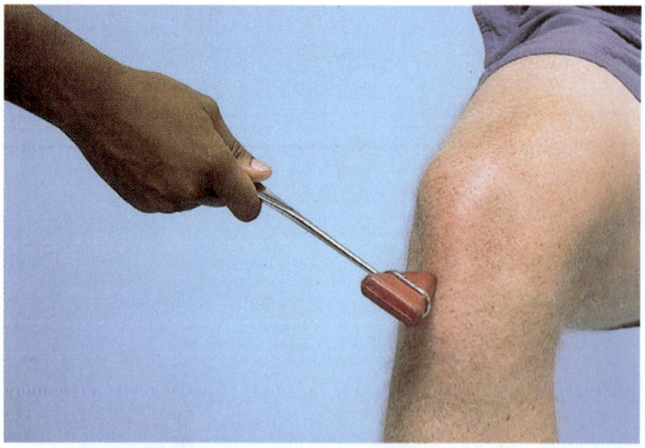

FIGURE 13-54. Quadriceps/patellar (L2, L3, L4) reflex—patient sitting.

There are two options for examining the supine patient. Supporting both knees at once allows you to assess small differences between quadriceps reflexes by repeatedly testing one reflex and then the other (Fig. 13-55). If supporting both legs is uncomfortable for you or the patient, you can place your supporting arm under the patient's leg (Fig. 13-56). Some patients find it easier to relax with this method.

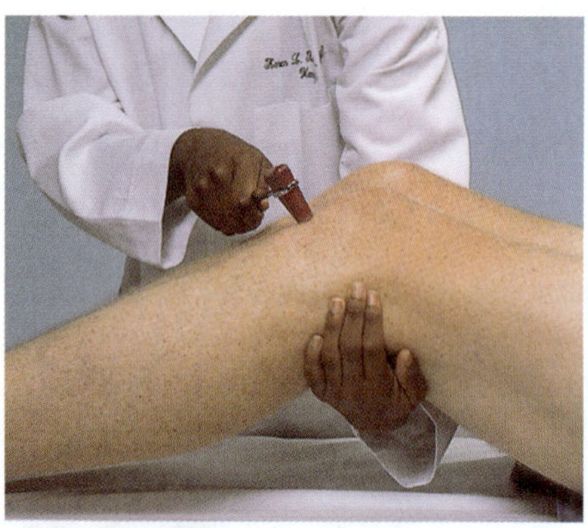

FIGURE 13-55. Quadriceps/patellar (L2, L3, L4) reflex—patient supine with both legs supported.

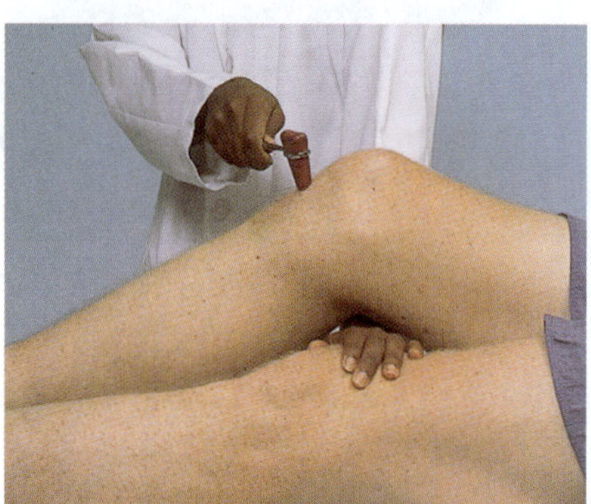

FIGURE 13-56. Quadriceps/patellar (L2, L3, L4) reflex—patient supine with one leg supported.

Achilles (Ankle) Reflex (Primarily S1). If the patient is sitting, partially dorsiflex the foot at the ankle. Persuade the patient to relax. Strike the Achilles tendon, and watch and feel for plantar flexion at the ankle (Fig. 13-57). Also note the speed of relaxation after muscular contraction.

The slowed relaxation phase of reflexes in *hypothyroidism* is often best detected during the ankle reflex.

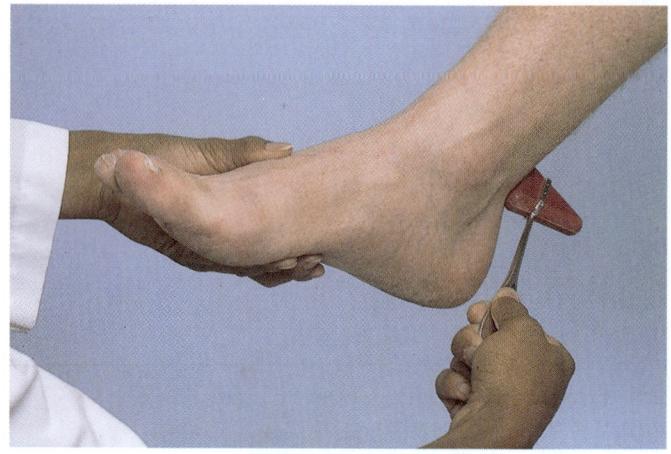

FIGURE 13-57. Achilles/ankle reflex (S1)—patient sitting.

When the patient is lying down, flex one leg at both hip and knee and rotate it externally so that the lower leg rests across the opposite shin. Then dorsiflex the foot at the ankle and strike the Achilles tendon (Fig. 13-58).

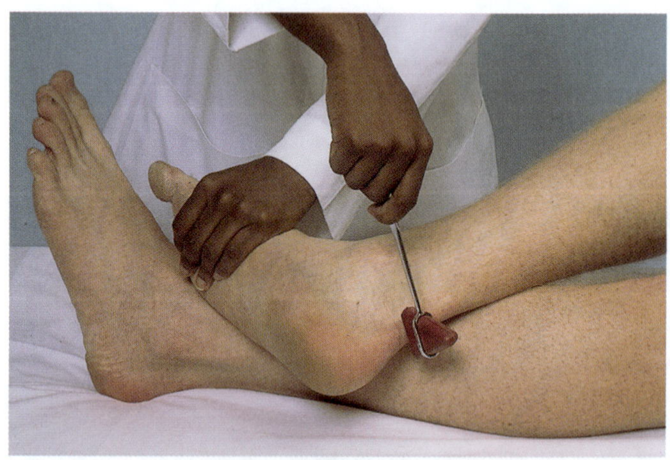

FIGURE 13-58. Achilles/ankle reflex (S1)—patient supine.

Clonus. If the reflexes seem hyperactive, test for ankle **clonus**. Support the knee in a partly flexed position. With your other hand, dorsiflex and plantar flex the foot a few times while encouraging the patient to relax, then sharply dorsiflex the foot and maintain it in dorsiflexion (Fig. 13-59). Look and feel for rhythmic oscillations between dorsiflexion and plantar flexion. Normally the ankle does not react to this stimulus and will remain held in dorsiflexion. There may be a few clonic beats if the patient is tense or has exercised.

Sustained clonus points to CNS disease affecting the corticospinal tract. Clonus must be present for a reflex to be graded 4 (see p. 330).

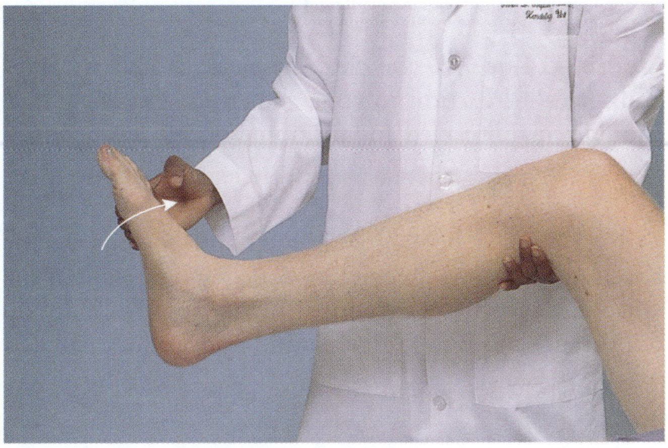

FIGURE 13-59. Testing for ankle clonus.

Other joints may display clonus. A sharp downward displacement of the patella, for example, may elicit patellar clonus in the extended knee. Spreading of reflexes to adjacent muscle groups can also indicate hyperreflexia, for example flexion of the fingers in response to testing the biceps reflex.

Cutaneous or Superficial Stimulation Reflexes

Abdominal Reflexes. Test the abdominal reflexes by lightly but briskly stroking each side of the abdomen, above (T8, T9, T10) and below (T10, T11, T12) the umbilicus in the directions illustrated (Fig. 13-60). Use a key, the wooden end of a cotton-tipped applicator, or the handle of your

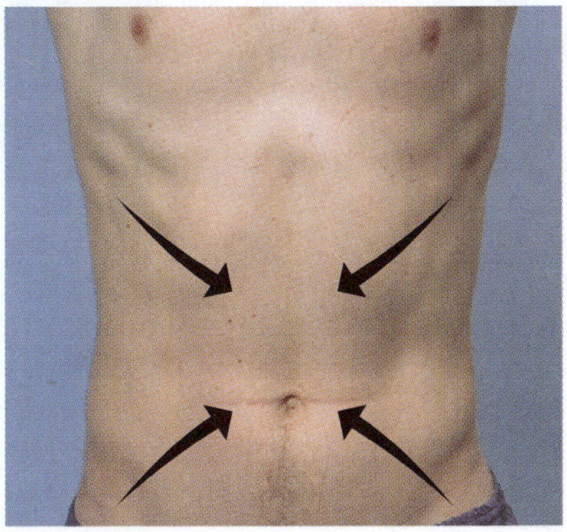

FIGURE 13-60. Direction of light touch while testing for abdominal reflexes.

reflex hammer. Note the contraction of the abdominal muscles and movement of the umbilicus toward the stimulus. If obesity or previous abdominal surgery masks the abdominal reflexes, retract the patient's umbilicus away from the side being tested with your finger and feel for the muscular contraction. Abdominal reflexes may be difficult to elicit. Asymmetry (left-to-right or above and below the umbilicus) is most compelling.

Abdominal reflexes may be absent in both central and peripheral nerve disorders.

Physiology OSCE Videos:
Superficial Reflexes

Plantar Response (Corticospinal Tract). Using a key or the wooden end of an applicator stick, stroke the lateral aspect of the sole from the heel to the ball of the foot, curving medially across the ball (Fig. 13-61). Use the lightest stimulus needed to provoke a response but increase firmness if necessary. Closely observe movement of the big toe, normally plantar flexion.

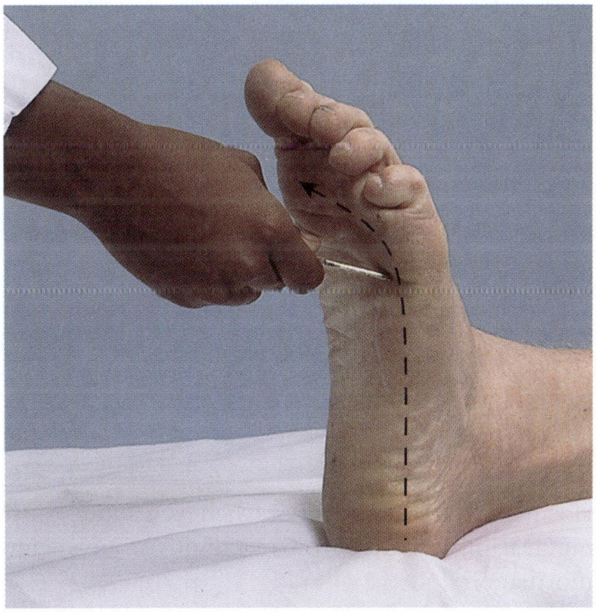

FIGURE 13-61. Testing the plantar response.

Dorsiflexion of the big toe is a *positive Babinski response* (Fig. 13-62), arising from a CNS lesion affecting the corticospinal tract (sensitivity ~50%; specificity 99%). The Babinski response can be transiently positive in unconscious states from drug or alcohol intoxication and during the postictal period following a seizure.

Some patients withdraw from this stimulus by flexing the hip and the knee. Hold the ankle, if necessary, to complete your observation. At times, it is difficult to distinguish withdrawal from a Babinski response.

Dorsiflexion of the big toe may be accompanied by fanning the other toes apart known as a positive Babinski response.

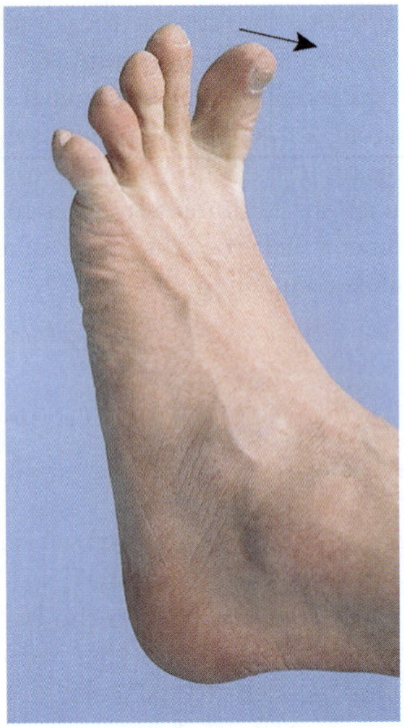

FIGURE 13-62. Abnormal plantar response (*Babinski* response). Note dorsiflexion of big toe.

Anal (Anocutaneous) Reflex. Using the broken end of an applicator stick, lightly stroke the anus on both sides. Watch for reflex contraction of the external anal sphincter. Detection of the reflex contraction is facilitated by placing a gloved finger in the anus during digital testing.

Loss of the anal (anocutaneous) reflex suggests a lesion in the S2–S3–S4 reflex arc, seen in cauda equina lesions.

SPECIAL TECHNIQUES

Meningeal Signs

Perform these maneuvers whenever you suspect meningeal inflammation from meningitis or subarachnoid hemorrhage.

Inflammation in the subarachnoid space causes resistance to movement that stretches the spinal nerves and meninges.

Although these meningeal signs have low specificity, specificity is increased if other signs and symptoms (fever, recent onset of headache) suggestive of meningitis are present.

The sensitivity of these maneuvers is reduced in the very old and very young, patients who have received analgesia, and patients with viral meningitis.

Nuchal Rigidity. First, make sure there is no injury or fracture to the cervical vertebrae or cervical cord. In trauma settings, this often requires radiologic evaluation. Then, with the patient supine, place your hands behind the patient's head and flex the neck forward, if possible until the chin touches the chest. Normally the neck is supple, and the patient can easily bend the head and neck forward.

Nuchal rigidity (neck stiffness with resistance to flexion) is found in ~84% of patients with acute bacterial meningitis and 21% to 86% of patients with subarachnoid hemorrhage. It is most reliably present in severe meningeal inflammation, but its overall diagnostic accuracy is low.

Brudzinski Sign. As you flex the neck, watch the hips and knees in reaction to your maneuver. Normally they should remain relaxed and motionless.

Flexion of both the hips and knees is a *positive Brudzinski sign.*

Kernig Sign. Flex the patient's leg at both the hip and the knee, and then slowly extend the leg and straighten the knee (Fig. 13-63). Discomfort behind the knee during full extension is normal but should not produce pain.

Pain and increased resistance to knee extension are a *positive Kernig sign.*

The frequency of Brudzinski and Kernig signs in patients with meningitis has a reported range of 5% to 60%. Sensitivity and specificity for Brudzinski and Kernig signs are reported as ~5% and 95% in limited study sets but are used in emerging scoring systems and merit more systematic investigation.

Meningitis may be present in older adult patients in the absence of these signs, and in those without meningitis, the Kernig sign was positive in 12% and the Brudzinski sign was positive in 8%.

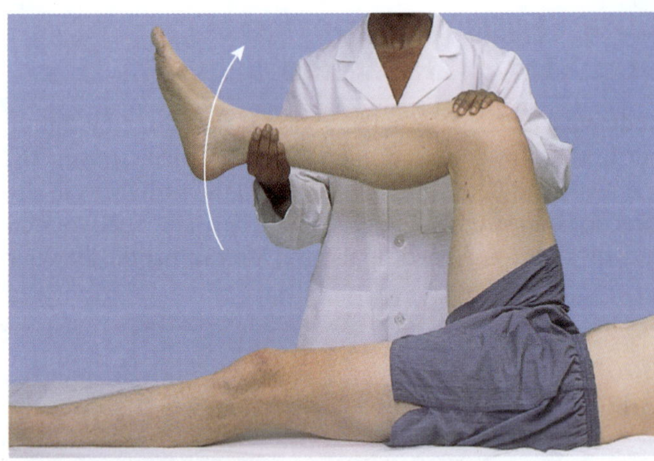

FIGURE 13-63. Testing for Kernig sign.

The mechanism of this sign is similar to the positive straight-leg raise test. Irritation or compression of a lumbar or sacral nerve root or the sciatic nerve causes radicular or sciatic pain radiating into the leg when the nerve is stretched by extending the leg.

Jolt Accentuation of Headache (JAH). Have the patient rotate their head side to side (as if nodding no) at a speed of 2 to 3 times per second. The test is positive if this maneuver worsens headache.

Although a positive JAH strongly increases the possibility of meningitis, a negative result is not able to rule out the presence of acute meningitis.

Lumbosacral Radiculopathy: Straight-Leg Raise

If the patient has low back pain that radiates down the thigh and leg, commonly called *sciatica* if in the sciatic nerve distribution, test straight-leg raising on each side in turn. Place the patient in the supine position. Raise the patient's relaxed and straightened leg, flexing the thigh at the hip (Fig. 13-64). Some examiners first raise the patient's leg with the knee flexed, then extend the leg.

See Table 15-4, Low Back Pain.

Compression of the spinal nerve root as it passes through the vertebral foramen causes a painful radiculopathy with associated muscle weakness and dermatomal sensory loss, commonly from a herniated disc. More than 95% of disc herniations in the lumbar spine occur at L4–L5 or L5–S1, where the spine angles sharply posterior. Look for ipsilateral leg wasting or weak ankle dorsiflexion, which make the diagnosis five times more likely.

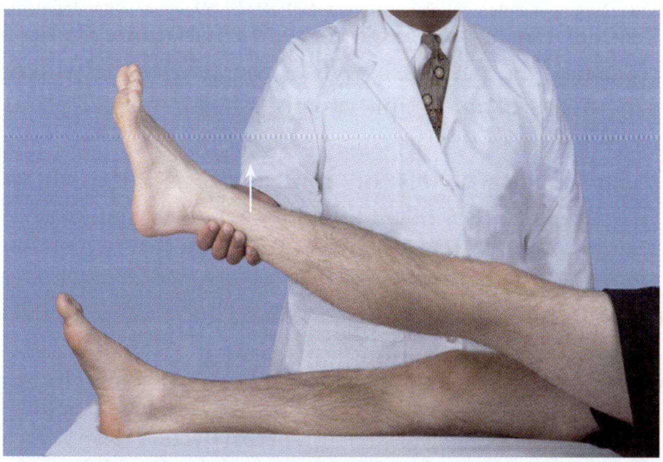

FIGURE 13-64. Testing for lumbosacral radiculopathy with the straight-leg raise.

Assess the degree of elevation at which pain occurs, the quality and distribution of the pain, and the effects of foot dorsiflexion. Tightness or discomfort in the buttocks or hamstrings is common during these maneuvers and should not be interpreted as "radiating pain" or a positive test.

Pain radiating into the ipsilateral leg is a *positive straight leg test* for *lumbosacral radiculopathy.* Foot dorsiflexion can further increase leg pain in *lumbosacral radiculopathy, sciatic neuropathy,* or both. Increased pain when the contralateral healthy leg is raised is a *positive crossed straight-leg raise sign.* These maneuvers stretch the affected nerve roots and sciatic nerve.

If positive, be sure to examine motor and sensory function and reflexes at the lumbosacral levels.

Sensitivity and specificity of positive ipsilateral straight-leg raise for lumbosacral radiculopathy in patients with sciatica are relatively low, with an LR of only 1.5. For the crossed straight-leg raise the LR is higher, 3.4.

Asterixis (Flapping Tremor)

Ask the patient to "stop traffic" by extending both arms, with wrists dorsiflexed and fingers spread (Fig. 13-65). Observe for abnormal "flapping" tremor at the wrist. Watch for 30 seconds, encouraging the patient to maintain this position.

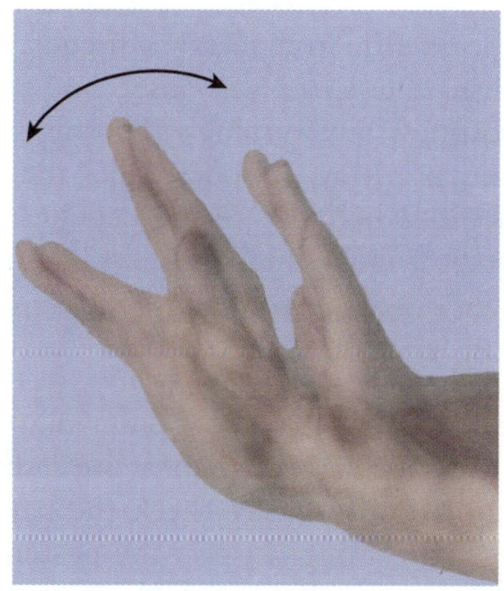

FIGURE 13-65. Testing for asterixis.

Sudden, brief loss of muscle tone manifest as nonrhythmic flexion of the hands and fingers followed by recovery indicates asterixis and suggests metabolic encephalopathy as seen in liver disease, uremia, and hypercapnia.

Asterixis is caused by abnormal function of the diencephalic motor centers that regulate agonist and antagonist muscle tone and maintain posture.

Assessing the Comatose Patient

Coma, a state of impaired arousal and awareness, signals a potentially life-threatening event affecting the two hemispheres, the brainstem, or both. Accurate assessment of the severity of the insult and its underlying cause is critical. Although arousal and awareness are interrelated, "a change in one is not always associated with a similar change in the other."

Arousal (wakefulness) depends on the ascending reticular activating system of the brainstem which projects through the thalamus to several areas of the cortex, which "processes, integrates, and gives context to the information provided to it thus generating awareness. Injury to any of these areas or their connections can result in impaired consciousness." The usual sequence of history, physical examination, and laboratory evaluation does not apply. Instead, you must:

- First assess and stabilize the ABCs (airway, breathing, and circulation)

Be familiar with the Glasgow Coma Scale. See Table 13-13, Glasgow Coma Scale.

- Assess the patient's level of consciousness
- Perform a neurologic examination. Identify any focal or asymmetric findings and determine if the cause of impaired consciousness is structural or metabolic.

See Table 13-14, Metabolic and Structural Coma.

- Obtain information from relatives, friends, or witnesses to establish the speed of onset and duration of unconsciousness, any warning symptoms, precipitating factors, or previous episodes, and the premorbid appearance and behavior of the patient. Any history of past medical and mental disorders is also important.

During your examination, remember two cardinal DON'Ts (Box 13-10).

Airway, Breathing, and Circulation. Brain injury significant enough to cause coma can compromise respiratory and circulatory function. Quickly check the patient's color and pattern of breathing. Inspect the posterior pharynx and listen over the trachea for stridor to make sure the airway is clear. If respirations are slowed or shallow, or if the airway is obstructed by secretions, consider options for maintaining the airway open while stabilizing the cervical spine.

Box 13-10. "Don'ts" When Assessing the Comatose Patient

- *Don't* dilate the pupils, which serve as an important clue to the underlying cause of coma (structural vs. metabolic) and may warn of life-threatening cerebral herniation syndromes.
- *Don't* flex the neck if there is any question of trauma to the head or neck. Immobilize the cervical spine and obtain imaging first to rule out fractures of the cervical vertebrae that could compress and damage the spinal cord.

See Table 13-15, Pupils in Comatose Patients.

See Table 10-4, Abnormalities in Rate and Rhythm of Breathing.

Assess the remaining vital signs: pulse, blood pressure, and temperature. If hypotension or hemorrhage is present, establish intravenous access and begin intravenous fluids. (Further emergency management and laboratory studies are beyond the scope of this text.)

Neurologic Evaluation of the Comatose Patient

Level of Consciousness. Level of consciousness primarily reflects the patient's capacity for arousal, or wakefulness. Testing targets the amount of stimulation required to arouse the patient as well as the activity the patient can then sustain. Think of this as your mental status examination in the comatose patient.

Five clinical levels of consciousness are listed in Box 13-11, with related techniques for examination.

Box 13-11. Maneuvers for Testing Level of Consciousness (Arousal) and Expected Patient Response

Level	Maneuvers for Testing Arousal	Expected Patient Response
Alertness	Speak to the patient in a normal tone of voice.	The alert patient opens the eyes, looks at you, and responds fully and appropriately to stimuli (arousal intact).
Lethargy	Speak to the patient in a *loud voice*. For example, call the patient's name or ask, "How are you?"	The lethargic patient appears drowsy but opens the eyes and looks at you, responds to questions, and then falls asleep.
Obtundation	Apply *tactile* stimulus by gently shaking the patient as if awakening a sleeper.	The obtunded patient opens the eyes and looks at you but responds to you slowly and is somewhat confused. Alertness and interest in the environment are decreased.
Stupor	Apply a *painful* stimulus (Fig. 13-66). For example, pinch a tendon, rub the sternum, or roll a pencil across a nail bed. (No stronger stimuli needed!)	The stuporous patient arouses from sleep only after painful stimuli. Verbal responses are slow or even absent. The patient lapses into an unresponsive state when the stimulus ceases. There is minimal awareness of self or the environment.
Coma	Apply repeated painful stimuli to the trunk and extremities.	A comatose patient remains unarousable with eyes closed. There is no evident response to inner need or external stimuli.

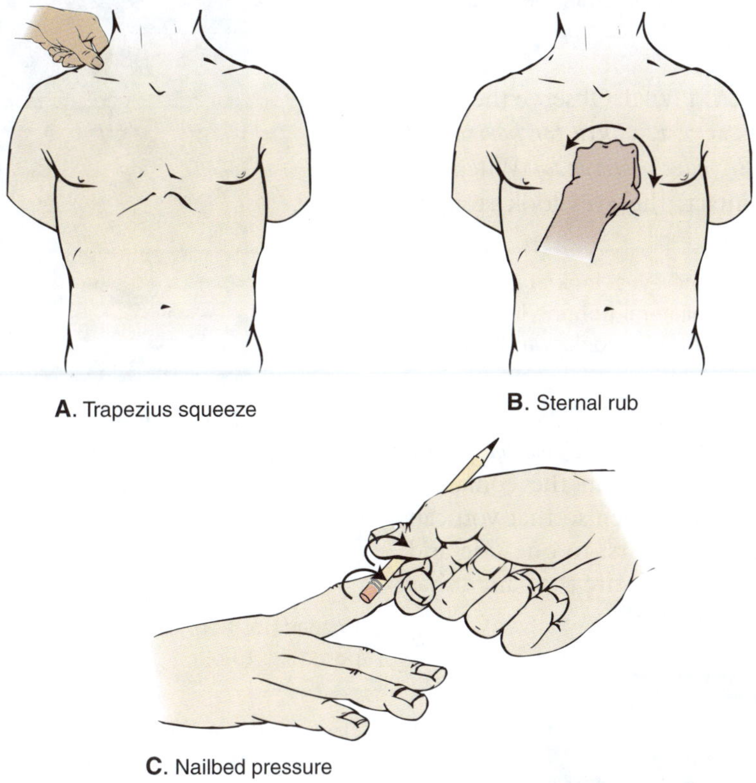

FIGURE 13-66. Maneuvers for testing arousal. **A:** Trapezius squeeze. **B:** Sternal rub. **C:** Nailbed pressure. (Modified from Morton PG, Fontaine DK. *Critical Care Nursing*. 11th ed. Wolters Kluwer; 2018, Fig. 36-5.)

Increase your stimuli in a stepwise manner, depending on the patient's response. When you examine patients with an altered level of consciousness, describe and record exactly what you see and hear. Imprecise use of terms such as lethargy, obtundation, stupor, or coma may mislead other examiners.

Respirations. Observe the rate, rhythm, and pattern of respiration. Because neural structures that govern breathing in the cortex and brainstem overlap with those that govern consciousness, abnormalities of respiration often occur in coma.

See Table 10-4, Abnormalities in Rate and Rhythm of Breathing.

Brainstem Reflexes. It is possible to assess the majority of the cranial nerves in the comatose patient by observing the patient and testing brainstem reflexes (Box 13-12). The presence or absence of these reflexes provides information about the health of the brainstem, helps localize structural causes of coma, and informs prognosis.

Determining prognosis after coma is complex and is complicated by use of therapeutic hypothermia. Research targets include clinical examination, EEG patterns, serum biomarkers, and imaging. Careful neurologic examination remains a mainstay of prognosis, especially after 72 hours.

Box 13-12. Assessing Cranial Nerves in a Comatose Patient

Examination Maneuver	Cranial Nerves Tested
Pupillary light reflex	II, III
Ocular position and movement	III, IV, VI
Oculocephalic reflex	III, IV, VI, VIII
Oculovestibular reflex with caloric stimulation	III, IV, VI, VIII
Corneal reflex	V, VII
Facial asymmetry, grimace in response to painful stimulus	VII
Gag reflex	IX, X

Pupillary Light Reflex (CNs II, III). Observe the size and equality of the pupils and test their reaction to light. The presence or absence of the light reaction is one of the most important signs distinguishing structural from metabolic causes of coma. The light reaction often remains intact in metabolic coma.

See Table 13-15, Pupils in Comatose Patients.

Structural lesions from stroke, abscess, or tumor mass may lead to asymmetrical pupils and loss of the light reaction.

Ocular Position and Movement (CNs II, IV, VI). Observe the position of the eyes and eyelids at rest. *Check for horizontal deviation of the eyes to one side (gaze preference).* When the oculomotor pathways are intact, the eyes look straight ahead.

In structural hemispheric lesions, the eyes "look at the lesion" in the affected hemisphere. In a unilateral pontine lesion or in seizure affecting one hemisphere, the eyes "look away" from the affected side.

Oculocephalic Reflex (CNs III, IV, VI, VIII). The *oculocephalic reflex* helps assess brainstem function in the comatose patient. Holding the upper eyelids open so that you can see the eyes, turn the head quickly, first to one side and then to the other (Fig. 13-67). Make sure the patient has no neck injury before performing this test.

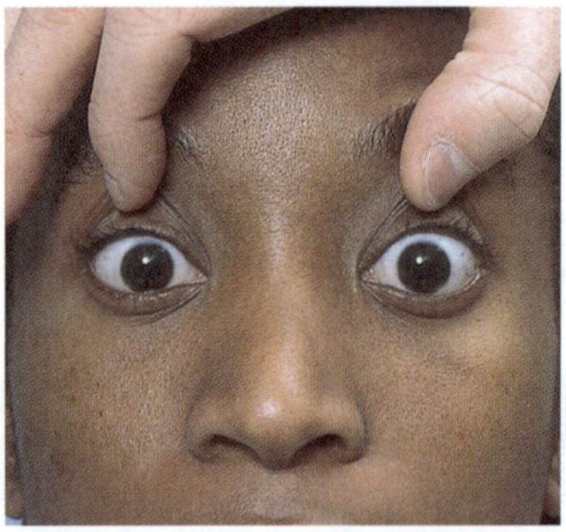

FIGURE 13-67. Testing the oculocephalic reflex (CNs III, IV, VI, VIII).

In a comatose patient with an intact brainstem, as the head is turned in one direction, the eyes move toward the opposite side (*doll's eye movements*), as shown in Figure 13-68.

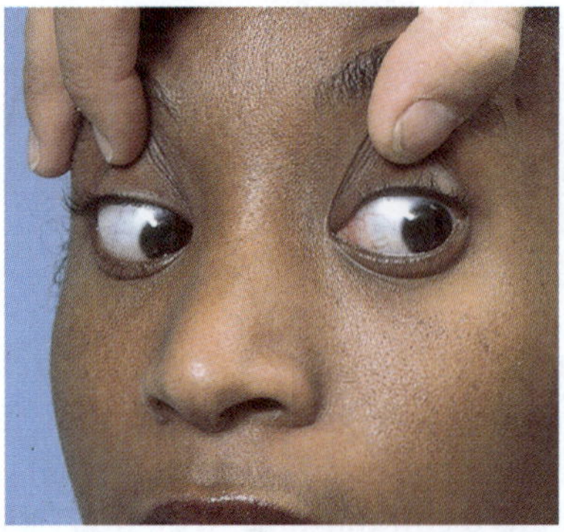

FIGURE 13-68. Oculocephalic reflex intact. Note movement of eyes toward left on head turn toward right (doll's eye movement).

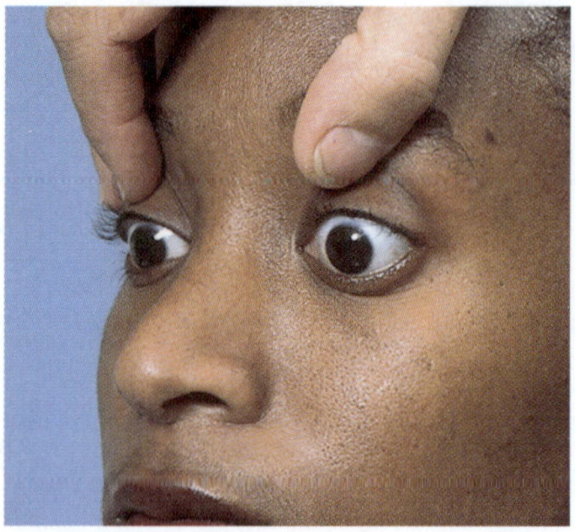

FIGURE 13-69. Oculocephalic reflex absent. Note loss of movement of eyes toward left on head turn toward right.

In a comatose patient with absent doll's eye movements, the eyes continue to look straight ahead, with no movement relative to head position. This is suspicious for a lesion of the midbrain or pons (Fig. 13-69).

Oculovestibular Reflex with Caloric Stimulation (CNs III, IV, VI, VIII). If the oculocephalic reflex is absent and you seek further testing of brainstem function, test the *oculovestibular reflex.* Note that this test is usually not performed in an awake patient.

Make sure the eardrums are intact and the ear canals clear. Elevate the patient's head to 30 degrees to perform the test accurately. Place a towel or basin under the ear to catch any water that spills over. With a large syringe, inject ice water through a small catheter that is lying in (but not plugging) the ear canal. Watch for deviation of the eyes in the horizontal plane. You may need to use up to 120 mL of ice water to elicit a response. In the comatose patient with an *intact brainstem,* the eyes drift *toward* the irrigated ear. Repeat on the opposite side, waiting 3 to 5 minutes, if necessary, for the first response to disappear.

No response to stimulation indicates brainstem injury.

Corneal Reflex (CN V, VII). Test the *corneal reflex.* Avoiding the eyelashes, lightly touch the cornea (not just the conjunctiva) with a fine wisp of cotton (Fig. 13-70). Inspect for blinking of both eyes, the normal reaction to this stimulus. In the comatose patient, the eyelids may need to be held open. The sensory limb of this reflex is carried by CN V, and the motor response by CN VII on both sides.

Corneal reflexes can also be assessed in the awake patient and may be useful if sensory testing seems unreliable. Ask the patient to look up and away from you and approach from the opposite side, out of the patient's

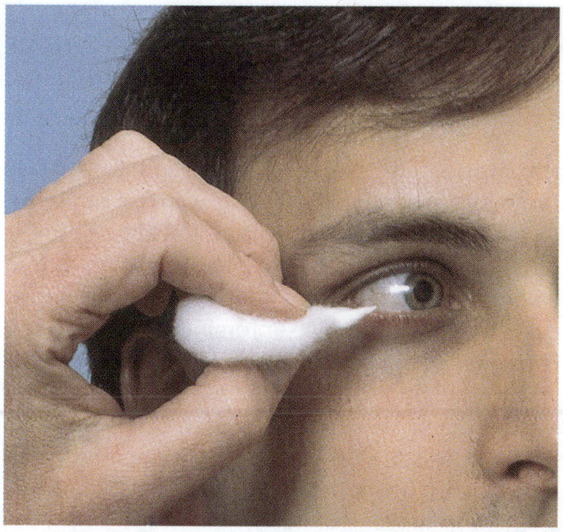

FIGURE 13-70. Testing the corneal reflex (CNs V, VII).

line of vision. If the patient is apprehensive, touching the conjunctiva first may be helpful. Contact lenses interfere with this testing.

Blinking is absent in both eyes in CN V lesions and on the side of weakness in lesions of CN VII.

Absent blinking and sensorineural hearing loss occur in *acoustic neuroma*.

Gag Reflex (CN IX, X). This reflex consists of elevation of the tongue and soft palate and constriction of the pharyngeal muscles. Using a cotton tipped applicator, stimulate the back of the throat lightly on each side in turn and observe the gag reflex. The gag reflex can also be tested in awake patients but may be diminished in many awake healthy people.

Unilateral absence of this reflex suggests a lesion of CN IX, and perhaps CN X.

Observe the patient's posture and movement. If there is no spontaneous movement, you may need to apply a painful stimulus (see Fig. 13-66). Classify the resulting pattern of movement as:

- *Normal–avoidant*—the patient purposefully pushes the stimulus away or withdraws
- *Stereotypic*—the stimulus evokes abnormal postural responses of the trunk and extremities
- *Flaccid paralysis or no response*—no response on one side suggests a corticospinal tract lesion

See Table 13-11, Abnormal Body Postures. Two stereotypic responses predominate in coma: decorticate rigidity and decerebrate rigidity.

Test muscle tone by grasping each forearm near the wrist and raising it to a vertical position. Note the position of the hand, which is usually only slightly flexed at the wrist (Fig. 13-71).

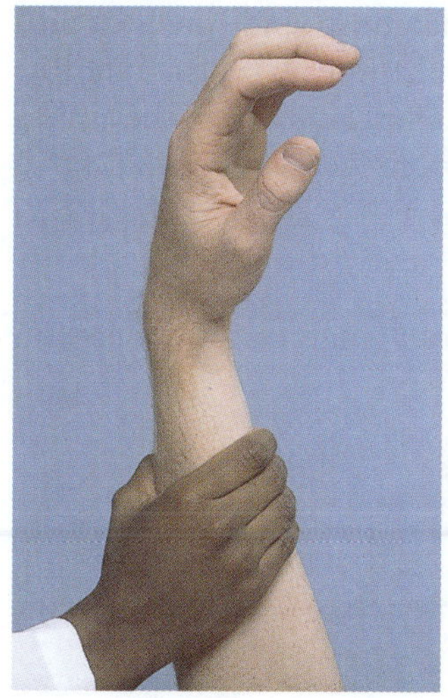

FIGURE 13-71. Testing muscle tone in the arm.

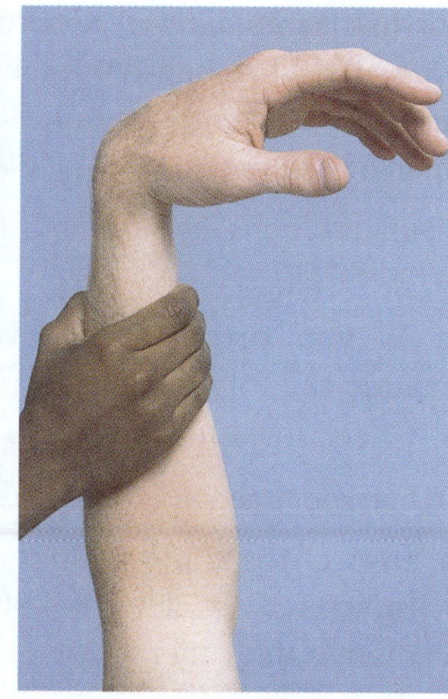

FIGURE 13-72. Arm tone flaccid. Note flexed wrist.

The hemiplegia of acute cerebral infarction is usually flaccid at first. The limp hand drops to form a right angle with the wrist (Fig. 13-72).

Then lower the arm to about 12 or 18 in off the bed and drop it. Watch how it falls. A normal arm drops somewhat slowly.

A flaccid arm drops rapidly, like a rock.

Support the patient's flexed knees. Then extend one leg at a time at the knee and let the leg fall (Fig. 13-73). Compare the speed with which each leg falls.

In acute hemiplegia, the flaccid leg falls more rapidly.

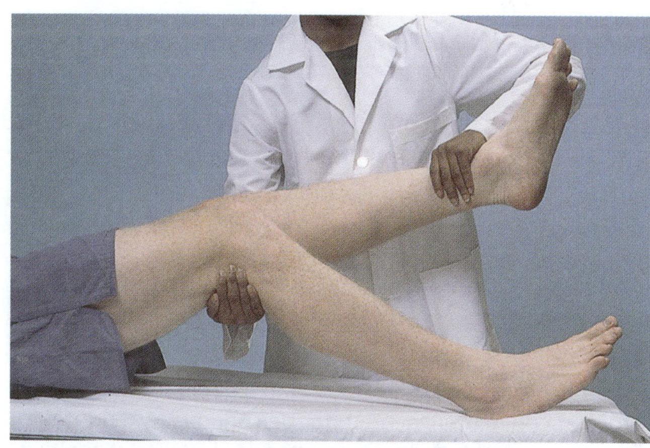

FIGURE 13-73. Testing muscle tone in the leg.

Flex both legs so that the heels rest on the bed and then release them. The normal leg returns slowly to its original extended position.

In acute hemiplegia, the weak leg falls rapidly into extension, with external rotation at the hip.

Further Examination. Coordination and gait cannot be tested. The sensory examination may be limited to response to painful stimuli. Reflexes can be tested just as in an awake patient. Test for meningeal signs if indicated.

Meningeal signs are suspicious for meningitis or subarachnoid hemorrhage.

As you proceed with your physical examination, include the following assessments.

- Check for unusual odors.

  Consider alcohol, liver failure, or uremia.

- Inspect for abnormalities of the skin, including color, moisture, evidence of bleeding disorders, needle marks, and other lesions.

  Note any jaundice, cyanosis, or the cherry red color of carbon monoxide poisoning.

- Inspect and palpate the scalp and skull for signs of trauma.

  Look for bruises, lacerations, or swelling.

- Examine the fundi carefully.

  Examine closely for papilledema, an important sign of elevated intracranial pressure.

- Inspect the ears and nose and examine the mouth and throat.

  Blood or cerebrospinal fluid in the nose or the ears suggests a skull fracture; otitis media suggests a possible brain abscess. Tongue injury suggests a seizure.

RECORDING YOUR FINDINGS

Note that initially you may use sentences to describe your findings; later you will use phrases. The style below contains phrases appropriate for most write-ups. Note the five components of the examination and write-up of the nervous system.

Recording the Nervous System Examination

"***Mental Status:*** Alert, relaxed, and cooperative. Thought process coherent. Oriented to person, place, and time. Speech is fluent, follows commands. Detailed cognitive testing deferred. ***Cranial Nerves:*** I—not tested; II through XII intact. ***Motor:*** Normal muscle bulk and tone. Strength 5/5 throughout. No pronator drift. Cerebellar—Rapid alternating movements (RAMs), finger-to-nose (F→N), heel-to-shin (H→S) intact. Gait with normal stance and stride. ***Sensory:*** Pinprick, light touch, position, and vibration intact. Romberg—maintains balance with eyes closed. ***Reflexes:*** 2+ and symmetric with plantar reflexes downgoing."

(continued)

Recording the Nervous System Examination (*continued*)

OR

"***Mental Status:*** The patient is alert and tries to answer questions but has difficulty finding words. ***Cranial Nerves:*** I—not tested; II—visual acuity intact; visual fields full; II, III—pupils are equal and reactive to light. III, IV, VI—extraocular movements intact; V—temporal and masseter strength intact, corneal reflexes present; VII—prominent right facial droop and flattening of right nasolabial fold, left facial movements intact; VIII—hearing intact bilaterally to whispered voice, IX, X—gag intact; XI—strength of sternocleidomastoid and trapezius muscles 5/5; XII—tongue midline. ***Motor:*** Normal bulk. Spasticity in the right arm and right leg. Strength in right biceps, triceps, iliopsoas, gluteals, quadriceps, hamstring, and ankle flexor and extensor muscles 3/5; strength in comparable muscle groups on the left 5/5. Right pronator drift present. Gait—unable to test. Cerebellar—unable to test on right due to right arm and leg weakness; RAMs, F→N, H→S intact on left. ***Sensory:*** decreased sensation to pinprick over right face, arm, and leg; intact on the left. Stereognosis and two-point discrimination not tested. Romberg—unable to test due to right leg weakness. ***Reflexes*** *(can record in two ways):*

	Biceps	Triceps	Brach	Knee	Ankle	Plantar
RT	++++	++++	++++	++++	++++	↑
LT	++	++	++	++	+	↓

OR

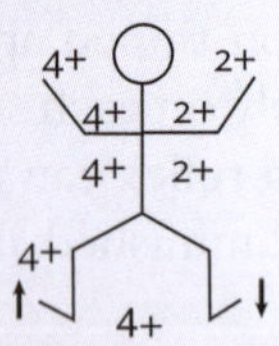

These findings are suspicious for left hemispheric cerebral infarction in the distribution of the left middle cerebral artery, with right-sided hemiparesis.

HEALTH PROMOTION AND COUNSELING: EVIDENCE AND RECOMMENDATIONS

Important Topics for Health Promotion and Counseling

- Preventing cerebrovascular disease
- Screening for asymptomatic carotid artery stenosis
- Screening for peripheral neuropathy
- Herpes zoster vaccination (see Chapter 6)
- Detecting the "three Ds": delirium, dementia, and depression (see Chapter 9, pp. 167–169)

Preventing Cerebrovascular Disease

Stroke is an acute brain injury that can be caused by cerebrovascular ischemia (blockage in blood vessels to the brain) or hemorrhage (blood vessel rupture). Ischemic stroke subtypes include (1) cardioembolic (e.g., from atrial fibrillation); (2) large vessel atheroembolic (e.g., from carotid artery stenosis); (3) small vessel disease (also called lacunar infarcts; related to hypertension and diabetes); (4) other, including cervical artery dissection or a hypercoagulable state; and (5) cryptogenic, when no cause is found. Hemorrhagic stroke subtypes include (1) intraparenchymal; (2) subarachnoid; which can be either aneurysmal or nonaneurysmal; (3) subdural; or (4) epidural. Dural venous sinus thrombosis can also lead to infarction of brain tissue that is frequently hemorrhagic. About 87% of all strokes results from ischemia, 10% from intracerebral hemorrhage, and 3% from subarachnoid hemorrhage.

Harms from stroke are often worsened because people do not recognize the warning signs of stroke and delay seeking medical care. Thrombolytic therapy is most effective in preventing permanent neurologic injury when administered within 4.5 hours of symptom onset. Interventional therapies (e.g., clot retrieval) are now also widely used also, if patients present early. The American Heart Association/American Stroke Association encourages people to seek immediate medical attention if they have the following signs after stroke (Box 13-13).

Box 13-13. AHA/ASA Stroke Attack Warning Signs

- Sudden numbness or weakness of the face, arm, or leg
- Sudden confusion, trouble speaking or understanding
- Sudden trouble seeing in one or both eyes
- Sudden trouble walking, dizziness, or loss of balance or coordination
- Sudden severe headache

One of the strongest risk factors for stroke is a TIA, an episode of neurologic dysfunction that resolves within 24 hours. Following a TIA, 3% to 10% of patients have a stroke within 2 days and 9% to 17% within 90 days. Overall, about 15% of all strokes are preceded by a TIA. Short-term stroke risk following a TIA is highest in those age 60 years and older and those having diabetes, focal symptoms of weakness or impaired speech, and symptoms lasting more than 10 minutes.

Box 13-14 shows potentially modifiable risk factors for stroke, many of which are also risk factors for coronary artery disease. Discussions about screening and behavioral interventions for these risk factors appear elsewhere in the textbook.

Box 13-14. Stroke Risk Factors—Primary Prevention for Ischemic Stroke

Potentially Modifiable Risk Factors	
Hypertension	Hypertension is the leading modifiable risk factor for both ischemic and hemorrhagic stroke. Pharmacologically reducing blood pressure significantly reduces stroke risk, particularly among African Americans and older adults.
Diabetes	Stroke risk is about doubled with diabetes, and 16% of patients with diabetes over age 65 will die of stroke. Achieving good blood pressure control and prescribing statins reduces stroke risk in diabetic patients, though the benefit of glycemic control is uncertain.
Atrial fibrillation	Atrial fibrillation increases the risk of ischemic stroke about fivefold, but risk can vary 20-fold among patients depending upon age; gender; and clinical conditions such as diabetes, vascular disease, hypertension, congestive heart failure, and previous cerebrovascular events. Antiplatelet agents and anticoagulants can reduce the risk for ischemic stroke. When considering antithrombotic therapy, experts recommend individual risk stratification into high-, moderate-, and low-risk groups to balance risk of stroke against risk of bleeding. All patients, however, with atrial fibrillation should be at least on aspirin (unless contraindicated), and all those except "low-risk" would benefit from escalation to anticoagulation (unless contraindicated).
Dyslipidemia	The associations between blood cholesterol levels and stroke incidence are inconsistent, though numerous studies have found high total cholesterol to be a risk factor for ischemic stroke. Statin treatment reduce the risk of all strokes by about 20% for patients with or at risk for atherosclerotic cardiovascular disease.

(continued)

Box 13-14. Stroke Risk Factors—Primary Prevention for Ischemic Stroke (*continued*)

Potentially Modifiable Risk Factors	
Smoking/tobacco use	Smoking is associated with a two- to fourfold increased risk of stroke compared to never smokers or former smokers who have quit for >10 years. Smoking cessation rapidly reduces the risk of stroke, but never to the level of never smokers.
Physical inactivity	Increased levels of physical activity are correlated with reduced stroke risk.
Chronic kidney disease	A low glomerular filtration rate is associated with an increased risk for stroke.
Weight	Obesity (body mass index >30 kg/m^2) is associated with a 64% increased risk for ischemic stroke. The effect of weight reduction on stroke risk has not been well evaluated.
Diet and nutrition	Higher consumption of red meat, sodium, or sugary or artificially sweetened beverages has been associated with increased stroke risk. Conversely, higher dietary intake of nuts, olive oil, fish, fruits, and vegetables is associated with a reduced risk for stroke.
Alcohol use	Heavy alcohol intake, by leading to hypertension, hypercoagulable states, atrial fibrillation, and reduced cerebral blood flow, is a risk factor for ischemic and hemorrhagic stroke. However, light or moderate alcohol consumption has been observed to have a protective against the risk of total and ischemic strokes.
Carotid artery disease	Medical therapy, including statins, antiplatelet agents, treatment of diabetes and hypertension, and smoking cessation, can reduce the risk of stroke in individuals with asymptomatic carotid artery stenosis. Endarterectomy has the biggest role in symptomatic (TIA or stroke) patients; thus, experts recommend carotid endarterectomy only for selected asymptomatic patients with carotid artery stenosis >60% (provided that the surgeon and center have very low perioperative risks for stroke and mortality).
Sickle cell disease	Stroke at an early age is a common manifestation of sickle cell disease (SCD); the prevalence is 11% by age 20. Periodic red cell transfusions can reduce stroke risk in these patients.
Obstructive sleep apnea	Sleep apnea is an independent risk factor for stroke, particularly in men. Stroke risk increases with increasing sleep apnea severity as measured by the number of respiratory events (cessation or air flow reduction) per hour. Sleep apnea is usually treated with continuous positive airway pressure (CPAP), although its effectiveness for reducing stroke risk is unknown.

Screening for Asymptomatic Carotid Artery Stenosis

Carotid duplex ultrasound can accurately and safely detect significant (60% to 99%) carotid artery stenosis and is widely used for evaluating symptomatic persons. Although asymptomatic carotid artery stenosis is a stroke risk, it accounts for only a small proportion of ischemic strokes.

Screening for Diabetic Peripheral Neuropathy

Diabetes mellitus causes several types of peripheral neuropathy. Many patients with diabetes are not aware they have neuropathy because they do not detect sensory loss because it is not painful to them, but they are still at risk for ulceration and injuries that may worsen and require amputation. Screening for neuropathy is therefore imperative. The most common neuropathy is distal symmetric polyneuropathy (DSPN), which is slowly progressive; often asymptomatic; and a risk factor for ulcerations, arthropathy, and amputation. DSPN accounts for about 75% of diabetic neuropathies, others include autonomic dysfunction, mononeuropathies, and polyradiculopathies. The prevalence of DSPN is estimated to be about 20% in patients with long-term type 1 diabetes and up to 50% among patients with long-term type 2 diabetes. Patients with symptomatic DSPN may report numbness; tingling; poor balance; or pain that is burning, stabbing, or electrical shock-like in the lower extremities. Maintaining tight glycemic control can prevent or delay the onset of neuropathy, particularly for patients with type 1 diabetes. Tight glycemic control alone is only modestly effective for patients with type 2 diabetes. The American Diabetes Association recommends routinely examining the feet of patients with diabetes, assessing for neuropathy by testing either temperature or pinprick sensation, proprioception, ankle reflexes, vibration perception (with a 128-Hz tuning fork), and plantar light touch sensation (with a 10-g monofilament) as well as checking for skin breakdown, poor circulation, and musculoskeletal abnormalities.

TABLE 13-1. Disorders of the Central and Peripheral Nervous Systems

Central Nervous System Disorders

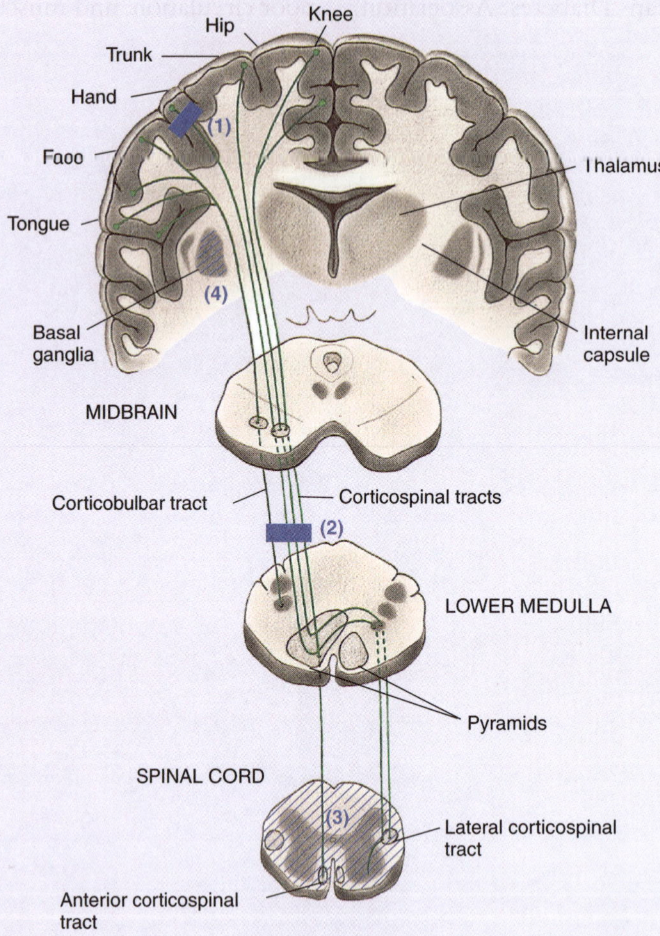

Location of Lesion	Typical Findings: Motor	Typical Findings: Sensory	Typical Findings: Deep Tendon Reflexes	Examples of Cause
Cerebral Cortex (1)	Chronic contralateral corticospinal-type weakness and spasticity; flexion is stronger than extension in the arm, plantar flexion is stronger than dorsiflexion in the foot, and the leg is externally rotated at the hip	Contralateral sensory loss in the face, limbs, and trunk on the same side as the motor deficits	↑	Cortical stroke
Brainstem (2)	Weakness and spasticity as above, plus CN deficits such as diplopia (from weakness of the extraocular muscles) and dysarthria	Variable depending on level of brainstem	↑	Brainstem stroke, MS plaque

(*continued*)

TABLE 13-1. Disorders of the Central and Peripheral Nervous Systems *(Continued)*

Location of Lesion	Typical Findings: Motor	Typical Findings: Sensory	Typical Findings: Deep Tendon Reflexes	Examples of Cause
Spinal Cord (3)	Weakness and spasticity as above, but often affecting both sides (when cord damage is bilateral), causing paraparesis or quadriparesis depending on the level of injury	Dermatomal sensory deficit on the trunk on one or both sides at the level of the lesion, and sensory loss from tract damage below the level of the lesion	↑	Trauma, spinal cord tumor
Subcortical Gray Matter: Basal Ganglia (4)	Slowness of movement (bradykinesia), rigidity, and tremor	Sensation not affected	Normal or ↓	Parkinsonism
Cerebellar (not illustrated)	Hypotonia, ataxia, nystagmus, dysdiadochokinesis, and dysmetria	Sensation not affected	Normal or ↓	Cerebellar stroke, brain tumor

(continued)

TABLE 13-1. Disorders of the Central and Peripheral Nervous Systems *(Continued)*

Peripheral Nervous System Disorders

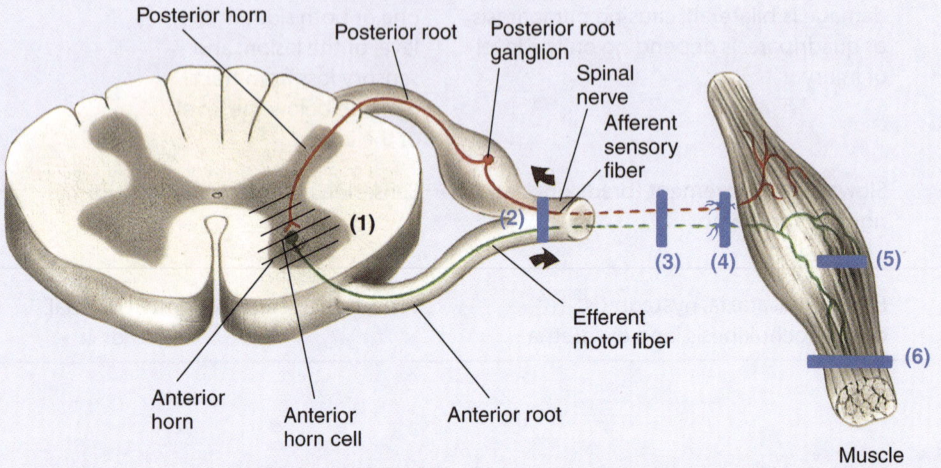

Location of Lesion	Typical Findings: Motor	Typical Findings: Sensory	Typical Findings: Deep Tendon Reflexes	Examples of Cause
Anterior Horn Cell (1)	Weakness and atrophy in a segmental or focal pattern; fasciculations	Sensation intact	↓	Polio, amyotrophic lateral sclerosis
Spinal Roots and Nerves (2)	Weakness and atrophy in a root-innervated pattern; sometimes with fasciculations	Corresponding dermatomal sensory deficits	↓	Herniated cervical or lumbar disc
Peripheral Nerve—Mononeuropathy (3)	Weakness and atrophy in a peripheral nerve distribution; sometimes with fasciculations	Sensory loss in the pattern of that nerve	↓	Trauma, compression (e.g., carpal tunnel syndrome)
Peripheral Nerve—Polyneuropathy (4)	Weakness and atrophy more distal than proximal; sometimes with fasciculations	Sensory deficits, commonly in stocking-glove distribution	↓	Peripheral polyneuropathy of alcoholism, diabetes
Neuromuscular Junction (5)	Fatigability more than weakness	Sensation intact	Normal	Myasthenia gravis
Muscle (6)	Weakness usually more proximal than distal; no fasciculations	Sensation intact	Normal or ↓	Muscular dystrophy

TABLE 13-2. Disorders of Speech

Disorders of speech fall into three groups affecting: (1) phonation of the voice, (2) the articulation of words, and (3) the production and comprehension of language.

- *Aphonia* refers to a loss of voice that accompanies disease affecting the larynx or its nerve supply. *Dysphonia* refers to less severe impairment in the volume, quality, or pitch of the voice. For example, a person may be hoarse or only able to speak in a whisper. Causes include laryngitis, laryngeal tumors, and unilateral vocal cord paralysis (CN X).
- *Dysarthria* refers to a defect in the muscular control of the speech apparatus (lips, tongue, palate, or pharynx). Words may be nasal, slurred, or indistinct, but the central symbolic aspect of language remains intact. Causes include motor lesions of the CNS or PNS, parkinsonism, and cerebellar disease.
- *Aphasia* refers to a disorder in producing or understanding language. It is often caused by lesions in the dominant cerebral hemisphere, usually the left.

Compared below are two common types of aphasia: (1) *Wernicke*, a fluent (receptive) aphasia, and (2) *Broca*, a nonfluent (or expressive) aphasia. There are other less common kinds of aphasia, which are distinguished by differing responses on the specific tests listed. Neurologic consultation is usually indicated.

	Wernicke Aphasia	Broca Aphasia
Qualities of Spontaneous Speech	Fluent; often rapid, voluble, and effortless. Inflection and articulation are good, but sentences lack meaning, and words are malformed (*paraphasias*) or invented (*neologisms*). The meaning of speech may be totally incomprehensible	Nonfluent; slow and broken, with few words and laborious effort. Inflection and articulation are impaired, but words are meaningful, with nouns, transitive verbs, and important adjectives. Small grammatical words are often dropped
Word Comprehension	Impaired	Fair to good
Repetition	Impaired	Impaired
Naming	Impaired	Impaired, though the patient recognizes objects
Reading Comprehension	Impaired	Fair to good
Writing	Impaired	Impaired
Location of Lesion	Posterior superior temporal lobe	Posterior inferior frontal lobe

Although it is important to recognize aphasia early in your encounter with a patient, integrate this information with your neurologic examination as you generate your differential diagnosis.

TABLE 13-3. Abnormalities of Gait and Posture

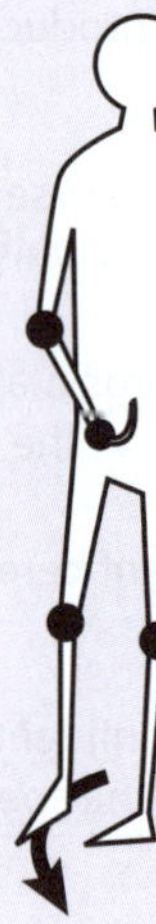

Spastic Hemiparesis

Spastic Hemiparesis

Seen in corticospinal tract lesions that cause poor control of flexor muscles during swing phase (for example, from stroke).

- Affected arm is flexed, immobile, and held close to the side, with elbow, wrists, and interphalangeal joints flexed.
- Affected leg extensors are spastic; ankles are plantar-flexed and inverted.
- Patients may drag toe, circle leg stiffly outward and forward (*circumduction*), or lean trunk to contralateral side to clear affected leg during walking.

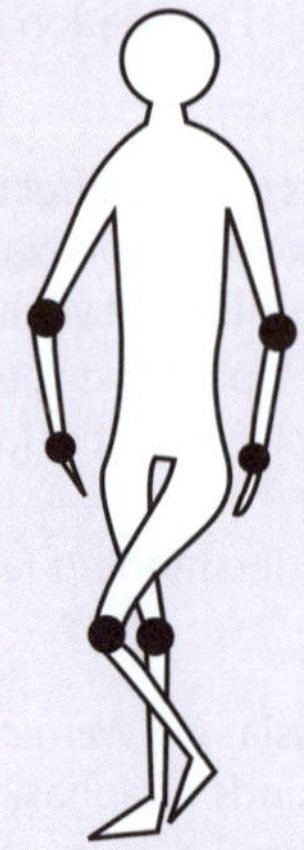

Scissors Gait

Seen in spinal cord disease, causing bilateral lower extremity spasticity, including adductor spasm.

- Gait is stiff. Patients advance each leg slowly, and the thighs tend to cross forward on each other at each step.
- Steps are short.
- Patients appear to be walking through water, and there may be compensating sway of the trunk away from the side of the advancing leg.
- Scissoring is seen in all spasticity disorders, most commonly cerebral palsy.

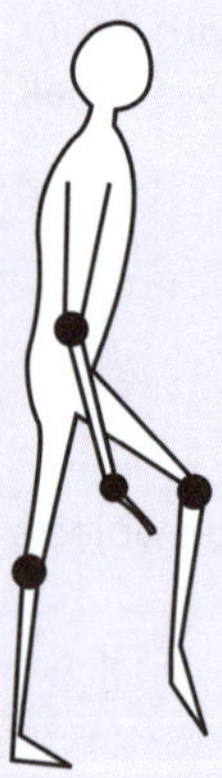

Steppage Gait

Steppage Gait

Seen in foot drop, usually secondary to peripheral nervous system disease.

- Patients either drag the feet or lift them high, with knees flexed, and bring them down with a slap onto the floor, appearing to be walking up stairs.
- Patients cannot walk on their heels.
- Gait may involve one or both legs.
- Tibialis anterior and toe extensors are weak.

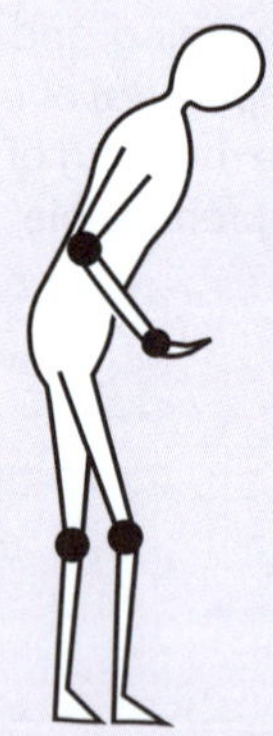

Parkinsonian Gait

Parkinsonian Gait

Seen in the basal ganglia defects of Parkinson disease.

- Posture is stooped, with flexion of head, arms, hips, and knees.
- Patients are slow getting started.
- Steps are short and shuffling, with involuntary hastening (*festination*).
- Arm swings are decreased, and patients turn around stiffly—"all in one piece."
- Postural control is poor (*anteropulsion* or *retropulsion*).

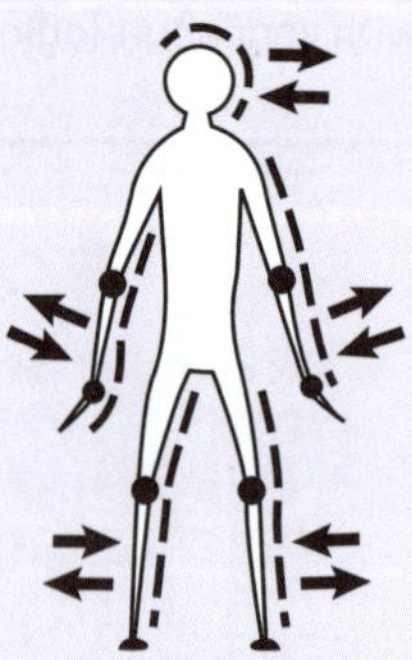

Cerebellar Ataxia

Seen in disease of the cerebellum or associated tracts.

- Gait is staggering and unsteady, with feet wide apart and exaggerated difficulty on turns.
- Patients cannot stand steadily with feet together, whether eyes are open or closed.
- Other cerebellar signs are present such as dysmetria, nystagmus, and intention tremor.

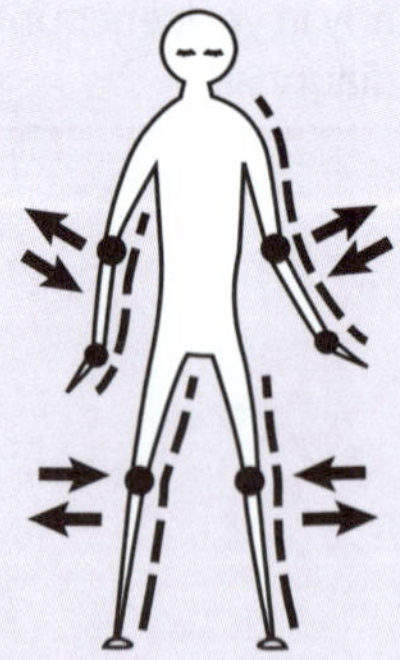

Sensory Ataxia

Sensory Ataxia

Seen in loss of position sense in the legs from polyneuropathy or posterior column damage.

- Gait is unsteady and wide based (with feet wide apart).
- Patients throw their feet forward and outward and bring them down, first on the heels and then on the toes, with a double tapping sound.
- Patients watch the ground for guidance when walking.
- With eyes closed, patients cannot stand steadily with feet together (positive Romberg sign), and the staggering gait worsens.

TABLE 13-4. Primary Headaches

Headaches are classified as *primary,* without underlying pathology, or *secondary*, with a serious underlying cause often warranting urgent attention. Secondary headaches are more likely to occur after age 50 with a sudden severe onset and should be ruled out before making the diagnosis of a primary headache. About 90% of headaches are primary headaches and fall into four categories: tension, migraine, cluster, and chronic daily headache. The features of tension, migraine, and cluster headaches are highlighted below. *Chronic daily headache* is not a diagnosis, but a category containing pre-existing headaches which have been transformed into more pronounced forms of migraines, chronic tension-type headaches, and medication-overuse headaches and last more than 15 days a month for more than 3 months. Risk factors include obesity, >1 headache a week, caffeine ingestion, overuse of headache medications >10 days a month such as analgesics, ergots, and triptans, and sleep and mood disorders.

	Tension	Migraines	Cluster
Process	Process unclear—possibly heightened CNS pain sensitivity. Involves pericranial muscle tenderness; etiology also unclear	Neuronal dysfunction, possibly of brainstem origin, involving low serotonin level, spreading cortical depression and trigeminovascular activation; types: with aura; without aura; variants	Process unclear—possibly hypothalamic then trigemino-autonomic activation
Lifetime Prevalence	Most common headache (40%); prevalence about 50%	10% of headaches; prevalence 18% of U.S. adults; affects ~15% of women, 6% of men	<1%, more common in men
Location	Usually bilateral; may be generalized or localized to the back of the head and upper neck or to the frontotemporal area	Unilateral in ~70%; bifrontal or global in ~30%	Unilateral, usually behind or around the eye or temple
Quality and Severity	Steady; pressing or tightening; nonthrobbing pain; mild to moderate intensity	Throbbing or aching, pain, moderate to severe in intensity; preceded by aura in up to 30%	Sharp, continuous, intense; severe in intensity
Timing			
Onset	Gradual	Fairly rapid, reaching a peak in 1–2 hrs	Abrupt; peaks within minutes
Duration	30 min to 7 days	4–72 hrs	15 min to 3 hrs
Course	Episodic; may be chronic	Recurrent—usually monthly, but weekly in ~10%; peak incidence early to mid-adolescence	Episodic, clustered in time, with several each day for 4–8 wks and then relief for 6–12 mo
	Tension	**Migraines**	**Cluster**
Associated Symptoms	Sometimes photophobia, phonophobia; scalp tenderness; nausea absent	Prodrome: nausea, vomiting, photophobia, phonophobia; aura in 30%; either visual (flickering, zig-zagging lines), or motor (paresthesias of hand, arm, or face, or language dysfunction)	Unilateral autonomic symptoms: lacrimation, rhinorrhea, miosis, ptosis, eyelid edema, conjunctival infection
Triggers/ Factors That Aggravate or Provoke	Sustained muscle tension, as in driving or typing; stress; sleep disturbances	Alcohol, certain foods, or stress may provoke; also menses, high altitude; aggravated by noise and bright light	During attack, sensitivity to alcohol may increase
Factors That Relieve	Possibly massage, relaxation	Quiet, dark room; sleep; sometimes transient relief from pressure on the involved artery	

Sources: Headache Classification Committee of the International Headache Society (IHS). *Cephalalgia.* 2013;33(9):629–808; Lipton RB et al. *Neurology.* 2004;63:427; Sun-Edelstein C et al. *Cephalalgia.* 2009;29:445; Lipton RB et al. *Headache.* 2001;41:646; Fumal A, Schoenen J. *Lancet Neurol.* 2008;7:70; Nesbitt AD, Goadsby PJ. *BMJ.* 2012;344:e2407.

TABLE 13-5. Secondary Headaches and Cranial Neuralgias

Type	Process	Location	Quality and Severity
Secondary Headaches			
Analgesic Rebound	Withdrawal of medication	Previous headache pattern	Variable
Headaches from Eye Disorders			
■ *Errors of Refraction (farsightedness and astigmatism, but not nearsightedness)*	Probably the sustained contraction of the extraocular muscles, and possibly of the frontal, temporal, and occipital muscles	Around and over the eyes; may radiate to the occipital area	Steady, aching, dull
■ *Acute Glaucoma*	Sudden increase in intraocular pressure (see p. 578)	Pain in and around one eye	Steady, aching, often severe
Headache from Sinusitis	Mucosal inflammation of the paranasal sinuses	Usually frontal sinuses above the eyes or over the maxillary sinus	Aching or throbbing, severity variable; consider possible migraine
Meningitis	Viral or bacterial infection of the meninges surrounding the brain and spinal cord	Generalized	Steady or throbbing, very severe
Subarachnoid Hemorrhage—"Thunderclap Headache"	Bleeding from a ruptured cerebral saccular aneurysm; rarely from AV malformation, mycotic aneurysm	Generalized	Very severe, "the worst of my life"
Brain Tumor	Mass lesion causing displacement of or traction on pain-sensitive arteries and veins or pressure on nerves	Variable, including lobes of brain, cerebellum, brainstem	Aching, steady, dull pain worse on awakening the better after several hours

Timing			Associated Symptoms	Factors That Aggravate or Provoke	Factors That Relieve
Onset	Duration	Course			
Variable	Depends on prior headache pattern	Depends on frequency of "mini-withdrawals"	Depends on prior headache pattern	Fever, carbon monoxide, hypoxia, withdrawal of caffeine, other headache triggers	Depends on cause
Gradual	Variable	Variable	Eye fatigue, "sandy" sensations in eyes, redness of conjunctiva	Prolonged use of the eyes, particularly for close work	Rest of the eyes
Often rapid	Variable, may depend on treatment	Variable, may depend on treatment	Blurred vision, nausea and vomiting; halos around lights, reddening of eye	Sometimes provoked by mydriatic drops	
Variable	Often daily several hours at a time, persisting until treatment	Often daily in a repetitive pattern	Local tenderness, nasal congestion, discharge, and fever	May be aggravated by coughing, sneezing, or jarring the head	Nasal decongestants, antibiotics
Fairly rapid, usually <24 hrs; may be sudden onset	Variable, usually days	Viral: usually <1 wk; bacterial: persistent until treatment	Fever, stiff neck, photophobia, change in mental status	—	Immediate antibiotics until diagnosis of bacterial or viral
Sudden onset; can be less than a minute	Variable, usually days	Varies according to presenting severity and level of consciousness; worst if initial coma	Nausea, vomiting, loss of consciousness, neck pain. Possible prior neck symptoms from "sentinel leaks"	Rebleeding, ↑ intracranial pressure, cerebral edema	Subspecialty treatments
Variable	Often brief; depends on location and rate of growth	Intermittent but may progress in intensity over a period of days	Seizures, hemiparesis, field cuts, personality changes. Also nausea, vomiting, vision change, gait change	May be aggravated by coughing, sneezing, or sudden movements of the head	Subspecialty treatments

(continued)

TABLE 13-5. Secondary Headaches and Cranial Neuralgias *(Continued)*

Type	Process	Location	Quality and Severity
Giant Cell (Temporal) Arteritis	Transmural lymphocytic vasculitis often involving multinucleated giant cells that disrupts the internal elastic lamina of large-caliber arteries	Localized near the involved artery, most often the temporal artery in those > age 50, women > men (2:1 ratio)	Throbbing, generalized, persistent; often severe
Postconcussion Headache	Follows mild acceleration–deceleration traumatic brain injury. May involve axonal, cerebrovascular autoregulatory, neurochemical injury	Often but not always localized to the injured area	Dull, aching, constant; may have features of tension and migraine headaches
Cranial Neuralgias			
Trigeminal Neuralgia (CN V)	Vascular compression of CN V, usually near entry to pons leading to focal demyelination, aberrant discharge. 10% with causative intracranial lesion	Cheek, jaws, lips, or gums; trigeminal nerve divisions 2 and 3 > 1	Shocklike, stabbing, burning; severe

Note: Blanks appear in this table when the categories are not applicable or not usually helpful in assessing the problem.

Sources: Headache Classification Committee of the International Headache Society (IHS). *Cephalalgia*. 2013;33(9):629–808; Schwedt TJ et al. *Lancet Neurol.* 2006;5:621; Van de Beek D et al. *N Engl J Med.* 2004;351:1849; Salvarini C et al. *Lancet*. 2008;372:234; Smetana GW, Shmerling RH. *JAMA*. 2002;287:92; Ropper AH, Gorson KC. *N Engl J Med.* 2007;356:166; American College of Physicians. Neurology—MKSAP 16. Philadelphia.

Timing			Associated Symptoms	Factors That Aggravate or Provoke	Factors That Relieve
Onset	**Duration**	**Course**			
Gradual or rapid	Variable	Recurrent or persistent over weeks to months	Tenderness over temporal artery, adjacent scalp; fever (in ~50%), fatigue, weight loss; new headache (~60%), jaw claudication (~50%), visual loss or blindness (~15%–20%), polymyalgia rheumatica (~50%)	Movement of neck and shoulders	Often steroids
Within 7 days of the injury up to 3 mo	Weeks to up to a year	Tends to diminish over time	Drowsiness, poor concentration, confusion, memory loss, blurred vision, dizziness, irritability, restlessness, fatigue	Mental and physical exertion, straining, stooping, emotional excitement, alcohol	Rest; medication
Abrupt, paroxysmal	Each jab lasts seconds but recurs at intervals of seconds or minutes	May recur daily for weeks to months then resolve; can be chronic progressive.	Exhaustion from recurrent pain	Touching certain areas of the lower face or mouth; chewing, talking, brushing teeth	Medication; neurovascular decompression

TABLE 13-6. Types of Stroke

Assessment of stroke requires careful history taking and a detailed physical examination, and should focus on three fundamental questions: What brain area and related vascular territory explain the patient's findings? Is the stroke ischemic or hemorrhagic? If ischemic, is the mechanism thrombosis or embolus? Stroke is a medical emergency, and timing is of the essence. Answers to these questions are critical to patient outcomes and use of antithrombotic therapies.

In *acute ischemic stroke,* ischemic brain injury begins with a central core of very low perfusion and often irreversible cell death. This core is surrounded by an *ischemic penumbra* of metabolically disturbed cells that are still potentially viable, depending on the restoration of blood flow and duration of ischemia. Because most irreversible damage occurs in the first 3–6 hrs after onset of symptoms, achieving reperfusion as early as possible provides the best outcomes, with recovery in up to 50% of patients treated within 3 hrs in some studies.

Clinical Features and Vascular Territories of Stroke

Clinical Finding	Vascular Territory	Additional Comments
Contralateral leg weakness	*Anterior circulation*—anterior cerebral artery (ACA)	The internal carotid arteries supply the anterior circulation, providing blood flow to the anterior and middle cerebral arteries
Contralateral face, arm > leg weakness, sensory loss, visual field loss, apraxia, aphasia (left MCA), or neglect (right MCA)	*Anterior circulation*—middle cerebral artery (MCA)	Largest vascular bed for stroke, so most common territory affected
Contralateral motor or sensory deficit without cortical signs (such as aphasia or neglect)	*Subcortical circulation*[a]—lenticulostriate deep-penetrating branches of MCA	Small vessel subcortical *lacunar infarcts* in internal capsule, thalamus, or brainstem. Five classical syndromes are seen: pure motor stroke (hemiplegia/hemiparesis), pure sensory stroke (hemianesthesia), ataxic hemiparesis, clumsy-hand/dysarthria syndrome, and mixed sensorimotor stroke
Contralateral visual field loss	*Posterior circulation*—posterior cerebral artery (PCA)	The paired vertebral arteries join to form the basilar artery, which supplies the posterior circulation. Bilateral PCA infarction causes cortical blindness but preserved pupillary light reaction.
Dysphagia, dysarthria, tongue/palate deviation, and/or ataxia with crossed sensory/motor deficits (= ipsilateral face with contralateral body)	*Posterior circulation*—Vertebral or basilar artery branches supplying the brainstem	
Oculomotor deficits and/or ataxia with crossed sensory/motor deficits	*Posterior circulation*—basilar artery	Complete basilar artery occlusion—"locked-in syndrome" with intact consciousness but with inability to speak and quadriplegia

[a]Learn to differentiate cortical from subcortical involvement. *Subcortical or lacunar syndromes* do not affect higher cognitive function, language, or visual fields.

Source: Reproduced with permission from Medical Knowledge Self-Assessment Program, 14th edition (MKSAP 14), Neurology. Philadelphia, PA: American College of Physicians; 2006:52–68. Copyright 2006, American College of Physicians.

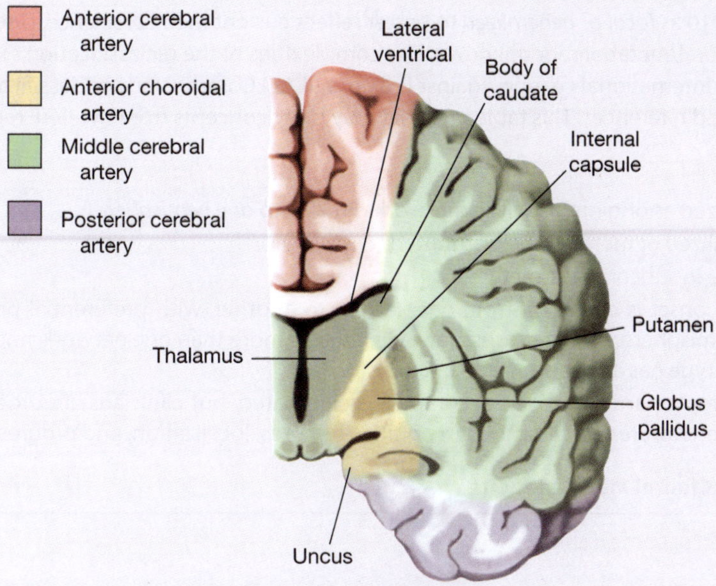
Anterior cerebral artery
Anterior choroidal artery
Middle cerebral artery
Posterior cerebral artery
Lateral ventrical
Body of caudate
Internal capsule
Putamen
Thalamus
Globus pallidus
Uncus

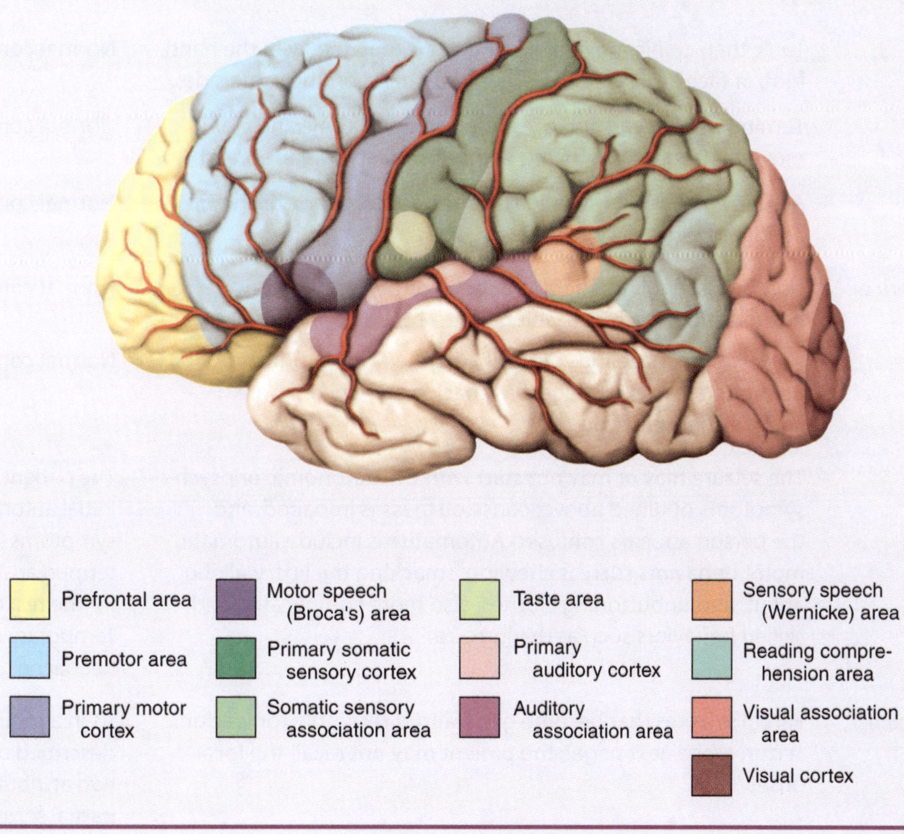
Prefrontal area
Premotor area
Primary motor cortex
Motor speech (Broca's) area
Primary somatic sensory cortex
Somatic sensory association area
Taste area
Primary auditory cortex
Auditory association area
Sensory speech (Wernicke) area
Reading compre-hension area
Visual association area
Visual cortex

TABLE 13-7. Seizure Disorders

Seizures were reclassified in 2010 as *focal* or *generalized* to better reflect current medical science. Underlying causes should be identified as genetic, structural/metabolic, or unknown. The complexities of the reclassification scheme are best explored by turning to the report of the International League Against Epilepsy (ILAE) Commission on Classification and Terminology, 2005–2009 and to more detailed references. This table presents only basic concepts from the ILAE report.

Focal Seizures

Focal seizures "are conceptualized as originating within networks limited to *one hemisphere*."

- They may be discretely localized or more widely distributed.
- Focal seizures may originate in subcortical structures.
- For each seizure type, ictal onset is *consistent* from one seizure to another, with preferential propagation patterns that can involve the contralateral hemisphere. In some cases, however, there is more than one network, and more than one seizure type, but each individual seizure type has a consistent site of onset."
- The distinction between simple partial and partial complex is eliminated, but clinicians are urged to recognize and describe "impairment of consciousness/awareness or other dyscognitive features, localization, and progression of ictal events."

Type	Clinical Manifestations	Postictal State
Focal Seizures without Impairment of Consciousness		
With observable motor and autonomic symptoms		
■ Jacksonian	Tonic then clonic movements that start unilaterally in the hand, foot, or face and spread to other body parts on the same side	Normal consciousness
■ Other motor	Turning of the head and eyes to one side, or tonic and clonic movements of an arm or leg without the Jacksonian spread	Normal consciousness
■ With autonomic symptoms	A "funny feeling" in the epigastrium, nausea, pallor, flushing, lightheadedness	Normal consciousness
With subjective sensory or psychic phenomena	Numbness, tingling; simple visual, auditory, or olfactory hallucinations such as flashing lights, buzzing, or odors	Normal consciousness
	Anxiety or fear; feelings of familiarity (déjà vu) or unreality; dreamy states; fear or rage; flashback experiences; more complex hallucinations	Normal consciousness
Focal Seizures with Impairment of Consciousness	The seizure may or may not start with the autonomic or psychic symptoms outlined above; consciousness is impaired, and the person appears confused Automatisms include automatic motor behaviors such as chewing, smacking the lips, walking about, and unbuttoning clothes; also more complicated and skilled behaviors such as driving a car	The patient may remember initial autonomic or psychic symptoms (which are then termed an *aura*), but is amnesic for the rest of the seizure. Temporary confusion and headache may occur
Focal Seizures That Become Generalized	Partial seizures that become generalized resemble tonic–clonic seizures (see next page); the patient may not recall the focal onset	As in a tonic–clonic seizure, described on the next page; two attributes indicate a partial seizure that has become generalized: (1) the recollection of an *aura,* and (2) a *unilateral* neurologic deficit during the postictal period

(*continued*)

TABLE 13-7. Seizure Disorders *(Continued)*

Generalized Seizures and Nonepileptic Seizures

Generalized seizures "are conceptualized as originating at some point within, and rapidly engaging, bilaterally distributed networks … that include cortical and subcortical structures, but do not necessarily include the entire cortex …"

- The location and lateralization are *not consistent* from one seizure to another.
- Generalized seizures can be asymmetric.
- They may begin with body movements, impaired consciousness, or both.
- If onset of tonic–clonic seizures begins after age 30 yrs, suspect either a partial seizure that has become generalized or a generalized seizure caused by a toxic or metabolic disorder.

Toxic and metabolic causes include withdrawal from alcohol or other sedative drugs, uremia, hypoglycemia, hyperglycemia, hyponatremia, drug toxicity, and bacterial meningitis.

Problem	Clinical Manifestations	Postictal (*Postseizure*) State
Generalized Seizures		
Tonic–Clonic (Grand Mal)[a]	The patient loses consciousness suddenly, sometimes with a cry, and the body stiffens into tonic extensor rigidity. Breathing stops, and the patient becomes cyanotic. A clonic phase of rhythmic muscular contraction follows. Breathing resumes and is often noisy, with excessive salivation. Injury, tongue biting, and urinary incontinence may occur.	Confusion, drowsiness, fatigue, headache, muscular aching, and sometimes the temporary persistence of bilateral neurologic deficits such as hyperactive reflexes and Babinski responses. The patient is amnestic about the seizure and aura.
Absence	A sudden brief lapse of consciousness, with momentary blinking, staring, or movements of the lips and hands but no falling. Two subtypes are: *typical absence*—lasts <10 sec and stops abruptly; *atypical absence*—may last >10 sec	No aura recalled. In typical absence, a prompt return to normal; in atypical absence, some postictal confusion
Myoclonic	Sudden, brief, rapid jerks, involving the trunk or limbs. Myoclonus has many potential causes, however, and is not always caused by seizure	Variable
Myoclonic Atonic (Drop Attack)	Sudden loss of consciousness with falling but no movements. Injury may occur	Either a prompt return to normal or a brief period of confusion
Nonepileptic Seizures (previously called pseudoseizures)		
May mimic seizures but are due to a conversion disorder (termed "Functional Neurologic Symptom Disorder" in *DSM-5*)	The movements may be complex and often do not follow a neuroanatomic pattern. Can sometimes be difficult to distinguish from epileptic seizure without EEG. It is not uncommon for a patient to have both epileptic and nonepileptic seizures.	Variable

[a] *Febrile convulsions* that resemble brief tonic–clonic seizures occur in infants and young children. They are usually benign but may also be the first manifestation of a seizure disorder.

Source: Adapted from Berg AT et al. *Epilepsia*. 2010;51(4):676–685.

TABLE 13-8. Tremors and Involuntary Movements

Tremors

Tremors are rhythmic oscillatory movements, which may be roughly subdivided into three groups: resting (or static) tremors, postural tremors, and intention tremors.

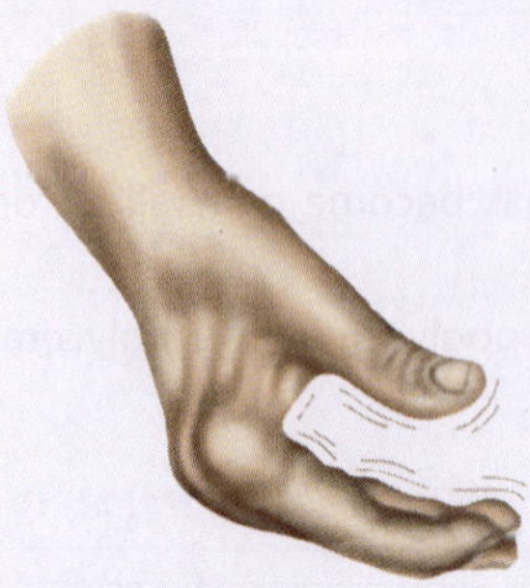

Resting (Static) Tremors

These tremors are most prominent at rest and may decrease or disappear with voluntary movement. Illustrated is the common relatively slow, fine pill-rolling tremor of parkinsonism, about 5/sec.

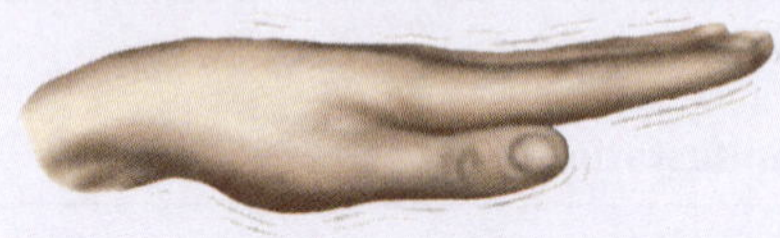

Postural Tremors

These tremors appear when the affected part is actively maintaining a posture. Examples include the fine rapid tremor of hyperthyroidism, the tremors of anxiety and fatigue, and benign essential (and often familial) tremor.

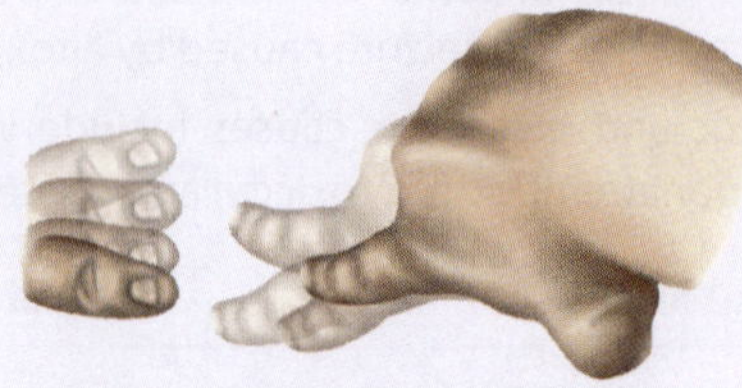

Intention Tremors

Intention tremors, absent at rest, appear with movement and get worse as the limb approaches the target. Seen in disorders affecting the cerebellum or its related tracts, such as multiple sclerosis or stroke.

Involuntary Movements

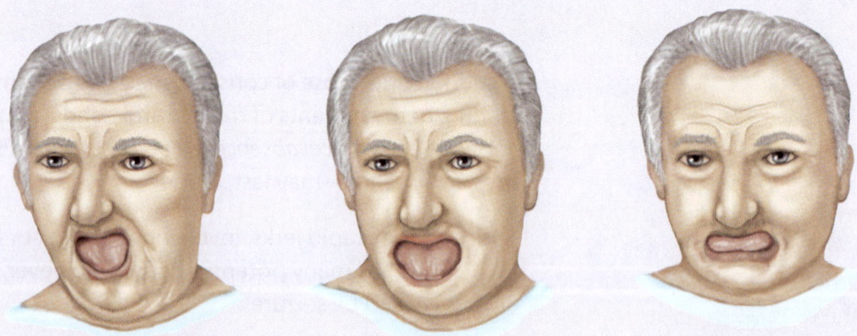

Oral–Facial Dyskinesias

Oral–facial dyskinesias are arrhythmic, repetitive, bizarre movements that chiefly involve the face, mouth, jaw, and tongue: grimacing, pursing of the lips, protrusions of the tongue, opening and closing of the mouth, and deviations of the jaw. The limbs and trunk are involved less often. These movements may be a late complication of antipsychotic or antiemetic drugs such as phenothiazines, termed *tardive* (late) dyskinesias. They also occur in long-standing psychoses, in some older adults, and in some edentulous persons.

(*continued*)

TABLE 13-8. Tremors and Involuntary Movements *(Continued)*

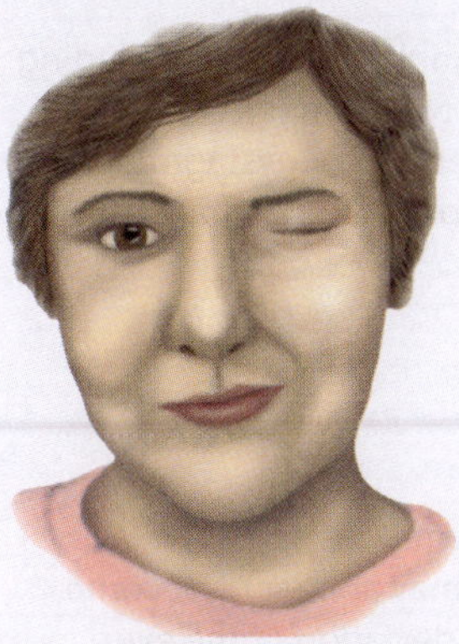

Tics

Tics are brief, repetitive, stereotyped, coordinated movements occurring at irregular intervals. Examples include repetitive winking, grimacing, and shoulder shrugging. Causes include Tourette syndrome and late effects of drugs such as phenothiazines.

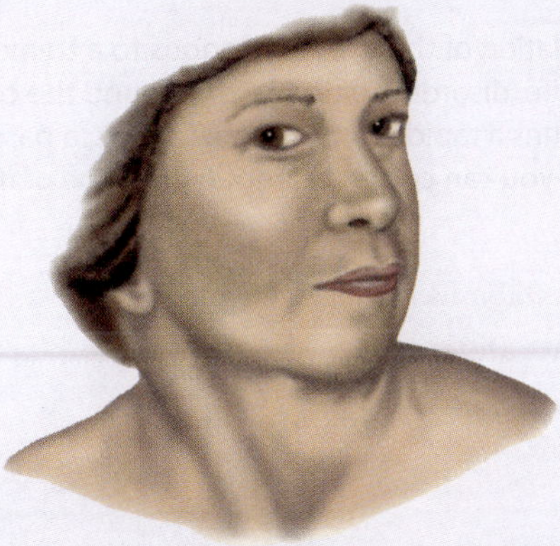

Dystonia

Dystonia causes irregular movements resembling athetosis or tremor. These are often accompanied by abnormal postures that limit voluntary movement and can at times be painful. Examples include writer's cramp, blephorospasm, and as illustrated, spasmodic torticollis.

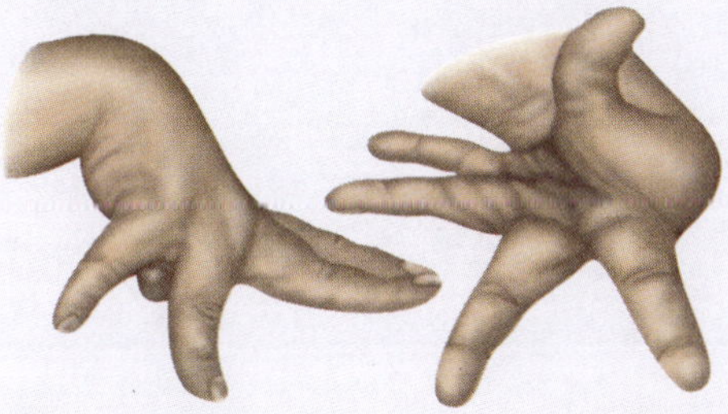

Athetosis

Athetoid movements are slower and more twisting and writhing than choreiform movements and have a larger amplitude. They most commonly involve the face and the distal extremities. Athetosis is often associated with spasticity. Causes include cerebral palsy.

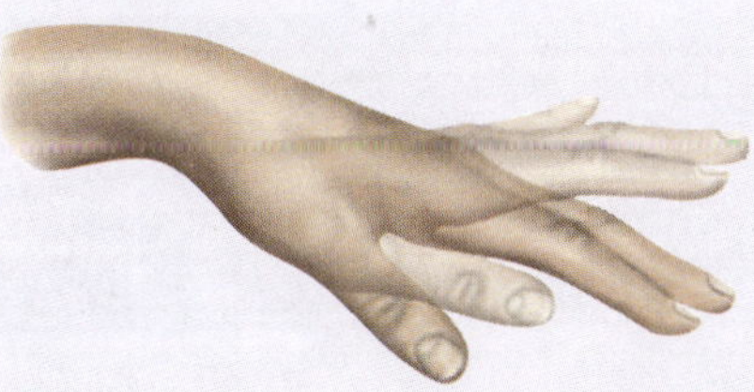

Chorea

Choreiform movements are brief, rapid, jerky, irregular, and unpredictable. They occur at rest or interrupt normal coordinated movements. Unlike tics, they seldom repeat themselves. The face, head, lower arms, and hands are often involved. Causes include Sydenham chorea (with rheumatic fever) and Huntington disease.

TABLE 13-9. Nystagmus

Nystagmus is a rhythmic oscillation of the eyes, analogous to a tremor in other parts of the body. It has multiple causes, including impairment of vision in early life, disorders of the labyrinth and the cerebellar system, and drug toxicity. Nystagmus occurs normally when a person watches a rapidly moving object (e.g., a passing train). Study the three characteristics of nystagmus described in this table so that you can correctly identify the type of nystagmus. Then refer to textbooks of neurology for differential diagnoses.

Direction of Gaze in which Nystagmus Appears

Example: Nystagmus on Right Lateral Gaze

Nystagmus Present (Right Lateral Gaze)

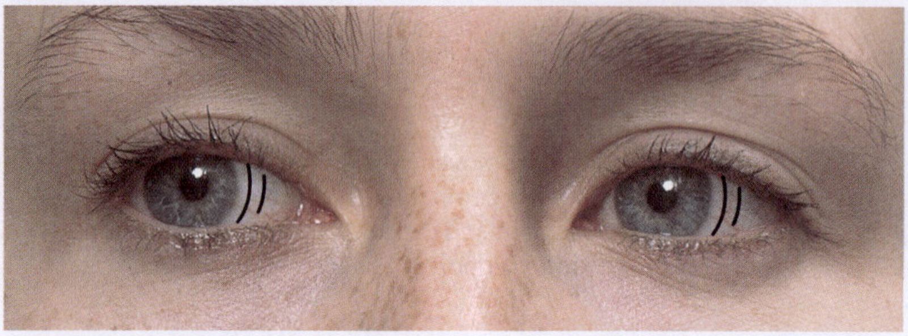

Although nystagmus may be present in all directions of gaze, it may appear or become accentuated only on deviation of the eyes (e.g., to the side or upward). On extreme lateral gaze, the normal person may show a few beats resembling nystagmus. Avoid making assessments in such extreme positions and *observe for nystagmus only within the field of full binocular vision.*

Nystagmus Not Present (Left Lateral Gaze)

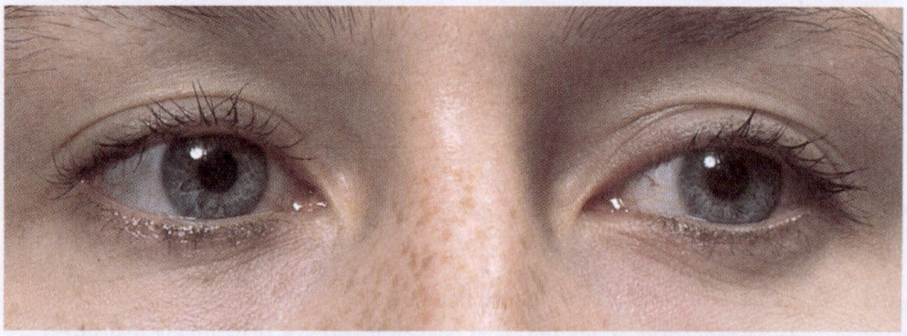

Direction of the Quick and Slow Phases

Example: Left-Beating Nystagmus—a Quick Jerk to the Left in Each Eye, then a Slow Drift to the Right

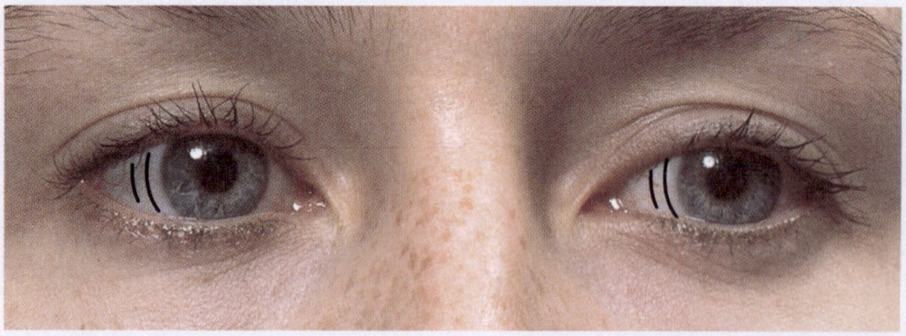

Nystagmus usually has both slow and fast movements but *is defined by its fast phase.* For example, if the eyes jerk quickly to the patient's left and drift back slowly to the right, the patient is said to have *left-beating nystagmus.* Occasionally, nystagmus consists only of coarse oscillations without quick and slow components, described as *pendular.*

(*continued*)

TABLE 13-9. Nystagmus *(Continued)*

Plane of the Movements

Horizontal Nystagmus

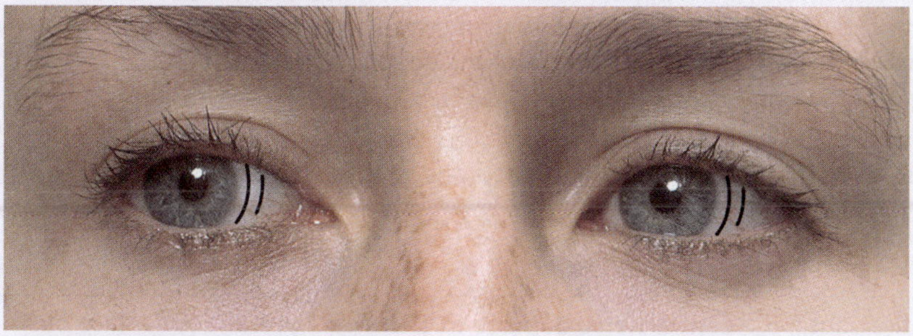

The movement of nystagmus may occur in one or more planes, namely horizontal, vertical, or rotary. It is the plane of the movements, not the direction of the gaze, that defines this variable.

Vertical Nystagmus

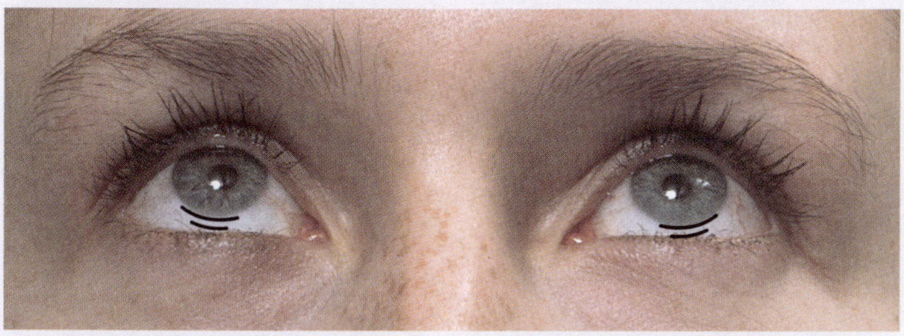

Rotary Nystagmus

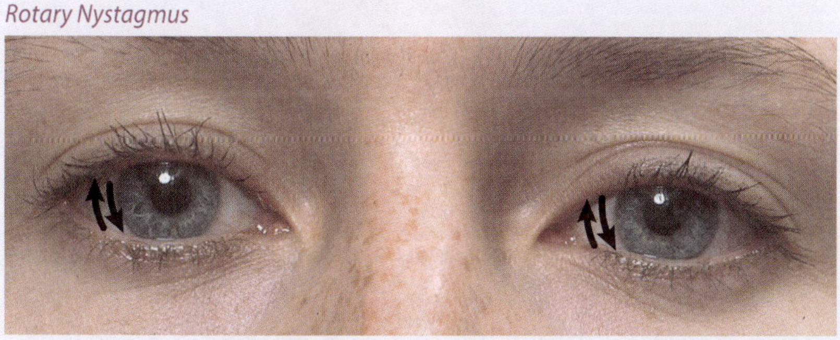

TABLE 13-10. Types of Facial Paralysis

Facial weakness or paralysis may result from either (1) a peripheral lesion of CN VII, the facial nerve, anywhere from its origin in the pons to its periphery in the face, or (2) a central lesion involving the upper motor neuron system between the cortex and the pons. A peripheral lesion of CN VII, exemplified here by a Bell palsy, is compared with a central lesion, exemplified by a left hemispheric cerebral infarction. These can be distinguished by their different effects on the upper portion of the face.

The lower portion of the face is normally controlled by upper motor neurons located on only one side of the cortex—the opposite side. *Left hemispheric damage to these pathways, as in stroke, weakens the right lower face.* The upper face, however, is controlled by pathways from both sides of the cortex. Even though the upper motor neurons on the left are destroyed, others on the right remain, and the right upper face continues to function fairly well.

CN VII—Peripheral Lesion

Peripheral nerve damage to CN VII paralyzes the entire right side of the face, including the forehead.

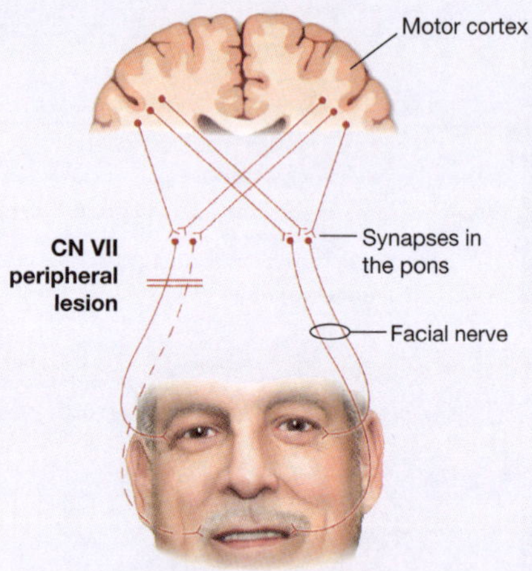

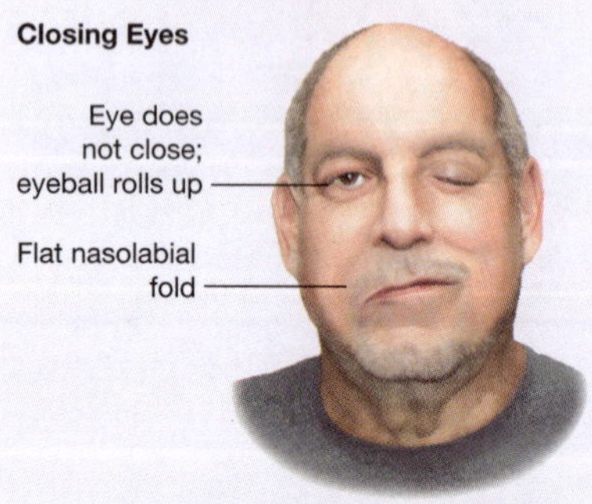

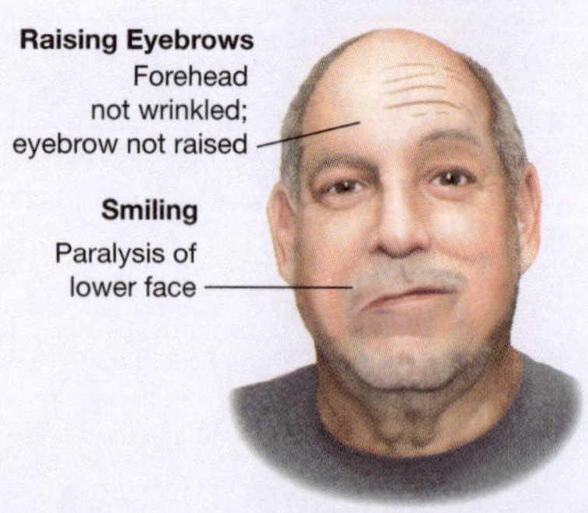

CN VII—Central Lesion

Central nerve damage to CN VII paralyzes the lower face but cortical innervation to the forehead is preserved.

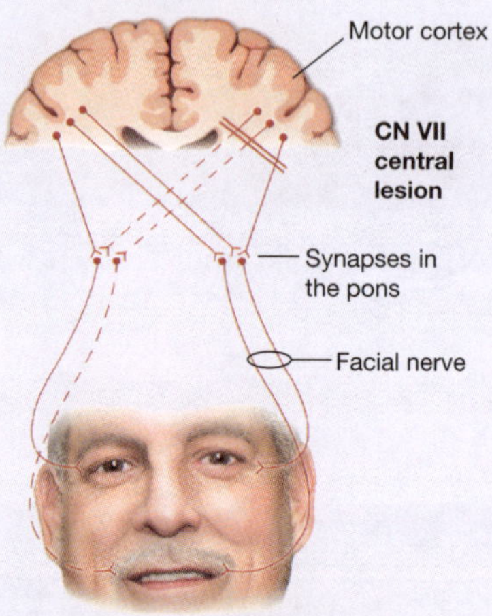

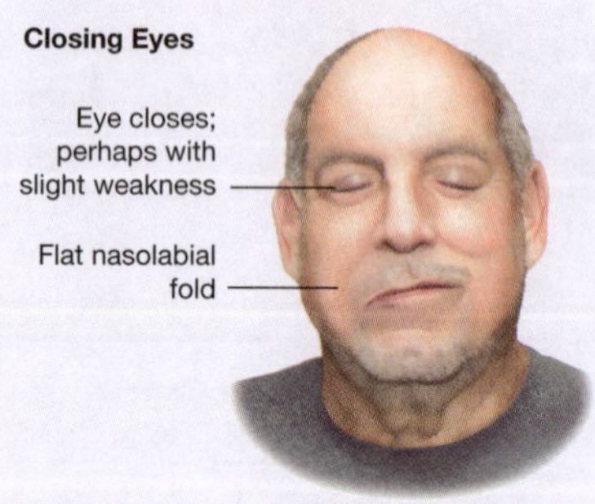

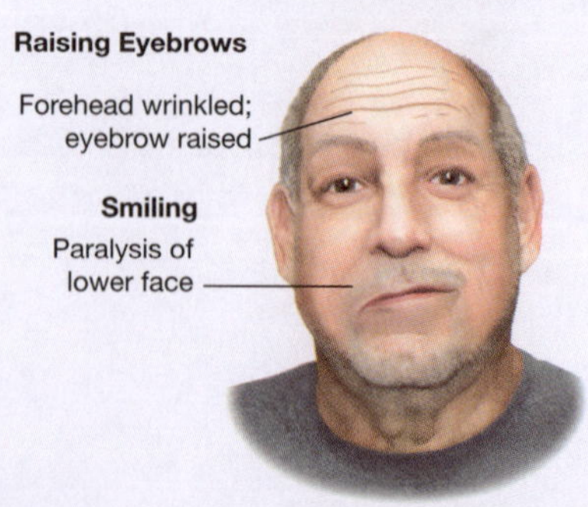

TABLE 13-11. Abnormal Body Postures

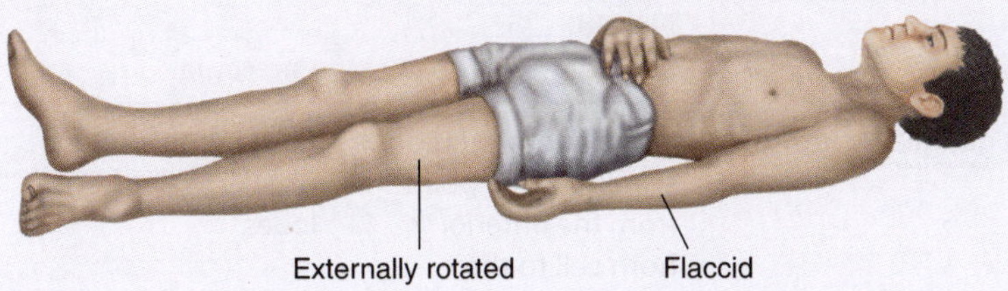

Hemiplegia (Early)

Sudden unilateral brain damage involving the corticospinal tract may produce a *hemiplegia* (one-sided paralysis), which is flaccid early in its course. Spasticity will develop later (see below). The paralyzed arm and leg are slack. They fall loosely and without tone when raised and dropped to the bed. Spontaneous movements or responses to noxious stimuli are limited to the opposite side. The leg may lie externally rotated. One side of the lower face may be paralyzed, and that cheek puffs out on expiration.

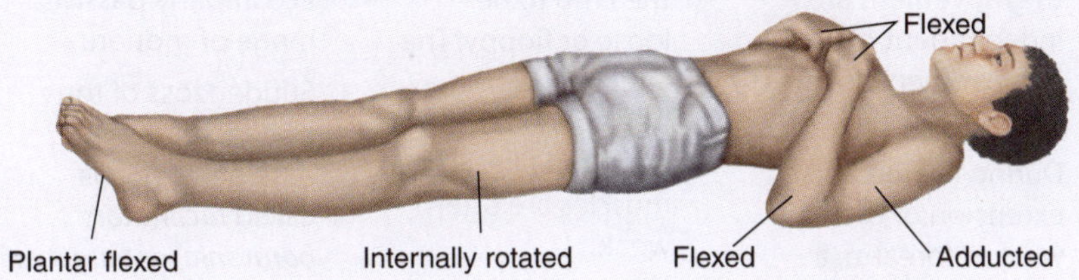

Decorticate Rigidity (Abnormal Flexor Response)

In *decorticate rigidity,* the upper arms are flexed tight to the sides with elbows, wrists, and fingers flexed. The legs are extended and internally rotated. The feet are plantar flexed. When seen bilaterally in a comatose patient, this implies a destructive lesion affecting the corticospinal tracts within or very near the cerebral hemispheres. This posture can also be seen unilaterally in a patient in the chronic recovery phase after a lesion of the corticospinal tract (chronic spastic hemiplegia), for example after stroke.

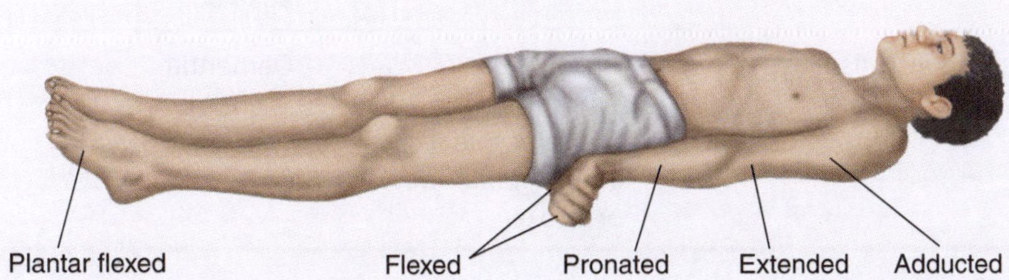

Decerebrate Rigidity (Abnormal Extensor Response)

In *decerebrate rigidity,* the jaws are clenched, and the neck is extended. The arms are adducted and stiffly extended at the elbows, with forearms pronated, wrists and fingers flexed. The legs are stiffly extended at the knees, with the feet plantar flexed. This posture may occur spontaneously or only in response to external stimuli such as light, noise, or pain. It is caused by a lesion in the diencephalon, midbrain, or pons, although may also arise from severe metabolic disorders such as hypoxia or hypoglycemia.

TABLE 13-12. Disorders of Muscle Tone

	Spasticity	Rigidity	Flaccidity (or Hypotonia)	Paratonia
Location of Lesion	Upper motor neuron or corticospinal tract systems	Basal ganglia system	Lower motor neuron system at any point from the anterior horn cell to the peripheral nerves, and in cerebellar disease	Both hemispheres, usually in the frontal lobes
Description	Increased muscle tone (*hypertonia*) is rate dependent. Tone increases when passive movement is rapid, and decreases when passive movement is slow. Tone is also greater at the extremes of the movement arc. During rapid passive movement, initial hypertonia may give way suddenly as the limb relaxes. This spastic "catch" and relaxation is known as "clasp-knife" resistance.	Increased resistance that persists throughout the movement arc, independent of rate of movement, is called *lead-pipe rigidity.* During flexion and extension of the wrist or forearm, a superimposed ratchet-like jerkiness is called *cogwheel rigidity* and can be due to underlying tremor.	Loss of muscle tone (*hypotonia*) causes the limb to be loose or floppy. The affected limbs may be hyperextensible or even flail-like. Flaccid muscles are often weak.	Sudden, irregular changes in tone accompany passive range of motion. Sudden loss of tone that increases the ease of motion is called *facilitatory paratonia, or mitgehen* (moving with). Sudden increase in tone making motion more difficult is called *oppositional paratonia, or gegenhalten* (holding against).
Common Cause	Stroke, especially late or chronic stage	Parkinsonism	Guillain–Barré syndrome; also initial phase of spinal cord injury (spinal shock) or stroke	Dementia

TABLE 13-13. Glasgow Coma Scale

Activity		Score
Eye Opening		
None	1 = Even to supraorbital pressure	
To pain	2 = Pain from sternum/limb/supraorbital pressure	
To speech	3 = Nonspecific response, not necessarily to command	
Spontaneous	4 = Eyes open, not necessarily aware	___
Motor Response		
None	1 = To any pain; limbs remain flaccid	
Extension	2 = Shoulder adducted and shoulder and forearm internally rotated	
Flexor response	3 = Withdrawal response or assumption of hemiplegic posture	
Withdrawal	4 = Arm withdraws to pain, shoulder abducts	
Localizes pain	5 = Arm attempts to remove supraorbital/chest pressure	
Obeys commands	6 = Follows simple commands	___
Verbal Response		
None	1 = No verbalization of any type	
Incomprehensible	2 = Moans/groans, no speech	
Inappropriate	3 = Intelligible, no sustained sentences	
Confused	4 = Converses but confused, disoriented	
Oriented	5 = Converses and is oriented	___
		TOTAL (3–15)*

***Interpretation:** Patients with scores of 3–8 usually are considered to be in a coma.

Source: Reprinted from Teasdale G, Jennett B. *Lancet*. 1974;304(7872):81–84. Copyright © 1974 Elsevier. With permission.

TABLE 13-14. Metabolic and Structural Coma

Although there are many causes of coma, most can be classified as either *structural* or *metabolic.* Findings vary widely in individual patients; the features listed are general guidelines rather than strict diagnostic criteria. Remember that *mental* disorders may mimic coma.

	Toxic—Metabolic	Structural
Pathophysiology	Arousal centers poisoned or critical substrates depleted	Lesion destroys or compresses brainstem arousal areas, either directly or secondary to more distant expanding mass lesions
Clinical Features		
■ Respiratory pattern	If regular, may be normal or hyperventilation	Irregular, especially Cheyne–Stokes or ataxic breathing
	If irregular, usually Cheyne–Stokes	Also with selected stereotypical patterns like "apneustic" respiration (peak inspiratory arrest) or central hyperventilation
■ Pupillary size and reaction	Equal, reactive to light. If *pinpoint* from opiates or cholinergics, you may need a magnifying glass to see the reaction	Unequal or unreactive to light (fixed) *Midposition, fixed*—suggests midbrain compression
	May be unreactive if *fixed and dilated* from anticholinergics or hypothermia	*Dilated, fixed*—suggests compression of CN III from herniation
■ Level of consciousness	Changes *after* pupils change	Changes *before* pupils change
Examples of Cause	Uremia, liver failure, hyperglycemia, hypoglycemia, alcohol, drugs, hypothyroidism, anoxia, ischemia, meningitis, encephalitis, hyperthermia, hypothermia	Epidural, subdural, or intracerebral hemorrhage; large cerebral infarction; tumor, abscess; brainstem infarct, tumor, or hemorrhage; cerebellar infarct, hemorrhage, tumor, or abscess

TABLE 13-15. Pupils in Comatose Patients

Pupillary size, equality, and light reactions are important signs in assessing the cause of coma and the region of the brain that is impaired. Keep in mind that unrelated pupillary abnormalities may precede coma, for example from use of miotic drops for glaucoma or mydriatic drops for viewing the ocular fundi (not recommended when assessing a comatose patient).

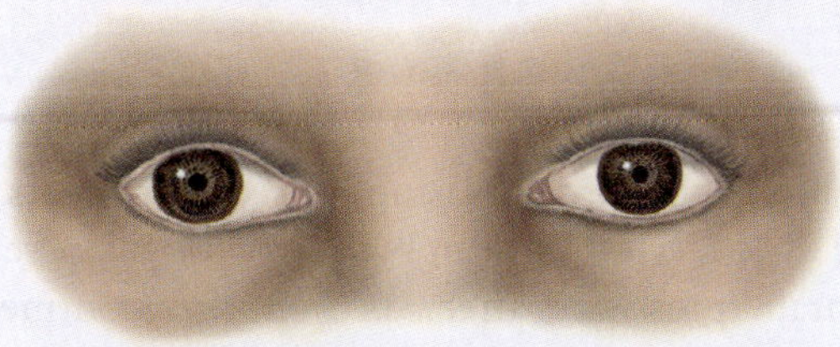

Small or Pinpoint Pupils

Bilaterally small pupils (1–2.5 mm) suggest damage to the sympathetic pathways in the hypothalamus, or metabolic encephalopathy, a diffuse failure of cerebral function that has many causes, including drugs. Light reactions are usually normal.

Pinpoint pupils (<1 mm) suggest a hemorrhage in the pons, or the effects of morphine, heroin, or other narcotics. The light reactions may be seen with a magnifying glass.

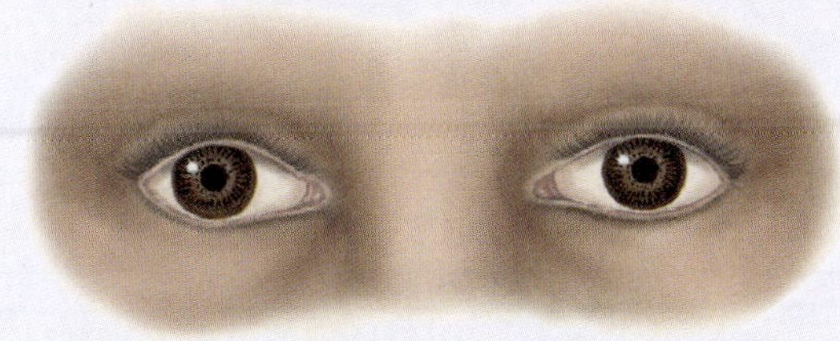

Midposition Fixed Pupils

Pupils that are in the *midposition or slightly dilated* (4–6 mm) and are *fixed to light* suggest structural damage in the midbrain.

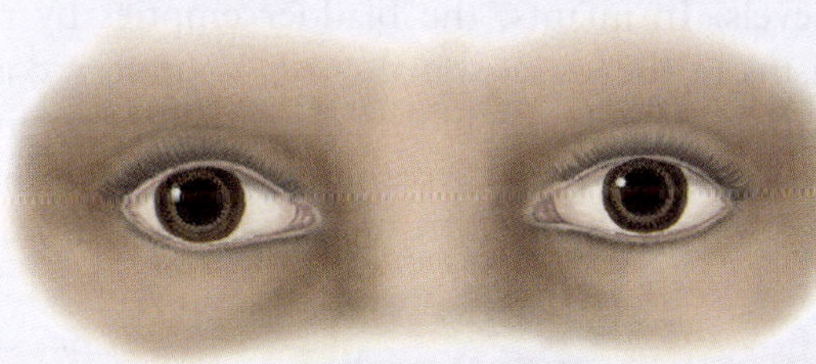

Large Pupils

Bilaterally fixed and dilated pupils may be due to severe anoxia and its sympathomimetic effects, as seen after cardiac arrest. They may also result from atropine-like agents, phenothiazines, or tricyclic antidepressants.

Bilaterally large reactive pupils may be due to cocaine, amphetamine, LSD, or other sympathetic nervous system agonists.

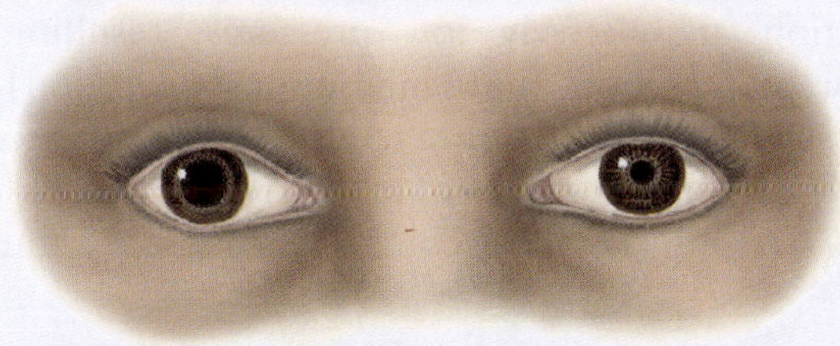

One Large Pupil

A pupil that is *fixed and dilated* warns of herniation of the temporal lobe, causing compression of the oculomotor nerve (CN III) and midbrain. A single large pupil can be seen in diabetic patients from infarction of CN III.

CHAPTER 14

Genitourinary System

ANATOMY AND PHYSIOLOGY

The genitourinary system starts at the kidneys which lie in the retroperitoneal cavity of the body at the level of T12–L3.

Urinary Bladder

The *urinary bladder* is a hollow reservoir with strong smooth muscle walls composed chiefly of *detrusor muscle*. It accommodates roughly 400 to 500 mL of urine filtered by the kidneys into the renal pelvis and the ureters.

Bladder expansion stimulates parasympathetic innervation at relatively low pressures, resulting in detrusor contraction and inhibition (relaxation) of the *internal urethral sphincter*, also under autonomic control. Voiding further requires relaxation of the *external urethral sphincter*, composed of striated muscle under voluntary control. Rising pressure triggers the conscious urge to void but can be overcome by increased intraurethral pressure that prevents incontinence. Intraurethral pressure is related to smooth muscle tone in the internal urethral sphincter; the thickness of the urethral mucosa; and, in women, sufficient support to the bladder and proximal urethra from pelvic muscles and ligaments to maintain proper anatomical relationships. Striated muscle around the urethra can also contract voluntarily to interrupt voiding (Fig. 14-1).

A distended bladder may be palpable above the symphysis pubis.

Neuroregulatory control of the bladder functions at several levels. In infants, the bladder empties by reflex mechanisms in the sacral spinal cord. Voluntary control of the bladder depends on higher centers in the brain and motor and sensory pathways connecting the brain and the reflex arcs of the sacral spinal cord. When voiding

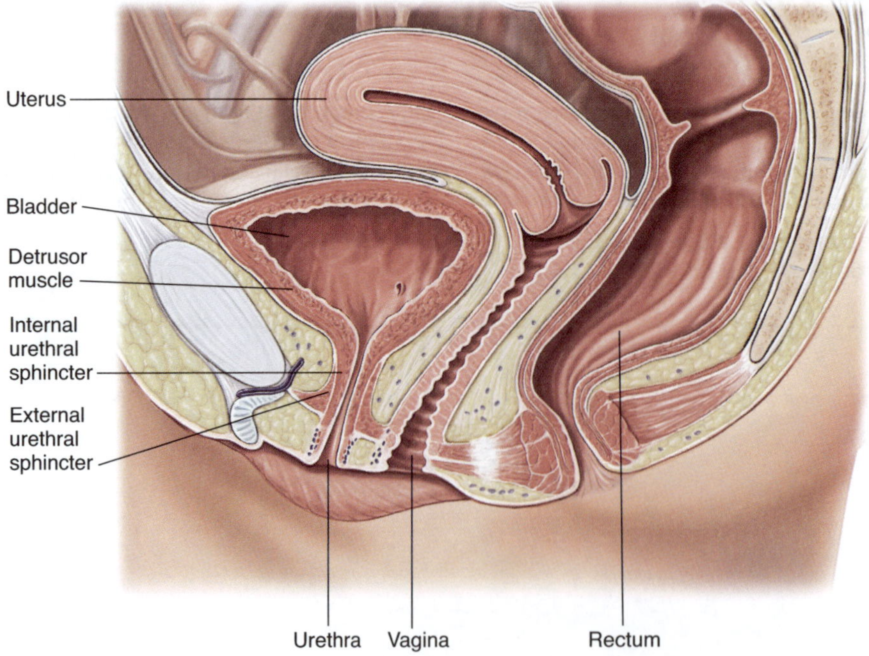

FIGURE 14-1. Female pelvic anatomy, sagittal section.

is inconvenient, higher centers in the brain can inhibit detrusor contractions until the capacity of the bladder, approximately 400 to 500 mL, is exceeded. The integrity of the sacral nerves that innervate the bladder can be tested by assessing perirectal and perineal sensation in the S2, S3, and S4 dermatomes (see p. 328).

Prostate

In the male, the prostate gland surrounds the urethra and lies next to the bladder outlet. The prostate gland is small during childhood, but, between puberty and approximately age 20 years, it increases roughly fivefold in size (to about the size of a chestnut). Prostate volume further expands as the gland becomes hyperplastic with age (see p. 384). The **base of the prostate gland** is the broad top and is directed upward near the inferior surface of the bladder. The greater part of this surface is directly continuous with the bladder wall (normally palpable during examination). The **apex of the prostate** is the pointed bottom of the gland and is in contact with the superior fascia of the urogenital diaphragm.

The prostate is divided into several lobes. The right and left *lateral lobes*, the main mass of the prostate, lie against the anterior rectal wall, where they are palpable as a rounded, heart shaped structure approximately 2.5 cm long. They are separated by a shallow *median sulcus* or groove, also palpable. The posteromedial part of the lateral lobes that can be palpated through the rectum during an examination is often referred to as the *posterior lobe*. Note that the *anterior* and *median* lobes of the prostate cannot be examined, as they are not in contact with the rectal wall. The *seminal vesicles*, shaped like rabbit ears above the prostate, are also not normally palpable.

Male Genitalia

Review the anatomy of the male genitalia (Fig. 14-2). The *shaft of the penis* is formed by three columns of vascular erectile tissue: the *corpus spongiosum*, containing the *urethra*, and two *corpora cavernosa*. The corpus spongiosum extends from the bulb of the penis to the cone-shaped *glans* with its expanded base, or *corona*. In an uncircumcised penis, the glans is covered by a loose, hood-like fold of skin called the *prepuce* or *foreskin*, where **smegma**, or secretions of the glans, may collect. The urethra is located in the ventral midline of the shaft of the penis; urethral abnormalities may sometimes be felt there. The urethra opens into the vertical slit-like urethral *meatus* located somewhat ventrally at the tip of the glans.

The *testes* are paired ovoid glands consisting primarily of seminiferous tubules and interstitial tissue, covered by

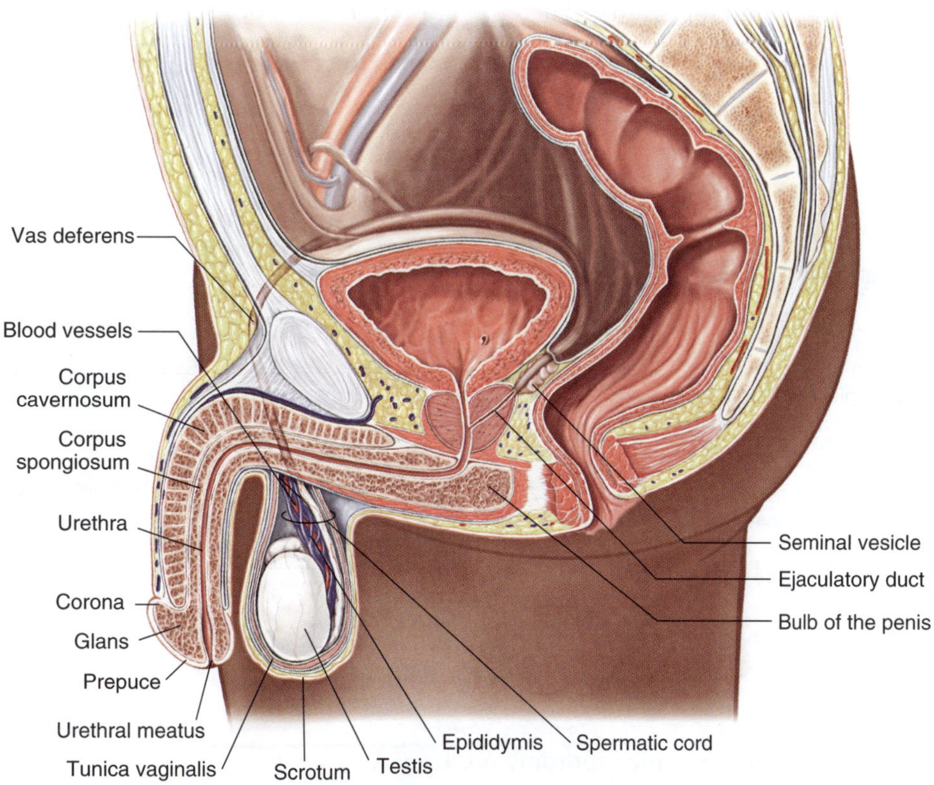

FIGURE 14-2. Anatomy of male genitalia, sagittal view.

a fibrous outer coating, the *tunica albuginea*. The testes are normally 1.5 to 2 cm in length for prepubertal boys and 4 to 5 cm post puberty. Surrounding or appended to the testes are several structures. The *scrotum* is a loose, wrinkled pouch of skin and underlying *tunica dartos (dartos muscle)*. It is divided into two compartments, each containing a *testis* or *testicle*. Covering the testis, except posteriorly, is the serous membrane of the *tunica vaginalis*, derived from the peritoneum of the abdomen and brought down into the scrotum during testicular descent through the deep internal inguinal ring. The *parietal layer* of the tunica vaginalis cloaks the anterior two-thirds of the testis, and the *visceral layer* lines the adjacent scrotum. On the posterolateral surface of each testis is the softer, comma-shaped *epididymis*, consisting of tightly coiled tubules emanating from the testis that become the *vas deferens*. The epididymis is normally separated from the testis by a palpable *sulcus* and provides a reservoir for storage, maturation, and transport of sperm.

If the peritoneal lining remains an open channel to the scrotum, it can give rise to an *indirect inguinal hernia*.

The parietal and visceral layers form a potential space for the abnormal fluid accumulation of a *hydrocele*.

During ejaculation, the *vas deferens*, a firm muscular cord-like structure, transports sperm from the tail of the epididymis along a somewhat circular route to the urethra. The vas ascends from the scrotal sac into the pelvic cavity through the *inguinal canal*, and then loops anteriorly over the ureter to the prostate behind the bladder. There, it merges with the *seminal vesicle* to form the *ejaculatory duct*, which traverses the prostate and empties into the urethra. Secretions from the vasa deferentia, the seminal vesicles, and the prostate all contribute to the *seminal fluid*. Within the scrotum, each vas is closely associated with blood vessels, nerves, and muscle fibers. These structures make up the *spermatic cord*.

Female Genitalia

Begin by reviewing the anatomy of the external female genitalia and the internal structure of the female pelvic organs.

Vulva. *Vulva* is the collective term for the external part of the female genitalia (Fig. 14-3). It consists of the *mons pubis*, a hair-covered fat pad overlying the symphysis pubis; the *labia majora*, rounded folds of adipose tissue forming the outer lips of the vagina; the *labia minora*, the thinner pinkish-red folds or inner lips that extend anteriorly to form the *prepuce*; and the *clitoris*. It also includes the *vestibule*, the boat-shaped fossa between the labia minora that surrounds the opening of the urethra, the *urethral meatus* anteriorly and the vaginal opening, the *introitus*, posteriorly. The vaginal opening may be partially occluded by a membrane, the *hymen*. The term *perineum* refers to the tissue between the introitus and the anus.

The openings of *Bartholin glands* are located posteriorly on both sides of the vaginal opening but are

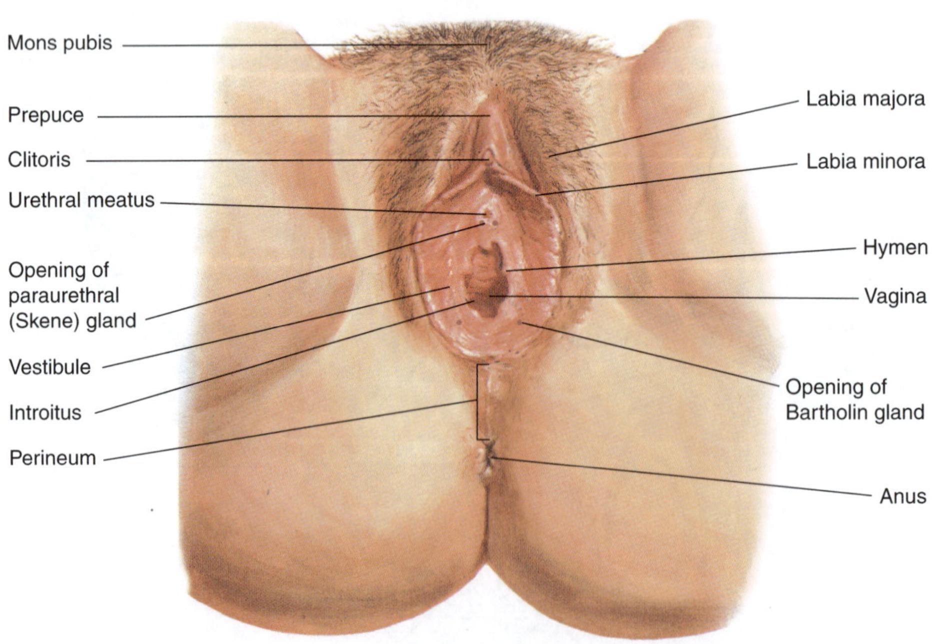

FIGURE 14-3. External female genitalia in the lithotomy position.

not usually visible (Fig. 14-4). The glands themselves are situated more deeply. Just posterior and adjacent to the urethral meatus on either side lie the openings of the *paraurethral (Skene) glands.*

See Table 14-1, Lesions of the Vulva, and Table 14-2, Bulges and Swelling of the Vulva, Vagina, and Urethra.

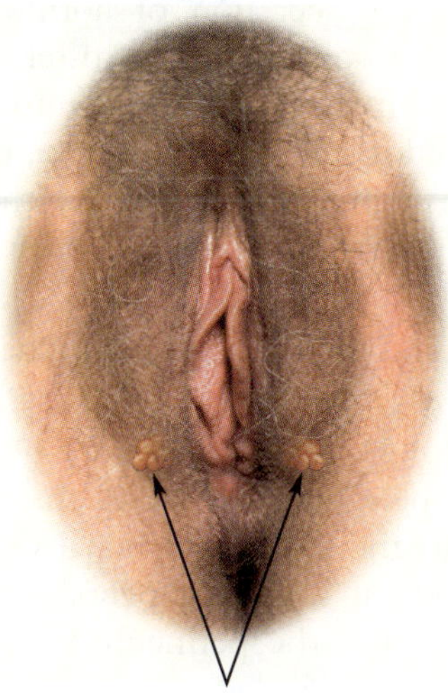

FIGURE 14-4. Bartholin glands.

Vagina. The *vagina* is a musculomembranous tube extending upward and posteriorly between the urinary bladder and urethra and the rectum. Its upper third lies at a horizontal plane and terminates in the cup-shaped *fornix.* The vaginal mucosa lies in transverse folds, or *rugae.*

The vaginal fornix lies at almost a right angle to the *cervix*, a firm, collagenous cylindrical organ with a central slit or depression, that is connected to the *uterus*, a thick-walled fibromuscular structure shaped like an inverted pear (Fig. 14-5). The cervix protrudes into the vagina, dividing the upper vagina into three recesses, the *anterior*, *posterior*, and *lateral fornices.*

Uterus. The vaginal surface of the cervix, the *ectocervix*, is seen easily with the help of a speculum (Fig. 14-6). At its center is a round, oval, or slit-like depression, the *external os* of the cervix, which marks the opening into the endocervical canal. The ectocervix is covered by plushy red *columnar epithelium* that surrounds the os and lines the endocervical canal and by shiny pink *squamous epithelium* continuous with the vaginal lining. The *squamocolumnar junction* forms the boundary between these two types of epithelium. During puberty, the broad band of columnar epithelium encircling the os, called *ectropion*, is gradually replaced by squamous epithelium. The squamocolumnar junction migrates toward the os, creating the *transformation zone.*

The squamocolumnar junction in the transformation zone is the area at risk for later dysplasia, which is sampled by the *Papanicolaou*, or *Pap, smear.*

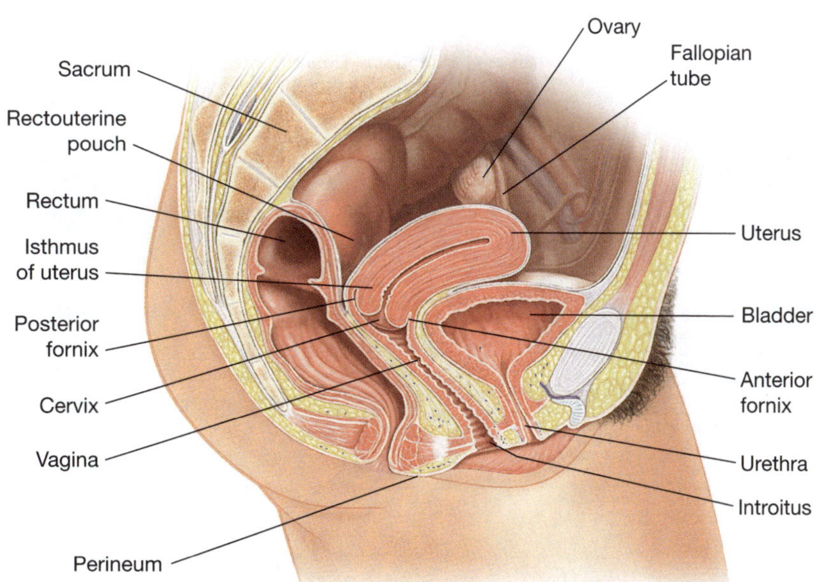

FIGURE 14-5. Pelvic anatomy, sagittal view.

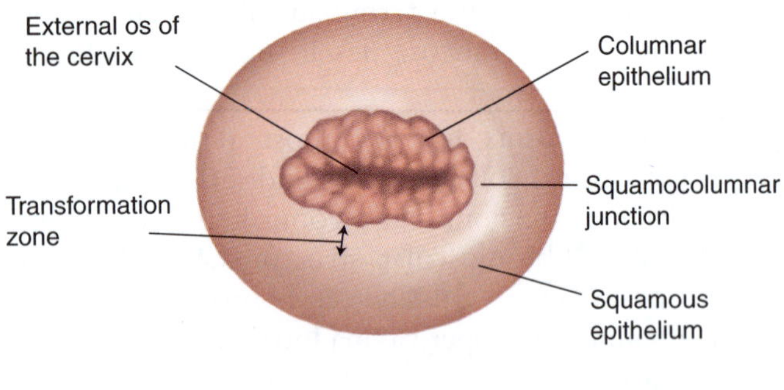

FIGURE 14-6. Cervical epithelia and transformation zone.

The cervix connects to the *isthmus*, or the lower portion of the uterus. Superior to the isthmus is the body of the uterus called the *corpus* and the upper portion of the uterus called the *fundus*. The uterine walls contain three layers: the *perimetrium*, with its serosal coating from the perineum; the *myometrium* of distensible smooth muscle; and the *endometrium*, the adherent inner coating. The uterine cavity is lined by the endometrium and connects inferiorly to the endocervical canal.

Adnexa. The term *adnexa*, Latin for "appendages," refers to the ovaries, fallopian tubes, and their supporting tissues. The two bilateral fallopian tubes insert into the uterine fundus. The *fallopian tube* has a fan-like tip, the *fimbria*, that extends to the *ovary* to each side of the uterus and collects the *oocyte* from the periovarian peritoneal cavity and conducts it to the uterine cavity (Fig. 14-7).

The two *ovaries* are almond-shaped glands that vary considerably in size but average approximately 3.5 × 2 × 1.5 cm from adulthood to menopause. The ovaries are palpable on pelvic examination in roughly half of women during the reproductive years. Normally, the fallopian tubes are not palpable.

The ovaries have two primary functions: the production of oocytes and the secretion of hormones, including estrogen, progesterone, and testosterone. Increased hormonal secretion during puberty stimulates the growth of the uterus and its endometrial lining, enlargement of the vagina, thickening of the vaginal epithelium, and the development of *secondary sex characteristics*, including the breasts and pubic hair.

The area behind the uterus is in the shape of a cul-de-sac called the *rectouterine pouch (pouch of Douglas)*. You can palpate this area on rectovaginal examination.

The greater pelvis, protected by the bony wings of the ilia, contains the lower abdominal viscera, and then narrows inferiorly at the lesser pelvis, which surrounds the pelvic cavity and the perineum. The anatomy and innervation of the pelvis and pelvic organs are complex, but they involve several common symptoms and disorders, so review the following text and figures carefully.

Pelvic Floor. The pelvic organs are supported by a sling of tissues composed of muscle, ligaments, and endopelvic fascia called the *pelvic floor*, which helps support the pelvic organs above the outlet of the lesser pelvis (Fig. 14-8). Pelvic floor muscles also aid in sexual function (*orgasm*), urinary and fecal continence, and stabilization of

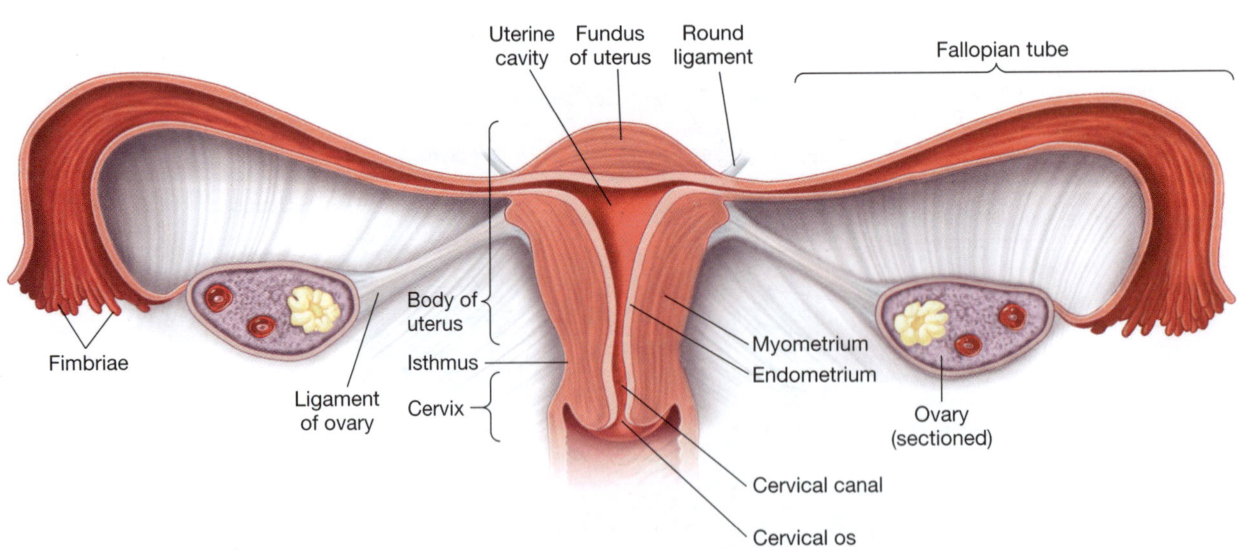

FIGURE 14-7. Uterus and adnexa, anterior cross-sectional view.

connecting joints. The pelvic floor consists of the pelvic diaphragm and the perineal membrane.

Weakness of the pelvic floor muscles may cause pain; urinary incontinence; fecal incontinence; and prolapse of the pelvic organs that can produce a *cystocele* (prolapse of the bladder into the vagina), *rectocele* (prolapse of the rectum into the vagina), or *enterocele* (prolapse of the bowel into the vagina).

See Table 14-2, Bulges and Swelling of the Vulva, Vagina, and Urethra.

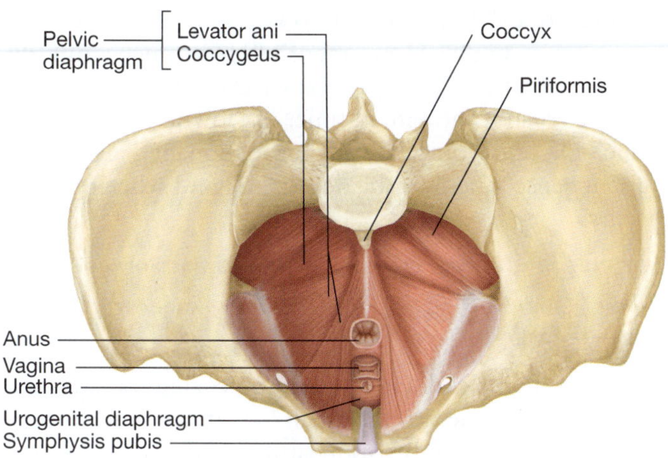

FIGURE 14-8. Pelvis and the pelvic floor, superior view.

- The *pelvic diaphragm* separates the pelvic cavity from the perineum and consists of the *levator ani* and the *coccygeal muscles*, which attach to the inner surface of the lesser pelvis.
- The *perineal membrane* is a triangular sheet of fibromuscular tissue that contains the bulbocavernosus and ischiocavernosus muscles, the superficial transverse perineal body, and the external anal sphincter. This membrane spans the *anterior triangle* that anchors the urethra, vagina, and perineal body to the ischiopubic rami.
- The urethra, vagina, and anorectum pass through the key-like opening in the center of the pelvic diaphragm, the *urogenital (levator) hiatus*.
- Inferior to the pelvic diaphragm is the third supporting structure, the *deep urogenital diaphragm*. This diaphragm includes the external urethral sphincter; the urethra; and the supporting deep transverse perineal muscle, which runs from the inferior ischium to the midline. Note the structures of the *posterior triangle*, principally the external anal sphincter muscle that encircles the rectum and the internal anal sphincter.
- The pelvic diaphragm is innervated by the sacral nerve roots S3–S5. The perineal membrane and the urogenital diaphragm are innervated by the pudendal nerve.

Loss of urethral support contributes to stress incontinence. Weakness of the perineal body from childbirth predisposes to rectoceles and enteroceles.

Lymphatics

Lymph drainage from the penis passes primarily to the deep inguinal and external inguinal nodes. Lymph vessels from the scrotum drain into the superficial inguinal lymph nodes. Lymphatic drainage from the testes parallels their venous drainage: The left testicular vein empties into the left renal vein, and the right testicular vein empties into the inferior vena cava. The connecting lumbar and preaortic lymph nodes in the abdomen are clinically undetectable.

When you find an inflammatory or suspect a possible malignant lesion on the penis, scrotum, or testes, assess the inguinal nodes carefully for enlargement or tenderness.

Lymph from the vulva and lower vagina drains into the inguinal nodes. Lymph from the internal genitalia, including the upper vagina, flows into the pelvic and abdominal lymph nodes, which are not palpable.

Male Sexual Development and Function

Gonadotropin-releasing hormone (GRH) from the hypothalamus stimulates pituitary secretion of *luteinizing hormone (LH)* and *follicle-stimulating hormone (FSH)*. LH acts on the interstitial Leydig cells to promote synthesis of *testosterone*, which is converted in target tissues to *5α-dihydrotestosterone (5α-DHT)*. It is 5α-DHT that triggers pubertal growth of the male genitalia; prostate; seminal vesicles; and secondary sex characteristics, such as facial and body hair, musculoskeletal growth, and enlargement of the larynx with its associated low-pitched voice. FSH regulates sperm production by the germ cells and Sertoli cells of the *seminiferous tubules*.

Male sexual function depends on normal levels of testosterone, arterial blood flow from the internal iliac artery to the internal pudendal artery and its penile artery and branches, and intact neural innervation from α-adrenergic and cholinergic pathways. Erection from venous engorgement of the corpora cavernosa results from two types of stimuli. Visual, auditory, and erotic cues trigger sympathetic outflow from higher brain centers to the T11–L2 levels of the spinal cord. Tactile stimulation initiates sensory impulses from the genitalia to the S2–S4 reflex arcs and the parasympathetic pathways through the pudendal nerve. Both sets of stimuli appear to increase levels of nitric oxide and cyclic guanosine monophosphate, resulting in local vasodilation.

HEALTH HISTORY: GENERAL APPROACH

The interview of patients presenting with symptoms concerning the genitourinary system requires a systematic approach.

Common or Concerning Symptoms

Urinary and Renal Disorders	Male Genitalia	Female Genitalia
■ Urinary symptoms, including suprapubic pain; dysuria, urgency, or frequency; nocturia or polyuria; urinary incontinence; hematuria Flank pain and ureteral colic	■ Penile discharge or lesions and scrotal or testicular pain, swelling, or lesions ■ Sexually transmitted infections	■ Menarche and menstruation ■ Abnormal bleeding ■ Menopause ■ Pelvic pain—acute and chronic ■ Vulvovaginal symptoms ■ Sexually transmitted infections (STIs) (see Chapter 6)
■ Weak urinary stream		■ Sexual health (see Chapter 3) ■ Pregnancy (see Chapter 24)

Taking a patient's sexual and genital health history can be an uncomfortable topic to address. Clinicians and educators recognize the importance of a robust education in sexual health, yet training and clinical expertise remain limited. It is important for a clinician to ensure that patients feel comfortable so that they are open and honest regarding their history and symptoms. This is accomplished by addressing questions in a respectful, direct, nonjudgmental, and sensitive way.

Adopt a systematic approach each time you obtain a patient's obstetric and gynecologic history. It is important to obtain the history in a relaxed and private setting because discussions related to obstetric and gynecologic issues may be difficult for some women. The history should be obtained with the patient fully clothed, particularly if you are meeting her for the first time. Ideally, the patient should be interviewed alone unless the patient specifically requests the presence of a caregiver, friend, or family member. Exceptions may also be made for children, adolescents, and women with cognitive impairments. However, even in these circumstances, it is desirable for the patient to have time to speak with you privately. In order to increase a patient's level of comfort, questions should be asked in an open-ended and nonjudgmental way. You may want to review effective communication and interpersonal skills as described in Chapter 2, pp. 32–36.

Urinary Symptoms

General questions include: "Do you have any difficulty passing urine?" "How often do you go?" "Do you have to get up at night? How often?" "How much urine do you pass at a time?" "Is there any pain or burning?" "Do you ever rush to urinate in time?" "Do you ever leak any urine? Or find yourself wet unintentionally?" Does the patient sense when the bladder is full and when voiding occurs?

See Table 14-3, Urinary Frequency, Nocturia, and Polyuria.

Involuntary voiding or lack of awareness suggests cognitive or neurosensory deficits.

Ask women if sudden coughing, sneezing, or laughing causes loss of urine. Roughly half of young women report this experience even before bearing children. Occasional leakage is not necessarily significant. Ask older men, "Do you have trouble starting your stream?" "Do you have to stand close to the toilet to void?" "Is there a change in the force or size of your stream, or straining to void?" "Do you hesitate or stop in the middle of voiding?" "Is there dribbling when you're through?"

Stress incontinence arises from decreased intraurethral pressure (see p. 368).

These problems are common in men with partial bladder outlet obstruction from benign prostatic hyperplasia (BPH) or urethral stricture.

Suprapubic Pain. Disorders in the urinary tract may cause pain in either the abdomen or the back. Bladder disorders may cause suprapubic pain.

In bladder infection, pain in the lower abdomen is typically dull and pressure-like. In sudden overdistention of the bladder, pain is often agonizing; in contrast, chronic bladder distention is usually painless.

Pain from sudden overdistention accompanies acute urinary retention.

Dysuria, Urgency, or Frequency. Infection or irritation of the bladder or urethra frequently leads to pain on urination, usually felt as a burning sensation. Some clinicians refer to this as *dysuria*. Women may report internal urethral discomfort, sometimes described as a pressure, or an external burning from the flow of urine across irritated or inflamed labia. Men typically feel a burning sensation proximal to the glans penis. In contrast, prostatic pain is felt in the perineum and occasionally in the rectum.

Painful urination accompanies *cystitis* (bladder infection), urethritis, and urinary tract infections, bladder stones, tumors, and, in men, acute prostatitis. Women report internal burning in urethritis, and external burning in vulvovaginitis.

Urgency. Other commonly associated urinary symptoms are *urgency*, an unusually intense and immediate desire to void, sometimes leading to involuntary voiding or urge incontinence, and *frequency*, or abnormally frequent voiding. Ask about any related fever or chills; blood in the urine; or any pain in the abdomen, flank, or back (see Fig. 14-9). Men with partial obstruction to urinary outflow often report hesitancy in starting the urine stream, straining to void, reduced caliber and force of the urinary stream, or dribbling as voiding is completed.

Urgency suggests urinary tract infection (UTI) or irritation from possible urinary calculi. Frequency is common in UTI and bladder neck obstruction. In men, painful urination without frequency or urgency suggests urethritis. Associated flank or back pain suggests pyelonephritis.

See Table 14-12, Abnormalities of the Prostate.

Polyuria and Nocturia. Two additional terms describe important changes in patterns of urination. *Polyuria* refers to a significant increase in 24-hour urine volume, roughly defined as exceeding 3 L. It should be distinguished from *urinary frequency*, which can be either high volume (*polyuria*) or low volume (*oliguria*). *Nocturia* refers to urinary frequency at night, sometimes defined as awakening the patient more than once; urine volumes may be large or small. Clarify the patient's daily total fluid intake and how much occurs in the evening.

Causes of polyuria include the high fluid intake of psychogenic polydipsia and poorly controlled diabetes, the decreased secretion of antidiuretic hormone (ADH) of central diabetes insipidus, and the decreased renal sensitivity to ADH of nephrogenic diabetes insipidus.

Urinary Incontinence. Up to 30% of older adults are concerned about *urinary incontinence*, an involuntary loss of urine that can be socially restricting and cause problems with hygiene.

If the patient reports incontinence, ask whether the patient is leaking small amounts of urine due to increased intraabdominal pressure from coughing, sneezing, laughing, or lifting. Or, following an urge to void, is there an involuntary loss of large amounts of urine? Is there a sensation of bladder fullness, frequent leakage, or voiding of small amounts but difficulty emptying the bladder?

See Table 14-4, Urinary Incontinence.

There are five broad categories of incontinence. In *stress* incontinence, increased abdominal pressure causes bladder pressure to exceed urethral resistance—there is poor urethral sphincter tone or poor support of bladder neck. In *urge* incontinence, urgency is followed by involuntary leakage due to uncontrolled detrusor contractions that overcome urethral resistance. In *overflow* incontinence, neurologic disorders or anatomic obstruction from pelvic organs or the prostate limit bladder emptying until the bladder becomes overdistended.

Bladder control involves complex neuroregulatory and motor mechanisms (see p. 368). Several central or peripheral nerve lesions affecting S2–S4 can affect normal voiding. Does the patient sense when the bladder is full? And when voiding occurs?

Functional incontinence arises from impaired cognition, musculoskeletal problems, or immobility. Combined stress and urge incontinence is called *mixed* incontinence.

In addition, the patient's functional status may affect voiding behaviors even when the urinary tract is intact. Is the patient mobile? Alert? Able to respond to voiding cues and reach the bathroom? Is alertness or voiding affected by medications?

Hematuria. Blood in the urine, or *hematuria*, is a major cause for concern. When visible to the naked eye, it is called *gross hematuria*; the urine may appear obviously bloody. Blood may be detected only during microscopic urinalysis, known as *microscopic hematuria*; smaller amounts of blood may tinge the urine with a pinkish or brownish cast. In women, be sure to distinguish menstrual blood from hematuria. If the urine is reddish, ask about medications that might discolor the urine. Test the urine with a dipstick and microscopic examination before you diagnose hematuria.

Myoglobin from rhabdomyolysis can also tinge the urine pink in the absence of red cells.

Flank Pain and Ureteral Colic. Disorders of the urinary tract may also cause kidney pain, often reported as flank pain, at or below the posterior costal margin near the costovertebral angle (CVA). It may radiate anteriorly toward the umbilicus. Kidney pain is a visceral pain usually produced by distention of the renal capsule and typically dull, aching, and steady. Ureteral colic is a dramatically different severe colicky pain radiating around the trunk into the lower abdomen and groin or possibly into the upper thigh, testicle, or labium (Fig. 14-9). Ureteral pain results from sudden distention of the ureter and the renal pelvis. Ask about any associated fever, chills, or hematuria.

Flank pain, fever, and chills signal acute pyelonephritis.

Renal or ureteral colic is caused by sudden obstruction of a ureter, for example, from renal or urinary stones or blood clots.

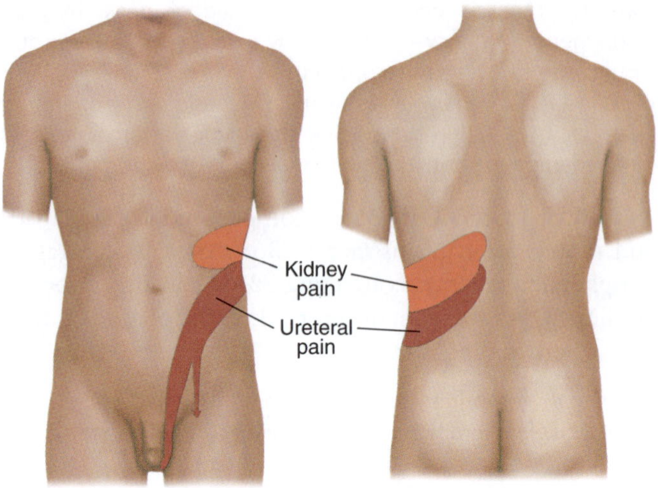

FIGURE 14-9. Radiation of renal and ureteral pain.

Weak Urinary Stream. In men, review the pattern of urination (see pp. 374–375). Does the patient have difficulty starting or holding back the urine stream? Is the flow weak? Does he have intermittency, or a stream that starts/stops during urination? What about frequent urination, especially at night? Is there any blood in the urine?

These genitourinary symptoms suggest BPH, especially in men older than 70 years.

The American Urological Association (AUA) Symptom Score helps quantify BPH severity and guide management decisions. See Table 14-5, BPH Symptom Score: American Urological Association.

Advanced prostate cancer can cause urinary symptoms and back pain.

Blood in the urine can be caused by BPH; urolithiasis; urinary tract infections; or prostate, bladder, or kidney cancer.

Also, in men, has there been sudden onset of irritative urinary tract symptoms (frequency, urgency, pain with urination), perineal and low back pain, malaise, fever, or chills?

These symptoms suggest possible acute prostatitis.

Penile Discharge or Lesions and Scrotal or Testicular Pain, Swelling, or Lesions

Ask about any discharge from the penis, dripping, or staining of underwear. If penile discharge is present, clarify the amount; color; and any fever, chills, rash, or associated symptoms.

Look for yellow penile discharge in gonorrhea and white discharge in nongonococcal urethritis from *Chlamydia*. See Table 14-6, Sexually Transmitted Infections of the Male Genitalia.

Rash, tenosynovitis, monoarticular arthritis, and even meningitis, not always with urogenital symptoms, occur in disseminated gonorrhea.

Inquire about sores or growths on the penis.

Look for an ulcer in syphilitic chancre and herpes, and multiple frond-like genital warts from human papillomavirus (HPV).

Ask about pruritus or intense itching. Look for excoriations made from scratching.

Suspect scabies or pediculosis pubis (lice) in a patient complaining of intense pruritus with evidence of penile or pubic excoriations.

Ask about swelling or pain in the scrotum or on the testicles.

Look for scrotal swelling in mumps orchitis, scrotal edema, and testicular cancer, and pain in testicular torsion, epididymitis, and orchitis.

See Table 14-7, Abnormalities of the Penis and Scrotum, and Table 14-8, Abnormalities of the Testis.

Sexually Transmitted Infections

Review any previous genital symptoms or past history of infection from herpes, gonorrhea, or syphilis.

Men who engage in high-risk sexual behaviors (multiple sex partners, condomless sex), use illicit drugs, or have a prior history of sexually transmitted infections (STIs) are at an increased risk of human immunodeficiency virus (HIV) infection and other STIs.

Because STIs may involve other areas of the body, explain to the patient that, "sexually transmitted infections can involve any body opening where you have sex. That's why it is important for me to know the kinds of sex you have had—anal, vaginal, or oral—in the past 3 months."

Infections from oral–penile transmission include gonorrhea, chlamydia, syphilis, and herpes. Symptomatic or asymptomatic proctitis may follow anal intercourse.

Ask about symptoms such as sore throat, diarrhea, rectal bleeding, and anal itching or pain.

Because many infected individuals do not have symptoms or risk factors, ask all patients, "Do you have any concerns about HIV infection?" and discuss the need for *universal testing for HIV*.

Look for evidence of other systemic illnesses as well as other symptoms such as fever, dysuria, skin rashes, joint pains (arthralgias or arthritis), and conjunctivitis.

Fever and dysuria in a man suggests acute prostatitis, acute pyelonephritis, disseminated gonococcal infection, syphilis, or postobstructive urinary tract infection. Characteristic skin rashes can be seen in reactive arthritis, gonococcemia, and secondary syphilis. Joint pains can be seen in systemic disseminated gonococcal infection. Conjunctivitis suggests reactive arthritis.

Menarche and Menses

Questions about *menarche, menstruation,* and *menopause* provide an opportunity to explore the patient's concerns and her attitude about her body. Learn to describe menstrual patterns, using the terms in Box 14-1.

Box 14-1. Menstrual History—Helpful Definitions

- *Menarche*—onset of menses
- *Dysmenorrhea*—pain with menses, often with bearing down, aching, or cramping sensation in the lower abdomen or pelvis
- *Premenstrual syndrome (PMS)*—a cluster of emotional, behavioral, and physical symptoms occurring 5 days before menses for three consecutive cycles
- *Amenorrhea*—absence of menses
- *Abnormal uterine bleeding*—bleeding between menses; includes infrequent, excessive, prolonged, or postmenopausal bleeding
- *Menopause*—absence of menses for 12 consecutive months, usually occurring between ages 48 and 55 years
- *Postmenopausal bleeding*—bleeding occurring 6 months or more after cessation of menses

Median age at menarche is relatively stable—between 12 and 13 years. Adolescent girls usually begin menstruation between ages 9 and 16 years, and it often takes ≥1 year for **menstrual cycles** to settle into a regular pattern. Environmental factors, including socioeconomic conditions, nutrition, and access to preventive health care, may influence the timing and progression of puberty. The interval between periods ranges roughly from 24 to 32 days; menstrual flow lasts from 3 to 7 days.

For the menstrual history, ask the patient her age at **menarche**, when her menses began. Ask when her *last menstrual period (LMP)* occurred, and, if possible, the one before that, called the *prior menstrual period (PMP)*. How often does she have periods, as measured by the interval between the first day of two successive periods? How regular or irregular are they? How long do they last? How heavy is the flow? Is it lighter or heavier than usual? What color is it? Flow can be assessed roughly by the number of pads or tampons used daily. Because women differ in their definitions of heavy, moderate, or light flow, ask the patient whether she usually soaks a pad or tampon, or spots it lightly. Further, does she use a pad and tampon at the same time? Does she have any bleeding between periods? Or after intercourse?

The dates of previous menstrual periods provide clues to possible pregnancy or menstrual irregularities.

Dysmenorrhea

Dysmenorrhea, or pain with menses, is reported by almost half of women patients. Ask whether the patient has any discomfort or pain before or during her periods. If so, what is it like, how long does it last, and does it interfere with usual activities? Are there other associated symptoms? Dysmenorrhea may be *primary*, without an organic cause, or *secondary*, with an organic cause.

Primary dysmenorrhea results from increased prostaglandin production during the luteal phase of the menstrual cycle, when estrogen and progesterone levels decline.

Causes of secondary dysmenorrhea include endometriosis, adenomyosis (endometriosis in the muscular layers of the uterus), pelvic inflammatory disease (PID), and endometrial polyps.

Premenstrual Syndrome. Premenstrual syndrome (PMS) includes emotional and behavioral symptoms such as depression, angry outbursts, irritability, anxiety, confusion, crying spells, sleep disturbance, poor concentration, and social withdrawal. Ask about signs such as bloating and weight gain, swelling of the hands and feet, and generalized aches and pains. *Criteria for diagnosis* are symptoms and signs in the 5 days prior to menses for at least three consecutive cycles, cessation of symptoms and signs within 4 days after onset of menses, and interference with daily activities.

Amenorrhea

Amenorrhea refers to the absence of periods. Absence of ever initiating periods is *primary amenorrhea*; cessation of periods after they have been established is *secondary amenorrhea*. Pregnancy, lactation, and menopause are physiologic causes of secondary amenorrhea.

Other causes of secondary amenorrhea include low body weight from any condition, including malnutrition, anorexia nervosa, stress, chronic illness, and hypothalamic–pituitary–ovarian dysfunction.

Abnormal Bleeding

Ask about any *abnormal bleeding*. "Do you have periods where the bleeding is quite heavier or the duration is longer than usual (**menorrhagia**)?" "Do you have bleeding or spotting in between your menstruation (**metrorrhagia**)?" "Do you have a combination of both (**menometrorrhagia**)?" The term **abnormal uterine bleeding** encompasses several of these patterns (Box 14-2).

Causes vary by age group and include pregnancy, cervical or vaginal infection or cancer, cervical or endometrial polyps or hyperplasia, fibroids, bleeding disorders, and hormonal contraception or replacement therapy.

Box 14-2. Patterns of Abnormal Bleeding

- Polymenorrhea, or less than 21-day intervals between menses
- Oligomenorrhea, or infrequent bleeding
- Menorrhagia, or excessive flow[a]
- Metrorrhagia, or intermenstrual bleeding
- Postcoital bleeding[b]

[a]Unlike the normal dark red menstrual discharge, (menorrhagia) tends to be bright red and may include "clots" (not true fibrin clots).

[b]Postcoital bleeding suggests cervical polyps or cancer or, in an older woman, atrophic vaginitis.

Menopause

Menopause typically occurs between ages 48 and 55 years, peaking at a median age of 51 years. It is defined as cessation of menses for 12 months, progressing through several stages of erratic cyclical bleeding. These stages of variable cycle length, often with vasomotor symptoms such as hot flashes, flushing, and sweating, represent *perimenopause*. The ovaries stop producing estradiol and progesterone, and estrogen levels drop significantly, although some testosterone synthesis persists. Pituitary secretion of LH and FSH gradually becomes markedly elevated. Low levels of estradiol remain detectable due to conversion of adrenal steroids in peripheral adipose tissue.

During the menopausal transition, women may experience mood shifts; changes in self-image; hot flashes from vasomotor changes; accelerated bone loss; increases in total and low-density lipoprotein cholesterol; and vulvovaginal atrophy with vaginal drying, dysuria, and dyspareunia. Studies suggest that only vasomotor symptoms, vaginal symptoms, and trouble sleeping are consistently linked to menopause. Urinary symptoms may occur in the absence of infection, due to atrophy of the urethra and urinary trigone.

Women may ask about alternative compounds and botanicals for relief of menopause-related symptoms. Most are poorly studied and not proven to be beneficial. Estrogen replacement relieves symptoms but poses other health hazards. Relatively few medications have been shown to affect symptoms (see p. 391).

Ask a middle-aged or older woman whether she has stopped menstruating. When? Continue with "How do (did) you feel about not having your periods anymore?" "Has this affected your life in either a positive or a negative way?" Did any symptoms accompany her transition to menopause?

Some women may have stopped menstruating before the age of 40 years. This "early menopause" (premature ovarian failure) is characterized by symptoms similar to menopause such as hot flashes, no period, and vaginal dryness. The average age of early onset is 27 years.

Always be sure to ask about any bleeding or spotting after menopause as this may be an early sign of cancer.

Causes of postmenopausal bleeding include endometrial cancer, hormone replacement therapy (HRT), and uterine and cervical polyps.

Pelvic Pain—Acute and Chronic

Acute pelvic pain in menstruating adolescent girls and women warrants immediate attention. The differential diagnosis is broad but includes life-threatening conditions such as ectopic pregnancy, ovarian torsion, and appendicitis.

As you identify onset, timing, features of the pain, and associated symptoms, you will need to consider infectious, gastrointestinal (GI), and urinary causes. Be sure to ask about STIs, recent insertion of an intrauterine device (IUD), and any symptoms in the sexual partner. A careful pelvic examination, with attention to vital signs, and testing for pregnancy will help narrow your diagnosis and guide further testing.

The most common cause of acute pelvic pain is PID, followed by ruptured ovarian cyst and appendicitis. STIs and recent IUD insertion are red flags for PID. Always rule out ectopic pregnancy first with serum or urine testing and possible ultrasound.

Also consider *mittelschmerz*, which is typically a mild unilateral pain lasting for a few hours to a few days arising at midcycle from ovulation, ruptured ovarian cyst, or tubo-ovarian abscess.

Chronic pelvic pain refers to pain that lasts for more than 6 months and does not respond to treatment. It accounts for approximately 10% of ambulatory referrals to gynecologists and 20% of hysterectomies. Risk factors are advancing age, prior pelvic surgery or trauma, parity and childbirth, clinical conditions (obesity, diabetes, multiple sclerosis, Parkinson disease), medications (anticholinergics, α-adrenergic blockers), and chronically increased intraabdominal pressure (chronic obstructive pulmonary disease, chronic constipation, obesity). Explore gynecologic, urologic, GI, musculoskeletal, and neurologic causes. The Pelvic Pain Assessment Form of the International Pelvic Pain Society, which includes screening questions for depression and physical and sexual abuse, as well as a pain map that women complete, is a helpful resource. Asking the woman to keep a daily pain journal, noting any changes in situational, dietary, or seasonal conditions, may also be useful.

Endometriosis, from retrograde menstrual flow and extension of the uterine lining outside the uterus, affects 50% to 60% of women and girls with pelvic pain. Other causes include PID; adenomyosis; and fibroids, which are tumors in the uterine wall or submucosal or subserosal surfaces arising from the smooth muscle cells of the myometrium.

Chronic pelvic pain is a red flag for a history of sexual abuse. Also consider pelvic floor spasm from myofascial pain with trigger points on examination (see pp. 388–389).

Vulvovaginal Symptoms

The most common vulvovaginal symptoms are *vaginal discharge* and *itching*. If the patient reports a discharge, inquire about its amount, color, consistency, and odor. Ask about any local *sores* or *lumps* in the vulvar area. Are they painful? Because patients vary in their understanding of anatomical terms, be prepared to try alternative phrasing such as "Any itching (or other symptoms) near your vagina? … between your legs? … where you urinate?"

See Table 14-1, Lesions of the Vulva, and Table 14-9, Vaginal Discharge.

PHYSICAL EXAMINATION: GENERAL APPROACH

Before beginning the examination, it is important to let the patient know that you will be examining the anorectal area, as this examination can be very sensitive and a source of discomfort. In men, the addition of the prostate assessment adds extra time to what may already be unwelcome. When deciding whether prostate examination is warranted, it is important to take health history and age into account. In young patients without any urinary complaints related to the prostate, anorectal and prostate examination is rarely indicated. In older patients who have symptoms consistent with BPH, a prostate examination should be part of the normal physical examination.

Although the rectal and prostate examination may cause discomfort, it is rarely painful. Thus, the approach to this section of the examination requires effective and constant communication about what is about to happen as well as the expected outcomes of the examination. Be sure to warn the patient about what he or she may feel—including pressure, wetness from the lubricant, possible discomfort, and the slow gentle movement of your examining finger.

Many students at the start of their training may feel uneasy about examining the male genitalia. "How will the patient react?" "Will he let me examine him?" "What if he develops an erection during the examination?" Explain to the patient what is involved and review each step of the examination so that he feels reassured and knows what to expect. When needed, request an assistant to accompany you. Occasionally, if the patient has an erection, explain that this is a normal response, finish your examination, and proceed with a calm demeanor. If the patient refuses the examination, try to explore his reasoning for refusal.

During the genital examination, the patient may be either standing or sitting but ensure that you expose only the areas you are examining at any given time to promote his comfort. For example, when the patient is supine, the gown should cover his chest and abdomen. Place a drape at the midthigh. Expose the genitalia and inguinal areas and make sure that you wear gloves at all times. When treating younger patients, it is important to review their sexual maturity rating so that you can more accurately document your findings on examination.

TECHNIQUES OF EXAMINATION

Key Components of the Genitourinary System Examination

- Examine the kidney and urinary bladder (see Chapter 12, Gastrointestinal System).
- Male genitalia examination
  - Inspect the skin, prepuce, and glans (ulcers, scars, nodules, inflammation).
  - Inspect the urethral meatus (discharge), and, if indicated, strip or "milk" the penile shaft.
  - Palpate the shaft of the penis (induration, tenderness).
  - Inspect the scrotum including skin, hair, and contour (lesion, swelling, veins, bulging masses, asymmetry).
  - Palpate each testis including the epididymis and spermatic cord (presence, size, shape, consistency, symmetry, tenderness, masses, nodules).
  - Examine the prostate.
- Female genitalia examination
  - Perform an external examination.
    - Assess sexual maturity (if adolescent).

(continued)

Key Components of the Genitourinary System Examination (*continued*)

- Inspect the mons pubis, labia, and perineum (inflammation, ulceration, discharge, swelling, nodules, any lesions).
- Perform an internal examination.
  - Inspect the cervix (color, position, surface characteristics, any ulcerations, nodules, masses, bleeding, discharge).
  - Inspect the vagina (masses, lesions, or abnormal discharge or bleedIng).
- Perform a bimanual examination.
  - Palpate the cervix (position, shape, consistency, regularity, mobility, tenderness).
  - Palpate the uterus (size, shape, consistency, mobility, any tenderness or masses).
  - Palpate the ovaries (size, shape, consistency, mobility, any tenderness).
  - Assess the pelvic floor muscles (strength and tenderness).
- Perform a rectovaginal examination (if indicated).

Male Genitalia: Penis

Inspection. Inspect the penis, including:

See Table 14-7, Abnormalities of the Penis and Scrotum.

- *Skin*. Inspect the skin on the ventral and dorsal surfaces and the base of the penis for excoriations or inflammation, lifting the penis when necessary.

Pubic or genital excoriations suggest *pediculosis pubis* (lice or crabs) or sometimes scabies in the pubic hair.

- *Prepuce* (foreskin). If present, retract the prepuce or ask the patient to retract it. This step is essential for the detection of chancres and carcinomas. *Smegma*, a cheesy, whitish material, may accumulate normally under the foreskin.

Phimosis is a tight prepuce that cannot be retracted over the glans. Paraphimosis is a tight prepuce that, once retracted, cannot be returned. Edema ensues.

- *Glans*. Look for any ulcers, scars, nodules, or signs of inflammation.

Balanitis is inflammation of the glans; *balanoposthitis* is inflammation of the glans and prepuce.

- *Urethral meatus*. Inspect the location of the urethral meatus.

Hypospadias is a congenital ventral displacement of the meatus on the penis, while *epispadias* is a congenital dorsal displacement (see p. 666).

Compress the glans gently between your index finger above and your thumb below (Fig. 14-10). This maneuver should open the urethral meatus and allow you to inspect it for spontaneous discharge. Normally, there is none.

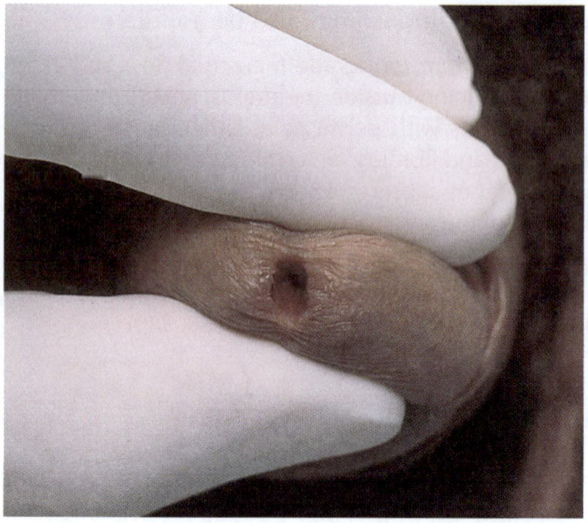

FIGURE 14-10. Gently compressing the glans to inspect the urethral meatus.

If the patient has reported a urethral discharge that you are unable to see, ask him to strip or "milk" the shaft of the penis from its base to the glans. Alternatively, do this yourself. This maneuver may expel some discharge from the urethral meatus for appropriate examination. Have a culture swab or glass slide and culture materials ready.

Purulent, cloudy or yellow discharge sometimes signals gonococcal urethritis; scanty white or clear discharge can signal nongonococcal urethritis. The quality of the discharge is a useful clue but is insufficient to diagnose a specific type of urethritis. A definitive diagnosis requires Gram stain and culture.

Palpation. *Palpate the shaft of the penis* between your thumb and first two fingers, noting any induration. Palpate any abnormality of the penis, noting any induration or tenderness.

On the dorsal side of the penis, plaques of Peyronie disease can sometimes be palpated under the skin on the right or left aspect of the shaft in the corpora cavernosa.

Urethral strictures most commonly occur in the proximal urethra, but induration or firmness along the ventral surface of the penis suggests a urethral stricture or possibly a carcinoma.

If you retract the foreskin, replace it before proceeding on to examine the scrotum.

Assessing Urethritis. To evaluate possible urethritis or inflammation of the paraurethral glands, insert your index finger into the vagina and milk the urethra gently outward from the inside (Fig. 14-11). Note any discharge from or about the urethral meatus. If present, culture it.

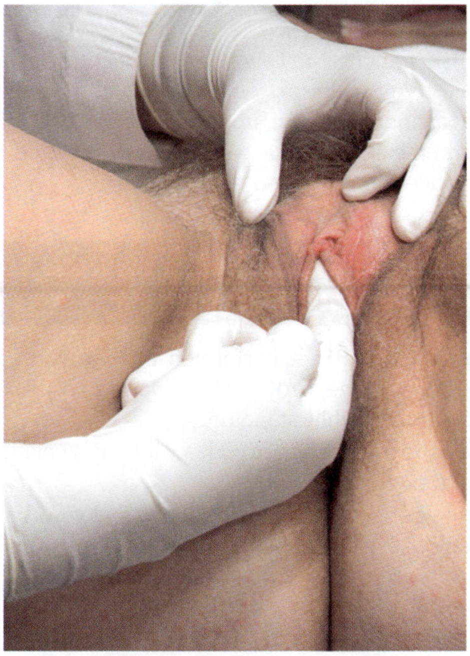

FIGURE 14-11. Milking the urethra.

Causes of urethritis include infection from *Chlamydia trachomatis* and *Neisseria gonorrhoeae*.

Scrotum and Scrotal Contents

Inspection. Inspect the scrotum, including:

See Table 14-7, Abnormalities of the Penis and Scrotum.

- *Skin.* Lift up the scrotum so that you can inspect its posterior surface. Note any lesions or scars. Inspect the pubic hair distribution.

Inspection may reveal scrotal nevi, hemangiomas, or telangiectasias as well as STIs including condyloma or ulcers from herpes and chancroid (painful) and syphilis and lymphogranuloma venereum (painless), with associated inguinal lymphadenopathy.

- *Scrotal contours.* Inspect for swelling, lumps, veins, bulging masses, or asymmetry of the left and right hemiscrotum.

A poorly developed scrotum on one or both sides suggests cryptorchidism (an undescended testicle). Common scrotal swellings include indirect inguinal hernias, hydroceles, scrotal edema, and, rarely, testicular carcinoma.

- *Inguinal areas.* Note any erythema, excoriation, or visible adenopathy.

Erythema and mild excoriation point to fungal infection, not uncommon in this moist area.

There may be dome-shaped white or yellow papules or nodules formed by occluded follicles filled with keratin debris of desquamated follicular epithelium. Such epidermoid cysts are common, frequently multiple, and benign (Fig. 14-12).

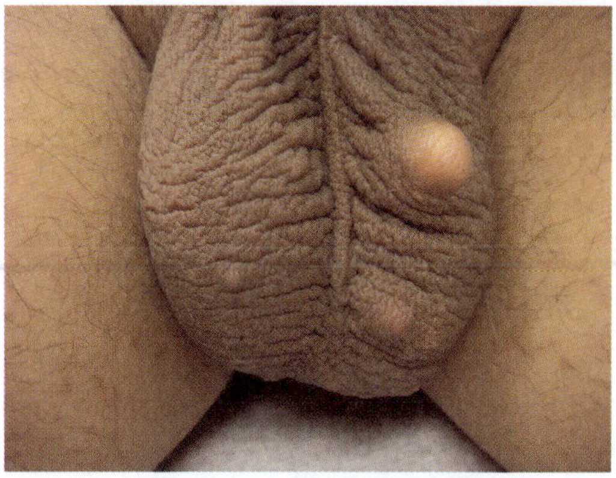

FIGURE 14-12. Benign scrotal epidermoid cysts. (From Goodheart H, Gonzalez M. *Goodheart's Photoguide to Common Pediatric and Adult Skin Disorders.* 4th ed. Wolters Kluwer; 2016, Fig. 30-28.)

Palpation. If using a one-handed technique, *palpate each testis and epididymis* between your thumb and first two fingers (Fig. 14-13). If using two hands, cradle the testis at both poles in the thumb and fingertips of both hands. Palpate the scrotal contents as you gently slide them back and forth from the fingertips of one hand to the other, without changing the position of your hands as they cup the scrotum. This technique is comfortable for the patient and allows a subtle controlled and accurate examination. The testes should be firm but not hard, descended, symmetric, or nontender, and they should also be without masses.

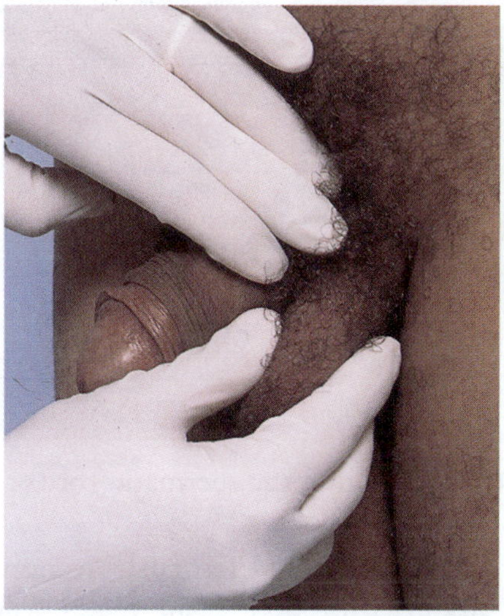

FIGURE 14-13. Palpating the testis and epididymis using one-handed technique.

See Table 14-8, Abnormalities of the Testis, and Table 14-10, Abnormalities of the Epididymis and Spermatic Cord.

Tender painful scrotal swelling is present in acute epididymitis, acute orchitis, testicular torsion, and strangulated inguinal hernias.

- For each testis, assess size, shape, consistency, and tenderness; feel for any nodules. Pressure on the testis normally produces a deep visceral pain.

  Any painless nodule on the testis raises the possibility of testicular cancer, a potentially curable cancer with a peak incidence between the ages 15 and 34 years. Recall that lymph drainage from the testes parallels retroperitoneal venous flow from the renal vein and inferior vena cava, the primary site of lymph node involvement in testicular cancer (see p. 390).

- Palpate the epididymis on the posterior surface of each testicle without applying excess pressure, which can cause discomfort. Normally, it should not be tender. The epididymis feels nodular and cord-like and should not be confused with an abnormal lump.
- Palpate each spermatic cord, including the vas deferens, between your thumb and fingers, from the epididymis to the external inguinal ring (Fig. 14-14). The vas deferens feels slightly stiff and tubular and is distinct from the accompanying vessels of the spermatic cord.

  The vas deferens, if chronically infected, may feel thickened or beaded. A cystic structure in the spermatic cord suggests a hydrocele of the cord.

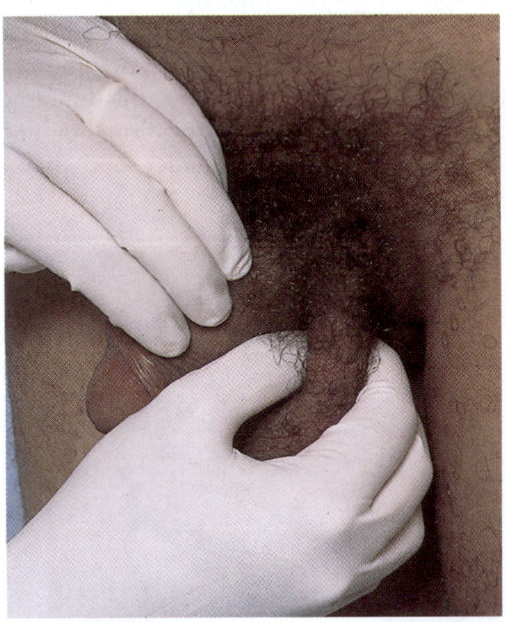

FIGURE 14-14. Palpating the spermatic cord.

Testicular Self-Examination. Testicular cancer is not common. About 1 of every 250 males will develop testicular cancer at some point during their lifetime. The clinician may wish to teach the testicular self-examination (TSE) to enhance a patient's health awareness and self-care, especially for high-risk patients. Box 14-3 provides instructions for TSE.

For high-risk patients, review the risk factors for testicular carcinoma: cryptorchidism, which confers a high risk for testicular carcinoma in the undescended testicle; history of carcinoma in the contralateral testicle; mumps orchitis; inguinal hernia; hydrocele in childhood; and positive family history.

Box 14-3. Patient Instructions for Testicular Self-Examination

This examination is best performed after a warm bath or shower. This way, the scrotal skin is warm and relaxed. It is best to do the test while standing.

- Standing in front of a mirror, check for any swelling on the skin of the scrotum.
- With the penis out of the way, gently feel your scrotal sac to locate a testicle. Examine each testicle separately.

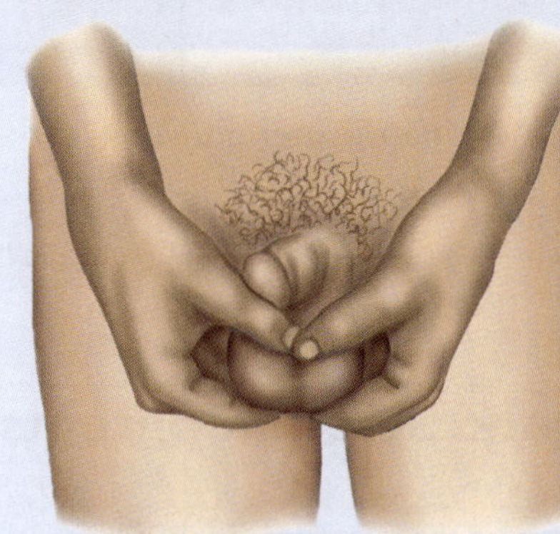

- Use one hand to stabilize the testicle. Using the fingers and thumb of your other hand, firmly but gently feel or roll the testicle between your fingers. Feel the entire surface. Find the epididymis. This is a soft, tube-like structure at the back of the testicle that collects and carries sperm and is not an abnormal lump. Check the other testicle and epididymis the same way.
- If you find a hard lump, an absent or enlarged testicle, a painful swollen scrotum, or any other differences that do not seem normal, do not wait. See your healthcare provider right away.

As noted by the American Cancer Society, "It's normal for one testicle to be slightly larger than the other, and for one to hang lower than the other. You should also know that each normal testicle has a small, coiled tube (epididymis) that can feel like a small bump on the upper or middle outer side of the testicle. Normal testicles also have blood vessels, supporting tissues, and tubes that carry sperm. Some men may confuse these with abnormal lumps at first. If you have any concerns, ask your doctor or clinician."

Patient with a Prostate. Choose one of several *suitable patient positions* for conducting the examination, with input from the patient when needed. Usually, the side-lying position (Fig. 14-15) with the hips and knees partially flexed is satisfactory and allows good visualization of the perianal and sacrococcygeal areas. Some clinicians ask the patient to stand and lean forward with the upper body resting across the examining table and hips flexed, although this can seem less dignified. In either position, your examining finger cannot reach the full length of the rectum.

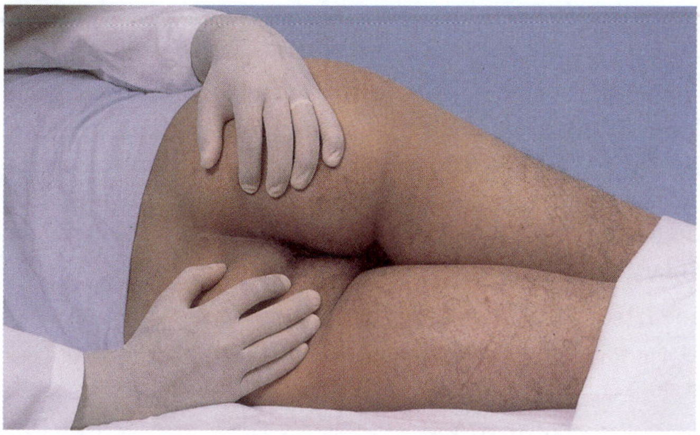

FIGURE 14-15. Positioning the patient on the left side for the anorectal examination.

Ask the patient to lie on his left side with his buttocks close to the edge of the examining table near you. Partially flexing the patient's hips and knees, especially in the upper leg, stabilizes his position and improves visibility. Drape the patient appropriately and adjust the light to ensure good visualization of the perirectal and anal area. Glove your hands and spread the buttocks apart.

- *Inspect the sacrococcygeal and perianal areas* for lesions, ulcers, inflammation, rashes, or excoriations. Adult perianal skin is normally more pigmented and somewhat coarser than the skin over the buttocks. Palpate any abnormal areas, noting masses or tenderness.

Anal and perianal lesions include symptomatic hemorrhoids, perianal abscesses/anal fistulas, anorectal, rashes, skin tags, anal fissures, and anal condylomas (warts). A linear crack or tear suggests anal fissure from large, hard stools, inflammatory bowel disease (IBD), or STIs. Consider pruritus ani if there is swollen, thickened, fissured perianal skin with excoriations.

- *Examine the anus and rectum* and *perform a digital rectal examination (DRE)*. First, inspect the anus noting any external lesions, masses, or areas of skin breakdown. Lubricate your gloved index finger, and explain to the patient that you are going to perform a DRE. The patient will feel some pressure but should not feel pain. Place the pad of your gloved and lubricated finger over the anus (Fig. 14-16A). The sphincter will initially tighten, and, as it gradually relaxes, gently insert your fingertip into the anal canal (Fig. 14-16B). Proceed in the general direction of the umbilicus. Palpate circumferentially noting any masses, areas of tenderness, or breaks in the mucosa.

A tender fluctuant mass with overlying redness and induration is suggestive of a perirectal/perianal abscess. These patients may or may not have accompanying systemic signs of infection such as fever or chills. Chronic abscesses with persistent drainage from an external opening on the skin surface represent a perirectal fistula. Fistulas may ooze blood, pus, or feculent mucus. Such patients should be referred to an appropriate specialist for further evaluation.

- *Ask the patient to squeeze the external anal sphincter* to assess muscular tone. Normally, the muscles of the anal sphincter close snugly around your finger. Initial resting tone reflects the integrity of the internal anal sphincter.

Sphincter tightness may occur with anxiety, inflammation, or scarring. Sphincter laxity occurs in neurologic diseases,

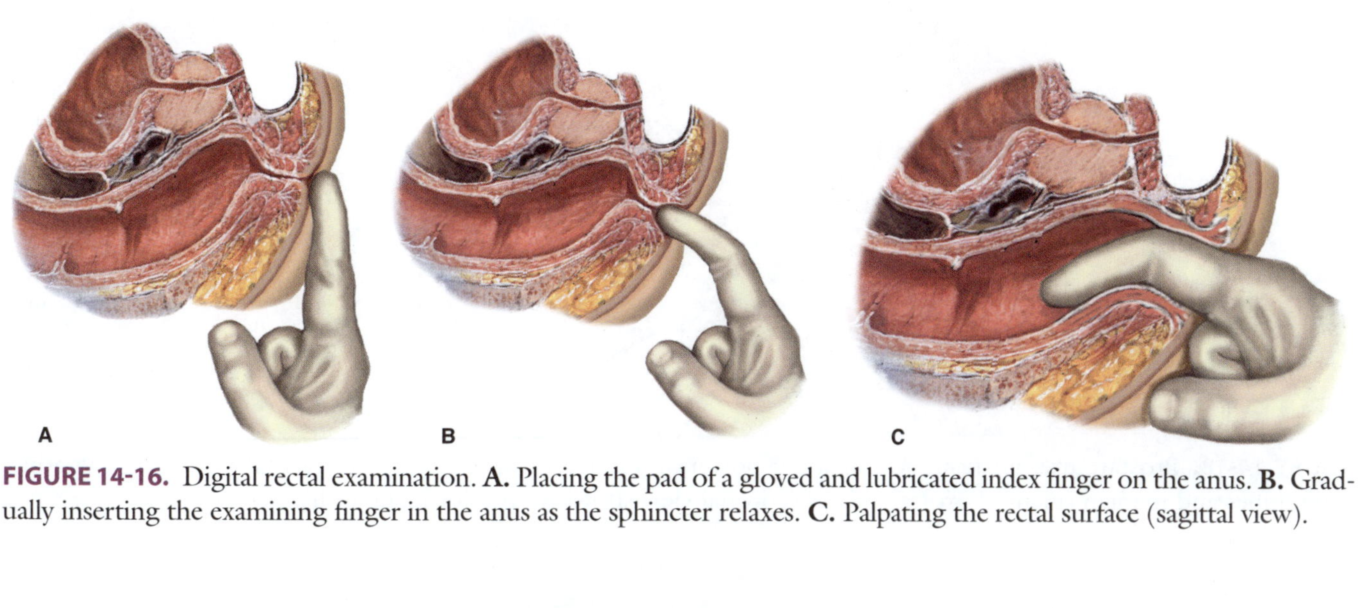

FIGURE 14-16. Digital rectal examination. **A.** Placing the pad of a gloved and lubricated index finger on the anus. **B.** Gradually inserting the examining finger in the anus as the sphincter relaxes. **C.** Palpating the rectal surface (sagittal view).

such as S2–S4 cord lesions, and signals possible changes in the urinary sphincter and detrusor muscle. Consider testing perianal sensation.

Occasionally, severe tenderness prevents entry and internal examination. Do not apply force. Instead, place your fingers on both sides of the anus, gently spread the orifice, and ask the patient to bear down.

Palpate the rectal surface. Insert your finger into the rectum as far as possible. Rotate your hand clockwise to palpate as much of the rectal surface as possible on the patient's right side, and then counterclockwise to palpate the surface posteriorly and on the patient's left side (see Fig. 14-16C). Note any masses with irregular borders suspicious for rectal cancer (Fig. 14-17), nodules, irregularities, or induration. To bring a possible lesion into reach, take your finger off the rectal surface, ask the patient to bear down, and palpate again.

See Table 14-11, Abnormalities of the Anus, Surrounding Skin, and Rectum.

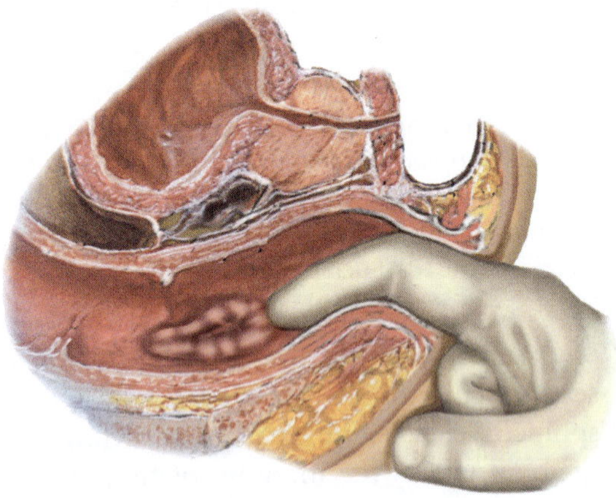

FIGURE 14-17. Palpable rectal cancer.

Palpate the prostate gland. Rotate your hand further counterclockwise so that your finger can examine the posterior surface of the prostate gland (Fig. 14-18A). By turning your body slightly away from the patient, you can feel this area more easily. Tell the patient that examining his prostate gland may prompt in him an urge to urinate.

Sweep your finger carefully over the prostate gland, identifying its lateral lobes and the groove of the **median sulcus** between them (Fig. 14-18B). Note the size, shape, mobility, and consistency of the prostate, and identify any nodules or tenderness. The normal prostate is rubbery and nontender, with no evidence of fixation to the surrounding tissues. Take note of any asymmetry, such as a difference in firmness or size between each lobe. If possible, extend your finger above the prostate to the region of the seminal vesicles and the peritoneal cavity and sweep the anterior wall. Note any nodules or tenderness. This can be difficult in patients with an enlarged prostate.

See Table 14-12, Abnormalities of the Prostate.

Findings include a rectal "shelf" of peritoneal metastases (see p. 406) or the tenderness of peritoneal inflammation.

Gently withdraw your finger, and wipe the anal area or give the patient a disposable absorbent paper. Note the appearance of any fecal matter on your glove.

Patient without a Prostate (Woman or Man with Prostatectomy). The rectum is usually examined after examining the female genitalia while the woman is in the lithotomy position. This position allows you to conduct the bimanual examination, delineate a possible adnexal or pelvic mass, and test the integrity of the rectovaginal wall, and may help you to palpate a cancer high in the rectum.

If only a rectal examination is needed, the lateral position is satisfactory and affords a better view to

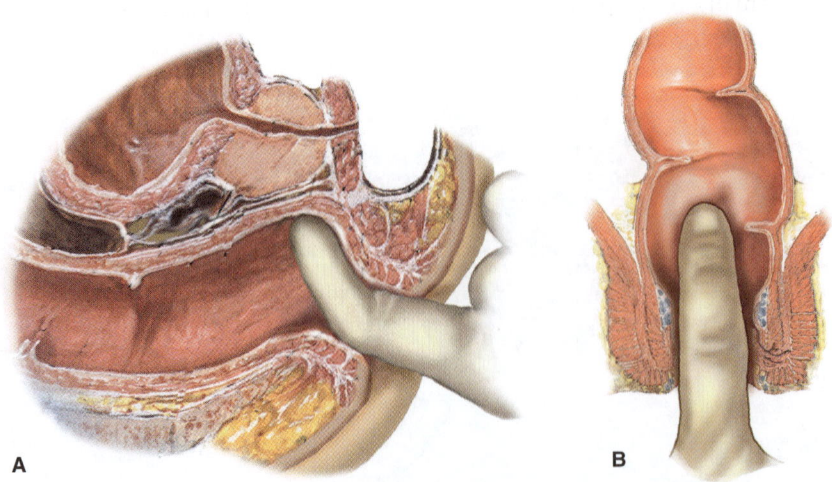

FIGURE 14-18. Prostate examination. **A.** Palpating posterior surface of prostate gland (sagittal view). **B.** Palpating lateral lobes and median sulcus of prostate gland (coronal view showing anterior rectal wall).

the perianal and sacrococcygeal areas. Use the same techniques for examination that you use for men. Note that the cervix is readily palpated through the anterior rectal wall. Sometimes, a retroverted uterus is also palpable. Do not mistake either of these, or a vaginal tampon, for a suspicious mass.

For those with prostatectomies, use the examining positions and techniques described above in "Patient with a Prostate."

Assess the Sexual Maturity of an Adolescent Patient. You can assess pubic hair during either the abdominal or the pelvic examination. Note its characteristics and distribution, and rate it according to the Tanner stages, described on p. 713.

Delayed puberty is often familial or related to chronic illness. It may also reflect disorders of the hypothalamus, anterior pituitary gland, or ovaries.

Female Genitalia

Box 14-4 provides tips for patients and clinicians to achieve a successful examination.

Box 14-4. Tips for a Successful Female Genitalia Examination

Patient	Examiner
■ Avoids intercourse, douching, or use of vaginal suppositories for 24 to 48 hours before examination ■ Empties her bladder before the examination ■ Lies supine, with head and shoulders elevated, and arms at her sides or folded across the chest to enhance eye contact and reduce tightening of abdominal muscles	■ Obtains permission; selects chaperone ■ Explains each step of the examination in advance ■ Drapes the patient from midabdomen to knees; depresses the drape between the knees to provide eye contact with patient ■ Avoids unexpected or sudden movements ■ Chooses a speculum that is the correct size ■ Warms the speculum with tap water ■ Monitors the comfort of the examination by watching the patient's face and obtaining verbal feedback ■ Uses excellent but gentle technique, especially when inserting the speculum

Examine the External Genitalia. Position yourself comfortably and let the patient know beforehand that you will be touching her genital area. Inspect the mons pubis, labia, and perineum. Separate the labia and inspect:

Excoriations or itchy, small, red maculopapules suggest *pediculosis pubis* (lice or "crabs"), often found at the bases of the pubic hairs.

- Labia minora
- Clitoris

An enlarged clitoris is seen in masculinizing endocrine disorders.

- Urethral meatus

Inspect for urethral caruncle, prolapse of the urethral mucosa (p. 394), and tenderness in interstitial cystitis.

- Vaginal opening, or introitus
  Note any inflammation, ulceration, discharge, swelling, or nodules. Palpate any lesions.

For descriptions of herpes simplex, Behçet disease, syphilitic chancre, and epidermoid cyst, see Table 14-1, Lesions of the Vulva.

- If the patient reports labial swelling, examine the Bartholin glands. Insert your index finger into the vagina near the posterior introitus (Fig. 14-19). Place your thumb outside the posterior part of the labium majus. Palpate each side in turn, at approximately the "4-o'clock" and "8-o'clock" positions, between your finger and thumb, checking for swelling or tenderness. Note any discharge exuding from the duct opening of the gland. If any is present, culture it.

A Bartholin gland may become acutely or chronically infected, resulting in swelling. See Table 14-2, Bulges and Swelling of the Vulva, Vagina, and Urethra.

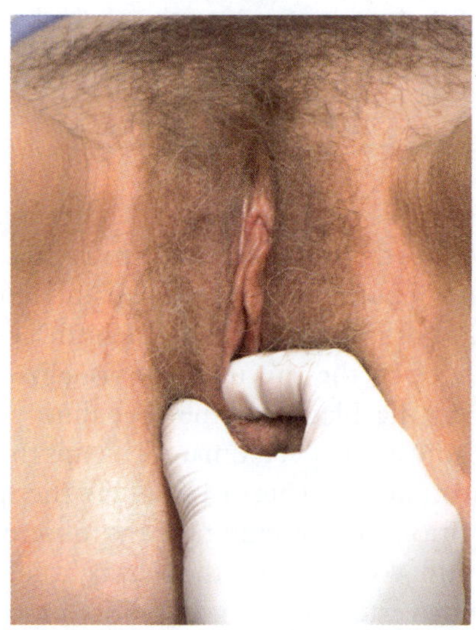

FIGURE 14-19. Palpating the Bartholin gland.

Internal Examination

Insert the Speculum. Select a speculum of appropriate size and shape, and moisten it with warm water. (Lubricants or gels may interfere with cytologic studies and bacterial or viral cultures so use them sparingly.) *Let the patient know you are about to insert the speculum and will be applying downward pressure.*

Gently separate the labia minora and introduce the closed speculum at approximately 30 degrees downward toward the cervix (Fig. 14-20). Some clinicians carefully enlarge the vaginal introitus by lubricating one finger with water and applying downward pressure at its lower margin, and then palpate the location of the cervix in order to angle the speculum more accurately.

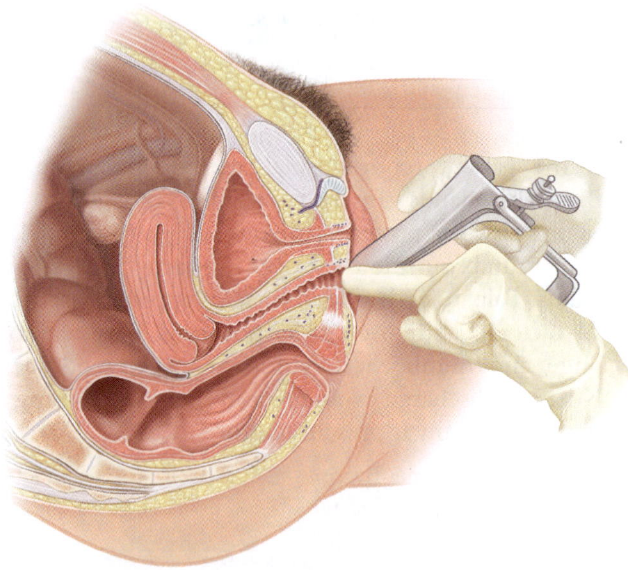

FIGURE 14-20. Gently inserting the vaginal speculum.

A yellowish discharge on the endocervical swab commonly represents mucopurulent cervicitis from *C. trachomatis, N. gonorrhoeae*, or *herpes simplex* (p. 393). Raised, friable, or lobed wart-like lesions are seen with condylomata or cervical cancer.

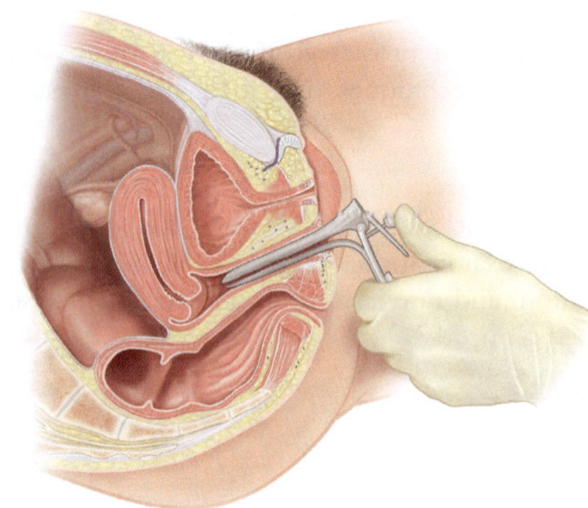

FIGURE 14-21. Inserting the speculum to its full length.

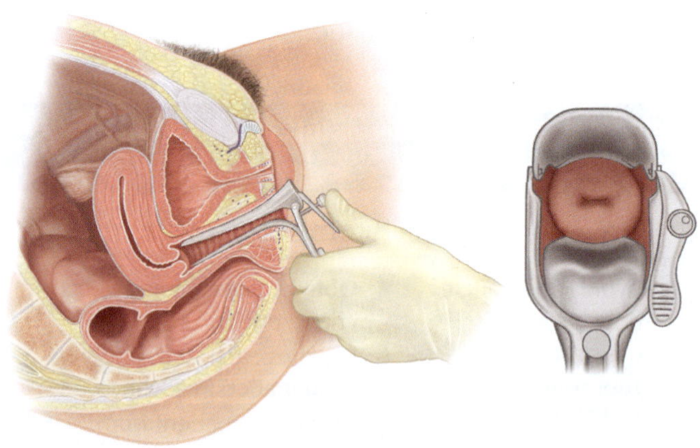

FIGURE 14-22. Visualizing the cervix.

Inspect the Cervix

After placing the speculum in the vagina, remove your fingers of your other hand from the introitus. Rotate the speculum into a horizontal position, maintaining pressure posteriorly, and insert it to its full length (Fig. 14-21). Then slowly open the speculum to visualize the cervix. Do not open the blades of the speculum prematurely. Rotate and adjust the speculum until it cups the cervix and brings it into full view (Fig. 14-22). Fix the speculum in its open position by tightening the thumbscrew. Position the light until you can see the cervix well. When the uterus is retroverted, the cervix points more anteriorly than illustrated. If you have difficulty finding the cervix, withdraw the speculum slightly and reposition it on a different slope. If a discharge obscures your view, wipe it away gently with a large cotton swab.

See Table 14-13, Variations in the Cervical Surface; Table 14-14, Shapes of the Cervical Os; and Table 14-15, Abnormalities of the Cervix.

Note the color of the cervix; its position and surface characteristics; and any ulcerations, nodules, masses, bleeding, or discharge. Inspect the cervical os for discharge.

Inspect the Vagina. Withdraw the speculum slowly while observing the vaginal walls. As the speculum clears the cervix, release the thumbscrew and maintain the open position of the speculum with your thumb. Inspect the vaginal walls for masses, lesions, or abnormal discharge or bleeding. Check for bulging in the vaginal wall. Remove either the upper or the lower blade of the speculum (or use a single-blade speculum) and ask the woman to bear down so that you can assess the location of vaginal wall relaxation or the degree of uterine prolapse.

Look for lateral displacement of the cervix in endometriosis involving the uterosacral ligaments.

See Table 14-9, Vaginal Discharge.

Vaginal discharge often accompanies infection from *Candida, Trichomonas vaginalis*, and bacterial vaginosis. Diagnosis depends on laboratory tests because the sensitivity and specificity of discharge characteristics are low. Vaginal cancer is rare; diethylstilbestrol (DES) exposure in utero and HPV infection are risk factors.

Use of the cervical broom and liquid-based cytology is increasingly common and can also be used to test for chlamydia and gonorrhea.

After inspection is completed, the speculum is gently closed and removed.

Use of the lower blade as a retractor during bearing down helps expose anterior vaginal wall defects such as cystoceles; likewise, use of the upper blade helps expose rectoceles. See Table 14-2, Bulges and Swelling of the Vulva, Vagina, and Urethra.

Obtain Specimens for Cervical Cytology (Pap Smears)

Cervical Cytology. Obtain one specimen from the endocervix and another from the ectocervix, or a combination specimen using the cervical brush ("broom"); see Box 14-5. For best results, the patient should not be menstruating. She should avoid intercourse and use of douches, tampons, contraceptive foams or creams, and vaginal suppositories for 48 hours before the examination. For sexually active women aged 26 years or younger, and for other asymptomatic women at an increased risk of infection, plan to culture the cervix routinely for *Chlamydia*.

Box 14-5. Obtaining the Pap Smear: Options for Specimen Collection

Cervical Broom

Many clinicians use a plastic brush tipped with a broom-like fringe to collect a single specimen containing both squamous and columnar epithelial cells. Rotate the tip of the brush in the cervical os, in a full clockwise direction, and then place the sample directly into a preservative so that the laboratory can prepare the slide (liquid-based cytology).

Alternatively, stroke each side of the brush on the glass slide. Promptly place the slide in a solution or spray with a fixative.

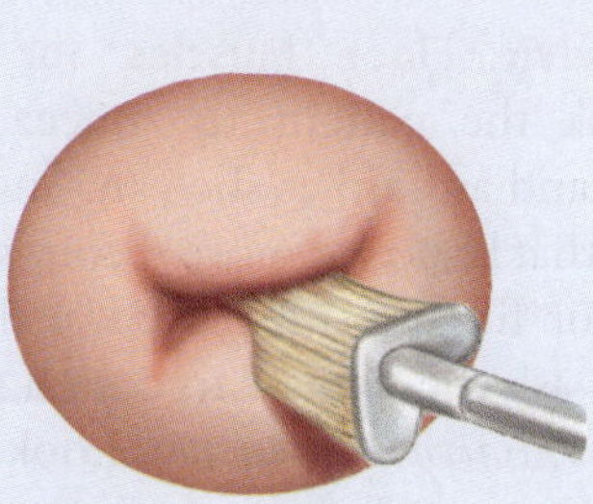

(continued)

Cervical Scrape

Place the longer end of the scraper in the cervical os. Press, turn, and scrape in a full circle, making sure to include the *transformation zone* and the *squamocolumnar junction*. Smear the specimen on a glass slide. Set the slide in a safe spot that is easy to reach. Note that doing the cervical scrape first reduces the presence of red blood cells, which sometimes appear after rotating the endocervical brush.

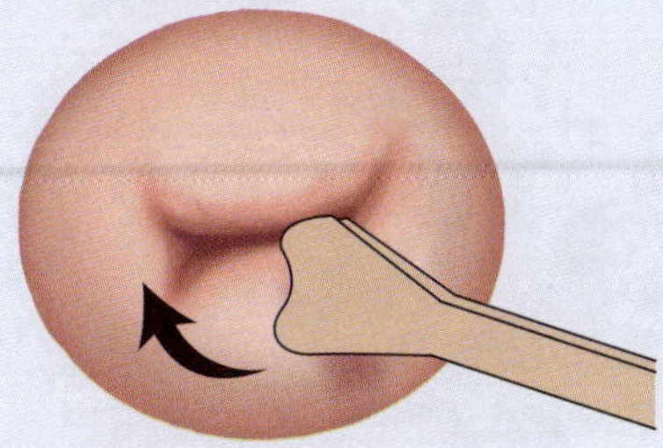

Endocervical Brush

Place the endocervical brush in the cervical os. Roll it between your thumb and index finger, clockwise and counterclockwise. Remove the brush and smear the glass slide using a gentle painting motion to avoid destroying any cells. Place the slide into an ether–alcohol solution at once, or spray it promptly with a special fixative.

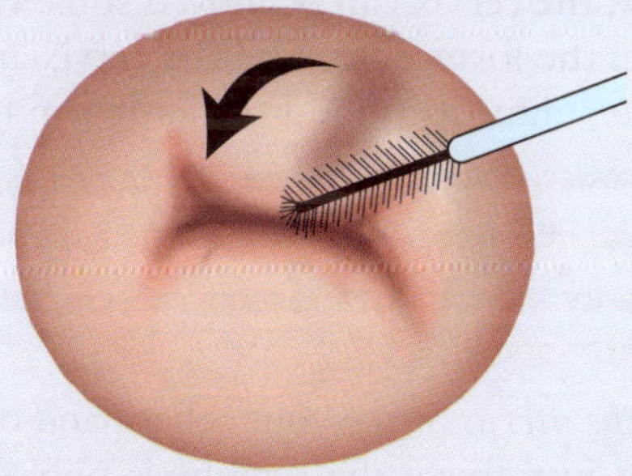

Note that for pregnant women, a cotton-tipped applicator, moistened with saline, is advised in place of the endocervical brush.

Perform a Bimanual Examination. Lubricate the index and middle fingers of one of your gloved hands, and, *from a standing position, insert your lubricated fingers into the vagina*, again exerting pressure primarily posteriorly. Your thumb should be abducted, your third and fourth fingers flexed into your palm (Fig. 14-23). Pressing inward on the perineum with your flexed fingers causes little, if any, discomfort and allows you to position your palpating fingers correctly. Note any lesions or tenderness in the vaginal wall, including the region of the urethra and the bladder anteriorly.

Stool in the rectum may simulate a rectovaginal mass, but, unlike a malignant mass, it can usually be dented by digital pressure. Rectovaginal examination confirms the distinction.

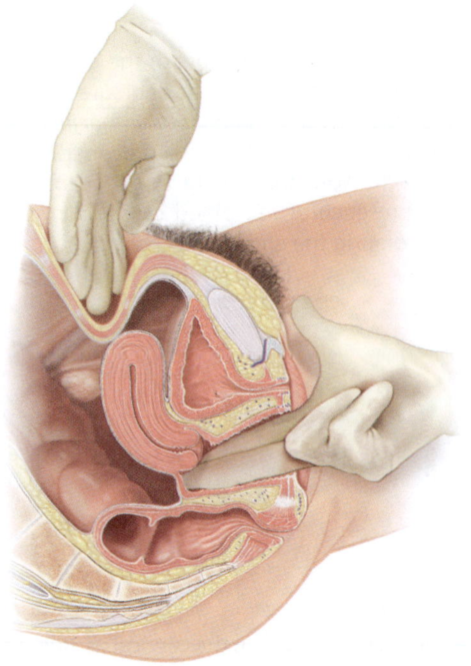

FIGURE 14-23. Performing a bimanual examination.

- *Palpate the cervix*, noting its position, shape, consistency, regularity, mobility, and tenderness. Normally, the cervix can be moved somewhat without pain. Feel the fornices around the cervix and note any nodularity, immobility, and tenderness in this area.

Cervical motion tenderness and/or adnexal tenderness are hallmarks of PID, ectopic pregnancy, and appendicitis.

Nodularity, immobility, and tenderness in the fornices may result from endometriosis.

- *Palpate the uterus.* Place your other hand on the lower abdomen just above the symphysis pubis. While you elevate the cervix and uterus with your pelvic hand, press your abdominal hand in and down, trying to grasp the uterus between your two hands (see Fig. 14-23). Note its size, shape, consistency, and mobility, and identify any tenderness or masses.

See Table 14-16, Positions of the Uterus, and Table 14-17, Abnormalities of the Uterus.

Uterine enlargement suggests pregnancy, uterine myomas (fibroids), or malignancy.

Nodules on the uterine surfaces suggest myomas (see p. 411).

If you cannot feel the uterus with either of these maneuvers, it may be tipped posteriorly. Slide your pelvic fingers into the posterior fornix and feel for the uterus butting against your fingertips. An obese or poorly relaxed abdominal wall may also prevent you from feeling the uterus even when it is located anteriorly.

See retroversion and retroflexion of the uterus (p. 410).

- *Palpate each ovary.* Place your abdominal hand on the right lower quadrant, and your pelvic hand in the right lateral fornix (Fig. 14-24). Press your abdominal hand in and down, trying to push the adnexal structures toward your pelvic hand. Try to identify the right ovary or any adjacent adnexal masses. By moving your hands slightly, slide the adnexal structures between your fingers, if possible, and note their size, shape, consistency, mobility, and tenderness. Repeat the procedure on the left side.

Within 3 to 5 years after menopause, the ovaries become atrophic and usually nonpalpable. In postmenopausal women, investigate a palpable ovary for possible ovarian cyst or ovarian cancer. Pelvic pain, bloating, increased abdominal size, and urinary tract symptoms are more common in women with ovarian cancer.

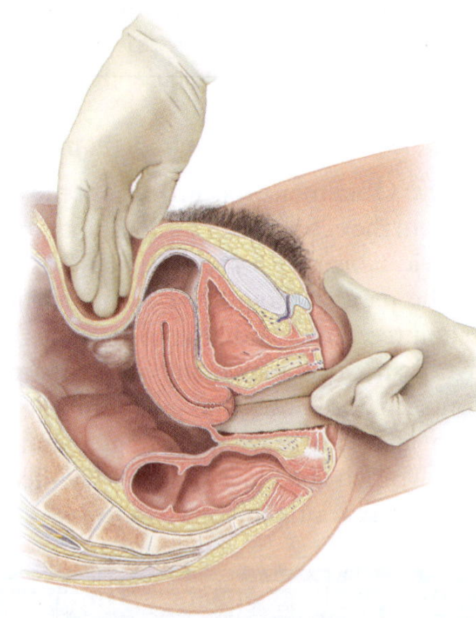

FIGURE 14-24. Palpating the ovaries.

Normal ovaries are somewhat tender. They are usually palpable in slender relaxed women, but are difficult or impossible to feel in women who are obese or tense.

Adnexal masses can also arise from a tubo-ovarian abscess; salpingitis, or inflammation of the fallopian tubes from PID; or ectopic pregnancy. Distinguish such a mass from a uterine myoma. See Table 14-18, Adnexal Masses.

Assess the Pelvic Floor Muscles for Strength and Tenderness. Ask the patient to squeeze around your fingers as long and as hard as she can. Snug compression of your fingers that lasts 3 or more seconds is full strength. Then, with your fingers still placed against the vaginal walls inferiorly, ask the patient to cough several times or to bear down (*Valsalva maneuver*). Look for any urinary leakage during increased abdominal pressure. Watch for abdominal muscle overrecruitment or tightening of the adductor or gluteal muscles.

Muscle weakness arises from aging, vaginal deliveries, and neurologic conditions and contributes to the urine leakage of stress incontinence during increased abdominal pressure. Overrecruitment with tightening, vaginal wall tenderness, and referred pain signal pelvic pain from pelvic floor spasm, interstitial cystitis, vulvodynia, and urethral spasm.

In patients with pelvic pain or vaginal wall tenderness, palpate the external pelvic floor muscles in a clockwise rotation to identify trigger points.

Trigger point tenderness in these muscles accompanies pelvic floor spasm and pelvic floor dysfunction from trauma, interstitial cystitis, and fibromyalgia. Pelvic floor disorders, present in ~25% of all women and ≥30% of older women, include urinary and fecal incontinence, pelvic organ prolapse, and other sensory and emptying abnormalities of the lower urinary and GI tracts.

Perform a Rectovaginal Examination, If Indicated. The rectovaginal examination (Fig. 14-25) has the following primary purposes: to palpate a retroverted uterus, the uterosacral ligaments, cul-de-sac, and adnexa; and to assess pelvic pathology.

Nodularity and thickening of the uterosacral ligaments occur in endometriosis, also pain with uterine movement.

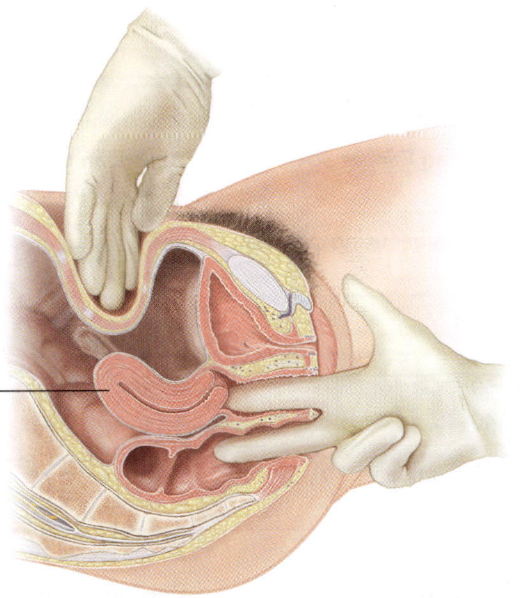

FIGURE 14-25. Examining the rectovaginal area.

After withdrawing your fingers from the bimanual examination, change your gloves and lubricate your fingers as needed. Slowly reintroduce your index finger into the vagina and your middle finger into the rectum. Ask the patient to strain down as you do this to relax her anal sphincter. Mention that this may stimulate an urge to move her bowels, but this will not occur. Apply pressure against the anterior and lateral walls with the examining fingers, and downward pressure with the hand on the abdomen.

Check the *rectal vault* for masses. If fecal blood testing is planned, change gloves to avoid contaminating fecal material with any blood provoked by collecting the Pap smear. After the examination, wipe off the external genitalia and rectum, or offer several pieces of soft, absorbent disposable paper to the patient so that she can do it herself.

RECORDING YOUR FINDINGS

Note that initially you may use sentences to describe your findings; later you will use phrases. The style below contains phrases appropriate for most write-ups.

Recording the Genitourinary System Examination

Male genitalia

"Circumcised penis. No penile discharge or lesions. No scrotal swelling or discoloration. Testes descended bilaterally, smooth, without masses. Epididymis is nontender. No inguinal or femoral hernias."

Or

"Uncircumcised penis; prepuce easily retractable. No penile discharge or lesions. No scrotal swelling or discoloration. Testes descended bilaterally; right testicle smooth; 1 × 1 cm firm nodule on left lateral testicle. It is fixed and nontender. Epididymis nontender. No inguinal or femoral hernias."

These findings are suspicious for *testicular carcinoma*.

Prostate

"Left lateral prostate lobe with 1 × 1 cm firm, hard nodule near the apex; right lateral lobe smooth; median sulcus obscured."

These findings are suspicious for prostate cancer.

Female genitalia

"No inguinal adenopathy. External genitalia without erythema, lesions, or masses. Vaginal mucosa pink. Cervix parous, pink, and without discharge. Uterus anterior, midline, smooth, and not enlarged. No adnexal tenderness. Pap smear obtained. Rectovaginal wall intact. Rectal vault without masses. Stool brown and negative for fecal blood."

Or

"Bilateral shotty inguinal adenopathy. External genitalia without erythema or lesions. Vaginal mucosa and cervix coated with thin white homogeneous discharge with mild fishy odor. After swabbing cervix, no discharge visible in the cervical os. Uterus midline; no adnexal masses. Rectal vault without masses. Stool brown and negative for fecal blood. pH of vaginal discharge >4.5."

These findings are consistent with bacterial vaginosis.

HEALTH PROMOTION AND COUNSELING: EVIDENCE AND RECOMMENDATIONS

Important Topics for Health Promotion and Counseling

- Testicular cancer
- Prostate cancer
- Cervical cancer
- Menopause and hormone replacement therapy
- Ovarian cancer

Testicular Cancer

A major risk factor for testicular cancer is cryptorchidism (undescended testicle), which confers a 3- to 17-fold increased cancer risk. Other risk factors include family history, Klinefelter syndrome, and HIV infection. About 70% of testicular cancers are localized at diagnosis; most are curable even when found at advanced stage. Seek medical attention for any of the following: a painless lump, swelling, or enlargement in either testicle; pain or discomfort in a testicle or the scrotum; breast growth or soreness; or a feeling of heaviness or a dull ache in the lower abdomen or the groin.

Prostate Cancer

Age, ethnicity, and family history are the strongest risk factors for prostate cancer. Prostate cancer is rare before age 40 years; however, incidence rates begin increasing rapidly after age 50 years, and the median age at diagnosis is 66 years. Family history of prostate cancer is associated with an increased cancer risk, particularly when multiple first-degree relatives have been diagnosed and/or the relative's cancer was early onset (age ≤55).

There is no convincing evidence that any lifestyle modification, such as consuming diets high in fruits and vegetables or increasing physical activity, can prevent prostate cancer. Similarly, there is no evidence that chemoprevention with dietary supplements such as the antioxidant vitamin E or the micronutrient selenium can prevent cancer. While chemoprevention with medications such as the 5α-reductase inhibitors (5-ARIs) finasteride and dutasteride does reduce the incidence of prostate cancer, there is no evidence as to whether they can reduce prostate cancer mortality.

The *prostate-specific antigen (PSA)* blood test is the primary prostate cancer screening test. Major professional organizations, including the U.S. Preventive Services Task Force, the American Cancer Society (ACS), and the AUA, have all issued guidelines in recent years, summarized in Box 14-6.

Box 14-6. Prostate Cancer Screening Guidelines

	United States Preventive Services Task Force (2018)	American Cancer Society (2012)	American Urological Association (2013)
Shared decision making	Yes	Yes (consider using decision aid)	Yes
Age to begin offering screening (years) ■ Average-risk ■ High-risk	 ■ 55 ■ No recommendation	 ■ 50 ■ 40–45	 ■ 55 ■ 40
Age to stop offering screening	69 years	Life expectancy <10 years	Life expectancy <10 years
Screening tests	PSA	PSA DRE (optional)	PSA DRE (optional)
Frequency of screening	No recommendation	Annual (biennial when PSA <2.5 ng/mL)	Every 2 years may be preferable
Biopsy referral criteria	No recommendation	PSA ≥4 ng/mL Abnormal DRE Individualized risk assessment for PSA levels 2.5 to 4 ng/mL	No specific PSA level, consider using biomarkers, imaging, and risk calculators to inform biopsy decisions

DRE, digital rectal examination; PSA, prostate-specific antigen.

Cervical Cancer

HPV, particularly types 16 and 18, is found in virtually all cervical cancers. It is sexually transmitted, and having multiple sexual partners and an earlier age of sexual activity are risk factors for developing cervical cancer. Other important risk factors include inadequate screening with the Pap smear, immunosuppression, long-term use of oral contraception, coinfection with *C. trachomatis*, previous cervical cancer or high-grade precancerous lesion, tobacco smoking, in utero exposure to DES, and having more than three full-term pregnancies.

HPV vaccination offers the opportunity to prevent cervical cancer and precancers. The only currently available HPV vaccine is the 9-valent vaccine, which targets HPV infections that can cause cervical, vulvar, vaginal, anal, and oropharyngeal cancers as well as most anogenital warts.

The routine vaccination for females and males beginning at age 11 or 12 years is recommended, though vaccinations can be first given at age 9 years. For persons being vaccinated before age 15 years, the recommendation is two doses of HPV vaccine within 6 to 12 months. For persons first being vaccinated at ages 15 to 26 years and immunocompromised persons ages 9 to 26 years, the recommendation is for three doses of HPV vaccine (0, 1 to 2, and 6 months). Vaccination is also recommended for all persons through age 26 years who were not previously adequately vaccinated. Vaccinated women should still get cervical cancer screening (see Box 14-7) and recognize that using condoms does not eliminate the risk of cervical HPV infection.

Widespread organized cervical screening with the Pap smear has contributed to significant declines in cervical cancer incidence and mortality since the 1960s. Pap smears can identify high-risk precancerous changes or early cancers that can be further evaluated and treated by gynecologists. Current guidelines on cervical cancer screening for average-risk women are shown in Box 14-7. The guidelines defined average risk as having no history of a high-grade, precancerous cervical lesion or cervical cancer; not being immunocompromised; and having no in utero exposure to DES. They recommended against screening women younger than age 21 years, average-risk women older than 65 years with adequate previous screening, and women who had undergone hysterectomy with removal of the cervix.

Box 14-7. Current Cervical Cancer Screening Guidelines for Average-Risk Women: USPSTF, ACS/ASCCP/ASCP, and ACOG

Variables	Recommendation
Age at which to begin screening	21 years
Screening method and interval	Ages 21–65 years: Cytology every 3 years *or* Ages 21–29 years: Cytology every 3 years Ages 30–65 years: Cytology plus HPV testing (for high-risk or oncogenic HPV types) every 5 years; HPV testing alone (age 25 or 30 years)
Age at which to end screening	Age >65 years, assuming three consecutive negative results on cytology or two consecutive negative results on cytology plus HPV testing within 10 years before cessation of screening, with the most recent test performed within 5 years
Screening after hysterectomy with removal of the cervix	Not recommended

ACOG, American College of Obstetricians and Gynecologists; ACS, American Cancer Society; ASCCP, American Society for Colposcopy and Cervical Pathology; ASCP, American Society for Clinical Pathology; HPV, human papillomavirus; USPSTF, U.S. Preventive Services Task Force.

Menopause and Hormone Replacement Therapy

Menopause may bring psychological and physiologic changes ranging from mood shifts to hot flashes to vaginal drying and bone loss. For many years, HRT with oral estrogen ± progestin was recommended to treat menopausal symptoms and protect against bone loss and cardiovascular disease events. However, the Women's Health Initiative, a large randomized, controlled trial investigating the use of postmenopausal HRT found that receiving hormones increased risks for cardiovascular disease events and breast cancer. The U.S. Preventive Services Task Force (USPSTF) recommends against the use of either estrogen alone (for women who have had a hysterectomy) or combined use of estrogen and progestin for preventing chronic conditions in postmenopausal women. However, the USPSTF recommendation did not address using HRT to treat menopausal symptoms. The American College of Obstetricians and Gynecologists (ACOG) advises individualized decision making regarding using HRT for menopausal symptoms based on a woman's symptom severity and risk–benefit ratio. Doses should be low, prescribed early in menopause, and for the shortest acceptable duration.

Ovarian Cancer

Ovarian cancer is associated with hereditary cancer syndromes such as mutations in the *BRCA1* or *BRCA2* genes, which increase risks for breast and ovarian cancers. Women with worrisome family histories should be referred to a genetic counselor. Women found to have a *BRCA* mutation might be advised to screen for ovarian cancer with transvaginal ultrasound, pelvic examination, or serum cancer antigen 125 testing. However, none of these screening methods have been proven effective in reducing ovarian cancer mortality. Chemoprevention or prophylactic surgery, though, might reduce ovarian cancer risk in women with a *BRCA* mutation.

TABLE 14-1. Lesions of the Vulva

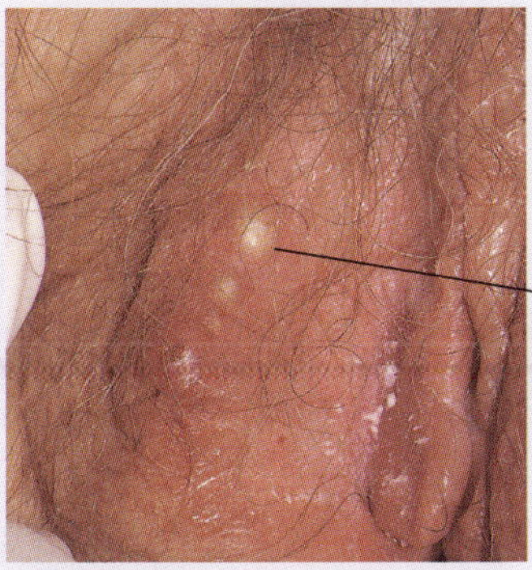

Epidermoid Cyst
A small firm round cystic nodule in the labia suggests an epidermoid cyst. These are yellowish in color. Look for the dark punctum marking the blocked opening of the gland.

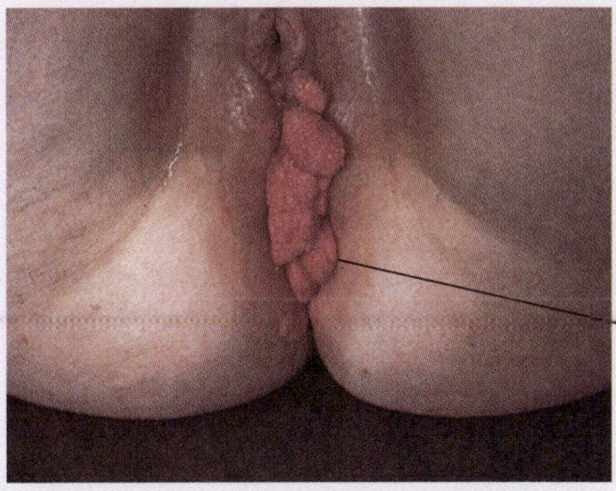

Venereal Wart (*Condyloma Acuminatum*)
Warty lesions on the labia and within the vestibule are often condyloma acuminata from infection with *human papillomavirus*.

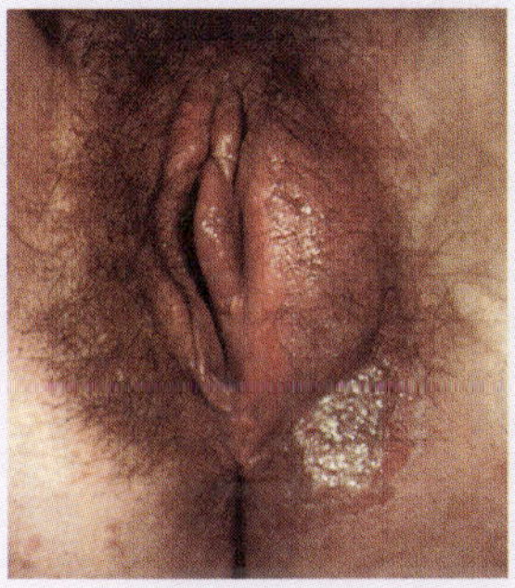

Syphilitic Chancre
This firm painless ulcer from primary syphilis forms ~21 days after exposure to *Treponema pallidum*. It may remain hidden and undetected in the vagina and heals regardless of treatment in 3–6 weeks.

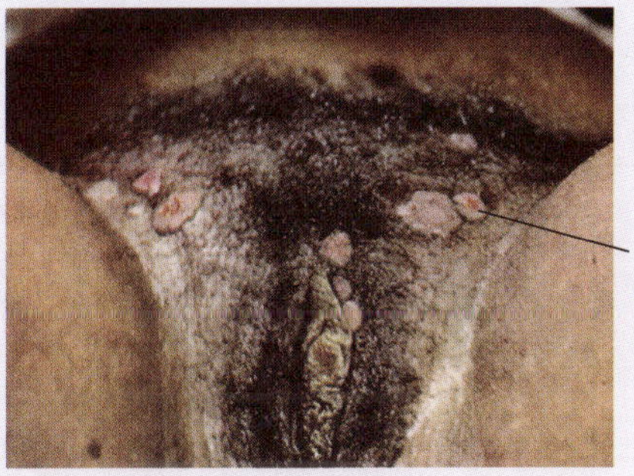

Secondary Syphilis (*Condyloma Latum*)
Large raised, round or oval, flat-topped gray or white lesions point to condylomata lata. These are contagious and, along with rash and mucous membrane sores in the mouth, vagina, or anus, are manifestations of secondary syphilis.

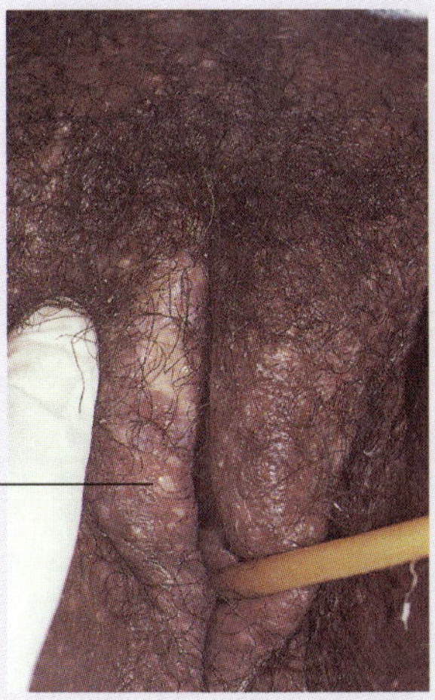

Genital Herpes
Shallow small painful ulcers on red bases are suspicious for infection from genital herpes simplex virus 1 or 2. Ulcers may take 2 to 4 weeks to heal. Recurrent outbreaks of localized vesicles, and then ulcers are common.

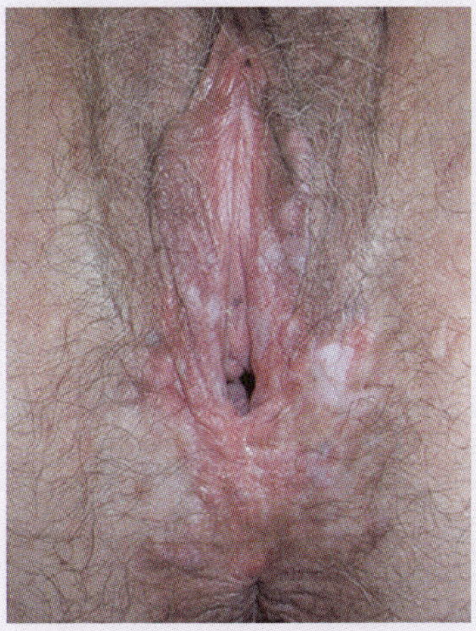

Carcinoma of the Vulva
An ulcerated or raised red vulvar lesion in an elderly woman may be a vulvar carcinoma, usually a squamous cell carcinoma arising on the labia.

TABLE 14-2. Bulges and Swelling of the Vulva, Vagina, and Urethra

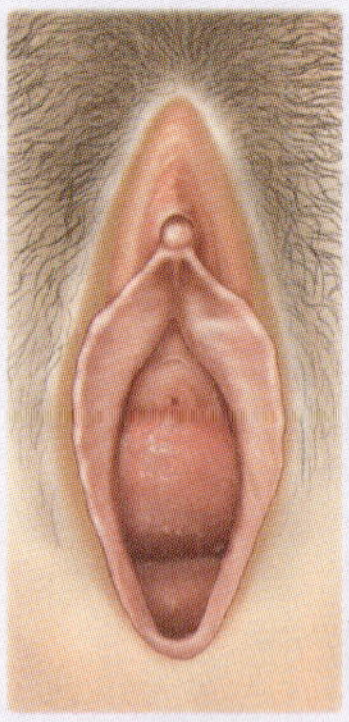

Cystocele

A cystocele is a bulge of the upper two-thirds of the anterior vaginal wall, together with the bladder above it. It results from weakened anterior supporting tissues.

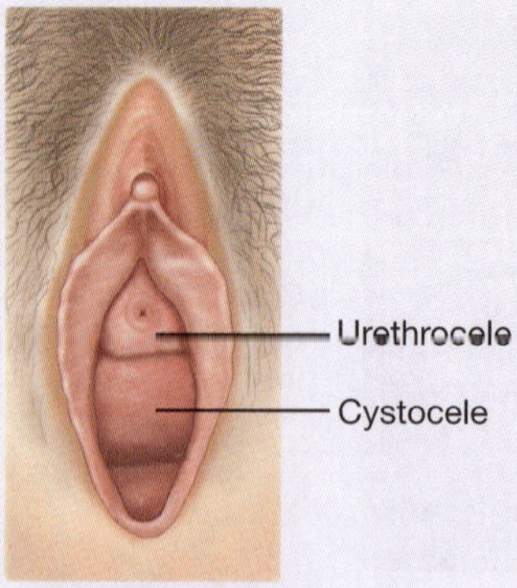

Cystourethrocele

When the entire anterior vaginal wall, together with the bladder and urethra, produces the bulge, a cystourethrocele is present. A groove sometimes defines the border between the urethrocele and the cystocele, but is not always present.

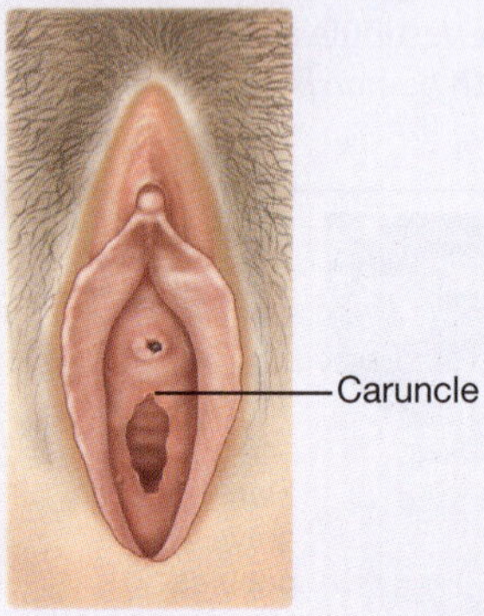

Urethral Caruncle

A urethral caruncle is a small red benign tumor visible at the posterior urethral meatus. It occurs chiefly in postmenopausal women and usually causes no symptoms. Occasionally, a carcinoma of the urethra is mistaken for a caruncle. To check, palpate the urethra through the vagina for thickening, nodularity, or tenderness, and palpate for inguinal lymphadenopathy.

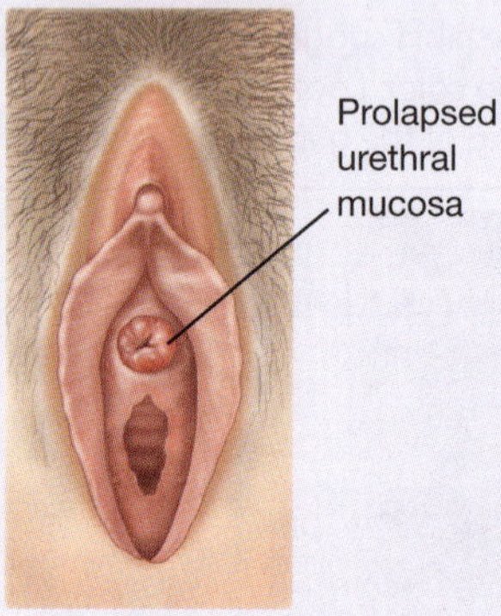

Prolapse of the Urethral Mucosa

Prolapsed urethral mucosa forms a swollen red ring around the urethral meatus. It usually occurs before menarche or after menopause. Identify the urethral meatus at the center of the swelling to make this diagnosis.

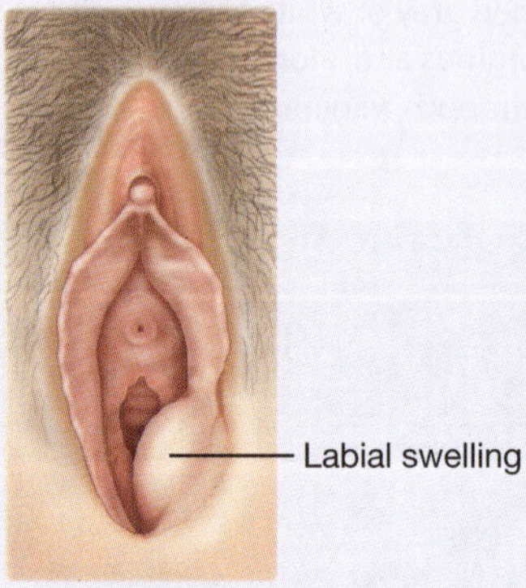

Bartholin Gland Infection

Causes of a Bartholin gland infection include trauma, gonococci, anaerobes such as *Bacteroides* and peptostreptococci, and *C. trachomatis*. Acutely, the gland appears as a tense, hot, very tender abscess. Look for pus emerging from the duct or erythema around the duct opening. Chronically, a nontender cyst is felt that may be large or small.

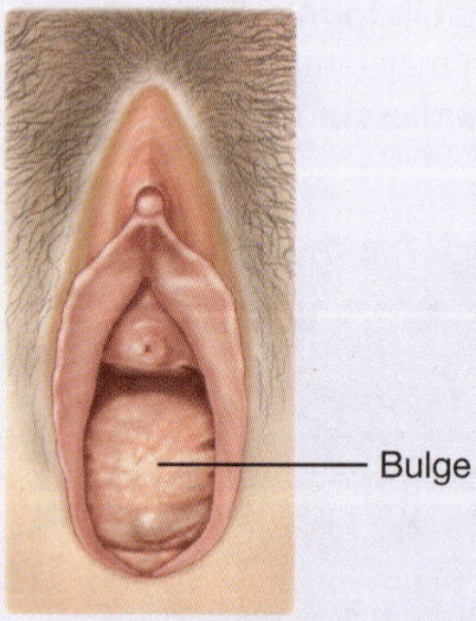

Rectocele

A rectocele is a herniation of the rectum into the posterior wall of the vagina, resulting from a weakness or defect in the endopelvic fascia.

TABLE 14-3. Urinary Frequency, Nocturia, and Polyuria

Problem	Mechanisms	Selected Causes	Associated Symptoms
Frequency	Decreased bladder capacity		
	Increased bladder sensitivity to stretch because of inflammation	Infection, stones, tumor, or foreign body in the bladder	Burning on urination, urinary urgency, sometimes gross hematuria
	Decreased elasticity of the bladder wall	Infiltration by scar tissue or tumor	Symptoms of associated inflammation (see above) are common
	Decreased cortical inhibition of bladder contractions	Motor disorders of the central nervous system, such as a stroke	Urinary urgency; neurologic symptoms such as weakness and paralysis
	Impaired bladder emptying with residual urine in the bladder		
	Partial mechanical obstruction of the bladder neck or proximal urethra	Most commonly, benign prostatic hyperplasia; also urethral stricture and other obstructive lesions of the bladder or prostate	Prior obstructive symptoms: hesitancy in starting the urinary stream, straining to void, reduced size and force of the stream, and dribbling during or at the end of urination
	Loss of S2–S4 innervation to the bladder	Neurologic disease affecting the sacral nerves or nerve roots (e.g., diabetic neuropathy)	Weakness or sensory defects
Nocturia			
With High Volumes	Most types of polyuria (see p. 375)		
	Decreased concentrating ability of the kidney with loss of the normal drop in nocturnal urine output	Chronic renal insufficiency due to a number of diseases	Possibly other symptoms of renal insufficiency
	Excessive fluid intake before bedtime	Habit, especially involving alcohol and coffee	
	Fluid-retaining, edematous states. Daytime accumulation of dependent edema that is excreted at night when the patient is supine	Heart failure, nephrotic syndrome, hepatic cirrhosis with ascites, chronic venous insufficiency	Edema and other symptoms of the underlying disorder; urinary output during the day may be reduced as fluid accumulates in the body tissues
With Low Volumes	Urinary frequency		
	Voiding while up at night without a real urge, a "pseudofrequency"	Insomnia	Variable
Polyuria	Deficiency of antidiuretic hormone (diabetes insipidus)	A disorder of the posterior pituitary and hypothalamus	Thirst and polydipsia, often severe and persistent; nocturia

(continued)

TABLE 14-3. Urinary Frequency, Nocturia, and Polyuria *(Continued)*

Problem	Mechanisms	Selected Causes	Associated Symptoms
	Renal unresponsiveness to antidiuretic hormone (nephrogenic diabetes insipidus)	A number of kidney diseases, including hypercalcemic and hypokalemic nephropathy; drug toxicity (e.g., from lithium)	Thirst and polydipsia, often severe and persistent; nocturia
	Solute diuresis		
	Electrolytes, such as sodium salts	Large saline infusions, potent diuretics, certain kidney diseases	Variable
	Nonelectrolytes, such as glucose	Uncontrolled diabetes mellitus	Thirst, polydipsia, and nocturia
	Excessive water intake	Primary polydipsia	Polydipsia tends to be episodic; thirst may not be present; nocturia is usually absent

TABLE 14-4. Urinary Incontinence[a]

Problem	Mechanisms	Symptoms	Physical Signs
Stress Incontinence			
The urethral sphincter is weakened so that transient increases in intraabdominal pressure raise the bladder pressure to levels that exceed urethral resistance.	In women, pelvic floor weakness and inadequate muscular and ligamentous support of the bladder neck and proximal urethra change the angle between the bladder and the urethra. Causes include childbirth and surgery. Local conditions affecting the internal urethral sphincter, such as postmenopausal atrophy of the mucosa and urethral infection, may also contribute. In men, stress incontinence may follow prostate surgery.	Momentary leakage of small amounts of urine with coughing, laughing, and sneezing while the person is in an upright position. Urine loss is unrelated to a conscious urge to urinate.	Stress incontinence may be demonstrable, especially if the patient is examined before voiding and in a standing position. Atrophic vaginitis may be evident. Bladder distention is absent.
Urge Incontinence			
Detrusor contractions are stronger than normal and overcome the normal urethral resistance. The bladder is typically small.	Decreased cortical inhibition of detrusor contractions from stroke, brain tumor, dementia, and lesions of the spinal cord above the sacral level.	Involuntary urine loss preceded by an urge to void. The volume tends to be moderate.	The small bladder is not detectable on abdominal examination.
	Hyperexcitability of sensory pathways, as in bladder infections, tumors, and fecal impaction.	Urgency, frequency, and nocturia with small to moderate volumes. If acute inflammation is present, pain on urination.	When cortical inhibition is decreased, mental deficits or motor signs of central nervous system disease are often present.
	Deconditioning of voiding reflexes, as in frequent voluntary voiding at low bladder volumes.	Possibly "pseudostress incontinence"—voiding 10 to 20 seconds after stresses such as a change of position, going upstairs or downstairs, and possibly coughing, laughing, or sneezing.	When sensory pathways are hyperexcitable, signs of local pelvic problems or a fecal impaction may be present.
Overflow Incontinence			
Detrusor contractions are insufficient to overcome urethral resistance, causing urinary retention. The bladder is typically flaccid and large, even after an effort to void.	Obstruction of the bladder outlet, as in benign prostatic hyperplasia or tumor. Weakness of the detrusor muscle associated with peripheral nerve disease at S2–S4 level. Impaired bladder sensation that interrupts the reflex arc, as in diabetic neuropathy.	When intravesicular pressure overcomes urethral resistance, continuous dripping or dribbling incontinence ensues. Decreased force of the urinary stream. Prior symptoms of partial urinary obstruction or other symptoms of peripheral nerve disease may be present.	Examination often reveals an enlarged, sometimes tender, bladder. Other signs include prostatic enlargement, motor signs of peripheral nerve disease, a decrease in sensation (including perineal sensation), and diminished to absent reflexes.

(continued)

TABLE 14-4. Urinary Incontinence[a] *(Continued)*

Problem	Mechanisms	Symptoms	Physical Signs
Functional Incontinence			
The patient is functionally unable to reach the toilet in time because of impaired health or environmental conditions.	Problems in mobility resulting from weakness, arthritis, poor vision, or other conditions. Environmental factors such as an unfamiliar setting, distant bathroom facilities, bed rails, or physical restraints.	Incontinence on the way to the toilet or only in the early morning.	The bladder is not detectable on examination. Look for physical or environmental clues as the likely cause.
Incontinence Secondary to Medications			
Drugs may contribute to any type of incontinence listed.	Sedatives, antipsychotics, anticholinergics, sympathetic blockers, and potent diuretics.	Variable. A careful history and chart review are important.	Variable.

[a]Patients may have more than one kind of incontinence.

TABLE 14-5. BPH Symptom Score: American Urological Association

Score or ask the patient to score each of the questions below. Higher scores (maximum 35) indicate more severe symptoms; scores ≤7 are considered mild and generally do not warrant treatment.

PART A	Not at All	Less Than 1 Time in 5	Less Than Half the Time	About Half the Time	More Than Half the Time	Almost Always	Total Points for Each Row
1. **Incomplete emptying:** Over the past month, how often have you had a sensation of not emptying your bladder completely after you finished urinating?	0	1	2	3	4	5	
2. **Frequency:** Over the past month, how often have you had to urinate again <2 hours after you finished urinating?	0	1	2	3	4	5	
3. **Intermittency:** Over the past month, how often have you stopped and started again several times when you urinated?	0	1	2	3	4	5	
4. **Urgency:** Over the past month, how often have you found it difficult to postpone urination?	0	1	2	3	4	5	
5. **Weak stream:** Over the past month, how often have you had a weak urinary stream?	0	1	2	3	4	5	
6. **Straining:** Over the past month, how often have you had to push or strain to begin urination?	0	1	2	3	4	5	
PART B	**None**	**1 Time**	**2 Times**	**3 Times**	**4 Times**	**5 Times**	**Points for Part B**
7. **Nocturia:** Over the past month, how many times did you most typically get up to urinate from the time you went to bed at night until the time you got up in the morning?	0	1	2	3	4	5	

TOTAL PARTS A and B (maximum 35)_____

Source: Adapted from Madsen FA, Bruskewitz RC. *Urol Clin North Am.* 1995;22(2):291–298. Copyright © 1995 Elsevier. With permission.

TABLE 14-6. Sexually Transmitted Infections of the Male Genitalia

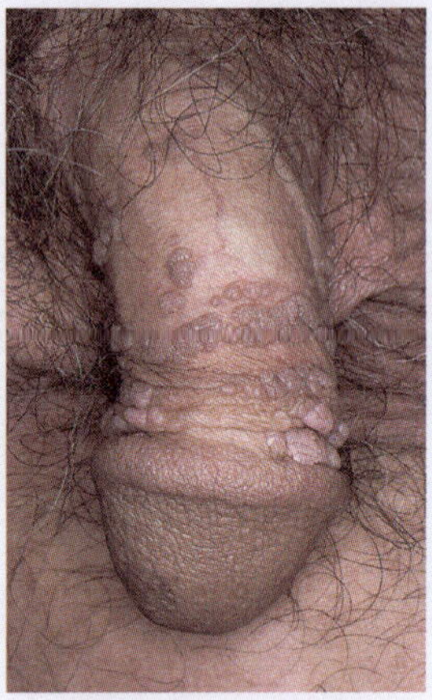

Genital Warts (Condylomata Acuminata)

- *Appearance:* Single or multiple papules or plaques of variable shapes; may be round, acuminate (pointed), or thin and slender. May be raised, flat, or cauliflower-like (verrucous).
- *Causative organism:* HPV, usually subtypes 6, 11; carcinogenic subtypes rare, approximately 5% to 10% of all anogenital warts. Incubation: Weeks to months; infected contact may have no visible warts.
- Can arise on penis, scrotum, groin, thighs, anus; usually asymptomatic, occasionally cause itching and pain.
- May disappear without treatment.

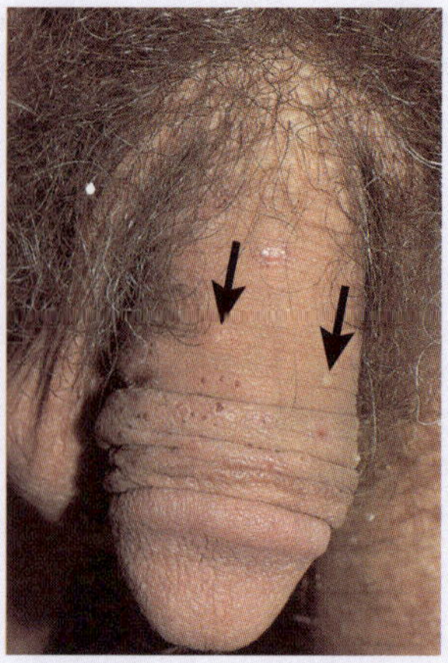

Genital Herpes Simplex

- *Appearance:* Small scattered or grouped vesicles, 1 to 3 mm in size, on glans or shaft of penis. Appear as erosions if vesicular membrane breaks.
- *Causative organism:* Usually *herpes simplex virus* 2 (90%), a double-stranded DNA virus. *Incubation:* 2 to 7 days after exposure.
- Primary episode may be asymptomatic; recurrence usually less painful, of shorter duration.
- Associated with fever, malaise, headache, arthralgias, local pain and edema, lymphadenopathy.
- Need to distinguish from genital herpes zoster (usually in older patients with dermatomal distribution) and candidiasis.

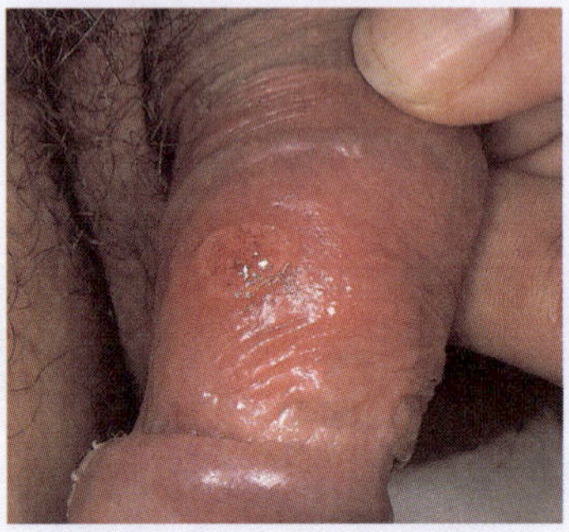

Primary Syphilis

- *Appearance:* Small red papule that becomes a chancre, a painless erosion up to 2 cm in diameter. Base of chancre is clean, red, smooth, and glistening; borders are raised and indurated. Chancre heals within 3 to 8 weeks.
- *Causative organism: Treponema pallidum*, a spirochete. Incubation: 9 to 90 days after exposure.
- May develop inguinal lymphadenopathy within 7 days; lymph nodes are rubbery, nontender, mobile.
- 20% to 30% of patients develop secondary syphilis while chancre still present (suggests coinfection with HIV).
- Distinguish from: genital herpes simplex; chancroid; granuloma inguinale from *Klebsiella granulomatis*.

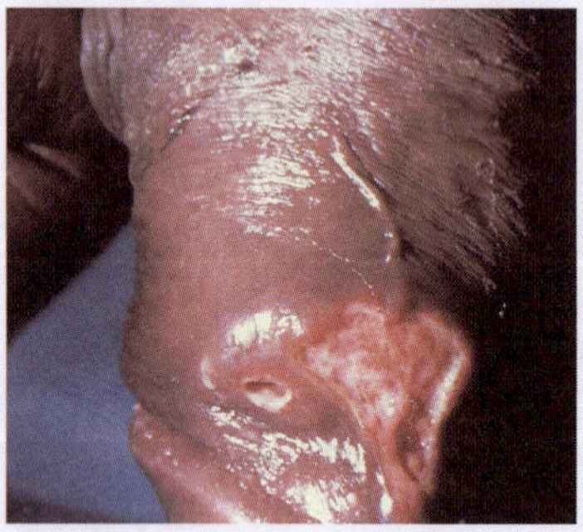

Chancroid

- *Appearance:* Red papule or pustule initially, and then forms a painful deep ulcer with ragged nonindurated margins; contains necrotic exudate, has a friable base.
- *Causative organism: Haemophilus ducreyi*, an anaerobic bacillus. *Incubation:* 3 to 7 days after exposure.
- Painful inguinal adenopathy; suppurative buboes in 25% of patients.
- Need to distinguish from: primary syphilis; genital herpes simplex; lymphogranuloma venereum, granuloma inguinale from *K. granulomatis*.

TABLE 14-7. Abnormalities of the Penis and Scrotum

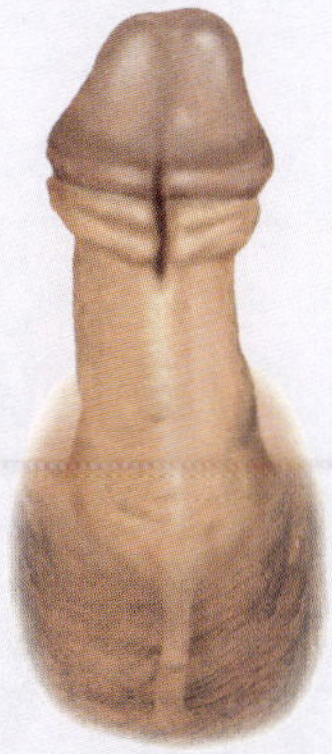

Hypospadias
A congenital displacement of the urethral meatus to the inferior surface of the penis. The meatus may be subcoronal, midshaft, or at the junction of the penis and scrotum (penoscrotal).

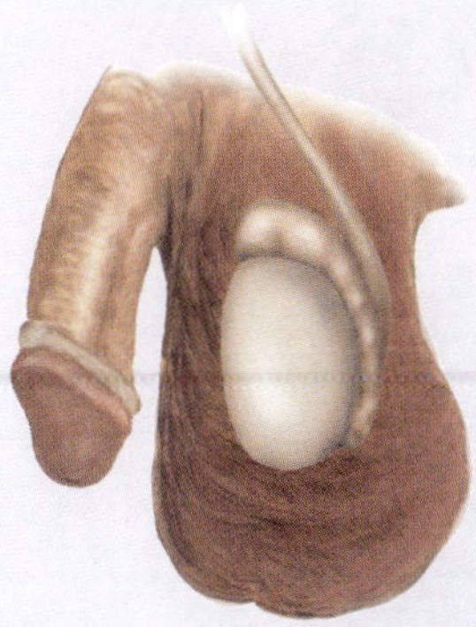

Scrotal Edema
Pitting edema may make the scrotal skin taut; seen in heart failure, liver failure, or nephrotic syndrome.

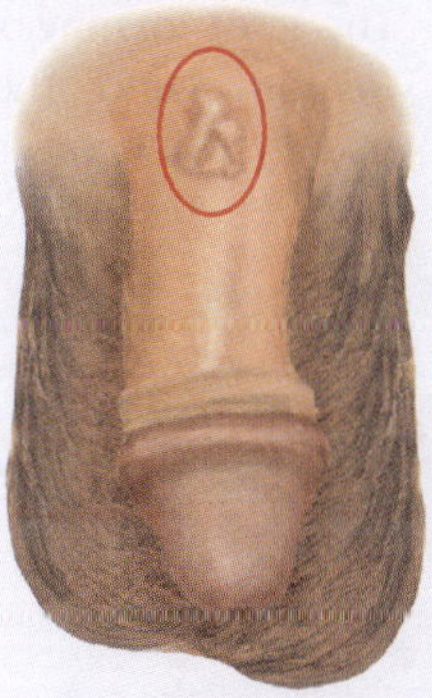

Peyronie Disease
Palpable, nontender, hard plaques are found just beneath the skin, usually along the dorsum of the penis. The patient complains of curved, painful erections.

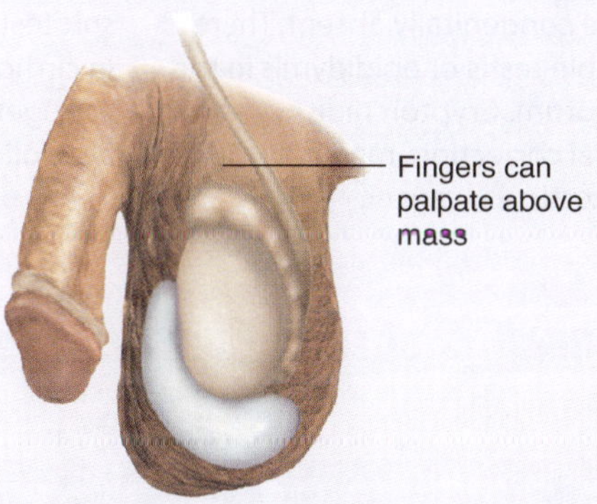

Hydrocele
A nontender, fluid-filled mass within the tunica vaginalis. It transilluminates, and the examining fingers can palpate above the mass within the scrotum.

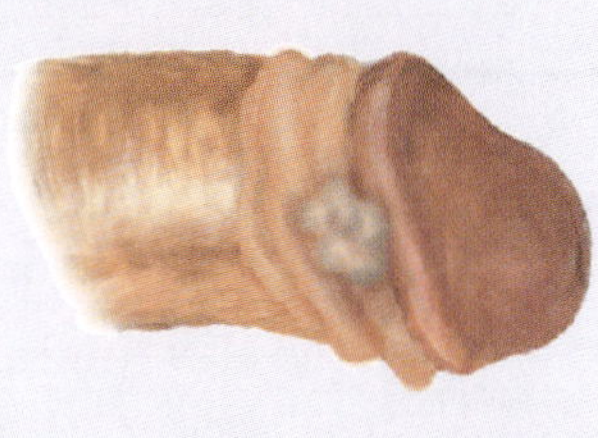

Carcinoma of the Penis
An indurated nodule or ulcer that is usually nontender. Limited almost completely to men who are not circumcised, it may be masked by the prepuce. Any persistent penile sore is suspicious.

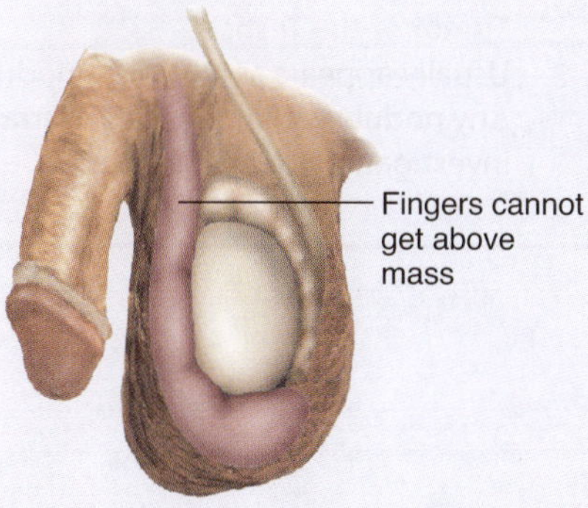

Scrotal Hernia
Usually an indirect inguinal hernia that comes through the external inguinal ring, so the examining fingers cannot get above it within the scrotum.

TABLE 14-8. Abnormalities of the Testis

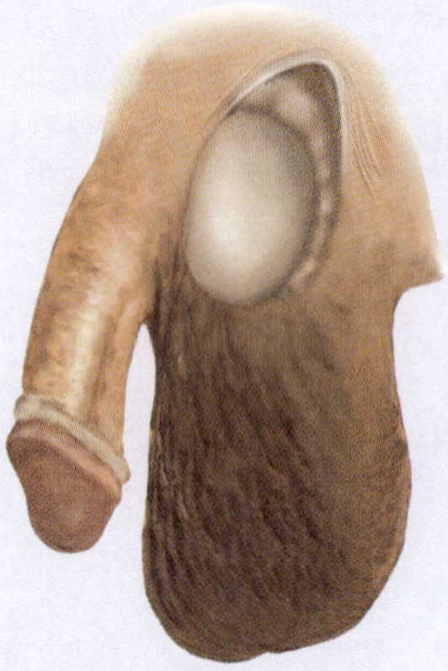

Cryptorchidism
The testis is atrophied and lies outside the scrotum in the inguinal canal or abdomen, or near the pubic tubercle; it may also be congenitally absent. There is no palpable testis or epididymis in the unfilled scrotum. Cryptorchidism, even with surgical correction, markedly raises the risk of testicular cancer.

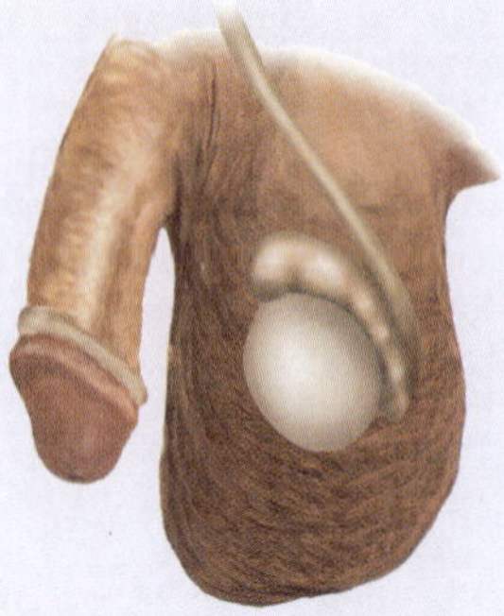

Small Testis
In adults, testicular length is usually ≤3.5 cm. Small firm testes usually ≤2 cm suggest Klinefelter syndrome. Small soft testes suggesting atrophy are seen in cirrhosis, myotonic dystrophy, use of estrogens, and hypopituitarism; may also follow severe orchitis.

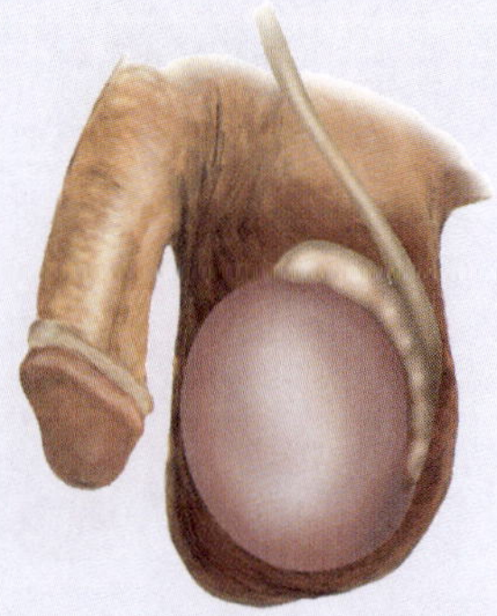

Acute Orchitis
The testis is acutely inflamed, painful, tender, and swollen. It may be difficult to distinguish from the epididymis. The scrotum may be reddened. Seen in mumps and other viral infections; usually unilateral.

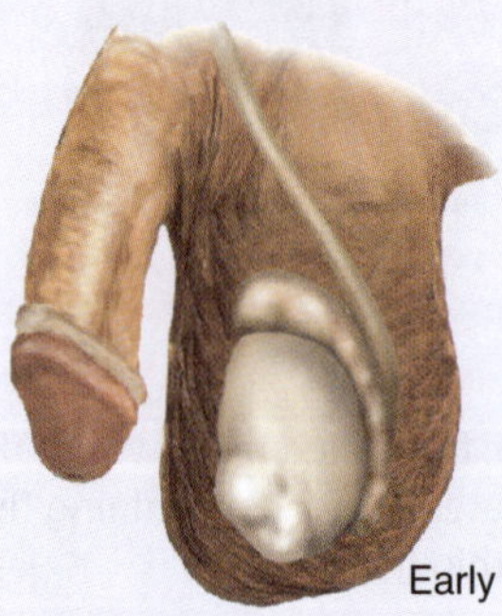

Early

Tumor of the Testis
Usually appears as a painless nodule. Any nodule within the testis warrants investigation for malignancy.

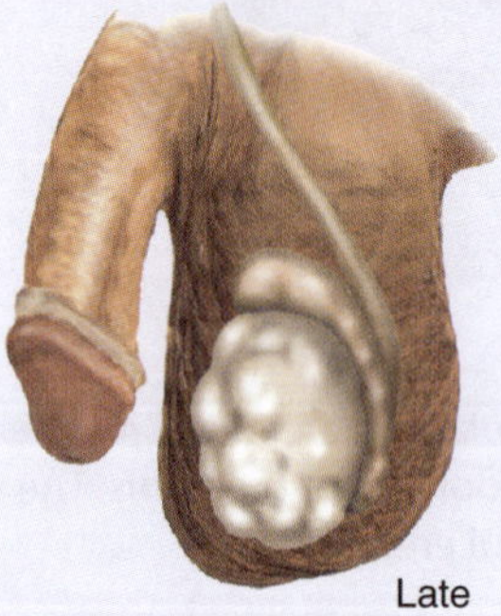

Late

As a testicular neoplasm grows and spreads, it may seem to replace the entire organ. The testicle characteristically feels heavier than normal.

TABLE 14-9. Vaginal Discharge

Discharge from a vaginal infection must be distinguished from a physiologic discharge. A physiologic discharge is clear or white, may contain white clumps of epithelial cells, and is not malodorous. To distinguish vaginal from cervical discharges, use a large cotton swab to wipe off the cervix. If no cervical discharge is present in the os, suspect a vaginal origin and consider the causes below. Note that the diagnosis of cervicitis or vaginitis hinges on careful collection and analysis of the appropriate laboratory specimens.

	Trichomonal Vaginitis	Candidal Vaginitis	Bacterial Vaginosis
	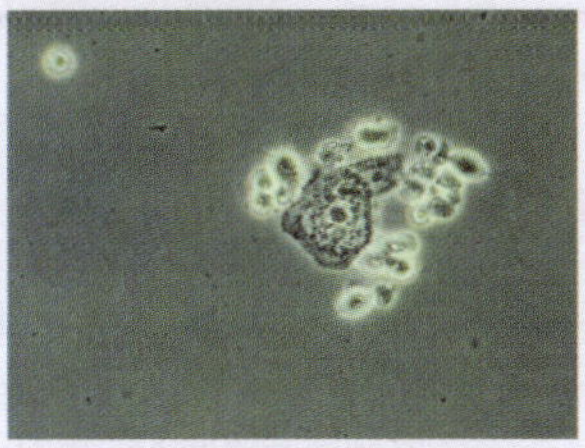	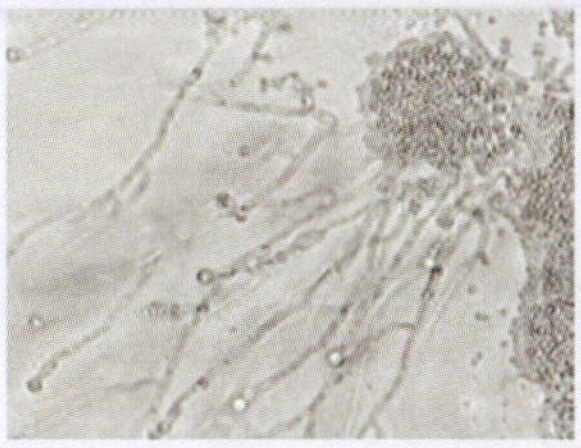	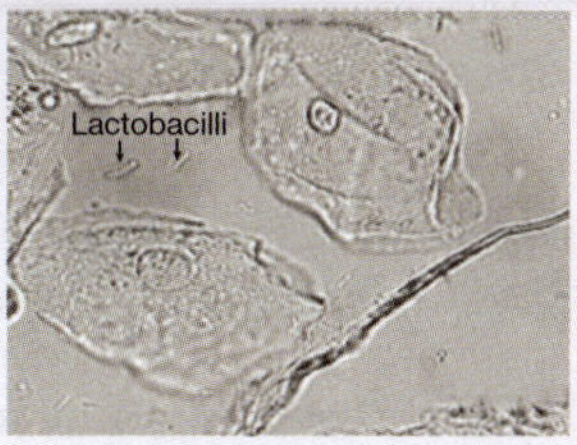
Cause	*Trichomonas vaginalis*, a protozoan; often but not always acquired sexually	*Candida albicans*, a yeast (normal overgrowth of vaginal flora); many factors predispose, including antibiotic therapy	Bacterial overgrowth probably from anaerobic bacteria; often transmitted sexually
Discharge	Yellowish green or gray, possibly frothy; often profuse and pooled in the vaginal fornix; may be malodorous	White and curdy; may be thin but typically thick; not as profuse as in trichomonal infection; not malodorous	Gray or white, thin, homogeneous, malodorous; coats the vaginal walls; usually not profuse, may be minimal
Other Symptoms	Pruritus (though not usually as severe as with *Candida* infection); pain on urination (from skin inflammation or possibly urethritis); dyspareunia	Pruritus; vaginal soreness; pain on urination (from skin inflammation); dyspareunia	Unpleasant fishy or musty genital odor; reported to occur after intercourse
Vulva and Vaginal Mucosa	Vestibule and labia minora may be erythematous; the vaginal mucosa may be diffusely reddened, with small red granular spots or petechiae in the posterior fornix; in mild cases, the mucosa looks normal	The vulva and even the surrounding skin are often inflamed and sometimes swollen to a variable extent; the vaginal mucosa is often reddened, with white tenacious patches of discharge; the mucosa may bleed when these patches are scraped off; in mild cases, the mucosa looks normal	The vulva and vaginal mucosa usually appear normal
Laboratory Evaluation	Scan saline wet mount for trichomonads	Scan potassium hydroxide (KOH) preparation for the branching hyphae of *Candida*	Scan saline wet mount for *clue cells* (epithelial cells with stippled borders); sniff for fishy odor after applying KOH ("whiff test"); test the vaginal secretions for pH >4.5

TABLE 14-10. Abnormalities of the Epididymis and Spermatic Cord

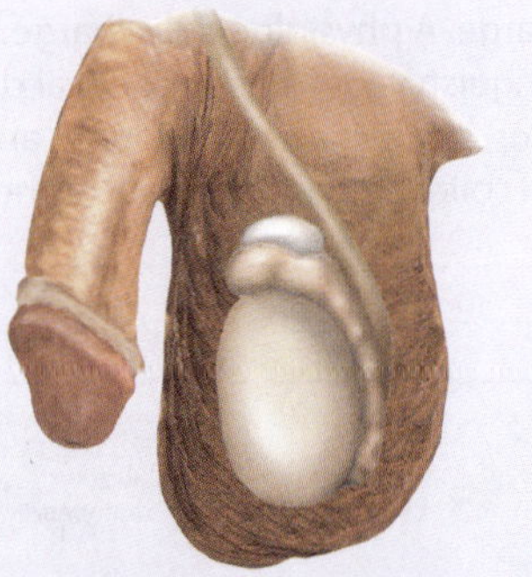

Spermatocele and Cyst of the Epididymis

A painless, movable cystic mass just above the testis suggests a spermatocele or an epididymal cyst. Both transilluminate. The former contains sperm, and the latter does not, but they are clinically indistinguishable.

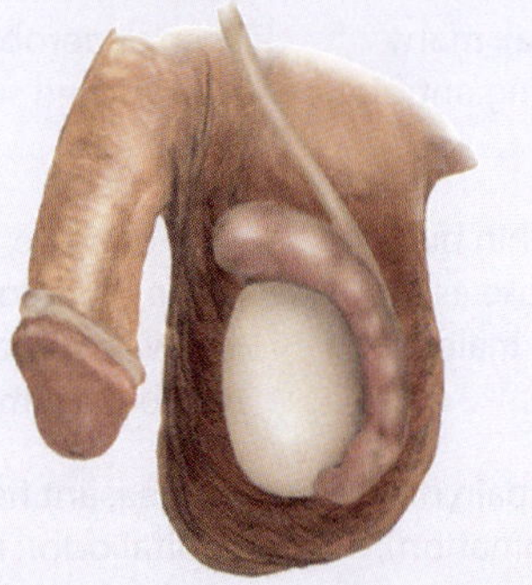

Acute Epididymitis

An acutely inflamed epididymis is indurated, swollen, and notably tender, making it difficult to distinguish from the testis. The scrotum may be reddened and the vas deferens inflamed. Causes include infection from *Neisseria gonorrhoeae*, *Chlamydia trachomatis* (younger adults), *Escherichia coli*, and *Pseudomonas* (older adults); trauma; and autoimmune disease. Barring urinary symptoms, urinalysis is often negative.

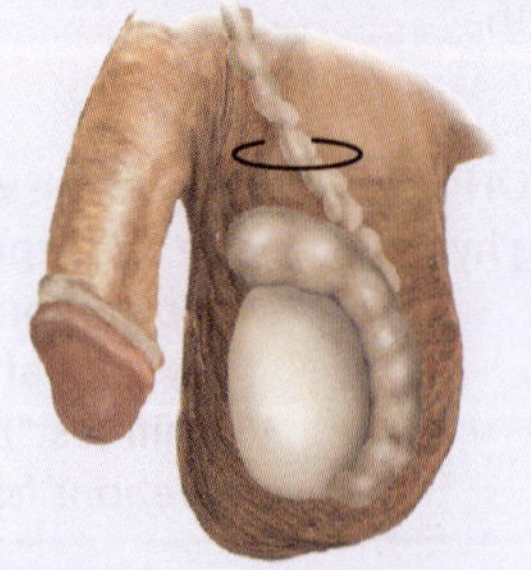

Tuberculous Epididymitis

The chronic inflammation of tuberculosis produces a firm enlargement of the epididymis, which is sometimes tender, with thickening or beading of the vas deferens.

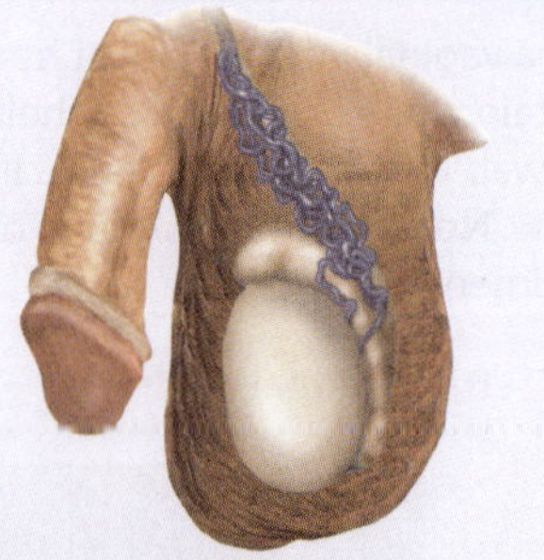

Varicocele of the Spermatic Cord

Varicocele refers to gravity-mediated varicose veins of the spermatic cord, usually found on the left. It feels like a soft "bag of worms" in the spermatic cord above the testis, and if prominent, appears to distort the contours of the scrotal skin. A varicocele collapses in the supine position, so examination should be both supine and standing. If the varicocele does not collapse when the patient is supine, suspect a left spermatic vein obstruction within the abdomen.

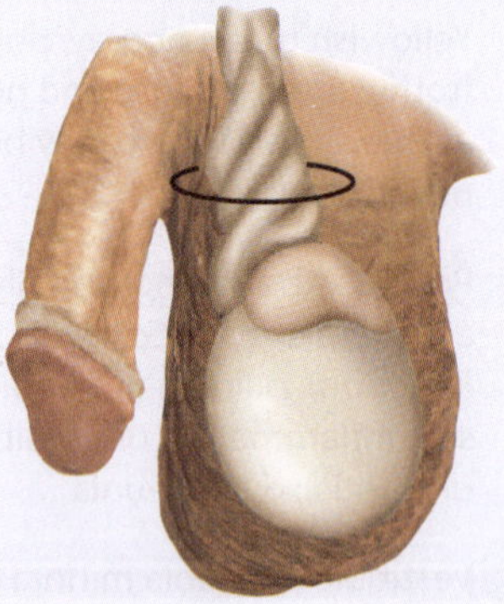

Testicular Torsion

Torsion, or twisting, of the testicle on its spermatic cord produces an acutely painful, tender, and swollen organ that is often retracted upward in the scrotum. The cremasteric reflex is nearly always absent on the affected side in boys or men with testicular torsion, though this can be difficult to assess during acute pain episodes. If the presentation is delayed, the scrotum becomes red and edematous. There is no associated urinary infection. Torsion is most common in neonates and adolescents but can occur at any age. It is a surgical emergency because of obstructed circulation and requires urgent surgical consultation.

TABLE 14-11. Abnormalities of the Anus, Surrounding Skin, and Rectum

Pilonidal Cyst and Sinus

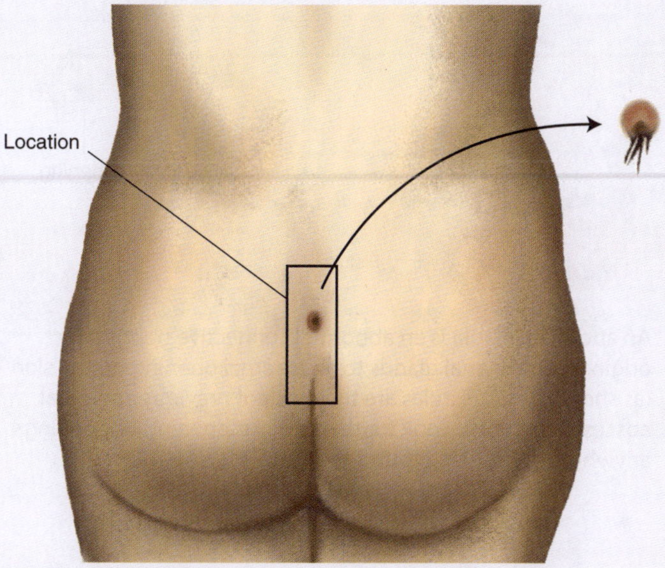

A pilonidal cyst is a fairly common, probably congenital, abnormality located in the midline natal cleft. Look for the opening of a sinus tract, sometimes with a small tuft of hair surrounded by a halo of erythema. Pilonidal cysts are generally asymptomatic, except for slight drainage, but abscess formation and secondary sinus tracts may occur.

External Hemorrhoids (*Thrombosed*)

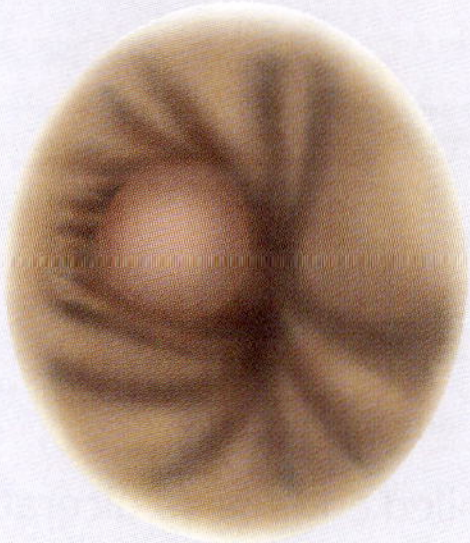

External hemorrhoids are dilated hemorrhoidal veins that originate below the pectinate line that are covered with skin. They seldom produce symptoms unless thrombosis occurs. Thrombosis causes acute local pain that increases with defecation and sitting. A tender, swollen, bluish, ovoid mass is visible at the anal margin.

Internal Hemorrhoids (*Prolapsed*)

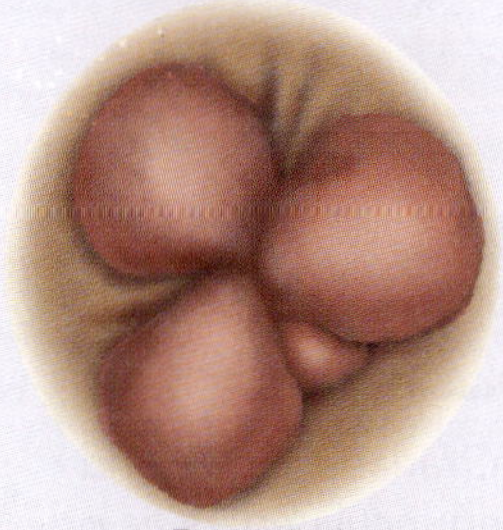

Internal hemorrhoids are enlargements of the normal vascular cushions located above the pectinate line, usually not palpable. They may cause bright red bleeding, especially during defecation. They may also prolapse through the anal canal and appear as reddish, moist, protruding masses, typically located in one or more of the positions illustrated.

Prolapse of the Rectum

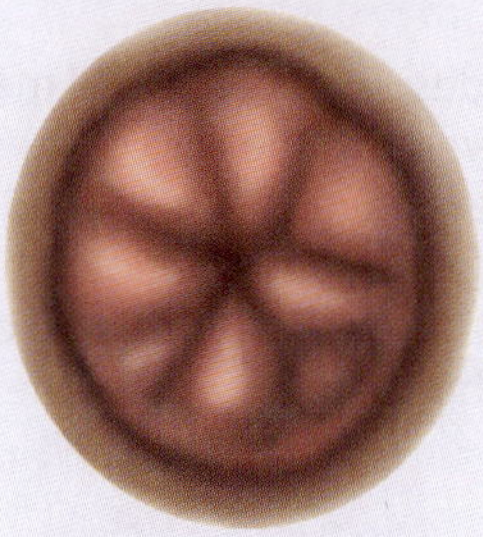

On straining for a bowel movement, the rectal mucosa, with or without its muscular wall, may prolapse through the anus, telescoping through the anal verge. A prolapse involving only mucosa is relatively small and shows radiating folds, as illustrated. When the entire bowel wall is involved, the prolapse is larger and covered by concentrically circular folds.

(*continued*)

TABLE 14-11. Abnormalities of the Anus, Surrounding Skin, and Rectum *(Continued)*

Anal Fissure

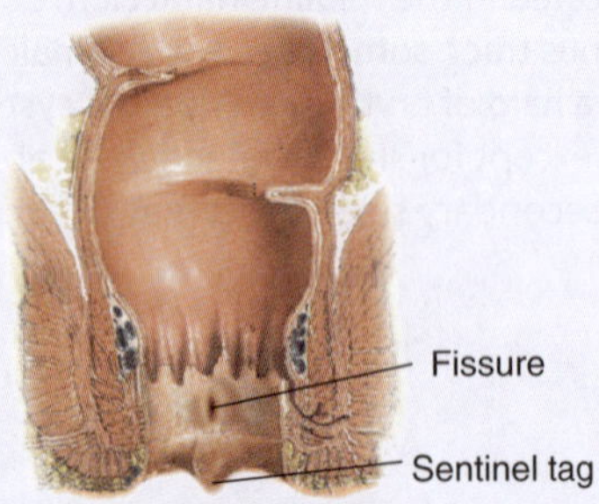

An anal fissure is a very painful tear/ulceration of the anoderm, found most commonly in the midline posteriorly, less commonly in the midline anteriorly. Its long axis lies longitudinally. There may be a swollen "sentinel" skin tag just below it. Gentle separation of the anal margins may reveal the lower edge of the fissure. The sphincter is spastic; the examination is painful. An examination under anesthesia may be necessary to fully characterize the lesion.

Anorectal Fistula

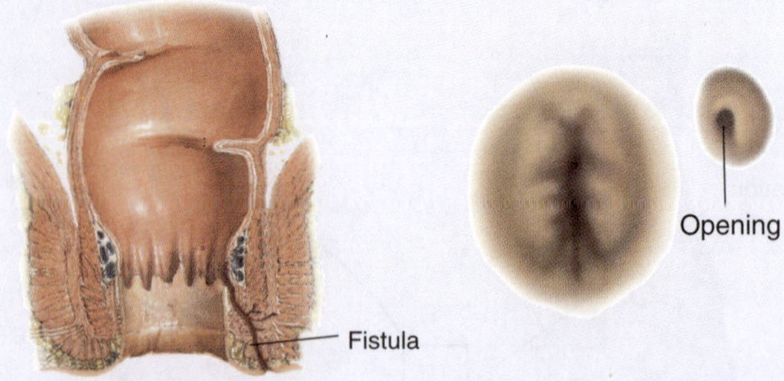

An anorectal fistula is an abnormal connective tract that originates from anal glands to an external opening on the skin (as shown here). Fistulas are the result of previous anorectal abscess/infections. Look for the fistulous opening or openings anywhere in the skin around the anus.

Polyps of the Rectum

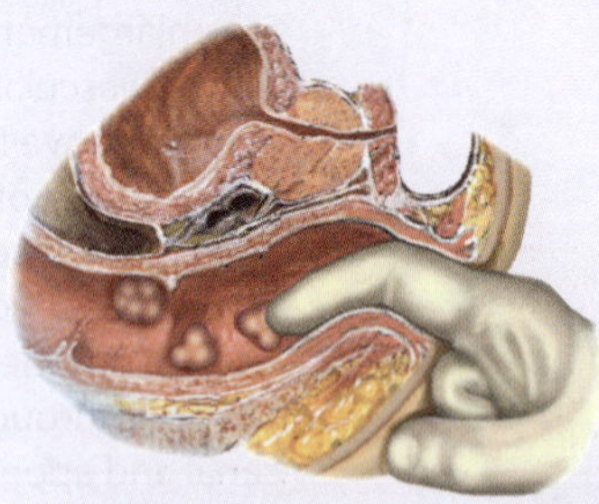

Polyps of the rectum are fairly common. Variable in size and number, they can develop on a stalk (pedunculated) or lie on the mucosal surface (sessile). They are soft and may be difficult or impossible to feel even when in reach of the examining finger. Endoscopy and biopsy are needed for differentiation of benign from malignant lesions.

Cancer of the Rectum

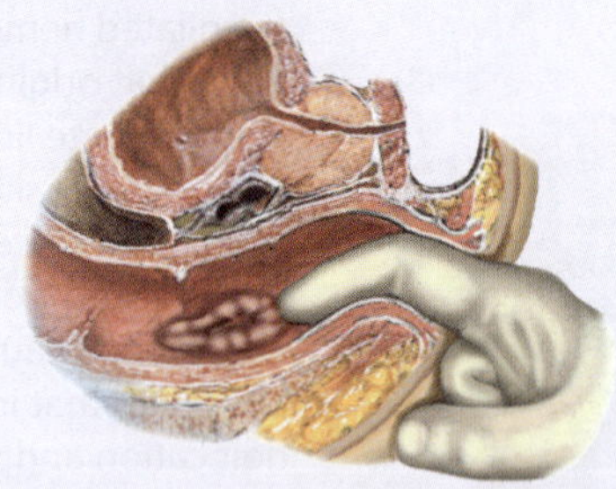

Illustrated here is the firm, nodular, rolled edge of an ulcerated cancer.

Rectal Shelf

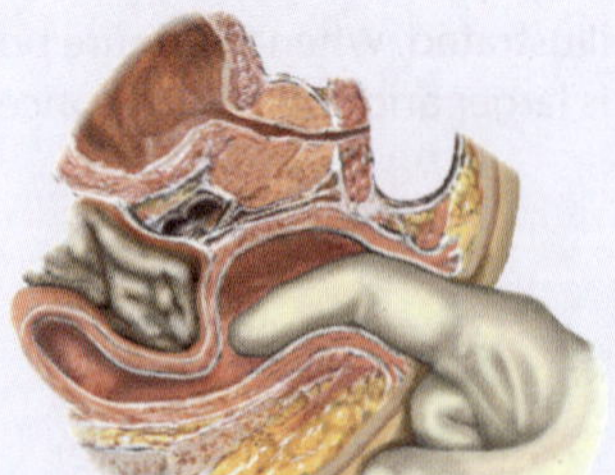

Widespread peritoneal metastases from any source may develop in the area of the peritoneal reflection anterior to the rectum. A firm to hard nodular rectal "shelf" may be just palpable with the tip of the examining finger. In a woman, this shelf of metastatic tissue develops in the rectouterine pouch, behind the cervix and the uterus.

TABLE 14-12. Abnormalities of the Prostate

Normal Prostate Gland

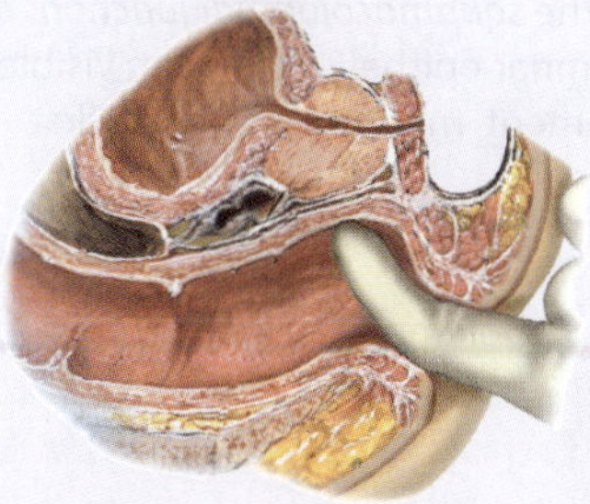

As palpated through the anterior rectal wall, the normal prostate is a rounded, heart-shaped structure approximately 2.5 cm long. The median sulcus can be palpated between the two lateral lobes. Only the posterior surface of the prostate is palpable. Anterior and central lesions, including those that obstruct the urethra, are not detectable by physical examination as they are not in contact with the rectal wall.

Prostatitis

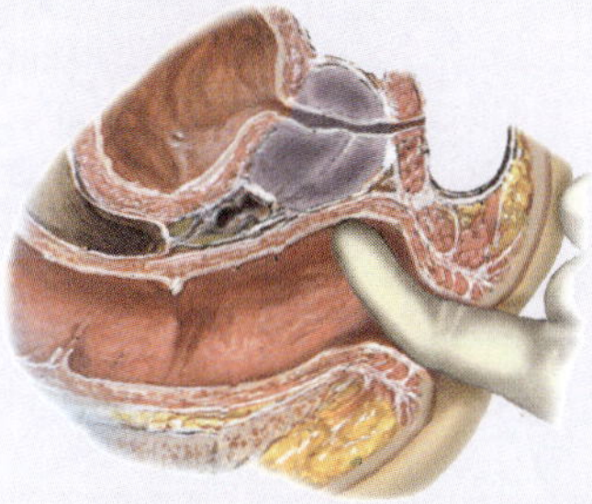

Acute bacterial prostatitis, illustrated here, presents with fever and urinary tract symptoms such as frequency, urgency, dysuria, incomplete voiding, and sometimes low back pain. The gland feels tender, swollen, "boggy," and warm. Examine it gently as it can be extremely tender and painful for the patient. More than 80% of infections are caused by gram-negative aerobes such as *Escherichia coli* and *Enterococcus* and *Proteus* spp. In men younger than age 35 years, consider sexual transmission of *Neisseria gonorrhea* and *Chlamydia trachomatis*.

Chronic bacterial prostatitis is associated with recurrent urinary tract infections, usually from the same organism. Men may be asymptomatic or have symptoms of dysuria or mild pelvic pain. The prostate gland may feel normal, without tenderness or swelling. Cultures of prostatic fluid usually show infection with *E. coli*.

It may be challenging to distinguish these conditions from the more common chronic pelvic pain syndrome, seen in up to 80% of symptomatic men who report obstructive or irritative symptoms on voiding but show no evidence of prostate or urinary tract infection. Physical examination findings are not predictable, but examination is needed to assess any prostate induration or asymmetry suggestive of more acute processes, benign prostatic hyperplasia (BPH), or carcinoma.

BPH

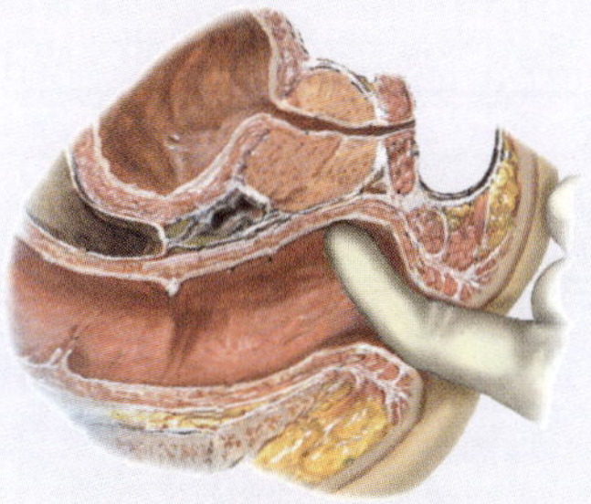

BPH is a nonmalignant enlargement of the prostate gland that increases with age, present in more than 50% of men by age 50 years. Symptoms arise both from smooth-muscle contraction in the prostate and bladder neck and from compression of the urethra by hypertrophied prostate tissue. They may be irritative (urgency, frequency, nocturia), obstructive (decreased stream, incomplete emptying, straining), or both, and are seen in more than one-third of men by age 65 years. The affected gland may be normal in size, or may feel symmetrically enlarged, smooth, and firm, though slightly elastic; there may be obliteration of the median sulcus and more notable protrusion into the rectal lumen. Because of the limited nature of the digital rectal examination, the severity of symptoms may not correlate with the examination findings.

Prostate Cancer

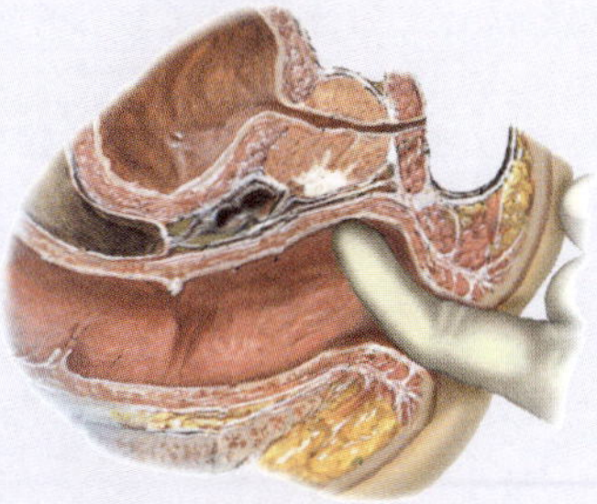

Prostate cancer is suggested by an area of hardness in the gland, such as a distinct hard nodule or firmness. As the cancer enlarges, it feels irregular and may extend beyond the confines of the gland. The median sulcus may be obscured. Hard areas in the prostate are not always malignant. They may also result from prostatic stones, chronic inflammation, and other conditions.

TABLE 14-13. Variations in the Cervical Surface

Two kinds of epithelia cover the cervix: (1) shiny pink *squamous epithelium*, which resembles the vaginal epithelium, and (2) deep red, plushy *columnar epithelium*, which is continuous with the endocervical lining. These meet at the *squamocolumnar junction*. When this junction is at or inside the cervical os, only squamous epithelium is seen. A ring of columnar epithelium is often visible to a varying extent around the os—the result of a normal process that accompanies fetal development, menarche, and the first pregnancy.[a]

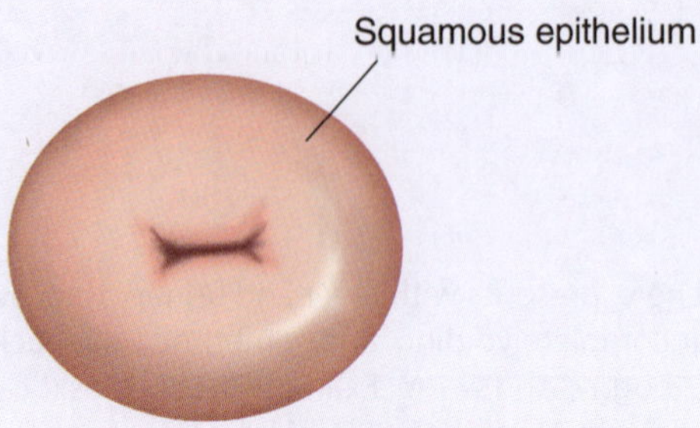

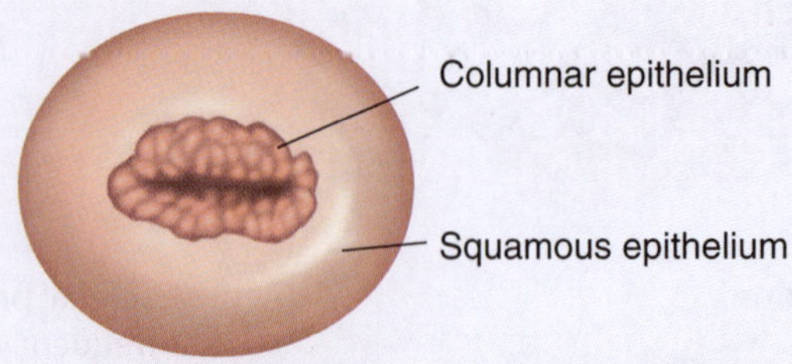

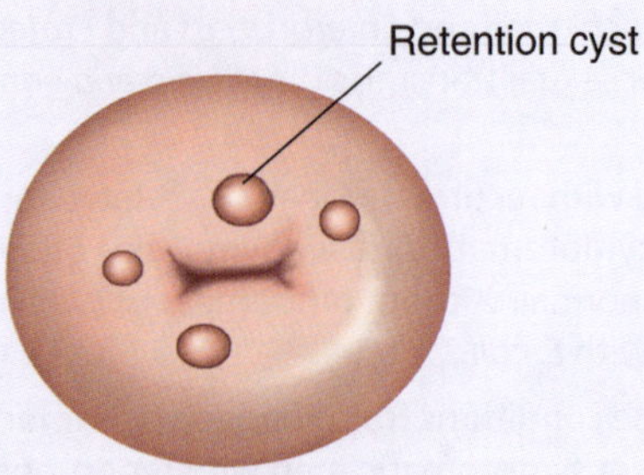

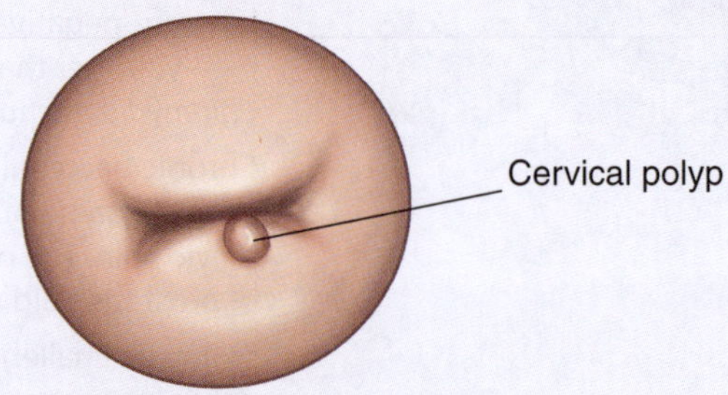

As estrogen stimulation increases during adolescence, all or part of this columnar epithelium is transformed into squamous epithelium by a process termed *metaplasia*. This change may block the secretions of columnar epithelium and cause *retention cysts*, also called *nabothian cysts*. These appear as translucent nodules on the cervical surface and have no pathologic significance.

A cervical polyp usually arises from the endocervical canal, becoming visible when it protrudes through the cervical os. It is bright red, soft, and rather fragile. When only the tip is seen, it cannot be differentiated clinically from a polyp originating in the endometrium. Polyps are benign but may bleed.

[a]Other terms for the columnar epithelium visible on the ectocervix are *ectropion*, *ectopy*, and *eversion*.

TABLE 14-14. Shapes of the Cervical Os

Normal

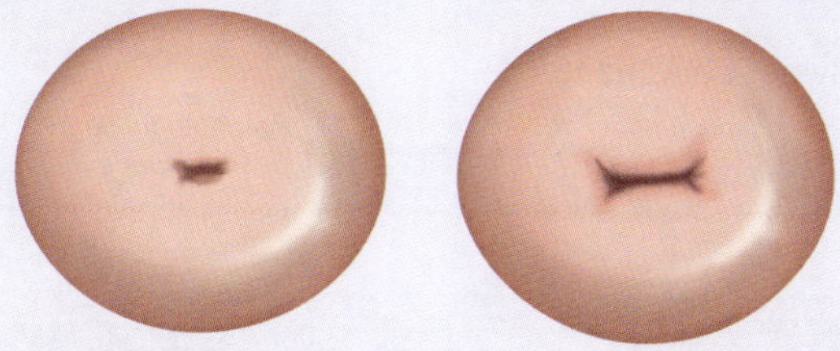

Oval Slit-like

Types of Lacerations from Delivery

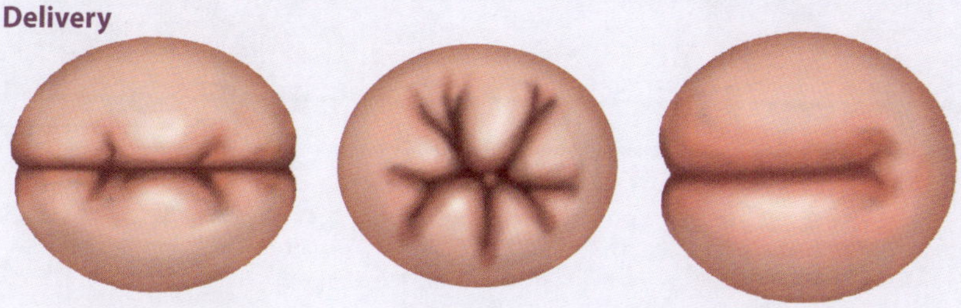

Bilateral transverse Stellate Unilateral transverse

TABLE 14-15. Abnormalities of the Cervix

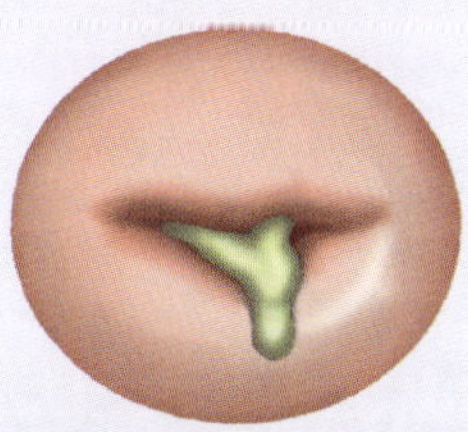

Mucopurulent Cervicitis

Mucopurulent cervicitis produces purulent yellow drainage from the cervical os, usually from *C. trachomatis*, *N. gonorrhoeae*, or herpes infection. These infections are sexually transmitted and may occur without symptoms or signs.

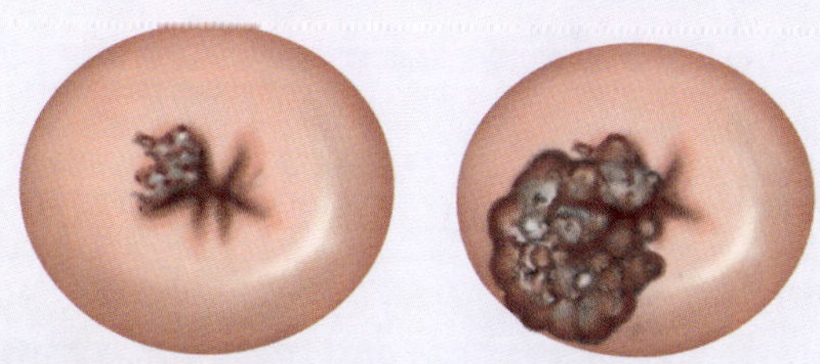

Carcinoma of the Cervix

Carcinoma of the cervix begins in an area of metaplasia. In its earliest stages, it cannot be distinguished from a normal cervix. In later stages, an extensive, irregular, cauliflower-like growth may develop. Early frequent intercourse, multiple partners, smoking, and infection with human papillomavirus increase the risk for cervical cancer.

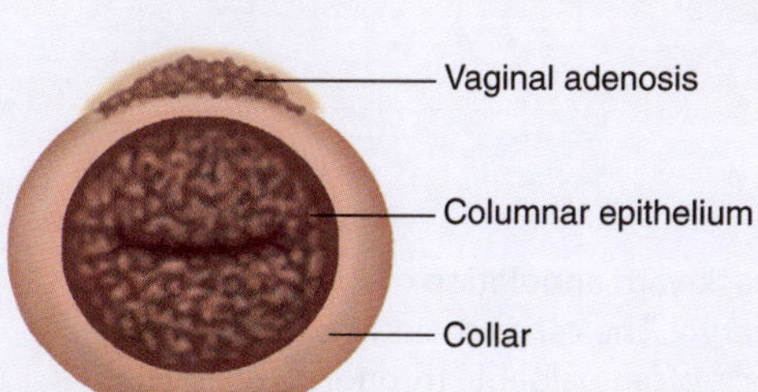

Fetal Exposure to Diethylstilbestrol (DES)

Daughters of women who took DES during pregnancy are at greatly increased risk for several abnormalities, including (1) columnar epithelium that covers most or all of the cervix, (2) vaginal adenosis (i.e., extension of this epithelium to the vaginal wall), and (3) a circular collar or ridge of tissue, of varying shapes, between the cervix and the vagina. Much less common is an otherwise rare carcinoma of the upper vagina.

TABLE 14-16. Positions of the Uterus

Retroversion and retroflexion are usually normal variants.

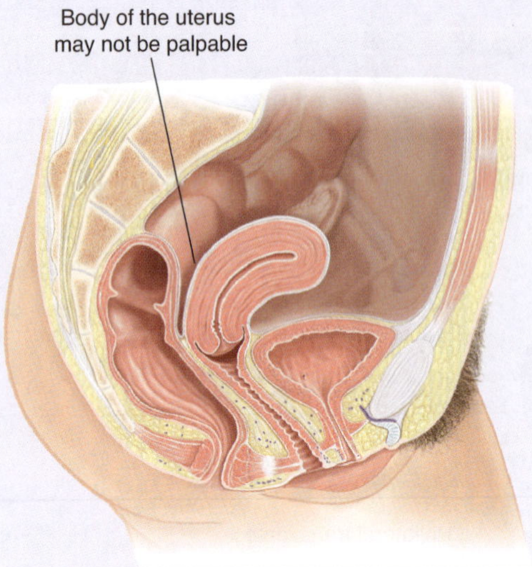

Moderate retroversion

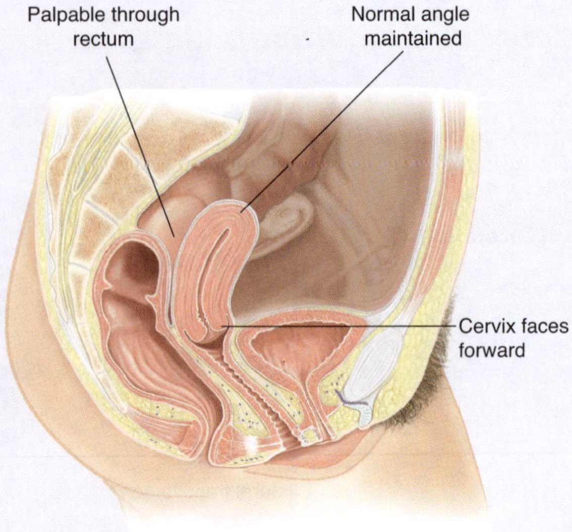

Marked retroversion

Retroversion of the Uterus

Retroversion of the uterus refers to a tilting backward of the entire uterus, including both the body and the cervix. It is a common variant occurring in approximately 20% of women. Early clues on pelvic examination are a cervix that faces forward and a uterine body that cannot be felt by the abdominal hand. In ***moderate retroversion***, the body may not be palpable with either hand. In ***marked retroversion***, the body can be felt posteriorly, either through the posterior fornix or through the rectum. A retroverted uterus is usually both mobile and asymptomatic. Occasionally, such a uterus is fixed and immobile, held in place by conditions such as endometriosis or PID.

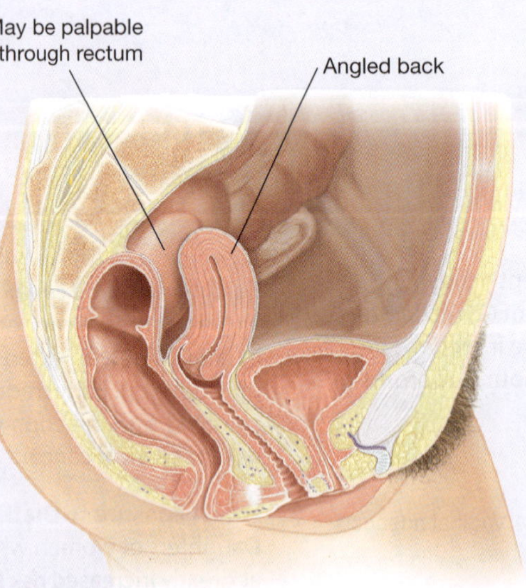

Retroflexion of the Uterus

Retroflexion of the uterus refers to a backward angulation of the body of the uterus in relation to the cervix. The cervix maintains its usual position. The body of the uterus is often palpable through the posterior fornix or through the rectum.

TABLE 14-17. Abnormalities of the Uterus

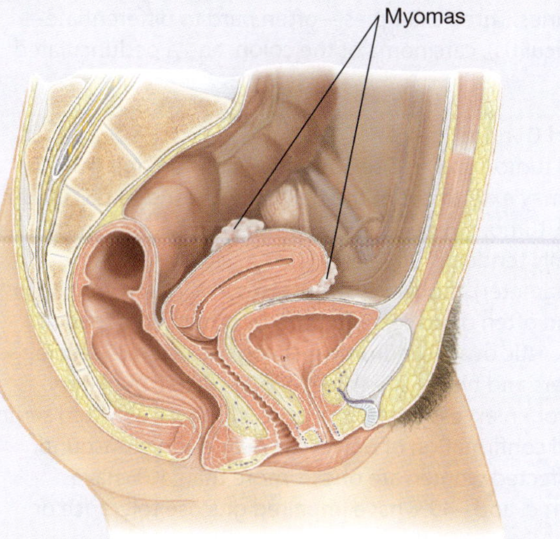

Myomas of the Uterus (Fibroids)

Myomas are very common benign uterine tumors. They may be single or multiple and vary greatly in size, occasionally reaching large proportions. They feel like firm irregular nodules that are continuous with the uterine surface. Occasionally, a myoma projecting laterally is confused with an ovarian mass; a nodule projecting posteriorly can be mistaken for a retroflexed uterus. Submucosal myomas project toward the endometrial cavity and are not palpable, although they may be suspected because of an enlarged uterus.

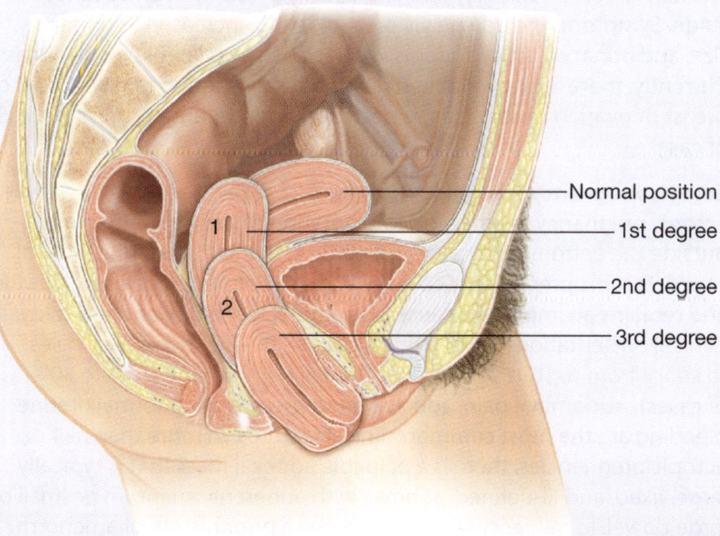

Prolapse of the Uterus

Prolapse of the uterus results from weakness of the supporting structures of the pelvic floor and is often associated with a cystocele and rectocele. In progressive stages, the uterus becomes retroverted and descends down the vaginal canal to the outside:

- In *first-degree prolapse*, the cervix is still well within the vagina.
- In *second-degree prolapse*, it is at the introitus.
- In *third-degree prolapse (procidentia)*, the cervix and vagina are outside the introitus.

TABLE 14-18. Adnexal Masses

Adnexal masses typically result from disorders of the fallopian tubes or ovaries. Three examples—often hard to differentiate—are described. Note that inflammatory disease of the bowel (such as diverticulitis), carcinoma of the colon, and a pedunculated myoma of the uterus may simulate an adnexal mass.

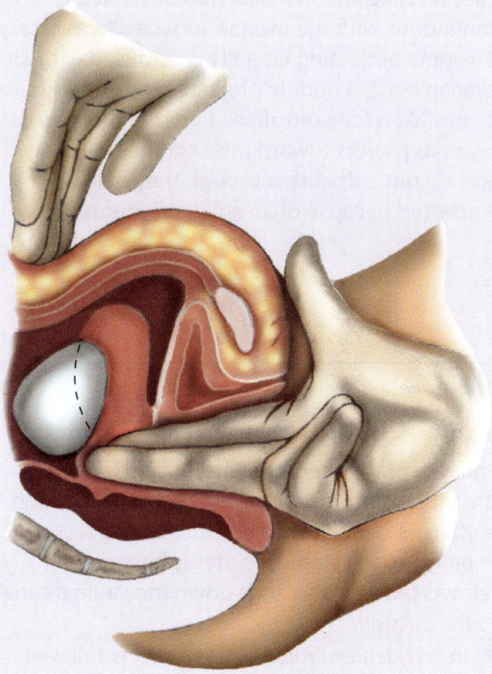

Ovarian Cysts and Ovarian Cancer

Ovarian cysts and tumors may cause adnexal masses on one or both sides. Later, they may extend out of the pelvis. Cysts tend to be smooth and compressible, tumors more solid and often nodular. Uncomplicated cysts are not usually tender.

Small (≤6 cm in diameter), mobile, cystic masses in a young woman are usually benign and often disappear after the next menstrual period.

Diagnosis of polycystic ovary syndrome rests on exclusion of several endocrine disorders and two of the three features listed: ovulatory dysfunction, androgen excess (hirsutism, acne, alopecia, elevated serum testosterone), and confirmation of polycystic ovaries on ultrasound. Roughly half of affected women are obese, more than 40% have metabolic syndrome, and ~40% have impaired glucose tolerance or diabetes.

Ovarian cancer is relatively rare and usually presents at an advanced stage. Symptoms include pelvic pain, bloating, increased abdominal size, and urinary tract symptoms; often there is a palpable ovarian mass. Currently, there are no reliable screening tests. A strong family history of breast or ovarian cancer is an important risk factor but occurs in only 5% of cases.

Ectopic Pregnancy, Including Rupture

Ectopic pregnancy results from implantation of the fertilized ovum outside the endometrial cavity, primarily in the fallopian tube (90% of cases). Ectopic pregnancy occurs in 1% to 2% of pregnancies worldwide and remains an important cause of maternal morbidity and mortality. Clinical presentation ranges from subacute, in ~80% to 90% of cases, to shock from rupture and intraperitoneal hemorrhage (10% to 30% of cases). Abdominal pain, adnexal tenderness, and abnormal uterine bleeding are the most common clinical features. In more than half of ectopic pregnancies, there is a palpable adnexal mass that is typically large, fixed, and ill-defined, at times with adherent omentum or small or large bowel. In milder cases, there may be a prior history of amenorrhea or other symptoms of a pregnancy.

Risk factors include tubal damage from PID, prior ectopic pregnancy, prior tubal surgery, age older than 35 years, presence of an IUD, subfertility (has altered tubal integrity), and assisted reproductive techniques.

Pelvic Inflammatory Disease

PID is due to "spontaneous ascension of microbes from the cervix or vagina to the endometrium, fallopian tubes, and adjacent structures." A total of 85% of cases involve STIs or bacterial vaginosis affecting the fallopian tubes (*salpingitis*) or the tubes and ovaries (*salpingo-oophoritis*), primarily *N. gonorrhoeae* and *C. trachomatis*. Hallmarks of acute disease are adnexal, cervical, and uterine compression tenderness. The diagnosis is imprecise, however—only 75% of patients have confirmed pathogens on tubal laparoscopy. If not treated, a tubo-ovarian abscess may ensue; 18% of treated patients report infertility after 3 years. Infection of the fallopian tubes and ovaries may also follow childbirth or gynecologic surgery.

CHAPTER 15

Musculoskeletal System

ANATOMY AND PHYSIOLOGY

Joints

To evaluate joint function, it is important to be familiar with the types of joints and how they articulate, or interconnect, and the role of bursae in easing joint movement (Box 15-1). Synovial, cartilaginous, and fibrous joints are the three primary types of joint articulation and each allows varying degrees of movement.

Box 15-1. Types of Joints

Type of Joint	Extent of Movement	Examples
Synovial	Freely movable	Knee, shoulder
Cartilaginous	Slightly movable	Vertebral bodies of the spine, symphysis pubis, sternomanubrial joint
Fibrous	Immovable	Skull sutures

Synovial Joints. The bones of these joints do not touch each other, and the joint articulations are *freely movable* within the limits of the surrounding ligaments (Fig. 15-1). The bones are covered by *articular cartilage*, which is composed of a collagen matrix containing charged ions and water that allows it to change shape in response to pressure or load, and separated by a *synovial cavity* that cushions joint movement. A *synovial membrane* lines the synovial cavity and secretes a small amount of viscous lubricating fluid called *synovial fluid*. This fluid also provides nutrition to the adjacent relatively avascular articular cartilage. The membrane pouches out at the edges before attaching at the margins of the articular cartilage to accommodate joint movement. Surrounding the joint is a fibrous *joint capsule*, which is strengthened by and in some cases continuous with ligaments extending from bone to bone.

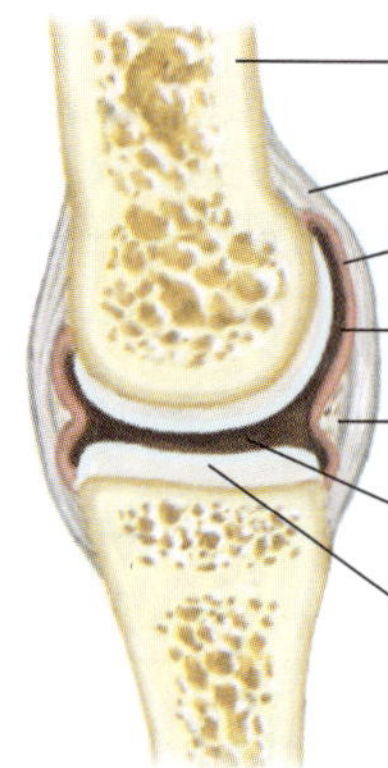

FIGURE 15-1. Synovial joint.

Many of the joints we examine are *synovial*, or movable, *joints* (Box 15-2). The shape of the articulating surfaces of synovial joints, as well as the surrounding soft tissues, determines the direction and extent of joint motion. Younger people and women tend to have increased soft tissue laxity, leading to increased range of motion ("double-jointed"). As you learn to examine the musculoskeletal system, focus on relating the anatomy of the joint to its movement. Knowing the underlying joint anatomy and allowable movement will help you assess possible diagnoses, especially degenerative disorders or possible trauma.

Spheroidal Joints. Spheroidal joints have a ball-and-socket configuration—a rounded, convex surface articulating with a concave cuplike cavity, allowing a wide range of rotatory movement, as in the shoulder and hip (Fig. 15-2).

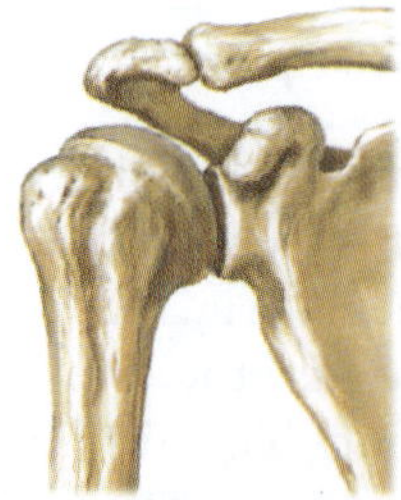

FIGURE 15-2. Spheroidal joint (ball and socket).

Box 15-2. Types of Synovial Joints

Type of Synovial Joint	Articular Shape	Movement	Examples
Spheroidal (ball and socket)	Convex surface in concave cavity	Wide-ranging–flexion, extension, abduction, adduction, rotation, circumduction	Shoulder, hip
Hinge	Flat, planar	Motion in one plane; flexion, extension	Interphalangeal joints of hand and foot; elbow
Condylar	Convex or concave	Movement of two articulating surfaces not dissociable	Knee; temporomandibular joint

Hinge Joints. Hinge joints are flat, planar, or slightly curved, allowing only a gliding motion in a single plane, as in flexion and extension of the elbow (Fig. 15-3).

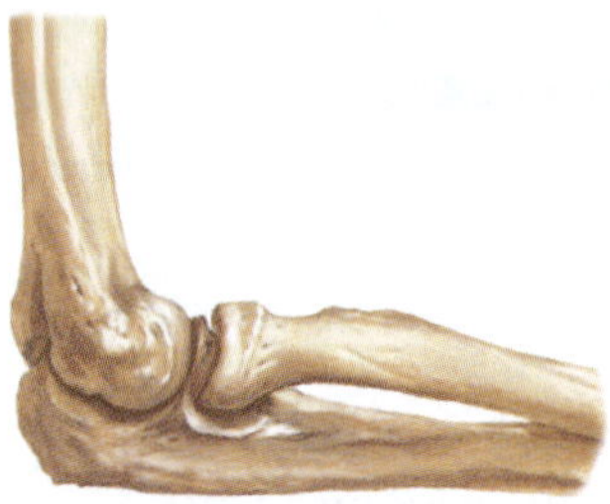

FIGURE 15-3. Hinge joint.

Condylar Joints. Condylar joints, such as the wrist joint, have articulating surfaces that are convex or concave (Fig. 15-4). These joints allow flexion, extension, rotation, and motion in the coronal plane.

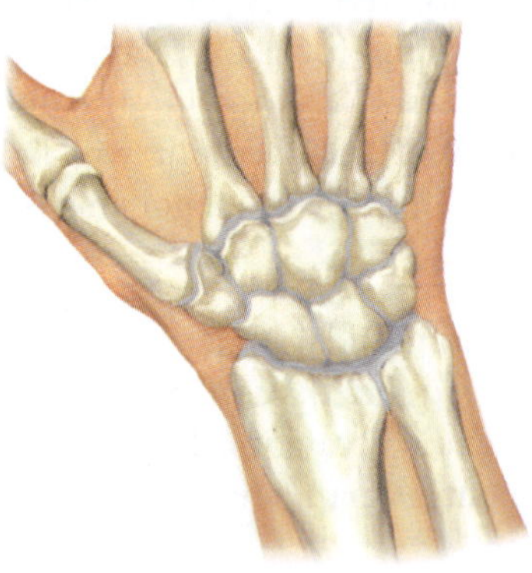

FIGURE 15-4. Condylar joints.

Cartilaginous Joints. Fibrocartilaginous discs separate the bony surfaces of these joints, which allow for a small amount of movement (Fig. 15-5). Examples include the intervertebral joints, the symphysis pubis, and the sternomanubrial joint. The surfaces of the bones on either side of the joint are covered with hyaline cartilage. The fibrocartilage at these joints is compressible and may assist with absorbing shock across a joint. An example is the *nucleus pulposus* at the center of each intervertebral disc that helps both with movement of the spine in all planes and acts to cushion shock through the spine.

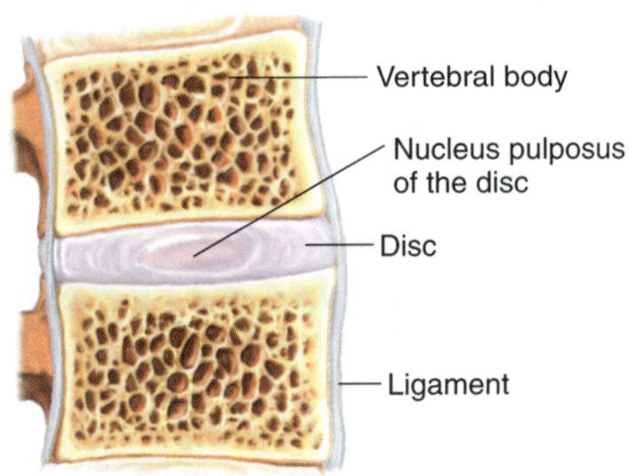

FIGURE 15-5. Cartilaginous joint.

Fibrous Joints. Fibrous joints, such as the sutures of the skull, have intervening layers of fibrous tissue or cartilage that hold the bones together (Fig. 15-6). The bones are almost in direct contact, which allows *no appreciable movement.*

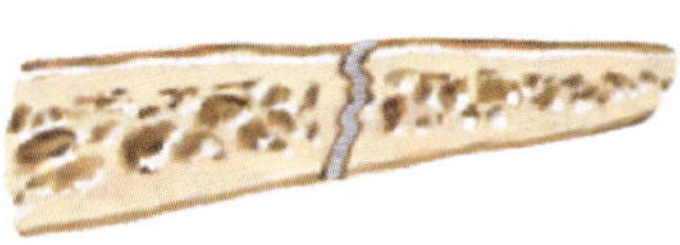

FIGURE 15-6. Fibrous joint.

Bursae

Bursae are roughly disc-shaped synovial sacs that facilitate joint action and allow adjacent muscles or muscles and tendons to glide over each other during movement with reduced friction. They can lie between the skin and the convex surface of a bone or joint, as in the prepatellar bursa of the knee or in areas where tendons or muscles rub against bone, ligaments, or other muscles and tendons, as in the subacromial bursa of the shoulder.

Articular and Extraarticular Joint Structures

Articular structures include the joint capsule and articular cartilage, the synovium and synovial fluid, intraarticular ligaments, and juxtaarticular bone. *Extraarticular structures* include periarticular **ligaments** (rope-like bundles of collagen fibers that connect bone to bone), **tendons** (bundles of collagen fibers that connect muscle to bone), bursae, muscle, fascia, nonarticular bone, nerves, and overlying skin.

Pathology of articular structures typically involves swelling and tenderness of the joint, crepitus, instability, "locking," or deformity and limits *both active and passive range of motion (ROM)* due to stiffness, mechanical blockage, or pain.

Pathology involving extraarticular structures rarely causes intraarticular joint swelling, instability, or joint deformity, typically involves "point or focal tenderness in regions adjacent to articular structures," and limits *active ROM only.*

HEALTH HISTORY: GENERAL APPROACH

Despite the distinct differences in the structures of the musculoskeletal system, joints share similar foundational components. All of these structures—bone, ligaments, cartilage, synovium, surrounding tendons and muscles, associated bursae, blood vessels, nerves, fat, and skin—may be injured by compression or stretching or seeded by infection or cancer. A careful history should elicit characteristic features of injury to each of these musculoskeletal structures.

Also, evaluating a musculoskeletal complaint requires a firm understanding of anatomy and how these anatomical structures relate and work with each other. Learn to visualize the joint's underlying anatomy. Visualization helps trigger the health interview questions you will ask and the examination techniques and maneuvers you will need to perform next to confirm what you are thinking as diagnostic possibilities.

Age may also provide clues to causes of joint pain. If *age <60 years,* consider repetitive strain or overuse syndromes, crystal-induced arthritis, rheumatoid arthritis (RA), psoriatic arthritis, reactive arthritis, and infectious arthritis. If *age >60 years,* look for osteoarthritis (OA), gout and pseudogout, polymyalgia rheumatica (PMR), osteoporotic fracture, and septic bacterial arthritis.

Common or Concerning Symptoms

- Joint pain
- Neck pain
- Low back pain

Joint Pain

Joint pain is a leading complaint of patients seeking health care. Begin by asking, "Do you have any joint pain?" Ask the patient to point to the pain. As you elicit the patient's story, you must diligently clarify the attributes of each symptom, including context, associations, and chronology. For pain and many other symptoms, understanding these essential characteristics, summarized as the seven attributes of a symptom, is critical (Box 15-3).

Generalized muscle "aches and pains" are called **myalgias. Arthralgia** is a joint pain without evidence of arthritis.

See Chapter 3, Health History, for the seven features of pain.

Box 15-3. Tips for Assessing Joint Pain

- Ask the patient to *"point to the pain,"* ideally with one finger if possible. This may save considerable time because many patients have trouble pinpointing pain location in words.
- Clarify and record when the pain started and the exact mechanism of injury to the best of the patient's memory, particularly if there is a history of trauma.
- Determine whether the pain is *articular* or *extraarticular, acute* (usually days to weeks) *or chronic* (usually months to years), *inflammatory* or *noninflammatory,* and *localized (monoarticular)* or *diffuse (polyarticular).*
- Clarify the attributes of each symptom, including context, associations, and chronology.
- Characterizing the pain using the seven attributes of a symptom is critical: *location, quality, quantity or severity, timing, onset, remitting or exacerbating factors, and associated manifestations.*

Location. Ask the patient which joints are painful. Ask the patient to point to the pain, ideally with one finger if possible. If pain is localized to only one joint, it is **monoarticular**. Joint pain may also involve two to four joints (**oligoarticular** or **pauciarticular**) or more than four (**polyarticular**). Often, the size and kind of joints involved provide major diagnostic clues.

Pain in a single joint suggests injury; monoarticular arthritis; or extraarticular causes like tendinitis, bursitis, or soft tissues injury.

Oligoarticular (pauciarticular) arthritis can result from infection (e.g., gonorrhea or rheumatic fever, connective tissue disease, and OA) among other causes.

Causes of polyarthritis include viral or inflammatory from RA, systemic lupus erythematosus (SLE), or psoriasis.

Spondyloarthropathies (e.g., psoriatic arthritis) often involve the spine, including sacroiliac joints and medium-to-large joints, such as the shoulders, hips, knees, and ankles. Smaller joint involvement, such as the wrists, fingers, and toes, is more consistent with RA and SLE.

If polyarticular, determine if there is a *pattern of involvement*. Does the pain migrate from joint to joint or steadily spread from one joint to multiple joints? Is the involvement *symmetric* (affecting similar joints on both sides of the body) or *asymmetric* (affecting different joints on different sides)? Is it *intermittent* or *constant* (fluctuating from mild, moderate, and/or severe)?

Rheumatic fever and gonococcal arthritis exhibit a migratory pattern of spread. In RA, the pattern is additive and progressive with symmetric involvement. Involvement is usually *asymmetric* in psoriatic, reactive, and inflammatory bowel disease (IBD) associated arthritis.

Does it *radiate* or travel anywhere else? Pain originating in the small joints of the hands and feet is often more sharply localized than pain in larger joints.

Pain from the hip joint can be particularly deceptive since true pain from the hip joint typically radiates to the groin, although it can also cause knee pain. Sacral/sacroiliac pain is often in the buttock, and trochanteric pain from bursitis or tendinitis can occur on the lateral thigh.

Quality. What is the pain like? Ask, "Can you describe the pain (what it feels like)?." Patients may describe the pain in many different ways including dull, gnawing, or stiff. Because of the complex nature of joint anatomy, pain quality does not often designate specific diagnostic possibilities compared to the other symptom attributes, such as onset/timing and location/pattern of involvement.

Severity. How bad is the pain? Ask for the severity rating on a scale of 1 to 10. In general, inflammatory causes of joint pain are considerably more painful than noninflammatory types. Different mechanisms appear to be involved—interleukins and tumor necrosis factor in inflammatory joint pain and prostaglandins, chemokines, and growth factors in noninflammatory pain.

Inflammatory disorders have many causes: infectious (e.g., *Neisseria gonorrhoeae* or *Mycobacterium tuberculosis*), crystal-induced (gout, pseudogout), immune-related (RA, SLE), reactive (rheumatic fever, reactive arthritis), or idiopathic.

In noninflammatory disorders, consider trauma (e.g., rotator cuff tear in the shoulder), overuse (bursitis, tendinitis), degenerative changes (OA), or fibromyalgia.

Onset and Timing. Onset is especially important. When did (does) the pain start? How long does it last? How often does it come? How long has the pain been present? Has the pain progressed slowly or fluctuated with periods of improvement and worsening? Does it vary over the course of a day and in what way?

Did the pain or discomfort develop rapidly over the course of a few hours as the result of a specific event or insidiously over weeks to months without an obvious cause? *Acute joint pain* typically lasts from days to weeks; *chronic pain* lasts for months to years.

Severe pain of rapid onset in a red swollen joint occurs in acute septic arthritis or crystal-induced arthritis (gout; calcium pyrophosphate deposition disease [CPPD]). In children, consider osteomyelitis in a bone contiguous to a joint.

See Table 15-1, Patterns of Pain in and Around the Joints.

Also ask about the setting in which the pain occurs and how the pain arose. Include environmental factors, personal activities, emotional reactions, and other circumstances that may have contributed to the occurrence of the pain. Was there an acute injury or overuse from repetitive motion of the same part of the body? If the pain comes from trauma, determine in detail the *mechanism of injury* or the specific series of events that caused the joint pain.

Remitting or Exacerbating Factors. Ask what aggravates or relieves the pain. What are the effects of exercise or physical activity, rest, medications and physical therapy? You may want to quantify the change in severity, if any, using the same rating scale of 1 to 10 to describe it initially.

In inflammatory joint disorders (e.g., RA), rest tends to worsen the pain, whereas activity improves it. In mechanical joint disorders (e.g., OA), activity tends to increase the pain and stiffness, and rest improves the symptoms.

Associated Manifestations

Inflammation. Ask about the four cardinal features of inflammation—*swelling, warmth,* and *redness,* in addition to *pain*. Several of these features are best assessed on examination, but patients can often guide you to points of inflammation and pain. Ask the patient if anything else accompanies the pain. Also ask about fever or chills.

Inflammation with high-grade fever and chills is usually seen in septic arthritis. Low-grade fever can be present in crystal-induced arthritis or inflammatory arthritis like RA.

Extraarticular pain occurs in inflammation of bursae (**bursitis**), tendons (**tendinitis**), or tendon sheaths (**tenosynovitis**) as well as in *sprains* from stretching or tearing of ligaments.

Note that the symptoms of *decreased joint movement* and *stiffness* can help you decide if the pain might be *articular.*

Limitation in Movement and Stiffness. Musculoskeletal **stiffness** refers to a perceived tightness or resistance to movement. Elicit any pattern of stiffness if present. Is it worse in the morning but gradually better with activity? Or is there an intermittent "**gel phenomenon**," namely brief periods of daytime stiffness following inactivity that usually last from 30 to 60 minutes then get worse again with movement?

Stiffness lasting more than 1 hour represents severe inflammation commonly seen in RA and PMR.

Morning stiffness that gradually improves with activity is more common in inflammatory disorders like RA and PMR. Intermittent stiffness or *gelling* that worsens over the course of the day is commonly seen in OA.

To assess *decreased* or *limited movement,* ask about changes in activity due to problems with the involved joint, for example, in the ability to walk, stand, lean over, sit or sit up, rise from a sitting position, pinch, grasp, turn a page, or open a door handle or jar. Common activities like combing hair, brushing teeth, eating, dressing, and bathing may also be affected.

Articular joint pain generally involves decreased *active* (joint movement performed by the patient) *and passive* (joint movement performed on the patient by the examiner) ROM with morning stiffness or "gelling." Periarticular joint pain involves periarticular tenderness and pain with active ROM, while passive ROM remains intact.

Associated Constitutional Symptoms and Systemic Manifestations from Other Organ Systems. Some joint problems have associated *constitutional symptoms* such as fever, chills, rash, fatigue, anorexia, weight loss, and weakness. Some joint disorders have systemic manifestations in other organ systems, which can provide important clues to diagnosis. Watch for the symptoms, signs, and disorders associated with these disorders. Ask about any family history of joint or muscle disorders.

Constitutional symptoms are common in inflammatory arthritides such as RA, SLE, and PMR. High fever and chills suggest an infectious cause.

See Table 15-2, Systemic Manifestations of Musculoskeletal Disorders.

Neck Pain

Neck pain is a common complaint, but it is essential to discern neck pain requiring immediate stabilization from pain resulting from the more common musculoskeletal causes. If the patient reports neck trauma, from a motor vehicle accident, for example, ask about neck tenderness and consider clinical decision rules that identify risk of cervical spine injury. Persistent pain after blunt trauma or a collision almost always warrants further evaluation.

See Table 15-3, Pains in the Neck.

Neck pain is usually self-limited without the need for treatment, but it is important to ask about radiation into the arm or scapular area, arm weakness, numbness, or paresthesias that could indicate impingement of the spinal cord or one of the spinal nerves.

Radicular pain signals spinal nerve compression and/or irritation. Any level can be affected, but the C6 and C7 levels are most common. Unlike low back pain, foraminal impingement from degenerative joint changes is more common (70% to 75%) than disc herniation (20% to 25%).

Low Back Pain

At least 60% of adults have low back pain at least once during their lifetime with prevalence and related disability peaking between ages 35 and 55. Begin by asking, "Where is your back pain?." Using open-ended questions, get a clear and complete picture of the problem, especially the location, radiation of the pain, specific exacerbating positions, and any prior history of trauma.

Medicine History Taking OSCE Video:
Low Back Pain

See Table 15-4, Low Back Pain.

Most guidelines categorize low back pain into three groups: nonspecific (>90%), nerve root entrapment with radiculopathy or spinal stenosis (~5%), and pain from a specific underlying disease (1% to 2%).

Nonspecific low back pain is usually from musculoligamentous injuries and age-related degenerative processes of the intervertebral discs and facet joints.

Note that the term "nonspecific low back pain" is preferred to "low back sprain or strain."

Determine if the pain is *on the midline* (over the spinous processes of the vertebrae) or *off the midline* (in the paraspinal muscles surrounding the spine).

For *midline back pain,* diagnoses can include: musculoligamentous injury; disc herniation; degenerative disc disease; degenerative disease of the facet joints of the spine; vertebral fracture or collapse; and, rarely, spinal cord metastases or epidural abscess. For *pain off the midline,* assess for muscle strain, myofascial pain (trigger points), sacroiliitis, greater trochanteric pain syndrome, and hip arthritis as well as for renal conditions like pyelonephritis or stones.

Is there radiation into the buttock or lower extremity? Is there any associated numbness, paresthesia or weakness?

Sciatica is radicular gluteal and posterior leg pain usually caused by impingement nerve roots at the L4–S1 root levels (see p. 332 for related neurologic findings). Up to 85% of cases are associated with a disc disorder, usually at L4–L5 or L5–S1 levels. Pain associated with forward flexion of the spine, straight-leg raise or seated slump maneuvers, or Valsalva or sneezing is suggestive of underlying disc disease. Leg pain that improves with lumbar forward flexion occurs in spinal stenosis.

In addition to asking for any limitation in movement and stiffness, it is important that you ask about associated bladder or bowel dysfunction. Elicit any other associated manifestations that may be warning signs or red flags for serious underlying systemic disease (Box 15-4).

Consider cauda equina syndrome from an S2–S4 midline disc herniation or tumor if there is bowel or bladder dysfunction (usually urinary retention with overflow incontinence), especially with saddle anesthesia or perineal numbness. Pursue immediate imaging and surgical evaluation.

Box 15-4. Red Flags for Low Back Pain from Underlying Systemic Disease

- Age <20 yrs or >50 yrs
- History of cancer
- Unexplained weight loss, fever, or decline in general health
- Pain lasting more than 1 mo or not responding to treatment
- Pain at night or present at rest
- History of intravenous drug use, addiction, or immunosuppression
- Presence of active infection or human immunodeficiency virus (HIV) infection
- Long-term steroid therapy
- Saddle anesthesia
- Bladder or bowel incontinence
- Neurologic symptoms or progressive neurologic deficit
- Lower extremity weakness

PHYSICAL EXAMINATION: GENERAL APPROACH

During the interview, the patient has shared his or her ability to carry out normal activities of daily living. Keep the patient's baseline level of function in mind as you perform the musculoskeletal examination. During the general survey, you have assessed the patient's general appearance, body proportions, and ease of movement. Now visualize the underlying anatomy of the joints and recall pertinent elements of the history, for example, the mechanism of injury if there is trauma and the time course of symptoms and specific functional limitation. Recall that the anatomical shape of each joint determines its ROM.

The detail needed for examining joints varies widely. On a screening examination of a patient who has no musculoskeletal complaints, it is adequate to inspect and observe the trunk and extremities for any visible abnormalities. You may also want to perform a complete active ROM with each joint. However, in a patient with specific musculoskeletal complaints, it is important to do a thorough musculoskeletal examination to delineate the extent of these abnormalities.

As you begin your examination, remind yourself to be systematic. The approach can be divided into three broad sections: visual inspection, palpation, and the evaluation of joint motion (Look, Feel and Move). This systematic approach can best be remembered by the mnemonic *IPROMS* ("*I promise...*"), which includes Inspection, Palpation of bony structures and related joint and soft tissue structures, assessment of Range Of Motion, and Special maneuvers to test specific movements.

1. Inspect: *Look*—evaluate visually for signs of deformity, swelling, scars, inflammation or muscle atrophy.
2. Palpate: *Feel*—use surface anatomy landmarks to localize points of tenderness or fluid collection.
3. Range of Motion: have the patient actively move the involved joints, then move them passively as the examiner.
4. Special Maneuvers: *Move*—perform stress maneuvers (if indicated) to evaluate joint stability and the integrity of ligaments, tendons, and bursae, especially if pain or trauma is present.

In addition, assess any areas of inflammation, especially tenderness, swelling, warmth, and redness, and, whenever possible, evaluate the neurologic and vascular integrity of the area by checking sensation, strength, and pulses.

Inspection

During inspection, *look* for **joint symmetry** of involvement. Is the change in joints on both sides of the body, or is the change only in one or two joints?

Acute involvement of only one joint suggests trauma, septic arthritis, or crystal-induced arthritis. RA is typically polyarticular and symmetrical.

Note any *deformities* or *malalignment of bones or joints.*

Malalignment can occur in Dupuytren contracture (p. 476), bow-legs (*genu varum*), or knock-knees (*genu valgum*), for example.

Use inspection to assess the *surrounding tissues,* noting skin changes, subcutaneous nodules, muscle atrophy, and location of tenderness if present.

Palpation

Use palpation to *feel* not only the musculoskeletal structures affected but also key anatomic landmarks nearby. This will help orient you as you try to visualize the underlying anatomy of the joints. This is particularly helpful when movement is limited since the anatomic shape of joints determine their ROM.

Also note any **crepitus**, an audible or palpable crunching during movement of tendons or ligaments over bone or areas of cartilage loss. It may occur in joints without pain and is more significant when associated with symptoms or signs.

Look for subcutaneous nodules in RA or rheumatic fever, effusion in trauma, and crepitus over inflamed joints in OA or over the inflamed tendon sheaths of tenosynovitis.

Box 15-5. Assessing the Four Signs of Inflammation

- **Swelling.** Palpable swelling may involve: (1) the synovial membrane, which can feel boggy or doughy; (2) effusion from excess synovial fluid within the joint space; or (3) soft tissue structures, such as bursae, tendons, and tendon sheaths.

Palpable bogginess or doughiness of the synovial membrane indicates synovitis, which is often accompanied by effusion. Palpable joint fluid is present in effusion. Tenderness over the tendon sheath is seen in tendinitis.

- **Warmth.** Use the backs of your fingers to compare the involved joint with its unaffected contralateral joint or with nearby tissues if both joints are involved.

Increased warmth can be seen in arthritis, tendinitis, bursitis, and osteomyelitis.

- **Redness.** Redness of the overlying skin is the least common sign of inflammation near the joints and is usually seen in more superficial joints like fingers, toes, and knees.

Diffuse tenderness and warmth over a thickened synovium suggest arthritis or infection; focal tenderness suggests injury and trauma.

- **Pain or tenderness.** Try to identify the specific anatomic structure that is tender.

Redness over a tender joint suggests acute inflammation of the joint or synovium, like in septic, crystal-induced, or rheumatoid arthritis.

Also inspect and palpate any joints with signs of *inflammation* (Box 15-5).

Range of Motion

There are two phases of **range of motion**: **active** (by the patient) and **passive** (by the examiner).

If patients have painful joints, *move* them gently or let patients demonstrate the movements themselves, showing you how they manage.

For injured joints with concern for fracture, consider an x-ray before attempting movement.

Test active and passive ROM and maneuvers to demonstrate *limitations in ROM* or *joint instability* from excess mobility of joint ligaments, called **ligamentous laxity**.

Decreased ROM is present in arthritis, joints with effusion, joints with tissue inflammation or surrounding fibrosis, or bony fixation (*ankylosis*).

Special Maneuvers

Certain special maneuvers or motions are performed during the musculoskeletal examination to evaluate underlying mechanisms of a patient's symptom, often pain, or an underlying structural abnormality such as a joint laxity or weakness. Again, a sound understanding of the anatomic structures is crucial. If you are performing a maneuver designed to reproduce pain, warn the patient beforehand and perform it with care. As you carefully perform the maneuver and the symptom is reproduced or the structural finding is observed, picture how the underlying structures contribute to what the patient is experiencing or what you are observing.

The special maneuvers of specific joints that can help identify common pathologic conditions will be described in the related sections to follow.

Other Examination Techniques

Finally, test *muscle strength* to aid in the assessment of joint function and ensure normal *sensation* and good *distal pulses*.

For these techniques, see Chapter 13, Nervous System, and Chapter 16, Peripheral Vascular System.

REGIONAL JOINT EXAMINATIONS

The following sections follow a head-to-toe sequence, beginning with the jaw and joints of the upper extremities and ending with the ankles and feet. Each section will include an overview of distinguishing anatomical and functional characteristics of the joint and examination techniques specific to that joint (IPROMS)—inspection, palpation of bony and soft tissue structures, ROM (the arc of measurable joint movement in a single plane), and special maneuvers for testing joint function and stability.

Temporomandibular Joint

The temporomandibular joint (TMJ) is the most active joint in the body, opening and closing up to 2,000 times a day (Figs. 15-7 and 15-8). It is formed by the fossa and articular tubercle of the temporal bone and the condyle of the mandible. It lies midway between the external acoustic meatus and the zygomatic arch.

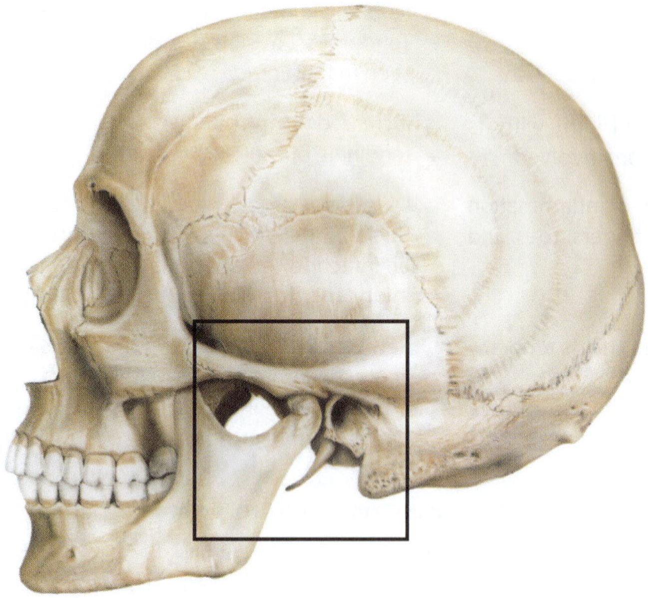

FIGURE 15-7. Area of temporomandibular joint in adult skull.

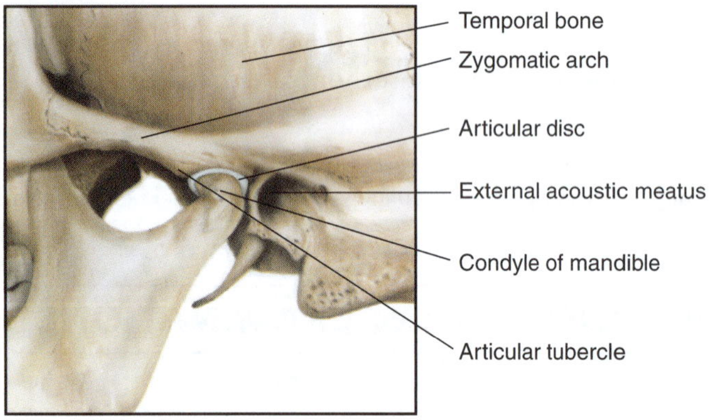

FIGURE 15-8. Temporomandibular joint, inset.

A fibrocartilaginous disc cushions the action of the condyle of the mandible against the synovial membrane and capsule of the articulating surfaces of the temporal bone. Therefore, it is a *condylar synovial joint*. The principal muscles opening the mouth are the *external pterygoids* (Fig. 15-9). Closing the mouth are the muscles innervated by cranial nerve V, the trigeminal nerve, including the *masseter*, the *temporalis*, and the *internal pterygoids*.

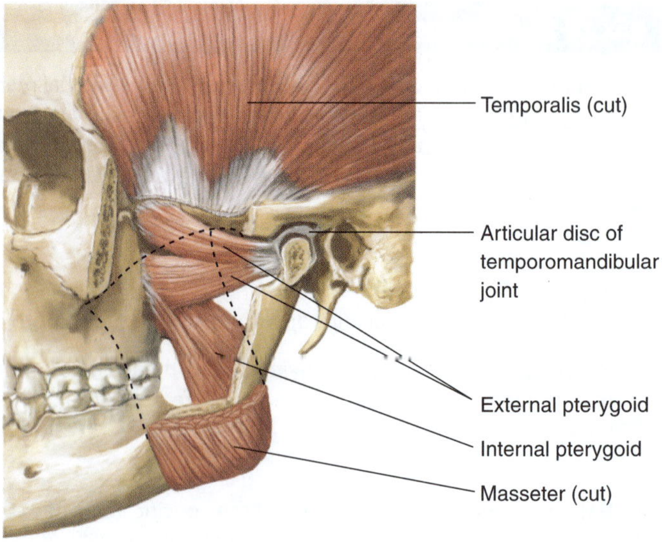

FIGURE 15-9. TMJ muscles.

Techniques of Examination

Key Components of the Temporomandibular Joint Examination

- Inspect the face and TMJ (swelling, redness).
- Palpate muscles of mastication (masseters, temporal muscles, pterygoid muscles).
- Assess range of motion: opening and closing; protrusion and retraction; and lateral, or side-to-side, motions.

Inspection. Inspect the face for symmetry. Inspect the TMJ for swelling or redness. Swelling may appear as a rounded bulge just anterior to the external auditory meatus.

Facial asymmetry is often seen in TMJ disorders. These disorders can have many etiologies. Typically, there is unilateral chronic pain with chewing, jaw clenching, or teeth grinding often accompanied by headache. Pain with chewing can also occur in trigeminal neuralgia and temporal arteritis.

Palpation. To locate and palpate the joint, place the tips of your index fingers just in front of the tragus of each ear and ask the patient to open his or her mouth (Fig. 15-10). The fingertips should drop into the joint spaces as the mouth opens. Note any swelling or tenderness. Snapping or clicking may be felt or heard in normal people and is not necessarily a sign of pathology.

Palpable crepitus or clicking is present in poor occlusion, meniscus injury, or synovial swelling from trauma.

Box 15-6. Range of Motion of the Temporomandibular Joint

Jaw Movement	Primary Muscles Affecting Movement	Patient Instructions
Opening	Inferior head of lateral pterygoid, anterior digastric, mylohyoid	"Open your mouth wide."
Closing	Masseter, anterior and middle temporalis, medial pterygoid, superior head lateral pterygoid	"Close your mouth."
Protrusion	Lateral pterygoid	"Move your lower jaw by sticking it out (jutting it out)."
Retraction (Retrusion)	Middle and posterior temporalis	"Move your lower jaw by moving it in toward you."
Side-to-side (Laterotrusion)	Ipsilateral middle and posterior temporalis, contralateral inferior head lateral pterygoid	"Move your lower jaw from side to side."

Swelling, tenderness, and decreased ROM signal TMJ inflammation or arthritis.

Patients who are unable to close their mouths may have dislocated the TMJ, which can happen with extreme mouth opening. More uncommonly, TMJ dislocation can be caused by trauma.

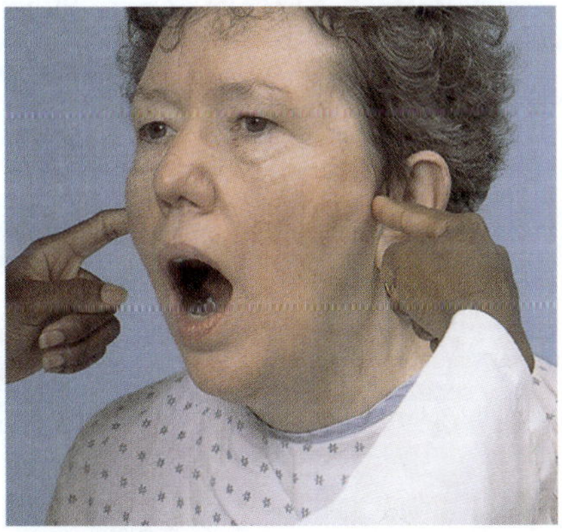

FIGURE 15-10. Palpating the TMJ while asking the patient to open and close mouth.

Palpate the *muscles of mastication* (see Fig. 15-9):

In TMJ syndrome, there is pain and tenderness with palpation.

- *Masseters*, externally at the angle of the mandible
- *Temporal muscles*, externally during clenching and relaxation of the jaw
- *Pterygoid muscles*, internally between the tonsillar pillars at the mandible (difficult to palpate)

Range of Motion. The TMJ has glide and hinge motions in its upper and lower portions, respectively. Grinding or chewing consists primarily of gliding movements in the upper compartments.

ROM is threefold: ask the patient to demonstrate *opening* and *closing*; *protrusion* and *retraction* (by jutting the mandible forward); and *lateral*, or *side-to-side*, motion (Box 15-6). Normally, as the mouth is opened wide, three fingers can be inserted between the incisors. During normal protrusion of the jaw, the bottom teeth can be placed in front of the upper teeth.

Shoulder Joint

The shoulder derives its mobility from a complex interconnected structure of three joints; three large bones; and three principal muscle groups, often referred to as the *shoulder girdle*. These structures are viewed as **dynamic stabilizers**, which are capable of movement, or **static stabilizers**, which are incapable of movement (Box 15-7).

Box 15-7. Shoulder Girdle Stabilizers

- *Dynamic stabilizers:* These consist primarily of the *SITS muscles of the rotator cuff* (**S**upraspinatus, **I**nfraspinatus, **T**eres minor, and **S**ubscapularis), which move the humerus and compress and stabilize the humeral head within the glenoid cavity. Other muscles, such as the biceps brachii, the latissimus dorsi, and pectoralis major also play a role in stabilizing the shoulder.
- *Static stabilizers:* These are the bony and ligamentous structures of the shoulder girdle including the labrum, the articular capsule, and the glenohumeral ligaments. The *labrum* is a fibrocartilaginous ring that surrounds the glenoid and deepens its socket, providing greater stability to the humeral head. The rotator cuff and glenohumeral ligaments strengthen the joint capsule and add to joint stability.

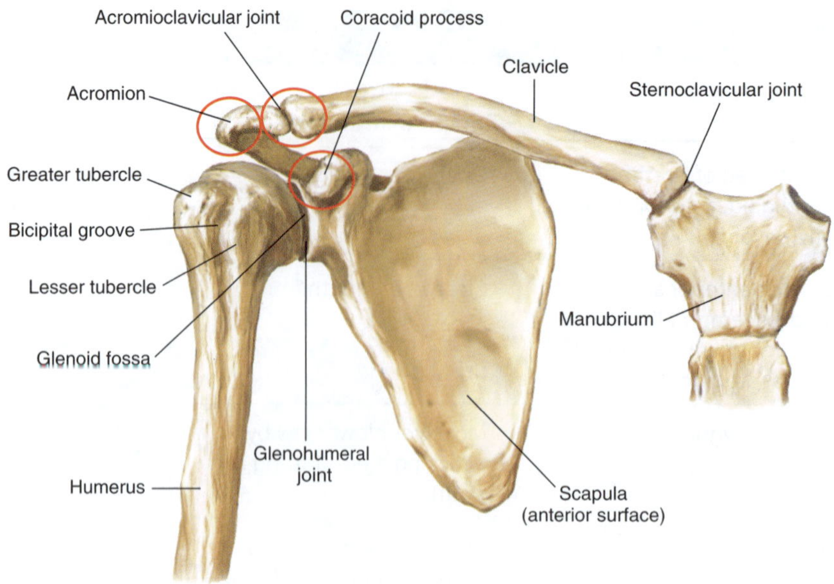

FIGURE 15-11. Anatomy of the right shoulder.

The bony structures of the shoulder include the humerus, the clavicle, and the scapula (Fig. 15-11). The scapula is anchored to the axial skeleton only by the sternoclavicular joint and inserting muscles, often called the *scapulothoracic articulation* because the sternoclavicular joint is not a true joint.

Identify the *manubrium,* the *sternoclavicular joint,* and the *clavicle.* Also identify the *tip of the acromion,* the *greater tubercle of the humerus,* and the *coracoid process,* which are important landmarks of shoulder anatomy.

Three different joints articulate at the shoulder:

- *Glenohumeral joint.* In this joint, the head of the humerus articulates with the shallow glenoid fossa of the scapula. This joint is deeply situated and normally not palpable. It is a ball-and-socket joint, allowing the arm its wide arc of movement.
- *Sternoclavicular joint.* The convex medial end of the clavicle articulates with the concave hollow in the upper sternum.
- *Acromioclavicular joint.* The lateral end of the clavicle articulates with the acromion process of the scapula.

Three groups of muscles attach at the shoulder:

Rotator cuff disorders are the most common cause of shoulder pain in primary care.

- The *scapulohumeral group* (Fig. 15-12) extends from the scapula to the humerus and includes the muscles inserting directly on the humerus, namely the *SITS muscles* of the rotator cuff:
  - *Supraspinatus*—originates on the posterior scapula superior to the scapular spine and runs above the glenohumeral joint; inserts on the greater tubercle
  - *Infraspinatus* and *Teres minor*—originate on the posterior scapula inferior to the scapular spine and cross the glenohumeral joint posteriorly; insert on the greater tubercle
  - *Subscapularis* (Fig. 15-13)—originates on the anterior surface of the scapula and crosses the joint anteriorly; inserts on the lesser tubercle

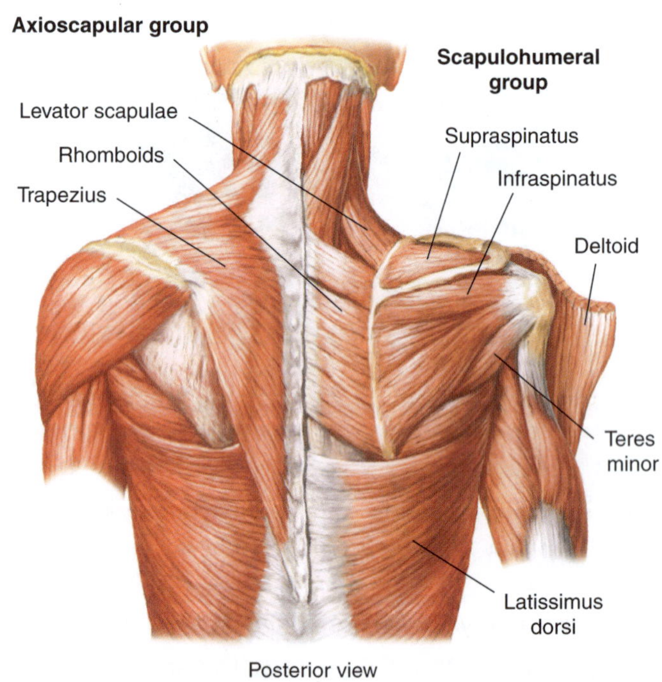

FIGURE 15-12. Axioscapular and scapulohumeral muscle groups.

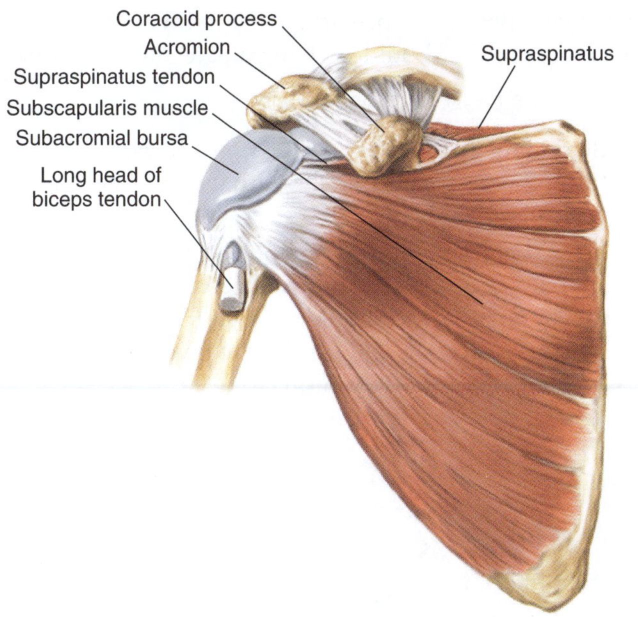

FIGURE 15-13. Anterior view of the right shoulder.

The scapulohumeral group abducts, internally and externally rotates the shoulder (hence the name *rotator cuff*) and depresses and rotates the head of the humerus (see Fig. 15-12).

- The *axioscapular group* attaches the scapula to the trunk and includes the trapezius, rhomboids, serratus anterior, and levator scapulae (see Fig. 15-12). These muscles rotate the scapula and pull the shoulder posteriorly.
- The *axiohumeral group* attaches the humerus to the trunk and includes the pectoralis major and minor and the latissimus dorsi (Fig. 15-14). These muscles rotate the shoulder internally and adduct the humerus.

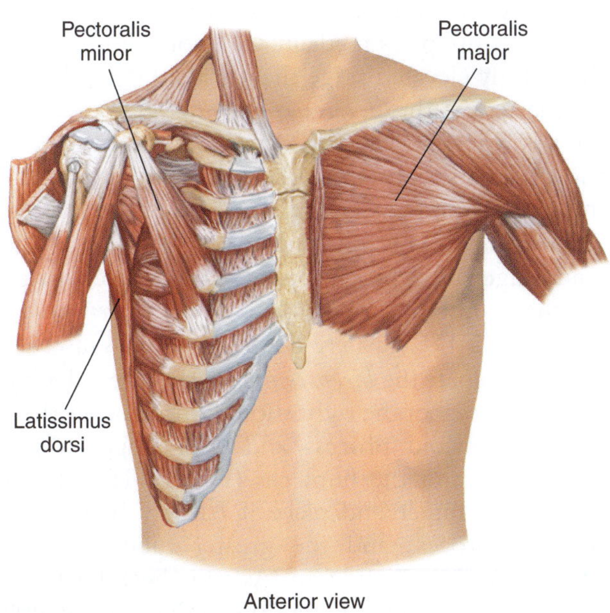

FIGURE 15-14. Axiohumeral muscle group.

The *biceps* and *triceps,* which connect the scapula to the bones of the forearm across the humerus, are also involved in shoulder movement, especially forward flexion (biceps) and extension (triceps).

Additional Structures. Surrounding the glenohumeral joint is a fibrous articular capsule formed by the tendon insertions of the rotator cuff and other capsular structures. The loose fit of the capsule allows the shoulder bones to separate and contributes to the shoulder's wide range of movement. The capsule is lined by a synovial membrane with two outpouchings—the *subscapular bursa* and the *synovial sheath of the tendon of the long head of the biceps.* The tendon of the long head of the biceps runs in the bicipital groove between the greater and lesser tubercles (see Fig. 15-13).

The principal bursa of the shoulder is the *subacromial subdeltoid bursa* and lies between the rotator cuff tendons and the acromion of the scapula, the acromioclavicular joint, the bicipital groove, and the deltoid muscle. Abduction of the shoulder compresses this bursa. Normally, the supraspinatus tendon and the subacromial subdeltoid bursa are not tender.

If the bursal surfaces are inflamed (subacromial subdeltoid bursitis), there may be tenderness just below the tip of the acromion, pain with abduction and rotation, and loss of smooth movement.

Techniques of Examination

Key Components of the Shoulder Joint Examination

- Inspect the shoulder and shoulder girdle anteriorly and the scapulae and related muscles posteriorly (swelling, deformity, atrophy, fasciculations, abnormal positioning).
- Palpate the sternoclavicular joint, clavicle, acromioclavicular joint, coracoid process, greater tubercle, biceps tendon, subacromial and subdeltoid bursae, and underlying palpable SITS muscles.
- Assess range of motion: flexion and extension, abduction and adduction, and internal and external rotations.
- Perform special maneuvers (if indicated): painful arc test, Neer test, Hawkins test, internal rotation lag test, external rotation lag test, drop arm test, external rotation resistance test, and empty can test.

Inspection. Inspect the shoulder and shoulder girdle anteriorly, then the scapulae and related muscles posteriorly.

Scoliosis may cause elevation of one shoulder. With anterior dislocation of the shoulder, the rounded lateral aspect of the shoulder appears flattened.

Note any swelling, deformity, muscle atrophy or **fasciculations** (fine tremors of the muscles), or abnormal positioning.

Atrophy of the supraspinatus and infraspinatus with increased prominence of scapular spine can appear within 2 to 3 weeks of a rotator cuff tear. Infraspinatus atrophy has been found to have a positive likelihood ratio (LR) of 2 for rotator cuff disease, making it an important finding if looking for a cuff tear.

Look for swelling of the joint capsule anteriorly or a bulge in the subacromial bursa under the deltoid muscle. Survey the entire upper extremity for color change, skin alteration, or unusual bony contours.

Swelling from synovial fluid accumulation is rare and must be significant before the glenohumeral joint capsule appears distended. Swelling in the acromioclavicular joint is easier to detect as the joint is more superficial.

When the shoulder muscles appear atrophic, inspect for scapular winging. Ask the patient to extend both arms and push against your hand or against a wall (Fig. 15-15). Observe the scapulae. Normally, they lie close to the thorax.

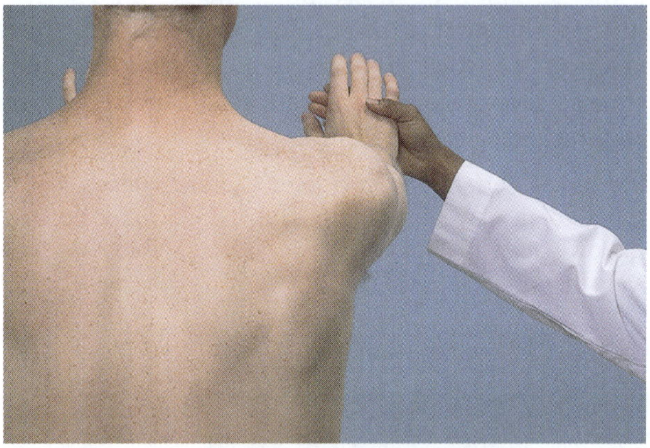

FIGURE 15-15. Testing for scapular winging.

In winging, the medial border of the scapula juts backward (Fig. 15-16), suspicious for weakness of the trapezius or serratus anterior muscle (seen in muscular dystrophy) or injury to the long thoracic nerve. In very thin individuals, the scapulae may appear "winged" even when the musculature is intact.

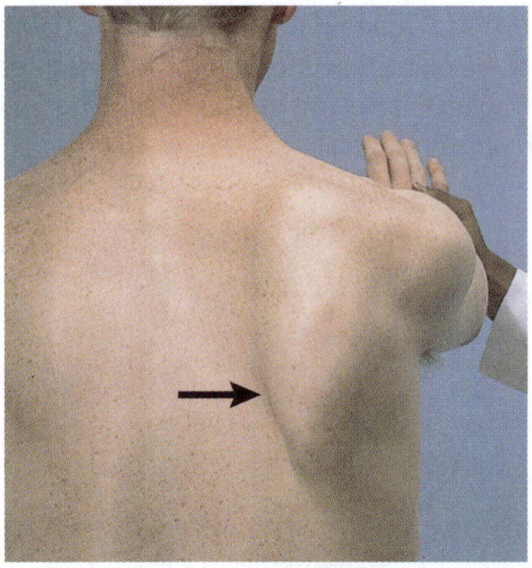

FIGURE 15-16. Scapular winging.

Palpation. Begin by palpating the bony contours and structures of the shoulder, then palpate any area of pain.

See Table 15-5, Painful Shoulders.

- Beginning medially, at the *sternoclavicular joint,* trace the clavicle laterally with your fingers to the *acromioclavicular joint.*
- From behind, follow the bony spine of the scapula laterally and upward until it becomes the acromion, the summit of the shoulder (Fig. 15-17A). Its upper surface is rough and slightly convex. Identify the anterior tip of the acromion.

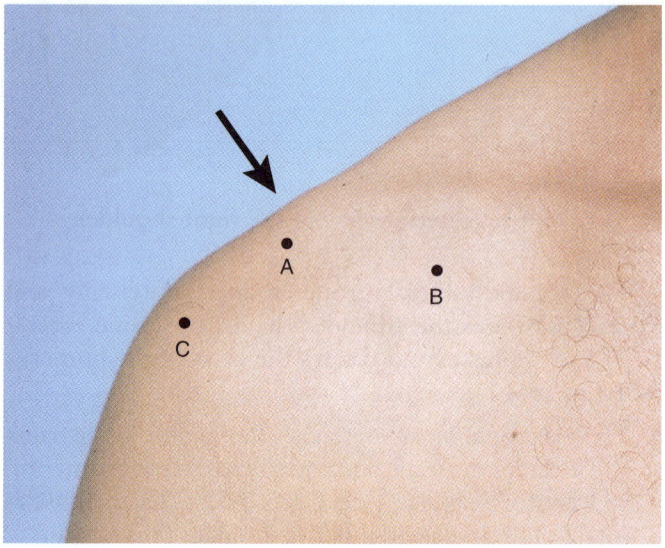

FIGURE 15-17. Surface anatomy landmarks for the right shoulder: acromion (**A**), coracoid process (**B**), and greater tubercle (**C**).

- With your index finger on top of the acromion, just behind its tip, press medially with your thumb to find the slightly elevated ridge that marks the distal end of the clavicle at the *acromioclavicular joint* (shown by the arrow in Fig. 15-17). Move your thumb medially and down a short step to the next bony prominence, the *coracoid process* (see Fig. 15-17B) of the scapula.
- With your thumb on the coracoid process, allow your fingers to fall on and grasp the lateral aspect of the humerus to palpate the *greater tubercle* (see Fig. 15-17C), where the SITS muscles insert.
- Next, to palpate the *biceps tendon* in the intertubercular *bicipital groove* of the right shoulder, keep your thumb on the coracoid process and your fingers on the lateral aspect of the humerus (Fig. 15-18). Remove your index finger and place it halfway between the coracoid process and the greater tubercle on the anterior surface of the arm. As you check for tendon tenderness, rolling the tendon under the fingertips may be helpful. You can also rotate the glenohumeral

joint externally, locate the muscle distally near the elbow, and track the muscle and its tendon proximally into the intertubercular groove.

See also bicipital tendinitis in Table 15-5, Painful Shoulders.

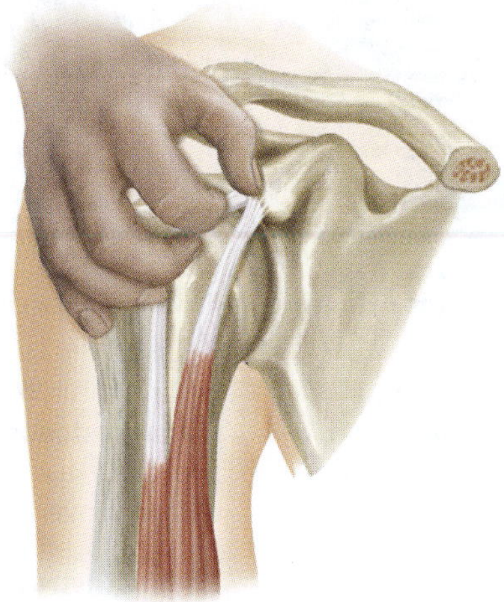

FIGURE 15-18. Palpating the bicipital tendon along the bicipital groove in the right shoulder.

- To examine the *subacromial subdeltoid bursa* and the *SITS muscles*, first passively extend the humerus by lifting the elbow posteriorly, which rotates these structures so that they are anterior to the acromion. Palpate carefully over the subacromial and subdeltoid bursae (Figs. 15-19 and 15-20).

Localized tenderness points to subacromial or subdeltoid bursitis, degenerative changes, or calcific deposits in the rotator cuff. Swelling may suggest a bursal tear that communicates with the articular cavity.

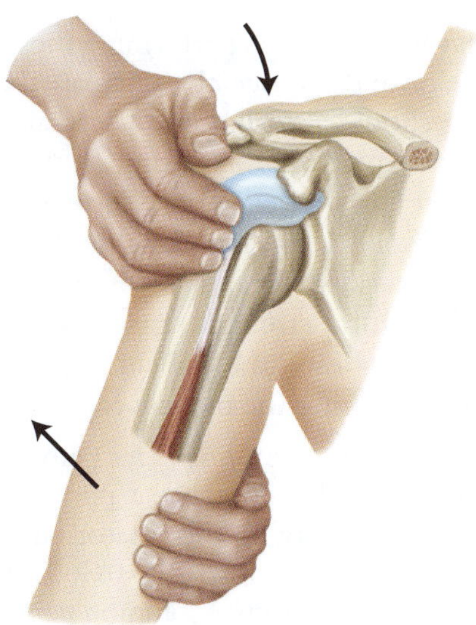

FIGURE 15-19. Extending the right humerus posteriorly to palpate the SITS muscle insertions and bursae.

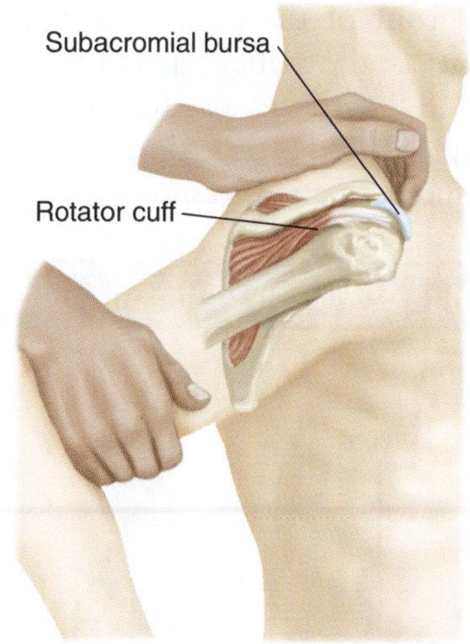

FIGURE 15-20. Palpating the subacromial bursa.

Tenderness over the SITS muscle insertions and inability to abduct the arm above shoulder level occurs in sprains; tears; and tendon rupture of the rotator cuff, most commonly the supraspinatus.

See Table 15-5, Painful Shoulders.

The underlying palpable SITS muscles are:
- Supraspinatus—directly under the acromion, also traceable from the muscle belly above the scapular spine posteriorly
- Infraspinatus—posterior to supraspinatus, also traceable from the muscle belly below the scapular spine
- Teres minor—posterior and inferior to the supraspinatus, difficult to palpate
- Subscapularis—inserts anteriorly from the medial side of the humerus onto the lesser tuberosity; external rotation is needed for indirect palpation through overlying muscles

- The fibrous articular capsule and the broad flat tendons of the rotator cuff are so closely associated that they must be examined simultaneously. Swelling in the capsule and synovial membrane is often best detected by looking down on the shoulder from above. Palpate the capsule and synovial membrane beneath the anterior and posterior acromion to check for injury or arthritis.

Tenderness and effusion suggest glenohumeral joint synovitis. If the margins of the capsule and synovial membrane are palpable, a moderate-to-large effusion is present. Minimal synovitis cannot be detected on palpation.

Range of Motion. The six cardinal movements of the shoulder girdle are flexion, extension, abduction, adduction, and internal and external rotation.

Restricted ROM occurs in bursitis, capsulitis, rotator cuff tears or sprains, and tendinitis.

Standing in front of the patient, watch for smooth fluid movement as the patient performs the motions listed in Box 15-8. Learn the specific muscles responsible for each motion. Note the clear simple instructions that prompt the requested patient response.

Box 15-8. Range of Motion of the Shoulder Joint

Flexion	Extension
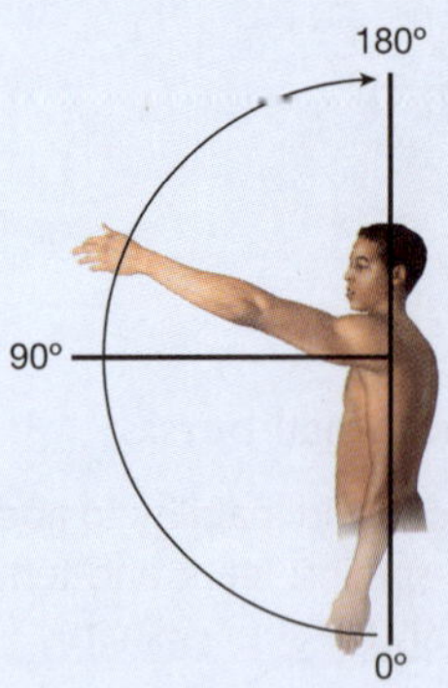	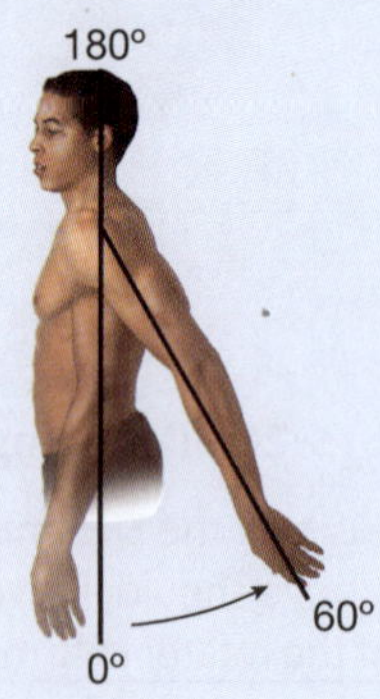
Principal Muscles Affecting Movement Anterior deltoid, pectoralis major (clavicular head), coracobrachialis, biceps brachii	**Principal Muscles Affecting Movement** Latissimus dorsi, teres major, posterior deltoid, triceps brachii (long head)
Patient Instructions "Raise your arms in front of you and overhead."	**Patient Instructions** "Raise your arms behind you."

Abduction	Adduction
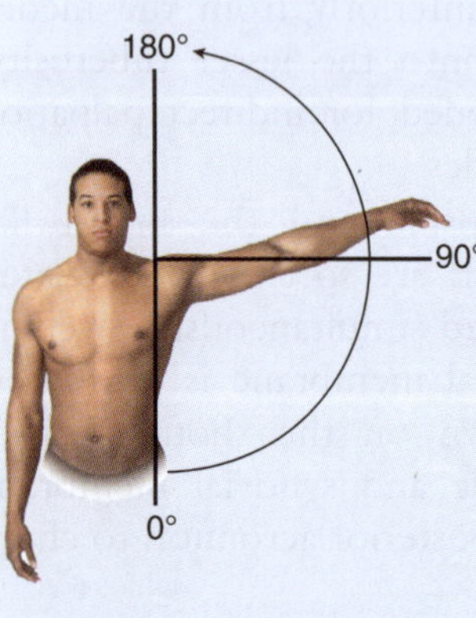	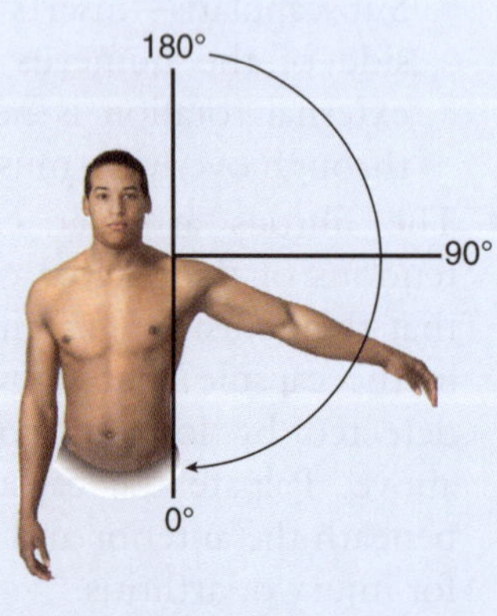
Principal Muscles Affecting Movement Supraspinatus, middle deltoid, serratus anterior (via upward rotation of the scapula)	**Principal Muscles Affecting Movement** Pectoralis major, coracobrachialis, latissimus dorsi, teres major, subscapularis
Patient Instructions "Raise your arms out to the side and overhead."	**Patient Instructions** "Cross your arm in front of your body."

(continued)

Internal Rotation	External Rotation
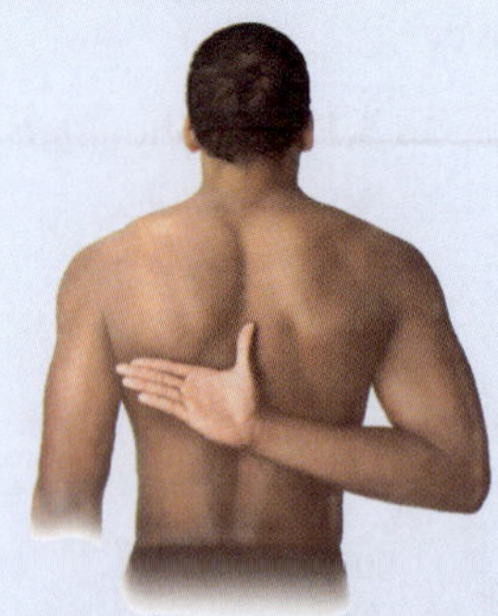	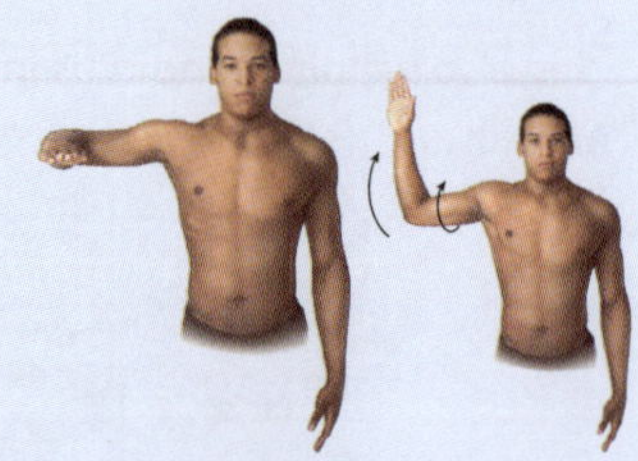
Principal Muscles Affecting Movement Subscapularis, anterior deltoid, pectoralis major, teres major, latissimus dorsi	**Principal Muscles Affecting Movement** Infraspinatus, teres minor, posterior deltoid, supraspinatus (especially with arm overhead)
Patient Instructions "Place one hand behind your back and try to touch your shoulder blade." Identify the highest midline spinous process the patient is able to reach.	**Patient Instructions** "Raise your arm to shoulder level; bend your elbow and rotate your forearm toward the ceiling." OR "Place one hand behind your neck or head as if you are brushing your hair."

Note that to test pure glenohumeral motion, the patient should raise the arms to shoulder level at 90°, with palms facing down. To test scapulothoracic motion, the patient should turn the palms up and raise the arms an additional 60°. The final 30° tests combined glenohumeral and scapulothoracic motion.

Special Maneuvers. Although performing these maneuvers takes supervision and practice, they increase the likelihood of identifying shoulder pathology. There are more than 150 different maneuvers for testing shoulder function (Box 15-9), but few are well studied. Five maneuvers that have the best likelihood ratios (LRs) and the narrowest confidence intervals are currently recommended: one pain provocation test, three strength tests, and one composite test. In composite tests, the patient experiences either pain or weakness during the maneuver.

- Pain provocation test: *painful arc test* (subacromial bursa and rotator cuff). This test has a positive LR of 3.7, which is the highest of all the rotator cuff maneuvers. It also has the best negative LR, 0.36, for ruling out rotator cuff disorders. Other common pain provocation tests are the *Neer* and *Hawkins* tests although their positive LRs are <2, so they are less diagnostic.

Box 15-9. Special Maneuvers for Examining the Shoulder Joint

Structure	Maneuver/ Type of Test	
Acromioclavicular Joint	*Crossover* or *crossed body adduction test.* Adduct the patient's arm across the chest. 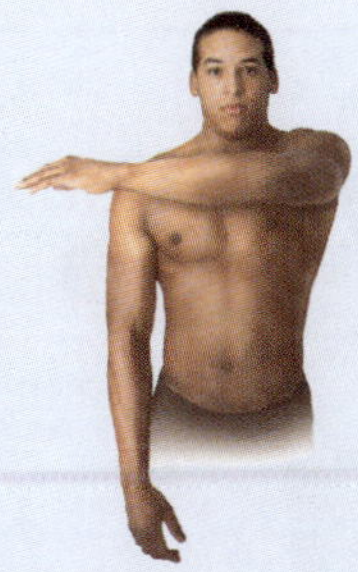	Pain with adduction is a positive test, with a positive LR of 3.7. Acromioclavicular joint tenderness and compression tenderness have low LRs so are not diagnostically helpful.
Overall Shoulder Rotation	*Apley scratch test.* Ask the patient to touch the opposite scapula using the two motions shown below. 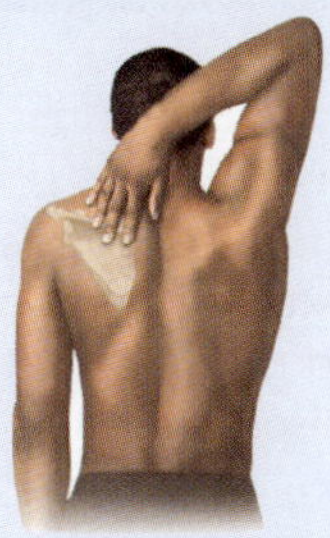 Tests abduction and external rotation. 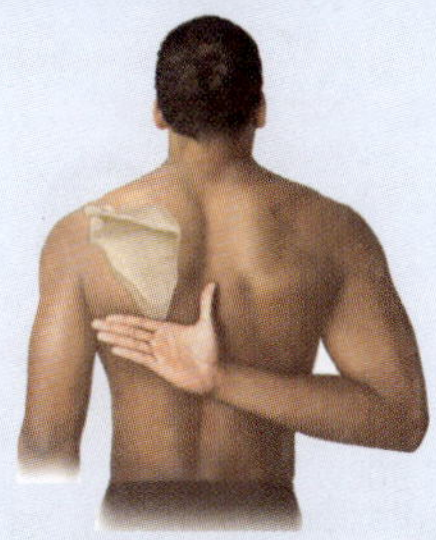 Tests adduction and internal rotation.	Pain during these maneuvers suggests a rotator cuff disorder or adhesive capsulitis.
Rotator Cuff *Pain Provocation Tests*	*Painful arc test.* Fully abduct the patient's arm from 0° to 180°. 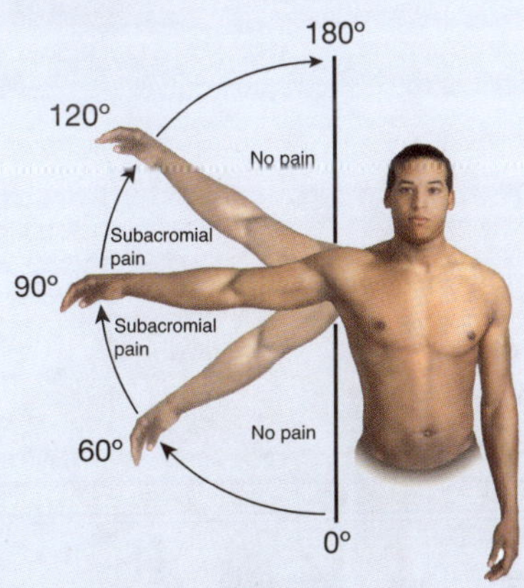	Shoulder pain from 60° to 120° is a *positive test* for a subacromial impingement/rotator cuff tendinitis disorder, with a positive LR 3.7 and a helpful negative LR of 0.36.
	Neer impingement sign. Press on the scapula to prevent scapular motion with one hand and raise the patient's arm with the other. This compresses the greater tuberosity of the humerus against the acromion. 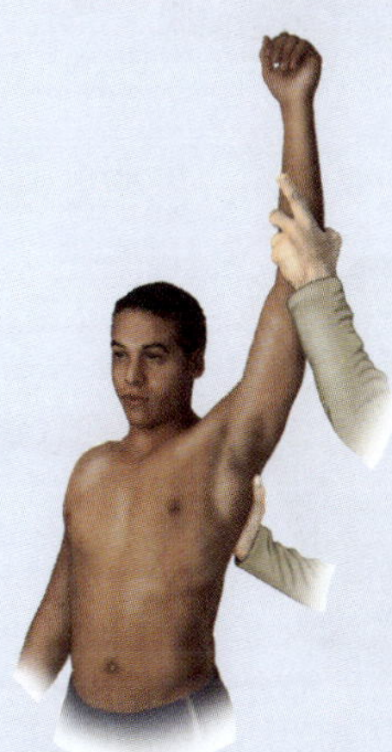	Pain during this maneuver is a *positive test* for a subacromial impingement/ rotator cuff tendinitis disorder, with a positive LR ~1.0 to 1.6. Compression of the rotator cuff muscles and tendons (most commonly the supraspinatus tendon) between the head of the humerus and the acromion causes *"impingement signs,"* or pain during shoulder movement.

(*continued*)

Box 15-9. Special Maneuvers for Examining the Shoulder Joint (*continued*)

Structure	Maneuver/ Type of Test		
	Hawkins impingement sign. Flex the patient's shoulder and elbow to 90° with the palm facing down. Then, with one hand on the forearm and one on the arm, rotate the arm internally. This compresses the greater tuberosity against the supraspinatus tendon and coracoacromial ligament.	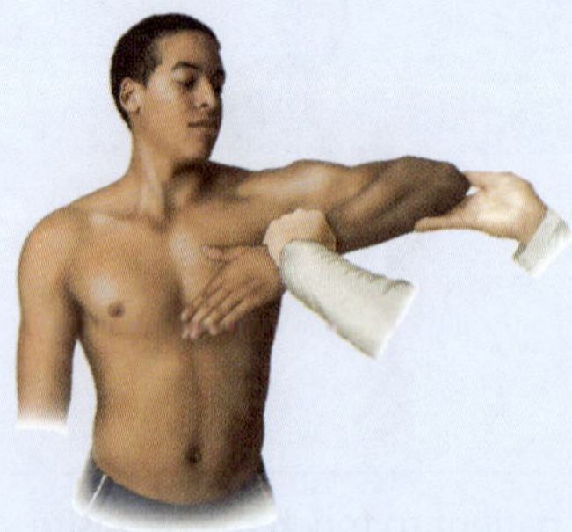	Pain during this maneuver is a *positive test* for supraspinatus impingement/ rotator cuff tendinitis, with a positive LR of ~1.5. When both the Hawkins and Neer signs are absent, the negative LR is helpful at 0.1.
Strength Tests	*External rotation lag test.* With the patient's arm flexed to 90° with palm up, rotate the arm into full external rotation and ask the patient to keep the arm in this position.	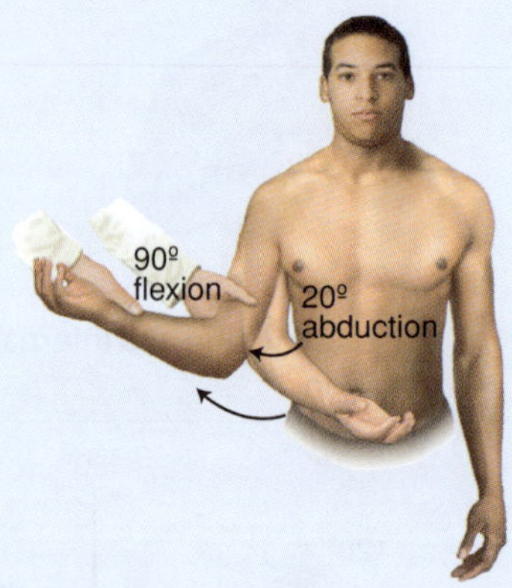	Inability of the patient to maintain external rotation is a *positive test* for supraspinatus and infraspinatus disorders, with a positive LR of 7.2.
	Internal rotation lag test (lift-off test). With you standing to the patient's rear, bring the dorsum of the hand behind the low back with the elbow flexed to 90°. Then grip the wrist and lift the hand off the back, which further internally rotates the shoulder. Ask the patient to keep the hand in this position as you release the wrist.	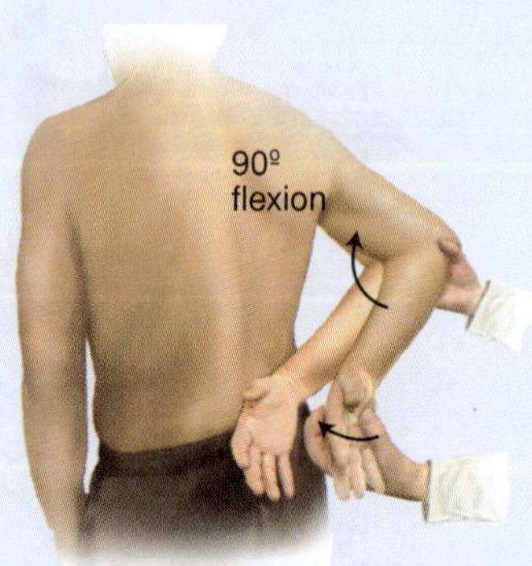	Inability of the patient to hold the hand in this position is a *positive test* for a subscapularis disorder, with a positive LR of 5.6 to 6.2 and an excellent negative LR of 0.04.
	Drop-arm test. Ask the patient to fully abduct the arm to shoulder level, up to 90°, and lower it slowly. Note that abduction above shoulder level, from 90° to 120°, reflects action of the deltoid muscle.	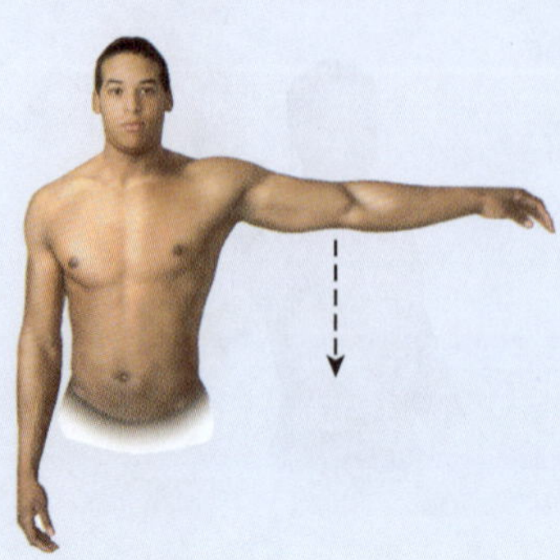	Weakness during this maneuver is a *positive test* for a supraspinatus rotator cuff tear or bicipital tendinitis, with a positive LR of 3.3.

(*continued*)

Box 15-9. Special Maneuvers for Examining the Shoulder Joint (*continued*)

Structure	Maneuver/ Type of Test		
Composite Tests	*External rotation resistance test.* Ask the patient to adduct and flex the arm to 90°, with the thumbs turned up. Stabilize the elbow with one hand and apply pressure proximal to the patient's wrist as the patient presses the wrist outward in external rotation.	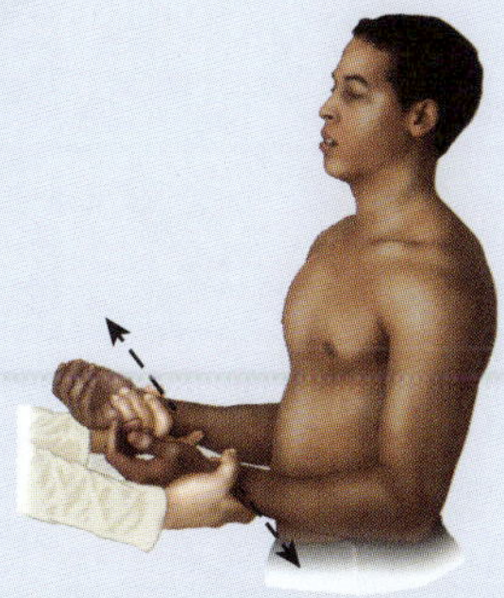	Pain or weakness during this maneuver is a *positive test* for an infraspinatus disorder, with a positive LR of 2.6 and negative LR of 0.49. Limited external rotation points to glenohumeral disease or adhesive capsulitis.
	Empty can test. Elevate the arms to 90° and internally rotate the arms with the thumbs pointing down, as if emptying a can. Ask the patient to resist as you place downward pressure on the arms.	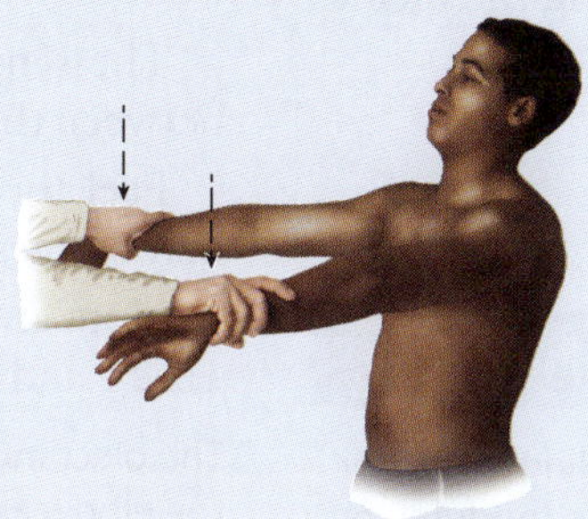	Inability of the patient to hold the arm fully abducted at shoulder level or control lowering the arm is a *positive test* for a suprasinatus rotator cuff tear, with a positive LR of 1.3.

- Strength tests: *internal rotation lag test* (subscapularis), *external rotation lag test* (supraspinatus and infraspinatus), and *drop arm test* (supraspinatus). These tests have positive LRs of 7.2, 5.6, and 3.3, respectively.
- Composite test: *external rotation resistance test* (infraspinatus). This test has a positive LR of 2.6. Another common composite test is the *empty can test.*

Elbow Joint

The elbow helps position the hand in space and stabilizes the lever action of the forearm. The elbow joint is formed by the humerus and the two bones of the forearm, the radius and the ulna (Fig. 15-21). Identify the medial and lateral epicondyles of the humerus and the olecranon process of the ulna.

These bones have three articulations: the *humeroulnar joint,* the *radiohumeral joint,* and the *radioulnar joint.* All three share a large common articular cavity and an extensive synovial lining.

Muscles traversing the elbow include the *biceps* and *brachioradialis* (flexion), the *brachialis,* the *triceps* (extension), the *pronator teres* (pronation), and the *supinator* (supination).

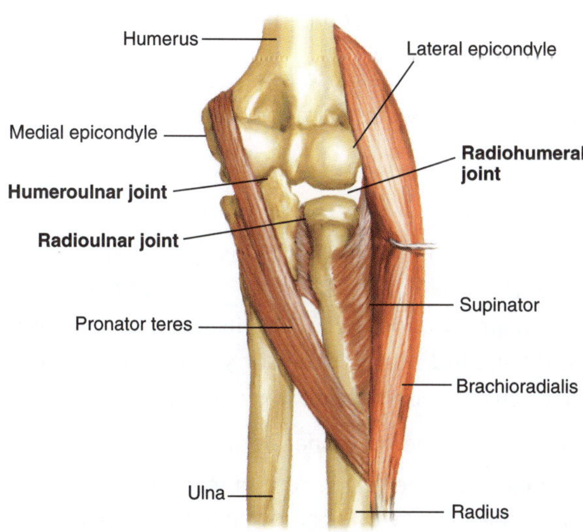

FIGURE 15-21. Anatomy of the left anterior elbow.

Note the location of the *olecranon bursa* between the olecranon process and the skin (Fig. 15-22). The bursa is not normally palpable but can swell and becomes tender when inflamed. The *ulnar nerve* runs posteriorly in the ulnar groove between the medial epicondyle and the olecranon process. The radial nerve is adjacent to the lateral epicondyle. On the ventral forearm, the *median nerve* is just medial to the brachial artery in the antecubital fossa.

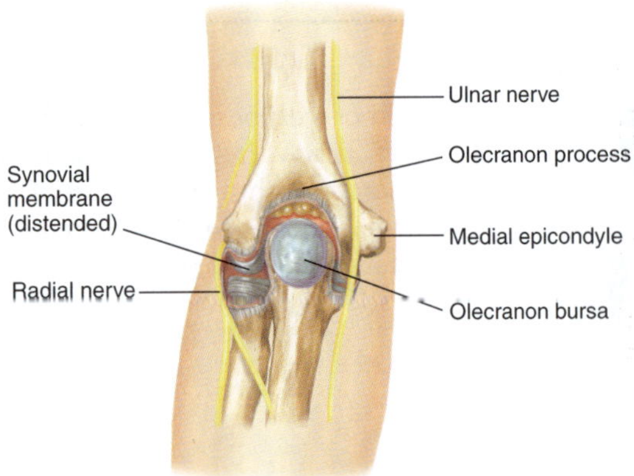

FIGURE 15-22. Left posterior elbow revealing the olecranon process and bursa.

Techniques of Examination

Key Components of the Elbow Joint Examination

- Inspect the contours of the elbow, including extensor surfaces of the ulna and olecranon process (nodules or swelling).
- Palpate the olecranon process and medial and lateral epicondyles (tenderness, warmth, displacement).
- Assess range of motion: flexion and extension and pronation and supination.
- Perform special maneuvers (if indicated): Cozen test, Mill test, and Maudsley test (lateral epicondylitis).

Inspection. Support the patient's forearm with your opposite hand so that the elbow is flexed to about 70°. Identify the medial and lateral epicondyles and the olecranon process of the ulna. Inspect the contours of the elbow, including the extensor surface of the ulna and the olecranon process. Note any nodules or swelling.

See Table 15-6, Swollen or Tender Elbows.

Swelling over the olecranon process is suspicious for olecranon bursitis (see p. 474). Inflammation of synovial fluid suggests arthritis.

Palpation. Palpate the olecranon process and press over the epicondyles for tenderness (Fig. 15-23).

Tenderness distal to the epicondyle is common in *lateral epicondylitis* (tennis elbow) and less common in *medial epicondylitis* (pitcher's or golfer's elbow).

Palpate the grooves between the epicondyles and the olecranon process, where the synovium is most easily examined. Normally the synovium and olecranon bursae are not palpable.

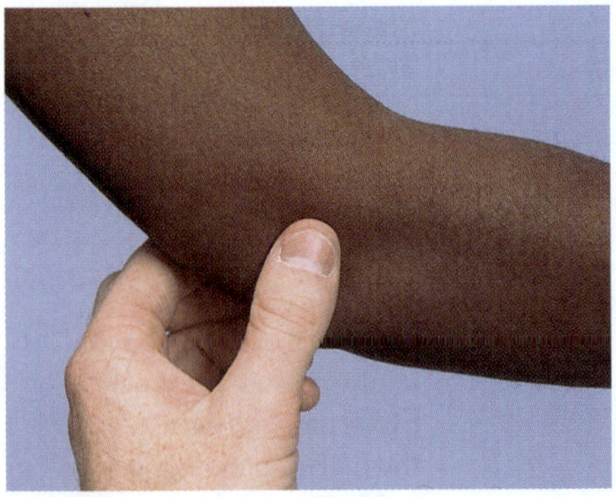

FIGURE 15-23. Palpating the epicondyles for tenderness.

The sensitive *ulnar nerve* can be palpated posteriorly between the olecranon process and the medial epicondyle.

Feel for warmth in the skin or around the joint that may suggest infection or underlying inflammation.

Note any displacement of the olecranon process (Figs. 15-24 and 15-25).

The olecranon is displaced posteriorly in posterior dislocation of the elbow and supracondylar fracture.

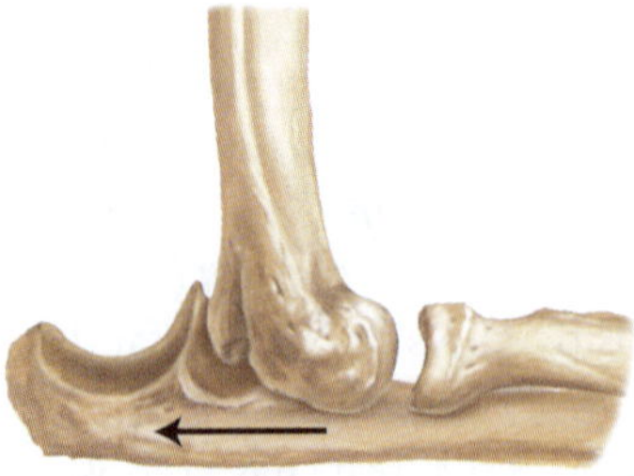

FIGURE 15-24. Posterior dislocation of the elbow.

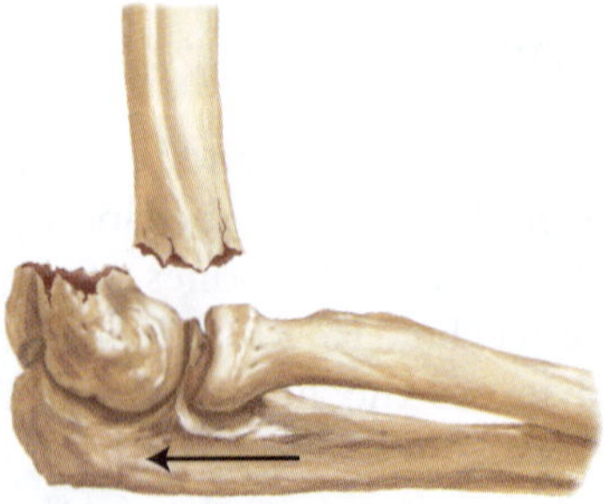

FIGURE 15-25. Supracondylar fracture of the elbow.

Range of Motion. ROM includes *flexion* and *extension* at the elbow and *pronation* and *supination* of the forearm, which also move the wrist and hand (Fig. 15-26). Note the specific muscles responsible for each motion and the instructions to the patient (Box 15-10).

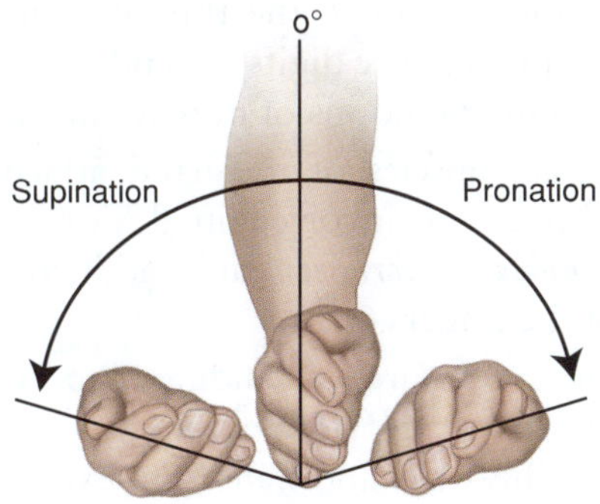

FIGURE 15-26. Elbow supination and pronation.

Pay attention to any clicking or crepitus that may suggest underlying arthritis, loose body within the joint, or possible damage to the radial head.

After injury, preservation of active ROM and full elbow extension makes fracture, intraarticular effusion, or hemarthrosis highly unlikely.

Box 15-10. Range of Motion of the Elbow Joint

Elbow Movement	Primary Muscles Affecting Movement	Patient Instructions
Flexion	Biceps brachii, brachialis, brachioradialis	"Bend your elbow."
Extension	Triceps brachii, anconeus	"Straighten your elbow."
Supination	Biceps brachii, supinator	"Turn your palms up, as if carrying a bowl of soup."
Pronation	Pronator teres, pronator quadratus	"Turn your palms down."

Special Maneuvers. Patients may often complain of pain at or around the bony prominence of the lateral epicondyle that often radiates down the forearm. A number of tests have been described that reproduce this pain along the lateral epicondyle and one such maneuver is the *Cozen test* (Fig. 15-27). Stabilize the patient's elbow and palpate the lateral epicondyle. Then ask the patient to pronate and extend the wrist against resistance. Pain should be reproduced along the lateral aspect of the elbow. Other maneuvers to reproduce the pain include passive stretching of the wrist extensors (*Mill test*) and resisted extension of the middle finger with the wrist extended (*Maudsley test*).

Reproduction of symptoms is characteristic of lateral epicondylitis. Infection and inflammatory or degenerative arthritis may also give rise to clinical signs mimicking lateral epicondylitis.

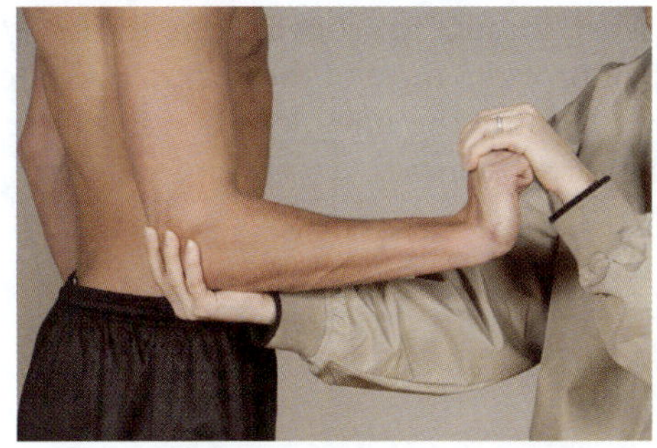

FIGURE 15-27. Testing for lateral epicondylitis or "tennis elbow" (Cozen test). (From Anderson MK. *Foundations of Athletic Training: Prevention, Assessment, and Management.* 6th ed. Wolters Kluwer; 2017, Fig. 18-11a.)

Wrist and Hand Joints

The wrists and hands form a complex unit of small highly active joints used almost continuously during waking hours. There is little protection from overlying soft tissue, increasing vulnerability to trauma and disability.

The wrist includes the *distal radius* and *ulna* and eight small *carpal bones* (Fig. 15-28). At the wrist, identify the bony tips of the radius and the ulna.

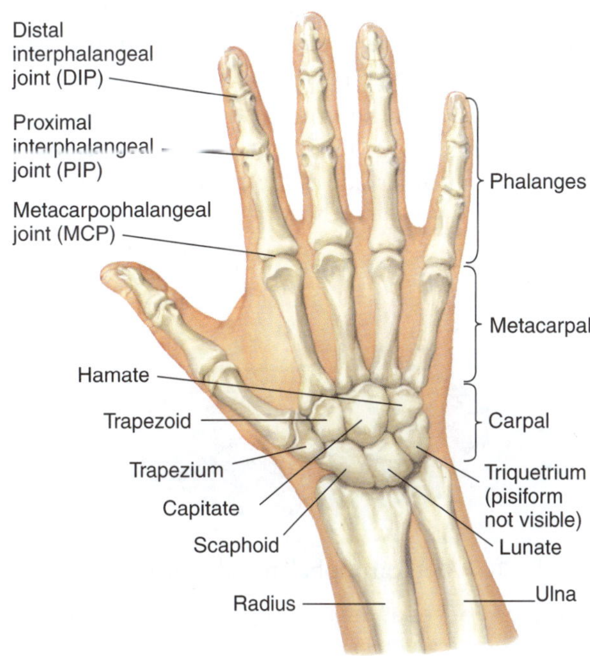

FIGURE 15-28. Anatomy of the right wrist and hand.

- The wrist joints include the *radiocarpal* or *wrist joint,* the *distal radioulnar joint,* and the *intercarpal joints* (Fig. 15-29). The joint capsule, articular disc, and synovial membrane of the wrist join the radius to the ulna and to the proximal carpal bones. On the dorsum of the wrist, locate the groove of the *radiocarpal joint.* This joint provides most of the flexion and extension at the wrist because the ulna does not articulate directly with the carpal bones.

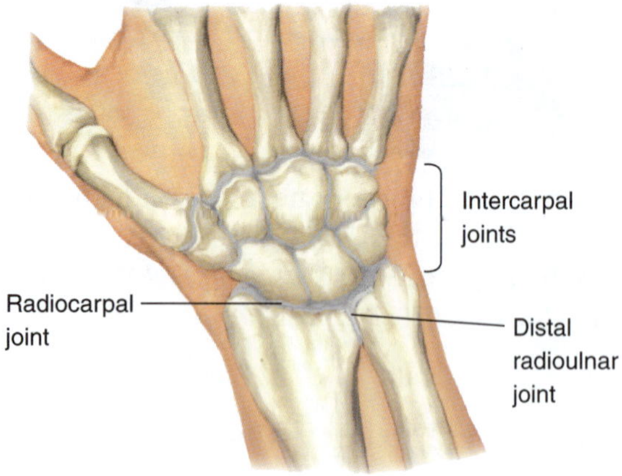

FIGURE 15-29. Joints of the right wrist.

Identify the *carpal bones* distal to the wrist joint; each of the five *metacarpals*; and the *proximal*, *middle*, and *distal phalanges.* Note that the thumb has only two phalanges.

The numerous joints of the wrist and hand make the hands unusually dexterous. The joints of the hand include the *metacarpophalangeal joints* (MCPs), the *proximal interphalangeal joints* (PIPs), and the *distal interphalangeal joints* (DIPs).

Flex the fingers and find the groove marking the MCP joint of each finger (Fig. 15-30). It is distal to the knuckle and is best felt on either side of the extensor tendon.

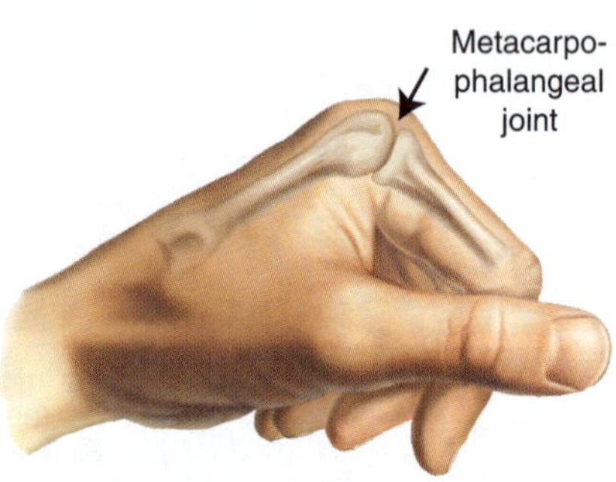

FIGURE 15-30. Metacarpophalangeal joints.

Degenerative changes at the first carpometacarpal joint of the thumb are more common in women.

Wrist flexion arises from the two carpal muscles, located on the radial and ulnar surfaces. Two radial and one ulnar muscle provide wrist extension. Supination and pronation are powered by muscle contraction in the forearm.

The thumb is powered by three muscles that form the thenar eminence and provide flexion, abduction, and opposition. The muscles of extension originate in the forearm and extend to the thumb along the radial margin. Movement in the digits depends on action of the flexor and extensor tendons of muscles in the forearm.

The intrinsic muscles of the hand attaching to the metacarpal bones are involved in flexion (*lumbricals*), abduction (*dorsal interossei*), and adduction (*palmar interossei*) of the fingers.

Soft tissue structures including tendons, tendon sheaths, and muscles are especially important to movement of the wrist and hand. Six extensor tendons and two flexor tendons pass across the wrist and hand to insert on the fingers. Through much of their course these tendons travel in tunnel-like *sheaths*, generally palpable only when swollen or inflamed.

Be familiar with the structures of the *carpal tunnel*, a channel beneath the palmar surface of the wrist and proximal hand (Fig. 15-31). The channel contains the sheath and flexor tendons for the thumb and fingers as well as the *median nerve.*

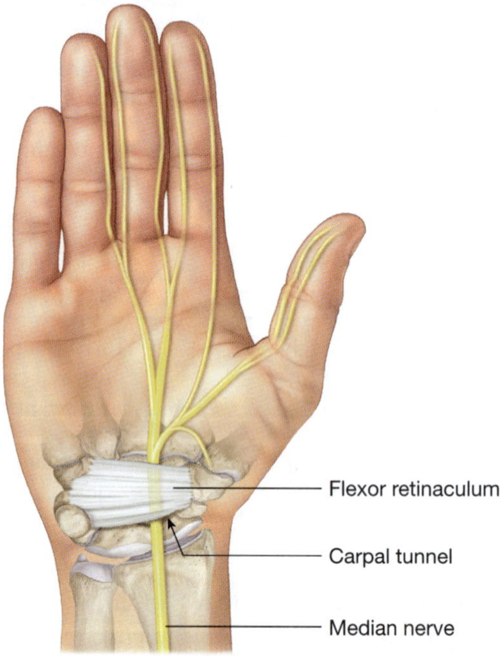

FIGURE 15-31. Carpal tunnel of the right hand.

Holding the tendons and tendon sheath in place is a transverse ligament, the *flexor retinaculum.* The median nerve lies between the flexor retinaculum and the tendon sheath. The median nerve provides sensation to the palm and the palmar surface of most of the thumb, the second and third digits, and half of the fourth digit. It also innervates the thumb muscles of flexion, abduction, and opposition.

Also learn the distribution of the median, radial, and ulnar nerve innervations of the wrist and hand (Figs. 15-32 and 15-33).

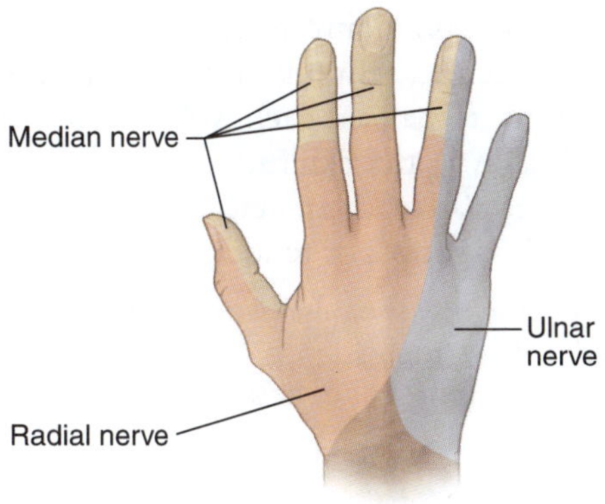

FIGURE 15-32. Peripheral innervation of the right hand (dorsal view).

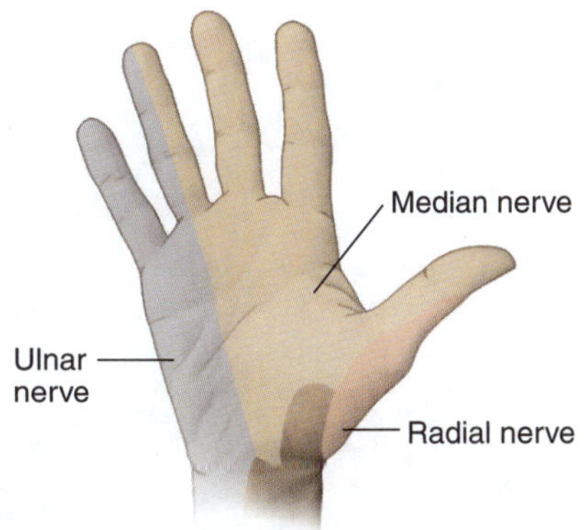

FIGURE 15-33. Peripheral innervation of the right hand (palmar view).

Techniques of Examination

Key Components of the Wrist Joint and Hand Examination

- Inspect position of the hands in motion and at rest; inspect the wrist, hand, and finger bones (swelling, deformities, angulation); thenar and hypothenar eminences (atrophy); and flexor tendons (thickening, contractures).
- Palpate the distal radius and ulna, radial styloid bone, and anatomic snuffbox (tenderness); the carpal bones (tenderness, excessive movement); the metacarpals and proximal, middle, and distal phalanges, wrist joint, MCPs, and PIPs (swelling, bogginess, tenderness).
- Assess range of motion. *Wrist:* flexion and extension, abduction (radial deviation) and adduction (ulnar deviation). *Fingers (MCP, PIP, DIP):* flexion and extension and abduction and adduction. *Thumb:* flexion and extension, abduction and adduction, and opposition.
- Perform special maneuvers (if indicated): hand grip strength, tests for thumb tenosynovitis (Finkelstein test), and nerve entrapment neuropathy (sensation, thumb abduction and opposition, Tinel sign, Phalen sign).

Inspection. Inspect the position of the hands in motion for smooth, natural movement. When the fingers are relaxed, they should be slightly flexed; the fingernail edges should be in parallel.

Guarded movement suggests injury. Flexor tendon damage causes abnormal finger alignment.

Inspect the palmar and dorsal surfaces of the wrist and hand carefully for swelling over the joints or signs of trauma.

Diffuse swelling is common in arthritis or infection. Local swelling may suggest a ganglion cyst or focal thickening of a tendon or tendon sheath as seen in *flexor tenosynovitis* (trigger finger). Laceration, puncture, injection marks, burn, or erythema result from trauma. See Table 15-7, Arthritis in the Hands, and Table 15-8, Swellings and Deformities of the Hands.

Note any deformities of the wrist, hand, or finger bones, as well as any angulation.

Heberden nodes (hard dorsolateral nodules on the DIP joints) and *Bouchard nodes* (hard dorsolateral nodules on the PIP joints) are common findings in OA. In RA, inspect for symmetric deformity in the PIP, MCP, and wrist joints. In later stages, you may see MCP subluxation and ulnar deviation. Of note, the DIP tends to be less affected in RA.

Observe the contours of the palm, namely the *thenar* and *hypothenar* eminences.

Thenar atrophy can occur in median nerve compression from carpal tunnel syndrome (sensitivity <50%; specificity >82% to 99%). In ulnar nerve compression, there is hypothenar atrophy.

Note any thickening of the flexor tendons or flexion contractures in the fingers.

Dupuytren flexion contractures occur in the third, fourth, and fifth fingers and arise from thickening of the palmar fascia. As mentioned earlier, trigger digits are caused by stenosing tenosynovitis.

Palpation. At the wrist, palpate the distal radius and ulna on the lateral and medial surfaces (Fig. 15-34). Palpate the groove of each wrist joint with your thumbs on the dorsum of the wrist, your fingers beneath it. Note any swelling, bogginess, or tenderness.

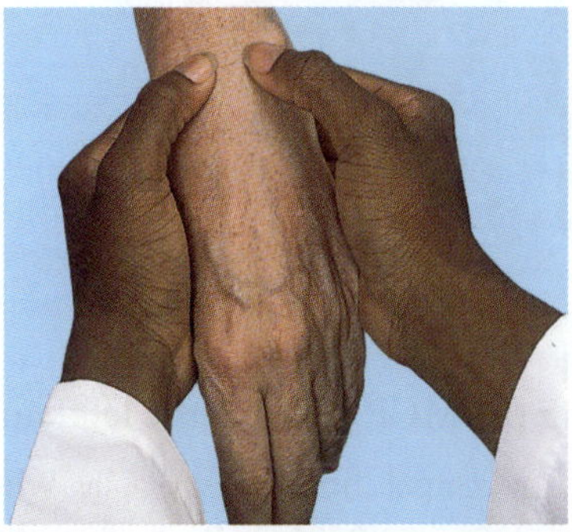

FIGURE 15-34. Palpating the left wrist joint.

Tenderness over the distal radius after a fall is suspicious for a Colles fracture. Bony step-offs may also suggest fracture.

In RA, there is often persistent bilateral swelling and/or tenderness.

Palpate the *radial styloid bone* and the *anatomic snuffbox*, a hollowed depression just distal to the radial styloid process formed by the abductor and extensor muscles of the thumb (Fig. 15-35). The "snuffbox" is more visible with abduction of the thumb.

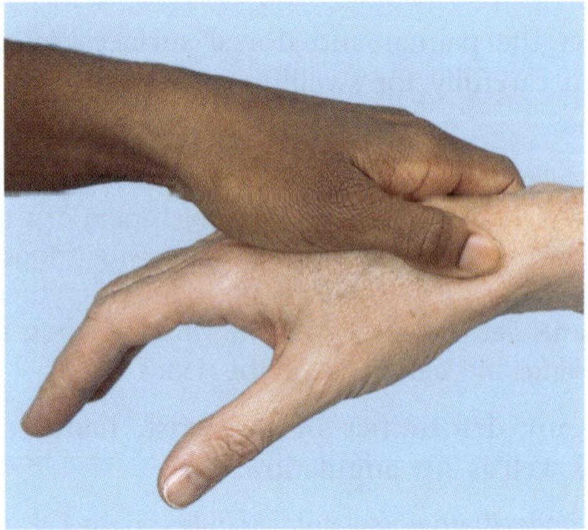

FIGURE 15-35. Palpating the anatomic snuffbox.

Tenderness over the extensor and abductor tendons of the thumb at the radial styloid occurs in de Quervain tenosynovitis and gonococcal tenosynovitis. See Table 15-9, Tendon Sheath, Palmar Space, and Finger Infections.

"Snuffbox" tenderness with the wrist in ulnar deviation and pain at the scaphoid tubercle are suspicious for occult scaphoid fracture. Poor blood supply increases risk of scaphoid bone avascular necrosis, making this a diagnosis that should not be missed.

Palpate the carpal bones lying distal to the wrist joint and then each of the metacarpals and the proximal, middle, and distal phalanges (Fig. 15-36). Attempt to move the carpal bones relative to each other. There should be little to no movement.

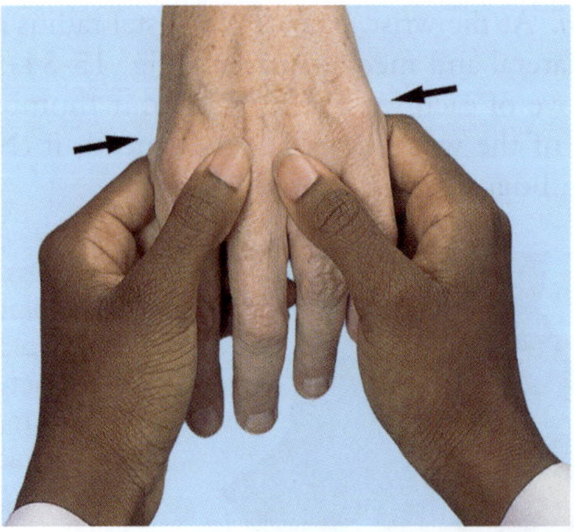

FIGURE 15-36. Palpating the MCP joints of the left hand.

Excessive movement of any carpal bones, especially when painful, may suggest underlying ligament laxity or disruption that can result from trauma.

Compress the MCP joints by squeezing the hand from each side between the thumb and fingers. Alternatively, use your thumb to palpate each MCP joint just distal to and on each side of the extensor tendons as your index finger feels the head of the metacarpal in the palm. Note any swelling, bogginess, or tenderness.

The MCPs are often boggy or tender in RA but are rarely involved in OA. Pain with compression also occurs in posttraumatic arthritis. Focal tenderness after trauma may suggest underlying fracture.

Now examine the fingers and thumb. Palpate the medial and lateral aspects of each PIP joint between your thumb and index finger, again checking for swelling, bogginess, bony enlargement, or tenderness. Using the same techniques, examine the DIP joints (Fig. 15-37).

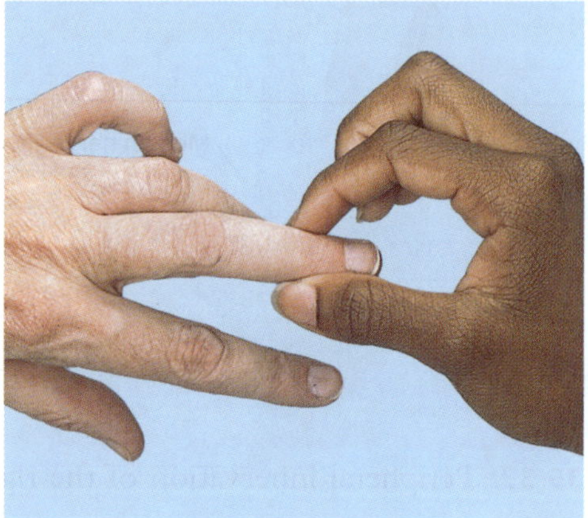

FIGURE 15-37. Palpating the DIP joints.

Bouchard nodes in the PIPs are a classic sign of OA. Heberden nodes, which are more common than Bouchard nodes, are similar bony swellings that develop in the DIPs of patients with OA (Fig. 15-38).

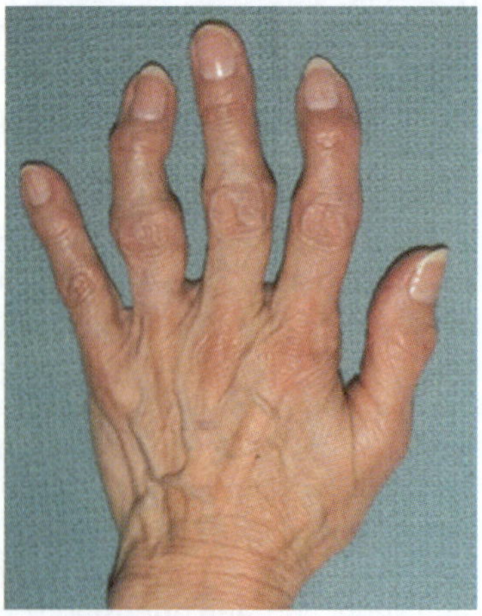

FIGURE 15-38. Heberden nodes (DIPs) and Bouchard nodes (PIPs) in a patient with classic hand osteoarthritis. (Modified from Ballantyne JC, et al. *Bonica's Management of Pain.* 5th ed. Wolters Kluwer; 2019, Fig. 34-3.)

Palpate along the tendons inserting on the thumb and fingers looking for tenderness, erythema, or inflammation. Examine for any focal thickening.

Tenderness and swelling occur in *tenosynovitis*, or inflammation of the tendon sheaths. De Quervain tenosynovitis involves the extensor and abductor tendons of the thumb as they cross the radial styloid in the first dorsal compartment of the wrist.

See Table 15-9, Tendon Sheath, Palmar Space, and Finger Infections.

Range of Motion: Wrist Joint. The specific muscles responsible for each movement are described in Box 15-11. During your examination, use clear instructions that prompt the patient to properly follow your directions to ensure you examine all active ROM. For techniques of testing wrist muscle strength, turn to Chapter 13, Nervous System.

Arthritis, tenosynovitis, and Dupuytren contracture all impair ROM (Figs. 15-39 and 15-40). See Table 15-8, Swellings and Deformities of the Hands.

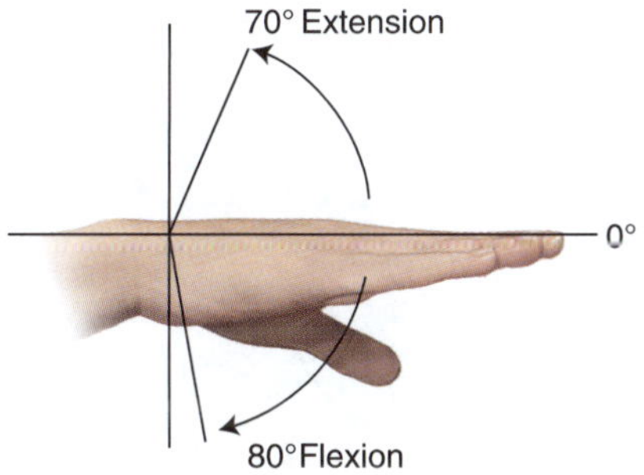

FIGURE 15-39. Wrist flexion and extension.

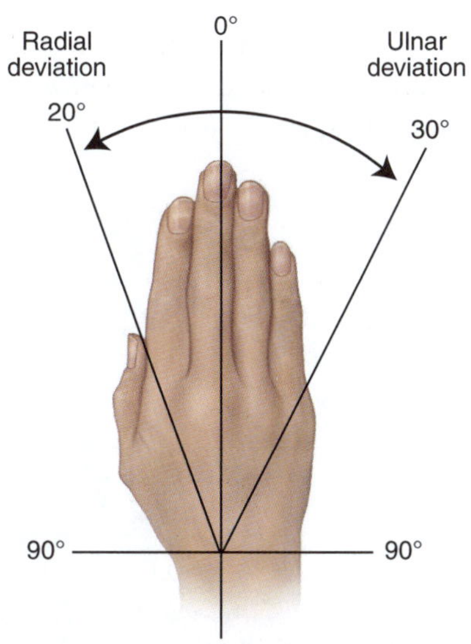

FIGURE 15-40. Wrist abduction (radial) and adduction (ulnar) deviation.

Box 15-11. Range of Motion of the Wrist Joint

Wrist Movement	Primary Muscles Affecting Movement	Patient Instructions
Flexion	Flexor carpi radialis, flexor carpi ulnaris	"With palms down, point your fingers toward the floor."
Extension	Extensor carpi ulnaris, extensor carpi radialis longus, extensor carpi radialis brevis	"With palms down, point your fingers toward the ceiling."
Adduction (ulnar deviation)	Flexor carpi ulnaris Extensor carpi ulnaris	"With palms down, move your fingers toward the midline."
Abduction (radial deviation)	Flexor carpi radialis Extensor carpi radialis longus and brevis Occasional contribution from abductor pollicis longus	"With palms down, move your fingers away from the midline."

See p. 431 for discussion of pronation and supination, which also involve the wrist and hand.

Range of Motion: Fingers and Thumb. Assess flexion, extension, abduction, and adduction of the fingers.

- *Flexion* and *extension* (Fig. 15-41). To test the lumbricals and finger flexor muscles, ask the patient to: "Bend your fingers and thumb into your palm and make a fist." To test *extension* of the finger extensor muscles, ask the patient to: "Straighten out your fingers and thumb." At the MCPs, the fingers may extend beyond the neutral position.

  Test the flexion and extension of the PIP and DIP joints. The fingers should open and close easily.

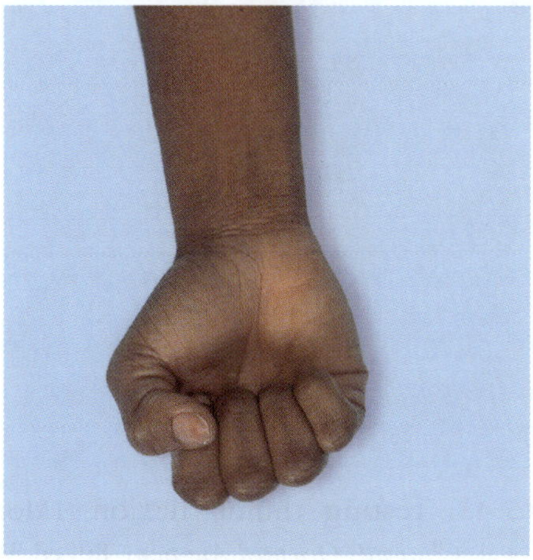

FIGURE 15-41. Testing finger flexion.

- *Abduction* and *adduction* (Fig. 15-42). Ask the patient to spread the fingers apart (abduction from dorsal interossei) and back together (adduction from palmar interossei). Check for smooth, coordinated movement.

Inspect for impaired hand movement or deformity in arthritis, trigger finger, and Dupuytren contracture as discussed previously.

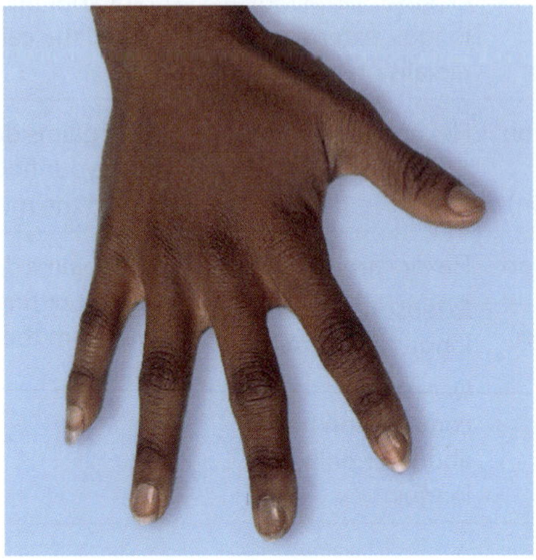

FIGURE 15-42. Testing finger abduction.

- At the *thumb*, assess *flexion, extension, abduction, adduction*, and *opposition*. Each of these movements is powered by a related muscle of the thumb.

Ask the patient to move the thumb across the palm and touch the base of the fifth finger to test *flexion* (Fig. 15-43) and then to move the thumb back across the palm and away from the fingers to test *extension* (Fig. 15-44).

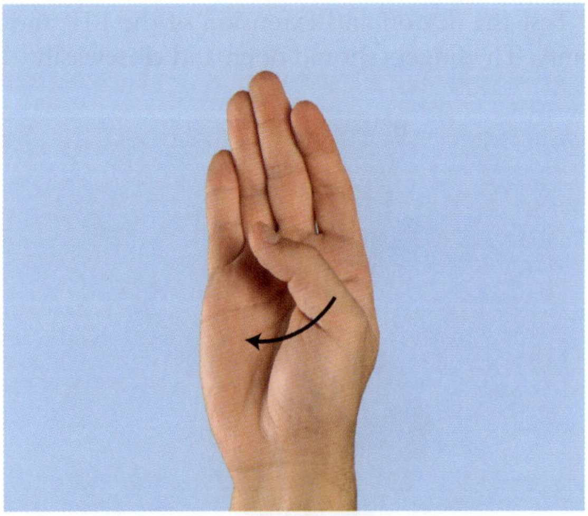

FIGURE 15-43. Testing thumb flexion. (Modified from Moore KL et al. *Clinically Oriented Anatomy.* 8th ed. Wolters Kluwer; 2018, Fig. 3-76.)

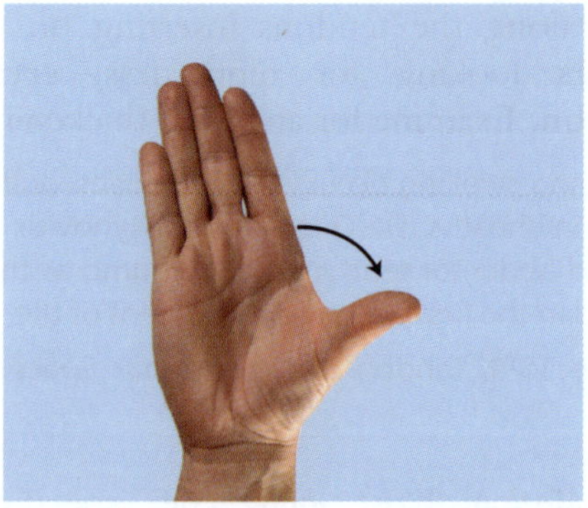

FIGURE 15-44. Testing thumb extension. (Modified from Moore KL et al. *Clinically Oriented Anatomy.* 8th ed. Wolters Kluwer; 2018, Fig. 3-76.)

- Next, ask the patient to place the fingers and thumb in the neutral position with the palm up, then have the patient move the thumb anteriorly away from the palm to assess *abduction* and back down for *adduction* (Fig. 15-45). To test *opposition*, or movements of the thumb across the palm, ask the patient to touch the thumb to each of the other fingertips (Fig. 15-46).

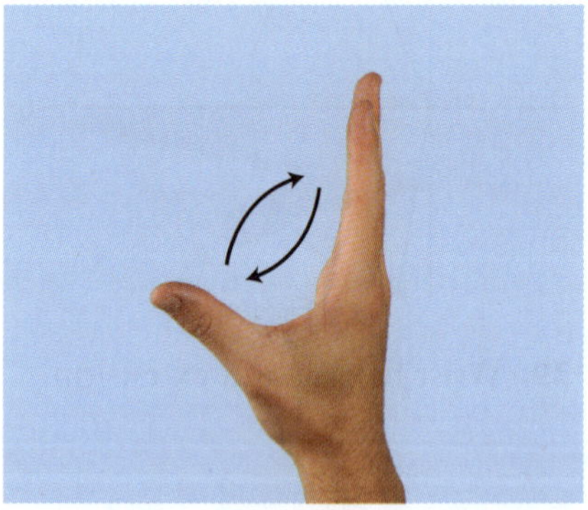

FIGURE 15-45. Testing thumb abduction and adduction. (Modified from Moore KL et al. *Clinically Oriented Anatomy.* 8th ed. Wolters Kluwer; 2018, Fig. 3-76.)

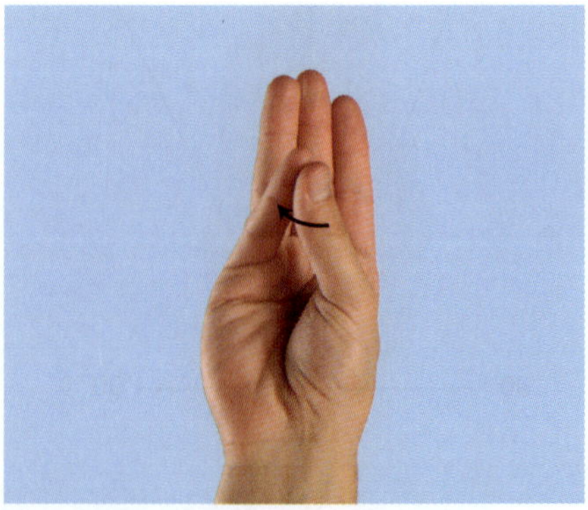

FIGURE 15-46. Testing thumb opposition. (Modified from Moore KL et al. *Clinically Oriented Anatomy.* 8th ed. Wolters Kluwer; 2018, Fig. 3-76.)

Special Maneuvers

Hand Grip Strength. Ask the patient to grasp your second and third fingers as tightly as possible (Fig. 15-47). This tests function of wrist joints, the finger flexors, and the intrinsic muscles and joints of the hand. It is always important to determine if weakness is related to pain or true inability to perform the desired action.

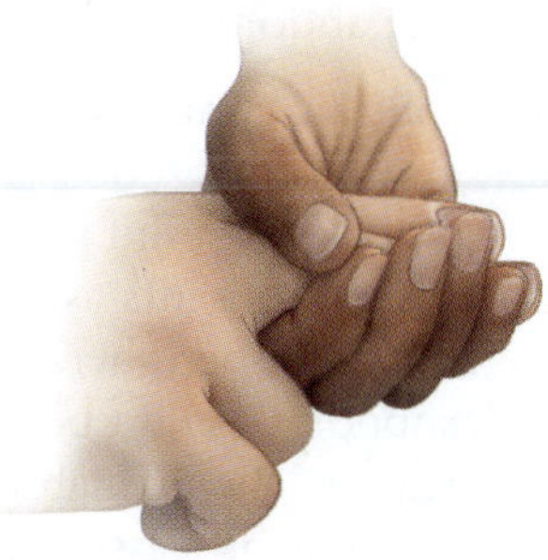

FIGURE 15-47. Testing hand grip strength.

Decreased grip strength is a positive test for weakness of the finger flexors and/or intrinsic muscles of the hand. It can also result from inflammatory or degenerative arthritis, carpal tunnel syndrome, epicondylitis, cervical radiculopathy and other nerve disorders of the arm and hand.

Grip weakness plus wrist pain are often present in de Quervain tenosynovitis.

Testing for Tenosynovitis. Ask the patient to grasp the thumb against the palm and then move the wrist toward the midline in ulnar deviation (*Finkelstein test*), as shown in Figure 15-48.

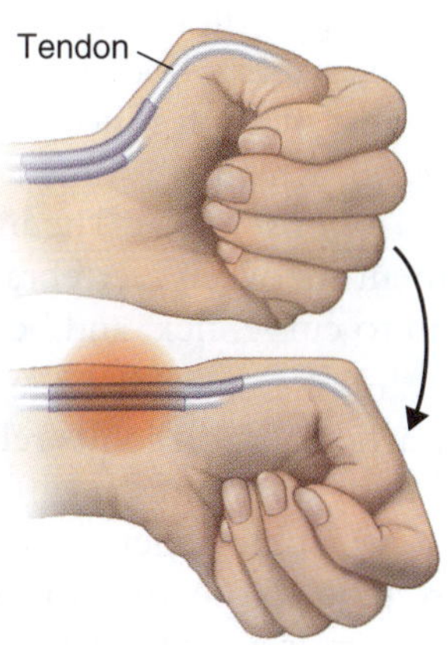

FIGURE 15-48. Testing for thumb tenosynovitis (Finkelstein test).

A full examination of the wrist and hand involves detailed testing of muscle strength and sensation, found in Chapter 13, Nervous System.

Pain during this maneuver identifies de Quervain tenosynovitis ("gamer's thumb") from inflammation of the abductor pollicis longus and extensor pollicis brevis tendons and tendon sheaths.

Tests for Nerve Entrapment Neuropathy (Thumb Abduction and Opposition, Tinel Sign, Phalen Sign). For complaints of nocturnal hand or arm numbness (*paresthesias*), dropping objects, inability to twist lids off jars, aching at the wrist or even the forearm, and numbness of the first three digits, test for *carpal tunnel syndrome,* the most common entrapment neuropathy, involving compression of the median nerve. Be aware that even though the first three fingers are usually involved, patients may report involvement of the whole hand.

Forceful repetitive handwork with prolonged wrist extension (such as keyboarding) and mail sorting, vibration, cold exposure, wrist anatomy, pregnancy, RA, diabetes, and hypothyroidism are risk factors for carpal tunnel syndrome.

Grossly assess the median, radial, and ulnar nerve sensory innervations in the wrist and hand (see Figs. 15-32 and 15-33). You can test sensation as follows:

- Pulp of the index finger—median nerve

  Decreased sensation in the median nerve territory is a common sign of *carpal tunnel syndrome* (sensitivity to pinprick and two-point discrimination <50%; specificity >85%; positive LR of hypalgesia is 3.1).

- Pulp of the fifth finger—ulnar nerve
- Dorsal web space of the thumb and index finger—radial nerve

To test *thumb abduction,* ask the patient to raise the thumb straight up away from the palm at a 90° angle from the hand as you apply downward resistance (Fig. 15-49). You can also test *thumb opposition* by asking the patient to touch the thumb to the fifth fingertip as you apply outward pressure against the base of the thumb.

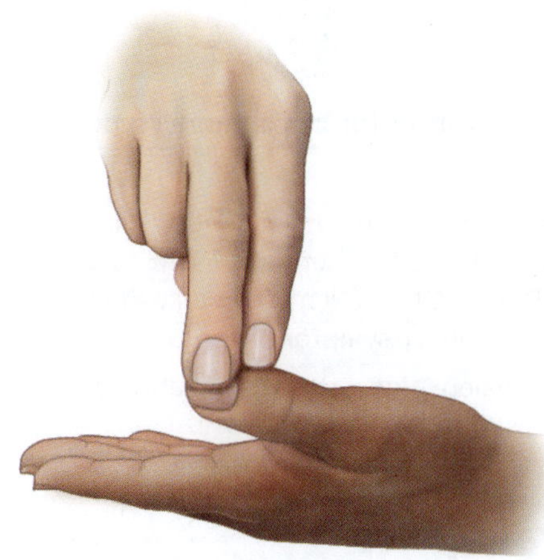

FIGURE 15-49. Testing for carpal tunnel syndrome (thumb abduction).

Weakness on thumb abduction or opposition is a *positive test.* The abductor pollicis longus is innervated only by the median nerve. The opponens pollicis is also only innervated by the median nerve.

Test the *Tinel sign* by repeatedly tapping over the course of the median nerve in the carpal tunnel, as shown in Figure 15-50.

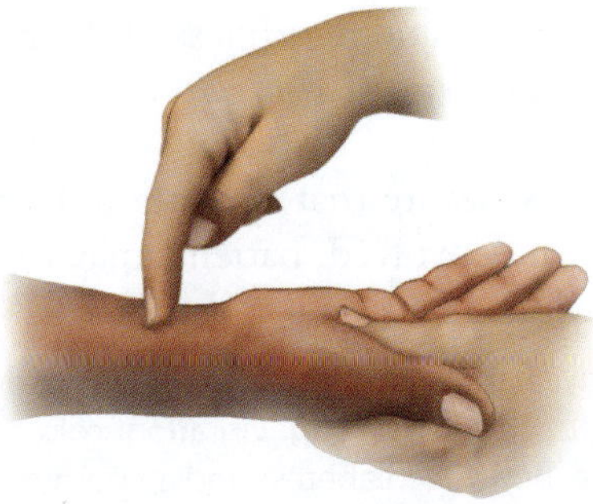

FIGURE 15-50. Testing for carpal tunnel syndrome (Tinel sign).

Shooting pain, aching, or worsening numbness in the median nerve distribution is a *positive test* (sensitivity 23% to 60%; specificity 64% to 91%; LR ≤1.5).

To test the *Phalen sign*, ask the patient to hold the wrists in full flexion and juxtaposing the dorsum of each hand against each other for 60 seconds with the elbows fully extended (Fig. 15-51). Alternatively, ask the patient to press the backs of both hands together to form right angles. These maneuvers compress the median nerve.

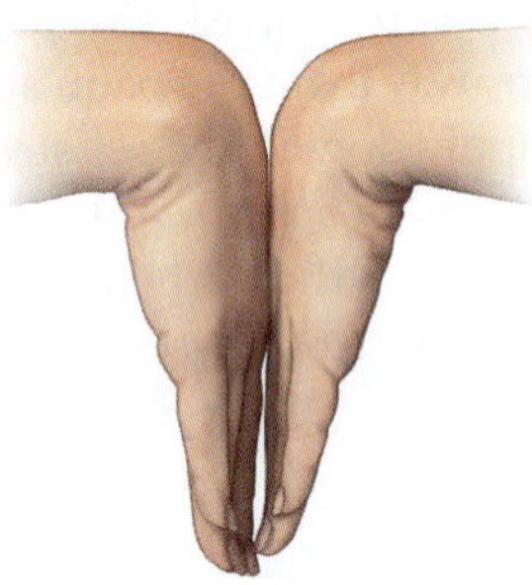

FIGURE 15-51. Testing for carpal tunnel syndrome (Phalen sign).

Numbness and tingling in the median nerve distribution within 60 seconds is a *positive test* (sensitivity 10% to 91%; specificity 33% to 86%; LR ≤1.5). Of note, it may not take a full 60 seconds for the patient to experience symptoms.

Tinel and Phalen signs do not reliably predict positive electrodiagnosis of carpal tunnel disease.

Vertebral Spine

The vertebral column, or spine, is the central supporting structure of the trunk and back. The *concave curves* of the cervical and lumbar spine and the *convex curves* of the thoracic and sacrococcygeal spine help distribute upper body weight to the pelvis and lower extremities and cushion the concussive impact of walking or running.

The complex mechanics of the back reflect the coordinated action of:

- Vertebrae and intervertebral discs
- An interconnecting system of ligaments between anterior vertebrae and posterior vertebrae, ligaments between the spinous processes, and ligaments between the lamina of two adjacent vertebrae
- Large superficial muscles, deeper intrinsic muscles, and muscles of the abdominal wall

The vertebral column contains 24 vertebrae stacked on the sacrum and coccyx (Box 15-12). A typical vertebra contains sites for joint articulations, weight bearing, and muscle attachments as well as foramina for the spinal nerve roots and peripheral nerves. Anteriorly, the *vertebral body* supports weight bearing. The posterior *vertebral arch* encloses the spinal cord. Review the location of the vertebral processes and foramina, with particular attention to:

- *Spinous process* projecting posteriorly in the midline and the two *transverse processes* (where muscles attach) at the junction of the *pedicle* and the *lamina*
- *Articular processes*—two on each side of the vertebra, one facing up and one facing down, at the junction of the pedicles and laminae, often called *articular facets*
- *Vertebral foramen* enclosing the spinal cord, the *intervertebral foramen* formed by the inferior and superior articulating process of adjacent vertebrae that create a channel for the spinal nerve roots to exit, and the *transverse foramen* for the vertebral artery in the cervical vertebrae only

The spine has slightly movable cartilaginous joints between the vertebral bodies and between the articular facets. Between the vertebral bodies are the *intervertebral discs* that each consist of a soft mucoid central core called the *nucleus pulposus*, which is rimmed by tough fibrous tissue called the *annulus fibrosis*. The intervertebral discs cushion movement between vertebrae and allow the vertebral column to curve, flex, and bend.

The flexibility of the spine is largely determined by the angle of the articular facet joints relative to the plane of the vertebral body and varies at different levels of the spine, with the lower spine generally being less moveable than the upper spine. Note that the vertebral column angles sharply posterior at the *lumbosacral junction* and becomes immovable.

The mechanical stress at this angulation contributes to the risk for disc herniation and subluxation/slippage (*spondylolisthesis*) of L5 on S1.

The *trapezius* and *latissimus dorsi* form the large, outer layer of muscles attaching to each side of the spine (Fig. 15-52). They overlie two deeper muscle layers: a layer attaching to the head, neck, and spinous processes

Box 15-12. Representative Cervical and Lumbar Vertebrae

C4–C5 Coronal and Lateral Views

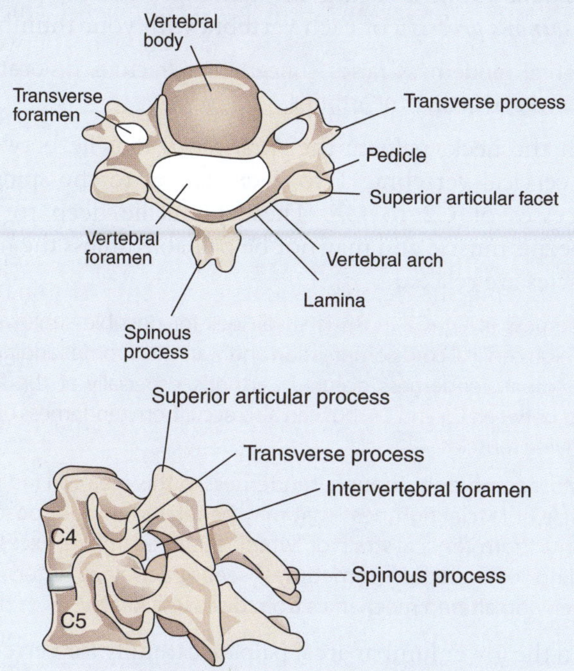

T12–L1 Coronal and Lateral Views

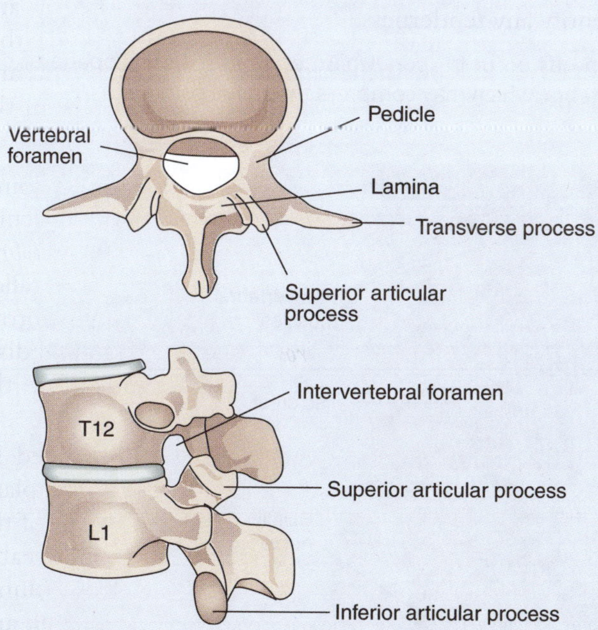

The proximity of the spinal cord and spinal nerve roots to their bony vertebral casing and the intervertebral discs makes them especially vulnerable to disc herniation, impingement from degenerative changes in the vertebrae and facets, and trauma.

(*splenius capitis, splenius cervicis,* and *sacrospinalis*) and a layer of smaller intrinsic muscles between vertebrae. A large group of paraspinal muscles (*iliocostalis, longissimus,* and *spinalis*) run vertically along the remainder of the spine and assist with stabilization, extension, and rotation of the spine. Muscles attaching to the anterior surface of the vertebrae, including the *psoas* muscle and muscles of the abdominal wall, assist with flexion and pelvic/hip stabilization.

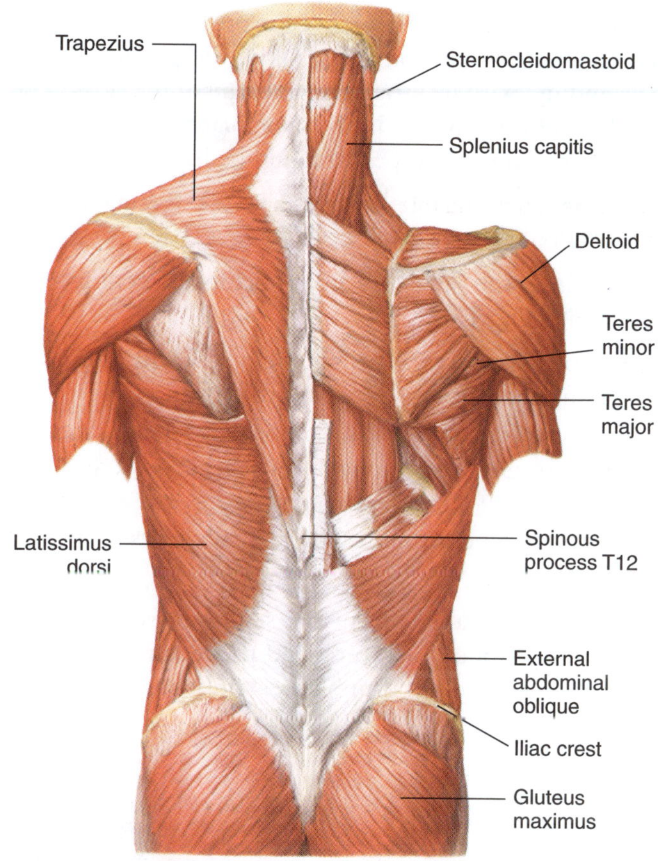

FIGURE 15-52. Muscles of the back.

Techniques of Examination

Key Components of the Vertebral Spine Examination

- Inspect posture; inspect cervical, thoracic, and lumbar curves laterally; and inspect upright spinal column, alignment of shoulders, iliac crests, and gluteal folds from posteriorly.
- Palpate vertebral spinous processes, facet joints, the sacroiliac joint, iliac crests, and posterior superior iliac spines (tenderness); paravertebral muscles (tenderness, spasm); and lumbosacral vertebrae (step-offs or slippage).
- Assess range of motion. *Cervical spine*: flexion and extension, rotation, and lateral bending. *Thoracolumbosacral spine*: flexion and extension, rotation, and lateral bending.
- Perform special maneuver (if indicated): cervical radiculopathy (Spurling test).

Inspection. Inspect the patient's *posture* when entering the room, including the position of both the neck and trunk. Assess the patient for erect position of the head, neck, and back; for smooth and coordinated neck movement; and for ease of gait.

Neck stiffness can signal arthritis, muscle strain, or other underlying pathology that should be pursued. In some cases, headache may be present.

Drape or gown the patient to expose the entire back for complete inspection. If possible, the patient should be standing, with feet together and arms at the sides. The head should be midline in the same plane as the sacrum, and the shoulders and pelvis should be level.

Lateral deviation and rotation of the head are seen in torticollis, often from contraction of the sternocleidomastoid muscle.

Viewing the patient from behind, identify the following (Fig. 15-53):

- Spinous processes, usually more prominent at C7 and T1 and more evident on forward flexion
- Paravertebral muscles on either side of the midline
- Iliac crests (A line drawn above the posterior iliac crests should cross the spinous process of L4.)
- Posterior superior iliac spines, usually marked by skin dimples

Inspect the patient from the side and from behind. Evaluate the spinal curvatures and the features discussed in Box 15-13. Note the curvatures' presence or absence. Also note any deviation of the spine from the midline. Observe any areas of abnormal prominence that may signal excessive curvature or underlying **scoliosis**.

Palpation. From a sitting or standing position, palpate the *spinous processes* of each vertebra with your thumb.

Vertebral tenderness raises concerns for fracture, dislocation, underlying infection, or arthritis.

In the neck, palpate the *facet joints* that lie between the cervical vertebrae 1 to 2 cm lateral to the spinous processes of C2 to C7. These joints lie deep to the trapezius muscle and may not be palpable unless the neck muscles are relaxed.

Tenderness at C1–C2 in RA is suspicious for possible subluxation and high cervical cord compression and warrants prompt additional assessment. Tenderness occurs in arthritis, especially at the facet joints between C5 and C6, but can also occur from tenderness of the overlying muscles.

Most commonly, though, tenderness in this area will indicate muscle or fascial tightness that may be related to poor posture, trauma (from cervical strain or "whiplash," for example), excessive loading of muscles (sometimes seen in weight lifters), or underlying altered mechanics from diseases like OA.

In the lower lumbar area, palpate carefully for vertebral "step-offs" to see if one spinous process seems unusually prominent (or recessed) in relation to the one above it. Identify any tenderness.

Step-offs occur in *spondylolisthesis,* or forward slippage of one vertebra, which may compress the spinal cord.

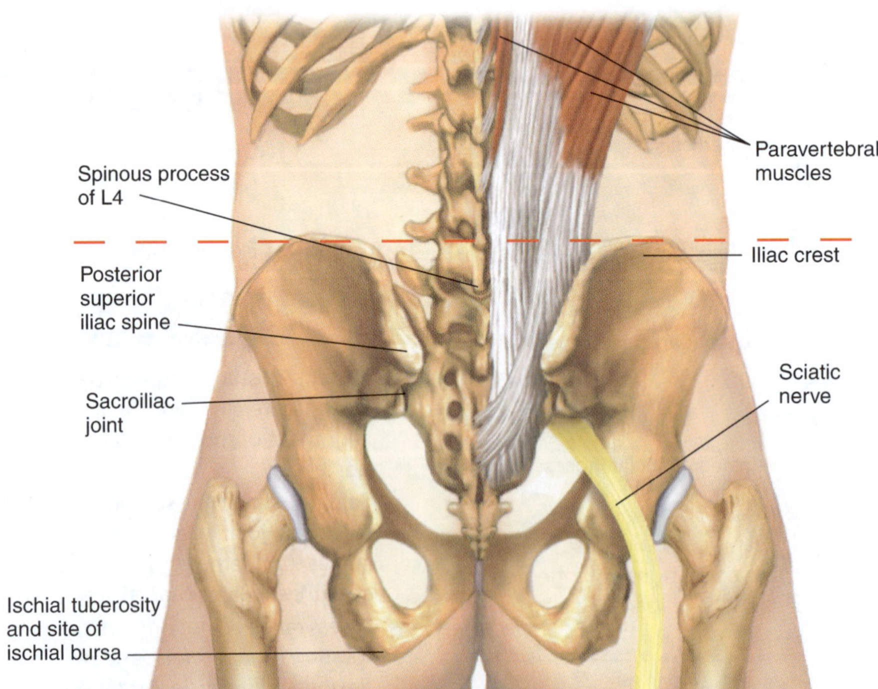

FIGURE 15-53. Anatomy of lower back.

Box 15-13. Inspection of the Vertebral Spine

View of Patient

From the Side
Inspect the cervical, thoracic, and lumbar curves.

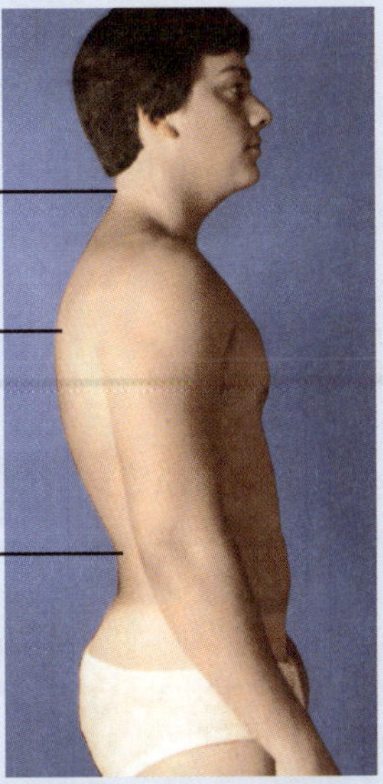

Increased thoracic kyphosis can occur with aging as the intervertebral discs lose height.

From Behind
Inspect the upright spinal column (an imaginary line should fall from C7 through the gluteal cleft).

Inspect the alignment of the shoulders, the iliac crests, and the skin creases below the buttocks (gluteal folds).

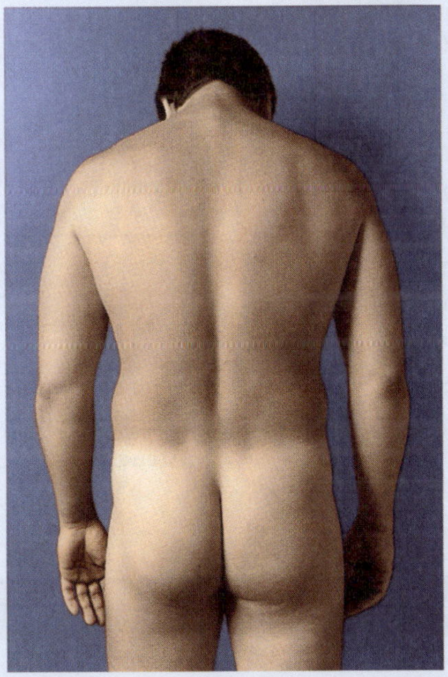

In scoliosis, lateral and rotatory curvature of the spine brings the head back to midline. Scoliosis often becomes evident during adolescence, before symptoms appear.

Unequal shoulder heights occur in scoliosis, the Sprengel deformity of the scapula from the attachment of an extra bone or band between the upper scapula and C7, and *"winging"* of the scapula from loss of long thoracic nerve innervation to the serratus anterior muscle and contralateral weakness of the trapezius (see p. 424).

Unequal heights of the iliac crests, or pelvic tilt, occur in unequal leg lengths, scoliosis, and hip abduction or adduction. Check if unequal leg lengths disappear when a block is placed under the shorter limb. "Listing" of the trunk to one side is seen with a herniated lumbar disc.

Inspect any skin markings, tags, or masses.

Birthmarks, port-wine stains, hairy patches, and lipomas often overlie bony defects such as those found in spina bifida.

Café-au-lait spots (discolored patches of skin), skin tags, and fibrous tumors are common in neurofibromatosis.

Palpate over the *sacroiliac joint*, often identified by the dimple overlying the posterior superior iliac spine several centimeters from the midline at the level of the gluteal cleft.

Tenderness over the sacroiliac joint is common in sacroiliitis and ankylosing spondylitis.

Palpate the *paravertebral muscles* for tenderness and spasm. Muscles in spasm feel firm and knotted and may be visible.

Spasm occurs in degenerative and inflammatory muscle disorders, overuse, prolonged contraction from abnormal posture, and anxiety.

Palpate for tenderness in any other areas suggested by the patient's symptoms. Check for pain radiation into the buttocks, perineum, or legs.

Herniated intervertebral discs, most common at L5–S1 or L4–L5, may cause tenderness of the spinous processes, intervertebral joints, paravertebral muscles, sacrosciatic notch, and sciatic nerve (Fig. 15-53).

Assess all low back pain for possible cauda equina compression, the most serious cause of pain, due to risk of limb paralysis or bladder/bowel dysfunction.

See Table 15-4, Low Back Pain.

Range of Motion: Cervical Spine. The neck is the most mobile portion of the spine, remarkable for its seven vertebrae supporting the 10- to 15-lb head. *Flexion* and *extension* occur primarily between the skull and C1, the atlas. *Rotation* primarily occurs at C1–C2, the axis. Finally, *lateral bending* primarily occurs at C2–C7.

Limited ROM can be caused by stiffness from arthritis, pain from trauma, and muscle spasm.

Review the specific muscles responsible for each movement and their related patient instructions (Box 15-14). Pay close attention to which of these movements, if any, reproduce your patient's symptoms, where those symptoms occur, and the characteristics of those symptoms.

Limited ROM generally signals underlying OA. However, sudden-onset limits in a patient's ROM generally warrant imaging, especially after trauma.

Assess for possible cervical cord or nerve root compression with any complaints or findings of neck, shoulder, or arm pain, numbness, or weakness. See Table 15-3, Pains in the Neck.

Box 15-14. Range of Motion of the Cervical Spine

Movement	Primary Muscles Affecting Movement	Patient Instructions
Flexion	Sternocleidomastoid, scalene, and prevertebral muscles	"Bring your chin to your chest."
Extension	Splenius capitis and cervicis and small intrinsic neck muscles	"Look up toward the ceiling."
Rotation	Sternocleidomastoid and small intrinsic neck muscles	"Look over one shoulder and then the other."
Lateral Bending	Scalenes and small intrinsic neck muscles	"Bring your ear to your shoulder."

Range of Motion: Thoracolumbosacral Spine. In Box 15-15, note the muscles responsible for each movement and instructions to the patient.

Box 15-15. Range of Motion of the Thoracolumbosacral Spine

Movement	Primary Muscles Affecting Movement	Patient Instructions
Flexion 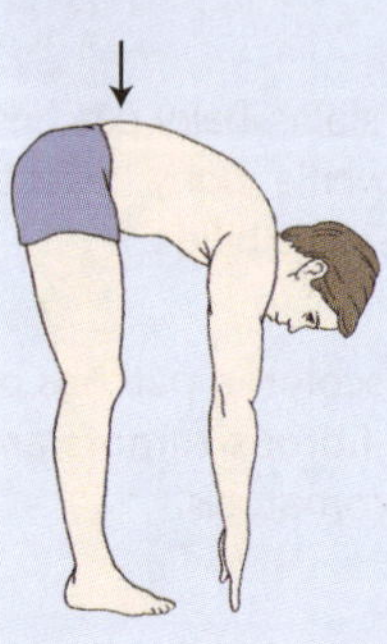	Psoas major, psoas minor, and quadratus lumborum; abdominal muscles attaching to the anterior vertebrae, such as the internal and external obliques and rectus abdominis	"Bend forward and try to touch your toes." Note the smoothness and symmetry of movement, the ROM, and the curve in the lumbar area. As flexion proceeds, the lumbar concavity should flatten out.

Deformity of the thorax on forward bending, especially when the height of the scapulae is unequal, suggests scoliosis.

Persistence of lumbar lordosis suggests decreased ROM at the lumbar spine and suggests muscle spasm or ankylosing spondylitis.

(*continued*)

Box 15-15. Range of Motion of the Thoracolumbosacral Spine (*continued*)

Movement	Primary Muscles Affecting Movement	Patient Instructions
Extension 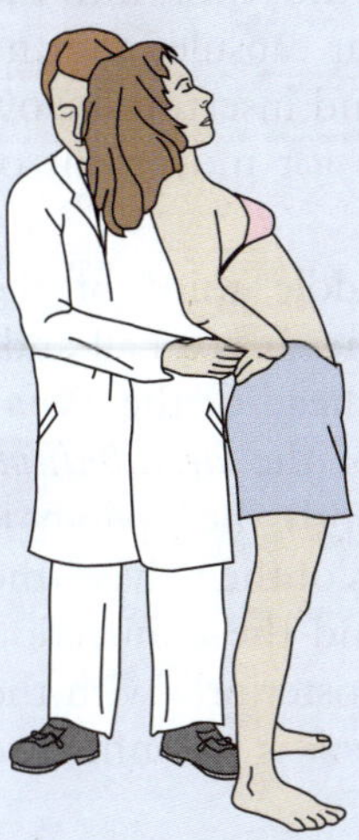	Deep intrinsic muscles of the back, such as the erector spinae, transversospinalis groups, iliocostalis, longissimus, and spinalis	"Bend back as far as possible." Support the patient by placing your hand on the posterior superior iliac spine, with your fingers pointing toward the midline.
Rotation 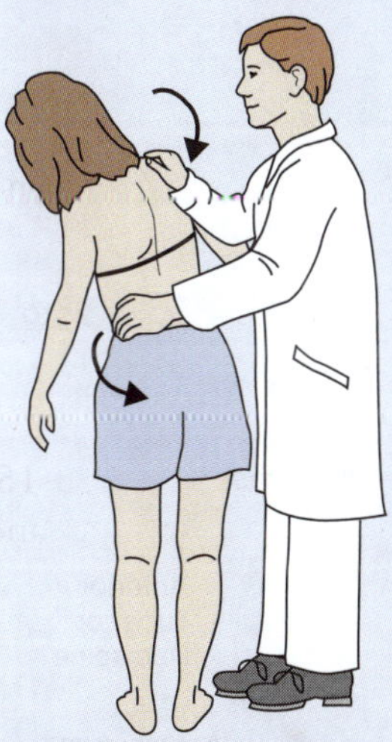	Abdominal muscles and intrinsic muscles of the back	"Rotate from side to side." Face the patient and stabilize the patient's pelvis by placing one hand on the patient's hip and the other on the opposite shoulder. Then rotate the trunk by pulling the shoulder anteriorly and then the hip posteriorly. Repeat these maneuvers for the opposite side.
Lateral Bending 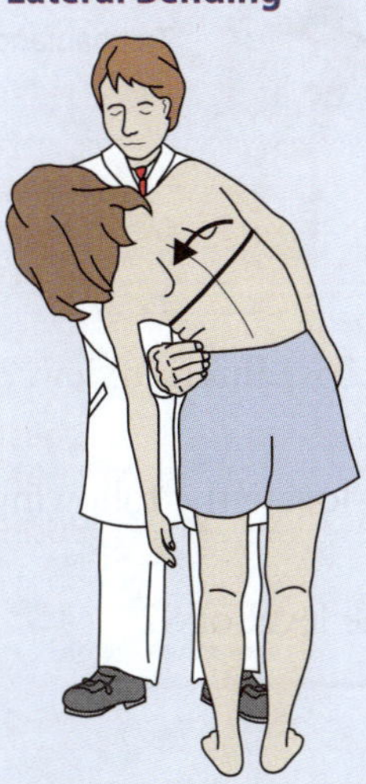	Abdominal muscles and intrinsic muscles of the back	"Bend to the side from the waist." Stabilize the patient's pelvis by placing your hand on the patient's hip. Repeat for the opposite side.

Decreased spinal mobility is common in OA and ankylosing spondylitis. It can also result from guarding if the patient is anticipating pain and feels unable or unwilling to move into painful positions.

If these maneuvers provoke pain or tenderness, particularly with radiation into the leg, proceed to careful neurologic testing of the lower extremities.

Possible causes include OA of the lumbar spine or hips, strain or sprain of the paraspinal muscles in the lower back, lumbosacral nerve root compression, lumbosacral spinal cord compression, or mass lesion. Infection in the hip, rectum, or pelvis may also cause symptoms. See Table 15-4, Low Back Pain.

It is also possible to assess the small facet joints of the spinal cord by having the patient rotate to one side and extend backward. If this reproduces the patient's pain, suspect underlying pathology of the facet joints.

See Chapter 13, Nervous System, for the Straight Leg Raise Test. Although helpful, this test is not pathognomonic of disc herniation.

Special Maneuver. To test for *cervical nerve root compression (Spurling test)* have the patient look over the shoulder and then up at the ceiling. Next, position yourself behind the patient and carefully apply downward pressure on the patient's head and check if the maneuver reproduces the neck pain with radiation to the same on the same side of the turned head (Fig. 15-54). Then use gentle traction following this test to release pressure.

The Spurling test is positive when the patient feels pain going down the arm on the same side the head is turned and indicates cervical nerve root involvement. Its sensitivity varies from moderate to high (38% to 97%), but it has a high specificity (89% to 100%).

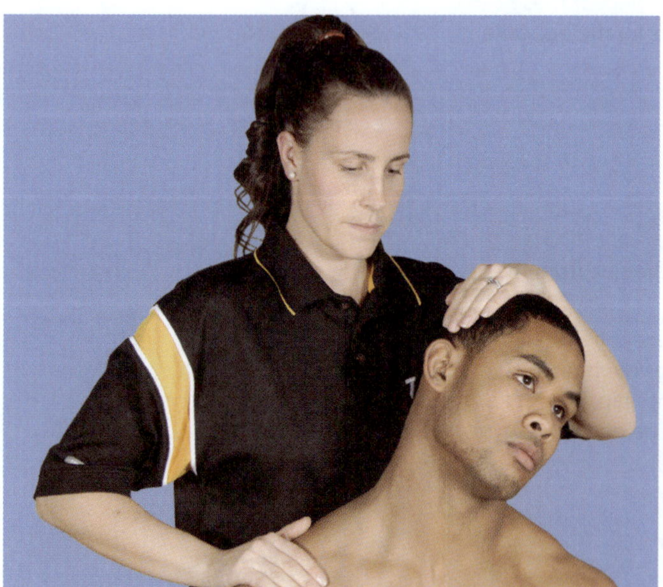

FIGURE 15-54. Positioning the patient's head and neck to test cervical nerve root compression (Spurling test). (From Anderson MK. *Foundations of Athletic Training: Prevention, Assessment, and Management.* 5th ed. Wolters Kluwer Health/Lippincott Williams & Wilkins; 2013, Fig. 11-22.)

Hip Joint

The hip joint is deeply embedded in the pelvis and is notable for its strength, stability, and wide ROM. The stability of the hip joint, essential for weight bearing, arises from the deep fit of the head of the femur into the acetabulum, its strong fibrous articular capsule, and the powerful muscles crossing the joint and inserting below the femoral head, providing leverage for movement of the femur.

The hip joint lies below the middle third of the inguinal ligament but in a deeper plane. It is a ball-and-socket joint. Note how the rounded head of the *femur* articulates with the cup-like cavity of the *acetabulum*. Because of its overlying muscles and depth, the hip joint is not readily palpable. Review the bones of the pelvis—the *ilium*, the *ischium*, and the *pubis*—and the connection inferiorly at the *symphysis pubis* and posteriorly with the *sacrum*. Recognize that the *acetabulum* is a confluence of all three bones of the pelvis.

On the *anterior surface of the hip*, locate the following bony structures (Fig. 15-55):

- Iliac crest at the level of L4
- Iliac tubercle
- Anterior superior iliac spine
- Greater trochanter
- Pubic tubercle
- Pubic symphysis

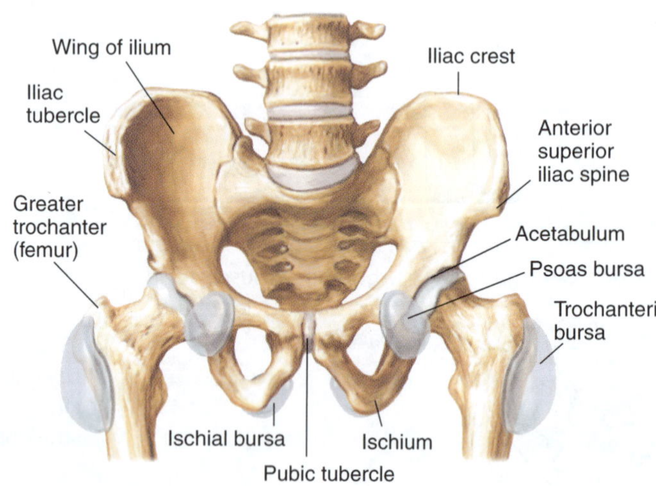

FIGURE 15-55. Anatomy of the pelvis, anterior view.

On the *posterior surface of the hip*, locate the following (Fig. 15-56):

- Posterior superior iliac spine at the level of S2
- Greater trochanter
- Ischial tuberosity
- Sacroiliac joint

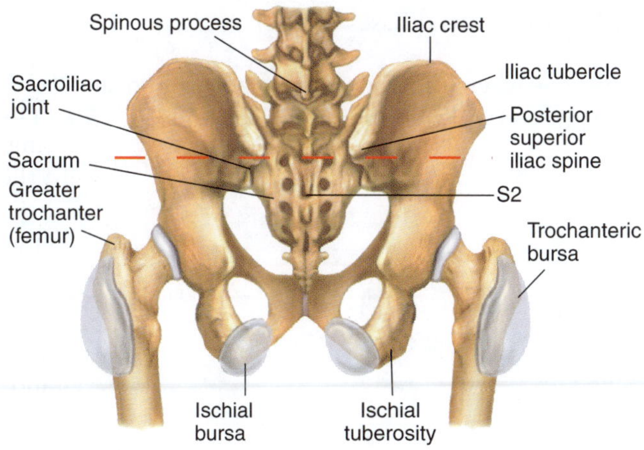

FIGURE 15-56. Anatomy of the pelvis, posterior view.

The location of S2 is approximately at the level of the posterior superior iliac spines (red dashed line in Fig. 15-56).

Four powerful *muscle groups* move the hip. Picture these groups as you examine patients and remember that to move the femur or any bone in a given direction, the muscle must cross the joint line.

The *flexor group* lies anteriorly and flexes the hip (Fig. 15-57). The primary hip flexor is the *iliopsoas*, a confluence of the *iliacus* and *psoas* muscles that originate at the iliac crest and on the lumbar spine, respectively, and extend to the lesser trochanter.

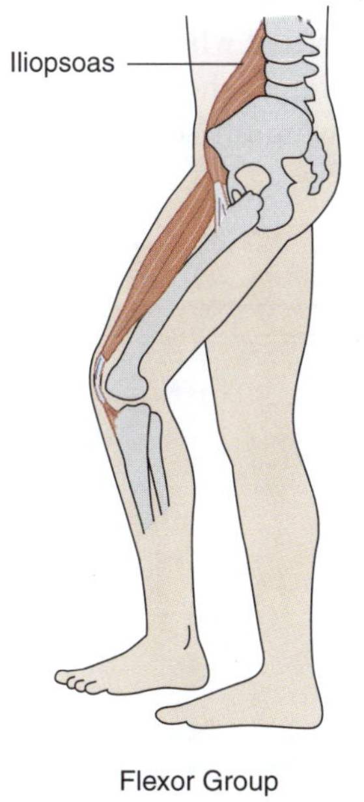

FIGURE 15-57. Flexor muscle group of the hip.

The *extensor group* lies posteriorly and extends the thigh (Fig. 15-58). The *gluteus maximus* is the primary extensor of the hip. It forms a band crossing from its origin along the medial pelvis to its insertion below the trochanter. The *hamstring muscles*, *adductor magnus*, and *gluteus medius* can also assist with hip extension.

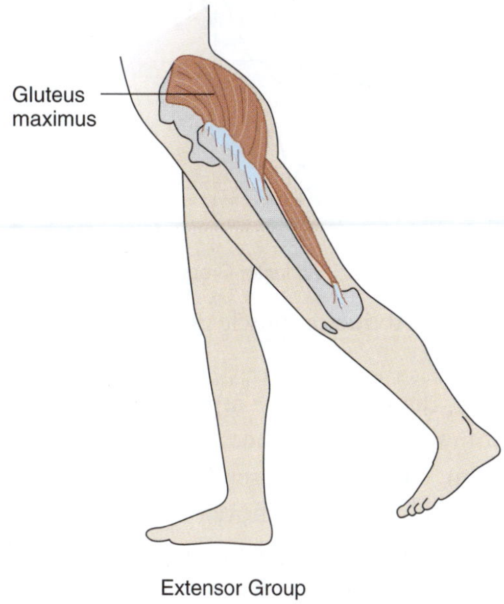

FIGURE 15-58. Extensor muscle group of the hip.

The *adductor group* is medial and pulls the thigh toward the body (Fig. 15-59). The muscles in this group arise from the rami of the pubis and ischium and insert on the posteromedial aspect of the femur.

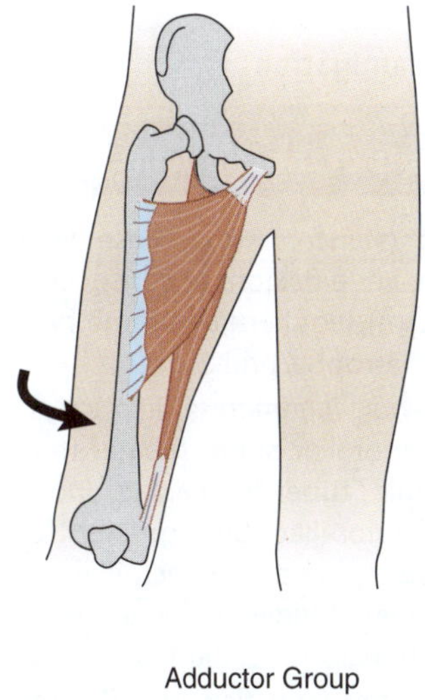

FIGURE 15-59. Adductor muscle group of the hip.

The *abductor group* is lateral and extends from the iliac crest to the greater trochanter, pulling the thigh away from the body (Fig. 15-60). This group includes the *gluteus medius* and *minimus*. These muscles help stabilize the pelvis during the stance phase of gait.

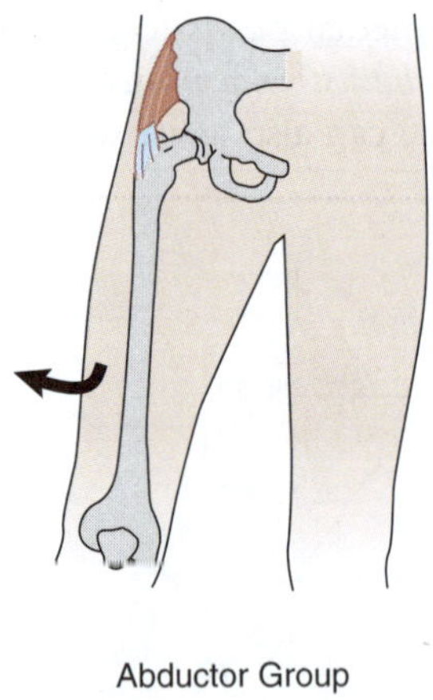

FIGURE 15-60. Abductor muscle group of the hip.

A strong, dense *articular capsule*, extending from the acetabulum to the femoral neck, encases and strengthens the hip joint. The capsule is reinforced by three overlying ligaments and lined with synovial membrane.

There are three principal bursae at the hip. Anterior to the joint is the *psoas bursa* (also termed *iliopectineal* or *iliopsoas bursa*), overlying the articular capsule and the psoas muscle. Next, find the bony prominence lateral to the hip joint called the *greater trochanter* of the femur. The large multilocular *trochanteric bursa* lies on its posterolateral surface. The *ischial* (or *ischiogluteal*) *bursa*, not always present, lies under the *ischial tuberosity*, and helps to accommodate the weight of the sitting position. Note its proximity to the sciatic nerve, as shown in Figure 15-64.

Techniques of Examination

Key Components of the Hip Joint Examination

- Inspect gait (stance, swing, base width, pelvis shift, stride length, knee flexion) and inspect the lumbar spine (lordosis, spasm), legs (length symmetry), and anterior and posterior hip (atrophy, bruising).
- Palpate *anterior landmarks:* iliac crest, iliac tubercle, anterior–superior iliac spine, greater trochanter of femur, and the pubic tubercle. Palpate *posterior landmarks:* posterior–superior iliac spine, greater trochanter laterally, ischial tuberosity, and the sacroiliac joint. Palpate the inguinal ligament (bulges, nodes, tenderness), psoas bursa, trochanteric bursa, and ischiogluteal bursa (tenderness).
- Assess range of motion: flexion and extension, abduction and adduction, and internal and external rotations.
- Perform special maneuvers (if indicated): groin strain (FABER or Patrick test) and flexion deformity (Kendall or Thomas test).

Inspection. Inspection of the hip begins with careful observation of the patient's gait when entering the room.

Observe the two phases of gait:

- *Stance*—when the foot is on the ground and bears weight (60% of the normal gait cycle) (Fig. 15-61)

Most hip problems appear during the weight-bearing stance phase.

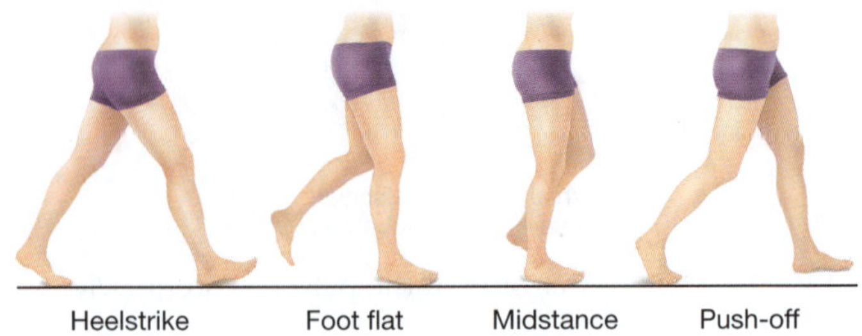

FIGURE 15-61. Stance phase of gait.

- *Swing*—when the foot moves forward and does not bear weight (40% of the normal gait cycle)

Inspect the gait for the width of the base, the shift of the pelvis, length of the stride, and flexion of the knee (Fig. 15-62). The width of the base should be 2 to 4 in from heel to heel. Normal gait has a smooth, continuous rhythm, achieved in part by contraction of the abductors of the weight-bearing limb. Abductor contraction stabilizes the pelvis and helps maintain balance by preventing the opposite hip from dropping during single stance. The knee should be slightly flexed throughout the stance phase, except when the heel strikes the ground to counteract motion at the ankle and during toe off just prior to starting swing phase.

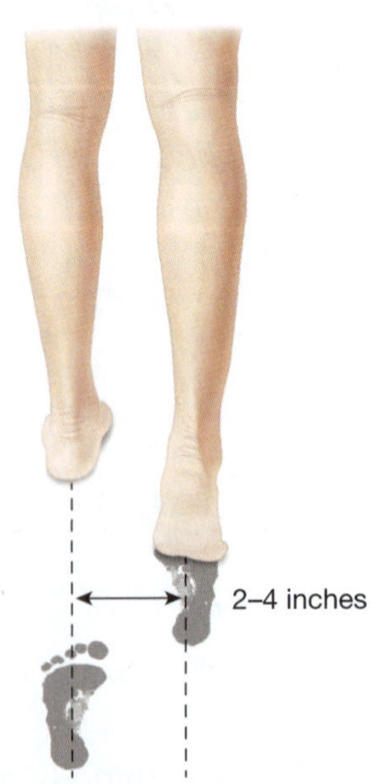

FIGURE 15-62. Inspecting the width of the base while ambulating.

A wide base suggests poor balance, which can result from lower extremity weakness, cerebellar disorders or osteoarthritis among other causes. Pain during weight bearing or examiner strike on the heel occurs in femoral neck stress fractures.

Abductor weakness, arthritis, unequal leg lengths, or chronic hip subluxation can cause the pelvis to drop on the opposite side and produce what appears to be a *waddling gait* also known as a *Trendelenburg gait.*

Lack of knee flexion or foot dorsiflexion makes the leg functionally longer and interrupts the smooth pattern of gait. The usual adaptation to this is circumduction of the longer leg (swinging the leg out to the side), but you may also observe *vaulting* (standing up on the toes of the stance phase foot during swing phase on the affected side to provide greater clearance).

Inspect the lumbar portion of the spine for the degree of lordosis.

Loss of lordosis can occur with paravertebral spasm, whereas excess lordosis may indicate a flexion deformity of the hip, spondylolisthesis, or compensation for altered center of gravity as seen in those who are obese or in those with severe kyphosis.

With the patient supine, assess the length of the legs for symmetry. (To measure leg length, see Special Techniques, p. 462.)

Leg shortening, and external rotation are common in hip fracture.

Inspect the anterior and posterior surfaces of the hip for any areas of muscle atrophy or bruising. The joint is too deeply situated to detect swelling.

Palpation. Palpate the surface landmarks of the hip anteriorly and posteriorly. Palpate structures as follows.

Anterior Landmarks. Identify the *iliac crest* at the upper margin of the pelvis at the level of L4. Follow the downward anterior curve and locate the *iliac tubercle,* marking the widest point of the crest. Continue tracking downward to the *anterior–superior iliac spine.* Place your thumbs on the anterior–superior spines and move your fingers downward and laterally from the iliac tubercles to the *greater trochanter* of the femur. Then move your thumbs medially and obliquely to the *pubic tubercle,* which lies at the same level as the greater trochanter.

Posterior Landmarks. Palpate the *posterior–superior iliac spine* directly underneath the visible dimples just above the buttocks (these may be difficult to find in overweight or obese patients). Placing your left thumb and index finger over the posterior superior iliac spine, next locate the *greater trochanter* laterally with your fingers at the level of the gluteal fold and place your thumb medially on the *ischial tuberosity.* The *sacroiliac joint* is not always palpable but may be tender. Note that an imaginary line along the posterior–superior iliac spines crosses the joint at S2 as shown in Figure 15-56.

Sacroiliac joint tenderness suggests sacroiliitis.

With the patient supine, ask the patient to place the heel of the leg being examined on the opposite knee. Then palpate along the *inguinal ligament,* which extends from the anterior–superior iliac spine to the pubic tubercle (Fig. 15-63).

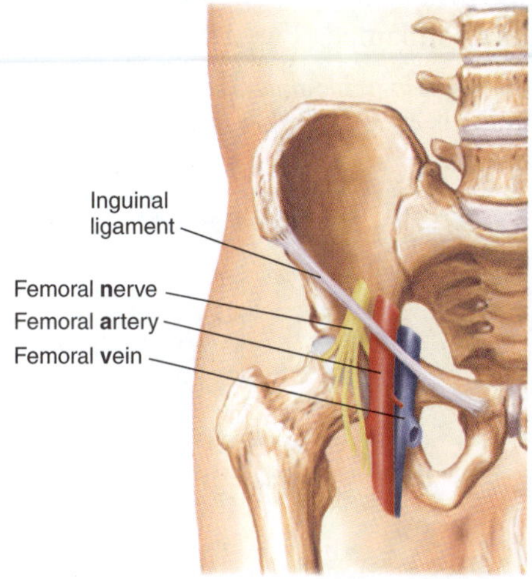

FIGURE 15-63. The inguinal ligament and N-A-V-E-L.

Bulges along the ligament suggest an inguinal hernia or, at times, an aneurysm, although these may be difficult to palpation unless they are significant.

Enlarged lymph nodes point to infection in the pelvis or lower extremity.

Causes of groin tenderness may include tendonitis/tendinopathy of the adductor or iliopsoas tendons, pubic symphysitis, femoral or inguinal hernias, synovitis of the hip joint, arthritis, bursitis, or possible psoas abscess.

Focal tenderness over the trochanter indicates greater trochanteric pain syndrome, which is rarely caused by bursitis and may indicate tendinopathy of the gluteus medius. Tenderness over the posterolateral surface of the greater trochanter occurs in localized tendinitis, muscle spasm from referred hip pain, and iliotibial band tendinitis.

The femoral nerve, artery, and vein bisect the overlying inguinal ligament with lymph nodes lying medially. The mnemonic **NAVEL** may help you remember the lateral-to-medial sequence of **N**erve–**A**rtery–**V**ein–**E**mpty space–**L**ymph node.

Anterior or inguinal pain, typically deep within the hip joint and radiating to the knee, points to intraarticular pathology. Pain radiating to the buttocks or posterior trochanteric region points to extraarticular causes.

Intraarticular causes include OA, osteonecrosis of the femoral head, femoroacetabular impingement, acetabular labral tears, and femoral neck stress fracture. Extraarticular causes include muscle strain or tendinopathy of the gluteus medius or iliopsoas tendons, sacroiliac disorders, and lumbar radiculopathy.

If the hip is painful, palpate the *psoas bursa* underneath the inguinal ligament. With the patient resting on one side and the hip flexed and internally rotated, palpate the *trochanteric bursa* lying over the greater trochanter (Fig. 15-64). Be aware that this bursa is rarely inflamed, and pain in this area is often secondary to injury to tendinous structures in the area. Normally, the *ischiogluteal bursa*, over the ischial tuberosity, is not palpable unless inflamed (Fig. 15-65).

Look for tenderness in *ischiogluteal bursitis* or "weaver's bottom"; because of the adjacent sciatic nerve, this may mimic sciatica.

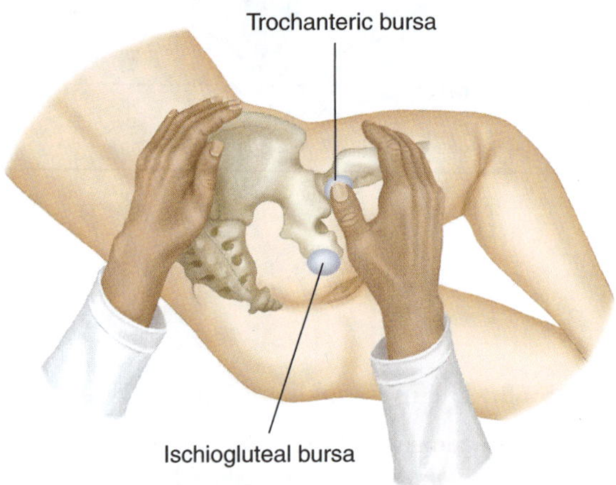

FIGURE 15-64. Palpating the trochanteric bursa.

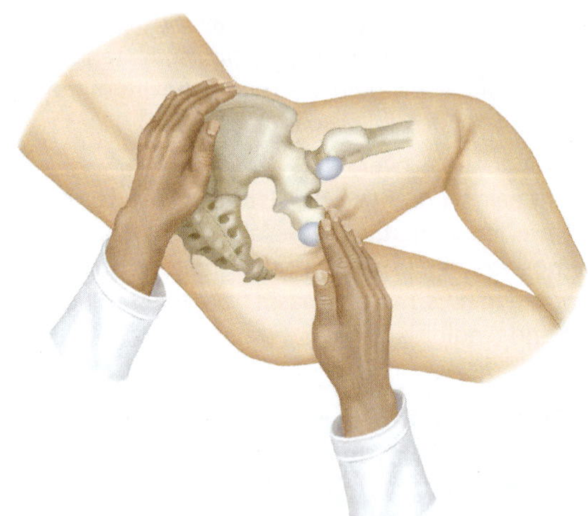

FIGURE 15-65. Palpating the ischiogluteal bursa.

Range of Motion. Assess hip ROM and the specific muscles responsible for each movement. Review the instructions to the patient (Box 15-16). Normal values for hip *flexion*, *abduction*, and *adduction* are 120°, 45°, and 20°, respectively.

Box 15-16. Range of Motion of the Hip Joint

Hip Movement	Primary Muscles Affecting Movement	Patient Instructions
Flexion	Iliopsoas and rectus femoris (especially when knee is in extension)	"Bring your knee to your chest and pull it against your abdomen."
Extension	Gluteus maximus, gluteus medius, adductor magnus, and hamstrings (especially when knee is in extension)	"Lie face down, then bend your knee and lift it up." OR "Lying flat, move your lower leg away from the midline and down over the side of the table."
Abduction	Gluteus medius and minimus, tensor fascia latae (TFL)	"Lying flat, move your lower leg away from the midline."
Adduction	Adductor brevis, adductor longus, adductor magnus, pectineus, and gracilis	"Lying flat, bend your knee and move your lower leg toward the midline."
External Rotation	Internal and external obturators, quadratus femoris, and superior and inferior gemelli	"Lying flat, bend your knee and turn your lower leg and foot across the midline."
Internal Rotation	Gluteus medius and minimus, TFL, and some assistance from the adductors	"Lying flat, bend your knee and turn your lower leg and foot away from the midline."

Flexion. With the patient supine, place your hand under the patient's lumbar spine. Ask the patient to bend each knee in turn up to the chest and pull it firmly against the abdomen (Fig. 15-66). Note that the hip can flex further when the knee is flexed because the hamstrings are relaxed. When the back touches your hand, indicating normal flattening of the lumbar lordosis, further flexion must arise from the hip joint itself. As the thigh is held against the abdomen, inspect the degree of flexion at the hip and knee.

Flexion deformity may be masked by an increase, rather than flattening, in lumbar lordosis and an anterior pelvic tilt as the patient extends the spine to compensate.

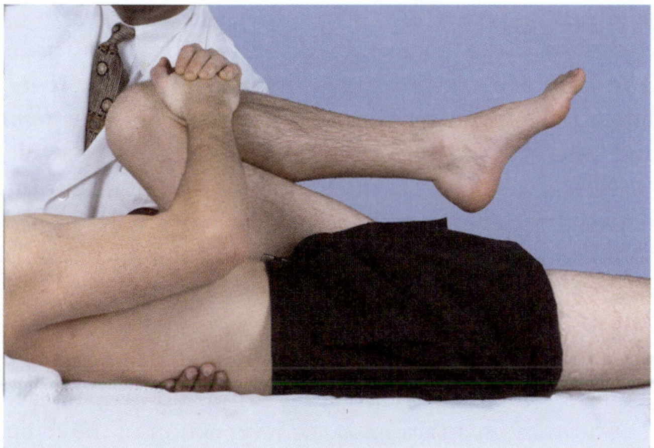

FIGURE 15-66. Testing hip flexion with flattening of lumbar lordosis against examiner's hand.

Extension. With the patient lying face down, extend the thigh toward you in a posterior direction. Alternatively, carefully position the supine patient near the edge of the table and extend the leg posteriorly.

Abduction. Stabilize the pelvis by pressing down on the opposite anterior–superior iliac spine with one hand. With the other hand, grasp the ankle and abduct the extended leg until you feel the iliac spine move (Fig. 15-67). This movement marks the limit of hip abduction.

Restricted abduction and internal and external rotation are common in hip OA. The LR for resisted external rotation due to pain is as high as 32.6. In general, pain with internal and external rotation signals pathology within the hip joint (intraarticular) since these movements result from significant movement of the femoral head against the acetabulum.

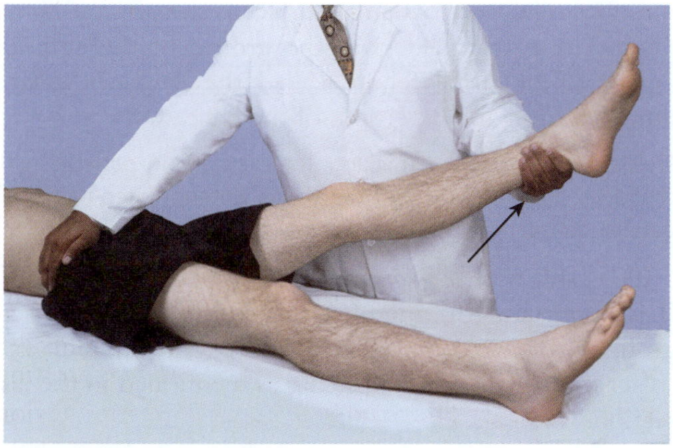

FIGURE 15-67. Testing left hip abduction.

Adduction. With the patient supine, stabilize the pelvis, hold one ankle, and move the leg medially across the body and over the opposite extremity (Fig. 15-68).

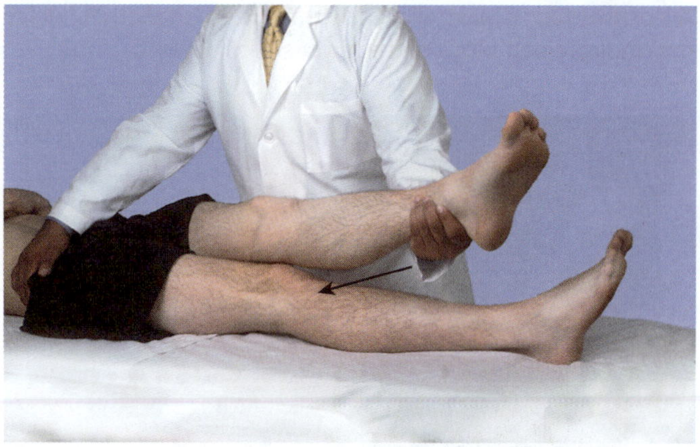

FIGURE 15-68. Testing left hip adduction.

External and Internal Rotation. Flex the leg to 90° at hip and knee, stabilize the thigh with one hand, grasp the ankle with the other, and swing the lower leg—*medially for external rotation at the hip* (Fig. 15-69) and *laterally for internal rotation.* Although confusing at first, it is the motion of the head of the femur in the acetabulum that identifies these movements.

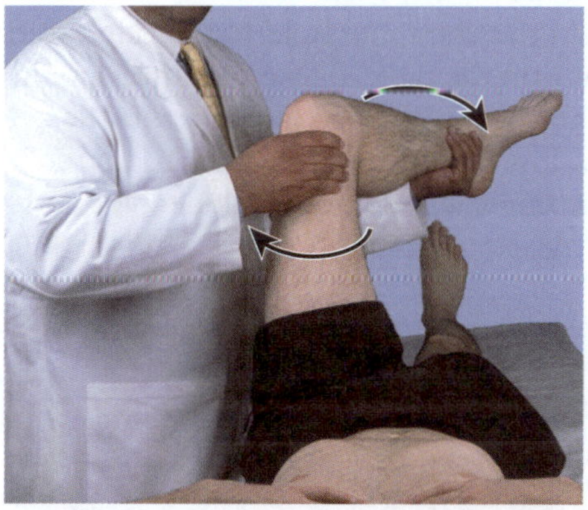

FIGURE 15-69. Testing internal and external rotation of the left hip.

Pain with maximal flexion and adduction and internal rotation or with abduction and external rotation with full extension can signal acetabular labral tear or femoroacetabular impingement.

Special Maneuvers. Often, the examiner must assist the patient with movements of the hip.

Test for Groin Strain. When groin strain is suspected due to a sudden forced abduction of the hip from sports injury that requires lateral movements or pivoting, you may test for reproducible pain with the *FABER (Flexion, ABduction, External Rotation)* or *Patrick test.* With the patient supine, position the leg into 90° of flexion and externally rotate and abduct it so that the ipsilateral ankle rests distal to the knee of the contralateral leg (Fig. 15-70).

A positive test is pain elicited with resisted adduction, which may indicate pathology of the hip or sacroiliac joint.

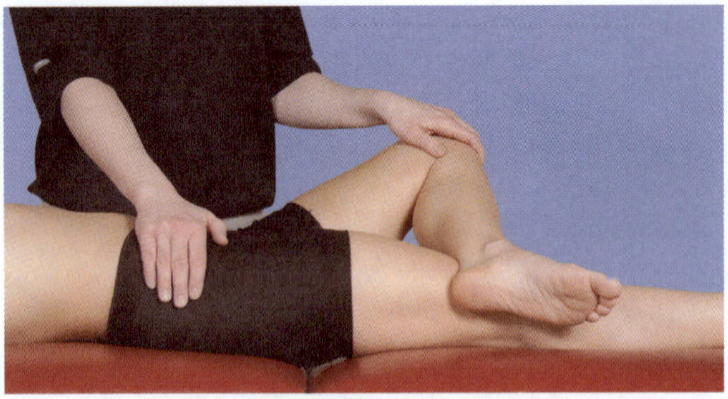

FIGURE 15-70. Testing for groin strain (FABER or Patrick test). (From Anderson MK. *Foundations of Athletic Training: Prevention, Assessment, and Management*. 6th ed. Wolters Kluwer; 2017, Fig. 16-19.)

Test for Hip Flexion Deformity. This can be tested using the *Kendall test*. Start with the patient in the sitting position with the patient's thighs half off the examining table. Then, ask the patient to lie down and flex the uninvolved leg toward the chest and hold just enough to flatten the lower back on the table. The other knee should be at the edge of the table with the knee free to flex. Normally, with the low back and sacrum flat on the table, the posterior thigh should touch the table, and the knee passively flexes.

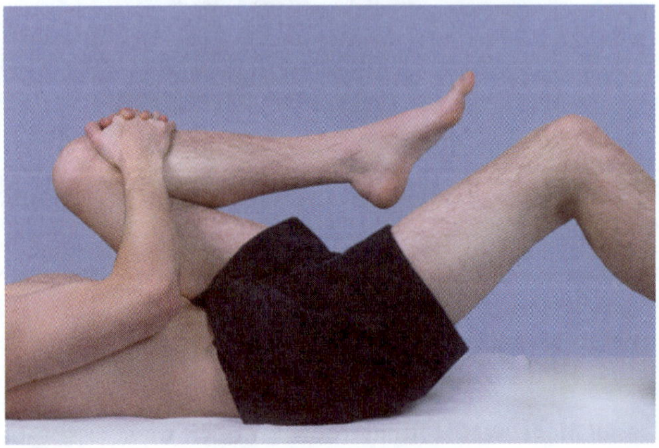

FIGURE 15-71. Positive flexion deformity of right hip (Kendall test).

When flexion deformity of the hip is present, the affected hip will rise off the table as the opposite hip is flexed. This is because the affected hip does not allow full hip extension and cannot maintain contact with the table as a result (Fig. 15-71).

When the leg flexed over the end of the table extends beyond 90°, it suggests rectus femoris shortening. If the extended leg is able to flex to 90° or more, but the thigh remains off the table, the test is suggestive for iliopsoas tightness.

Knee Joint

The knee joint is the largest joint in the body. It is a hinge joint involving three bones: the *femur*, the *tibia*, and the *patella (or knee cap)*, with three articular surfaces, two between the femur and the tibia and one between the femur and the patella. Note how the two rounded condyles of the femur rest on the relatively flat *tibial plateau*.

There is no inherent stability in the knee joint itself, making it dependent on a complex of ligaments and tendons to hold the articulating femur and tibia in place. This feature, in addition to the lever action of the femur on the tibia and the lack of padding from overlying fat or muscle, can predispose the knee to injury.

Learn the bony landmarks in and around the knee. These will guide your examination of this complicated joint (Fig. 15-72).

- Medial surface: Identify the *adductor tubercle*, the *medial epicondyle* of the femur, and the *medial condyle* of the tibia.
- Anterior surface: Identify the *patella*, which rests on the anterior articulating surface of the femur midway between the epicondyles, embedded in the tendon of the quadriceps muscle. This tendon continues below the knee joint as the *patellar tendon*, which inserts distally on the *tibial tuberosity*.
- Lateral surface: Find the *lateral epicondyle* of the femur, the *lateral condyle* of the tibia, and the head of the *fibula*.

Two condylar *tibiofemoral joints* are formed by the convex curves of the medial and lateral condyles of the femur as they articulate with the concave condyles of the tibia. The third articular surface is the *patellofemoral joint*. The patella slides on the groove of the anterior aspect of the distal femur, called the *trochlear groove*, during flexion and extension of the knee.

Problems with patellar tracking, for example, in patients with shallower grooves can lead to arthritis, anterior knee pain, and patellar dislocation in severe cases.

Powerful *muscle groups* move and support the knee. It is important to remember that both of these muscle groups also have components that cross the hip joint and so act to flex and extend the hip as mentioned in the last section.

- *Quadriceps femoris* is made up of four muscle bellies that extend the knee and cover the anterior, medial, and lateral aspects of the thigh (Fig. 15-73).

  In women, quadriceps contraction often exerts a more lateral pull (Q angle) that alters patellar tracking, contributing to anterior knee pain.

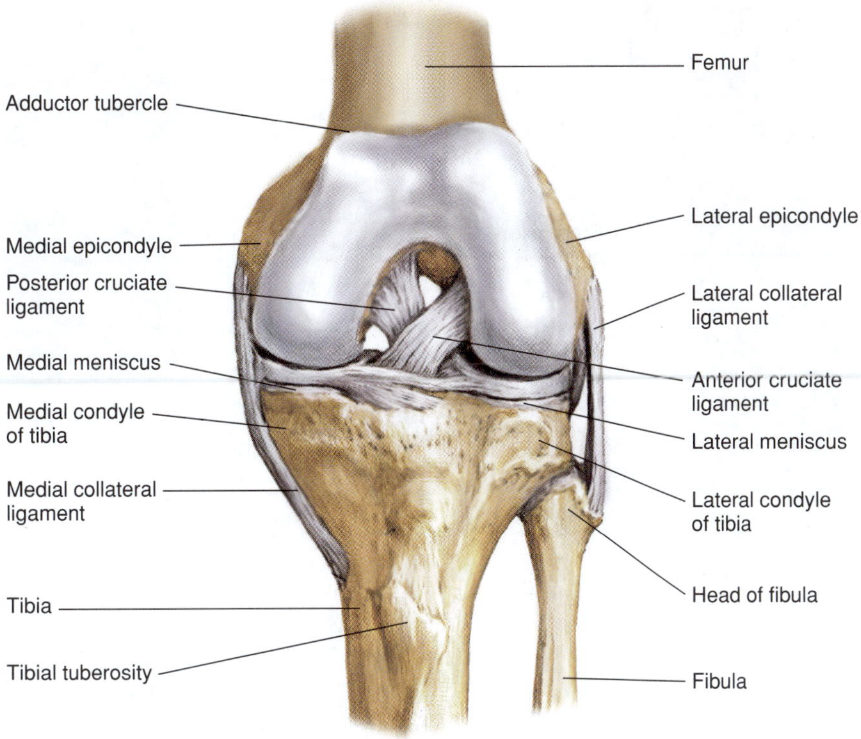

FIGURE 15-72. Anatomy of the left knee, anterior view.

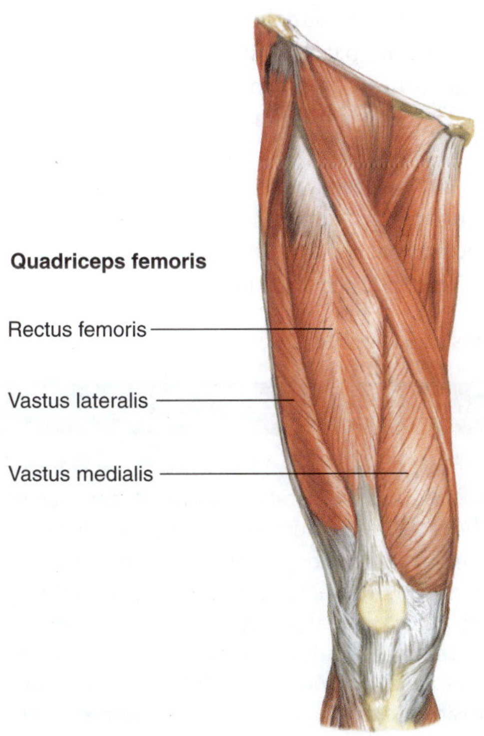

FIGURE 15-73. Quadriceps femoris—anterior view of right lower extremity.

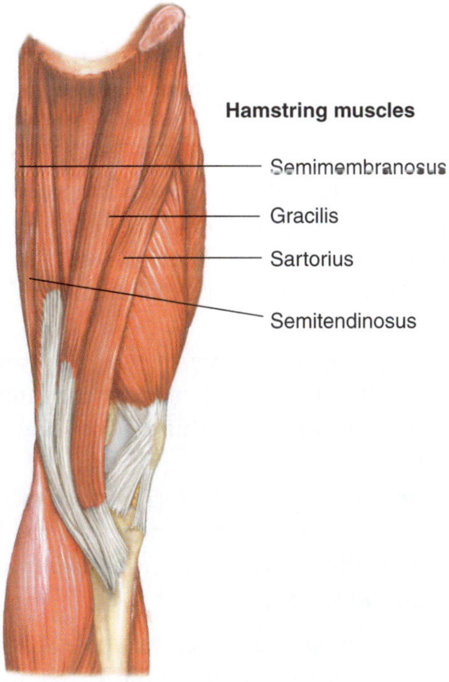

FIGURE 15-74. Hamstring muscles—posterior view of right lower extremity.

- *Hamstring muscles* lie on the posterior aspect of the thigh and flex the knee (Fig. 15-74).

The menisci and two important pairs of ligaments, the collaterals and the cruciates, are crucial to stability of the knee. Learn the location of these structures (Fig. 15-75; also see Fig. 15-72).

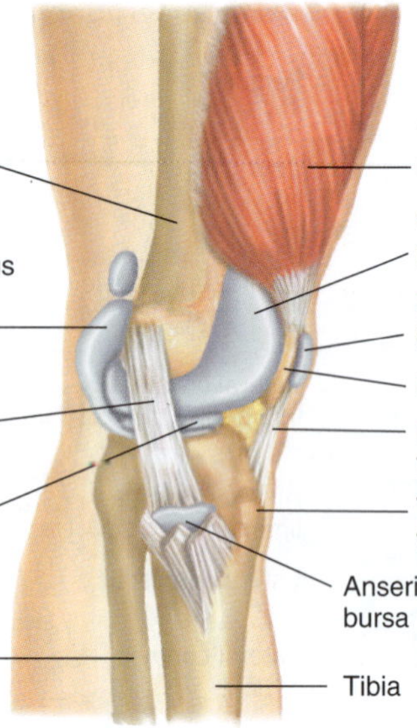

FIGURE 15-75. Menisci and ligaments of the left knee—medial view.

- *Medial and lateral menisci* cushion the action of the femur on the tibia. These crescent-shaped fibrocartilaginous discs add a cup-like surface to the relatively flat tibial plateau. They are often difficult to specifically palpate.
- *Medial collateral ligament (MCL),* not easily palpable because of its broad and flat shape, is a ligament connecting the medial femoral epicondyle to the medial condyle of the tibia. The medial portion of the MCL also attaches to the medial meniscus.
- *Lateral collateral ligament (LCL)* connects the lateral femoral epicondyle and the head of the fibula. The MCL and LCL provide medial and lateral stability to the knee joint.
- *Anterior cruciate ligament (ACL)* crosses obliquely from the anterior medial tibia to the lateral femoral condyle, preventing the tibia from sliding forward on the femur.
- *Posterior cruciate ligament (PCL)* crosses from the *posterior* tibia and lateral meniscus to the medial femoral condyle, preventing the tibia from slipping backward on the femur.

You will not be able to palpate the ACL and PCL since they lie transversely within the knee joint. They are crucial to the anteroposterior stability of the knee.

Inspect the concavities that are usually evident adjacent and superior to each side of the patella, known as the *infrapatellar space* (Fig. 15-76). Occupying these areas is the synovial cavity of the knee, one of the largest joint cavities in the body. It additionally contains the *infrapatellar fat pad* (also known as *Hoffa's fat pad*) and the *infrapatellar bursa.*

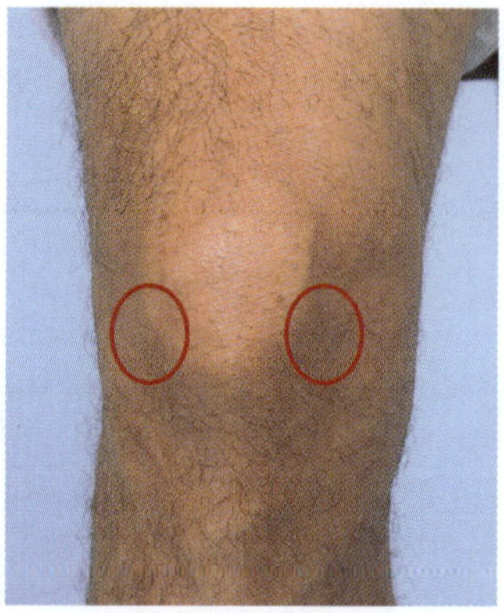

FIGURE 15-76. Infrapatellar spaces of the right knee occupied by the synovial cavity.

Although the synovium is not normally palpable, these areas may become swollen and tender when the joint is inflamed or injured.

This cavity includes an extension 6 cm above the upper border of the patella, lying upward and deep to the quadriceps muscle, called the *suprapatellar recess.* This recess also lies adjacent to the *suprapatellar fat pad* and *suprapatellar bursa.* The joint cavity covers the anterior, medial, and lateral surfaces of the knee as well as the condyles of the femur and tibia posteriorly.

Several *bursae* lie near the knee. The *prepatellar bursa* lies between the patella and the overlying skin. The *anserine bursa* lies 1 to 2 cm below the knee joint on the medial surface, proximal and medial to the attachments of the medial hamstring muscles on the proximal tibia. It cannot be palpated due to these overlying tendons. Now identify the large *semimembranosus bursa* that communicates with the joint cavity, also on the posterior and medial surfaces of the knee.

Techniques of Examination

Key Components of the Knee Joint Examination

- Inspect gait (knee flexion) and inspect the knee including hollows around the patella (alignment, contour, swelling) and the quadriceps muscles (atrophy, bruising).
- Palpate the tibiofemoral joint (tenderness, ridges). *Medial compartment*: medial femoral condyle, adductor tubercle, medial tibial plateau, and MCL. *Lateral compartment:* lateral femoral condyle, lateral tibial plateau, and LCL. *Patellofemoral compartment*: patella, patellar tendon, tibial tuberosity, prepatellar bursa, anserine bursa, and popliteal fossa.
- Assess range of motion: flexion and extension.
- Perform special maneuvers (if indicated): McMurray test (meniscus), abduction or valgus test (MCL), adduction or varus test (LCL), anterior drawer sign or Lachman test (ACL), and posterior drawer sign (PCL). Effusions: bulge sign, balloon sign, and balloting the patella.

Learn to examine the following structures: the medial and lateral menisci, the LCL and MCL, the ACL and PCL, and the patellar tendon. The ACL and PCL are not palpable but are tested by special maneuvers. Palpation and testing of these structures are especially helpful in primary care diagnosis.

Inspection. Inspect the *gait* for a smooth rhythmic flow as the patient enters the room. The knee should be extended at heel strike and mildly flexed at all other phases of swing and stance.

Stumbling or "giving way" of the knee during heel strike suggests quadriceps weakness or abnormal patellar tracking.

Check the alignment and contours of the knees. Observe for any atrophy of the quadriceps muscles.

Bow-legs (**genu varum**) and *knock-knees* (**genu valgum**) are common. Quadriceps atrophy can signal hip girdle weakness in older adults.

Inspect the normal hollows around the patella; loss of these hollows can be a sign of swelling in the knee joint and suprapatellar recess. Note any other swelling in or around the knee and which structure it may be related to.

Swelling over the patella occurs in prepatellar bursitis (housemaid's knee). Swelling over the tibial tubercle suggests infrapatellar or, if more medial, anserine bursitis.

Palpation. Ask the patient to sit on the edge of the examining table with the knees hanging relaxed in flexion. In this position, bony landmarks are more visible, and the muscles, tendons, and ligaments are more relaxed, making them easier to palpate. Pay special attention to any areas of tenderness. Pain is a common complaint in knee problems, and localizing the structure causing pain as precisely as possible is important for accurate evaluation and narrowing your differential diagnosis.

- Palpate the *tibiofemoral joint*. Facing the knee, place your thumbs in the soft tissue depressions on either side of the *patellar tendon*. Identify the groove of the tibiofemoral joint. Note that the inferior pole of the patella generally lies at the tibiofemoral joint line in this flexed position. As you press your thumbs downward, you can feel the edge of the tibial plateau. Follow it medially and laterally until you are stopped by the converging femur and tibia. By moving your thumbs upward toward the midline to the top of the patella, you can follow the articulating surface of the femur against the tibia and identify the margins of the joint, which should be palpated for pain.

  Note any irregular bony ridges along the joint margins.

  Bony enlargement at the joint margins, genu varum deformity, and stiffness lasting ≤30 minutes are typical findings in *OA* (LRs 11.8, 3.4, and 3.0, respectively). Crepitus is also common but not diagnostic.

- Palpate the *medial meniscus*. Press on the medial soft tissue depression along the upper edge of the tibial plateau with the tibia slightly internally rotated. Place the knee in slight flexion and palpate the *lateral meniscus* along the lateral joint line.

  A medial meniscus tear can manifest as joint line point tenderness and is common after trauma and requires prompt further evaluation. It is important to recognize that individuals with OA may end up with chronic tears of the meniscus related to abnormal biomechanics and loading of the knee.

- Palpate the *medial joint compartment* (Fig. 15-77) of the tibiofemoral joint with the knee flexed on the examining table to approximately 90°. Pay special attention to any areas of pain or tenderness. Medially, move your thumbs upward to palpate the *medial femoral condyle*. The *adductor tubercle* is posterior to the medial femoral condyle. Move your thumbs downward to palpate the *medial tibial plateau*.

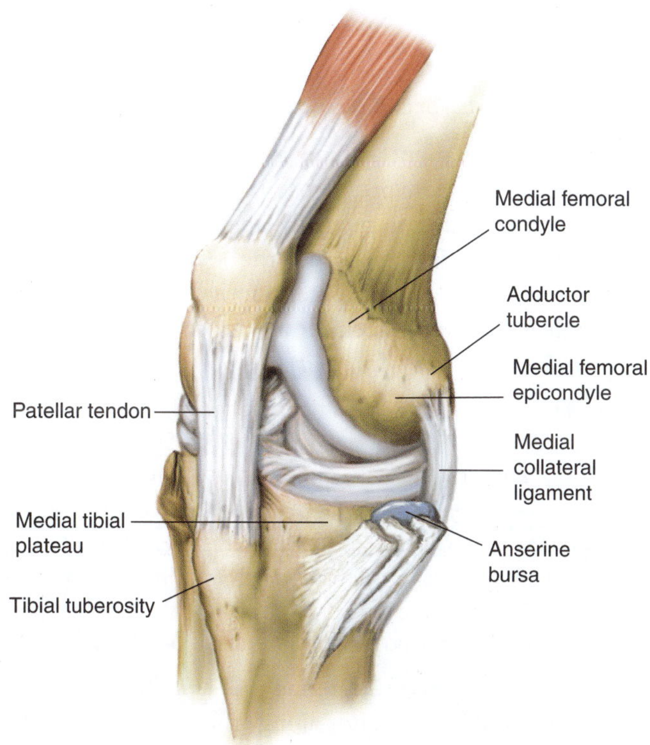

FIGURE 15-77. Structures in the medial compartment of the right knee.

Also medially, palpate along the joint line and identify the *MCL*, which connects the medial epicondyle of the femur to the medial condyle and superior medial surface of the tibia (in flexion, the course may be more posterior than you anticipate). Palpate along this broad, flat ligament from its origin to insertion.

- Now palpate the *lateral joint compartment* of the tibiofemoral joint in the same position, again paying attention to any areas of pain or tenderness. Lateral to the patellar tendon, move your thumbs upward to palpate the *lateral femoral condyle* and downward to palpate the *lateral tibial plateau*. When the knee is flexed, the femoral epicondyle is lateral to the tibial condyle.

MCL tenderness after injury is suspicious for an MCL tear. LCL injuries are less frequent. When either is injured, search for injury to the other ligaments and soft tissues of the knee that are also often affected.

Also, on the lateral surface, ask the patient to cross one leg so that the ankle rests on the opposite knee and find the *LCL*, a firm cord that runs from the lateral femoral epicondyle to the head of the fibula.

- Then palpate the *patellofemoral joint compartment*. Locate the patella and trace the patellar tendon distally until you palpate the tibial tuberosity. Ask the patient to extend the knee to make sure the patellar tendon is intact.

Tenderness over the tendon or inability to extend the knee suggests a partial or complete tear of the patellar tendon.

With the patient supine and the knee extended, compress the *patella* against the underlying femur, and gently move it medially and laterally, assessing for crepitus and pain. Ask the patient to tighten the quadriceps as the patella moves distally in the trochlear groove. Check for a smooth sliding motion (*patellofemoral grinding test*).

Pain and crepitus arise from the roughened undersurface of the patella as it articulates with the femur. Similar pain may occur when using the stairs or getting up from a chair.

Pain with compression and patellar movement during quadriceps contraction occur in chondromalacia. Two of three findings are most diagnostic of the *patellofemoral pain syndrome:* pain with quadriceps contraction, pain with squatting, and pain with palpation of the posteromedial/or lateral patellar border.

- Palpate for any thickening or swelling in the *suprapatellar recess* and along the margins of the patella (Fig. 15-78). Start 10 cm above the superior border of the patella, well above the recess, and feel the soft tissues between your thumb and fingers. Note any muscular tenderness. Move your hand distally in progressive steps, trying to identify fluid or swelling in the recess if present. Continue your palpation along the sides of the patella. Note any tenderness or increased warmth.

Swelling around the patella may point to synovial thickening or effusion of the knee joint (Fig. 15-79).

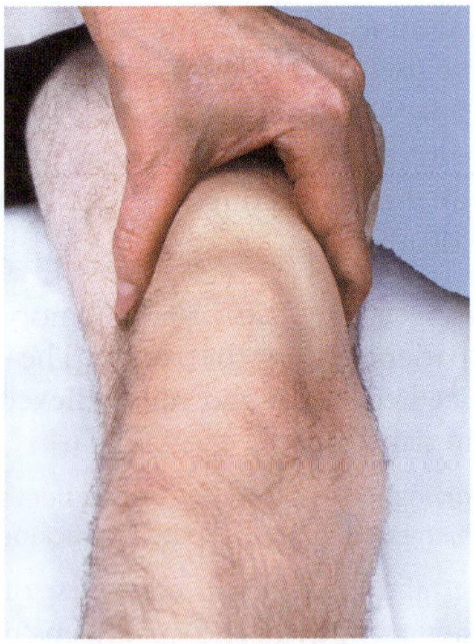

FIGURE 15-78. Palpating the suprapatellar pouch of the left knee.

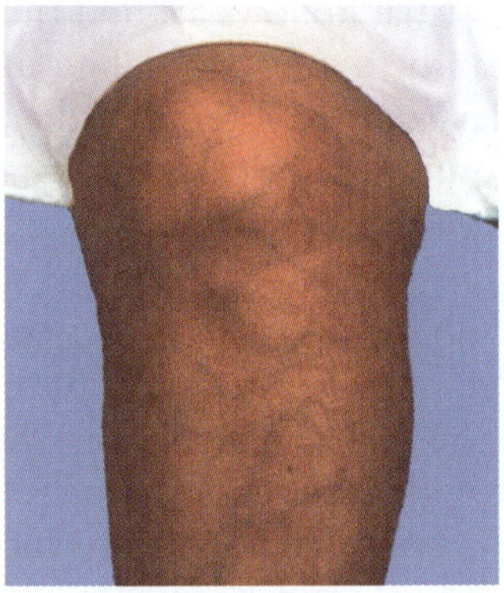

FIGURE 15-79. Effusion of the knee joint.

Thickening, bogginess, or warmth often occurs with synovitis. Nontender effusions are common in OA.

- Check three other bursae for bogginess or swelling. Palpate the *prepatellar bursa*. Palpate over the *anserine bursa* on the posteromedial side of the knee between the MCL and the tendons inserting on the medial tibial plateau. On the posterior surface, with the leg extended, check the medial aspect of the *popliteal fossa*.

Prepatellar bursitis is often triggered by excessive kneeling.

Anserine bursitis can be seen in running, valgus knee deformity, or OA.

A popliteal or "Baker" cyst can result from distention of the gastrocnemius semimembranosus bursa from underlying arthritis or trauma.

See examination techniques for gross assessment of knee joint effusions, p. 457.

Range of Motion. Now assess knee ROM; refer to Box 15-17 for specific muscles responsible for each movement and for instructions to the patient.

Box 15-17. Range of Motion of the Knee Joint

Knee Movement	Primary Muscles Affecting Movement	Patient Instructions
Flexion	Hamstring group: biceps femoris, semitendinosus, and semimembranosus	"Bend your knee."
Extension	Quadriceps: rectus femoris, vastus medialis, lateralis, and intermedius	"Straighten your leg."

Crepitus with flexion and extension can signal patellofemoral OA, a probable precursor of knee OA.

Special Maneuvers. You will often need to test ligamentous stability and integrity of the medial and lateral menisci, the MCL and LCL, the patellar tendon, and the ACL and PCL, particularly when there is a history of trauma or knee pain (Box 15-18). Always examine both knees and compare findings.

ACL tears are notably more frequent in women, attributed to ligamentous laxity related to estrogen cycling and to differences in anatomy and neuromuscular control. ACL injury prevention programs are now common, especially for young women playing high school or college sports who are especially vulnerable to these sorts of injuries.

Box 15-18. Special Maneuvers for Examining the Knee

Structure	Maneuver
Medial Meniscus and Lateral Meniscus 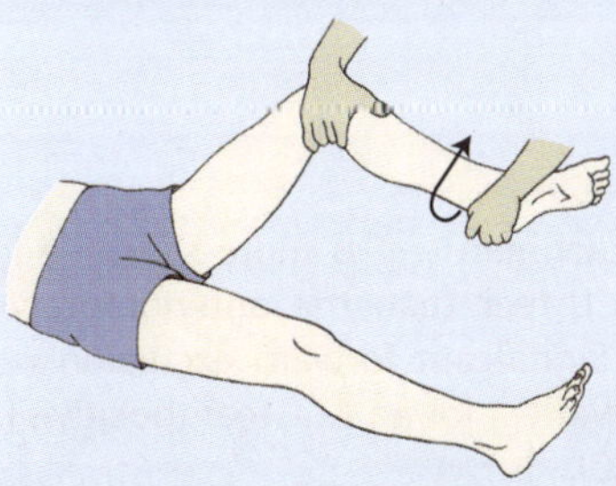	**McMurray Test.** With the patient supine, grasp the heel and flex the knee. Cup your other hand over the knee joint with fingers and thumb along the medial joint line. From the heel, externally rotate the lower leg, then push on the lateral side to apply a valgus stress on the medial side of the joint. At the same time, slowly extend the lower leg in external rotation. The same maneuver with internal rotation of the foot stresses the lateral meniscus. If a click is felt or heard at the joint line during flexion and extension of the knee, or if tenderness is noted along the joint line, further assess the meniscus for a tear.
Medial Collateral Ligament (MCL) 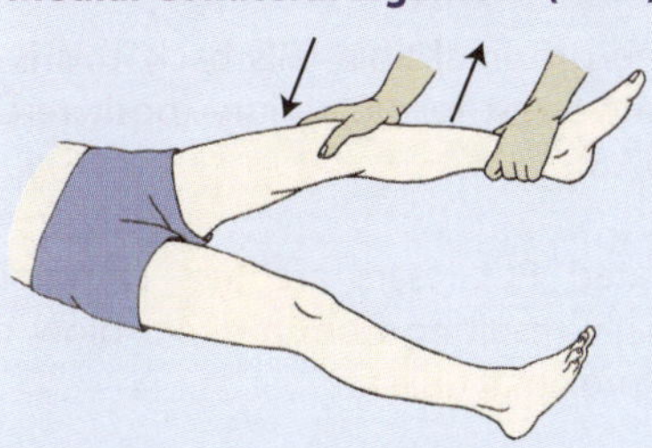	**Abduction (or Valgus) Stress Test.** With the patient supine and the knee slightly flexed, move the thigh about 30° laterally to the side of the table. Place one hand against the lateral knee to stabilize the femur and the other hand around the medial ankle. Push medially against the knee and pull laterally at the ankle to open the knee joint on the medial side (*valgus stress*). Feel for excessive widening of the joint and lack of endpoint that may signal the ligament is no longer intact.

A palpable click or pop along the medial or lateral joint line is a positive test for a tear of the posterior portion of the medial meniscus (positive LR of 4.5). The tear may displace meniscal tissue causing "locking" on full knee extension or movement of the loose tissue causing clicking.

Pain or a gap in the medial joint line is a positive test for an MCL injury (sensitivity 79% to 89%; specificity 49% to 99%).

(*continued*)

Box 15-18. Special Maneuvers for Examining the Knee (*continued*)

Structure	Maneuver	
Lateral Collateral Ligament (LCL) 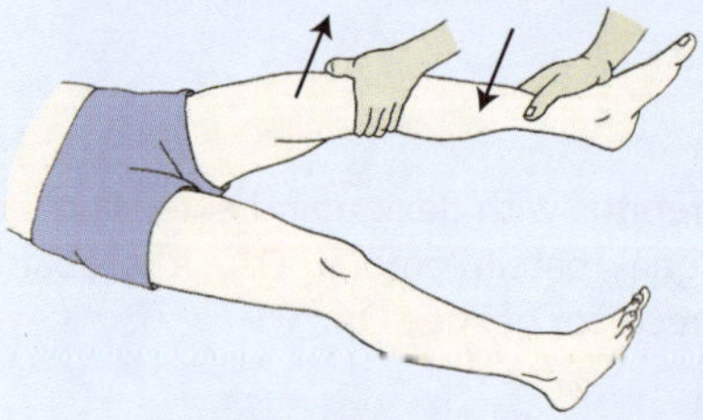	**Adduction (or Varus) Stress Test.** With the thigh and knee in the same position, change your position so that you can place one hand against the medial surface of the knee and the other around the lateral ankle. Push laterally against the knee and pull medially at the ankle to open the knee joint on the lateral side (*varus stress*). Feel for excessive widening of the joint and lack of endpoint that may signal the ligament is no longer intact.	Pain or a gap in the lateral joint line points is a positive test for LCL injury (less common than MCL injuries).
Anterior Cruciate Ligament (ACL) **Note:** With all ACL testing, PCL testing should also be done. This is because a torn PCL will allow the tibia to sag backward relative to the femur. As a result, an anterior drawer or Lachman test may feel positive, but actually reflect drawing the tibia forward into normal position in the setting of a torn PCL. 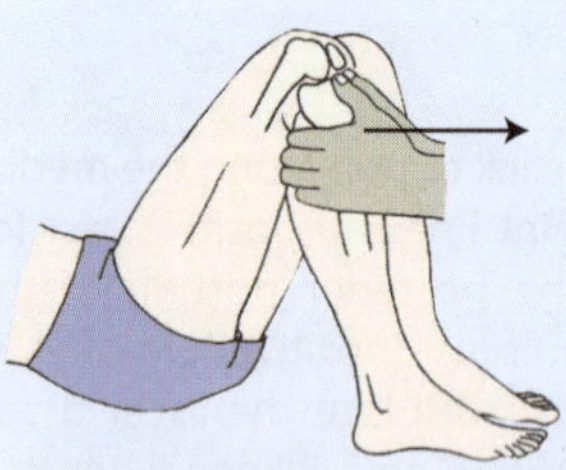	**Anterior Drawer Sign.** With the patient supine, hips flexed, and knees flexed to 90° and feet flat on the table, cup your hands around the knee with the thumbs on the medial and lateral joint line and the fingers on the medial and lateral insertions of the hamstrings. Sit on the patient's foot to ensure it does not move during the maneuver. Draw the tibia forward and observe if it slides forward (like a drawer) from under the femur. Compare the degree of forward movement with that of the opposite knee. The knee should have a firm endpoint with minimal movement. Lack of a firm endpoint with excessive movement may indicate the ACL is no longer intact.	A few degrees of forward movement are normal if equally present on the opposite side. A forward jerk showing the contours of the upper tibia is a positive test, or anterior drawer sign, with a positive LR of 11.5 for an ACL tear. ACL injuries result from knee hyperextension, direct blows to the knee, and twisting or landing on an extended hip or knee.
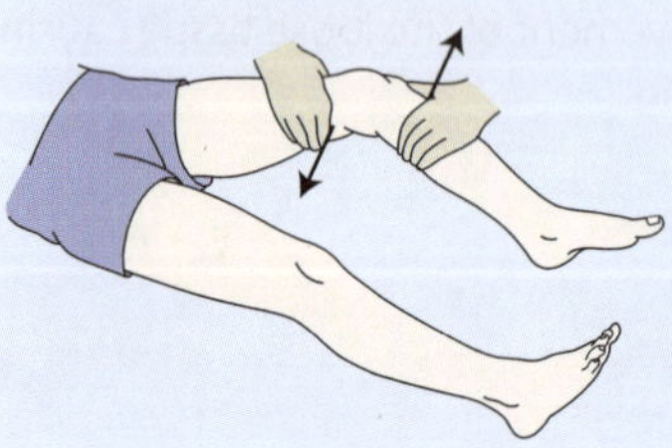	**Lachman Test.** Place the knee in 15° of flexion and mild external rotation. Grasp the distal femur on the lateral side with one hand and the proximal tibia on the medial side with the other. With the thumb of the tibial hand on the joint line, forcefully and simultaneously pull the tibia forward and the femur back. Estimate the degree of forward excursion. There should be a firm endpoint to any forward movement. Lack of a firm endpoint with excessive movement may indicate the ACL is no longer intact.	The Lachman test is more sensitive for an ACL tear than the anterior drawer sign. Significant forward excursion is a positive test for an ACL tear (positive LR of 17.0).
Posterior Cruciate Ligament (PCL) 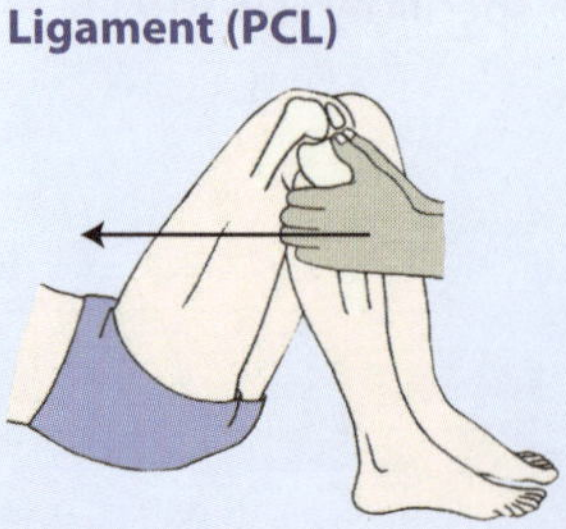	**Posterior Drawer Sign.** Position the patient and place your hands in the positions described for the anterior drawer test. Sit on the patient's foot to minimize foot movement. Push the tibia posteriorly and observe the degree of backward movement in the femur. There should be minimal posterior movement and excursion of the tibia relative to the femur. Excessive movement suggests an insufficient or torn PCL.	If the proximal tibia falls back, this is a positive test for PCL injury (positive LR of 97.8). Isolated PCL tears are less common, usually resulting from a direct blow to the proximal tibia.

Special Techniques: Tests for Knee Joint Effusions

Learn to apply three tests for approximating the amount of fluid in the knee joint: the bulge sign, the balloon sign, and balloting the patella.

Bulge Sign (for Minor Effusions). With the knee extended, place the left hand above the knee and apply pressure on the suprapatellar recess to displace or "milk" fluid downward (Fig. 15-80). Stroke downward on the medial aspect of the knee and apply pressure to force fluid into the lateral area (Fig. 15-81). Tap the knee just behind the lateral margin of the patella with the right hand (Fig. 15-82).

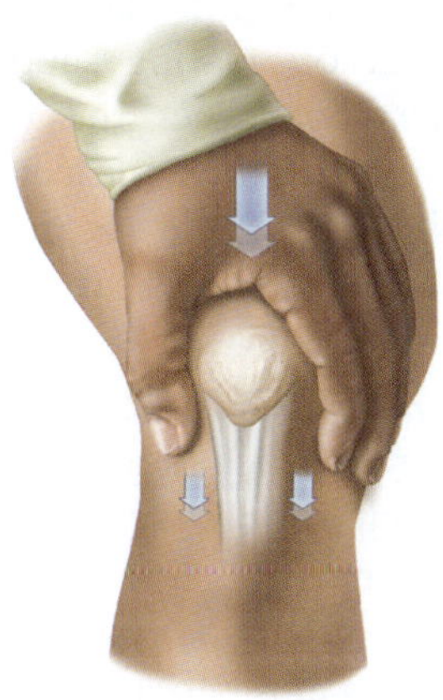

FIGURE 15-80. Bulge sign—Step 1: Displace ("milk") fluid downward from suprapatellar recess.

A bulge on the medial side between the patella and the femur is a *positive test* for effusion.

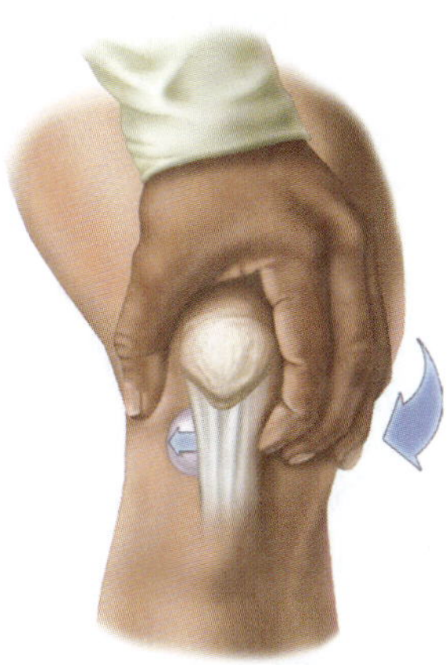

FIGURE 15-81. Bulge sign—Step 2: Then force fluid to lateral area by applying pressure on medial aspect of knee.

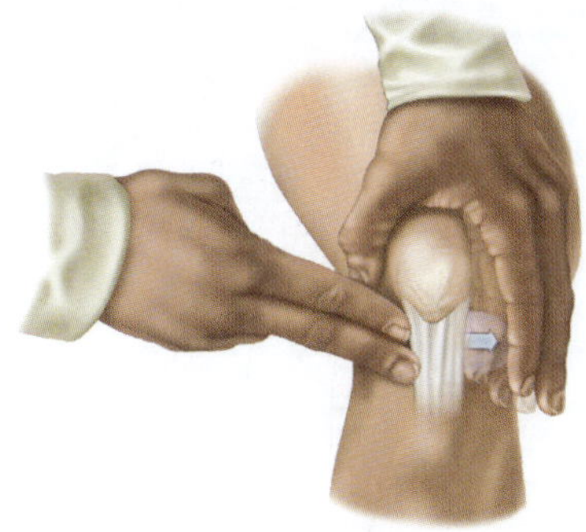

FIGURE 15-82. Bulge sign—Step 3: Tap the bulge formed by accumulated fluid on the lateral margin of the patella.

Balloon Sign (for Major Effusions). Place the thumb and index finger of your right hand on each side of the patella; with the left hand, compress the suprapatellar recess against the femur (Fig. 15-83). Palpate for fluid ejected or "ballooning" into the spaces next to the patella under your right thumb and index finger.

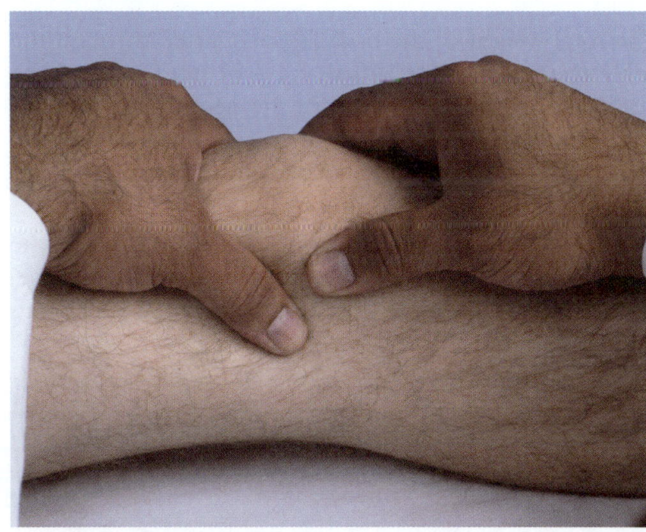

FIGURE 15-83. Displacing fluid from suprapatellar recess downward while compressing both sides of the knee to observe patella "balloon up" (balloon sign).

A palpable fluid wave is a *positive test* or "balloon sign." A palpable returning fluid wave into the suprapatellar recess further confirms a major effusion, present in knee fractures (LR 2.5).

Balloting of the Patella (for Major Effusions). To assess large effusions, you can also compress the suprapatellar pouch and "ballotte" or push the patella sharply against the femur (Fig. 15-84). Watch for fluid returning to the suprapatellar pouch and feel for movement of the patella within the underlying effusion.

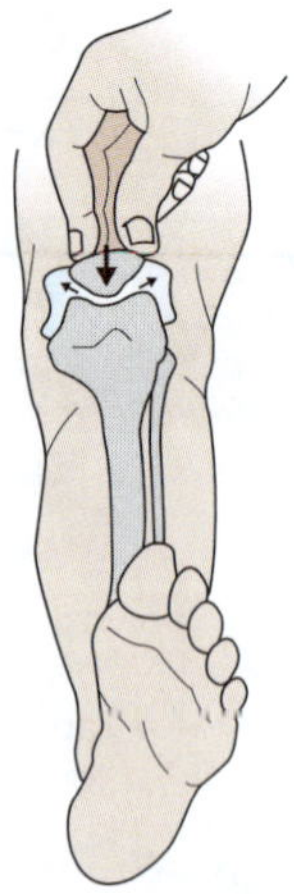

FIGURE 15-84. Pushing sharply (balloting) the patella against femur in fluid-filled knee.

A palpable fluid wave returning into the recess is also a *positive test* for a major effusion.

A palpable patellar click with compression may also occur but yields more false positives.

Ankle Joint and Foot

The total weight of the body is transmitted through the ankle to the foot. The ankle and foot must balance the body and absorb the impact of the heel strike and gait. Despite thick padding along the toes, sole, and heel and stabilizing ligaments at the ankles, the ankle and foot are frequent sites of sprain and bony injury.

The ankle is a hinge joint formed by the *tibia,* the *fibula,* and the *talus.* The tibia and fibula act as a mortise, with the tibia and fibula cradling the talus and stabilizing side-to-side movement.

The principal joints of the ankle are the *tibiotalar joint,* between the tibia and the talus, and the *subtalar (talocalcaneal) joint* (Fig. 15-85).

Note the principal landmarks of the ankle: the *medial malleolus,* the bony prominence at the distal end of the tibia, and the *lateral malleolus,* at the distal end of the fibula. Lodged under the talus and jutting posteriorly is the *calcaneus,* or heel bone.

An imaginary line, the *longitudinal arch,* spans the foot, extending from the calcaneus of the hind foot along the tarsal bones of the midfoot (see cuneiform, navicular, and cuboid bones in Fig. 15-86) to the forefoot metatarsals and toes. The *heads of the metatarsals* are palpable in the ball of the foot. In the forefoot, identify the *metatarsophalangeal joints,* proximal to the webs of the toes, and the *PIP and DIP joints* of the toes.

Movement at the ankle joint is limited to dorsiflexion and plantar flexion. *Plantar flexion* is powered by the gastrocnemius, the soleus, and plantaris, with the tibialis posterior and toe flexors playing supporting roles. The strong *Achilles tendon* attaches the gastrocnemius and soleus muscles to the posterior calcaneus. The *dorsiflexors* include the tibialis anterior and the toe extensors. They lie prominently on the anterior surface, or *dorsum,* of the ankle, anterior to the malleoli.

Muscles in the *lateral compartment* are responsible for *eversion* of the foot and include the fibularis longus and fibularis brevis, which run under the lateral malleolus and move the foot outward.

Muscles in the *medial compartment* of the foot are responsible for *inversion* of the foot (heel bows inward) and include the tibialis posterior and anterior muscles. The tibialis posterior runs just behind the medial malleolus with the toe extensors.

Ligaments extend from each malleolus onto the foot.

- Medially, the triangle-shaped *deltoid ligament* fans out from the inferior surface of the medial malleolus to the talus and proximal tarsal bones, protecting against stress from eversion (heel bows outward).

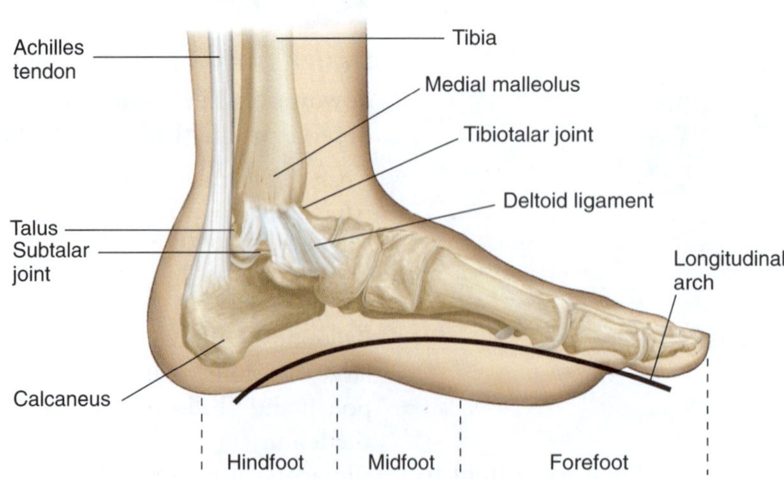

FIGURE 15-85. Anatomy of left ankle, medial view.

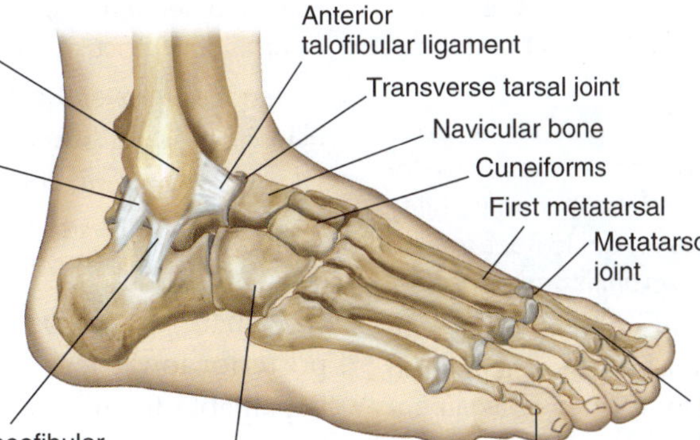

FIGURE 15-86. Anatomy of right ankle, lateral view.

- Laterally, the three ligaments are less substantial with higher risk for injury from inversion injuries. They include the *anterior talofibular ligament* (often most at risk), the *calcaneofibular ligament*, and the *posterior talofibular ligament* (see Fig. 15-85).

The plantar fascia inserts on the medial tubercle of the calcaneus.

Techniques of Examination

Key Components of the Ankle Joint and Foot Examination

- Inspect the ankle and foot (deformities, nodules, swelling, calluses, corns).
- Palpate the ankle joint (bogginess, swelling, tenderness), Achilles tendon (nodules, tenderness), calcaneus, plantar fascia (spurs, tenderness), medial and lateral ankle ligaments, medial and lateral malleolus (tenderness, swelling, ecchymoses), metatarsophalangeal (MTP) joints (tenderness), metatarsals (tenderness, abnormalities), gastrocnemius, and soleus (defect, tenderness, swelling).
- Assess range of motion: flexion (plantar flexion) and extension (dorsiflexion), and inversion and eversion.
- Perform special maneuvers (if indicated). *Tests for joint integrity*: tibiotalar, subtalar or talocalcaneal, talocrural, transverse tarsal, and metatarsophalangeal. Test for Achilles tendon integrity.

Inspection. Observe all surfaces of the ankles and feet, noting any deformities, nodules, swelling, calluses, or corns.

See Table 15-10, Abnormalities of the Feet, and Table 15-11, Abnormalities of the Toes and Soles.

Palpation. With your thumbs, palpate the anterior aspect of each *ankle joint*, noting any bogginess, swelling, or tenderness (Fig. 15-87).

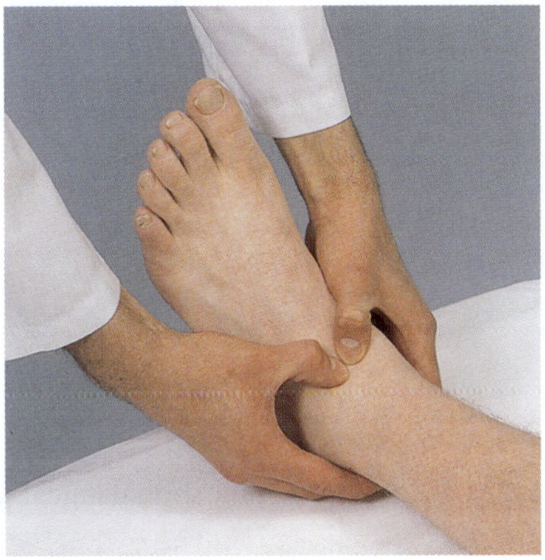

FIGURE 15-87. Palpating the left anterior ankle joint.

Localized tenderness is often present in arthritis, ligamentous injury, bony injury or infection.

Feel along the *Achilles tendon* for nodules and tenderness.

Check for rheumatoid nodules, which can be seen along the Achilles. Focal thickening and tenderness in the Achilles tendon are commonly found in Achilles tendinitis, bursitis, or partial tear from trauma.

Palpate the *heel*, especially the posterior and inferior calcaneus, and the plantar fascia for tenderness.

Bone spurs are common on the calcaneus and may not be pathologic.

Focal heel tenderness at the attachment site of the plantar fascia is typical of plantar fasciitis. Risk factors are anatomic (overpronation, flat feet), improper footwear, excessive use, and overtraining with overstriding in prolonged heel-strike exercise. Presence or absence of a heel spur does not change the diagnosis.

Palpate for tenderness over the *medial* and *lateral ankle ligaments* and the *medial* and *lateral malleolus*, especially in cases of trauma. In trauma, the distal tips of the tibia and fibula should also be palpated.

Most ankle sprains involve foot inversion and injury to the weaker lateral ligaments (anterior talofibular and calcaneofibular), with overlying tenderness, swelling, and ecchymosis.

After trauma, pain in the malleolar zone plus either bone tenderness over the posterior aspects of either malleolus (or over the navicular or base of the fifth metatarsal) or an inability to bear weight for four steps is suspicious for ankle fracture and warrants radiography (known as the *Ottawa ankle and foot rules*).

Watch also for tenderness and excessive movement with compression of the tibia and fibula toward each other, which may signal damage to the anterior-inferior tibiofibular ligament and a high ankle sprain.

Palpate the *metatarsophalangeal (MTP) joints* for tenderness (Fig. 15-88). Compress the forefoot between the thumb and fingers. Exert pressure just proximal to the heads of the first and fifth metatarsals.

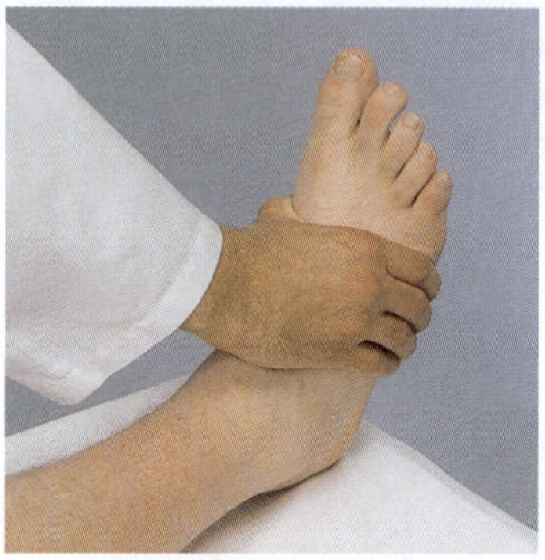

FIGURE 15-88. Palpating metatarsophalangeal joints.

Tenderness along the posterior medial malleolus is seen in posterior tibial tendinitis. This can also be seen along the lateral malleolus with fibularis longus or brevis tendinitis.

Acute inflammation with tenderness and erythema of the first MTP joint is common in gout.

Palpate the heads of the five metatarsals and the grooves between them with your thumb and index finger (Fig. 15-89). Place your thumb on the dorsum of the foot and your index finger on the plantar surface. Move the metatarsal heads relative to each other, evaluating both for increased laxity and pain with motion.

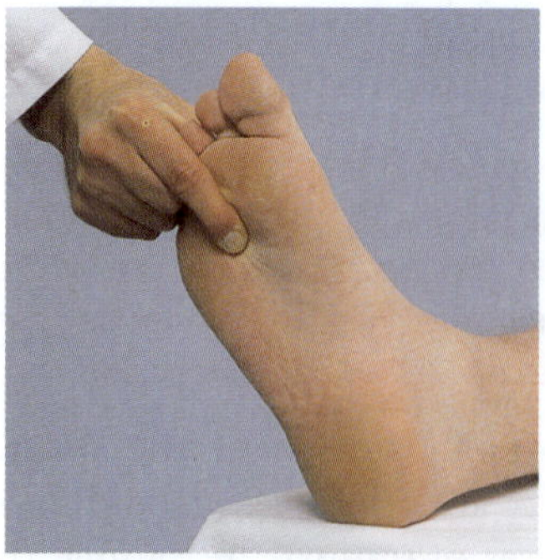

FIGURE 15-89. Palpating the metatarsal heads and grooves.

Pain and tenderness, called *metatarsalgia,* occurs in trauma, arthritis, and vascular compromise.

Tenderness over the third and fourth metatarsal heads on the plantar surface is suspicious for Morton neuroma (see p. 478).

Forefoot abnormalities like hallux valgus, metatarsalgia, and Morton neuroma are more common in those who wear high-heeled shoes and shoes with narrow or pointed toe boxes.

Palpate the *gastrocnemius* and *soleus* muscles on the posterior lower leg. Their common tendon, the *Achilles*, is palpable from about the lower third of the calf to its insertion on the calcaneus.

A defect in the muscles, tenderness, and swelling may signal a ruptured Achilles tendon.

Tenderness and thickening of the tendon, at times with a protuberant posterolateral bony process of the calcaneus, suggests Achilles tendinitis.

Range of Motion. Assess *flexion* and *extension* at the tibiotalar (ankle) joint. In the foot, assess *inversion* and *eversion* at the subtalar and transverse tarsal joints. The ankle should normally have about 20° of dorsiflexion and about 50° of plantar flexion from neutral. The foot has about 35° of inversion and about 25° of eversion from neutral (Box 15-19).

Box 15-19. Range of Motion of the Ankle Joint and Foot

Ankle and Foot Movement	Primary Muscles Affecting Movement	Patient Instructions
Ankle Flexion (Plantar Flexion)	Gastrocnemius, soleus, plantaris, and tibialis posterior	"Point your foot toward the floor."
Ankle Extension (Dorsiflexion)	Tibialis anterior, extensor digitorum longus, and extensor hallucis longus	"Point your foot toward the ceiling."
Inversion	Tibialis posterior and anterior	"Turn the sole of your foot inward or toward your midline."
Eversion	Fibularis longus and brevis	"Turn the sole of your foot outward or away from your midline."

Special Maneuvers. Perform the following maneuvers to determine joint integrity.

Testing Integrity of the Ankle (tibiotalar) Joint. Dorsiflex and plantar flex the foot at the ankle.

Pain during movements of the ankle and the foot helps to localize possible arthritis.

Testing Integrity of the Subtalar (Talocalcaneal) Joint. Stabilize the ankle with one hand, grasp the heel with the other, and invert and evert the foot by turning the heel inward then outward in a maneuver called the *talar tilt test* (Figs. 15-90 and 15-91).

Excessive movement suggests laxity from ligamentous injury.

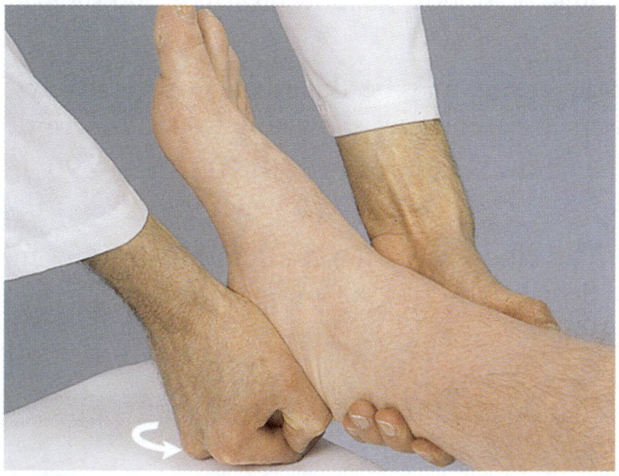

FIGURE 15-90. Testing integrity of subtalar (talocalcaneal) joint by inverting the heel.

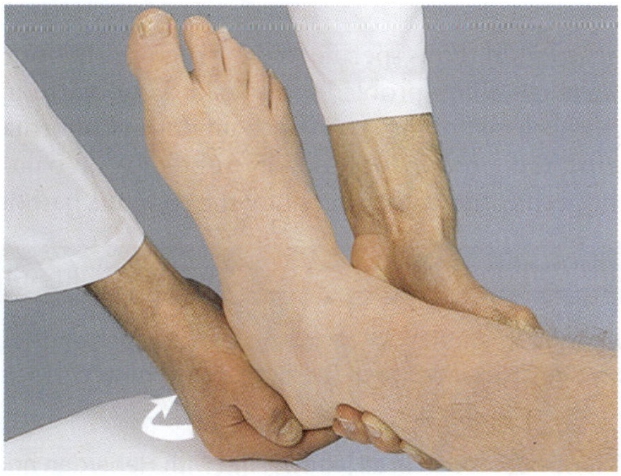

FIGURE 15-91. Testing integrity of subtalar (talocalcaneal) joint by everting the heel.

Testing Integrity of the Talocrural Joint. Grasp the anterior part of the lower leg with one hand and the posterior portion of the heel with the other. From this position, attempt to draw the heel forward under the tibia. You should feel a hard end point.

Excessive movement or lack of a hard end point suggests injury to the anterior talofibular ligament.

Closely observe which movements are most uncomfortable for your patient. An arthritic joint frequently causes pain when moved in any direction, whereas a ligamentous sprain produces pain when the ligament is stretched. For example, often, ankle sprain inversion with plantar flexion of the foot causes pain, whereas eversion with plantar flexion is relatively pain free.

Testing Integrity of the Transverse Tarsal Joint. Stabilize the heel and invert and evert the forefoot (Figs. 15-92 and 15-93).

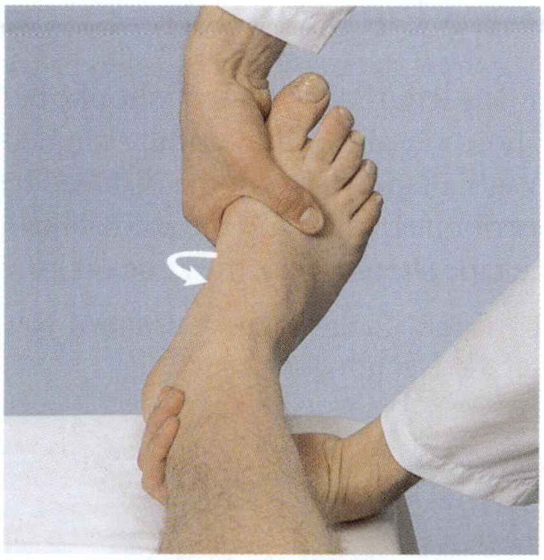

FIGURE 15-92. Testing integrity of transverse tarsal joint by inverting the forefoot.

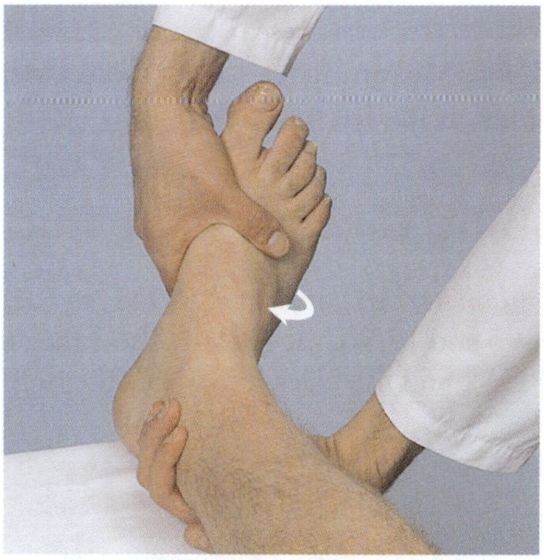

FIGURE 15-93. Testing integrity of transverse tarsal joint by everting the forefoot.

Testing Integrity of Metatarsophalangeal Joints. Move the proximal phalanx of each toe up and down.

Pain may suggest acute synovitis. Instability occurs in chronic synovitis and claw-toe deformity.

Testing Integrity of the Achilles Tendon. To test its integrity, place the patient prone with the knee and ankle flexed at 90°, or, alternatively, ask the patient to kneel on a chair. Squeeze the calf and watch for plantar flexion at the ankle.

Absent plantar flexion is a *positive test* for Achilles tendon rupture. Sudden severe pain "like a gunshot" with ecchymosis from the calf into the heel and a flat-footed gait with absent "toe-off" may all be present.

SPECIAL TECHNIQUES

Measuring Leg Length

To measure leg length, the patient should be relaxed in the supine position and symmetrically aligned with legs extended. With a tape, measure the distance between the anterior superior iliac spine and the medial malleolus (Fig. 15-94). The tape should cross the knee on its medial side.

Measured leg length is the same in scoliosis in spite of the appearance of a leg-length discrepancy.

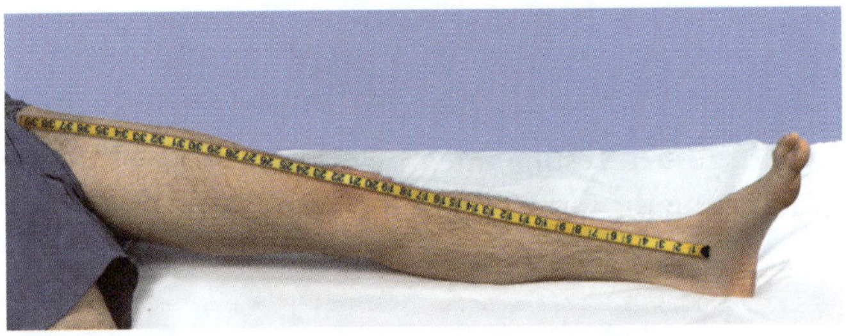

FIGURE 15-94. Measuring leg length from anterior superior iliac spine to medial malleolus.

Describing Limited Joint Motion

Use a *goniometer* to measure ROM in degrees. In Figures 15-95 and 15-96, the red lines show the range of the patient's ROM, and the black lines show the normal range.

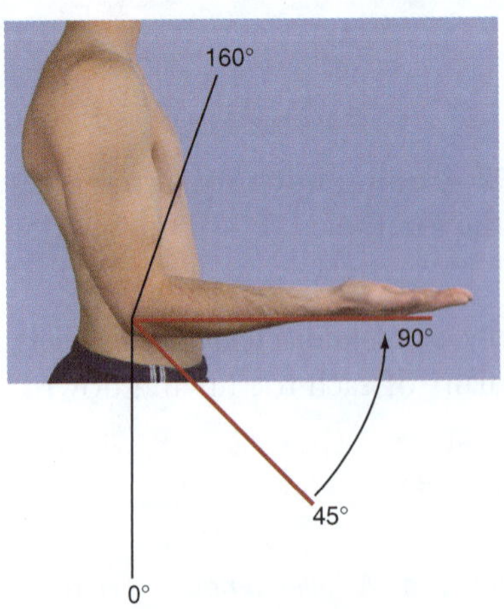

FIGURE 15-95. Normal (*black*) and patient's measured (*red*) range of motion of elbow flexion.

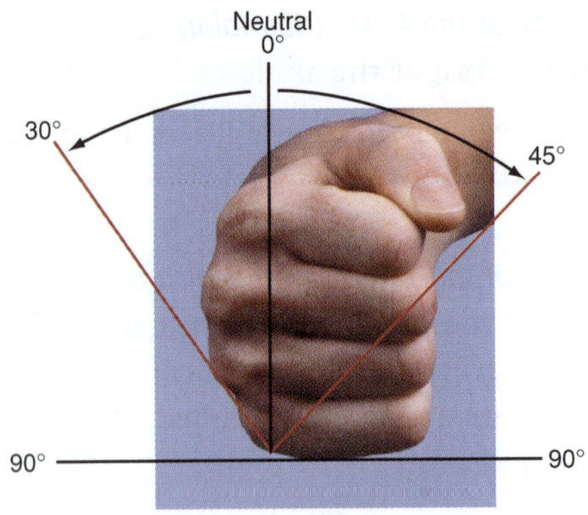

FIGURE 15-96. Normal (*black*) and patient's measured (*red*) range of motion of elbow pronation and supination.

Observations may be described in several ways. The numbers in parentheses show abbreviated descriptions.

A. The elbow flexes from 45° to 90° (45° → 90°),

-or-

The elbow has a flexion deformity of 45° and can be flexed farther to 90° (45° → 90°).

B. Supination at elbow = 30°
(0° → 30°)
Pronation at elbow = 45°
(0° → 45°)

RECORDING YOUR FINDINGS

Use anatomical terms specific to the structure and function of individual joint problems to make your write-up of musculoskeletal findings more meaningful and informative. Describe the precise location of pathology or pain and which specific movements replicate the patient's pathology.

Recording the Musculoskeletal System Examination

"Full range of motion in all joints of the upper and lower extremities. No evidence of swelling or deformity."

OR

"Full range of motion in all joints. Hand with Heberden nodes at the DIP joints, Bouchard nodes at PIP joints. Mild pain with flexion, extension, and rotation of both hips. Full range of motion in the knees, with moderate crepitus. No effusion but bony enlargement along the tibiofemoral joint line bilaterally. Both feet with hallux valgus at the first MTP joints."

These findings suggest OA.

OR

"Right knee with moderate effusion and tenderness over medial meniscus along the joint line. Moderate laxity of ACL on Lachman test. Moderate laxity with joint gapping noted on MCL stress testing. PCL and LCL intact with stress testing—no

(continued)

Recording the Musculoskeletal System Examination (*continued*)

posterior drawer sign or tenderness with varus stress. Patellar tendon intact without tenderness with patient able to extend lower extremity without difficulty. Hamstring tendons with no tenderness to palpation. Good range of motion without significant pain in the hip and ankle. No other deformity or swelling."

These findings suggest injury tear of the medial meniscus, MCL and ACL, possibly from sports injury or trauma and require prompt evaluation.

Keep in mind that strength should be evaluated across all joints of concern and documented as part of your examination. Strength testing is addressed separately (for these techniques, see Chapter 13, Nervous System).

HEALTH PROMOTION AND COUNSELING: EVIDENCE AND RECOMMENDATIONS

Important Topics for Health Promotion and Counseling

- Low back pain
- Osteoporosis
- Preventing falls

Each joint has specific vulnerabilities to trauma and wear. Staying active, eating well, avoiding obesity, and learning to independently manage disease when it arises all help protect and preserve well-functioning joints and muscles and prevent or delay the onset of arthritis, chronic back pain, and osteoporosis.

Low Back Pain

Most patients with acute low back pain get better within 6 weeks; however, about one-third of patients may have persistent moderate intensity pain 1 year later, some with substantial disability. Clinical guidelines emphasize nonpharmacologic approaches for patients with nonspecific acute low back pain symptoms, including reassurance, staying active, heat, massage, acupuncture, and spinal manipulation therapy. Recommended pharmacologic treatments include nonsteroidal anti-inflammatory drugs and smooth muscle relaxants. Factors associated with poor outcomes include inappropriate beliefs that low back pain is a serious clinical condition, maladaptive pain-coping behaviors (avoiding work, movement, or other activities for fear of causing back damage), multiple nonorganic physical examination findings, psychiatric disorders, poor general health, high levels of baseline functional impairment, and low work satisfaction.

Appropriate treatments for chronic low back pain include those for acute low back pain as well as back exercises, multidisciplinary rehabilitation programs, mindfulness-based stress reduction, and behavioral therapy. The American College of Physicians cites evidence supporting duloxetine and tramadol as second-line pharmacologic therapies, though noting that opioids should be used cautiously, given their adverse effects and risks for abuse. Treatment for acute lumbosacral radicular pain will depend upon the underlying cause and extent of neurologic deficits.

Psychosocial factors, now called "yellow flags," strongly affect the course of low back pain. Ask about anxiety, depression, and work stress. Assess any maladaptive coping, inappropriate fears or beliefs, or tendency to somatization.

Osteoporosis

Osteoporosis is characterized by markedly decreased bone mineral density (BMD). The prevalence increases with age and varies by race/ethnicity. Half of all postmenopausal women sustain an osteoporosis-related fracture during their lifetime; 25% develop vertebral deformities; and 15% suffer hip fractures that increase risk of chronic pain, disability, loss of independence, and mortality.

The majority of fragility fractures actually occur among osteopenic adults. Box 15-20 shows common risk factors for osteoporosis.

Box 15-20. Risk Factors for Osteoporosis

- Postmenopausal status in women
- Age ≥50 yrs
- Prior fragility fracture
- Low body mass index
- Low dietary calcium
- Vitamin D deficiency
- Tobacco and excessive alcohol use
- Immobilization
- Inadequate physical activity
- Osteoporosis in a first-degree relative, particularly with history of fragility fracture
- Clinical conditions such as thyrotoxicosis, celiac sprue, IBD, cirrhosis, chronic renal disease, organ transplantation, diabetes, HIV, hypogonadism, multiple myeloma, anorexia nervosa, and rheumatologic and autoimmune disorders
- Medications such as oral and high-dose inhaled corticosteroids, anticoagulants (long-term use), aromatase inhibitors for breast cancer, methotrexate, selected antiseizure medications, immunosuppressive agents, proton-pump inhibitors (long-term use), and androgen deprivation therapy for prostate cancer

Osteoporosis screening is recommended for women age ≥65 years and for younger women whose 10-year fracture risk equals or exceeds that of an average-risk 65-year-old white woman. Screen all men age 70 and older and selectively screen men ages 50 to 69 based on risk factor profiles.

Bone strength depends on bone quality, bone density, and overall bone size. Because there is no direct measure of bone strength, BMD—which provides roughly 70% of bone strength—is used as a reasonable surrogate. Dual-energy x-ray absorptiometry (DEXA) scanning of the lumbar spine and femoral neck is the optimal standard for measuring BMD, diagnosing osteoporosis, and guiding treatment decisions. DEXA measurement of BMD at the femoral neck is considered the best predictor of hip fracture.

Bone mass peaks by age 30 years. Bone loss from age-related declines in estrogen and testosterone is initially rapid, then slows and becomes continuous.

The World Health Organization (WHO) scoring criteria for *T scores* and *Z scores,* measured in standard deviations (SDs), are used worldwide (Box 15-21). A 1.0 SD decrease in BMD is associated with a twofold increased risk for a fragility fracture.

Box 15-21. World Health Organization Bone Density Criteria

- **Osteoporosis:** T score < −2.5 (>2.5 SDs below the young adult mean)
- **Osteopenia:** T score between −1.0 and −2.5 (1.0 to 2.5 SDs below the young adult mean)

Bone densitometry scoring also includes Z scores representing comparisons with age-matched controls. These measurements are useful for determining whether bone loss is caused by an underlying disease or condition.

Use the Fracture Risk Assessment (FRAX®) calculator. The FRAX® calculator generates a 10-year osteoporotic fracture risk based on age; gender; weight; height; parental hip fracture history; use of glucocorticoids; presence of RA or conditions associated with secondary osteoporosis; current tobacco use; heavy alcohol use; and, when available, femoral neck BMD. The FRAX® calculator also provides a 10-year hip fracture risk. The website for the FRAX® calculation tool is https://www.sheffield.ac.uk/FRAX/. FRAX® has been validated for black/African American, Hispanic, and Asian women in the United States and has calculated fracture risks that are continent- and country-specific.

A previous low-impact fracture from standing height or lower is the greatest risk factor for subsequent fracture.

A *10-year osteoporotic fracture risk threshold of 8.4%* is recommended when considering BMD screening in women ages 50 to 64 years. Screening decisions for women in this age range should account for menopausal status, clinical judgment, and patient preferences and values.

Calcium and Vitamin D. *Calcium* is an essential mineral for the development, growth, and maintenance of bone as well as for muscle and vascular function, nerve transmission, and hormonal secretion.

Humans acquire *vitamin D* from sunlight, food, and dietary supplements. Vitamin D from the skin and diet is metabolized in the liver to 25-hydroxyvitamin D (25[OH]D), the best determinant of vitamin D status. Serum 25[OH]D is then metabolized in the kidneys to 1,25-dihydroxyvitamin D (1,25[OH]$_2$D), the most active form of vitamin D. Without vitamin D, less than 25% of dietary calcium is absorbed. Parathyroid hormone (PTH) enhances renal tubular absorption of calcium and stimulates the conversion of 25[OH]D to 1,25[OH]$_2$D. PTH also activates osteoblasts, which lay down new bone matrix, and indirectly stimulates osteoclasts, which dissolve bone matrix.

The dietary intake recommendations for calcium and vitamin D is shown in Box 15-22. Serum 25[OH]D levels of 20 ng/mL are sufficient to maintain bone health and warned of potential adverse effects with levels above 50 ng/mL.

Box 15-22. Recommended Dietary Intakes of Calcium and Vitamin D for Adults (Institute of Medicine 2010)

Age Group	Calcium (Elemental) mg/d	Vitamin D IU/d
19–50 yrs	1,000	600
51–70 yrs		
Women	1,200	600
Men	1,000	600
71 and older	1,200	800

There are two main forms of calcium supplements, calcium carbonate and calcium citrate. Supplements contain variable amounts of elemental calcium. Calcium carbonate is less expensive and should be consumed with food. Calcium citrate is absorbed more easily in individuals with reduced levels of stomach acid and can be taken with or without food. Calcium absorption depends on the total amount consumed at one time—absorption diminishes at higher doses. Patients taking daily doses ≥1,000 mg should split the amount into two or more doses over the day. Vitamin D supplements are available in two forms, D_2 (ergocalciferol) and D_3 (cholecalciferol); D_3 increases serum 25(OH)D levels more effectively than D_2.

Antiresorptive agents inhibit osteoclast activity and slow bone remodeling, allowing better mineralization of bone matrix and stabilization of the trabecular microarchitecture. Currently used agents include bisphosphonates and selective estrogen-receptor modulators (SERMs). Bisphosphonates are considered the first-line therapy for osteoporosis. SERMs have been shown to reduce vertebral fractures. Bisphosphonates have been linked to the rare occurrence of osteonecrosis of the jaw and atypical femur fractures, and SERMs increase the risk for thromboembolic events. Estrogen is no longer considered a first-line treatment due to associated risks of breast cancer and vascular thrombosis. Calcitonin is no longer a preferred treatment because it is considered relatively ineffective and has been associated with an overall increased risk for malignancy.

Anabolic agents such as teriparatide, a PTH analog, stimulate bone formation by acting primarily on osteoblasts but require daily subcutaneous administration and monitoring for hypercalcemia. PTH is reserved for patients with severe osteoporosis (T scores < -3.5 or < -2.5 with a fragility fracture) or those who have failed or not tolerated other therapies. Randomized placebo-controlled trials have shown that PTH treatment significantly reduces radiographic vertebral and nonvertebral fractures in postmenopausal osteoporotic women. Side effects include leg cramps, dizziness, and nausea.

The receptor activator of NFκB ligand (RANKL) inhibitor denosumab is a monoclonal antibody that binds RANKL receptors and blocks osteoclast activity.

Falls are the leading cause of fatal and nonfatal injuries among older adults. Risk factors for falls include increasing age, impaired gait and balance, postural hypotension, loss of strength, medication use, comorbid illnesses, depression, cognitive impairment, environmental hazards, and visual deficits.

Exercise or physical therapy is recommended to prevent falls among at-risk community-dwelling adults ages 65 and older. Personalized decision making regarding *multifactorial fall-prevention interventions* for at-risk community-dwelling adults ages 65 and older is recommended. This needs to be begin with comprehensive assessment of modifiable fall risk factors and then offering appropriate multidisciplinary interventions (Box 15-23). Daily vitamin D supplementation to prevent falls is not advised at present.

Box 15-23. Stopping Elderly Accidents, Deaths, and Injuries (STEADI) Initiative: Key Features for Clinical Practice

- Screen *all* community-dwelling older adults about risk for falls.
  - "Did you fall in the past year?" If *yes*, how many times? "Were you injured?"
  - "Do you feel unsteady when standing or walking?"
  - "Do you worry about falling?"
- Do a gait, strength, and balance assessment with the Timed Get Up and Go test in patients if they say *yes* to any question.
- *Identify high-risk older adults,* namely, those with a gait, strength, or balance problem and at least two falls or at least one fall with an injury.
- In *high-risk older adults,* conduct a multifactorial risk assessment, including:
  - Review of the *Stay Independent* brochure (available at https://www.cdc.gov/steadi/pdf/STEADI-Brochure-StayIndependent-508.pdf)
  - A falls history and medication review
  - Physical examination including assessment of visual acuity, postural dizziness/hypotension, a cognitive screen, inspection of the feet and use of footwear, and use of mobility aids
- Implement individualized interventions, including physical therapy and follow-up in 30 days.

TABLE 15-1. Patterns of Pain in and Around the Joints

Problem	Process	Common Locations	Pattern of Spread	Onset	Progression and Duration
Rheumatoid Arthritis	Chronic inflammation of *synovial membranes* with secondary erosion of adjacent cartilage and bone and damage to ligaments and tendons	Hands—initially small joints (PIP and MCP joints), feet (MTP joints), wrists, knees, elbows, ankles	Symmetrically additive: progresses to other joints while persisting in initial joints	Usually insidious; human leukocyte antigen (HLA) and non-HLA genes account for >50% of risk of disease; involves proinflammatory cytokines	Often chronic (in >50%), with remissions and exacerbations
Osteoarthritis *(Degenerative Joint Disease)*	Degeneration and progressive loss of joint *cartilage* from mechanical stress, with damage to underlying bone and formation of new bone at the cartilage margins	Knees, hips, hands (distal, sometimes PIP joints), cervical and lumbar spine, and wrists (first carpometacarpal joint); also joints previously injured or diseased	Additive; however, may involve only one joint.	Usually insidious; genetics may account for >50% of risk of disease; repetitive injury and obesity increase risk; surgical intervention is also a risk factor	Slowly progressive with temporary exacerbations after periods of overuse
Gouty Arthritis					
Acute Gout	An inflammatory reaction to microcrystals of monosodium urate	Base of the big toe (the first MTP joint), the instep or dorsa of feet, the ankles, knees, and elbows	Early attacks usually confined to one joint	Sudden; often at night; often after injury, surgery, fasting, or excessive food or alcohol intake	Occasional isolated attacks lasting days up to 2 wks; they may get more frequent and severe, with persisting symptoms
Chronic Tophaceous Gout	Multiple local accumulations of sodium urate in the joints and other tissues (*tophi*), with or without inflammation	Feet, ankles, wrists, fingers, and elbows	Additive, not as symmetric as RA	Gradual development of chronicity with repeated attacks	Chronic symptoms with acute exacerbations
Polymyalgia Rheumatica	A disease of unclear etiology in people older than age 50 yrs, especially women; overlaps with giant cell arteritis	Muscles of the hip, shoulder girdle, and neck; symmetric		Insidious or abrupt, even appearing overnight	Chronic but ultimately self-limiting
Fibromyalgia Syndrome	Widespread musculoskeletal pain and tender points. Central pain sensitivity syndrome that may involve aberrant pain signaling and amplification	Multiple specific and symmetric "tender points," often unrecognized until examined; especially in the neck, shoulders, hands, low back, and knees	Shifts unpredictably or worsens in response to immobility, excessive use, or exposure to cold	Variable	Chronic, with "ups and downs"

Associated Symptoms				
Swelling	**Redness, Warmth, and Tenderness**	**Stiffness**	**Limitation of Motion**	**Generalized Symptoms**
Frequent swelling of synovial tissue in joints or tendon sheaths; also subcutaneous nodules	Tender, often warm, but seldom red	Prominent, often for an hour or more in the mornings, also after inactivity	Often develops; affected by associated joint contractures and subluxation, bursitis, and tendinopathy	Weakness, fatigue, weight loss, and low-grade fever are common
Small joint effusions may be present, especially in the knees; also bony enlargement	Possibly tender, seldom warm, and rarely red. Inflammation may accompany disease flares and progression	Frequent but brief (usually 5–10 min), in the morning and after inactivity	Often develops	Usually absent
Present, within and around the involved joint, usually in men (have higher serum urate levels); often polyarticular later in course	Exquisitely tender, hot, and red	Not evident	Motion is limited primarily by pain	Fever may be present; also consider also septic arthritis
Present as tophi in joints, bursae, and subcutaneous tissues; check ears and extensor surfaces for tophi	Tenderness, warmth, and redness may be present during exacerbations	Present	Present	Possibly fever; patients may also develop renal failure and renal stones
Swelling and edema may be present over dorsum of hands, wrists, feet	Muscles often tender, but not warm or red	Prominent, especially in the morning	Pain restricts movement, especially in shoulders	Malaise, depression, anorexia, weight loss, and fever, but no true weakness
None	Multiple specific and symmetric tender "trigger points," often not recognized until the examination	Present, especially in the morning—often confused with inflammatory conditions	Absent, though stiffness is greater at the extremes of movement	Sleep disturbance, usually with fatigue on awakening; overlaps with depression and other pain syndromes

TABLE 15-2. Systemic Manifestations of Musculoskeletal Disorders

Musculoskeletal Disorder	Associated Systemic Manifestation
Systemic lupus erythematosus	Butterfly (malar) rash on the cheeks
Psoriatic arthritis	Scaly plaques, especially on extensor surfaces, and pitted nails
Dermatomyositis	Heliotrope rash on the upper eyelid
Gonococcal arthritis	Papules, pustules, or vesicles with reddened bases on the distal extremities
Lyme disease (erythema chronicum migrans)	Expanding erythematous "target" or "bull's eye" patch early in an illness
Sarcoidosis, Behçet disease (erythema nodosum)	Painful subcutaneous nodules especially in pretibial area
Vasculitis	Palpable purpura
Serum sickness, drug reaction	Hives
Reactive arthritis (often with urethritis and/or uveitis)	Erosions or scaling on the penis and crusted scaling papules on the soles and palms
Arthritis of rubella	Maculopapular rash
Dermatomyositis, systemic sclerosis	Nailfold capillary changes
Hypertrophic osteoarthropathy	Clubbing of the fingernails (see p. 124)
Reactive arthritis, Behçet syndrome, ankylosing spondylitis	Red, burning, and itchy eyes (conjunctivitis), eye pain and blurred vision (uveitis)
RA, IBD, vasculitis	Scleritis
Acute rheumatic fever or gonococcal arthritis	Preceding sore throat
RA (usually painless); Behçet disease	Oral ulcerations
RA; systemic sclerosis	Pneumonitis; interstitial lung disease
IBD, scleroderma, reactive arthritis from *Salmonella*, *Shigella*, *Yersinia*, *Campylobacter*	Diarrhea, abdominal pain, cramping
Reactive arthritis, gonococcal arthritis	Urethritis
Lyme disease with central nervous system involvement	Mental status change, facial or other weakness, sensory changes, radicular pain

IBD, inflammatory bowel disease; RA, rheumatoid arthritis.

TABLE 15-3. Pains in the Neck

Patterns	Possible Causes	Physical Signs
Mechanical Neck Pain		
Aching pain in the cervical paraspinal muscles and ligaments with associated muscle spasm and stiffness and tightness in the upper back and shoulder, lasting up to 6 wks. No associated radiation, paresthesias, or weakness. Headache may be present.	Mechanism poorly understood, possibly sustained muscle contraction in the setting of weakness and poor biomechanics. Associated with poor posture, stress, poor sleep, poor head position during activities such as computer use, watching television, and driving.	Local muscle tenderness, pain on movement. No neurologic deficits. Possible trigger points in fibromyalgia. Torticollis if prolonged abnormal neck posture and muscle spasm.
Mechanical Neck Pain—Whiplash/Cervical Strain		
Mechanical neck pain with aching paracervical pain and stiffness, often beginning the day after injury. Occipital headache, dizziness, malaise, and fatigue may be present. Chronic whiplash syndrome if symptoms last more than 6 mo (20–40% of injuries).	Musculoligamentous sprain or strain from forced hyperflexion/ hyperextension injury to the neck, as in rear-end collisions.	Localized paracervical tenderness, decreased neck range of motion, perceived weakness of the upper extremities. Causes of cervical cord compression such as fracture, herniation, head injury, or altered consciousness are excluded.
Cervical Radiculopathy—From Nerve Root Compression		
Sharp burning or tingling pain in the neck and one arm, with associated paresthesias and/or weakness that follow a neurologic (dermotomal/ myotomal) pattern.	Dysfunction of cervical spinal nerve, nerve roots, or both from foraminal encroachment of the spinal nerve (~75%) or herniated cervical disc (~25%). Rarely from tumor, syrinx, or multiple sclerosis. Mechanisms may involve hypoxia of the nerve root and dorsal ganglion and release of inflammatory mediators.	C7 nerve root affected most often (45%–60%), with weakness in triceps and finger flexors and extensors. C6 nerve root involvement also common, with weakness in biceps, brachioradialis, wrist extensors.
Cervical Myelopathy—From Cervical Cord Compression		
Neck pain with bilateral weakness and paresthesias in both upper and lower extremities, often with urinary frequency. Hand clumsiness, palmar paresthesias, and gait changes may be subtle. Neck flexion often exacerbates symptoms.	Usually from cervical spondylosis, defined as cervical degenerative disc disease from spurs, degenerative thickening of the ligamentum flavum, and/or disc herniation; also from cervical stenosis from osteophytes, ossification of ligamentum flavum, and RA. Large central or paracentral disc herniation may also compress cord.	Hyperreflexia; clonus at the wrist, knee, or ankle; extensor plantar reflexes (positive Babinski signs); positive Hoffman sign; and gait disturbances. May also see *Lhermitte sign:* neck flexion with resulting sensation of electrical shock radiating down the spine. Confirmation of cervical myelopathy warrants urgent neck immobilization and neurosurgical evaluation.

TABLE 15-4. Low Back Pain

Patterns	Possible Causes	Physical Signs
Mechanical Low Back Pain		
Aching pain in the lumbosacral area; may radiate into the buttock or posterior thigh. Signifies anatomic or functional abnormality in absence of neoplastic, infectious, or inflammatory disease. Usually acute (<3 mo), idiopathic, benign, and self-limiting. Represents 97% of symptomatic low back pain. Commonly work related and occurring in patients 30–50 yrs. Risk factors include heavy lifting, poor conditioning and obesity.	Often arises from muscle and ligament injuries (~70%) in the setting of underlying weakness and poor biomechanics. Can be age-related intervertebral disc or facet disease (~4%). Causes also include herniated disc (~4%), spinal stenosis (~3%), compression fractures (~4%), and spondylolisthesis (2%).	Paraspinal muscle or facet tenderness, pain with back movement, loss of normal lumbar lordosis. Motor, sensory, and reflex findings are normal. In osteoporosis, check for thoracic kyphosis, percussion tenderness over a spinous process, or fractures in the thoracic spine or hip.
Sciatica (Radicular Low Back Pain)		
Shooting pain often below the knee, commonly into the lateral leg (L5) or posterior calf (S1). Typically accompanies low back pain, often with associated paresthesias and weakness. Bending, sneezing, coughing, straining during bowel movements can worsen the pain. When the sciatic nerve is irritated by the piriformis muscle, it is termed *piriformis syndrome.*	Sciatic pain is sensitive, ~95%, and specific, ~88%, for disc herniation. Usually from herniated intervertebral disc with compression or traction of nerve root(s) in people ages 50 yrs or older. L5 and S1 roots are involved in ~95% of disc herniations; root or spinal cord compression from neoplastic conditions in fewer than 1% of cases. Tumor or midline disc herniation may cause bowel or bladder dysfunction with leg weakness called *cauda equina syndrome* (S2–S4) because it compresses the cauda equina.	Calf wasting, weak ankle dorsiflexion, absent ankle jerk, positive crossed straight-leg raise (pain in affected leg when healthy leg tested). May see decreased or increased reflexes depending on the level of herniation, but most commonly decreased. Negative straight-leg raise makes diagnosis unlikely. Ipsilateral straight-leg raise sensitive, about 65%–98%, but not specific, about 10%–60%. In piriformis syndrome the hallmark is marked tenderness over the piriformis in the buttock as the sciatic nerve crosses near or through it. Symptoms may be reproduced with *FAIR* or sometimes *FADIR* test (***F**lexion, **AD**duction, **I**nternal **R**otation)*

(continued)

TABLE 15-4. Low Back Pain *(Continued)*

Patterns	Possible Causes	Physical Signs
Lumbar Spinal Stenosis		
Neurogenic claudication with gluteal and/or lower extremity pain and/or fatigue that may occur with or without back pain. Pain is provoked by lumbar extension (as in walking uphill) due to reduced space in the lumbar spine from degenerative changes in the spinal canal. Positive LR is >6.0 if pain is absent when seated, improved with bending forward, or present in both buttocks and legs. Positive LR is <4.0 if gait is wide-based and Romberg test is abnormal.	Arises from hypertrophic degenerative disease of one or more vertebral facets and thickening of the ligamentum flavum, causing narrowing of the spinal canal centrally or in lateral recesses. More common after age 60 yrs.	Posture may be flexed forward to reduce symptoms, with lower extremity weakness and hyporeflexia. Thigh pain typically occurs after 30 sec of lumbar extension. Straight-leg raise is usually negative.
Chronic Back Stiffness	Ankylosing spondylitis, an inflammatory polyarthritis, most common in men younger than 40 yrs. Diffuse idiopathic hyperostosis (*DISH*) affects men more than women, usually age ≥50 yrs. OA is also possible.	Findings depend on the underlying etiology. Decreased range of motion in the spine (flexion, extension, rotation).
Nocturnal Back Pain, Unrelieved by Rest	Consider metastatic malignancy to the spine from cancer of the prostate, breast, lung, thyroid, and kidney, and multiple myeloma.	Loss of the normal lumbar lordosis, muscle spasm, limited anterior and lateral flexion. Lateral immobility of the spine, especially in thoracic area improves with exercise. Pain with percussion over the spine.
Pain Referred from the Abdomen or Pelvis		
Usually a deep, aching pain; the level varies with the source. Accounts for ~2% of low back pain.	Peptic ulcer, pancreatitis, pancreatic cancer, chronic prostatitis, endometriosis, dissecting aortic aneurysm, retroperitoneal tumor, and other causes.	Variable with the source. Local vertebral tenderness may be present. Spinal movements are not painful, and range of motion is not affected. Look for signs of the primary disorder.

TABLE 15-5. Painful Shoulders

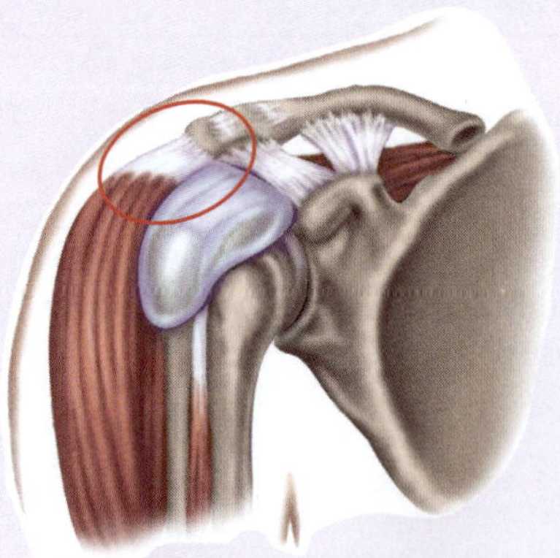

Rotator Cuff Tendinitis (Impingement Syndrome)

Repeated shoulder motion, for example, from throwing or swimming, can cause edema and hemorrhage followed by inflammation, most commonly involving the supraspinatus tendon. Acute, recurrent, or chronic pain may result, often aggravated by activity. Patients report sharp catches of pain, grating, and weakness when lifting the arm overhead. When the supraspinatus tendon is involved, *tenderness is maximal just below the tip of the acromion*. In older adults, bone spurs on the undersurface of the acromion may contribute to symptoms.

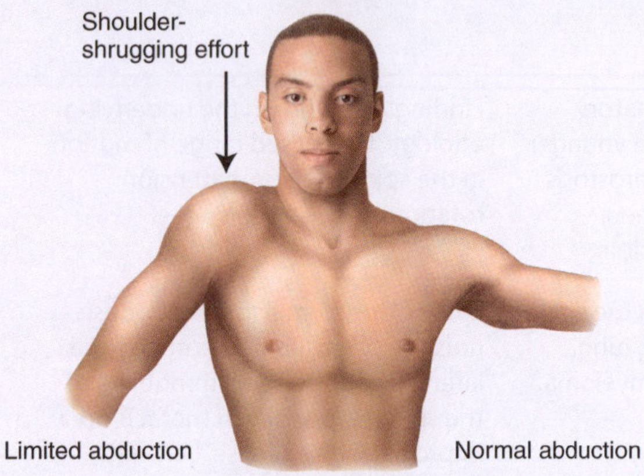

Rotator Cuff Tears

The rotator cuff muscles and tendons compress the humeral head into the concave glenoid fossa and strengthen arm movement—the subscapularis in internal rotation, the supraspinatus in elevation, and the infraspinatus and teres minor in external rotation. Injury from a fall, trauma, or repeated impingement against the acromion and the coracoacromial ligament may cause a partial- or full-thickness tear of tendons in the rotator cuff, especially in older patients. Patients complain of chronic shoulder pain, night pain, or catching and grating when raising the arm overhead. Weakness or tears of the tendons usually start in the supraspinatus tendon and progress posteriorly and anteriorly. Look for atrophy of the deltoid, supraspinatus, or infraspinatus muscles related to disuse from pain or retraction in the setting of a complete tear. Palpate anteriorly over the anterior greater tuberosity of the humerus to check for a defect in muscle attachment and below the acromion for crepitus during arm rotation. In a complete tear, active abduction and forward flexion at the glenohumeral joint are severely impaired, producing a characteristic shrug of the shoulder when trying to raise the arm and a positive "drop arm" test when trying to lower the arm (see p. 428).

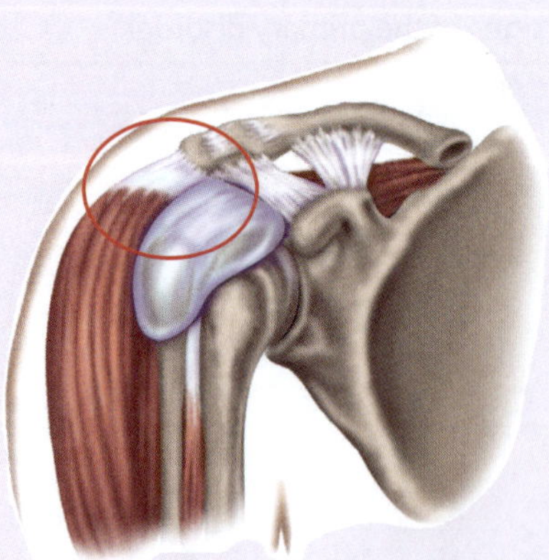

Calcific Tendinitis

Calcific tendinitis is a degenerative process in the tendon associated chronic tendon injury with improper healing that leads to the deposition of calcium salts. The supraspinatus tendon is usually involved. Acute disabling attacks of shoulder pain may occur, usually in patients ages ≥30 yrs, especially in women. The arm is held close to the side, and all motions are severely limited by pain. Tenderness is maximal below the tip of the acromion when the supraspinatus is involved. The subacromial/ subdeltoid bursa, which overlies the supraspinatus tendon, may also be inflamed. Chronic less severe pain may also occur.

(continued)

TABLE 15-5. Painful Shoulders *(Continued)*

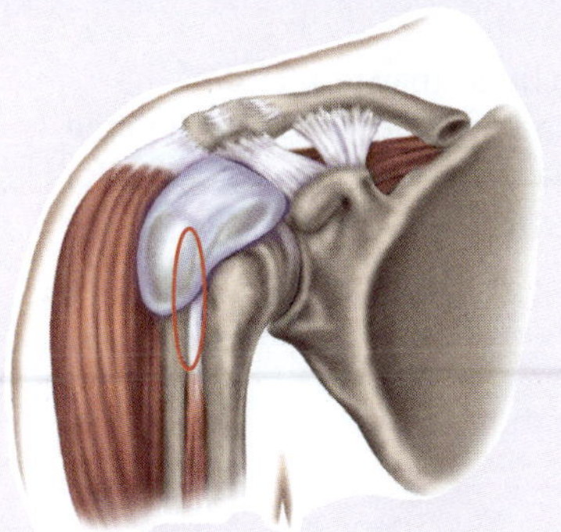

Bicipital Tendinitis
Inflammation of the long head of the biceps tendon and tendon sheath causes anterior shoulder pain resembling and often coexisting with rotator cuff tendinitis. Both conditions may involve impingement injury. Tenderness is maximal in the bicipital groove. Externally rotate and abduct the arm to separate this area from the subacromial tenderness of supraspinatus tendinitis. With the patient's arm at the side, elbow flexed to 90°, ask the patient to supinate the forearm against your resistance. Increased pain in the bicipital groove confirms this condition. Pain during resisted forward flexion of the shoulder with the elbow extended ("Speed's test") is also characteristic.

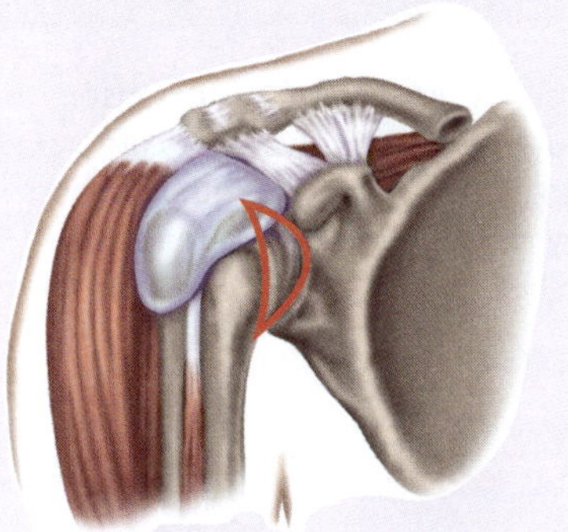

Adhesive Capsulitis (Frozen Shoulder)
Adhesive capsulitis refers to fibrosis of the glenohumeral joint capsule, manifested by diffuse, dull, aching pain in the shoulder and progressive restriction of active and passive range of motion, especially in external rotation, with localized tenderness. The condition is usually unilateral and occurs in people ages 40–60 yrs. There is often an antecedent disorder of the shoulder or another condition (such as myocardial infarction) that has decreased shoulder movements. The disorder may take 6 mo to 2 yrs to resolve. Stretching exercises and steroid injection may help.

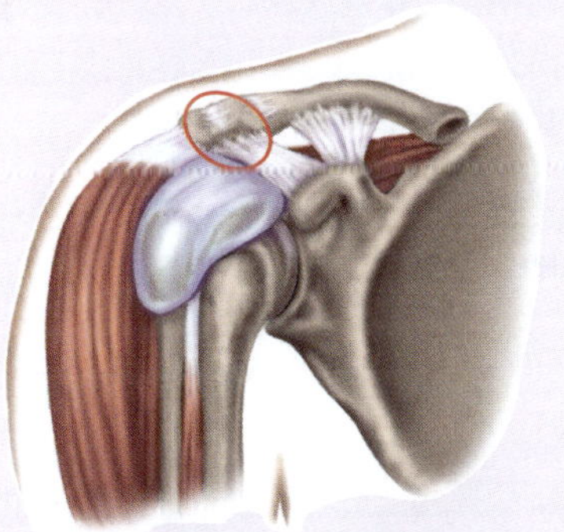

Acromioclavicular Arthritis
Acromioclavicular arthritis is relatively common, usually arising from prior direct injury to the shoulder girdle with resulting degenerative changes. Tenderness is localized over the acromioclavicular joint. Patients report pain with movements of the scapula and arm abduction. The cross-arm test may be positive.

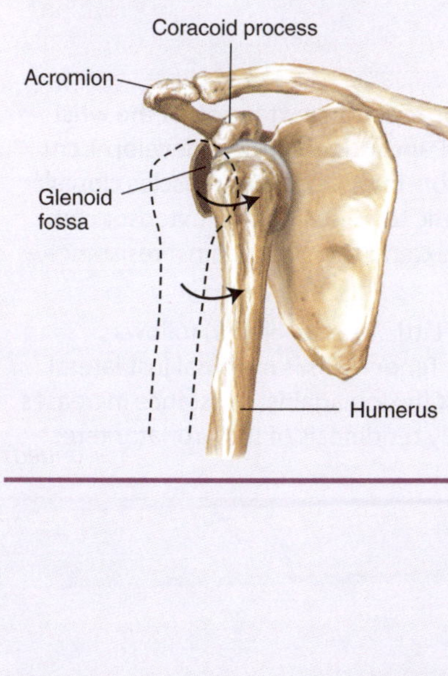

Anterior Dislocation of the Humerus
Shoulder instability from anterior subluxation or dislocation of the humerus usually results from a fall or forceful throwing motion. Recurrent episodes can become common unless treated or the precipitating motion avoided. The shoulder seems to "slip out of the joint" when the arm is abducted and externally rotated, causing a positive apprehension test for anterior instability when the examiner places the arm in this position. Any shoulder movement may cause pain, and patients hold the arm in a neutral position. The rounded lateral aspect of the shoulder appears flattened. Dislocations may also be inferior, posterior (relatively rare), and multidirectional.

TABLE 15-6. Swollen or Tender Elbows

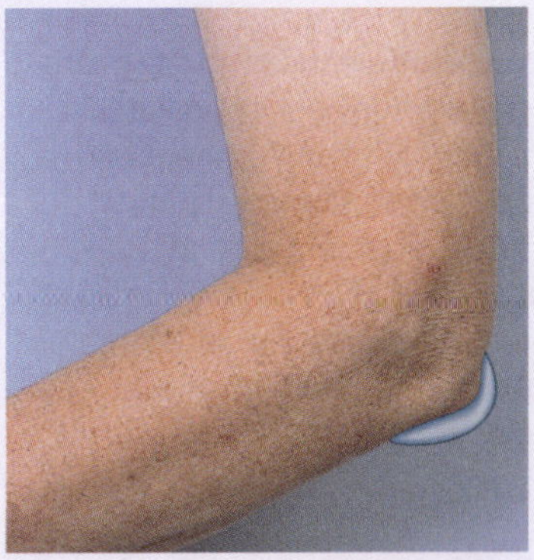

Olecranon Bursitis

Swelling and inflammation of the olecranon bursa may result from trauma, gout, or rheumatoid arthritis (RA). The swelling is superficial to the olecranon process and may reach 6 cm in diameter. Consider aspiration for both diagnosis and symptomatic relief.

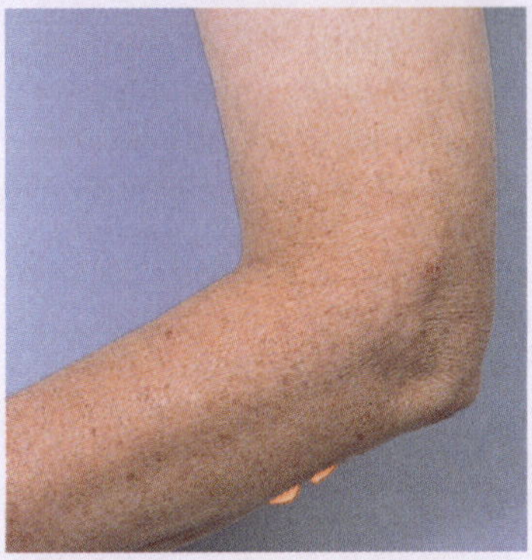

Rheumatoid Nodules

Subcutaneous nodules may develop at pressure points along the extensor surface of the ulna in patients with RA or acute rheumatic fever. They are firm and nontender. They are not attached to the overlying skin but may be attached to the underlying periosteum. They can develop in the area of the olecranon bursa, but often occur more distally.

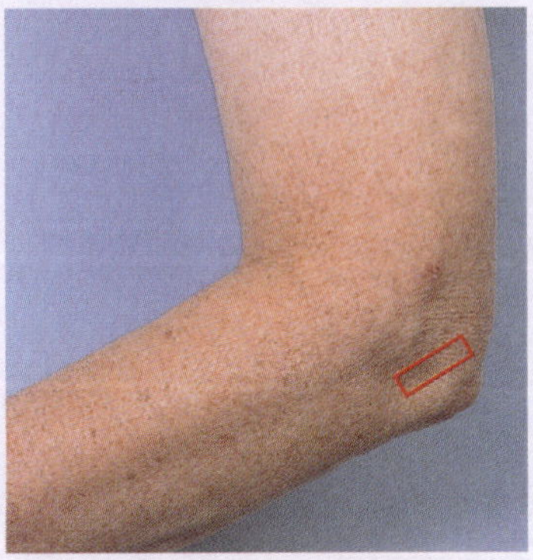

Arthritis of the Elbow

Synovial inflammation or fluid is felt best in the grooves between the olecranon process and the epicondyles on either side. Palpate for a boggy, soft, or fluctuant swelling and for tenderness. Causes include RA, gout and pseudogout, osteoarthritis, and trauma. Patients report pain, stiffness, and restricted motion.

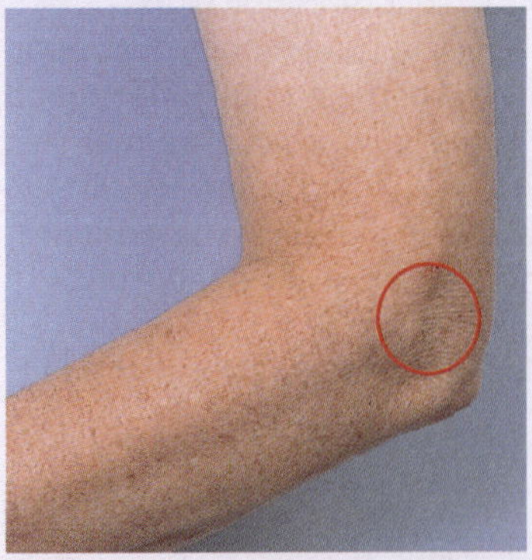

Epicondylitis

Lateral epicondylitis (tennis elbow) follows repetitive extension of the wrist or pronation–supination of the forearm. Pain and tenderness develop 1 cm distal to the lateral epicondyle and possibly in the extensor muscles close to it. The pain is most often caused by chronic tendinosis of the extensor carpi radialis brevis. When the patient tries to extend the wrist against resistance, pain increases.

Medial epicondylitis (pitcher's, golfer's, or Little League elbow) follows repetitive wrist flexion such as throwing. Tenderness is maximal just lateral and distal to the medial epicondyle. Wrist flexion against resistance increases the pain. The pain is most often caused by tendinosis of the pronator teres or flexor carpi radialis.

TABLE 15-7. Arthritis in the Hands

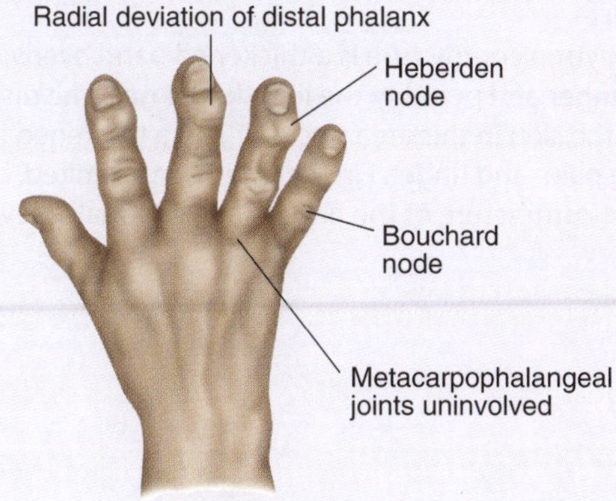

Osteoarthritis (Degenerative Joint Disease)
Heberden nodes on the dorsolateral aspects of the distal interphalangeal (DIP) joints from bony overgrowth of osteoarthritis (OA). Usually hard and painless, they affect middle-aged or older adults and are often associated with arthritic changes in other joints. Flexion and deviation deformities may develop. *Bouchard nodes* on the proximal interphalangeal (PIP) joints are less common. The metacarpophalangeal (MCP) joints are generally spared.

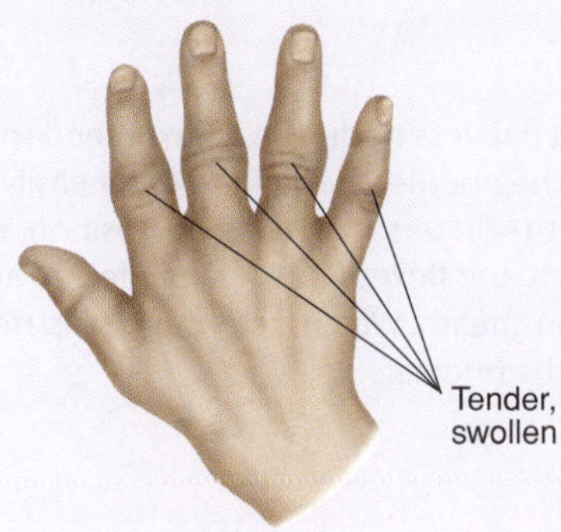

Acute Rheumatoid Arthritis
Tender, painful, stiff joints in *RA,* usually with symmetric involvement on both sides of the body. The DIP, MCP, and wrist joints are the most frequently affected. Note the fusiform or spindle-shaped swelling of the PIP joints in acute disease.

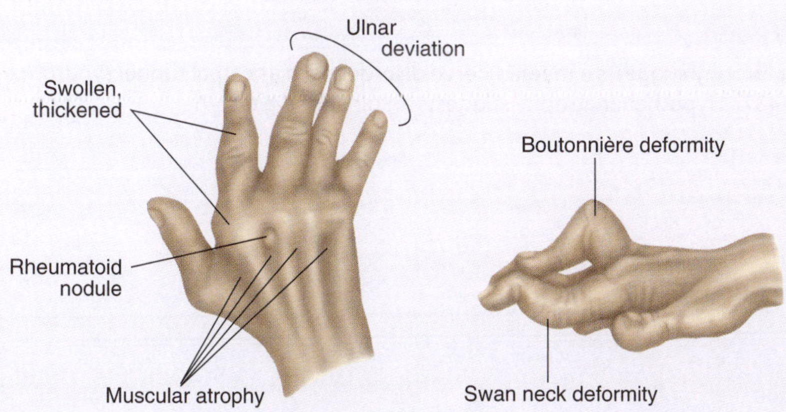

Chronic Rheumatoid Arthritis
In chronic disease, note the swelling and thickening of the MCP and PIP joints. Range of motion becomes limited, and fingers may deviate toward the ulnar side. The interosseous muscles atrophy. The fingers may show *"swan neck" deformities* (hyperextension of the PIP joints with fixed flexion of the DIP joints) related to inflammatory destruction of the joints and supporting ligaments. Less common is a *boutonnière deformity* (persistent flexion of the PIP joint with hyperextension of the DIP joint). Rheumatoid nodules are seen in the acute or the chronic stage.

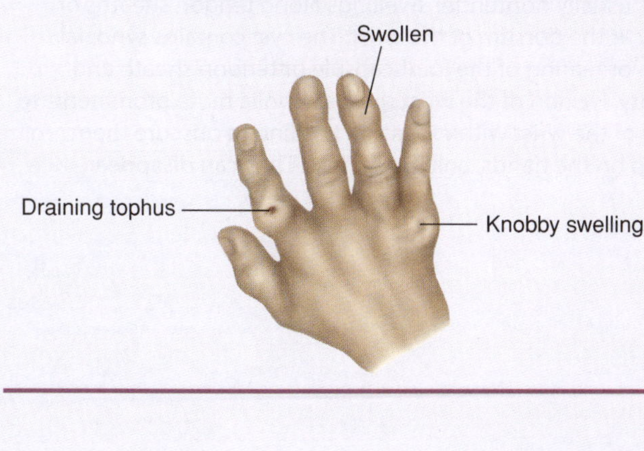

Chronic Tophaceous Gout
Urate crystal deposits, often with surrounding inflammation, cause deformities in subcutaneous tissues, bursae, cartilage, and subchondral bone that mimic rheumatoid arthritis (RA) and OA. Joint involvement is usually less symmetric than in RA. Acute inflammation may be present. Knobby swellings around the joints ulcerate and discharge white chalk-like urates.

TABLE 15-8. Swellings and Deformities of the Hands

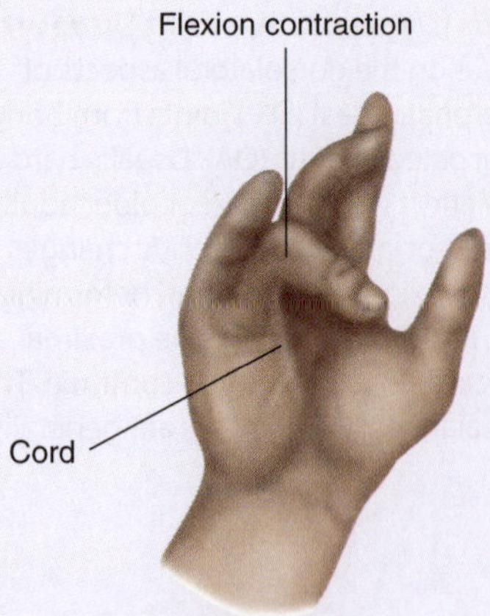

Dupuytren Contracture

The first sign of a Dupuytren contracture is a thickened band overlying the flexor tendon of the fourth finger and possibly the little finger near the distal palmar crease. Subsequently, the skin in this area puckers, and a thickened fibrotic cord develops between the palm and finger. Finger extension is limited, but flexion is usually normal. Flexion contracture of the fingers may gradually develop.

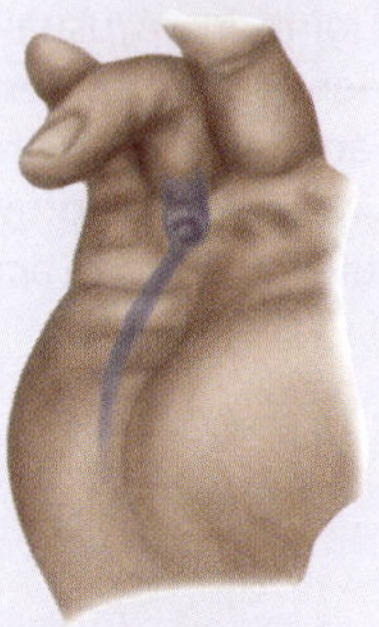

Trigger Finger

Trigger finger is caused by a painless nodule in a flexor tendon in the palm, near the metacarpal head. The nodule is too big to enter easily into the tendon sheath during extension of the fingers from a flexed position. With extra effort or assistance, the finger extends and flexes with a palpable and audible snap as the nodule pops into the tendon sheath. Watch, listen, and palpate the nodule as the patient flexes and extends the fingers.

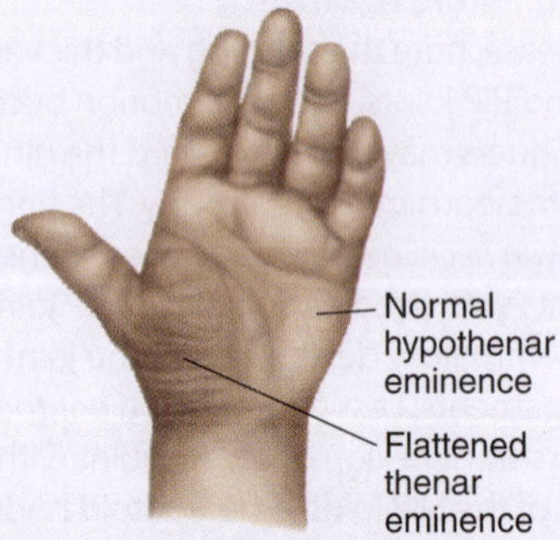

Thenar Atrophy

Thenar atrophy suggests a median nerve disorder such as carpal tunnel syndrome (see p. 437). Hypothenar atrophy suggests an ulnar nerve disorder.

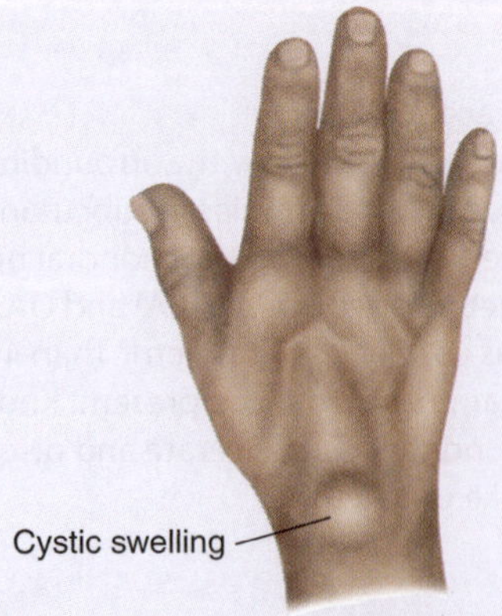

Ganglion

Ganglia are cystic, round, usually nontender swellings along tendon sheaths or joint capsules, frequently at the dorsum of the wrist. The cyst contains synovial fluid arising from erosion or tearing of the joint capsule or tendon sheath and trapped in the cystic cavity. Flexion of the wrist makes ganglia more prominent if present on the dorsum of the wrist with extension tending to obscure them. Ganglia may also develop on the hands, ankles and feet. They can disappear spontaneously.

TABLE 15-9. Tendon Sheath, Palmar Space, and Finger Infections

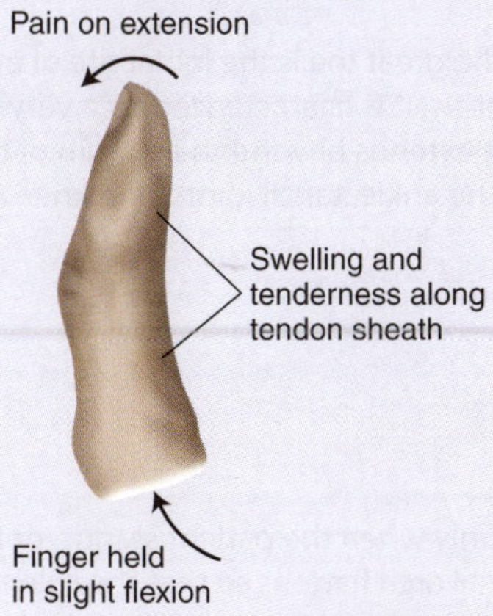

Acute Tenosynovitis

Inflammation of the flexor tendon sheaths, acute tenosynovitis, may follow local injury, overuse, or infection. Unlike arthritis, tenderness and swelling develop not in the joint but along the course of the tendon sheath. In the fingers, this often occurs from the distal phalanx to the level of the metacarpophalangeal joint. The finger is held in slight flexion since finger extension is very painful. Tenosynovitis can result from inflammation related to injury or irritation of the sheath or from infection. Causative infectious agents include *Staphylococcus* and *Streptococcus species,* disseminated gonorrhea, and *Candida albicans.*

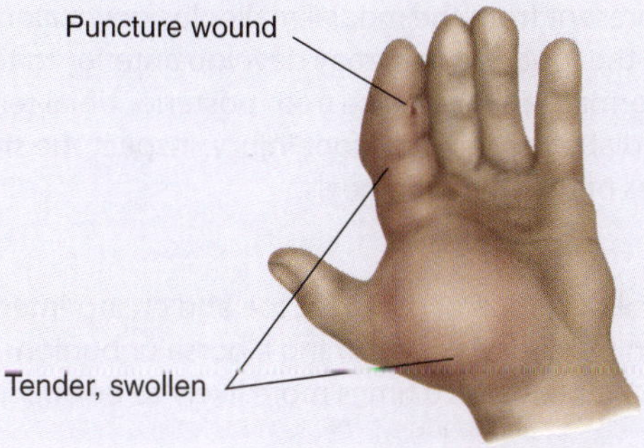

Acute Tenosynovitis and Thenar Space Involvement

Infectious tenosynovitis of the fingers may extend from the tendon sheath into the adjacent fascial spaces within the palm. Infections of the index finger and thenar space are illustrated. Early diagnosis and treatment are important.

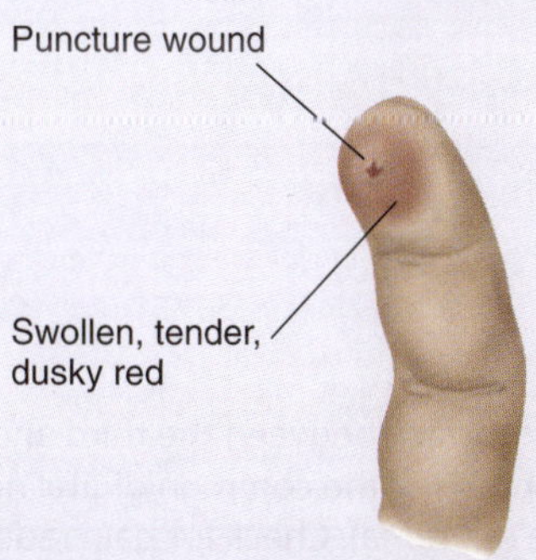

Felon

Injury to the fingertip may result in infection of the enclosed fascial spaces of the distal pulp or phalanx pad of the fingertip, usually from *Staphylococcus aureus.* Severe pain, localized tenderness, swelling, and dusky redness are characteristics. Early diagnosis and treatment, usually incision and drainage, are important for preventing abscess formation. If vesicles are present, consider herpetic whitlow instead, usually seen in health care workers exposed to herpes simplex virus in human saliva (rare when universal precautions are used).

TABLE 15-10. Abnormalities of the Feet

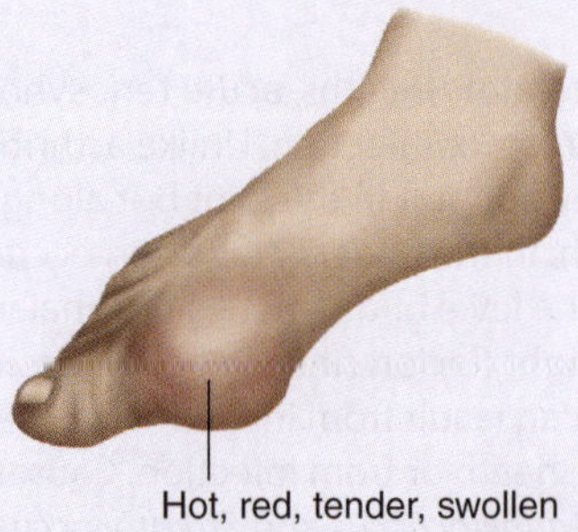

Acute Gouty Arthritis

The metatarsophalangeal joint of the great toe is the initial site of attack in 50% of the episodes of acute gouty arthritis. It is characterized by a very painful and tender, hot, dusky red swelling that extends beyond the margin of the joint. It is easily mistaken for a cellulitis. The ankle, tarsal joints, and knee are also commonly involved.

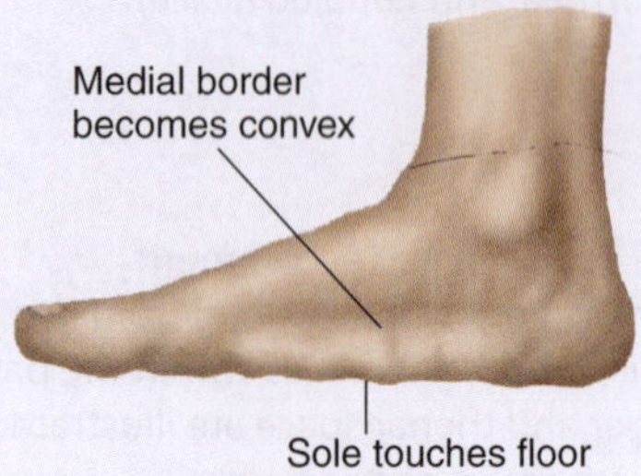

Flat Feet

Signs of flat feet may be apparent only when the patient stands, or they may become permanent. The longitudinal arch flattens so that the sole approaches or touches the floor. The normal concavity on the medial side of the foot becomes convex. Tenderness may be present from the medial malleolus down along the medial plantar surface of the foot. Swelling may develop anterior to the malleoli. Flat feet may be a normal variant or arise from posterior tibial tendon dysfunction, seen in obesity, diabetes, and prior foot injury. Inspect the shoes for excess wear on the inner sides of the soles and heels.

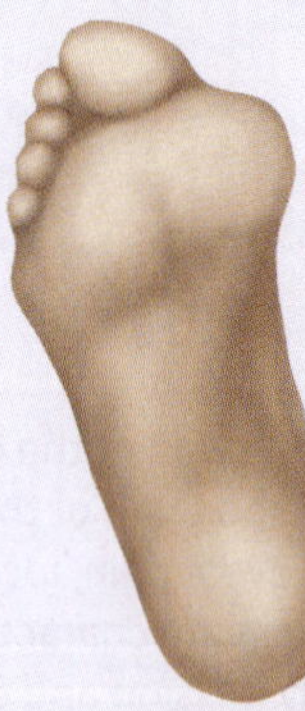

Hallux Valgus

In hallux valgus, there is lateral deviation of the great toe and enlargement of the head of the first metatarsal on its medial side, forming a bursa or bunion. This bursa may become inflamed. Women are 10 times more likely to be affected than men.

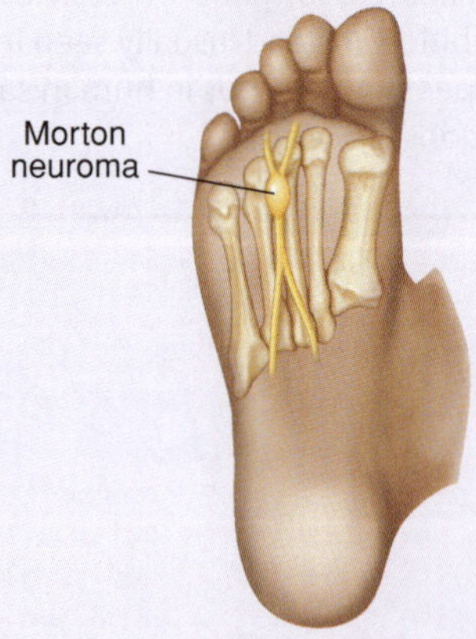

Morton Neuroma

Look for tenderness over the plantar surface between the third and fourth metatarsal heads, from perineural fibrosis of the common digital nerve due to repetitive nerve irritation (not a true neuroma). Check for pain radiating to the toes when you press on the plantar interspace and squeeze the metatarsals with your other hand. Symptoms include hyperesthesia, numbness, aching, and burning from the metatarsal heads into the third and fourth toes.

TABLE 15-11. Abnormalities of the Toes and Soles

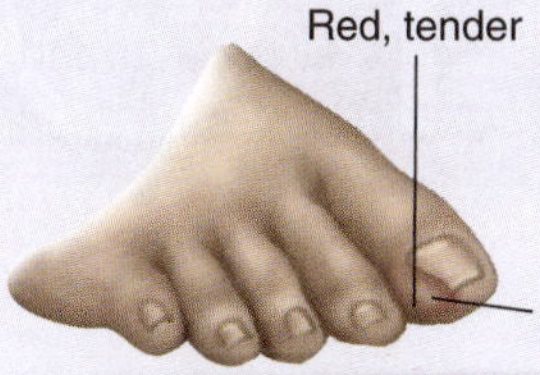

Ingrown Toenail
The sharp edge of a toenail may dig into and injure the lateral nail fold, resulting in inflammation and infection. A tender, reddened, overhanging nail fold, sometimes with granulation tissue and purulent discharge, results. The great toe is most often affected.

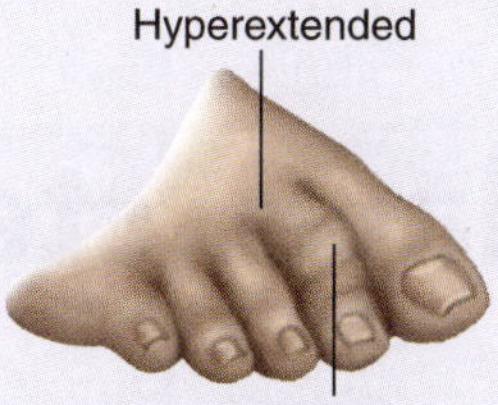

Hammer Toe
Usually involving the second toe, a hammer toe is characterized by hyperextension at the metatarsophalangeal joint with flexion at the proximal interphalangeal (PIP) joint. A corn frequently develops at the pressure point over the PIP joint.

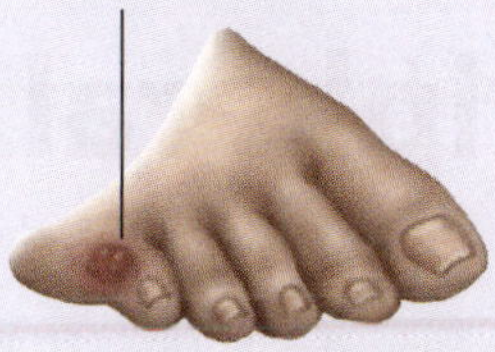

Corn
A corn is a painful conical thickening of skin that results from recurrent pressure on normally thin skin. The apex of the cone points inward and causes pain. Corns characteristically occur over bony prominences such as the fifth toe. When located in moist areas such as pressure points between the fourth and fifth toes, they are called *soft corns.*

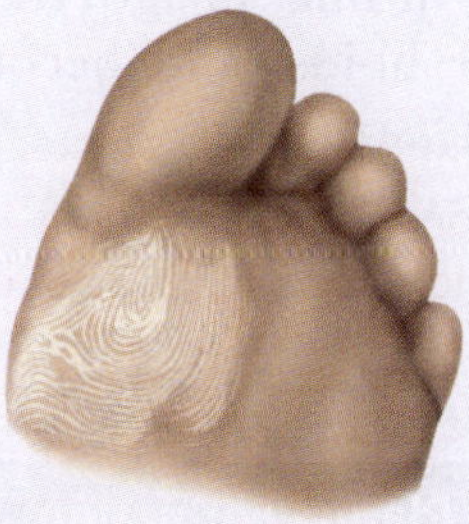

Callus
Like a corn, a callus is an area of greatly thickened skin that develops in a region of recurrent pressure. Unlike a corn, a callus involves skin that is normally thick, such as the sole, and is usually painless. If a callus is painful, suspect an underlying plantar wart.

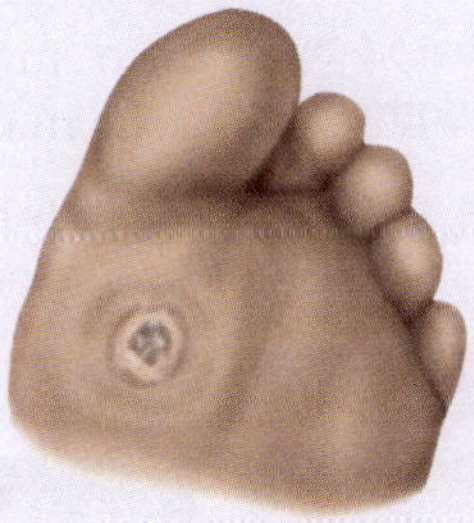

Plantar Wart
A plantar wart is a hyperkeratotic lesion caused by human papillomavirus, located on the sole of the foot. It may look like a callus. Look for the characteristic small dark spots that give a stippled appearance to a wart. Normal skin lines stop at the wart's edge. It is tender if pinched side to side, whereas a callus is tender to direct pressure.

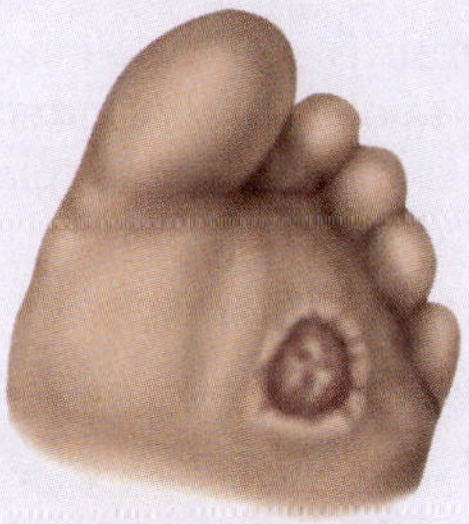

Neuropathic Ulcer
When pain sensation is diminished or absent, as in diabetic neuropathy, neuropathic ulcers may develop at pressure points on the feet. Although often deep, infected, and indolent, they are painless because of the sensory disruption that often leads to their formation. Underlying osteomyelitis and amputation may ensue. Early detection of loss of sensation using a nylon filament is the standard of care in diabetes.

CHAPTER

16

Peripheral Vascular System

ANATOMY AND PHYSIOLOGY

Arterial System

Arteries contain three concentric layers of tissue: the *intima*, the *media*, and the *adventitia* (Figs. 16-1 and 16-2). The internal elastic membrane borders the intima and the media; the external elastic membrane separates the media from the adventitia.

Atherosclerosis is a chronic inflammatory disease initiated by injury (i.e., smoking or hypertension) to vascular endothelial cells, provoking atheromatous plaque formation.

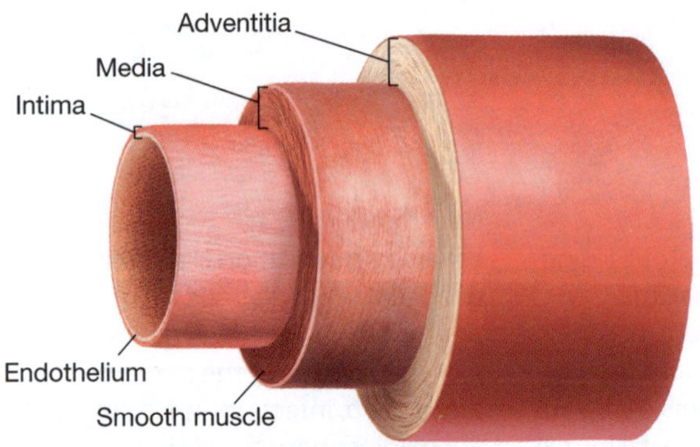

FIGURE 16-1. Anatomy of arteries.

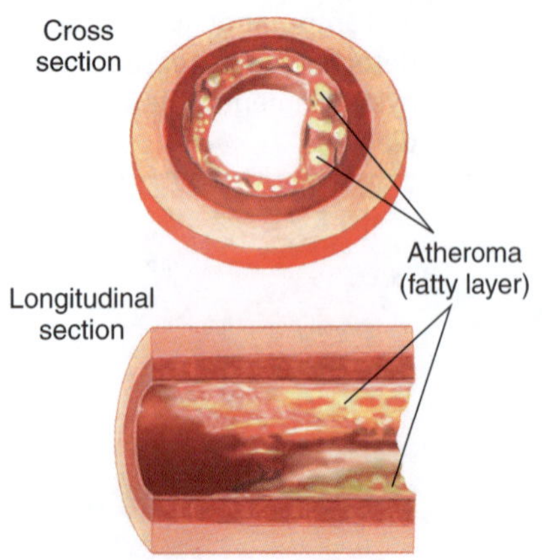

FIGURE 16-2. Atherosclerotic plaque.

Intima. The innermost layer of all blood vessels is the intima, a single continuous lining of endothelial cells with remarkable metabolic properties. Atherosclerotic plaque formation begins in the intima, where circulating cholesterol particles, especially low-density lipoproteins (LDLs), are exposed to proteoglycans from the extracellular matrix, undergo oxidative modification, and trigger a local inflammatory response that attracts mononuclear phagocytes (Box 16-1). Once in the intima, phagocytes mature into macrophages, ingest lipids, and become *foam cells* that develop into fatty streaks.

There is increasing emphasis on plaque activation, in addition to luminal stenosis, as a major precipitant of ischemia and infarction.

Box 16-1. Atherosclerotic Plaque Formation

- In atherosclerotic plaques, there is a proliferation of smooth muscle cells and extracellular matrix that breaches the endothelial lining.
- Atherosclerotic plaques contain a fibrous cap of smooth muscle cells that overlies a necrotic lipid-rich core, vascular cells, and a wide range of immune cells and prothrombotic molecules.
- Inflammatory mediators that alter collagen repair and cap fibrosis are increasingly implicated in plaque rupture and plaque erosion, which expose thrombogenic factors in the plaque core to coagulation factors in the blood, resulting in overlying thrombus formation.
- If in the coronary arteries, these thrombi can result in acute myocardial infarction. If in the carotid arteries, the thrombi can dislodge and travel to the brain, resulting in stroke.

Media. The media is composed of smooth muscle cells with elastic properties to accommodate blood pressure and flow. Its inner and outer boundaries consist of elastic fibers, or elastin, and are called *internal* and *external elastic laminae*, or membranes. The media receives its blood supply from small blood vessels called the *vasa vasorum*.

Adventitia. The outer layer of the artery is the adventitia, the connective tissue containing nerve fibers and the vasa vasorum.

Arterial Branching. Arteries must respond to the variations in cardiac output during systole and diastole. Their anatomy and size vary according to their distance from the heart. The aorta and its immediate branches are large, highly elastic arteries, such as the common carotid and iliac arteries. These arteries course into medium-sized muscular arteries, such as the coronary and renal arteries. The elastic recoil and smooth muscle contraction and relaxation in the media of large- and medium-sized arteries contribute to the propagation of blood flow and arterial pulsatile flow. Medium-sized arteries divide into small arteries less than 2 mm in diameter and even smaller arterioles with diameters from 20 to 100 μm (sometimes termed "microns"). *Arterioles* are known as the "resistance vessels," as their smooth muscle tone is a principal determinant of *systemic vascular resistance*, a major component of blood pressure. From the arterioles, blood flows into the vast network of *capillaries*, each the diameter of a single red blood cell, only 7 to 8 μm across. Capillaries have an endothelial cell lining, but no media, facilitating rapid diffusion of oxygen and carbon dioxide.

If an artery is obstructed, anastomoses between branching networks of smaller arteries can increase in size over time to form collateral circulation that perfuses structures distal to the occlusion.

Arterial Pulses. Arterial pulses are palpable in arteries lying close to the body surface.

Pulses in the Arms and Hands. In the arms, locate pulsations in the arteries shown in Figure 16-3:

- The *brachial artery* at the bend of the elbow just medial to the biceps tendon
- The *radial artery* on the lateral flexor surface
- The *ulnar artery* on the medial flexor surface, although overlying tissues may obscure pulsations in the ulnar artery

Two vascular arches within the hand interconnect the radial and ulnar arteries, doubly protecting circulation to the hand and fingers from arterial occlusion.

Pulses in the Abdomen. In the abdomen, locate the pulsations of the *aorta* in the epigastrium (Fig. 16-4). Not palpable are its three important deeper branches, the celiac trunk and the superior and inferior mesenteric arteries, which perfuse the important organs of the abdominal cavity.

- Celiac trunk: esophagus, stomach, proximal duodenum, liver, gallbladder, pancreas, spleen (foregut)

Despite the rich collateral network that protects the three abdominal branches against hypoperfusion, occlusion of the mesenteric arteries can result in acute mesenteric ischemia, a potentially life-threatening condition.

- Superior mesenteric artery: small intestine—jejunum, ileum, cecum; large intestine—ascending and transverse colon, right splenic flexure (midgut)
- Inferior mesenteric artery: large intestine—descending and sigmoid colon, proximal rectum (hindgut)

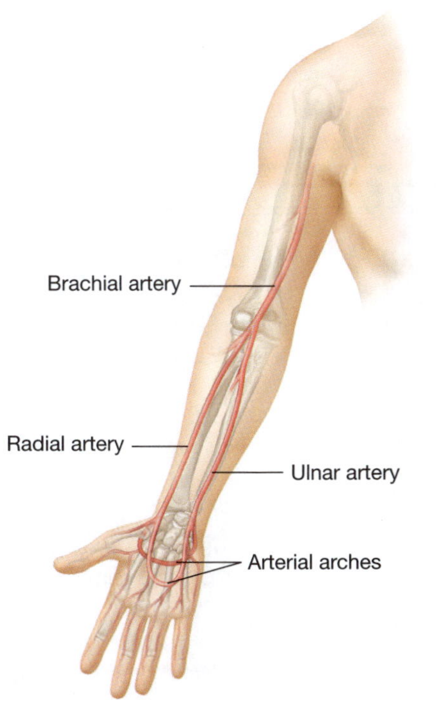

FIGURE 16-3. Arteries of the arm.

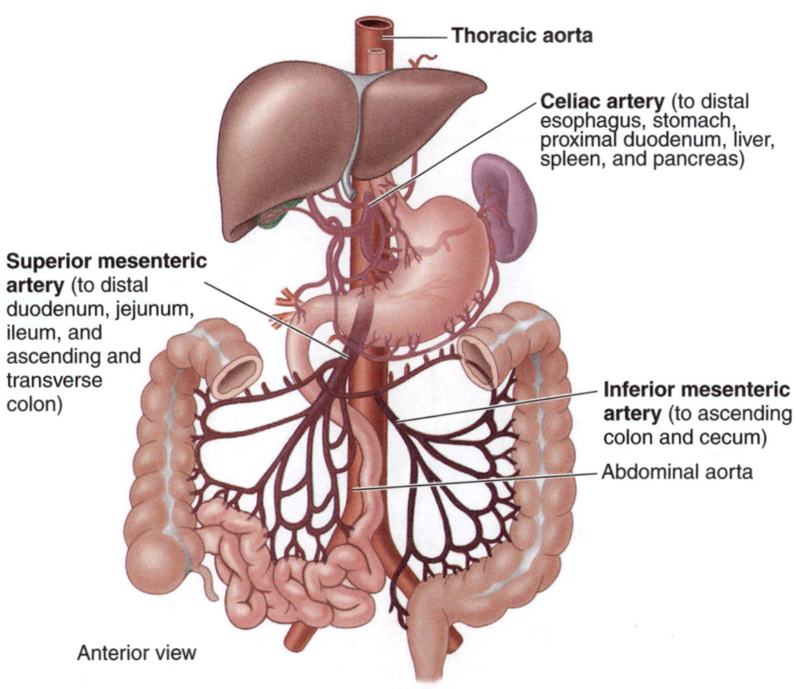

FIGURE 16-4. Abdominal aorta and its branches.

Pulses in the Legs. As shown in Figure 16-5, in the legs, palpate pulsations in:

- The *femoral artery* just below the inguinal ligament, midway between the anterior superior iliac spine and the symphysis pubis
- The *popliteal artery*, an extension of the femoral artery that passes medially behind the femur, palpable just behind but deep in the knee
- The *posterior tibial (PT) artery* that lies behind the medial malleolus of the ankle; an interconnecting arch between its two chief arterial branches protects circulation to the foot
- The *dorsalis pedis (DP)* artery on the dorsum of the foot just lateral to the extensor tendon of the big toe

Venous System

Unlike arteries, veins are thin walled and highly distensible, with a capacity for containing up to two-thirds of circulating blood flow. The venous intima consists of nonthrombogenic endothelium. The peripheral veins contain *unidirectional valves* that promote venous return to the heart. The media contains circumferential rings of elastic tissue and smooth muscle that change vein caliber in response to even minor changes in venous pressure. The smallest veins, or *venules*, drain capillary beds and form interconnecting venous plexuses, such as the prostatic and the rectal venous plexuses.

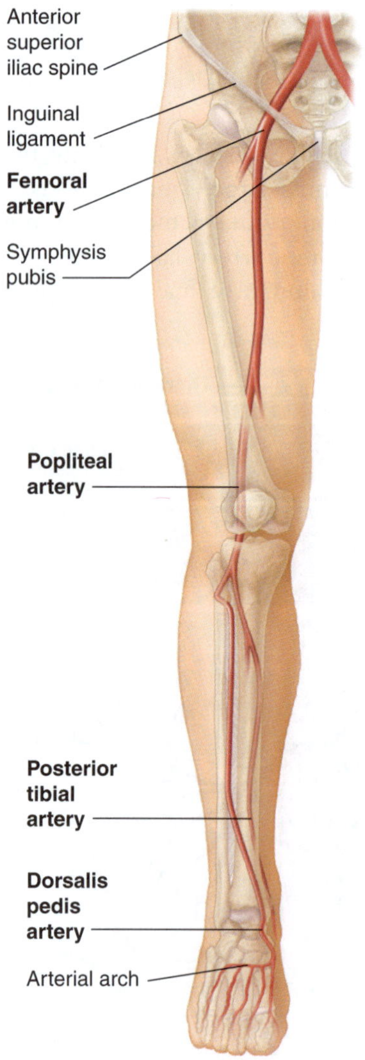

FIGURE 16-5. Arteries of the leg.

Veins from the arms, upper trunk, and head and neck drain into the *superior vena cava*, which empties into the right atrium. Veins from the abdominal wall, liver, lower trunk, and legs drain into the *inferior vena cava*. Veins from the abdominal viscera drain into the *portal vein*, which drains through the liver. The portal vein, at the confluence of the nutrient-rich superior mesenteric and splenic veins, supplies ~75% of the blood flow to the liver, supplemented by oxygenated blood from the hepatic artery. Blood from these vessels flows into the hepatic sinusoids, then drains into the hepatic veins that empty into the inferior vena cava. Because of their weaker wall structure, the leg veins are susceptible to irregular dilatation, compression, ulceration, and invasion by tumors, and, as such they warrant special attention.

Deep and Superficial Venous Systems of the Legs. The deep veins of the legs carry approximately 90% of the venous return from the lower extremities. They are well supported by surrounding tissues. In contrast, the superficial veins are subcutaneous, with relatively poor tissue support (Fig. 16-6).

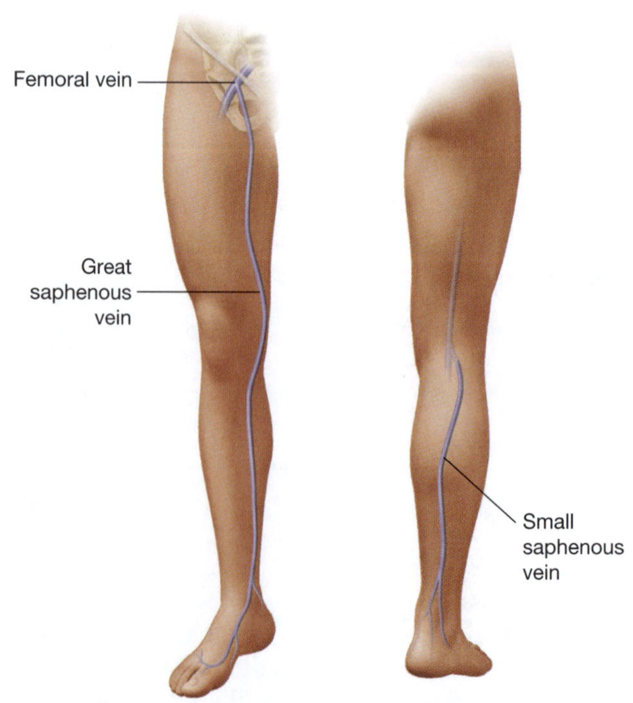

FIGURE 16-6. Superficial veins of the leg.

They include:

- The *great saphenous vein*, which originates on the dorsum of the foot, passes just anterior to the medial malleolus, continues up the medial aspect of the leg, and joins the femoral vein of the deep venous system below the inguinal ligament
- The *small saphenous vein*, which begins on the lateral side of the foot, passes upward along the posterior calf, and joins the deep venous system in the popliteal fossa

Anastomotic veins connect the two saphenous veins and are readily visible when dilated. *Bridging or perforating veins* connect the superficial system with the deep system (Fig. 16-7).

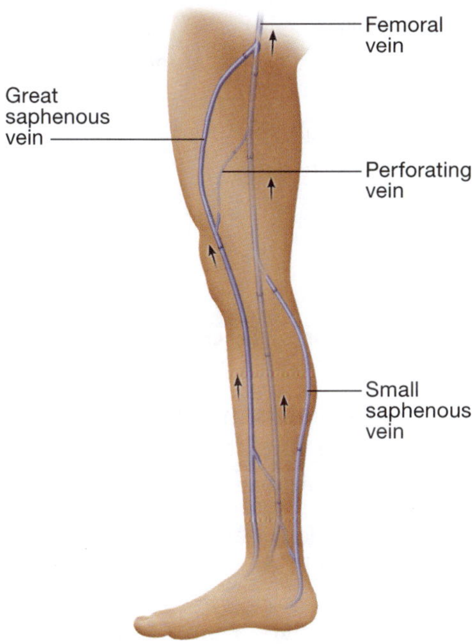

FIGURE 16-7. Deep, superficial, and perforating veins of the leg.

When competent, the one-way valves of the deep, superficial, and perforating veins propel blood toward the heart, preventing pooling, venous stasis, and backward flow. Additionally, contraction of the calf muscles during walking serves as a venous pump, also propelling blood upward against gravity.

Lymphatic System

The lymphatic system is an extensive vascular network that drains lymph fluid from body tissues and returns it to the venous circulation. Networks of lymphatic capillaries, the *lymphatic plexuses*, originate in the extracellular spaces, where the capillaries collect tissue fluid, plasma proteins, cells, and cellular debris via their porous endothelium. The lymphatic capillaries continue centrally as thin vascular channels, then as collecting ducts, and empty into the major veins at the neck. The *right lymphatic duct* drains fluid from the right side of the head, neck, thorax, and right upper limb and empties into the junction of the right internal jugular and the right subclavian veins. The *thoracic duct* collects lymph fluid from the rest of the body and empties into the junction of the left internal jugular and the left subclavian veins. Lymph fluid transported through these channels is filtered through lymph nodes interposed along the way.

Lymph Nodes. See Chapter 8, Lymph Nodes in General Examination.

HEALTH HISTORY: GENERAL APPROACH

You should approach a person presenting with signs and symptoms relating to the peripheral vascular system with the goal of *determining the integrity of the system*, which, as previously described, consists of arteries, veins, and lymphatics. It will be important for you to ask directed questions to distinguish nonspecific complaints—such as pain or weakness—from neurologic or musculoskeletal etiologies in an attempt to narrow the differential diagnosis. Questions such as (1) how rapidly the symptoms began and (2) what activity the person was doing (if any) when the symptoms started, while still important, are less helpful in the peripheral vascular system. In an effort to distinguish these complaints, try to determine the *perfusion* of the extremity in question, as musculoskeletal and neurologic disorders should not alter the extremity's blood supply. Symptoms related to the peripheral vascular system are usually worsened when the oxygen consumption exceeds the supply such as during exertion. Specific questions for the extremities that can aid you in determining perfusion include asking about color; throbbing or pulsatile quality; temperature; hair loss (especially for chronic complaints); symptoms provoked by exertion; and any swelling, ulceration, or gangrene.

Common or Concerning Symptoms

- Pain and/or swelling of legs or arms
- Cramping in legs on exertion with relief with rest (intermittent claudication)
- Cold, numbness, pallor or discoloration in the legs; hair loss
- Abdominal, flank, or back pain

Peripheral Arterial Disease

Peripheral arterial disease (PAD) is generally defined as atherosclerotic disease distal to the aortic bifurcation, although some guidelines also include the abdominal aorta. Detection is doubly important because PAD is both a marker for cardiovascular morbidity and mortality and a harbinger of functional decline. Risk of death from myocardial infarction (MI) and stroke triples in adults with PAD.

Pain or Swelling in Legs or Arms. Presenting symptoms almost always involve pain, swelling, and/or discoloration in the area of arterial distribution. Pain in the extremities can also arise from the skin, musculoskeletal system, or nervous system. It may also be referred, like the pain of MI that radiates to the left arm.

See Table 16-1, Painful Peripheral Vascular Disorders and Their Mimics.

- Ask about any pain or cramping in the legs that occurs at rest and during exertion.

  Symptomatic limb ischemia with exertion is usually atherosclerotic PAD. Pain with walking or prolonged standing, radiating from the spinal area into the buttocks, thighs, lower legs, or feet, is neurogenic claudication.

- Is the pain relieved by resting within 10 minutes (*intermittent claudication*)?
- Is there associated swelling in the legs or arms with the pain?

Because most patients with PAD report minimal symptoms, inquire about two common types of atypical leg pain from PAD that occur prior to critical limb ischemia: *leg pain on exertion and rest* (exertional pain that can begin at rest), and *exertional leg pain/carry on* (exertional pain that does not stop the patient from walking). Ask specifically about the PAD warning signs that follow, particularly in patients age ≥50 years and those with PAD risk factors, especially smoking, but also diabetes, hypertension, elevated cholesterol, African American ethnicity, and coronary artery disease (CAD). Note that these risk factors are the same as the risk factors for CAD. Atherosclerosis is a systemic arterial illness. When the symptoms or risk factors described in Box 16-2 are present, pursue careful examination and testing with the ankle–brachial index (ABI) (see also p. 490).

Only 10% of patients have the classic features of leg pain with exertion relieved by rest. Another 30% to 50% have atypical leg pain, and up to 60% are asymptomatic. Asymptomatic patients can have significant functional impairment that limits or slows walking to avoid symptoms as PAD is progressing.

Box 16-2. Peripheral Arterial Disease: Warning Signs

- Fatigue, aching, numbness, or pain that limits walking or exertion in the legs; if present, identify the location
- Erectile dysfunction
- Any poorly healing or nonhealing wounds of the legs or feet
- Any pain present when at rest in the lower leg or foot and changes when standing or supine
- Abdominal pain after meals and associated food fear and weight loss
- Any first-degree relatives with an abdominal aortic aneurysm

Symptom location suggests the site of arterial ischemia based on the artery's perfusion:

- Buttock, hip: aortoiliac
- Genitalia presenting as erectile dysfunction: aortoiliac–pudendal
- Thigh: common femoral or aortoiliac
- Upper calf: superficial femoral
- Lower calf: popliteal
- Foot: tibial or peroneal

Cold, Numbness, Pallor or Discoloration in the Legs/Hair Loss

- Ask also about coldness, numbness, discoloration or pallor in the legs or feet.
- Ask about loss of hair over the anterior tibial surfaces.

Hair loss over the anterior tibiae points to decreased arterial perfusion. "Dry" or brown-black ulcers from **gangrene** may ensue.

Abdominal, Flank, or Back Pain. Clarifying abdominal complaints related to the vasculature is difficult; however, they still relate to the perfusion of the organ systems. The acute onset of symptoms in the abdomen should raise the concern of arterial thrombosis. Symptoms here can also be related to oxygen supply–demand mismatch. For example, if the symptoms are provoked when the patient is eating (and thus, the abdominal viscera need a greater oxygen supply), the symptoms likely result from arterial pathology. This can evoke fear of eating (**food fear**) or progress to anorexia.

An expanding hematoma from an abdominal aortic aneurysm (AAA) may cause symptoms by compressing the bowel, aortic branch arteries, or the ureters. Prevalence of AAAs in first-degree relatives is 15% to 28%.

These symptoms suggest mesenteric ischemia from arterial embolism, arterial or venous thrombosis, bowel volvulus or strangulation, or hypoperfusion. Failure to detect acute symptoms can result in bowel necrosis and even death.

- Ask about abdominal, flank, or back pain, especially in older smokers. Is there unusual constipation or distention? Inquire about urinary retention, difficulty voiding, erectile dysfunction, and renal colic.

If the pain is relieved by sitting and bending forward, or if there is bilateral buttock or leg pain, the etiology is more likely to be spinal stenosis.

- If there is persistent abdominal pain, ask about any *food fear* (patients do not want to eat because they experience the pain), weight loss, or dark stool.

Food fear and weight loss suggest chronic intestinal ischemia of the celiac or superior or inferior mesenteric arteries.

Peripheral Venous Disease (or Venous Thromboembolism)

Thromboembolic disorders of the peripheral venous system in the lower extremities are also. In addition, DVT in the upper extremity now represents about 10% of the cases of DVT, reflecting complications from increased placement of central venous catheters, cardiac pacemakers, and defibrillators. Most patients present with unilateral or asymmetric swelling of the extremities.

- *In patients with central venous catheters*, ask about arm discomfort, pain, paresthesias, and weakness.

These symptoms point to upper extremity DVT, most commonly from catheter-associated thrombosis. Most patients are asymptomatic with thrombosis detected on routine screening.

- Ask about pain or swelling in the calf or leg.

Because individual clinical features have poor diagnostic value, experts recommend use of well-validated formal clinical scoring systems like the Wells Clinical Score and the Geneva Score for all patients with suspected DVT.

PHYSICAL EXAMINATION: GENERAL APPROACH

As with the clinical interview, we aim to examine the integrity of the arterial, venous, and lymphatic systems of the extremities and abdomen. We do this by ensuring pulses are equal throughout the extremities and that the perfusion of the extremities is intact. It is wise to progress through the examination in a top-down fashion, examining the carotid arteries, then upper extremities, followed by the abdomen, followed by the lower extremities. In doing so, compare and contrast the (1) quality of pulses, (2) size of the arteries, (3) temperature of the extremities, (4) hair patterns of the extremities, and (5) presence or absence of edema from *side to side*. When examining the abdomen, always consider palpating the abdominal aorta. If you discover a pulsatile mass, you may have uncovered an AAA, a potentially life-threatening disease. As you intensify your focus on the peripheral vascular system, recall that PAD is often asymptomatic and underdiagnosed, leading to significant morbidity and mortality.

TECHNIQUES OF EXAMINATION

Key Components of the Peripheral Vascular System

Arms:
- Inspect the upper extremities (size, symmetry, swelling, venous pattern, color).
- Palpate the upper extremities (radial pulse, brachial pulse, epitrochlear lymph nodes).

Abdomen:
- Palpate the inguinal lymph nodes (size, consistency, discreteness, any tenderness).
- Inspect and palpate the abdomen (aortic width and pulsation).
- Auscultate the abdomen (aortic, renal, and femoral bruits).

Legs:
- Inspect the lower extremities (size, symmetry, swelling, venous pattern, skin color, temperature, ulcers, hair loss).
- Palpate the lower extremities (femoral pulse, popliteal pulse, dorsalis pedis pulse, posterior tibial pulse, temperature, swelling, edema).

In addition, review the techniques for assessing blood pressure, the carotid artery, the aorta, and the renal and femoral arteries on the pages indicated below.
- Measure the blood pressure in both arms (see Chapter 8).
- Palpate the carotid upstroke, auscultate for bruits (see Chapter 11).
- Palpate the aorta and assess its maximal diameter (see Chapter 12).

Arms

Inspection. Inspect both arms from the fingertips to the shoulders. Note:

- Size, symmetry, and any swelling

Swelling from lymphedema of the arm and hand may follow axillary node dissection and radiation therapy.

- Venous pattern
- Color of the skin and nail beds and the texture of the skin

Visible venous collaterals, swelling, edema, and discoloration signal upper extremity DVT.

Palpation. Palpate for the *radial pulses*, *brachial pulses*, and one or more of the *epitrochlear lymph nodes*.

Bounding carotid, radial, and femoral pulses are present in aortic regurgitation.

Pulsus parvus refers to weak pulses, usually seen with atherosclerotic PVD, while **pulsus tardus** refers to sluggish pulses, usually occurring in the setting of aortic stenosis or low cardiac output.

If an artery is widely dilated, it is aneurysmal.

Palpate the radial pulse with the pads of your fingers on the flexor surface of the lateral wrist (Fig. 16-8). Partially flexing the patient's wrist may help you feel this pulse. Compare the pulses in both arms.

In Raynaud disease, wrist pulses are typically normal, but spasm of more distal arteries causes episodes of sharply demarcated pallor of the fingers, as shown in Figure 16-9.

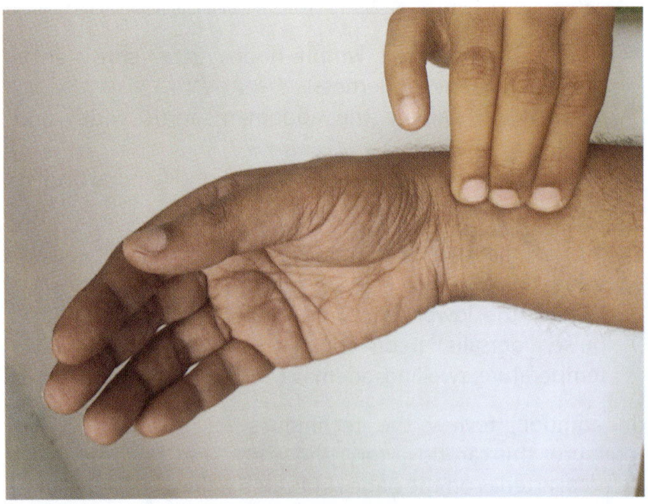

FIGURE 16-8. Palpating the radial pulse.

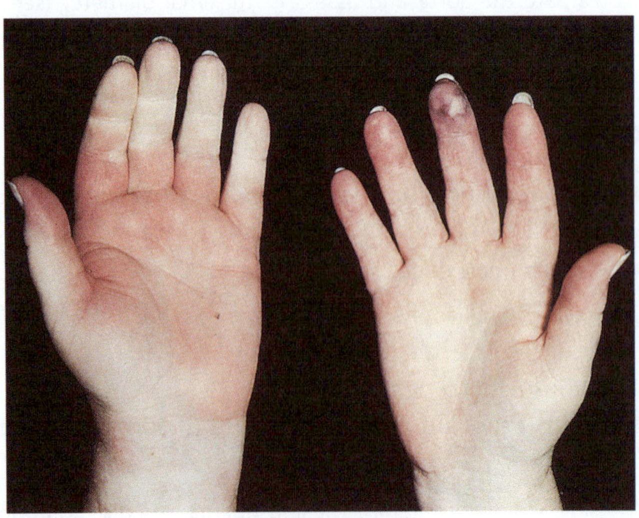

FIGURE 16-9. Raynaud disease.

Palpate the brachial pulses. Flex the patient's elbow slightly and palpate the artery just medial to the biceps tendon at the antecubital crease (Fig. 16-10). The brachial pulse can also be palpated higher in the arm in the groove between the biceps and triceps muscles.

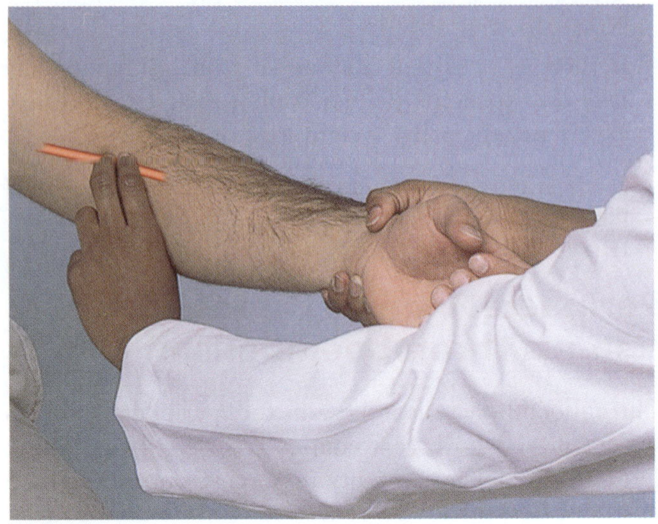

FIGURE 16-10. Palpating the brachial pulse.

Capillary refill time in the digits of >5 seconds has low sensitivity and specificity and is not considered diagnostically helpful.

Palpate one or more epitrochlear nodes. See Chapter 8, Lymph Nodes in General Examination.

Abdomen

For techniques of examination of the abdominal aorta, see Chapter 12, Gastrointestinal System, p. 276. In brief, listen for aortic, renal, and femoral bruits. Palpate and estimate the width of the abdominal aorta in the epigastric area by measuring the aortic width between two fingers, especially in older adults and smokers due to higher risk of AAA. Assess for a pulsatile mass.

Note that an inguinal mass suspicious for an incarcerated hernia is often diagnosed as an AAA at surgery.

Palpation. *Palpate the superficial inguinal nodes*, including both the horizontal and the vertical groups. Note their size, consistency, and discreteness, and note any tenderness. Nontender, discrete inguinal nodes up to 1 cm or even 2 cm in diameter are commonly palpable in healthy people.

Legs

The patient should be supine and draped so that the external genitalia are covered and the legs fully exposed. Stockings, leggings, or socks should be removed.

Inspection. Inspect both legs from the groin and buttocks to the feet. Note:

- Their *size and symmetry*—Inspect and compare the thighs, calves, and ankles for symmetry. Note their relative size. It is wise to use a tape ruler to measure the circumference of the thighs, calves, and ankles. Normally, the difference in calf circumference is <3 cm. Measure and compare other areas of asymmetry, if needed, including the thighs and ankles.

Calf asymmetry >3 cm increases the LR for DVT to >2. Also consider muscle tear or trauma, Baker cyst (posterior knee), and muscular atrophy.

- Any *swelling or edema*—Unilateral or bilateral? Extent of swelling?

Local swelling, redness, warmth, and a subcutaneous cord signal superficial thrombophlebitis, an emerging risk factor for DVT. Asymmetric warmth and redness over the calf signal cellulitis.

Unilateral calf and ankle swelling, and edema suggest venous thromboembolism (VTE) from DVT, chronic venous insufficiency from prior DVT, or incompetent venous valves; or it may be lymphedema. If you detect unilateral swelling or edema, *measure the calves* 10 cm below the tibial tuberosity. Bilateral edema is present in heart failure, cirrhosis, and nephrotic syndrome. Venous distention suggests a venous cause of edema.

- *Venous pattern and any venous enlargement*—Inspect the saphenous system for *varicosities*. If present, ask the patient to stand, which allows any varicosities to fill with blood and makes them visible; these changes are easily missed when the patient is supine (Fig. 16-11). Palpate along any varicosities to check for thrombophlebitis.

Edema may obscure the veins, tendons, and bony prominences (Fig. 16-12).

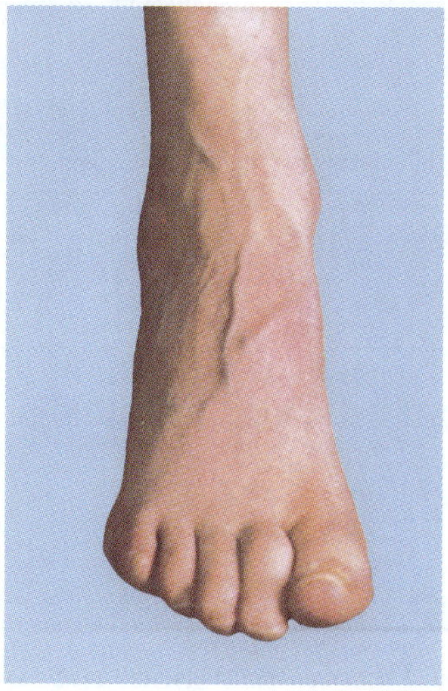

FIGURE 16-11. Note the prominent veins.

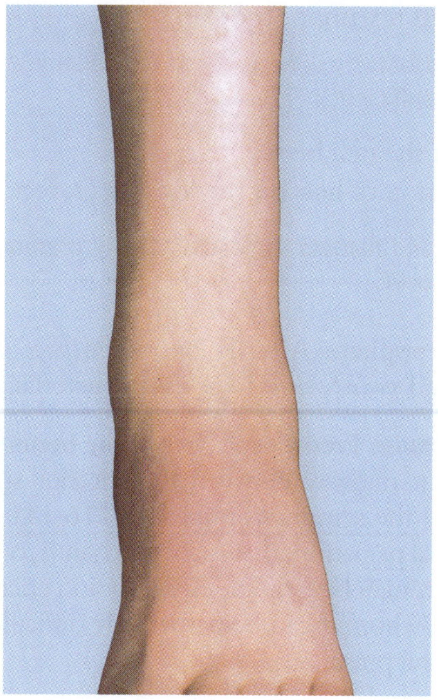

FIGURE 16-12. Pretibial edema.

Varicose veins are dilated and tortuous. Their walls may feel somewhat thickened (Fig. 16-13). See also Table 16-2, Chronic Insufficiency of Arteries and Veins.

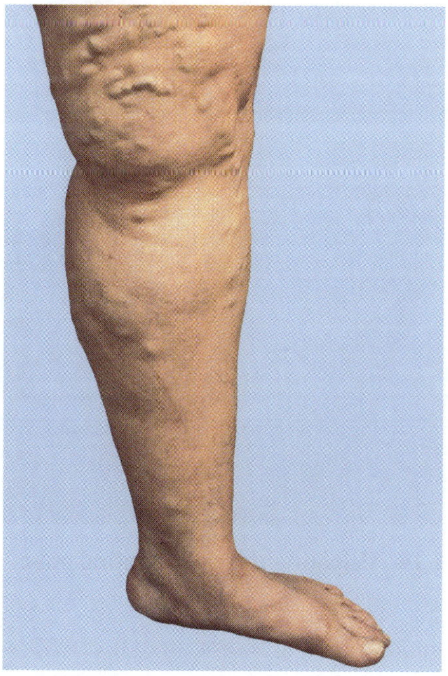

FIGURE 16-13. Varicose veins.

- Any *pigmentation*, *rashes*, *scars*, or *ulcers*

Ulcers or sores on the feet raise the likelihood ratio (LR) of peripheral vascular disease to 7. See Table 16-3, Common Ulcers of the Ankles and Feet.

Brownish discoloration or ulcers just above the malleolus suggest *chronic venous insufficiency*.

- Color and texture of the skin

Thickened, brawny skin suggests lymphedema and advanced venous insufficiency.

- Color of the nail beds
- Distribution of hair on the lower legs, feet, and toes

Atrophic and hairless skin is commonly present in PAD but not diagnostic.

Palpation: Peripheral Arterial Pulses. *Palpate the femoral, popliteal,* and *pedal pulses* to assess the arterial circulation.

- *Femoral pulse.* Press deeply, below the inguinal ligament and about midway between the anterior superior iliac spine and the symphysis pubis (Fig. 16-14). As in deep abdominal palpation, the use of two hands, one on top of the other, may be helpful, especially in patients who are obese, in whom it can be particularly difficult to palpate the femoral pulse.

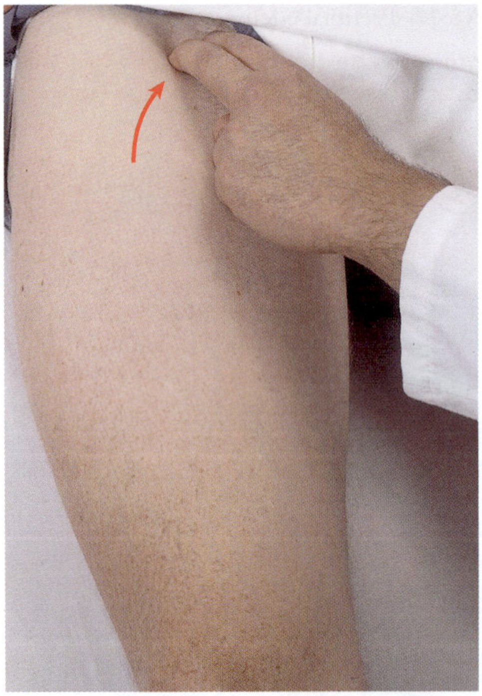

FIGURE 16-14. Palpating the right femoral pulse.

If the femoral pulse is absent, the LR of PAD is >6. If the occlusion is at the aortic or iliac level, all pulses distal to the occlusion are typically affected and may cause postural color changes.

An exaggerated, widened femoral pulse suggests the pathologic dilatation of a *femoral aneurysm.*

- *Popliteal pulse.* The patient's knee should be somewhat flexed, with the leg relaxed. Place the fingertips of both hands so that they just meet in the midline behind the knee and press them deeply into the popliteal fossa (Fig. 16-15). The popliteal pulse is more difficult to find than other pulses. It is deeper and feels more diffuse.

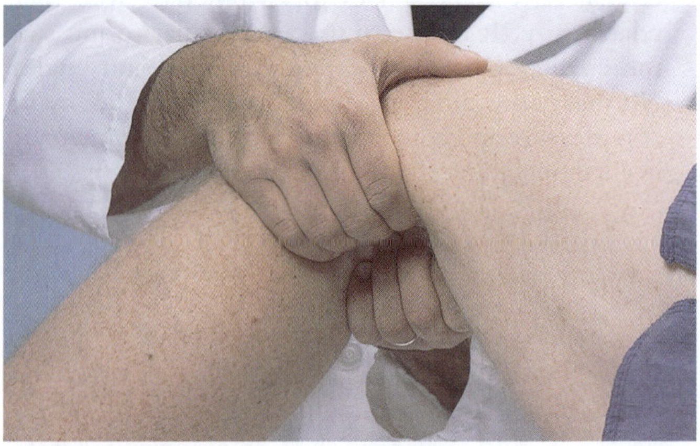

FIGURE 16-15. Palpating the popliteal pulse.

An exaggerated, widened popliteal pulse suggests a popliteal artery aneurysm. Popliteal and femoral aneurysms are uncommon. They are usually from atherosclerosis and occur primarily in men age ≥50 years.

If you cannot palpate the popliteal pulse with this approach, try with the patient prone. Flex the patient's knee to about 90°, let the lower leg relax against your shoulder or upper arm, and press your two thumbs deeply into the popliteal fossa (Fig. 16-16).

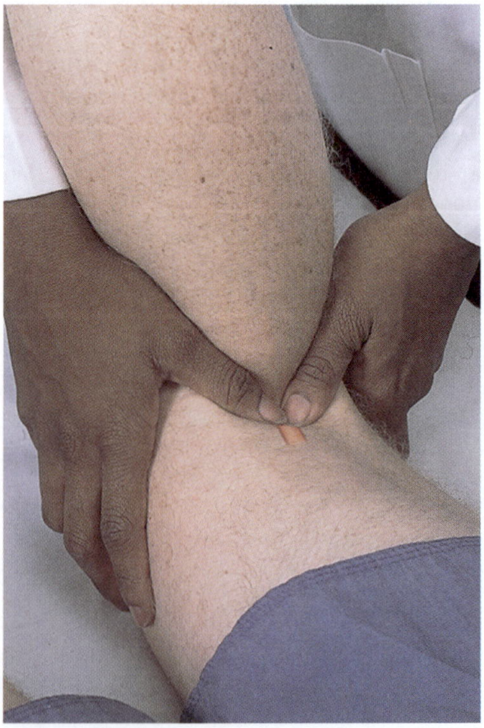

FIGURE 16-16. Deeply palpating the popliteal fossa, prone position.

- *Dorsalis pedis pulse.* Palpate the dorsum of the foot (not the ankle) just lateral to the extensor tendon of the great toe (Fig. 16-17). The DP artery may be congenitally absent or branch higher in the ankle. If you cannot feel a pulse, explore the dorsum of the foot more laterally.

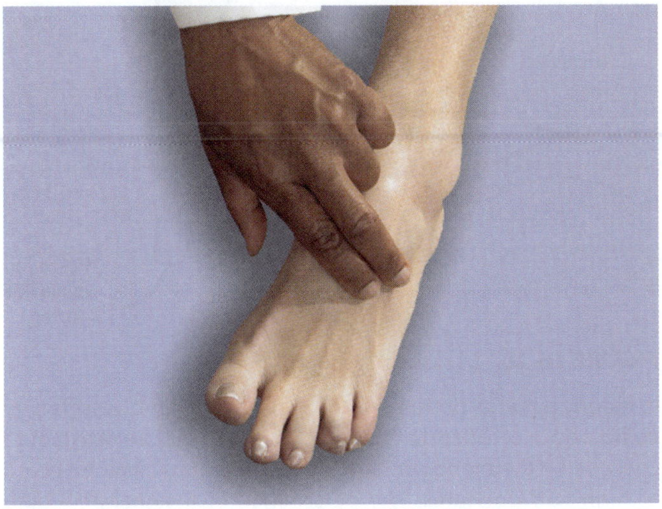

FIGURE 16-17. Palpating the dorsalis pedis pulse.

Absent pedal pulses with normal femoral and popliteal pulses raise the LR of PAD to >14.

- *Posterior tibial pulse.* Curve your fingers behind and slightly below the medial malleolus of the ankle (Fig. 16-18). This pulse may be hard to feel in a swollen or a thick ankle due to surrounding fat (Box 16-3).

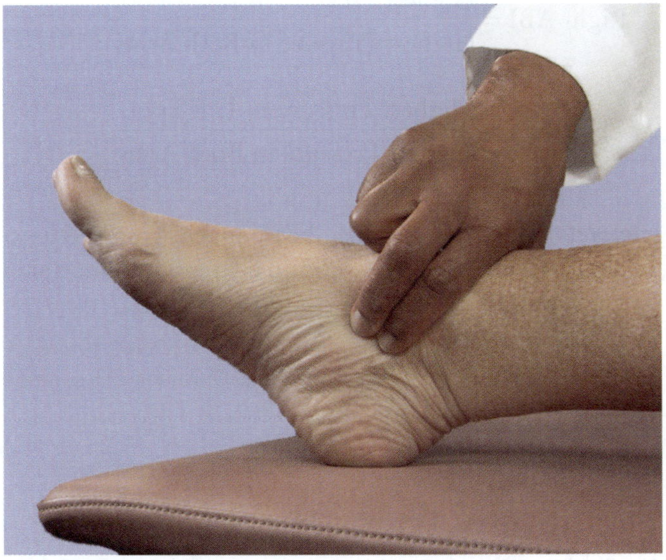

FIGURE 16-18. Palpating the posterior tibial pulse.

Acute arterial occlusion from embolism or thrombosis causes pain and numbness or tingling. The limb distal to the occlusion becomes cold, pale, and pulseless. Pursue emergency treatment.

Box 16-3. Tips for Palpating Difficult Pulses

1. Position your body and examining hand comfortably; awkward positions decrease tactile sensitivity.
2. Once your hand is positioned properly, linger and vary the pressure of your fingers to pick up a weak pulsation. If unsuccessful, explore the area gently but more deliberately.
3. Think of the position and depth of the pulse. A pulse may require several fingers or may require two hands to properly palpate.
4. Do not mistake the patient's pulse with your own pulsating fingertips. If needed, count your own heart rate and compare it to the patient's. The rates are usually different. Your carotid pulse is convenient for this comparison.
5. In some cases, it is helpful to compare the pulse you are trying to palpate with the patient's carotid or radial pulse simultaneously.

Assess the temperature of the feet and legs with the backs of your fingers. Compare one side with the other.

Asymmetric coolness of the feet has a positive LR of >6 for PAD.

Poikilothermia is the relative hypothermia of one extremity as compared with another. It is usually seen in peripheral vascular disease.

Palpation: Peripheral Veins. If swelling or edema is present, palpate for pitting edema.

Palpate for any venous tenderness or cords, which can accompany a DVT.

- Palpate the inguinal area just medial to the femoral pulse for tenderness of the femoral vein.

A painful, pale, swollen leg, together with tenderness in the groin over the femoral vein, suggests deep *iliofemoral thrombosis.* Risk of PE in proximal vein thrombosis is 50%.

- Next, with the patient's leg flexed at the knee and relaxed, palpate the calf. With your fingerpads, gently compress the calf muscles against the tibia and search for any tenderness or cords.

Only half of patients with DVT in the calf have tenderness or venous cords, and absence of calf tenderness does not rule out thrombosis. Note that the *Homan sign,* discomfort behind the knee with forced dorsiflexion on the foot, is neither sensitive nor specific, and discredited by Homan himself.

SPECIAL TECHNIQUES

Assessing for Peripheral Arterial Disease

Ankle–Brachial Index. If the patient presents with history and examination findings suspicious of peripheral vascular disease, such as pain, claudication, numbness, weakness, weak to absent dorsalis pedis and posterior tibial pulses, or pallor of distal extremities, then measuring the *ankle–brachial index (ABI)* is an important diagnostic technique. The ABI is the ratio of blood pressure measurements in the foot and arm. This noninvasive method is simple, reproducible, and accurate at detecting the decreased blood pressure distal to an arterial stenosis. It is often used to assess PAD.

Measuring Brachial Pressure. The patient should be resting in the supine position for 10 minutes. Place a blood pressure cuff on the arm (Fig. 16-19), then apply ultrasound gel over the brachial pulse. Using the transducer of a handheld vascular Doppler, locate the brachial pulse. Inflate the cuff to 20 mm Hg above the last audible pulse. Deflate the cuff slowly (approximately 1 mm Hg/sec) and record the pressure at which the pulse becomes audible again. Obtain two measures in each arm and record the average as the brachial pressure in that arm.

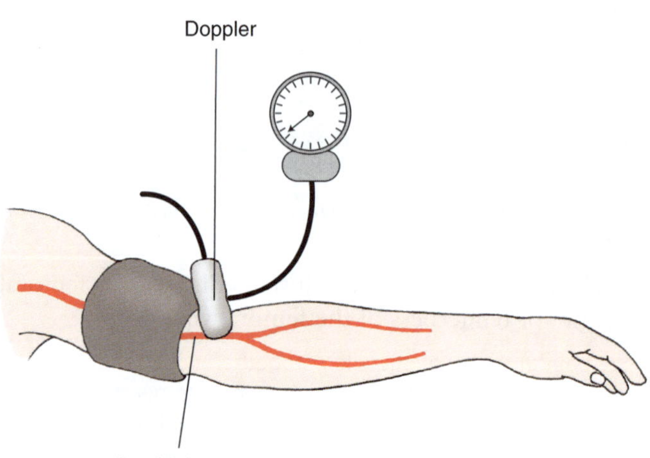

FIGURE 16-19. Measuring the brachial pressure.

Measuring Ankle Pressures. Now place the blood pressure cuff on the ankle proximal to the malleoli (Fig. 16-20), then apply ultrasound gel over the dorsalis pedis artery. Using the transducer of a handheld vascular Doppler, locate the DP pulse. Inflate the cuff to 20 mm Hg above the last audible pulse. Deflate the cuff slowly (approximately 1 mm Hg/sec) and record the pressure at which the DP pulse becomes audible again. Repeat the previous steps for the posterior tibial artery. Then repeat both measurements (DP and PT) on the opposite leg.

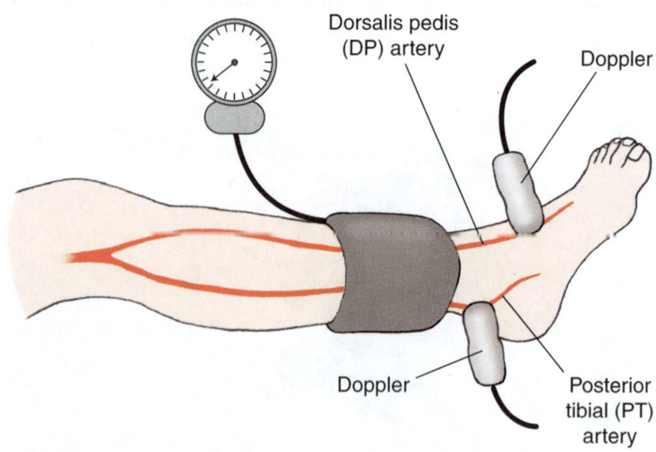

FIGURE 16-20. Measuring the ankle pressure.

In elderly patients or those with diabetes, the limb vessels may be fibrotic or calcified. In this case, the vessel may be resistant to collapse by the blood pressure cuff, and a signal may be heard at high cuff pressures. The persistence of a signal at a high pressure in these individuals results in an artifactually elevated blood pressure value.

Calculating the ABI. An ABI is calculated for each leg. The ABI value is determined by taking the higher pressure of the two arteries at the ankle, divided by the brachial arterial systolic pressure. Calculated ABI values should be recorded to two decimal places.

$$\text{Right ABI} = \frac{\text{Highest Pressure in Right Foot}}{\text{Highest Pressure in Both Arms}}$$

$$\text{Left ABI} = \frac{\text{Highest Pressure in Left Foot}}{\text{Highest Pressure in Both Arms}}$$

Interpreting the ABI. Normal ABI ranges from 0.90 to 1.40 because the pressure is normally higher in the ankle than the arm.

Values >1.40 suggest a noncompressible calcified vessel. A value <0.90 is considered diagnostic of PAD; values <0.5 suggest severe PAD.

Evaluating Arterial Perfusion of the Hand

If you suspect arterial insufficiency in the arm or hand, try to palpate the *ulnar pulse* as well as the radial and brachial pulses. Press deeply on the flexor surface of the medial wrist (Fig. 16-21). Partially flexing the patient's wrist may help you. The pulse of a normal ulnar artery may not be palpable.

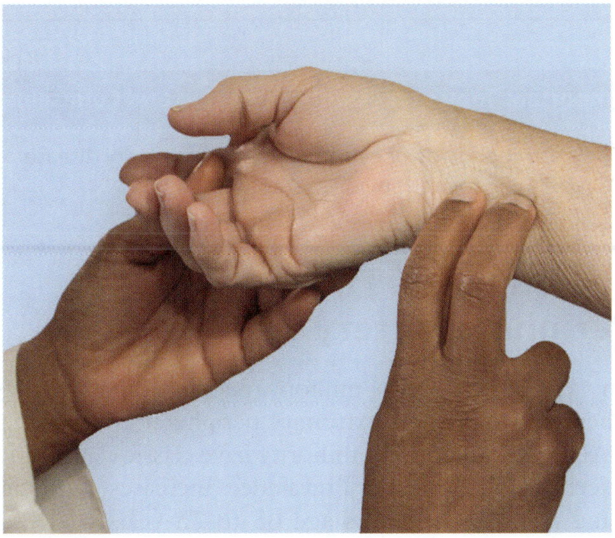

FIGURE 16-21. Palpating the ulnar pulse.

Arterial occlusive disease is much less common in the arms than in the legs. Absent or diminished pulses at the wrist occur in acute embolic occlusion and in *Buerger disease,* or *thromboangiitis obliterans.*

Allen Test. The **Allen test** compares patency of the ulnar and radial arteries. It also ensures patency of the ulnar artery before puncturing the radial artery for blood samples. The patient should rest with hands in lap, palms up.

Ask the patient to make a tight fist with one hand; then compress both radial and ulnar arteries firmly between your thumbs and fingers (Fig. 16-22).

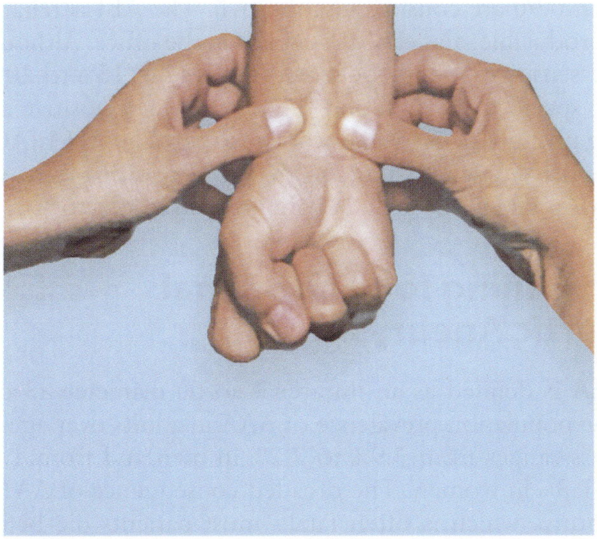

FIGURE 16-22. Compressing both the radial and ulnar arteries.

Next, ask the patient to open the hand into a relaxed, slightly flexed position (Fig. 16-23). The palm is pale.

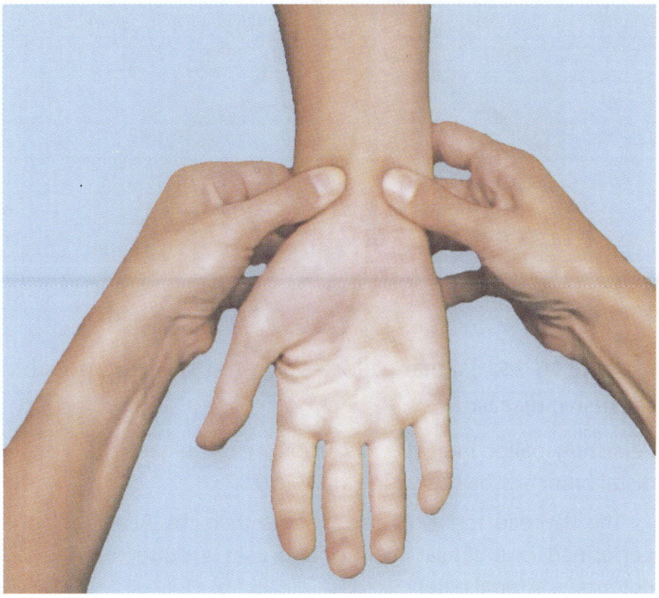

FIGURE 16-23. Pallor when hand relaxed.

Release your pressure over the ulnar artery. If the ulnar artery is patent, the palm flushes within about 3 to 5 seconds (Fig. 16-24).

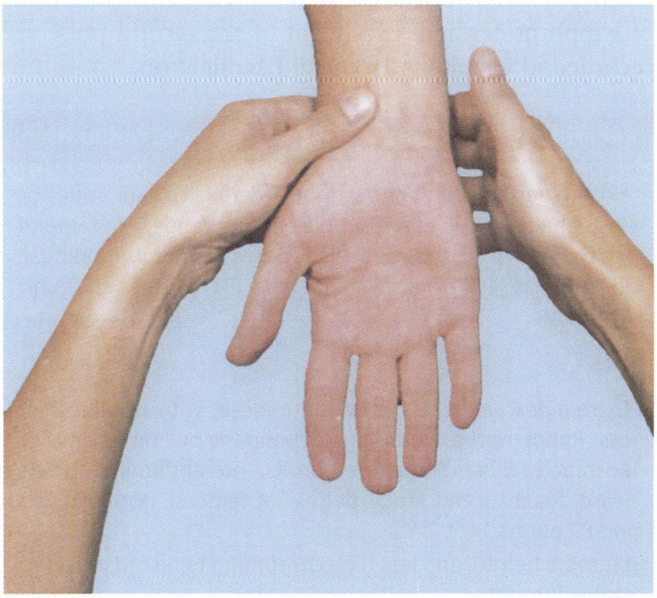

FIGURE 16-24. Palmar flushing—Allen test showing patent arterial circulation.

Extending the hand fully may cause **pallor** and a falsely positive test.

Test patency of the radial artery by releasing the radial artery while still compressing the ulnar artery.

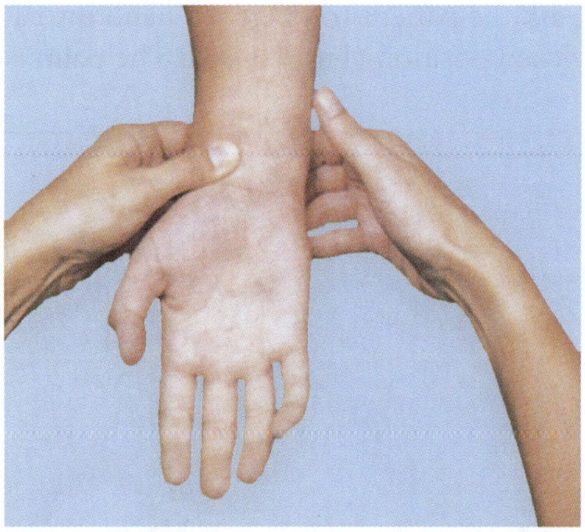

FIGURE 16-25. Palmar pallor—Allen test showing possible occlusive disease.

Persisting pallor indicates occlusion of the ulnar artery or its distal branches, as shown in Figure 16-25.

The Barbeau test is more objective than the Allen test. It is performed in a similar manner and uses a pulse oximeter to determine arterial patency.

RECORDING YOUR FINDINGS

Note that initially you may use sentences to describe your findings; later you will use phrases. Written descriptions of lymph nodes and assessment of the carotid pulse are recorded in Chapter 8, General Examination.

Recording the Peripheral Vascular System Examination

"Extremities are warm and without edema. No varicosities or stasis changes. Calves are supple and nontender. No femoral or abdominal bruits. Brachial, radial, femoral, popliteal, dorsalis pedis (DP), and posterior tibial (PT) pulses are 2+ and symmetric."

OR

"Extremities are pale below the midcalf, with notable hair loss. Rubor noted when legs dependent but no edema or ulceration. Bilateral femoral bruits; no abdominal bruits heard. Brachial and radial pulses 2+; femoral, popliteal, DP, and PT pulses 1+."*

It is more helpful and less time consuming to record pulses in a table format:

	Radial	Brachial	Femoral	Popliteal	Dorsalis Pedis	Posterior Tibial
RT	2+	2+	1+	1+	1+	1+
LT	2+	2+	1+	1+	1+	1+

*These findings suggest atherosclerotic peripheral arterial disease.

HEALTH PROMOTION AND COUNSELING: EVIDENCE AND RECOMMENDATIONS

Important Topics for Health Promotion and Counseling

- Screening for lower extremity peripheral artery disease
- Screening for abdominal aortic aneurysm

Screening for Lower Extremity Peripheral Artery Disease

An estimated 200 million people globally have atherosclerotic lower extremity peripheral artery disease (PAD), although only a minority have classic claudication (exertional calf pain). Prevalence increases with age, rising from 8% of adults age 65 to 75 years to 18% of adults 75 years of age and older. Prevalence is higher in low-income and middle-income countries than in high-income countries. Risk factors for PAD include age ≥65 years, risk factors for atherosclerosis (diabetes, tobacco use, hyperlipidemia, hypertension), and known atherosclerotic disease in another vascular area (coronary, carotid, subclavian, renal, or mesenteric artery or abdominal aortic aneurysm).

Detecting PAD is important because it is both a marker for cardiovascular morbidity and mortality and a harbinger of functional decline. Risk of death from myocardial infarction and stroke triples in adults with PAD. PAD can be detected noninvasively using the ankle–brachial index (ABI). The ABI is the ratio of blood pressure measurements in the foot and arm. Values less than 0.90 are considered abnormal. The ABI is reliable, reproducible, and easy to perform in the office. Although the sensitivity of an abnormal ABI is low (15% to 20%), the specificity is 99%, and the test has high positive and negative predictive values (both >80%). The AHA/ACC practice guideline suggests that it is reasonable to use ABI to screen for PAD in patients with risk factors.

Screening for Abdominal Aortic Aneurysm

AAA is defined as an infrarenal aortic diameter ≥3 cm. The population prevalence of AAA in adults over age 50 years ranges from 3.9% to 7.2% in men and from 1.0% to 1.3% in women. The dreaded consequence of AAA is rupture, which is often fatal—most patients die before reaching a hospital. The chances of rupture and mortality increase dramatically when the aortic diameter exceeds 5.5 cm. The strongest risk factors for AAA are older age, male sex, smoking, and family history; potential risk factors include history of other vascular aneurysms, taller height, CAD, cerebrovascular disease, atherosclerosis, hypertension, and hyperlipidemia.

AAAs are detectable with abdominal ultrasound, which is a noninvasive, inexpensive, and accurate (sensitivity 94% to 100%; specificity 98% to 100%) screening test. Palpation is not sensitive enough to be recommended for screening. Because symptoms are uncommon, and screening can reduce AAA-related mortality by about 50% over 13 to 15 years, it is recommended that one-time abdominal ultrasound screening of men aged 65 to 75 years who have smoked more than 100 cigarettes in a lifetime to be undertaken.

TABLE 16-1. Painful Peripheral Vascular Disorders and Their Mimics

Problem	Process	Location of Pain
Arterial Disorders		
Raynaud Phenomenon: Primary and Secondary	*Raynaud phenomenon, primary:* Episodic reversible vasoconstriction in the fingers and toes, usually triggered by cold temperatures (capillaries are normal); no definable cause *Raynaud phenomenon, secondary:* symptoms/signs related to autoimmune diseases—scleroderma, systemic lupus erythematosus, mixed connective tissue disease; cryoglobulinemia; also, to occupational vascular injury; drugs	Distal portions of one or more fingers Pain is usually not prominent unless fingertip ulcers develop; numbness and tingling are common
Peripheral Arterial Disease	Atherosclerotic disease leading to obstruction of peripheral arteries causing exertional claudication (muscle pain relieved by rest) and atypical leg pain; may progress to ischemic pain at rest	Usually calf muscles, but also occurs in the buttock, hip, thigh, or foot, depending on the level of obstruction; rest pain may be distal in the toes or forefoot
Acute Arterial Occlusion	Embolism or thrombosis	Distal pain, usually involving the foot and leg
Venous Disorders *(Lower Extremity)*		
Superficial Phlebitis and Superficial Vein Thrombosis	Involves inflammation of a superficial vein (*superficial phlebitis*), at times with venous thrombosis (*superficial vein thrombosis* when clot confirmed by imaging)	Pain and tenderness along the course of a superficial vein, most often in the saphenous system
Deep Venous Thrombosis (DVT)	DVT and PE are disorders of venous thromboembolic disease (VTE); DVTs are distal, limited to the deep calf veins, or proximal, in the popliteal, femoral, or iliac veins	Classically, painful or painless calf swelling with erythema; signs correlate poorly with site of thrombosis
Chronic Venous Insufficiency (Deep)	More severe form of chronic venous disease, with chronic venous engorgement from venous occlusion or incompetent venous valves	Diffuse aching of the leg(s), skin erythema which slowly progresses to brownish discoloration
Thromboangiitis Obliterans *(Buerger Disease)*	Inflammatory nonatherosclerotic occlusive disease of small- to medium-sized arteries and veins, especially in smokers; occluding thrombus spares the blood vessel wall	Often digit or toe pain progressing to ischemic ulcerations

Timing	Factors That Aggravate	Factors That Relieve	Associated Manifestations
Relatively brief (minutes), but recurrent	Exposure to cold, emotional upset	Warm environment	*Primary:* Distinct digital color changes of pallor, cyanosis, and hyperemia (redness); no necrosis *Secondary:* More severe, with ischemia, necrosis, and loss of digits; capillary loops are distorted
May be brief if relieved by rest; if there is *rest pain,* may be persistent and worse at night	Exercise such as walking; if *rest pain,* leg elevation and bedrest	Rest usually stops the pain in 1–3 min; *rest pain* may be relieved by walking (increases perfusion), sitting with legs dependent	Local fatigue, numbness, progressing to cool dry hairless skin, trophic nail changes, diminished to absent pulses, pallor with elevation, ulceration, gangrene (see p. 491)
Sudden onset; associated symptoms may occur without pain			Coldness, numbness, weakness, absent distal pulses
An acute episode lasting days or longer	Immobility, venous stasis and chronic venous disease, venous procedure (such as IV cannula placement), obesity	Supportive care, walking; measures prompted by further testing	Local induration, erythema; if palpable nodules or cords, consider superficial or deep vein thrombosis, both associated with significant risk of DVT and PE
Often hard to determine due to lack of symptoms; one-third of untreated calf DVTs extend proximally	Immobilization or recent surgery, lower extremity trauma, pregnancy or postpartum state, hypercoagulable state (e.g., nephrotic syndrome, malignancy)	Antithrombotic and thrombolytic therapy	Asymmetric calf diameters more diagnostic than palpable cord or tenderness over femoral triangle; high risk of PE (50% with proximal DVT)
Chronic, increasing as the day wears on	Prolonged standing, sitting with legs dependent	Limb elevation, walking	Chronic edema, pigmentation, swelling, and possibly ulceration, especially if advanced age, pregnancy, increased weight, prior history, or trauma
Ranges from brief recurrent to chronic persistent pain	Exercise	Rest; smoking cessation	May progress to gangrene at tips of digits; can move proximally, with migratory phlebitis and tender nodules along blood vessels; usually involves at least two limbs

(*continued*)

TABLE 16-1. Painful Peripheral Vascular Disorders and Their Mimics *(Continued)*

Problem	Process	Location of Pain
Compartment Syndrome	Pressure builds from trauma or bleeding into one of the four major muscle compartments between the knee and ankle; each compartment is enclosed by fascia that limits expansion to accommodate increasing pressure	Tight, bursting pain in calf muscles, usually in the anterior tibial compartment, sometimes with overlying dusky red skin
Acute Lymphangitis	Acute infection, usually from *Streptococcus pyogenes* or *Staphylococcus aureus,* spreading up the lymphatic channels from distal portal of entry such as skin abrasion, ulcer, or dog bite	An arm or a leg
Mimics (Primarily of Acute Superficial Thrombophlebitis)		
Acute Cellulitis	Acute bacterial infection of the skin and subcutaneous tissues, most commonly from beta-hemolytic streptococci (erysipelas) and *S. aureus*	In the arms, legs, or elsewhere
Erythema Nodosum	Painful raised, bilateral erythematous lesions from inflammation of subcutaneous fat tissue, seen in systemic conditions such as pregnancy, sarcoidosis, tuberculosis, streptococcal infections, inflammatory bowel disease, medications (oral contraceptives)	Anterior pretibial surfaces of both lower legs; can also appear on extensor arms, buttocks, and thighs

Timing	Factors That Aggravate	Factors That Relieve	Associated Manifestations
Several hours if acute (pressure must be relieved to avert necrosis); during exercise if chronic	*Acute:* Anabolic steroids; surgical complication; crush injury *Chronic:* Occurs with exercise	*Acute:* Surgical incision to relieve pressure *Chronic:* Avoiding exercise; ice, elevation	Tingling, burning sensations in calf; muscles may feel tight, full; numbness, paralysis if unrelieved
An acute episode lasting day or longer			Red streak(s) on the skin, with tenderness, enlarged, tender lymph nodes, and fever
An acute episode lasting days or longer			Erythema, edema, and warmth *Erysipelas:* Lesion raised and demarcated from skin; involves upper dermis, lymphatics *Cellulitis:* Involves deeper dermis, adipose tissue; may include enlarged, tender lymph nodes and fever
Pain associated with a series of lesions over 2–8 wk			2–5-cm lesions, initially elevated, bright red then fade to violet or red-brown; do not ulcerate; often with polyarthralgia, fever, malaise

TABLE 16-2. Chronic Insufficiency of Arteries and Veins

	Chronic Arterial Insufficiency (*Advanced*)	Chronic Venous Insufficiency (*Advanced*)
	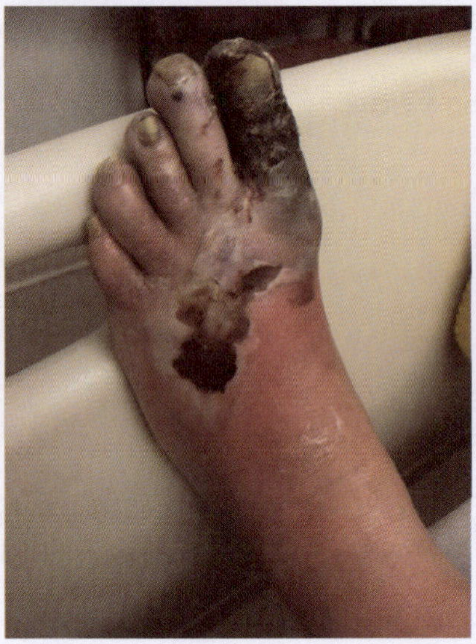	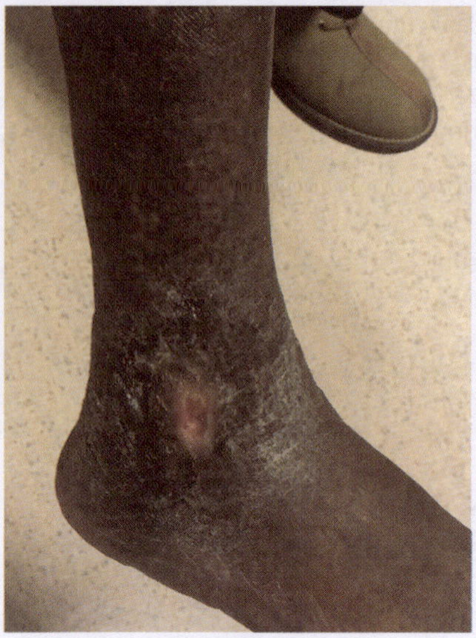
Pain	Intermittent claudication, progressing to pain at rest	Often painful
Mechanism	Tissue ischemia	Venous stasis and hypertension
Pulses	Decreased or absent	Normal, though may be difficult to feel through edema
Color	Pale, especially on elevation; dusky red on dependency	Normal, or cyanotic on dependency; petechiae and then brown pigmentation appear with chronicity
Temperature	Cool	Normal
Edema	Absent or mild; may develop as the patient tries to relieve rest pain by lowering the leg	Present, often marked
Skin Changes	Trophic changes: thin, shiny, atrophic skin; loss of hair over the foot and toes; nails thickened and ridged	Often brown pigmentation around the ankle, stasis dermatitis, and possible thickening of the skin and narrowing of the leg as scarring develops
Ulceration	If present, involves toes or points of trauma on feet	If present, develops at sides of ankle, especially medially
Gangrene	May develop	Does not develop

Source of photos: Courtesy of Daniel Han, MD.

TABLE 16-3. Common Ulcers of the Ankles and Feet

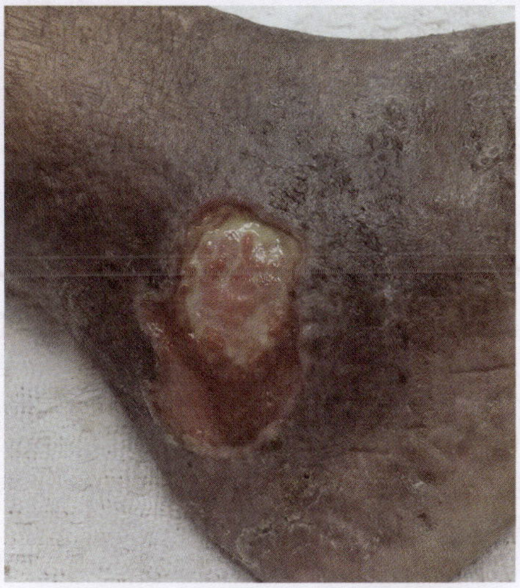

Chronic Venous Insufficiency

This condition usually appears over the medial and sometimes the lateral malleolus. The ulcer contains small, painful granulation tissue and fibrin; necrosis or exposed tendons are rare. Borders are irregular, flat, or slightly steep. Pain affects quality of life in 75% of patients. Associated findings include edema, reddish pigmentation and purpura, venous varicosities, the eczematous changes of stasis dermatitis (redness, scaling, and pruritus), and at times cyanosis of the foot when dependent. Gangrene is rare.

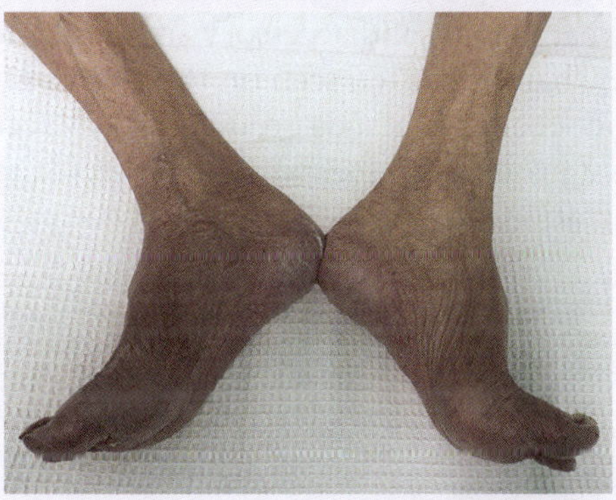

Arterial Insufficiency

This condition occurs in the toes, feet, or possibly areas of trauma (e.g., the shins). Surrounding skin shows no callus or excess pigment, although it may be atrophic. Pain often is severe unless masked by neuropathy. May be accompanied by gangrene, along with decreased pulses, trophic changes, foot pallor on elevation, and dusky rubor on dependency.

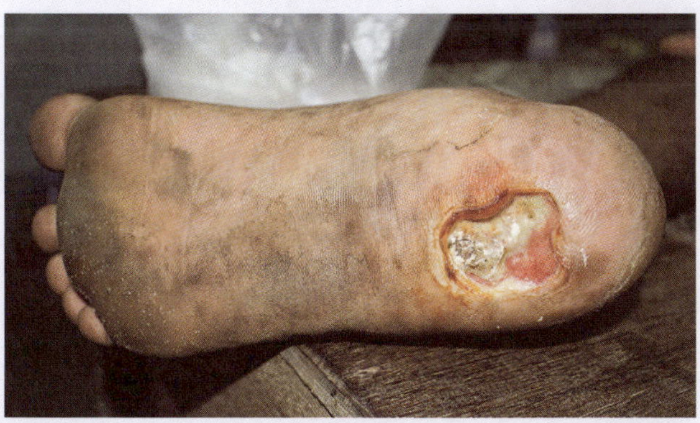

Neuropathic Ulcer

This condition develops in pressure points of areas with diminished sensation; seen in diabetic neuropathy, neurologic disorders, and Hansen disease. The surrounding skin is calloused. There is no pain, so the ulcer may go unnoticed. In uncomplicated cases, there is no gangrene. Associated signs include decreased sensation and absent ankle jerks.

Source of photos: *Chronic Venous Insufficiency*—Shutterstock photo by Casa nayafana; *Arterial Insufficiency*—Shutterstock photo by Alan Nissa; *Neuropathic Ulcer*—Shutterstock photo by Zay Nyi Nyi.

CHAPTER 17

Breasts and Axillae

ANATOMY AND PHYSIOLOGY

Female Breast

Anatomy. The female breast lies against the anterior thoracic wall, extending from the clavicle and second rib down to the sixth rib, and from the sternum across to the midaxillary line. The breast overlies the *pectoralis major* and, at its inferior and lateral margins, the *serratus anterior* (Fig. 17-1).

The *glandular tissue* of the breast is divided into 15 to 20 segments, or *lobes*, which converge in a radial fashion as *lactiferous ducts* and *sinuses* before opening on the surface of the nipple and areola. Each lactiferous duct drains a lobe that is made up of 20 to 40 smaller *lobules*, which consist of milk-secreting tubuloalveolar glands. Adipose tissue surrounds the breast, predominantly in the superficial and peripheral areas.

The surface of the *areola* has small, rounded elevations formed by *sebaceous glands* (called **Montgomery glands**), sweat glands, and accessory areolar glands (Fig. 17-2). A few hairs are often seen on the areola. During pregnancy, the sebaceous glands produce an oily secretion that serves as a protective lubricant for the areola and nipple during lactation.

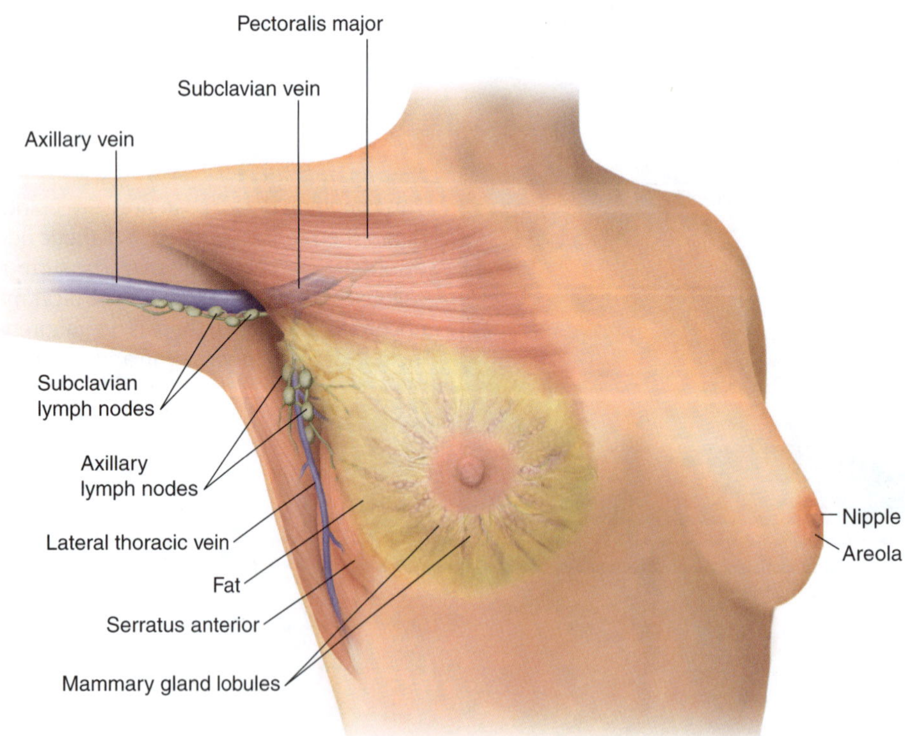

FIGURE 17-1. Female breast.

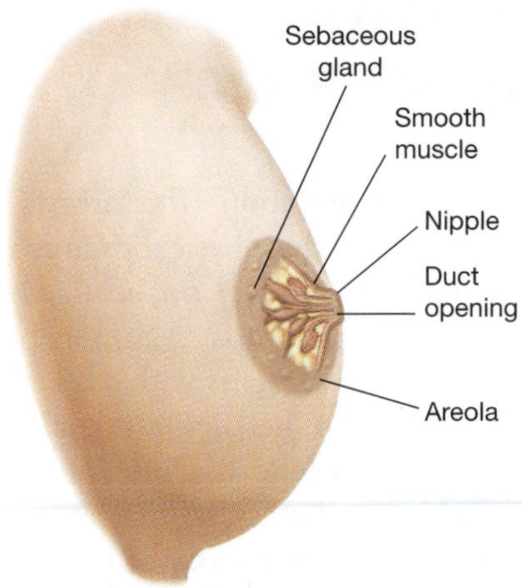

FIGURE 17-2. Nipple and areola.

There are two fascial layers of the breast. The *superficial fascia* lies deep to the dermis, and the *deep fascia* lies anterior to the pectoralis major muscle. The breast is attached to the skin by suspensory **Cooper ligaments**, fibrous bands that travel through the breast and insert perpendicular to the dermis (Fig. 17-3).

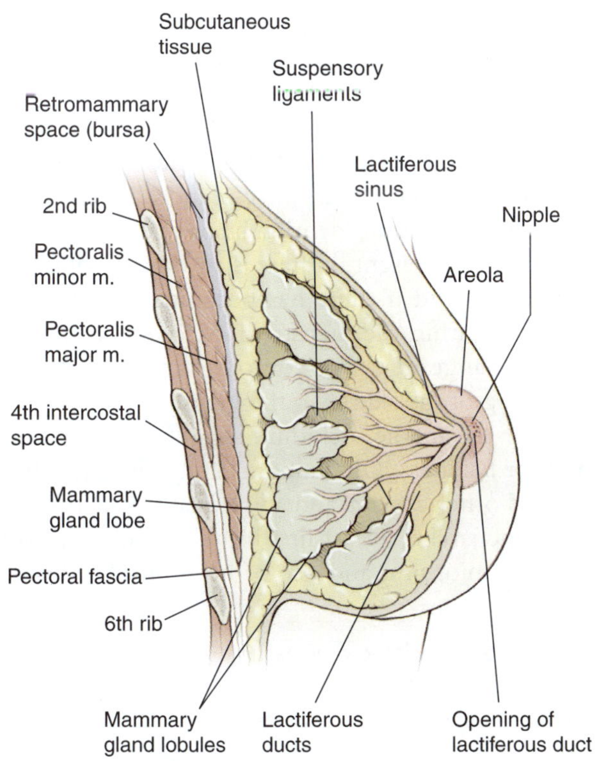

FIGURE 17-3. Sagittal section of female breast. (From Tank PW. *Grant's Dissector*. 15th ed. Wolters Kluwer Health/Lippincott Williams & Wilkins; 2013, Fig. 2-6.)

Occasionally, one or more extra or **supernumerary nipples** are located along the "milk line" (Fig. 17-4). Usually, only a small nipple and areola are present, often mistaken for a common mole. They may be familial, and, in the absence of associated glandular tissue, there is little evidence of association with other congenital anomalies. Those containing glandular tissue occasionally show increased pigmentation, swelling, tenderness, or even lactation during puberty, menstruation, or pregnancy and can be associated with other congenital anomalies, mainly renal and thoracic. Treatment is recommended if there is diagnostic ambiguity, cosmetic concerns, or possible pathology.

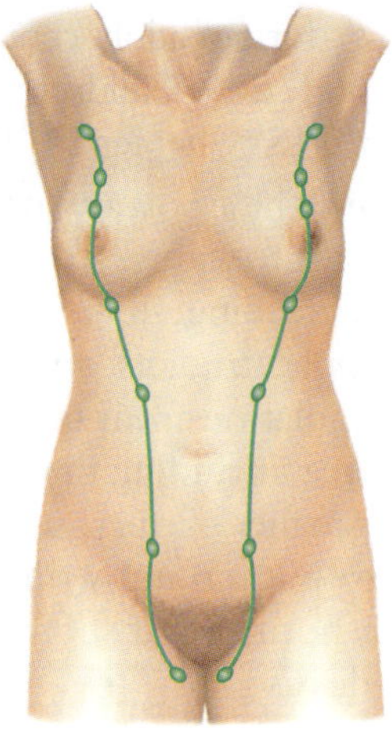

FIGURE 17-4. Milk lines.

To describe clinical findings, the breast is often divided into four quadrants based on horizontal and vertical lines crossing at the nipple (Fig. 17-5). A fifth area, the axillary tail of breast, sometimes termed the *"tail of Spence,"* extends laterally across the anterior axillary fold. Alternatively, findings can be localized as the time on the face of a clock (e.g., 3 o'clock) and the distance in centimeters from the nipple.

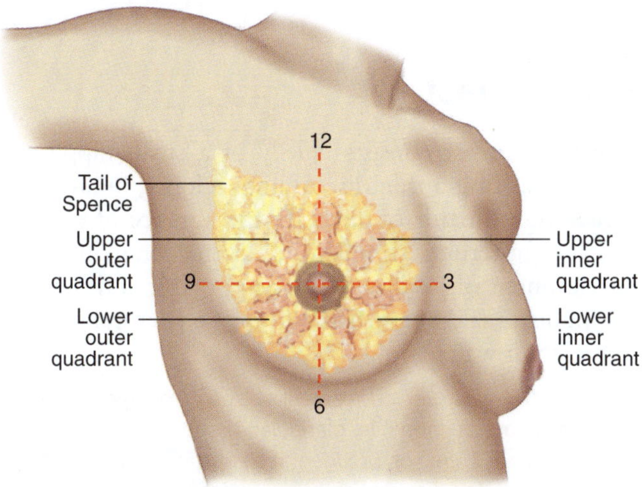

FIGURE 17-5. Breast quadrants and tail of Spence.

Physiology. The female breast is a hormonally sensitive tissue, responsive to the changes of monthly cycling and aging. The adult breast may be soft, but it often feels granular, nodular, or lumpy. This uneven texture is normal *physiologic nodularity.* It is often bilateral and may occur throughout the breast or only in some areas. The nodularity may increase before menses, a time when breasts often enlarge and become tender or even painful. In addition, the composition of the breast varies with age, nutritional status, pregnancy, exogenous hormone use, and other factors. After menopause, there is atrophy of glandular tissue, and a notable decrease in the number of lobules. For breast changes during adolescence and pregnancy, see p. 713 (Chapter 23, Children: Infancy through Adolescence) and p. 743 (Chapter 24, Pregnant Woman).

Both the nipple and the areola are supplied with smooth muscle that contracts to express milk from the ductal system during breastfeeding. Rich sensory innervation, especially in the nipple, triggers *milk letdown* following neurohormonal stimulation from infant sucking. Tactile stimulation of the area, including the breast examination, makes the nipple smaller, firmer, and more erect and causes the areola to pucker and wrinkle. These smooth muscle reflexes are normal and should not be mistaken for signs of breast disease.

Axilla

The axilla is a pyramidal structure defined by the axillary vein superiorly, the latissimus dorsi muscle laterally, and the serratus anterior muscle medially. Three important nerves course through the axilla; these include the thoracodorsal nerve, the long thoracic nerve, and the intercostobrachial nerve. The *thoracodorsal nerve* supplies the latissimus dorsi muscle, while the *long thoracic nerve* innervates the serratus anterior muscle. The *intercostobrachial nerve* is a sensory nerve that innervates the skin of the axilla and upper medial arm.

Male Breast

The male breast consists chiefly of a small nipple and areola overlying a thin disc of undeveloped breast tissue consisting primarily of ducts. In the absence of estrogen and progesterone stimulation, ductal branching and development of lobules are lacking, and it is difficult to distinguish male breast tissue from the pectoralis muscle of the chest wall.

Some men develop benign breast enlargement from **gynecomastia**, a proliferation of palpable glandular tissue generally defined as more than 2 cm, or *pseudogynecomastia*, an accumulation of subareolar fat. Causes of gynecomastia include increased estrogen, decreased testosterone, and medication side effects.

HEALTH HISTORY: GENERAL APPROACH

You can elicit concerns about the breasts during the history or later during the physical examination. Ask if the patient has had any *lumps, pain, or nipple discharge* of her breasts. These are the most common breast-related complaints. If a patient presents with a breast complaint, it is important to determine the nature and duration of the problem. If a patient reports a lump or pain, ask about the location within the breast, so that your examination can focus on this area. Always ask if the problem occurs, or is worse, at certain times of the menstrual cycle, since many benign breast complaints are related to hormonal changes. This may also be a good time to enhance her awareness of screening guidelines.

Common or Concerning Symptoms

- Breast lump or mass
- Breast discomfort or pain
- Nipple discharge

Breast Lump or Mass

Palpable lumps or nodularity and premenstrual enlargement and tenderness are common. If your patient reports a lump or mass, identify the precise location, how long it has been present, if there is any history of trauma, if it is tender, and if there has been any change in size or variation within the menstrual cycle. Ask if there has been any change in breast contour, dimpling, swelling, or puckering of the skin over the breasts. Also, ask about changes of the nipple including skin changes, itchiness, redness, or flakiness. Obtaining a family history of breast cancer and other cancers and additional risk factors, such as age at menarche, age at first birth, age at menopause, prior breast biopsies, and use of hormonal medications are also important.

Lumps may be physiologic or pathologic, ranging from cysts and fibroadenomas to breast cancer. See Table 17-1, Common Breast Masses, and Table 17-2, Visible Signs of Breast Cancer.

Breast Discomfort or Pain

Breast pain alone (**mastodynia** or **mastalgia**) is not typically a sign of breast cancer. Determine if the pain is *diffuse* (defined as involving >25% of the breast) or *focal* (involving <25% of the breast), *cyclic* (pain that occurs prior to menses and generally resolved at the completion of the menstrual period) or *noncyclic*, or related to medications.

Medications associated with breast pain include hormone replacement therapy; psychotropic drugs such as selective serotonin reuptake inhibitors; and haloperidol spironolactone, and digoxin.

Nipple Discharge

Ask about any discharge from the nipples and when it occurs. It is important to differentiate *physiologic discharge* from *pathologic discharge*. Physiologic hypersecretion is seen in pregnancy, lactation, chest wall stimulation, sleep, and stress. If the discharge is spontaneous, note its color, quantity, and frequency of occurrence.

Nipple discharge is more likely to be pathologic when it is bloody or serous, unilateral, spontaneous, associated with a mass, and occurring in women age ≥40 years. True *galactorrhea*, or the discharge of milk-containing fluid unrelated to pregnancy or lactation, is most commonly caused by hyperprolactinemia.

PHYSICAL EXAMINATION: GENERAL APPROACH

As in any examination, you should begin by taking a courteous, gentle approach. The best time for breast examination in a patient who is still menstruating is 5 to 7 days *after* the onset of menstruation because breasts tend to swell and become more nodular before menses from increasing estrogen stimulation. For postmenopausal women and for men, any time is appropriate. Nodules appearing during the premenstrual phase should be re-evaluated after the onset of menstruation.

Let patients know that an adequate breast examination, especially inspection, initially requires full exposure of both breasts. However, later in the examination, you may cover one breast while you are examining the other. It is also important to let patients know that you will be asking them to assume various positions to properly examine specific areas of the entire breast including the tail, periphery, and axilla. Warming hands under warm water or by rubbing together is also a nice gesture. It is advisable that you adopt a standardized approach, especially for palpation, and to use a systemic up-and-down search pattern, varying palpation pressure, and a circular motion with the fingerpads in the breast examination.

TECHNIQUES OF EXAMINATION

Key Components of the Breasts and Axillae Examination

In women:

- Inspect the breasts in four views: arms at sides, arms over head, arms pressed against hips, and leaning forward (skin appearance, size, symmetry, contour, nipple characteristics).
- Palpate the breasts (consistency, tenderness, nodules, nipple for color, consistency, and quantity of any discharge).
- Inspect the axillae (rash, irritation, infection, unusual pigmentation).
- Palpate the axillary nodes (size, shape, delimitation, mobility, consistency, and any tenderness).

In men:

- Inspect the nipple and areola (nodules, swelling, ulceration).
- Palpate the areola and breast tissue (nodules).

Female Breast

Inspection. Inspect the breasts and nipples with the patient in the sitting position and disrobed to the waist (Fig. 17-6). A thorough examination of the breasts includes careful inspection for skin changes, symmetry, contours, and retraction in four views—arms at sides, arms over head, arms pressed against hips, and leaning forward. When examining an adolescent girl, assess her breast development according to the Tanner sex maturity ratings (see Chapter 23, Children: Infancy through Adolescence).

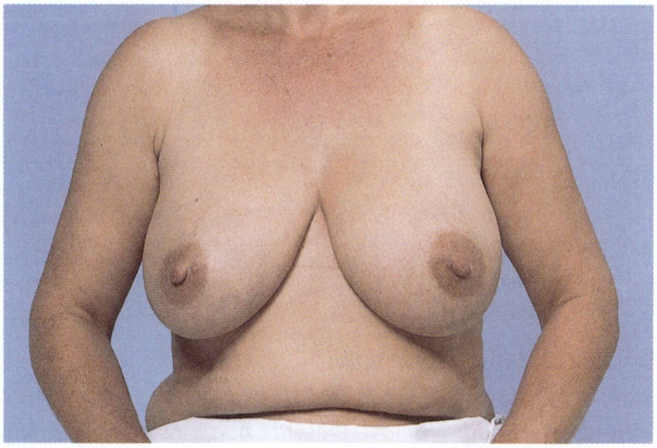

FIGURE 17-6. Inspection with arms at sides.

Arms at Sides. Note the clinical features listed below.

- *Appearance of the skin*, including:
  - Color

Redness suggests local infection or inflammatory carcinoma.

- Skin thickness and prominence of pores, which may accompany lymphatic obstruction.

  Thickening and prominent pores **(peau d'orange)** suggest breast cancer.

- *Size and symmetry of the breasts.* Some differences in the size of the breasts and areolae are common and usually normal.
- *Contour of the breasts.* Look for changes such as masses, dimpling, or flattening. Compare one side with the other.

  Flattening of the normally convex breast suggests cancer. See Table 17-2, Visible Signs of Breast Cancer.

- *Characteristics of the nipples.* Note size and shape, direction in which they point, any rashes or ulceration, or any discharge.

  Asymmetry due to change in nipple direction suggests an underlying cancer. Eczematous changes with rash, scaling, or ulceration on the nipple extending to the areola occurs in **Paget disease of the breast**, associated with underlying ductal or lobular carcinoma. (See Table 17-2, Visible Signs of Breast Cancer)

Occasionally, the nipple is ***inverted,*** or points inward, depressed below the areolar surface. It may be enveloped by folds of areolar skin, as shown in Figure 17-7, but can be moved out from its sulcus. It is usually a normal variant of no clinical consequence, except for possible difficulty when breastfeeding.

A nipple pulled inward, tethered by underlying ducts signals nipple retraction from a possible underlying cancer. The retracted nipple may be depressed, flat, broad, or thickened.

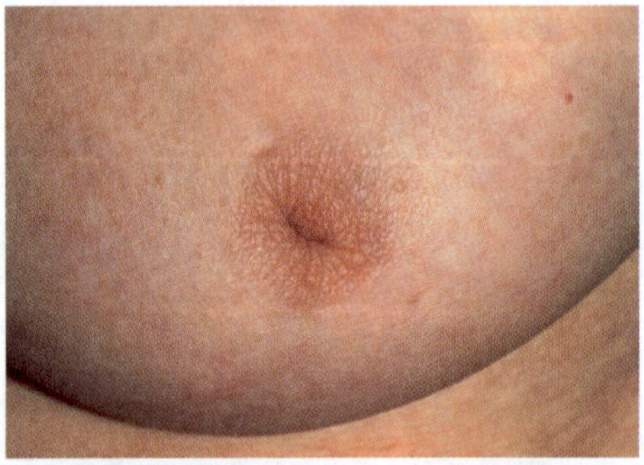

FIGURE 17-7. Inverted nipple.

Arms Over Head; Hands Pressed Against Hips; Leaning Forward. To bring out dimpling or retraction that may otherwise be invisible, ask the patient to raise her arms over her head (Fig. 17-8), then press her hands against her hips to contract the pectoral muscles (Fig. 17-9). Inspect the breast contours carefully in each position. If the breasts are large or pendulous, it may be useful to have the patient stand and lean forward (Fig. 17-10), supported by the back of the chair or the examiner's hands.

Breast dimpling or retraction in these positions suggests an underlying cancer. Cancers with fibrous strands attached to the skin and fascia over the pectoral muscles may cause inward dimpling of the skin during muscle contraction.

Occasionally, these signs accompany benign conditions such as posttraumatic fat necrosis or mammary duct ectasia but should always be further evaluated.

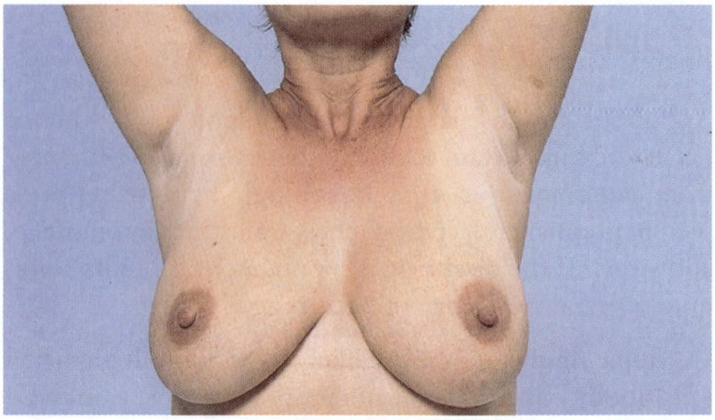

FIGURE 17-8. Inspection with arms overhead.

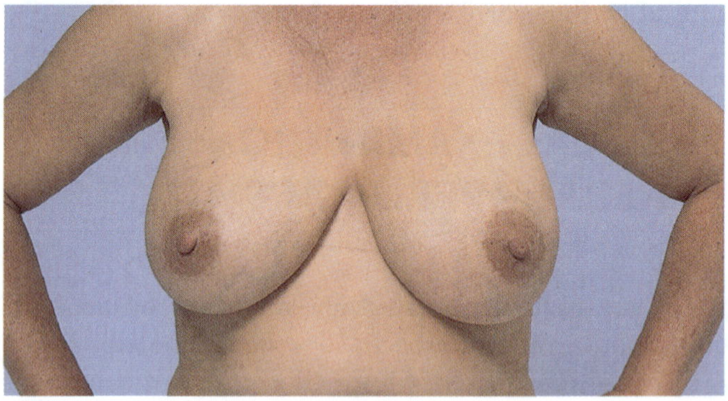

FIGURE 17-9. Inspection with hands pressed against hips.

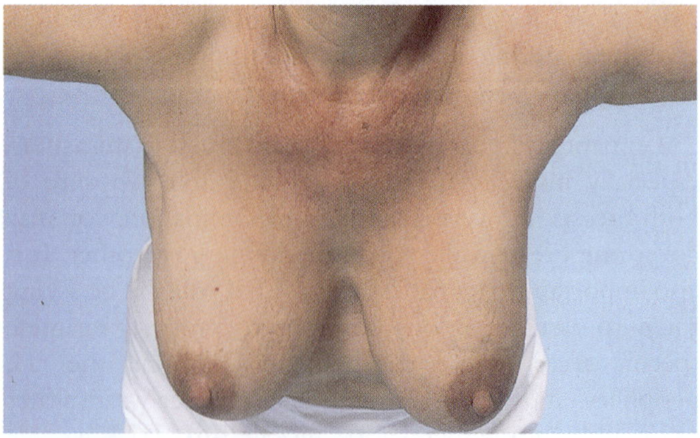

FIGURE 17-10. Inspection while leaning forward.

This position may reveal asymmetry or retraction of the breast, areola, or nipple that is not otherwise visible, suggesting an underlying cancer. (See Table 17-2, Visible Signs of Breast Cancer.)

Palpation. Palpation is best performed with the patient supine, thus flattening the breast tissue. Palpate the rectangular area extending from the clavicle to the inframammary fold or bra line and from the midsternal line to the posterior axillary line and well into the axilla to ensure that you examine the tail of the breast.

A thorough examination takes at least 3 minutes for each breast. Use the *pads* of the second, third, and fourth fingers, keeping the fingers slightly flexed. It is important to be *systematic*. The *vertical strip pattern* shown in Figure 17-11 is currently the best validated technique for detecting breast masses. Palpate in *small, concentric circles* applying light, medium, and deep pressure at each examining point. Press more firmly to reach the deeper tissues of a large breast. Examine the entire breast, including the periphery, tail, and axilla.

When pressing deeply on the breast, a normal rib can be mistaken for a hard breast mass.

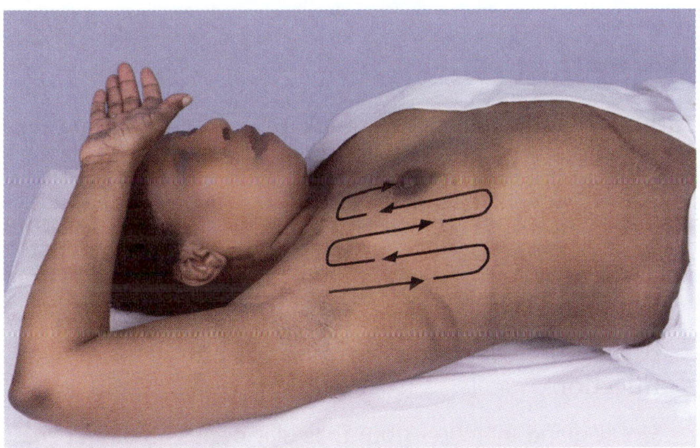

FIGURE 17-11. Vertical strip pattern, lateral breast.

Palpating the Lateral Breast. To examine *the lateral portion of the breast,* ask the patient to roll onto the opposite hip, placing her hand on her forehead but keeping the shoulders pressed against the bed or examining table. This flattens the lateral breast tissue. Begin palpation in the axilla, moving in a straight line down to the bra line, then move the fingers medially and palpate in a vertical strip up the chest to the clavicle. Continue in vertical overlapping strips until you reach the nipple, then reposition the patient to flatten the medial portion of the breast.

Nodules in the tail of the breast in the axilla (the tail of Spence) are sometimes mistaken for enlarged axillary lymph nodes.

Palpating the Medial Breast. To examine *the medial portion of the breast,* ask the patient to lie with her shoulders flat against the examining table, and then slide up her flexed elbow until it is at the level of her shoulder (Fig. 17-12). Palpate in a straight line down from the nipple to the bra line, then back to the clavicle, continuing in vertical overlapping strips to the midsternum.

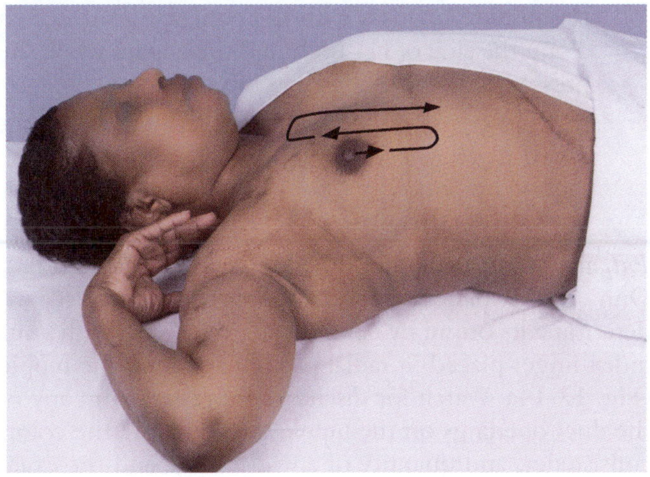

FIGURE 17-12. Vertical strip pattern, medial breast.

Examine the breast tissue carefully for:

- *Consistency of the tissues.* Normal consistency varies widely, depending on the proportions of firmer glandular tissue and soft fat. Physiologic nodularity may be present, increasing before menses. Note the firm inframammary ridge, which is the transverse ridge of compressed tissue along the lower margin of the breast, especially in large breasts. This ridge is sometimes mistaken for a tumor.

  Tender subareolar cords suggest mammary duct ectasia, a benign but sometimes painful condition of dilated ducts with surrounding inflammation and, at times, with associated masses.

- *Tenderness* that may occur prior to menses.

  Check for cysts and inflamed areas; some cancers may be tender.

- *Nodules.* Palpate carefully for any lump or mass that is qualitatively different from or larger than the rest of the breast tissue. This is sometimes called a dominant mass that may be pathologic when evaluated by mammogram, aspiration, or biopsy. Assess and describe the characteristics of any nodule:

  See Table 17-1, Common Breast Masses.

  - *Location*—by quadrant or clock, with centimeters from the nipple
  - *Size*—in centimeters
  - *Shape*—round or cystic, disc-like, or irregular in contour
  - *Consistency*—soft, firm, or hard
  - *Delimitation*—well circumscribed or not

  Hard irregular poorly circumscribed nodules, fixed to the skin or underlying tissues, strongly suggest cancer.

- *Tenderness*
- *Mobility*—in relation to the skin, pectoral fascia, and chest wall. Gently move the breast near the mass and watch for dimpling. Next, try to move the nodule or mass with the patient's arm relaxed along the side of her body and then again while she presses her hand against her hip.

A mobile mass that becomes fixed when the arm relaxes is attached to the ribs and intercostal muscles; if fixed when the hand is pressed against the hip, it is attached to the pectoral fascia.

Palpate each nipple, noting its elasticity (Fig. 17-13). Only if the patient reports nipple discharge, try to determine its origin by compressing the areola with your index finger placed in radial positions around the nipple (Fig. 17-14). Watch for discharge expressed from any of the duct openings on the nipple surface. Note the color, consistency, and quantity of any discharge and the exact location(s) where it appears.

Thickening of the nipple and loss of elasticity suggest an underlying cancer.

Milky discharge unrelated to a prior pregnancy and lactation is nonpuerperal **galactorrhea.** Causes include hyperthyroidism, pituitary prolactinoma, and dopamine antagonists, including psychotropics and phenothiazines.

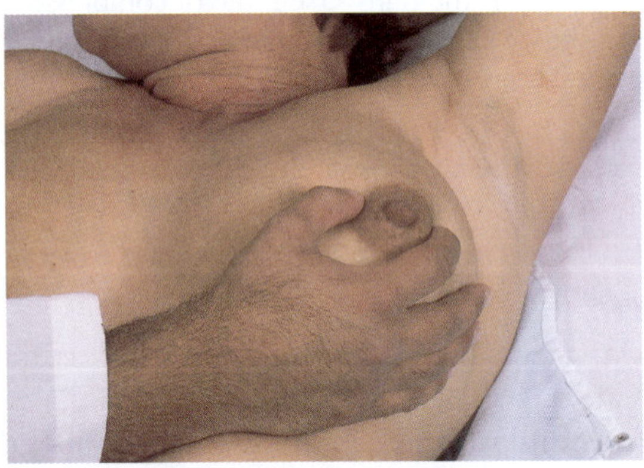

FIGURE 17-13. Palpating the nipple.

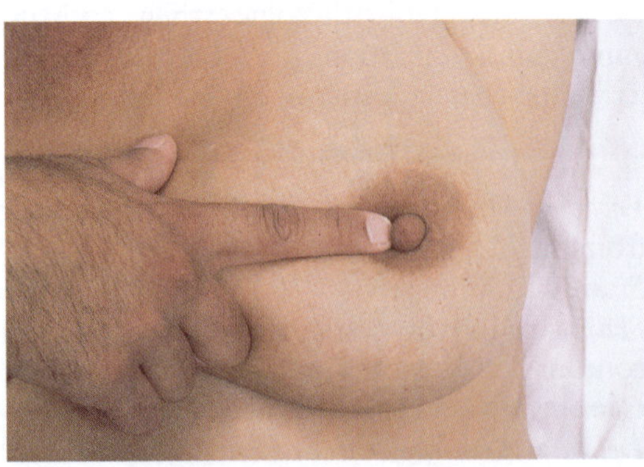

FIGURE 17-14. Compressing the areola for nipple discharge.

Spontaneous unilateral bloody discharge from one or two ducts warrants further evaluation for intraductal papilloma, shown in Figure 17-15, ductal carcinoma in situ, or Paget disease of the breast. Clear, serous, green, black, or nonbloody discharges that are multiductal are usually benign.

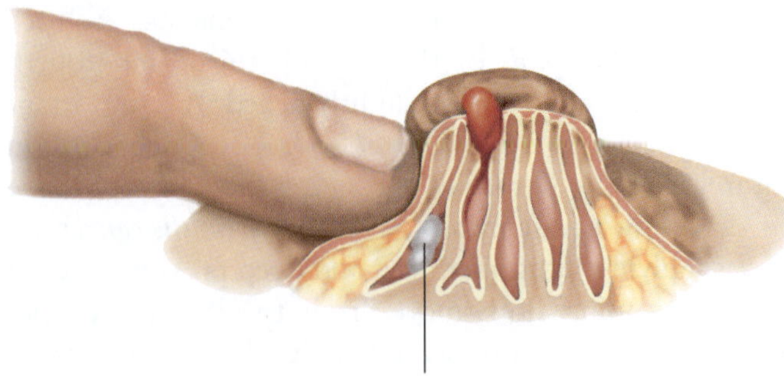

FIGURE 17-15. Intraductal papilloma.

Axillae

Although the axillae may be examined with the patient lying down, a sitting position is preferable.

Inspection. Inspect the skin of each axilla, noting evidence of:

- Rash
- Irritation
- Infection

Sweat gland infection from follicular occlusion (*hidradenitis suppurativa*) may be present.

- Unusual pigmentation

Deeply pigmented velvety axillary skin suggests **acanthosis nigricans**—associated with diabetes; obesity; polycystic ovary syndrome; and, rarely, malignant paraneoplastic disorders.

Palpation

Axillae. See Chapter 8, Lymph Nodes in General Examination.

Male Breast

Examination of the male breast may be brief but is important. *Inspect the nipple and areola* for nodules, swelling, or ulceration. *Palpate the areola and breast tissue* for nodules. If the breast appears enlarged (>2 cm), distinguish between the soft fatty enlargement of obesity (*pseudogynecomastia*) and the benign firm disc of glandular enlargement (*gynecomastia*). Breast tissue in gynecomastia is often tender.

Gynecomastia arises from an imbalance of estrogens and androgens, sometimes drug related; it is not a risk factor for male breast cancer. A hard, irregular, eccentric, or ulcerating painless dominant mass suggests breast cancer.

SPECIAL TECHNIQUES

Examination After Mastectomy or Breast Reconstruction

The woman with a mastectomy warrants special care on examination.

Inspection. Inspect the mastectomy scar and axilla carefully for any masses, unusual nodularity, or signs of inflammation or infection. Lymphedema may be present in the axilla and upper arm from lymph drainage interrupted by surgery.

Masses, nodularity, and change in color or inflammation, especially in the incision line, suggest recurrence of breast cancer.

Palpation. Palpate gently along the scar—these tissues may be unusually sensitive or numb. Palpate the breast tissue and incision lines bordering the breast augmentation or reconstruction areas. Use a circular motion with two or three fingers. Pay special attention to the upper outer quadrant and axilla. Note any enlarged lymph nodes.

RECORDING YOUR FINDINGS

Note that initially you may use sentences to describe your findings; later you will use phrases.

Recording the Breasts and Axillae Examination

"Breasts symmetric and smooth without nodules or masses. Nipples without discharge." (Axillary adenopathy usually included in section on Lymph Nodes in General Examination.)

OR

"Breasts pendulous with diffuse fibrocystic changes. Single firm 1 × 1 cm mass, mobile, and nontender, with overlying peau d'orange appearance in right breast, upper outer quadrant at 11 o'clock, 2 cm from the nipple."

These findings suggest possible breast cancer.

HEALTH PROMOTION AND COUNSELING: EVIDENCE AND RECOMMENDATIONS

Important Topics for Health Promotion and Counseling

- Breast cancer screening

Breast Cancer in Women

Breast cancer is the most commonly diagnosed cancer in the world and the leading cause of cancer death among women. About 80% of new breast cancer diagnoses occur after age 50, with a median age at diagnosis of 62. The probability of being diagnosed with breast cancer increases with age (Box 17-1).

Box 17-1. Probability of Developing Invasive Female Breast Cancer by Age Intervals[a]

Current Age (years)	10-Year Probability (%)
20	0.1 (1 in 1,567)
30	0.5 (1 in 220)
40	1.5 (1 in 68)
50	2.3 (1 in 43)
60	3.4 (1 in 29)
70	3.9 (1 in 25)
Lifetime Risk	12.4 (1 in 8)

[a]Probability is for women who are breast cancer free at the beginning of the age interval.

The strongest risk factors for breast cancer in women are increasing age, first-degree family members diagnosed with breast cancer (especially two or more diagnosed at an early age), inherited genetic mutations, personal history of breast cancer or ductal or lobular carcinoma in situ, biopsy-confirmed precancerous lesions, relatively denser breasts on mammography, high-dose radiation to the chest at a young age, and high levels of endogenous hormones.

A number of breast cancer risk assessment tools can be used to help women determine their personal risk of developing breast cancer (Box 17-2). One of the most commonly used tools is the National Cancer Institute's Breast Cancer Risk Assessment Tool (also known as the

Gail model), which incorporates age, race/ethnicity, personal history of breast cancer or ductal or lobular carcinoma in situ, chest radiation, genetic mutations, first-degree relatives with breast cancer, previous breast biopsy results, age at menarche, and age at first delivery.

Box 17-2. Calculators for Assessing Risk of Breast Cancer

- Gail model: http://www.cancer.gov/bcrisktool/
- Centers for Disease Control and Prevention Division of Cancer Prevention and Control—Know BRCA Tool: https://www.knowbrca.org/

Healthy behaviors that may reduce breast cancer risk include physical activity, consuming diets high in fruits and vegetables, and limiting alcohol. The U.S. Preventive Services Task Force (USPSTF) issued a grade B recommendation for using a risk tool to screen women for BRCA gene mutations if they have a family history of breast, ovarian, tubal, or peritoneal cancers. BRCA gene mutations account for up to 10% of all breast cancers. Women who screen positive should be referred to genetic counselors and considered for BRCA testing. Women with BRCA mutations can consider more intensive screening strategies (see below) and prophylactic bilateral mastectomy or chemoprophylaxis to prevent breast cancer. Women at high risk for breast cancer can also take selective estrogen-receptor modulators (SERMs), such as tamoxifen and raloxifene, which are used to treat breast cancers, to reduce their risk of developing invasive breast cancer. However, taking SERMs also increases the risks of thromboembolic events and endometrial cancer. Aromatase inhibitors are another class of breast cancer treatment medications that have been shown effective for preventing breast cancer in high-risk postmenopausal women, but their use is not currently approved by the U.S. Food and Drug Administration for this indication.

Recommendations for breast cancer screening vary based on a women's age and risk for breast cancer. Mammography is the primary screening modality for breast cancer. Concerning findings on mammography may be further evaluated with special mammographic views, breast ultrasound, magnetic resonance imaging (MRI), or digital breast tomosynthesis (DBT). Box 17-3 shows that the greatest mortality benefits are for women in their 60s, while women in their 40s are most likely to have false-positive results.

Box 17-4 shows the breast cancer screening recommendations for mammography, clinical breast examination, and breast self-examination issued by the USPSTF, the American Cancer Society, and the American College of Obstetricians and Gynecologists. Providers may want to perform clinical breast examinations or instruct women on performing breast self-exams when women are at very high risk for breast cancer. Breast self-examination, in combination with education efforts to address breast cancer, may also be advisable for women in limited-resource settings.

Evidence guiding screening practices for higher-risk women is limited. Experts suggest that women with moderately increased risk due to increased breast density or a family history of one or two relatives with breast cancer could reasonably consider beginning screening at an earlier age, screening annually, and screening with DBT. Women at very high risk due to genetic mutations are recommended to undergo annual screening beginning 10 years before the youngest family member was diagnosed (though not before age 30) using mammography and MRI. Women who received thoracic radiation are advised to begin annual screening with mammography and MRI 10 years after completing radiation, but not before age 30.

Box 17-3. Benefits and Harms of Screening Mammography by Age Ranges, Average-Risk Women

Age Group (Years)	Breast Cancer Mortality: Relative Risk (95% CI)	Deaths Prevented over 10 Yrs (95% CI)[a]	False-Positive Test Results (*n*)[a]	Breast Biopsies (*n*)[a]
40–49	0.92 (0.75–1.02)	3 (0–9)	1,212	164
50–59	0.86 (0.68–0.97)	8 (2–17)	932	159
60–69	0.67 (0.51–1.28)	21 (11–32)	808	165
70–74	0.80 (0.51–1.28)	13 (0–32)	696	175
50–69	0.78 (0.68–0.95)	13 (6–20)	—	—

[a]Per 10,000 women screened for 10 yrs.

Source: Adapted from Nelson HD et al. *Ann Intern Med.* 2016;164:244–255; Nelson HD... et al. *Ann Intern Med.* 2016;164:256–267.

Box 17-4. Recommendations for Breast Cancer Screening in Average-Risk Women

Organization	Mammography	Clinical Breast Examination	Breast Self-Examination
U.S. Preventive Services Task Force—average-risk women	50–74 yrs—biennially <50 yrs—individualize screening based on patient specific factors ≥75 yrs—insufficient evidence to assess the balance of benefits and harms	Insufficient evidence to assess the additional benefits and harms beyond screening mammography	Recommends against teaching breast self-examination, supports breast self-awareness
American Cancer Society—average-risk women (2015)	40–45 yrs—optional annual screening 45–54 yrs—annual screening ≥55 yrs—biennial screening with option to continue annual screens Continue screening if good health and life expectancy ≥10 yrs	Not recommended	Not recommended; encourages breast self-awareness
American College of Obstetricians and Gynecologists	Offer screening starting at age 40 yrs Screening should be every 1 or 2 yrs based on a shared decision-making process Continue screening until at least age 75	May be offered in context of a shared decision-making process every 1–3 yrs for women aged 25–39 yrs and annually for women 40 yrs and older	Not recommended, but women should be counseled about breast self-awareness

Sources: Siu AL, U.S. Preventive Services Task Force. *Ann Intern Med*. 2016;164:279–296; Oeffinger KC… et al. *JAMA*. 2015;314:1599–1614; *Obstet Gynecol*…. 2017;130:241–243.

MALE BREAST CANCER

Men are more likely to present at advanced stage than women because the diagnosis is often not suspected, and screening is not recommended for men. Risk factors include increasing age, radiation exposure, BRCA gene mutations, Klinefelter syndrome, testicular disorders, alcohol use, liver disease, diabetes, and obesity.

TABLE 17-1. Common Breast Masses

The three most common breast masses are *fibroadenoma* (a benign tumor), *cysts,* and *breast cancer.* The clinical characteristics of these masses are listed below. However, any breast mass should be carefully evaluated and usually warrants further investigation by ultrasound, aspiration, mammography, or biopsy.

The masses depicted below are large for purposes of illustration. *Fibrocystic changes,* not illustrated, are also commonly palpable as nodular, rope-like densities in women aged 25–50 yrs. They may be tender or painful. They are considered benign and not a risk factor for breast cancer.

	Fibroadenoma	Cysts	Cancer
	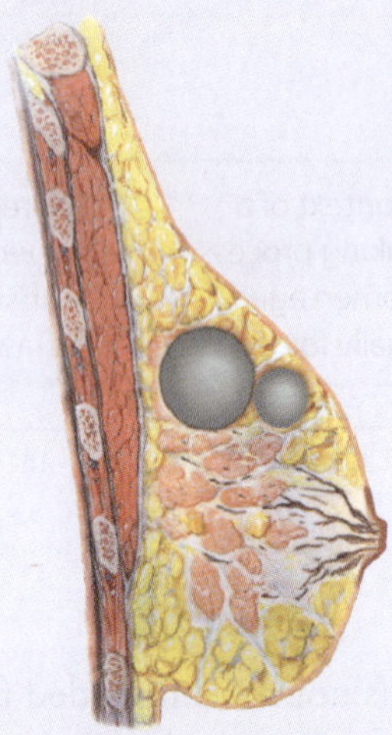	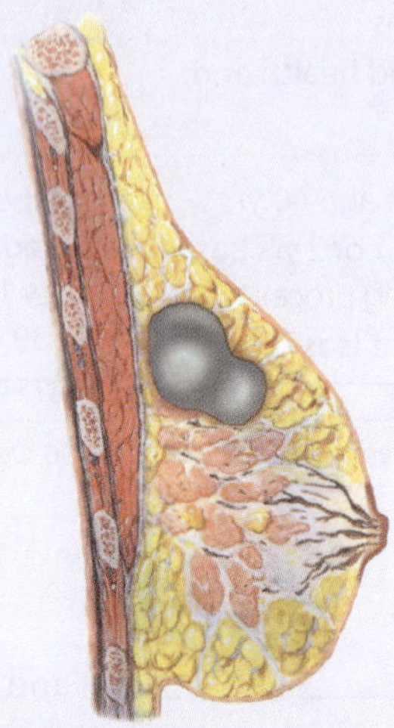	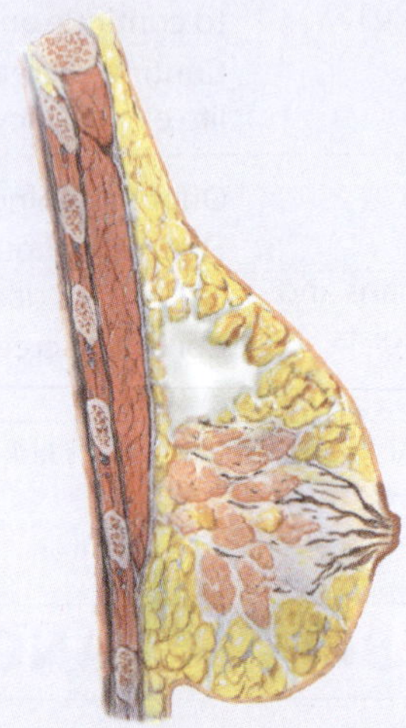
Usual Age (in Years)	15–25 yrs, usually puberty and young adulthood, but up to age 55 yrs	30–50 yrs, regress after menopause except with estrogen therapy	30–90 yrs, most common over age 50 yrs
Number	Usually single, may be multiple	Single or multiple	Usually single, although may coexist with other nodules
Shape	Round, disc-like, or lobular; typically small (1–2 cm)	Round	Irregular or stellate
Consistency	May be soft, usually firm	Soft to firm, usually elastic	Firm or hard
Delimitation	Well delineated	Well delineated	Not clearly delineated from surrounding tissues
Mobility	Very mobile	Mobile	May be fixed to skin or underlying tissues
Tenderness	Usually nontender	Often tender	Usually nontender
Retraction Signs	Absent	Absent	May be present

TABLE 17-2. Visible Signs of Breast Cancer

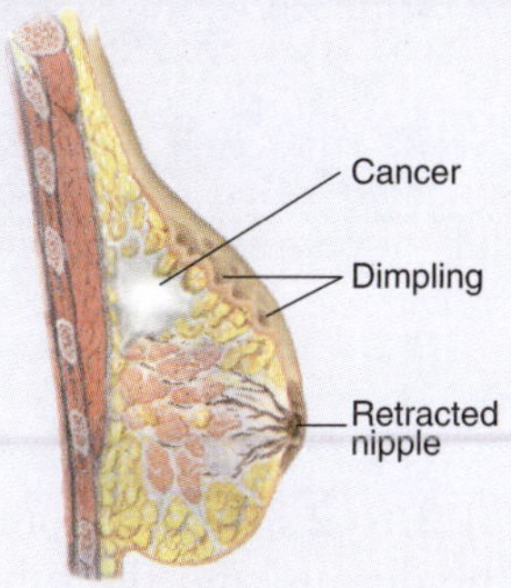

Retraction Signs

As breast cancer advances, it causes fibrosis (scar tissue). Shortening of this tissue produces *dimpling, changes in contour,* and *retraction or deviation of the nipple.* Other causes of retraction include fat necrosis and mammary duct ectasia.

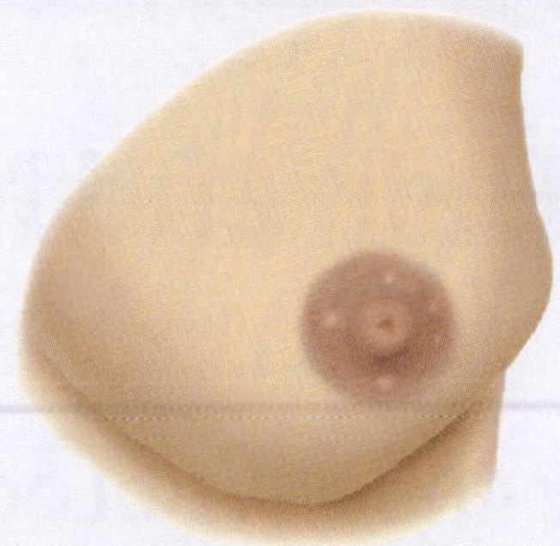

Abnormal Contours

Look for any variation in the normal convexity of each breast and compare one side with the other. Special positioning may again be useful. Shown here is marked flattening of the lower outer quadrant of the left breast.

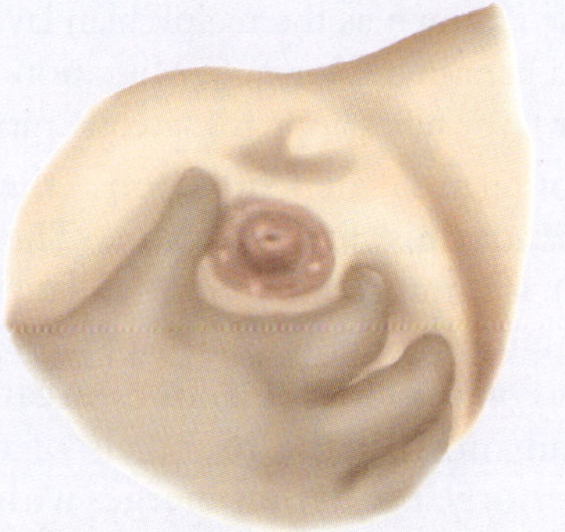

Skin Dimpling

Look for this sign with the patient's arm at rest, during special positioning, and on moving or compressing the breast, as illustrated here.

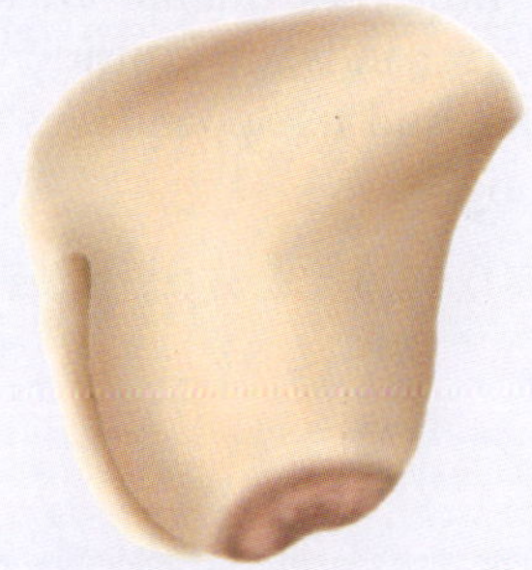

Nipple Retraction and Deviation

A retracted nipple is flattened or pulled inward, as illustrated here. It may also be broadened and feels thickened. When involvement is radially asymmetric, the nipple may deviate or point in a different direction from its normal counterpart, typically toward the underlying cancer.

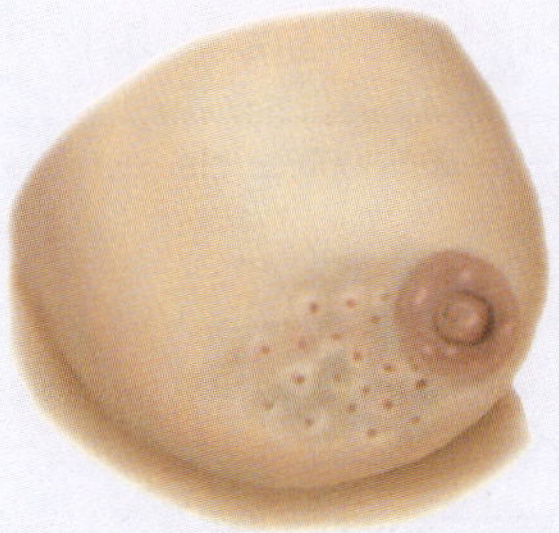

Edema of the Skin

Edema of the skin is produced by lymphatic blockade. It appears as thickened skin with enlarged pores—the so-called *peau d'orange* (orange peel) *sign.* It is often seen first in the lower portion of the breast or areola.

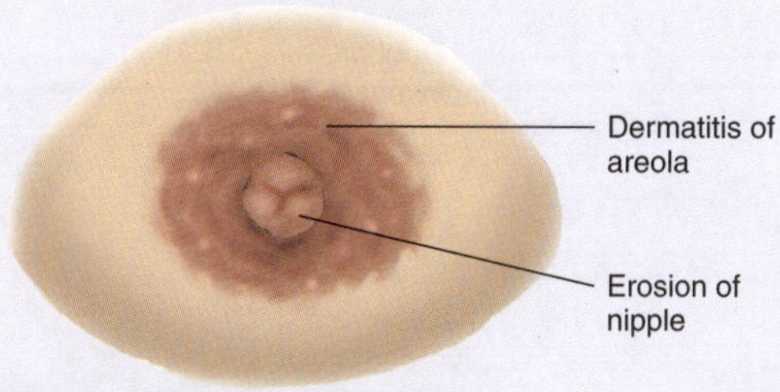

Paget Disease of the Nipple

This uncommon form of breast cancer usually starts as a scaly, eczema-like lesion on the nipple that may weep, crust, or erode. A breast mass may be present. Suspect Paget disease in any persisting dermatitis of the nipple and areola. Often (>60%) presents with an underlying in situ or invasive ductal or lobular carcinoma.

CHAPTER

18

Skin, Hair, and Nails

ANATOMY AND PHYSIOLOGY

The skin keeps the body in homeostasis despite daily assaults from the environment. It retains body fluids while protecting underlying tissues from microorganisms, harmful substances, and radiation. It modulates body temperature and synthesizes vitamin D. Hair, nails, and sebaceous and sweat glands are considered appendages of the skin. The skin and its appendages undergo many changes during aging.

See Chapter 25, Older Adult, p. 764, to review skin changes with aging.

Skin

The skin is the heaviest single organ of the body, accounting for approximately 16% of body weight and covering an area of roughly 1.2 to $2.3/m^2$. It contains three layers: the epidermis, the dermis, and the subcutaneous tissues (Fig. 18-1).

The most superficial layer, the **epidermis,** is a thin avascular keratinized epithelium consisting of two layers: an outer horny *stratum corneum* of dead keratinized cells and an inner cellular layer, the *stratum basale* and the *stratum spinosum,* also known as the malpighian layer, where both melanin and keratin are formed. Migration from the inner to the outer layer takes approximately 1 month.

The epidermis depends on the underlying vascularized dermis for nutrition. The **dermis** is a dense layer of interconnecting collagen and elastic fibers containing epidermal appendages such as *pilosebaceous glands* (oil glands), sweat glands, hair follicles, and most of the terminals of the cutaneous nerves. Inferiorly, the dermis merges with *subcutaneous* fatty tissue, or *adipose* tissue.

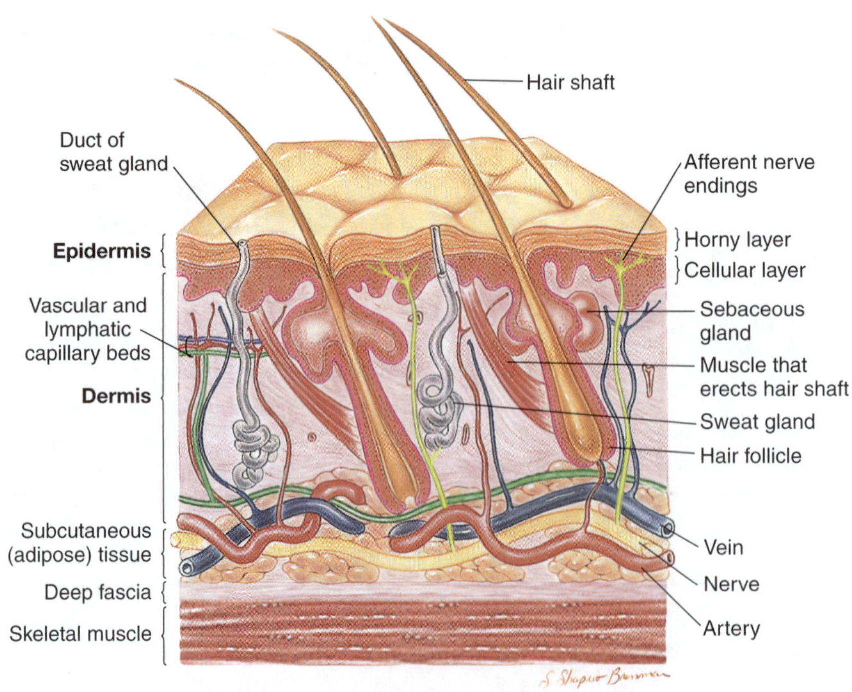

FIGURE 18-1. Structure of skin and subcutaneous tissue.

Normal skin color depends on the amount and type of melanin but is also influenced by underlying vascular structures, changing hemodynamics, and changes in carotene and bilirubin.

The amount of *melanin,* a brownish pigment, is genetically determined and increased by exposure to sunlight. Hemoglobin in the red blood cells transports oxygen in the form of *oxyhemoglobin,* a bright red pigment in the arteries and capillaries that causes reddening of the skin. After passing through the capillary bed and releasing oxygen to the tissues, the darker bluer pigment of *deoxyhemoglobin* circulates in the veins. The scattering of light through the turbid superficial layers of the skin or blood vessels also makes the veins look bluer and less red than circulating venous blood.

Pallor indicates anemia.

Cyanosis, a blue color, can indicate decreased oxygen in the blood or decreased blood flow in response to a cold environment.

Carotene, a yellow pigment, is found in the subcutaneous fat and heavily keratinized areas such as the palms and soles. *Bilirubin,* a yellow-brown pigment, arises from the breakdown of heme in the red blood cells.

Jaundice, or yellowing of the skin, results from increased bilirubin.

Hair

Adults have two types of hair: **vellus hair,** which is short, fine, inconspicuous, and relatively unpigmented, and **terminal hair**, which is coarser, thicker, more conspicuous, and usually pigmented. Scalp hair and eyebrows are examples of terminal hair.

Nails

Nails protect the distal ends of the fingers and toes. The firm rectangular and usually curving *nail plate* gets its pink color from the vascular *nail bed* to which the plate is firmly attached (Figs. 18-2 and 18-3). Note the whitish moon, or *lunula,* and the free edge of the nail plate. Roughly one-fourth of the nail plate, the *nail root,* is covered by the proximal nail fold. The **cuticle** extends from the fold and, functioning as a seal, protects the space between the fold and the plate from external moisture. *Lateral nail folds* cover the sides of the nail plate. Note that the angle between the proximal nail fold and nail plate is normally less than 180 degrees.

Fingernails grow approximately 0.1 mm daily; toenails grow more slowly.

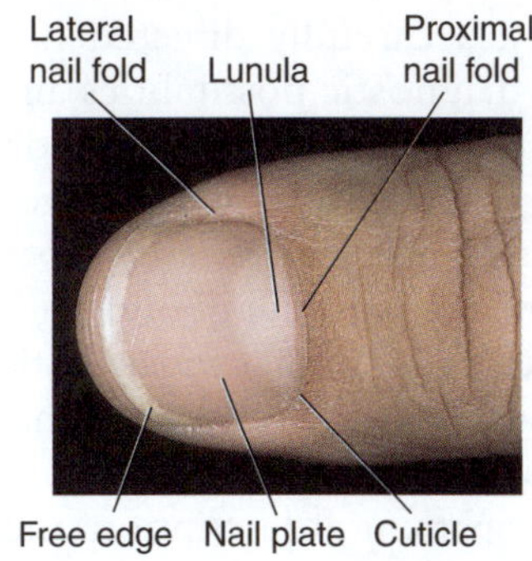

FIGURE 18-2. Surface structures of the fingernail.

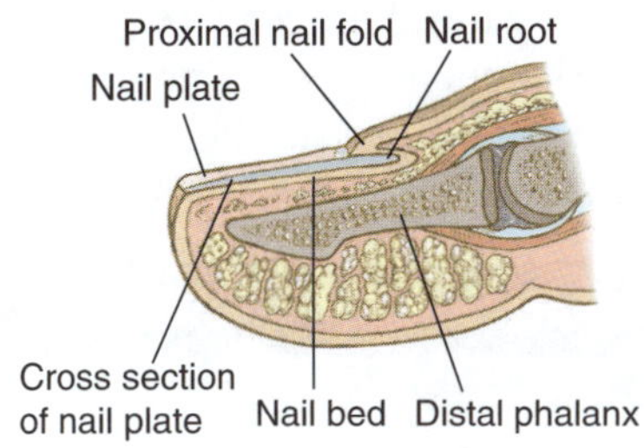

FIGURE 18-3. Cross-section of fingertip.

Pilosebaceous Glands and Sweat Glands

Pilosebaceous glands (*oil glands*) produce a fatty substance secreted onto the skin surface through the hair follicles. These glands are present on all skin surfaces except the palms and soles.

Sweat glands are of two types: eccrine and apocrine. The **eccrine sweat glands** are widely distributed, open directly onto the skin surface, and help to control body temperature by their sweat production. In contrast, the **apocrine sweat glands** are found chiefly in the axillary and genital regions and usually open into hair follicles. Bacterial decomposition of apocrine sweat is responsible for adult body odor.

HEALTH HISTORY: GENERAL APPROACH

As with any other system in the body, the diagnosis of skin diseases involves a thorough history and examination. Understanding symptoms that accompany skin lesions such as itching or pain may help in the clinical diagnosis. Since clinical diagnosis is paramount in dermatology, a carefully directed history will help you refine the diagnostic possibilities and may assist in identifying further investigations or address issues that may be important for optimal management. Certain relevant aspects of skin disease processes such as duration, evolution, periodicity, and prior episodes of a similar type are often familiar to the patient; therefore, a careful interview to obtain this information is critical. Similarly, if lesions are not visible, then diagnosis may depend on the patient's description and recollection. It is also important to obtain the patient's medical history since a number of systemic diseases may have cutaneous features and manifestations. Any exposures related during a careful history (e.g., dietary items, cosmetics, work chemicals, sunlight, medications, foreign travel) may potentially be important causes of dermatologic diseases.

Common or Concerning Symptoms

- Lesions
- Rashes and itching (pruritus)
- Hair loss and nail changes

Lesions

A **lesion** is any single area of altered skin. It may be solitary or multiple. Look for lesions suggesting melanoma, basal cell carcinoma (BCC), or squamous cell carcinoma (SCC) throughout the skin examination regardless of the patient's skin color. Detecting skin cancer at an early stage can increase the likelihood of successful treatment. Start by asking if the patient is concerned about any new lesions: "Have you noticed any changes in your skin? . . . your hair? . . . your nails?" "Have you had any growths? . . . sores? . . . lumps?" If the patient reports a new lesion, it is important to pursue the patient's personal and family history of skin cancer. Note the type, location, and date of any past skin cancer and ask about regular self-skin examination and use of sunscreen. Also ask "Has anyone in your family had a skin cancer removed? If so, who? Do you know what type of skin cancer—BCC, SCC, or melanoma?" Document the response even if the patient does not know which type and counsel the patient about skin cancer prevention.

Rashes and Itching (Pruritus)

A **rash** is a widespread eruption of lesions. For complaints of rash, ask about itching (*pruritus*), the most important symptom when assessing rashes. Does itching precede the rash or follow the rash? For itchy rashes, ask about seasonal allergies with itching and watery eyes, asthma, and atopic dermatitis, often accompanied by rash on the inside of the elbows and knees in childhood. Can the patient sleep all night or does itching wake up the patient? For rashes, it is important to find out what type of moisturizer or over-the-counter products have been applied.

Causes of generalized itching, without apparent rash, include dry skin; pregnancy; uremia; jaundice; lymphomas and leukemia; drug reactions; and, less commonly, polycythemia vera and thyroid disease.

Also ask about dry skin, which can cause itching and rash, especially in children with atopic dermatitis and older adults, due to loss of the natural moisture barrier in the epidermis.

Encourage use of moisturizers to replace the lost moisture barrier.

Hair Loss and Nail Changes

Patients often report hair loss or nail changes spontaneously. For *hair loss*, ask if hair is thinning or shedding and, if so, where. If shedding, does the hair come out at the roots or break along the hair shafts? Ask about hair care practices like frequency of shampooing and use of dyes, chemical relaxers, or heating appliances. See Table 18-8, for normal patterns of hair loss in men and women and counsel affected patients appropriately.

Be familiar with common nail changes such as onychomycosis, habit tic deformity, and melanonychia, shown in Table 18-9.

The most common causes of diffuse hair thinning are male and female pattern baldness.

Hair shedding at the roots is common in telogen effluvium and alopecia areata. Hair breaks along the shaft suggest damage from hair care or tinea capitis.

DESCRIBING SKIN LESIONS

It is important to use specific terminology to describe skin lesions and rashes. Good descriptions include each of the following elements: number, size, color, shape, texture, primary lesion, location, and configuration.

For example, for seborrheic keratosis, examine this record: "Multiple 5-mm to 2-cm tan to brown, oval, stuck-on, flat-topped verrucous plaques on the back and abdomen, following skin tension lines." Note the description of each element: *number*, multiple; *size*, 5 mm to 2 cm; *color*, tan to brown; *shape*, oval; *texture*, flat-topped verrucous; *primary lesion*, plaques; *location*, on the back and abdomen; and *configuration*, following skin tension lines.

When screening moles for melanomas, clinicians often describe these lesions using the ABCDE-EFG method (*see* Box 18-4 and Table 18-6). A lesion is described as it relates to its: **A**symmetry (of one side of mole compared to the other); **B**order irregularity especially if ragged, notched, or blurred; **C**olor variations (more than two colors, especially blue-black, white, or red); **D**iameter >6 mm; **E**volving or changing rapidly in size, symptoms, or morphology; **E**levation; **F**irmness to palpation and; progressive **G**rowing over several weeks.

Review the ABCDE-EFG method and photographs in Box 18-4, and Table 18-6, Brown Lesions: Melanoma and Its Mimics, which provide additional helpful identifiers and comparisons of benign brown lesions with melanoma (Fig. 18-4).

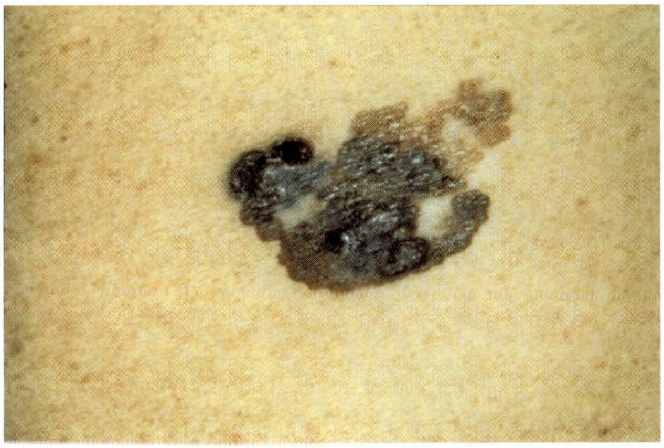

FIGURE 18-4. Melanoma with all the classic features of the ABCD method: **A**symmetry, **B**order irregularity, **C**olor variation, and **D**iameter >6 mm. (From DeVita VT, et al. *DeVita, Hellman, and Rosenberg's Cancer: Principles & Practice of Oncology*. 11th ed. Wolters Kluwer; 2019, Fig. 92.3, part c.)

Primary Lesion

Primary skin lesions are those that develop as a direct result of, and therefore are most characteristic of, the disease process. Review the descriptions of these primary lesions so you can identify these in your patients (Figs. 18-5 to 18-13). Primary lesions are flat, raised, or fluid filled.

See Table 18-1, Describing Primary Skin Lesions: Flat, Raised, and Fluid-Filled; Table 18-2, Additional Primary Lesions: Pustules, Furuncles, Nodules, Cysts, Wheals, Burrows; and Table 18-3, Dermatology Safari: Benign Skin Lesions. See Table 18-7, Vascular and Purpuric Lesions of the Skin.

A **macule** is a circumscribed flat area of change in color of the skin <1 cm in diameter.

Examples include freckles, flat moles, and port-wine stains and the rashes of rickettsial infections, rubella, and measles.

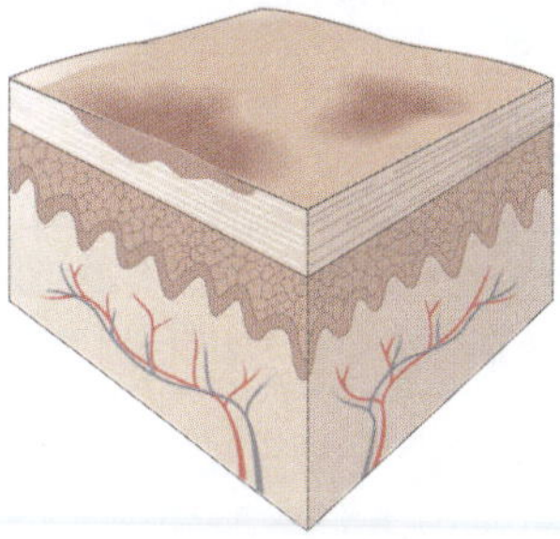

FIGURE 18-5. Macule. (Modified from Kronenberger J, Ledbetter J. *Lippincott Williams & Wilkins' Comprehensive Medical Assisting*. 5th ed. Wolters Kluwer; 2016; Fig. 28-2.)

A **patch** is a circumscribed flat area of change in color of the skin >1 cm in diameter.

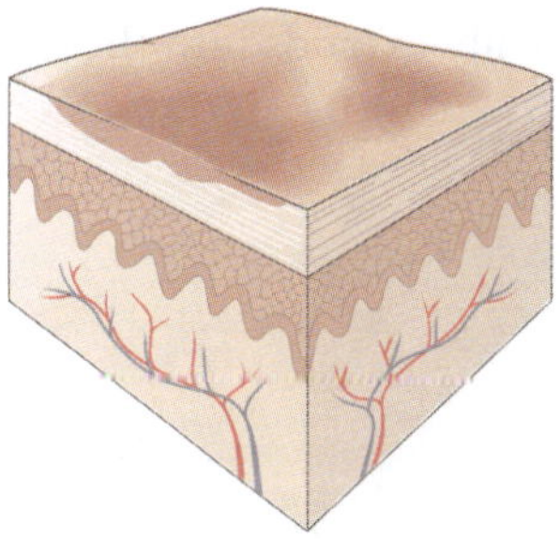

FIGURE 18-6. Patch. (Modified from Kronenberger J, Ledbetter J. *Lippincott Williams & Wilkins' Comprehensive Medical Assisting*. 5th ed. Wolters Kluwer; 2016, Fig. 28-2.)

A **papule** is a small solid elevation of the skin <1 cm in diameter.

Examples include nevi, warts, lichen planus, insect bites, seborrheic keratoses, actinic keratoses, some lesions of acne, and skin cancers.

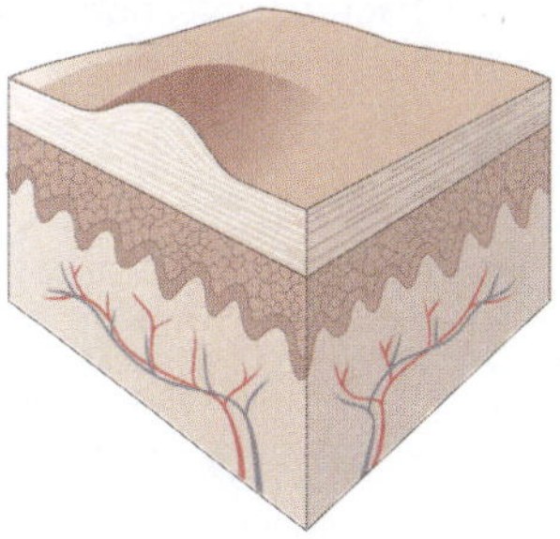

FIGURE 18-7. Papule. (Modified from Kronenberger J, Ledbetter J. *Lippincott Williams & Wilkins' Comprehensive Medical Assisting*. 5th ed. Wolters Kluwer; 2016, Fig. 28-2.)

A **plaque** is a large flatter elevation of the skin, sometimes formed by papules coalescing.

Lesions of psoriasis and granuloma annulare commonly form plaques.

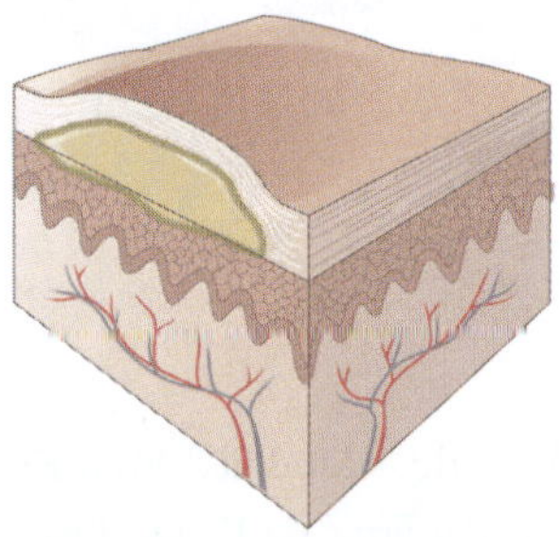

FIGURE 18-8. Plaque. (Modified from Kronenberger J, Ledbetter J. *Lippincott Williams & Wilkins' Comprehensive Medical Assisting*. 5th ed. Wolters Kluwer; 2016, Fig. 28-2.)

A **nodule** is a solid elevation of the skin >1 cm in diameter that usually extends into the deeper skin layers.

Examples include cysts, lipomas, and fibromas.

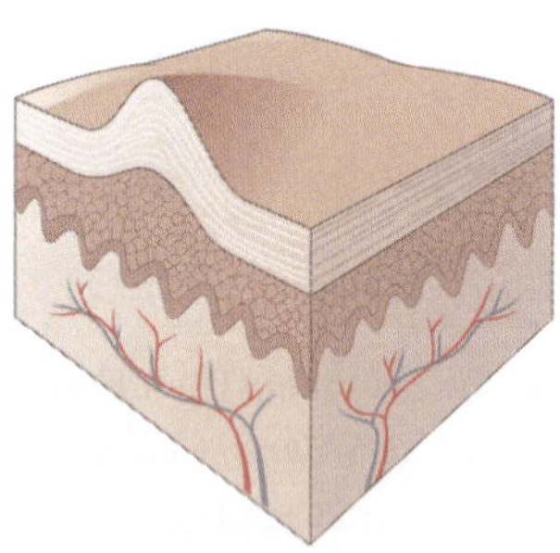

FIGURE 18-9. Nodule. (Modified from Kronenberger J, Ledbetter J. *Lippincott Williams & Wilkins' Comprehensive Medical Assisting*. 5th ed. Wolters Kluwer; 2016, Fig. 28-2.)

A **pustule** is a small circumscribed elevation of the epidermis filled with purulent fluid.

Pustules are common in bacterial infections and folliculitis.

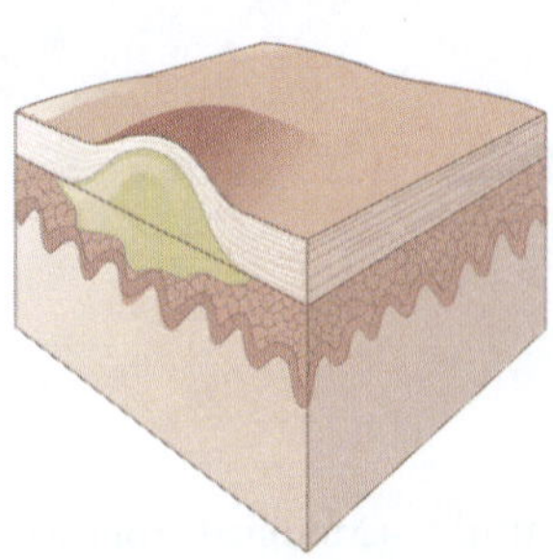

FIGURE 18-10. Pustule. (Modified from Kronenberger J, Ledbetter J. *Lippincott Williams & Wilkins' Comprehensive Medical Assisting*. 5th ed. Wolters Kluwer; 2016, Fig. 28-2.)

A **vesicle** is a small circumscribed elevation of the epidermis containing clear fluid <1 cm in diameter.

Vesicles are characteristic of herpes infections, acute allergic contact dermatitis, and some autoimmune blistering disorders such as dermatitis herpetiformis.

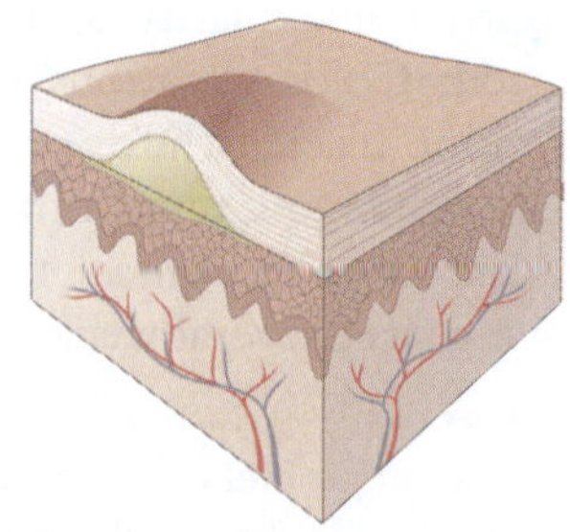

FIGURE 18-11. Vesicle. (Modified from Kronenberger J, Ledbetter J. *Lippincott Williams & Wilkins' Comprehensive Medical Assisting*. 5th ed. Wolters Kluwer; 2016, Fig. 28-2.)

A **bulla** is a circumscribed elevation of the epidermis containing clear fluid >1 cm in diameter.

Classic autoimmune bullous diseases include pemphigus vulgaris and bullous pemphigoid.

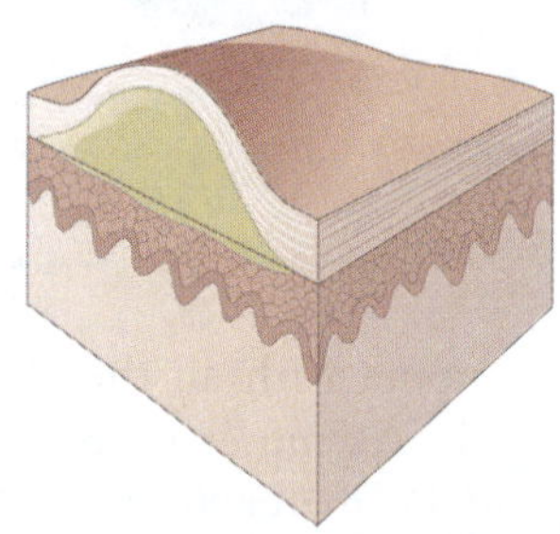

FIGURE 18-12. Bulla. (Modified from Kronenberger J, Ledbetter J. *Lippincott Williams & Wilkins' Comprehensive Medical Assisting*. 5th ed. Wolters Kluwer; 2016, Fig. 28-2.)

A **wheal** is a circumscribed, raised lesion consisting of dermal edema and is also known as *hives* or *urticaria*. Wheals typically last <24 hours.

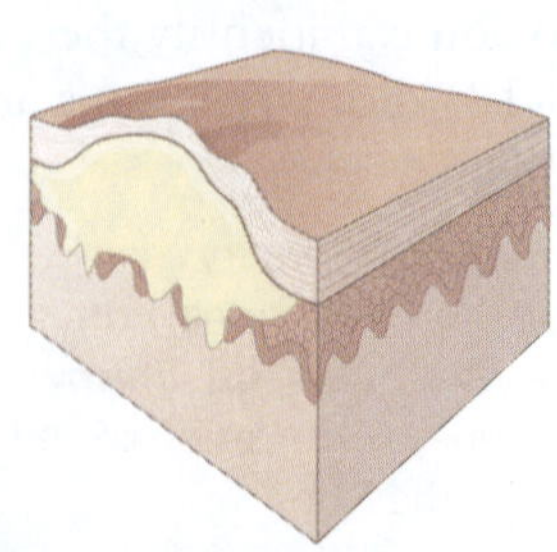

FIGURE 18-13. Wheal. (Modified from Kronenberger J, Ledbetter J. *Lippincott Williams & Wilkins' Comprehensive Medical Assisting*. 5th ed. Wolters Kluwer; 2016, Fig. 28-2.)

Wheals are a common manifestation of hypersensitivity to drugs; stings or bites; autoimmunity; and, less commonly, physical stimuli including temperature, pressure, and sunlight.

Other primary lesions include **erosions** (loss of epidermal or mucosal epithelium), **ulcers** (deeper loss of the epidermis and at least the upper dermis), **petechiae** (nonblanchable punctate foci of hemorrhage), **purpura** (nonblanchable, raised and palpable), and **ecchymoses** (nonblanchable, larger areas or purpura).

Size

Measure with a ruler in millimeters or centimeters. For oval lesions, measure in the long axis, then perpendicular to the axis.

Number

Lesions can be solitary (single) or multiple. If multiple, record how many. Also consider estimating the total number of the type of lesion you are describing.

Distribution

Distribution refers to how the skin lesions are scattered or spread out. It is important to note if particular body parts are affected (e.g., palms or soles, scalp, mucosal membranes, flexures or skin folds, extensor surfaces); whether distribution is random or patterned, symmetric or asymmetric and whether the lesions are confined to sun-exposed or in protected skin. Be as specific as possible. For single lesions, measure their distance from other landmarks (e.g., 1 cm lateral to left oral commissure).

Psoriasis frequently affects the scalp, extensor surfaces of the elbows and knees, umbilicus, and the gluteal cleft.

Lichen planus frequently arises on the wrists, forearms, genitals, and lower legs.

Vitiligo may be patchy and isolated or may group around the distal extremities and face, particularly around the eyes and mouth.

Discoid lupus erythematosus has characteristic lesions on sun-exposed skin of the face, especially the forehead, nose, and the ear.

Hidradenitis suppurativa involves skin containing a high density of apocrine glands, including the axillae, groin, and under the breasts.

Configuration

Configuration is the shape of single lesions and the arrangement of groups of lesions. Some descriptive terms to learn are *linear* or *striate* (straight line); *annular* (ring-like, with central clearing); *nummular* or *discoid* (coin-shaped, no central clearing); *target*, *bull's eye*, or *iris* (rings with central duskiness); and *serpiginous* or *gyrate* (having linear, branched, and curving elements).

Examples are herpes zoster with unilateral and dermatomal vesicles; herpes simplex, with grouped vesicles or pustules on an erythematous base; tinea pedis with annular lesions; and poison ivy allergic contact dermatitis with linear lesions.

Texture

Palpate the lesion to see if it is smooth, fleshy, *verrucous* or warty, or scaly (fine, keratotic, or greasy scale).

Scaling can be greasy, like seborrheic dermatitis or seborrheic keratoses, dry and fine like tinea pedis, or hard and keratotic like actinic keratoses or SCC.

Color

Use your imagination and be creative. Refer to a color wheel, if needed. There are many shades of tan and brown, but start with tan, light brown, and dark brown if you are having trouble.

- Use "skin-colored" to describe a lesion that is the same shade as the patient's skin.
- Other common colors are black, orange, yellow, and purple and shades of blue, silver, and gray.
- For red lesions or rashes (**erythema**), blanch the lesion by pressing it firmly with your finger or a glass slide to see if the redness temporarily lightens then refills.

Blanchable lesions are erythematous and suggest inflammation. Nonblanching lesions such as petechiae, purpura, and vascular structures (cherry angiomas, vascular malformations) are not erythematous, but rather bright red, purple, or violaceous. They are nonblanching because blood has extravasated out from the capillaries into the surrounding tissues.

See Tables 18-4 to 18-6 for rough, pink, and brown lesions and their mimics.

See Table 18-7, Vascular and Purpuric Lesions of the Skin.

PHYSICAL EXAMINATION: GENERAL APPROACH

When skin lesions are seen, inspect and palpate all lesions. Learn to describe each lesion accurately, using the terminology specified previously. Changing moles, a history of skin cancer, and other risk factors all warrant a full-body skin examination.

Lighting, Equipment, and Dermoscopy

Make sure there is adequate lighting. Good overhead ambient lighting or natural light from windows is usually adequate. You may wish to add a strong light source if the room is dark. You will also need a small ruler or tape measure. In addition, a small magnifying glass allows you to examine lesions more closely. These tools help you document important features of skin lesions, such as size, shape, color, and texture.

The use of a **dermoscope** is an increasingly useful office practice for deciding whether a melanocytic lesion is benign or malignant. This handheld device provides cross-polarized or unpolarized light to visualize patterns of pigmentation or vascular structures (Fig. 18-14).

With adequate clinician training, use of dermoscopy improves the sensitivity and specificity of differentiating melanomas from benign lesions.

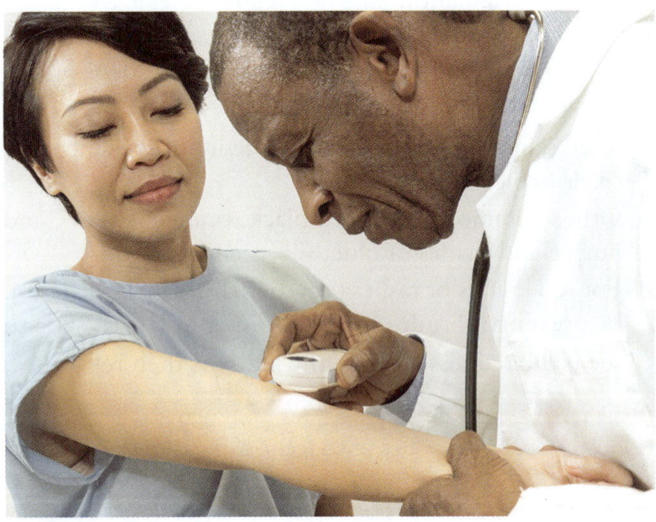

FIGURE 18-14. Using a dermoscope to examine skin lesions.

Patient Gown

Ask the patient to change into a gown with the opening in the back and clothes removed except for underwear (Fig. 18-15). This is the first requirement for the skin examination. Ask permission to expose the area to be examined before moving the gown to see each area. You may say, "I'd like to separate the gown to look at your back now. Is that okay?" Do this for every part of the body. Also ask if the patient would like to have a chaperone present, especially when examination of the genital areas is anticipated.

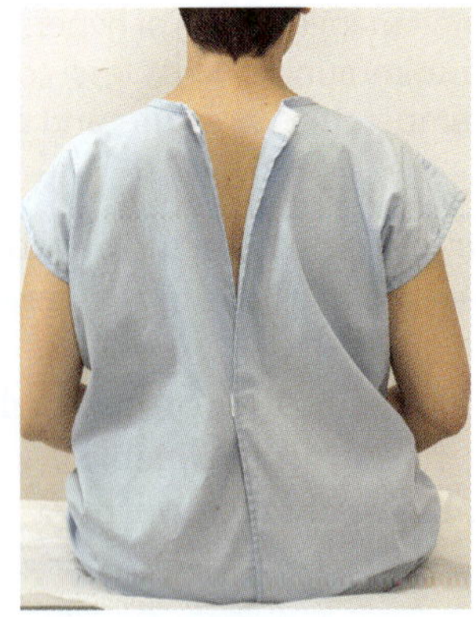

FIGURE 18-15. The patient gown should open in the back.

Handwashing

Before beginning the examination, cleanse your hands thoroughly. It is important for you to palpate lesions for texture, firmness, and scaliness. Because frequent handwashing increases the risk of irritant contact dermatitis, dermatologists recommend using hand sanitizers, which are less drying than soap and water. Explain to the patient that cleansing your hands ensures hygiene and an optimal examination. It is best to restrict use of gloves to touching wounds rather than throughout the examination so that the patient feels accepted. The power of professional and caring human touch can be therapeutic, especially for patients with stigmatizing diseases like psoriasis and HIV.

TECHNIQUES OF EXAMINATION

Key Components of the Full-Body Skin Examination

Patient Position—Seated

- Inspect the hair and scalp (distribution, texture, and quantity).
- Inspect the head and neck, including forehead, eyebrows, eyelids, eyelashes, conjunctivae, sclerae, nose, ears, cheeks, lips, oral cavity, chin, and beard.
- Inspect the upper back.
- Inspect the shoulders, arms, and hands including palpation of fingernails.
- Inspect the chest and abdomen.
- Inspect the anterior thighs and legs.
- Inspect the feet and toes including soles, interdigital areas, and toenails.

Patient Position—Standing

- Inspect the lower back.
- Inspect the posterior thighs and legs.
- Inspect the breasts, axillae, and genitalia including axillary and pubic hair.

(continued)

Key Components of the Full-Body Skin Examination (*continued*)

Alternative positioning is having the patient supine then prone. The systematic flow of examination from head to foot anteriorly to posteriorly remains.

Standard Technique: Patient Position—Seated Then Standing

Choose one of two patient positions for performing the full-body skin examination. The patient can be seated or can lie supine, then prone. Plan to examine the skin in the same order every time, so you are less likely to skip part of the examination. With the *patient seated* on the examining table, stand in front of the patient and adjust the table to a comfortable height. Start by examining the *hair* and *scalp* (Fig. 18-16). Note the distribution, texture, and quantity of hair. Then, using your fingers or a cotton-tipped applicator, separate the hair to examine the scalp from one side to the other.

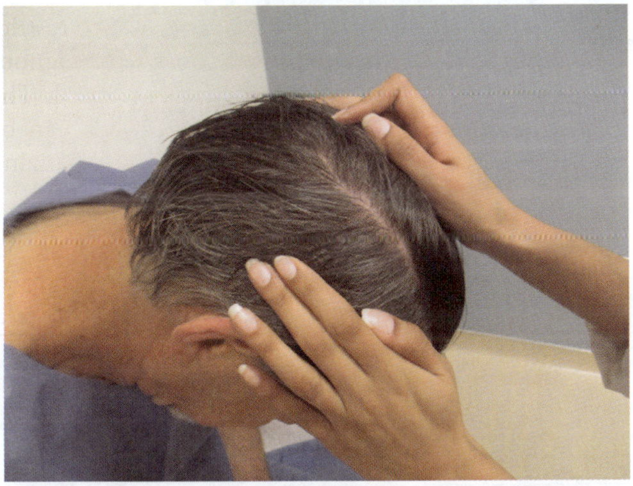

FIGURE 18-16. Parting the hair to expose the scalp.

Alopecia, or hair loss, can be diffuse, patchy, or total. Male and female pattern hair loss are normal with aging. Focal patches may be lost suddenly in alopecia areata. Refer scarring alopecia to a dermatologist.

Sparse hair is seen in hypothyroidism; fine, silky hair in hyperthyroidism. See Table 18-8, Hair Loss.

Now inspect the *head* and *neck*, including the forehead, eyes (including eyelids, conjunctivae, and sclerae), nose, ears, cheeks, lips, oral cavity, and chin (Figs. 18-17 to 18-19). Examination should also include inspection of terminal hair of the eyebrows, eyelashes, and beard.

Look for signs of BCC on the face. See Table 18-5, Pink Lesions: Basal Cell Carcinoma and Its Mimics.

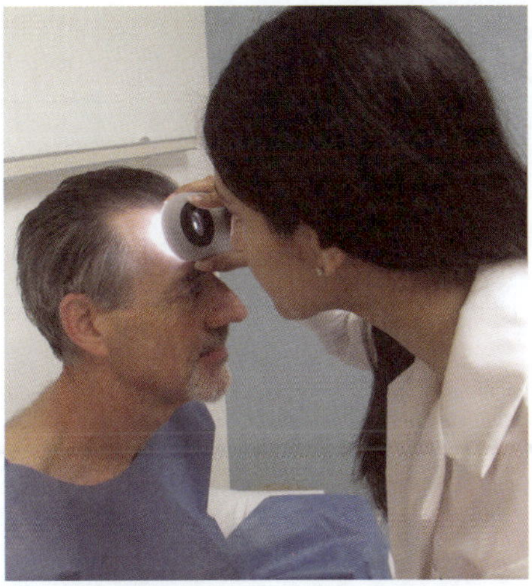

FIGURE 18-17. Inspecting a lesion in the forehead with a dermoscope.

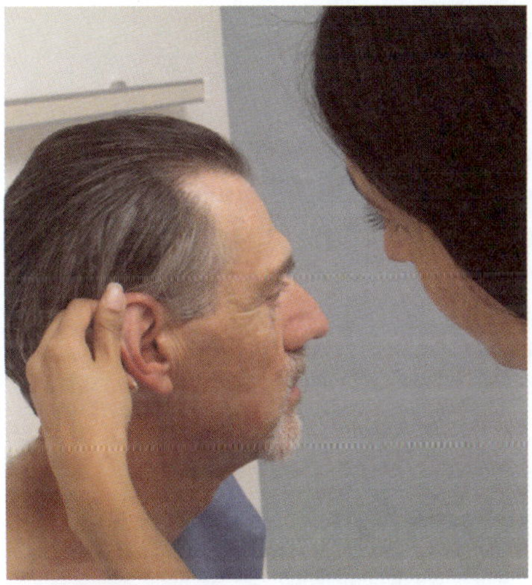

FIGURE 18-18. Inspecting the face and ears.

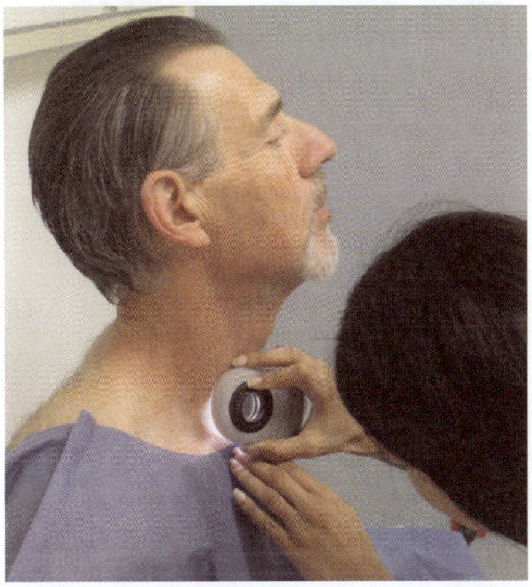

FIGURE 18-19. Inspecting an anterior neck lesion with a dermoscope.

Now ask the patient to lean forward, ask permission before opening the gown, and then inspect the *upper back* (Fig. 18-20).

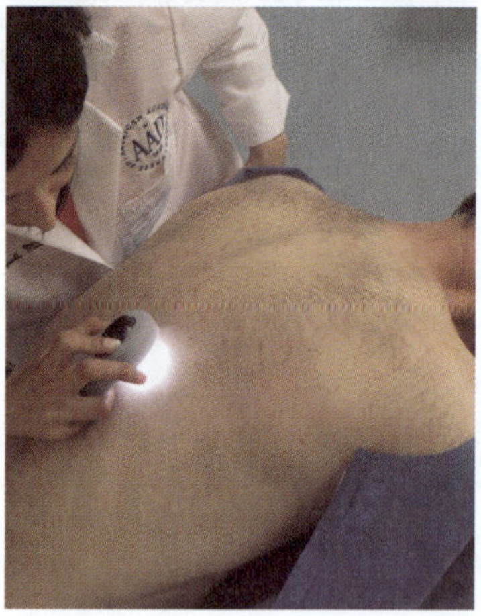

FIGURE 18-20. Inspecting a lesion in the back with the patient leaning forward.

Now inspect the *shoulders, arms,* and *hands* (Fig. 18-21). Inspect and palpate the *fingernails* (Fig. 18-22). Note their color, shape, and any lesions. Longitudinal bands of pigment are normal in people with darker skin.

See Table 18-9, Findings in or Near the Nails.

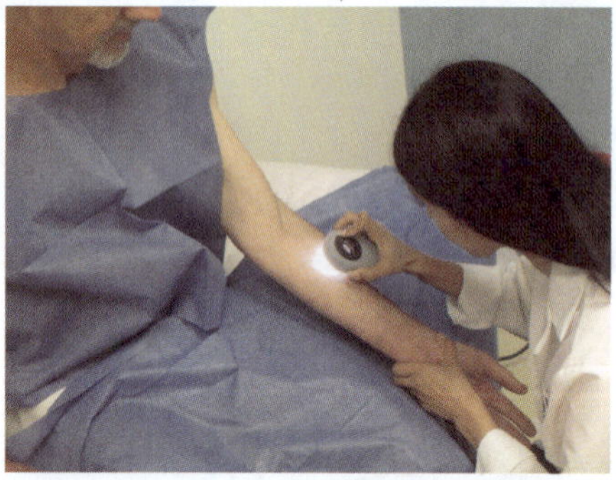

FIGURE 18-21. Inspecting an arm lesion with a dermoscope.

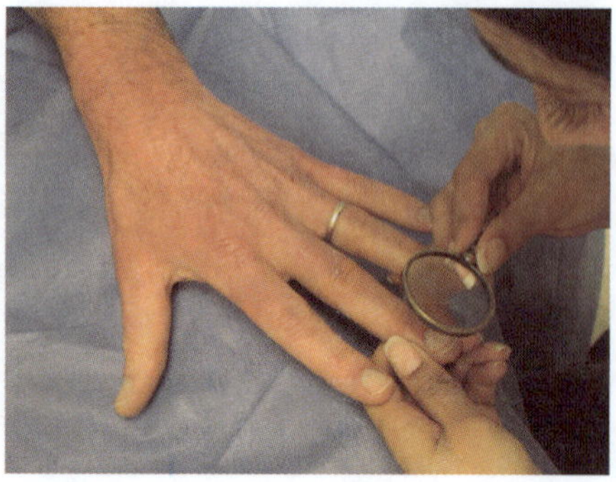

FIGURE 18-22. Inspecting the hands with a magnifying lens and palpating the fingernails.

Now inspect the *chest* and *abdomen* (Fig. 18-23), preparing the patient by saying, "Let's look at your upper chest and then your stomach area." The patient will generally help by lowering or raising the gown to expose these areas and covering up when you are finished (Fig. 18-24). You may want to inspect the *axillae* at this point or integrate them later in the examination of the *breasts* in a female patient.

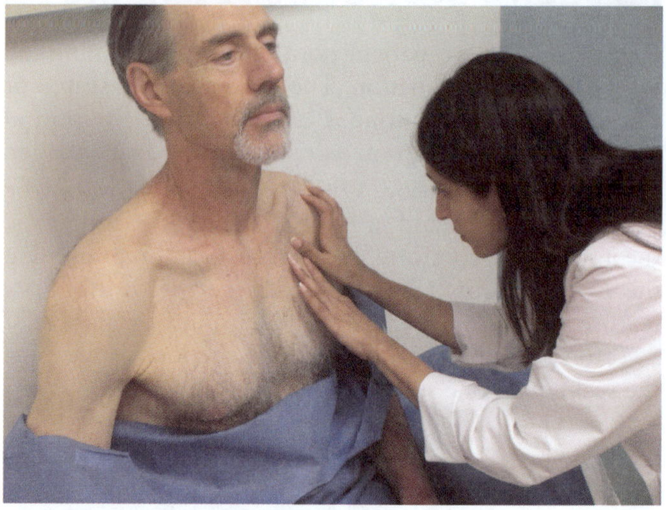

FIGURE 18-23. Inspecting the anterior chest.

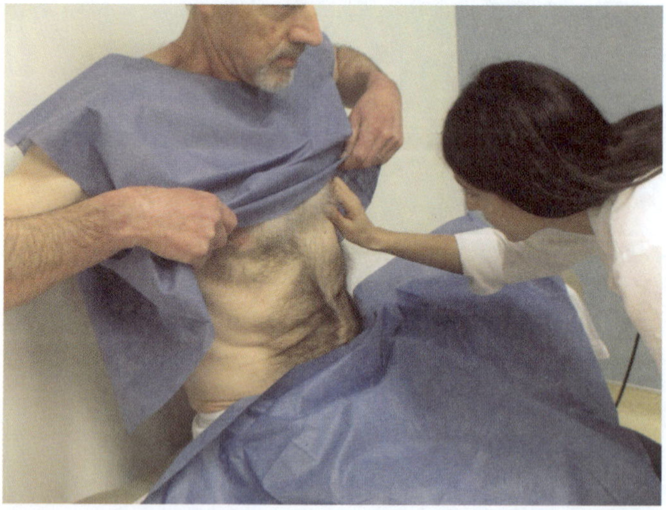

FIGURE 18-24. Inspecting the abdomen.

Now let the patient know that you will be inspecting the *anterior thighs* and *legs* (Fig. 18-25). You and the patient can work together to expose the skin in these areas, moving down to the *feet* and *toes* (Fig. 18-26). Inspect and palpate the *toenails*, and inspect the *soles* and areas between the toes (Figs. 18-27 and 18-28).

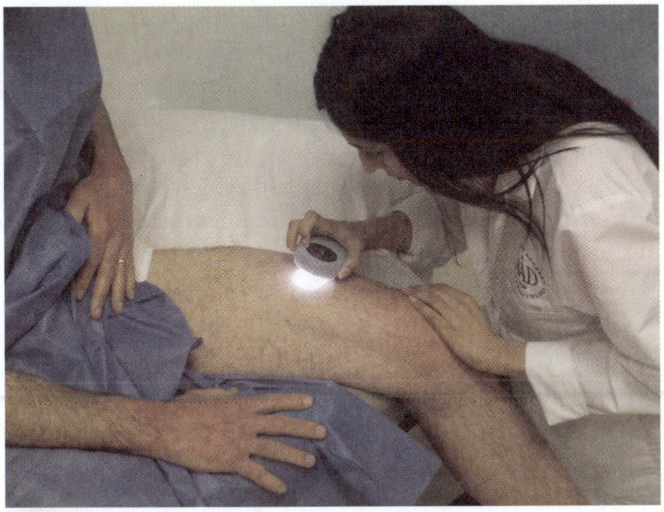

FIGURE 18-25. Inspecting a thigh lesion with a dermoscope.

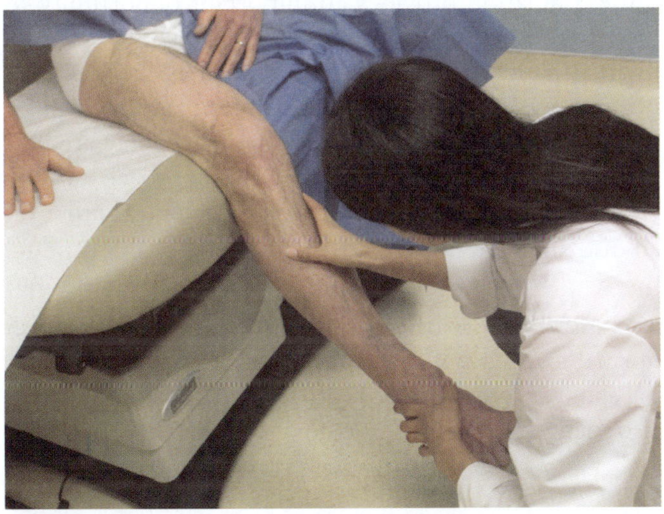

FIGURE 18-26. Inspecting the anterior legs.

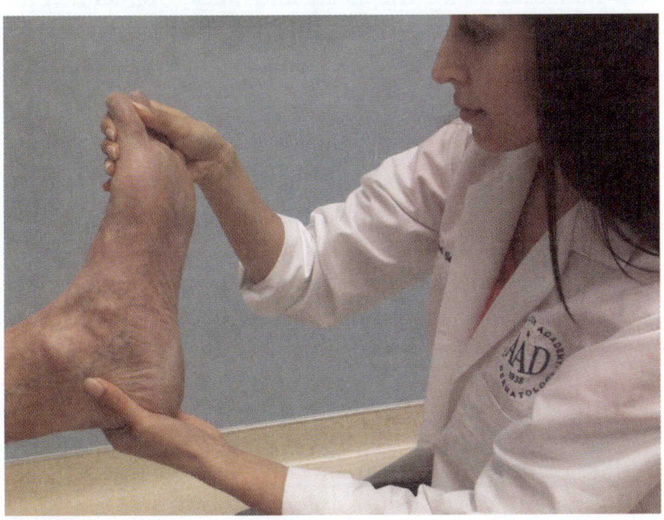

FIGURE 18-27. Inspecting the soles and heels of the feet.

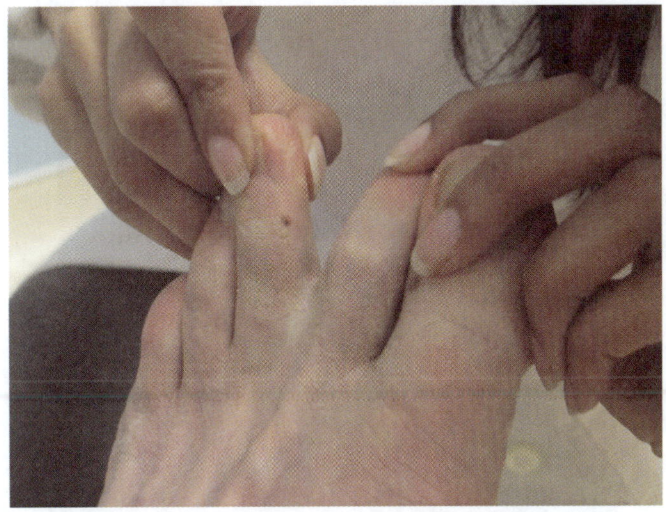

FIGURE 18-28. Inspecting the interdigital areas between toes.

Now ask the patient to stand so that you can inspect the *lower back* and *posterior legs* (Figs. 18-29 and 18-30). If needed, ask the patient to uncover the buttocks (Fig. 18-31). Examination of the *breasts* and *genitalia* may be saved for last. These examinations are described in other chapters. Remember to consider patient comfort, modesty, and use of a chaperone during these examinations. Examination should also include inspection of the *axilla* and hair in the *pubic area*.

See Chapter 17, Breasts and Axillae, p. 503; Chapter 14, Genitourinary System, p. 380.

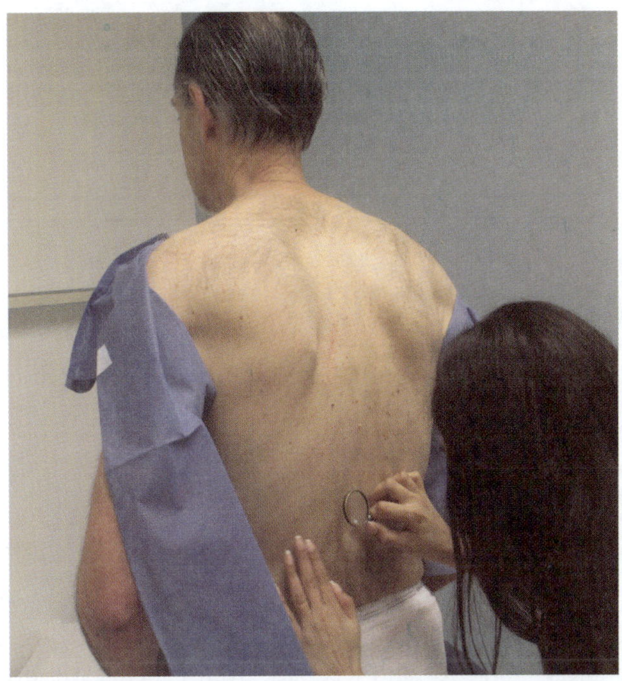

FIGURE 18-29. Inspecting lower back with the patient standing.

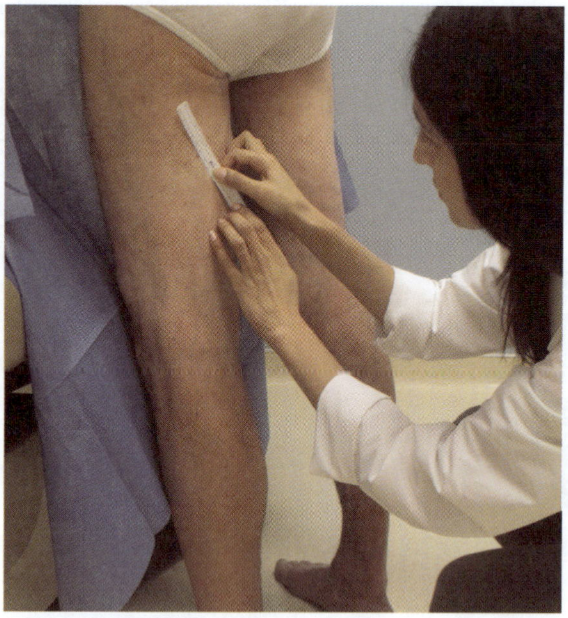

FIGURE 18-30. Determining the size of a lesion with a tape measure in the posterior thigh.

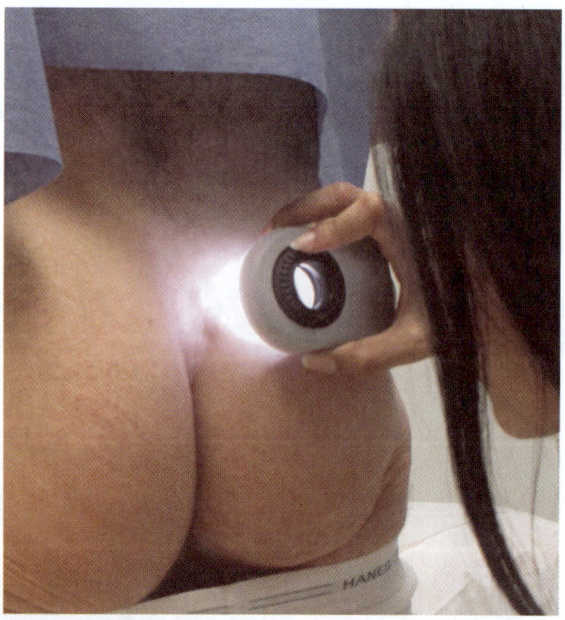

FIGURE 18-31. Inspecting a lesion in the gluteal area.

Alternative Technique: Patient Position—Supine Then Prone

Some clinicians prefer this positioning for more thorough examinations, although patients may feel it is more "clinical." Practice and feedback from patients will give you a sense of patient preferences. Start with the patient *supine,* lying flat on the examination table. As with the seated position, start by inspecting the *scalp, face,* and *anterior neck.* Next, move to the *shoulders, arms,* and *hands;* then to the *chest* and *abdomen; anterior thighs;* and *lower legs, feet,* and, if appropriate, the *genitalia.* As noted previously, ask permission when moving the gown to expose different areas, and explain which areas you will be examining next so that the patient feels more involved in the examination.

Now ask the patient to turn over to the *prone* position, lying face down. Look at the *posterior scalp, posterior neck, back, posterior thighs, legs, soles of the feet,* and *buttocks* (if appropriate).

Integrated Skin Examinations

Try to integrate aspects of the full-body skin examination into your routine physical examination. Integrating the skin examination into your general physical examination provides an important opportunity to look for melanomas and other skin cancers, especially in areas patients find hard to see, such as the back and posterior legs. It will also save you time and contribute to earlier detection of skin cancers, when they are easier to treat. Begin implementing this approach early in your training on each patient you examine, whether on an outpatient or inpatient basis. Instead of documenting what is not present on the skin, document what is present. This is the best way to learn to distinguish normal skin lesions from abnormal lesions and potential skin cancers. As noted earlier, systemic illnesses have also many associated skin manifestations.

See Table 18-10, Systemic Diseases and Associated Skin Findings.

For example, you can pursue an *integrated skin examination:*

- When examining the head and neck. Remember to inspect closely for skin cancers as well as common benign lesions such as acne, which can become scarring.

  See Table 18-11, Acne Vulgaris: Primary and Secondary Lesions.

- When examining the sun-exposed areas that are readily accessible such as the arms and hands, look for sun damage, actinic keratoses, and SCCs as well as normal findings. Educate the patient about such findings as solar lentigines and seborrheic keratoses.

  See Table 18-12, Signs of Sun Damage.

- When auscultating the lungs posteriorly, remove the shirt or open the gown and fully inspect the back for normal moles versus possible melanomas.

  See Risk Factors for Melanoma on p. 526.

SPECIAL TECHNIQUES

Patient Instructions for the Skin Self-Examination

The American Academy of Dermatology (AAD) recommends regular self-examination of the skin using the techniques illustrated in Box 18-1. The patient will need a full-length mirror, a handheld mirror, and a well-lit room that provides privacy. Teach the patient the *ABCDE-EFG method* for assessing moles. Help them to identify melanomas by looking at photographs of benign and malignant nevi on easy-to-access websites, handouts, or tables in this chapter.

Review the ABCDE-EFG criteria on pp. 526–527.

Box 18-1. Patient Instructions for Skin Self-Examination

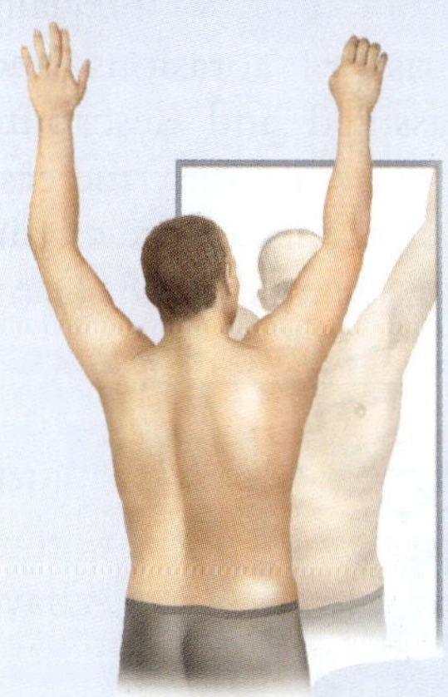

Examine your body front and back in the mirror, then look at right and left sides with your arms raised.

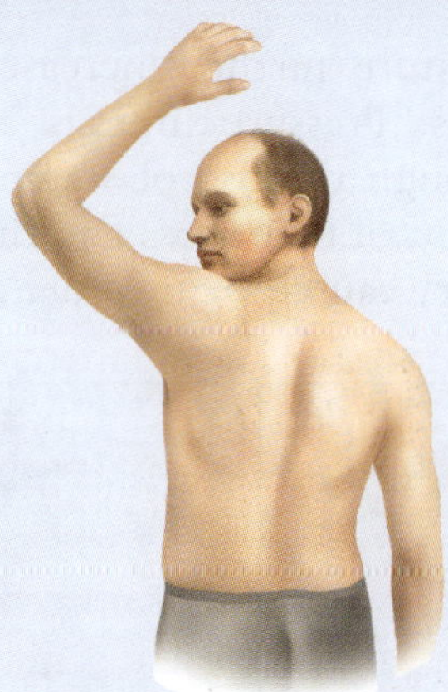

Bend elbows and look carefully at forearms, underarms, and palms.

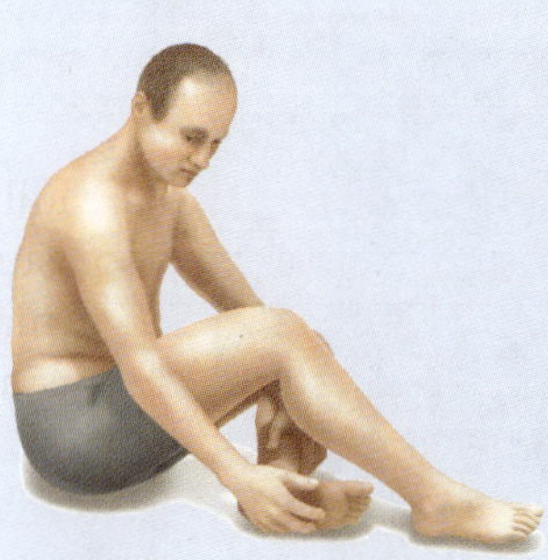

Look at the backs of your legs and feet, the spaces between your toes, and the soles.

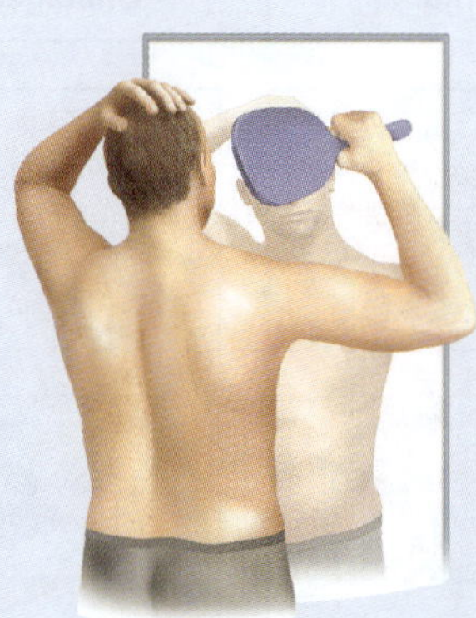

Examine the back of your neck and scalp with a hand mirror. Part hair for a closer look.

(continued)

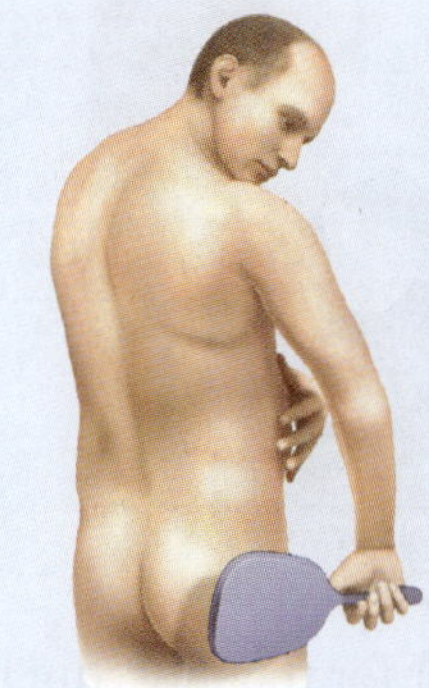

Finally, check your back and buttocks with a hand mirror.

Examining the Patient with Hair Loss

Based on the patient's history, start by examining the hair to determine the overall pattern of hair loss or hair thinning. Inspect the *scalp* for erythema, scaling, pustules, tenderness, bogginess, and scarring. Look at the width of the hair part in various sections of the scalp.

To examine the hair for shedding from the roots, perform a *hair pull test* by gently grasping 50 to 60 hairs with your thumb and index and middle fingers, pulling firmly away from the scalp (Fig. 18-32). If all the hairs have telogen bulbs, the most likely diagnosis is *telogen effluvium*.

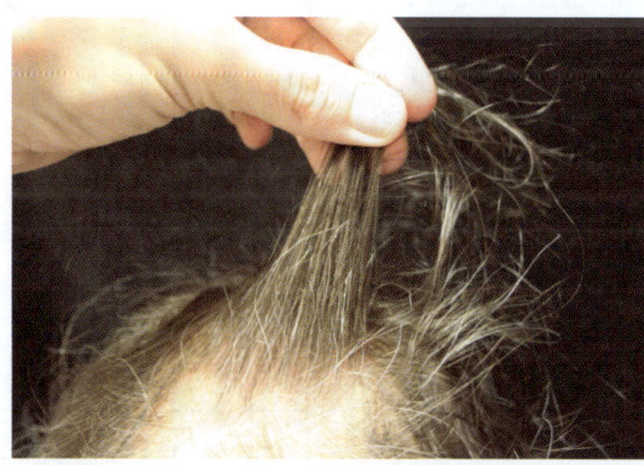

FIGURE 18-32. Examining the hair for shredding from the roots (hair pull test).

To examine the hair for fragility, perform the *tug test* by holding a group of hairs in one hand, pulling along the hair shafts with the other (Fig. 18-33); if any hairs break, it is abnormal. Most (97%) hair loss is nonscarring, but any scarring, namely shiny spots without any hair follicles on close examination with a magnifying glass, should prompt referral to dermatology for scalp biopsy.

Possible internal causes of diffuse nonscarring hair shedding in young women are iron deficiency anemia and hyper- or hypothyroidism.

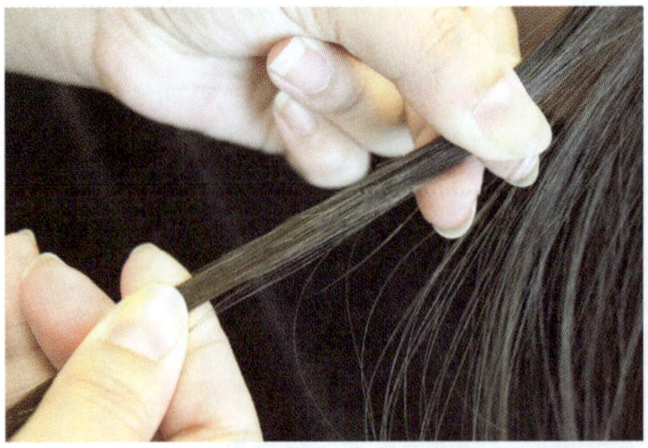

FIGURE 18-33. Examining the hair for fragility (tug test).

Evaluating the Bedbound Patient

People confined to bed, especially when they are emaciated, elderly, or neurologically impaired, are particularly susceptible to skin damage and ulceration. **Pressure injuries** or **ulcers** result from sustained compression that obliterates arteriolar and capillary blood flow to the skin and from shear forces created by body movements. When a person slides down in bed from a partially sitting position, for example, or is dragged rather than lifted up after being supine, rough movement can distort the soft tissues of the buttocks and close off the arteries and arterioles. Friction and moisture further increase the risk of abrasions and sores. Pressure injuries are classified and described through the use of staging systems that describe the extent of tissue loss and the physical appearance of the injury caused by pressure and/or shear (Box 18-2).

Box 18-2. Revised Pressure Injury Staging System

The new revised staging system uses the term *injury* instead of *ulcer* and denotes stages using Arabic numerals rather than Roman numerals (Fig. 18-34).

- *Stage 1:* Intact skin with a localized area of nonblanchable erythema, which may appear differently in darkly pigmented skin.
- *Stage 2:* Partial-thickness loss of skin with exposed dermis
- *Stage 3:* Full-thickness skin loss, in which adipose (fat) is visible in the ulcer and granulation tissue and rolled wound edges, is often present.
- *Stage 4:* Full-thickness skin and tissue loss with exposed or directly palpable fascia, muscle, tendon, ligament, cartilage, or bone in the ulcer.
- *Unstageable:* Full-thickness skin and tissue loss in which the extent of tissue damage within the ulcer cannot be confirmed because it is obscured by **slough** or **eschar**.
- *Deep tissue pressure injury:* Persistent nonblanchable deep red, maroon, or purple discoloration.

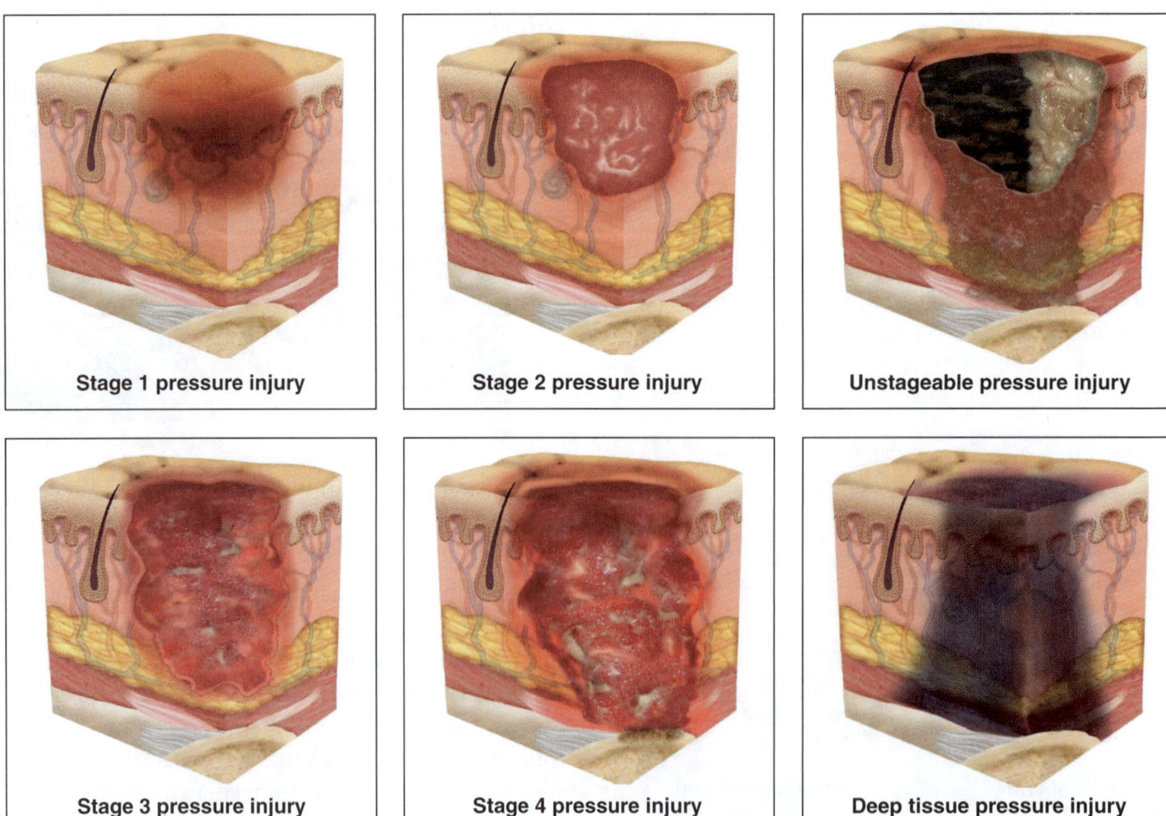

FIGURE 18-34. Pressure injury stages. (Modified from Nettina SM. *Lippincott Manual of Nursing Practice*. 11th ed. Wolters Kluwer; 2019, Fig. 9-3.)

Local redness of the skin warns of impending necrosis, although some deep pressure sores develop without antecedent redness.

Fever, chills, and pain suggest underlying osteomyelitis.

See Table 18-13, Pressure, Injuries.

Assess every susceptible patient by carefully inspecting the skin that overlies the sacrum, buttocks, greater trochanters, knees, and heels. Roll the patient onto one side to best see the low back and gluteal area. Inspect closely for skin breaks and injuries. Any pressure injuries should be thoroughly inspected for signs of infection (drainage, odor, cellulitis, or necrosis).

RECORDING YOUR FINDINGS

Note that initially you may use sentences to describe your findings; later you will use phrases. The examples below contain phrases appropriate for most write-ups.

For more details about this terminology, turn to Techniques of Examination, p. 518.

Use specific terms to describe skin lesions and rashes, including:

- *Number*—solitary or multiple; estimate of total number
- *Size*—measured in millimeters or centimeters
- *Color*—including erythematous if blanching; if nonblanching, vascular-like cherry angiomas and vascular malformations, petechiae, or purpura
- *Shape*—circular, oval, annular, nummular, or polygonal
- *Texture*—smooth, fleshy, verrucous or warty, keratotic; greasy if scaling
- *Primary lesion*—flat, a macule or patch; raised, a papule or plaque; or fluid filled, a vesicle or bulla (may also be erosions, ulcers, nodules, ecchymoses, petechiae, and palpable purpura)
- *Distribution/Location*—including measured distance from other landmarks
- *Configuration*—grouped, annular, linear

Recording the Skin, Hair, and Nails Examination

"Skin warm and dry. Nails without clubbing or cyanosis. Approximately 20 brown, round macules on upper back, chest, and arms; are all symmetric in pigmentation, none suspicious. No rash, petechiae, or ecchymoses."

These are normal nevi and perfusion without any rashes or suspicious lesions.

OR

"Marked facial pallor, and circumoral cyanosis. Palms cold and moist. Cyanosis in nail beds of fingers and toes. Numerous palpable purpura on lower legs bilaterally."

These findings suggest central cyanosis and vasculitis.

(continued)

OR

"Scattered stuck-on verrucous plaques on back and abdomen. More than 30 small round brown macules with symmetric pigmentation on back, chest, and arms. Single 1.2 × 1.6 cm asymmetric dark brown and black plaque with erythematous, uneven border, on left upper arm."

These findings suggest normal seborrheic keratoses and benign nevi, but also a possible malignant melanoma.

OR

"Facial plethora. Skin icteric. Many telangiectatic mats on chest and abdomen. Single 5-mm pearly papule with rolled border on left zygomatic cheek. Nails with clubbing but no cyanosis."

These findings suggest probable end-stage liver disease and incidental BCC.

HEALTH PROMOTION AND COUNSELING: EVIDENCE AND RECOMMENDATIONS

Important Topics for Health Promotion and Counseling

- Skin cancer prevention
- Skin cancer screening including melanoma

Epidemiology

Melanoma is the fifth most frequently diagnosed cancer in men and the sixth most frequently diagnosed cancer in women. The estimated lifetime risk of being diagnosed with melanoma is 1 in 44 (2.3%). Nonmelanoma skin cancers are rarely fatal, causing only about 2,000 deaths each year.

For discussion and examples of types of skin cancers, turn to Table 18-4, Rough Lesions: Actinic Keratoses, Squamous Cell Carcinoma, and Their Mimics; Table 18-5, Pink Lesions: Basal Cell Carcinoma and Its Mimics; and Table 18-6, Brown Lesions: Melanoma and Its Mimics.

Sun and ultraviolet (UV) radiation exposure are the strongest risk factors for developing nonmelanoma skin cancer. People who tan poorly or freckle or burn easily with sun exposure are most at risk; other risk factors include receiving immunosuppressive therapy for organ transplants and arsenic exposure. Melanoma risk factors are listed in Box 18-3. The *Melanoma Risk Assessment Tool,* developed by the National Cancer Institute, is available at http://www.cancer.gov/melanomarisktool. This tool assesses an individual's 5-year risk of developing melanoma based on geographic location, gender, race, age, history of blistering sunburns, complexion, number and size of moles, freckling, and sun damage. The tool is not intended for patients with a personal history of skin cancer or a family history of melanoma.

Box 18-3. Risk Factors for Melanoma

- Personal or family history of previous melanoma
- ≥50 common moles
- Atypical or large moles, especially if dysplastic
- Red or light hair
- *Solar lentigines* (acquired brown macules on sun-exposed areas)
- Freckles (inherited brown macules)
- Ultraviolet radiation from heavy sun exposure, sunlamps, or tanning booths
- Light eye or skin color, especially skin that freckles or burns easily
- Severe blistering sunburns in childhood
- Immunosuppression from human immunodeficiency virus (HIV) or from chemotherapy
- Personal history of nonmelanoma skin cancer

Skin Cancer Prevention

Increasing lifetime sun exposure correlates directly with increasing risk of skin cancer. Intermittent sun exposure appears to be more harmful than chronic exposure, particularly during childhood and adolescence. The best defense against skin cancer is to avoid UV radiation exposure by limiting time in the sun, avoiding midday sun, using sunscreen, and wearing sun-protective clothing with long sleeves and hats with wide brims. Advise patients to avoid indoor tanning, especially children, teens, and young adults.

Signs of chronic sun damage include numerous *solar lentigines* on the shoulders and upper back, many melanocytic nevi, solar elastosis (yellow, thickened skin with bumps, wrinkles, or furrowing), cutis rhomboidalis nuchae (leathery thickened skin on the posterior neck), and actinic purpura. See Table 18-12, Signs of Sun Damage.

The International Agency for Research on Cancer has classified UV-emitting tanning devices as "carcinogenic to humans." Ever use of sunbeds is associated with an increased risk for all skin cancers, particularly among those using sunbeds before age 35, and the risk for melanoma increases with each additional tanning session.

Use of indoor tanning beds, especially before age 35 years, increases risk of melanoma by as much as 75%.

Advise patients to use at least sun protective factor (SPF) 30 and broad-spectrum protection. New U.S. Food and Drug Administration labeling guidelines in 2011 make it easy to see these features on all bottles of sunscreen. The AAD recommends using sunscreen to cover all exposed skin whenever going outside, even on cloudy days. Sunscreen should be reapplied every 2 hours when outdoors and after being in the water.

Skin Cancer Screening

The AAD encouraged persons at high risk for melanoma to ask a dermatologist how often to receive a clinical skin examination. The AAD further recommended that individuals perform regular skin self-examinations and see a dermatologist for any new or suspicious spots and spots that are changing, itching, or bleeding. The American Cancer Society (ACS) does not have a screening guideline for skin cancer but highlighted the importance of regular skin examinations for people at increased risk for skin cancer. The ACS also noted that many clinicians perform routine skin examinations and encouraged patients to perform self-examinations.

Patients who have a clinical skin examination within the 3 years prior to a melanoma diagnosis have thinner melanomas than those who did not have a clinical skin examination. Both new and changing nevi should be closely examined, as at least half of melanomas arise de novo from isolated melanocytes rather than pre-existing nevi. Also consider "opportunistic screening" as part of the complete physical examination for patients with significant sun exposure and patients over age 50 years without a previous skin examination or who live alone.

Detecting melanoma requires knowledge of how benign nevi change over time, often going from flat to raised or acquiring additional brown pigment.

Turn to Tables 18-4 through 18-6 showing rough, pink, and brown nevi and their mimics.

Screening for Melanoma: The ABCDEs

Clinicians should apply the ABCDE method (Box 18-4) when screening moles for melanoma (this does not apply for nonmelanocytic lesions like seborrheic keratoses). The sensitivity of this tool for detecting melanoma ranges from 43% to 97%, and specificity ranges from 36% to 100%; diagnostic accuracy depends on how many criteria are used to define abnormality. If two or more of these features are present, biopsy should be considered. The most sensitive is E, for evolution or change. Pay close attention to nevi that have changed rapidly based on objective evidence.

Review the ABCDE-EFG rule and photographs in Box 18-4. Also see Table 18-6, Brown Lesions: Melanoma and Its Mimics, which provide additional helpful identifiers and comparisons of benign brown lesions with melanoma.

Patient Screening: The Skin Self-Examination. The AAD and the ACS recommend regular skin self-examination based on expert opinion. Instruct patients with risk factors for skin cancer and melanoma, especially those with a history of high sun exposure, prior or family history of melanoma, and ≥50 moles or >5 to 10 atypical moles, to perform regular skin self-examinations.

See Box 18-1, Patient Instructions for Skin Self-Examination.

Approximately half of melanomas are initially detected by patients or their partners.

Box 18-4. The ABCDE Rule

The ABCDE method has been used for many years to teach clinicians and patients about features suspicious for melanoma. If two or more of these are present, risk of melanoma increases, and biopsy should be considered. Some have suggested adding EFG to help detect aggressive nodular melanomas.

- Elevated
- Firm to palpation
- Growing progressively over several weeks

	Melanoma	Benign Nevus
Asymmetry Of one side of mole compared to the other	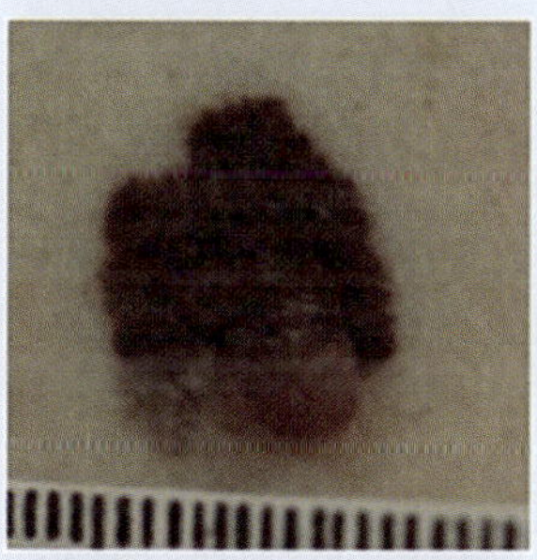	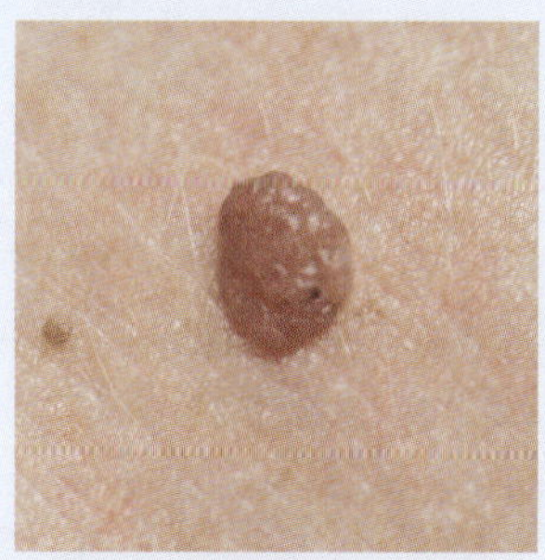
Border irregularity Especially if ragged, notched, or blurred	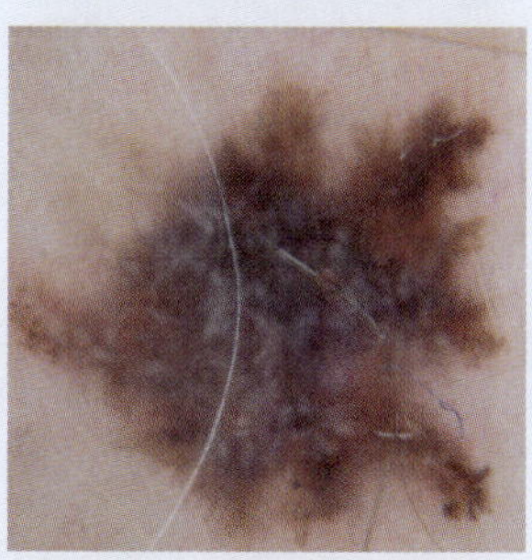	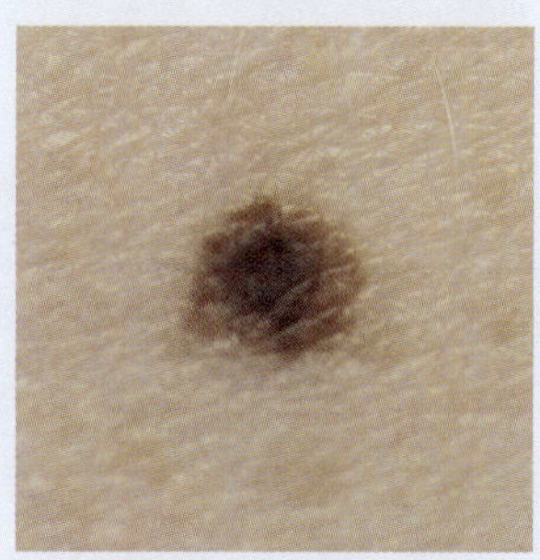
Color variations More than two colors, especially blue-black, white (loss of pigment due to regression), or red (inflammatory reaction to abnormal cells)	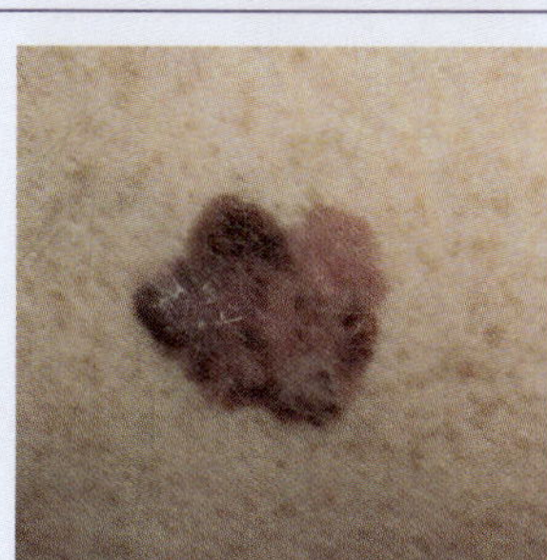	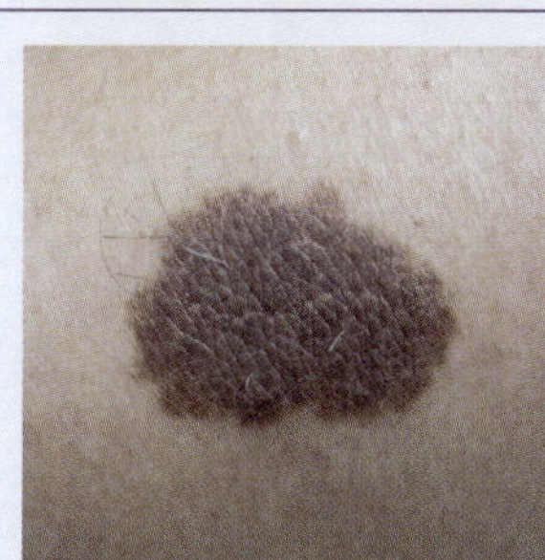

With the exception of a homogenous blue color in a blue nevus, blue or black color within a larger pigmented lesion is especially concerning for melanoma.

(continued)

Box 18-4. The ABCDE Rule (*continued*)

Diameter >6 mm Approximately the size of a pencil eraser

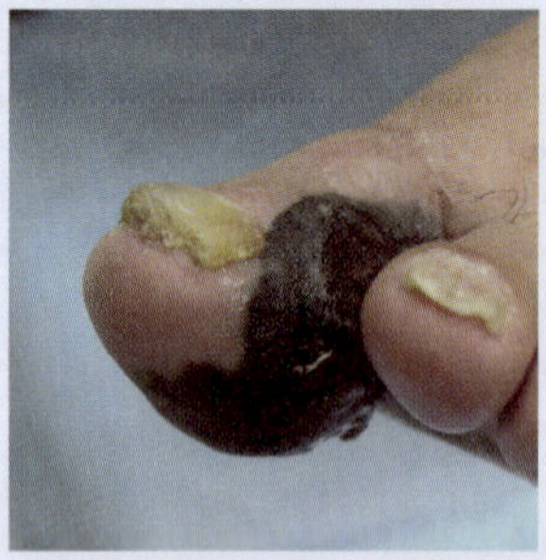

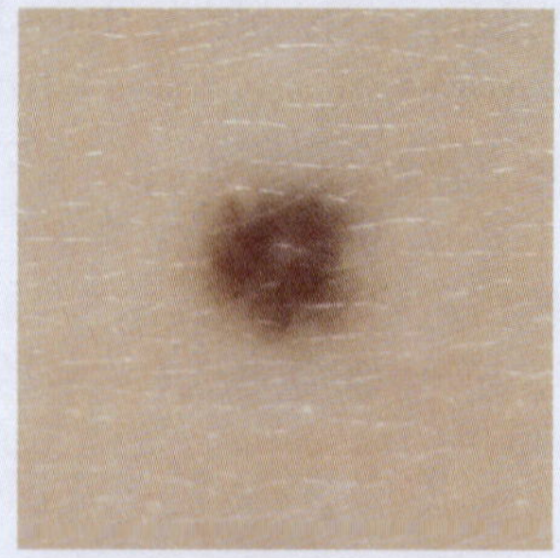

Early melanomas may be <6 mm, and many benign lesions are >6 mm.

Evolving Or changing rapidly in size, symptoms, or morphology

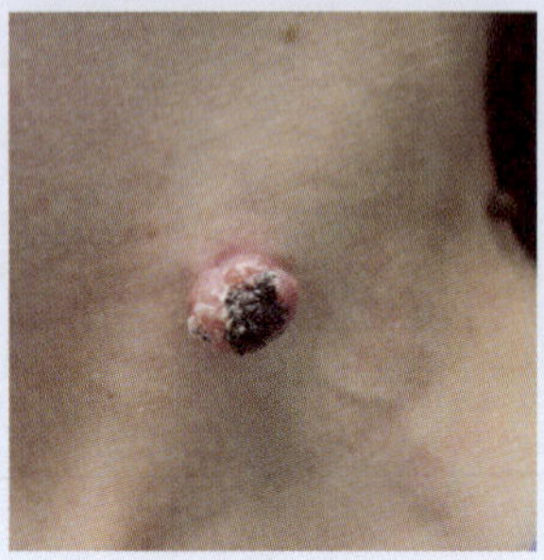

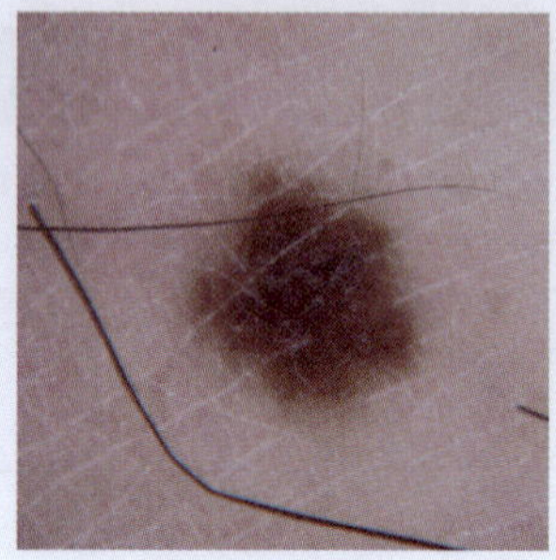

Evolution, or change, is the most sensitive of these criteria. A reliable history of change may prompt biopsy of a benign-appearing lesion.

TABLE 18-1. Describing Primary Skin Lesions: Flat, Raised, and Fluid-Filled

Describe skin lesions accurately, including number, size, color, texture, shape, primary lesion, location, and configuration. *This table identifies common primary skin lesions and includes classic descriptions of each lesion with the diagnosis in italics.*

FLAT SPOTS

If you run your finger over the lesion but do not feel the lesion, the lesion is *flat*. If a flat spot is small (<1 cm), it is a *macule*. If a flat spot is larger (>1 cm), it is a ***patch***.

Macules (flat, small)

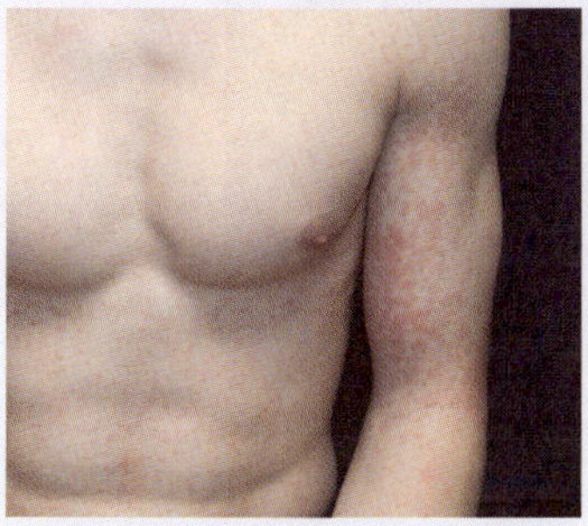

Multiple 3–8-mm erythematous confluent round macules on chest, back, and arms; *morbilliform drug eruption*

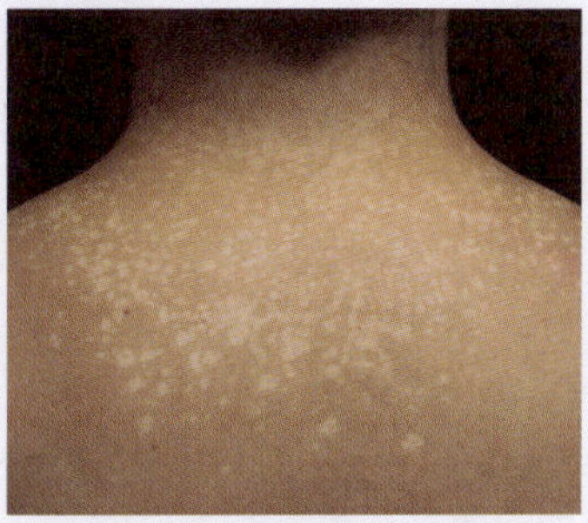

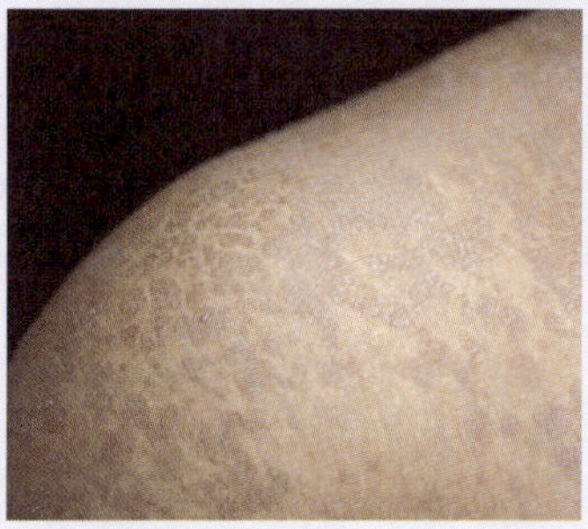

Multiple 2–5-mm hypopigmented, hyperpigmented, or tan round to oval macules on upper neck and back, upper chest, and arms with slight inducible scale on scraping (*tinea versicolor*)

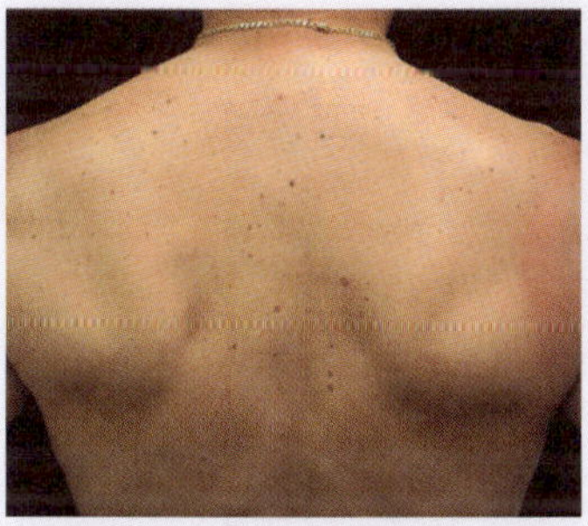

Multiple scattered 2–4-mm round and oval brown macules, symmetrically pigmented, on back and chest with reticular pattern on dermoscopy; *benign melanocytic nevi*

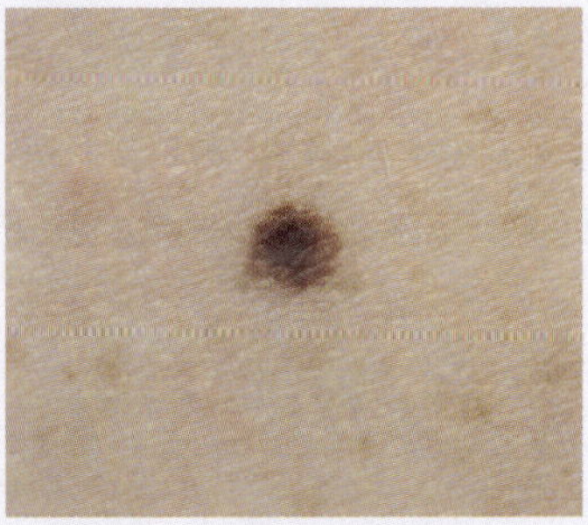

Solitary 6-mm dark brown round symmetric macule on upper back; *benign melanocytic nevus*

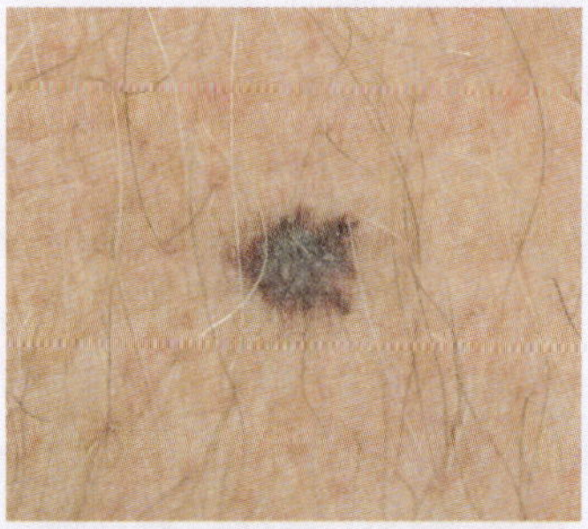

Solitary dark brown, blue-gray, and red 7-mm macule with irregular borders and fingerlike projections of pigment, on right forearm; *malignant melanoma*

Patches (flat, large)

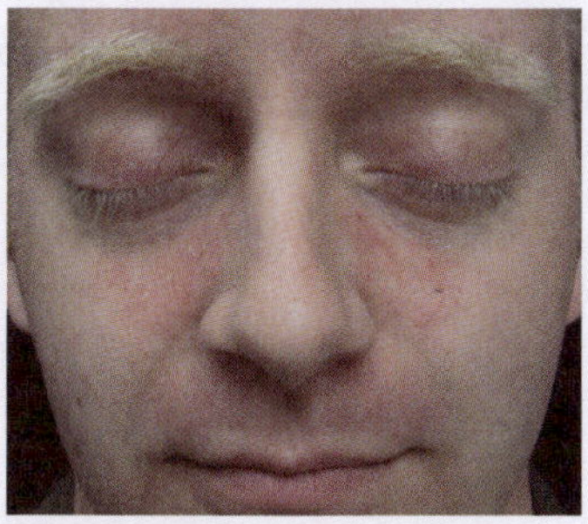

Bilaterally symmetric erythematous patches on central cheeks and eyebrows, some with overlying greasy scale; *seborrheic dermatitis*

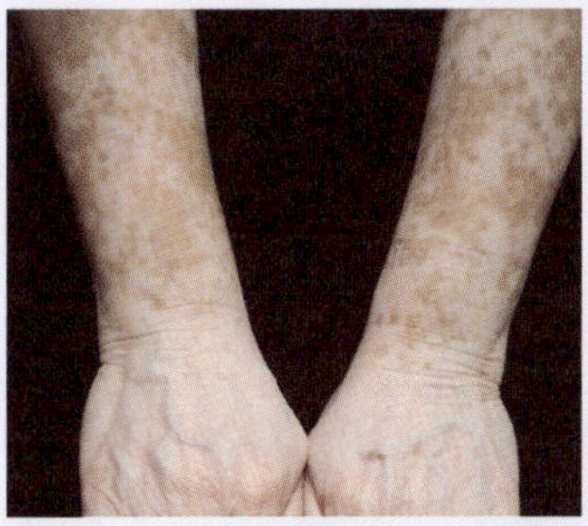

Large confluent completely depigmented patches on dorsal hands and distal forearms; *vitiligo*

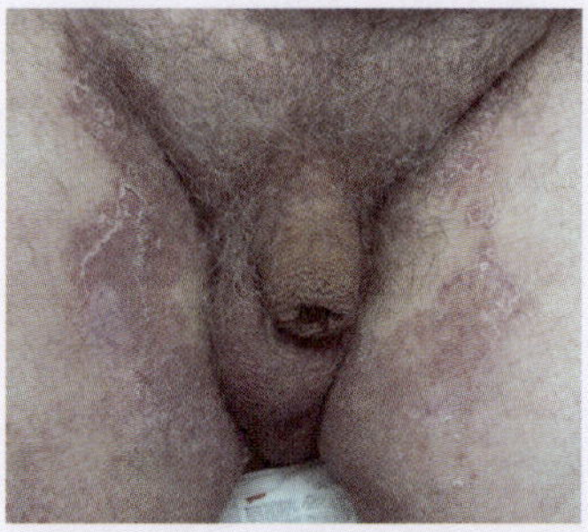

Bilateral erythematous, geographic patches with peripheral scaling, on inner thighs bilaterally, sparing the scrotum; *tinea cruris*

(*continued*)

TABLE 18-1. Describing Primary Skin Lesions: Flat, Raised, and Fluid-Filled *(Continued)*

RAISED SPOTS

If you run your finger over the lesion and it is palpable above the skin, it is *raised.* If a raised spot is small (<1 cm), it is a *papule*. If a raised spot is larger (>1 cm), it is a *plaque*.

Papules (raised, small)

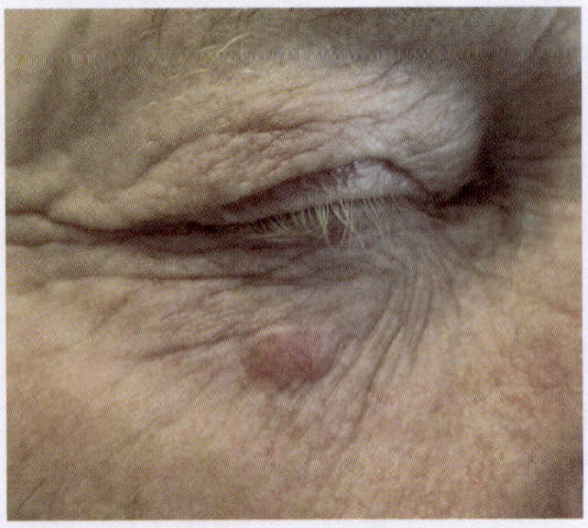

Solitary 7-mm oval pink pearly papule with overlying telangiectasias on right nasojugal fold; *basal cell carcinoma*

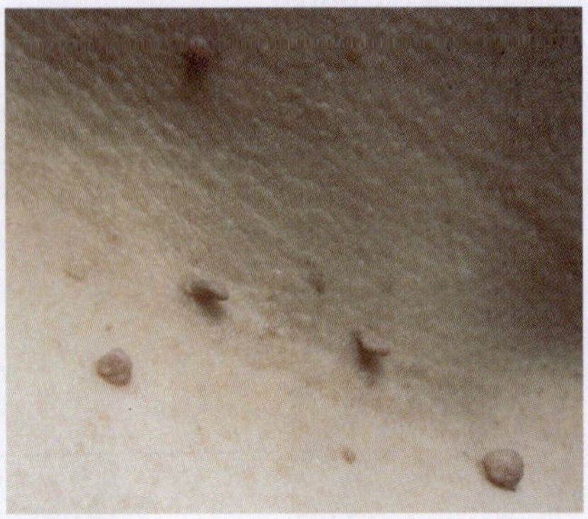

Multiple 2–4-mm soft, fleshy skin-colored to light brown papules on lateral neck and axillae in skin folds; *skin tags*

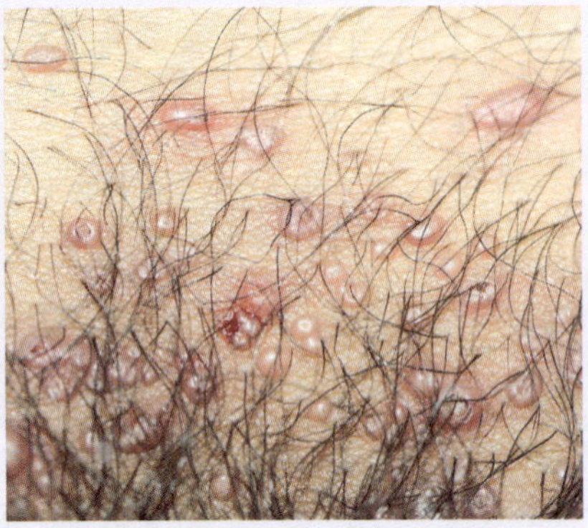

Multiple 3–5-mm pink firm smooth-domed papules with central umbilications, in mons pubis, and on penile shaft; *molluscum contagiosum*

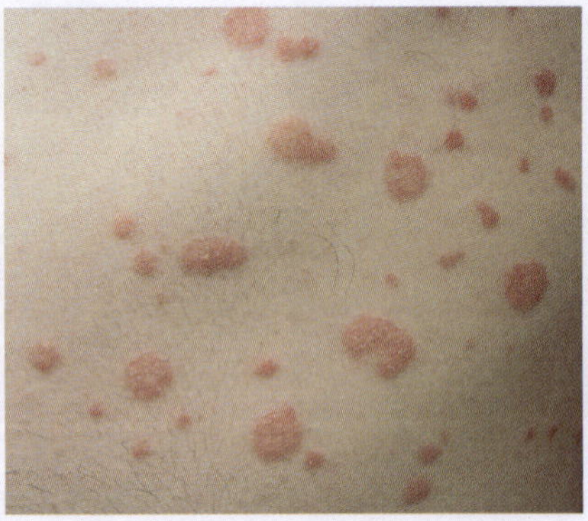

Scattered erythematous round drop-like, flat-topped well-circumscribed scaling papules and plaques on trunk; *guttate psoriasis*

(continued)

TABLE 18-1. Describing Primary Skin Lesions: Flat, Raised, and Fluid-Filled *(Continued)*

Plaques (raised, large)

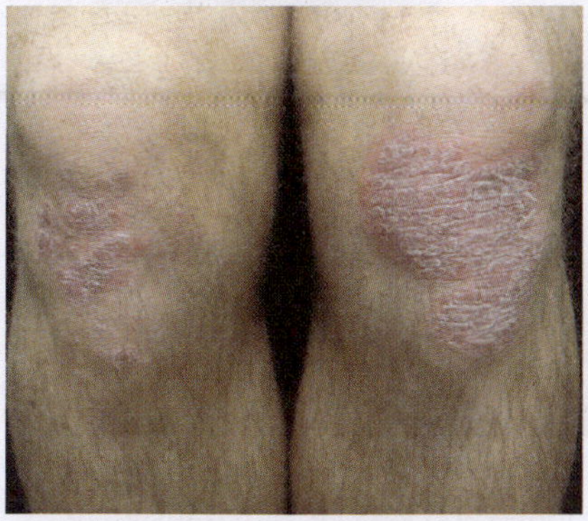

Scattered erythematous to bright pink well-circumscribed flat-topped plaques on extensor knees and elbows, with overlying silvery scale; *plaque psoriasis*

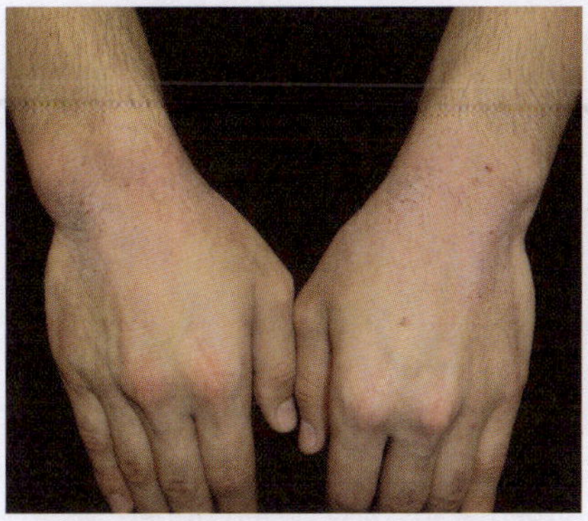

Bilateral erythematous, lichenified (thickened from rubbing) poorly circumscribed plaques on flexor wrists, antecubital fossae, and popliteal fossae; *atopic dermatitis*

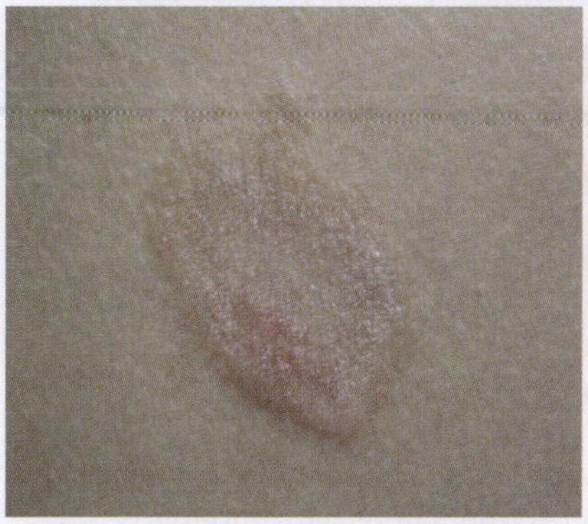

Single, oval, flat-topped superficial erythematous to skin-colored plaque on right abdomen; *herald patch of pityriasis rosea*

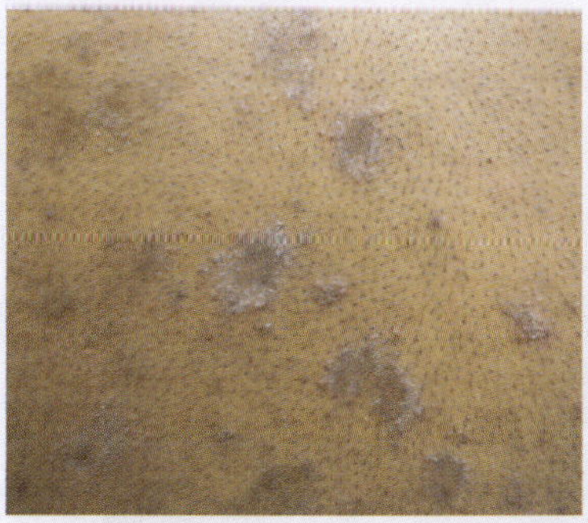

Multiple round to oval scaling violaceous plaques on abdomen and back; *pityriasis rosea*

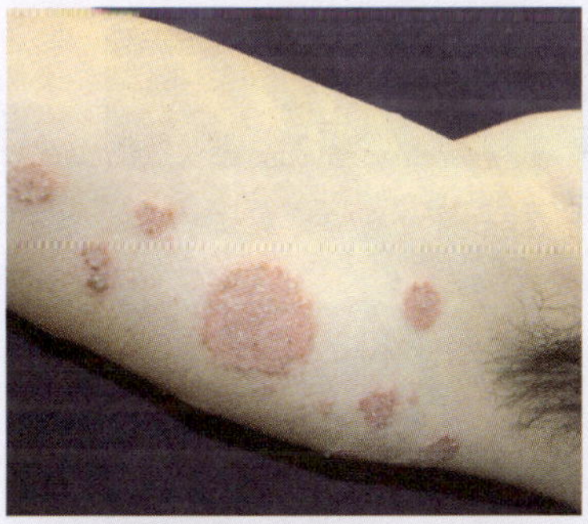

Multiple round coin-like eczematous plaques on arms, legs, and abdomen, with overlying dried transudate crust; *nummular dermatitis*

(continued)

TABLE 18-1. Describing Primary Skin Lesions: Flat, Raised, and Fluid-Filled *(Continued)*

FLUID-FILLED LESIONS

If the lesion is raised, filled with fluid, and small (<1 cm), it is a *vesicle*. If a fluid-filled spot is larger (>1 cm), it is a *bulla*.

Vesicles (fluid-filled, small)

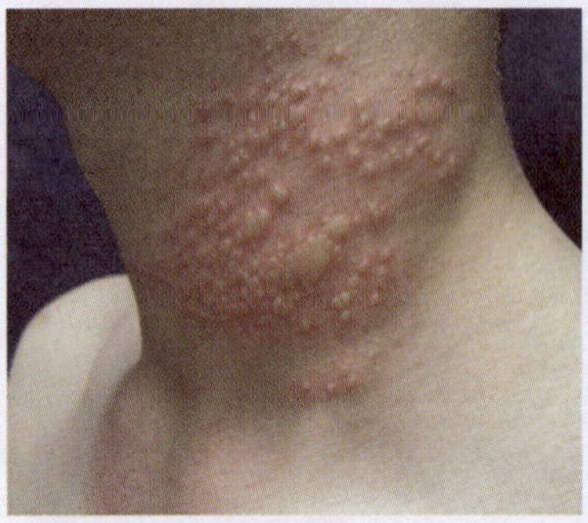

Multiple 2–4-mm vesicles and pustules on erythematous base, grouped together on left neck; *herpes simplex virus*

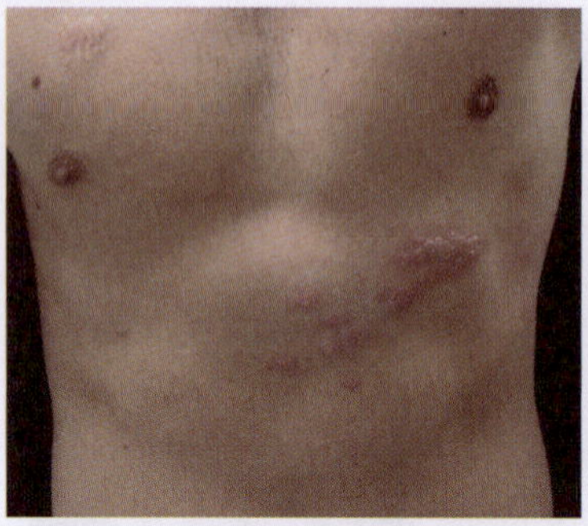

Grouped 2–5-mm vesicles on erythematous base on left upper abdomen and trunk in a dermatomal distribution that does not cross the midline; *herpes zoster, or* shingles

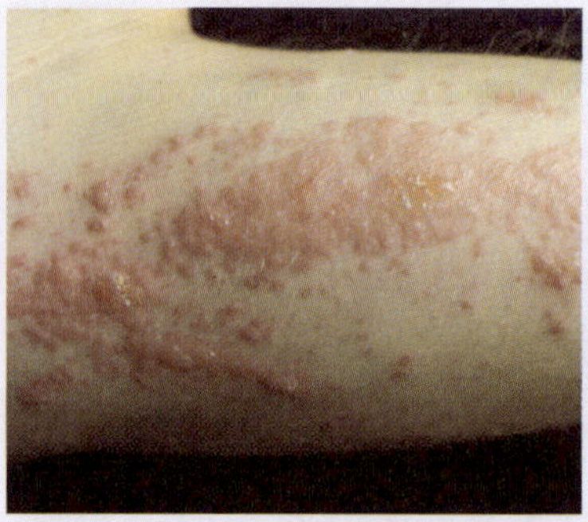

Scattered 2–5-mm erythematous papules and vesicles with transudate crust, some with linear arrays, on forearms, neck, and abdomen; *rhus dermatitis* or *allergic contact dermatitis* from poison ivy

Bullae (fluid-filled, large)

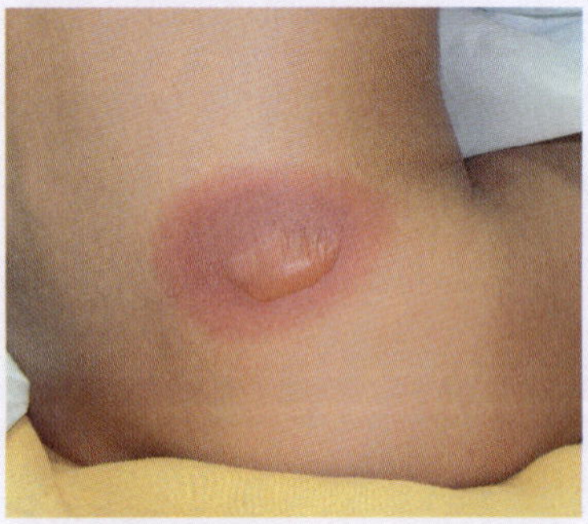

Solitary 8-cm dusky oval patch with smaller inner violaceous patch and central 3.5-cm tense bulla, on right posterior lower back; *bullous fixed drug eruption*

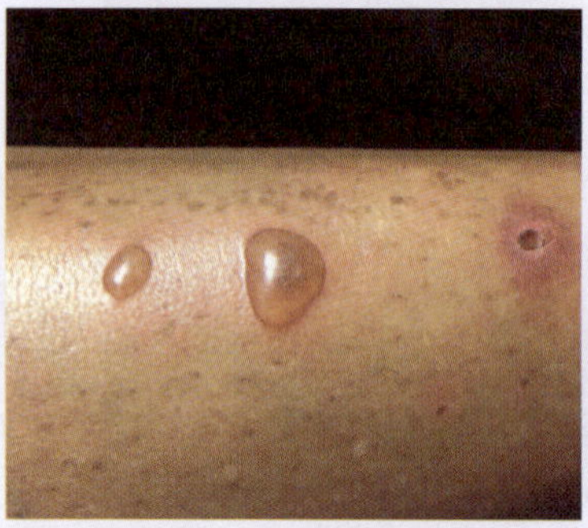

Several tense bullae on lower legs; *insect bites*

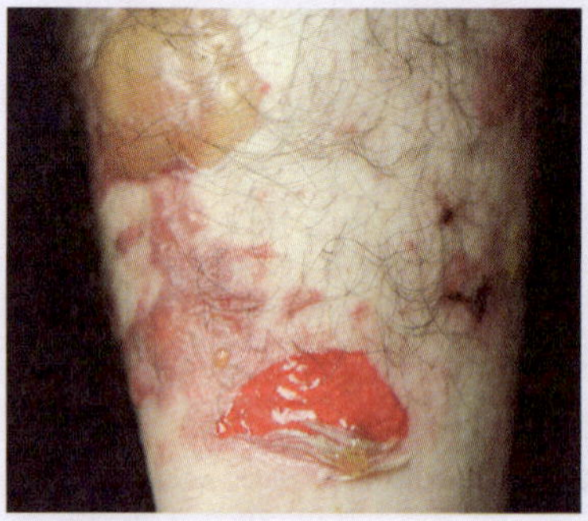

Many vesicles and tense bullae up to 4 cm, some having unroofed and left large (4-cm) erosions, on lower legs bilaterally up to the line of the top of combat boots; *an inherited skin fragility disorder*

TABLE 18-2. Additional Primary Lesions: Pustules, Furuncles, Nodules, Cysts, Wheals, Burrows

Pustule: Small palpable collection of neutrophils or keratin that appears white

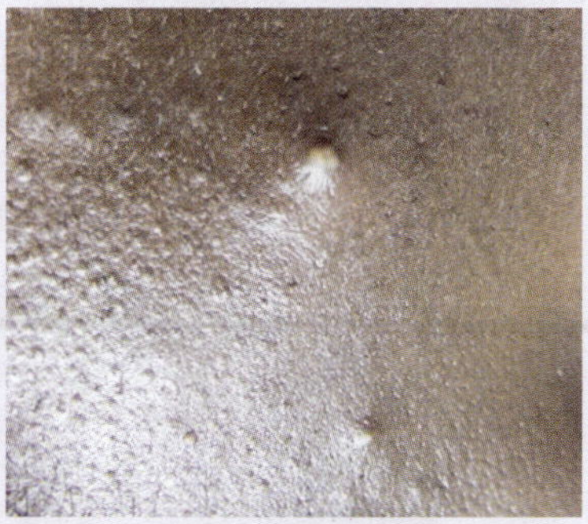

~15–20 pustules and acneiform papules on buccal and parotid cheeks bilaterally; *acne vulgaris*

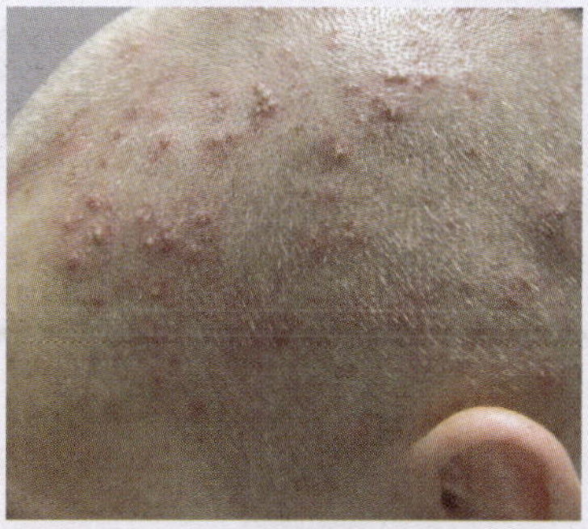

~30 2–5-mm erythematous papules and pustules on frontal, temporal, and parietal scalp; *bacterial folliculitis*

Furuncle: Inflamed hair follicle; multiple furuncles together form a *carbuncle*

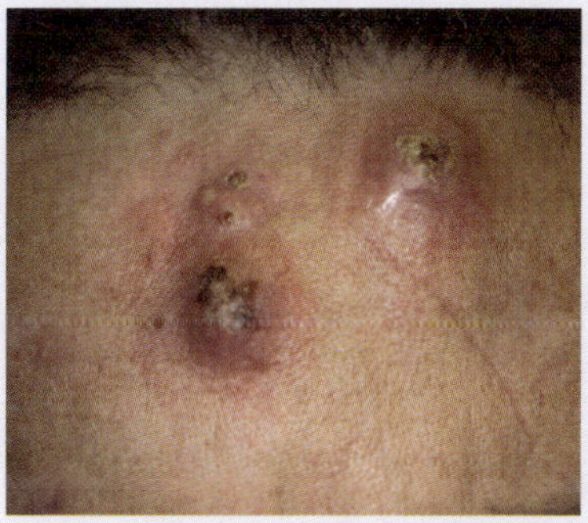

Two large (2-cm) furuncles on forehead, without fluctuance; *furunculosis* (Note: fluctuant deep infections are *abscesses*)

Nodule: Larger and deeper than a papule

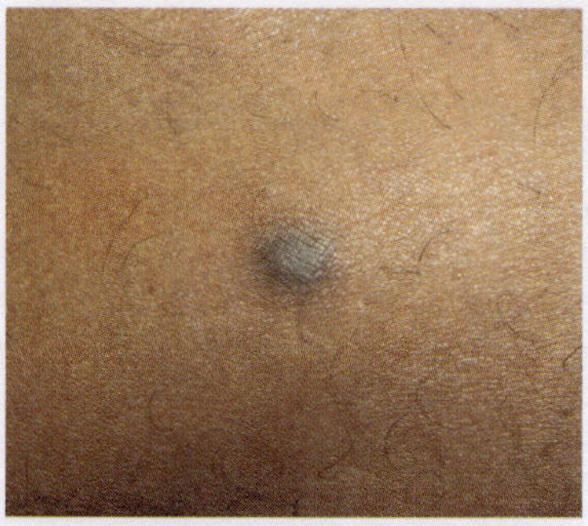

Solitary blue-brown 1.2-cm firm nodule with positive dimple sign and hyperpigmented rim on left lateral thigh; *dermatofibroma*

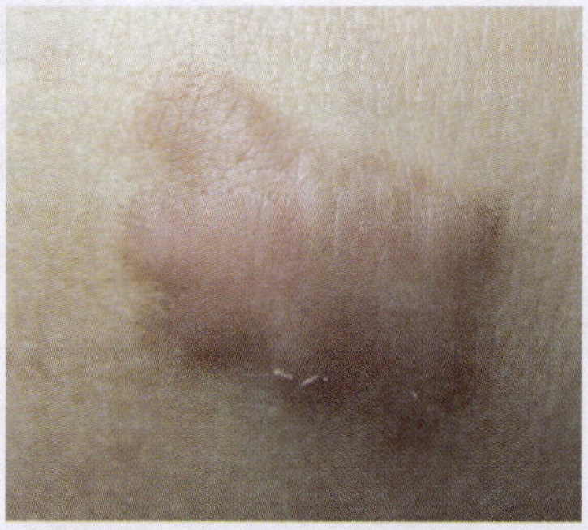

Solitary 4-cm pink and brown scar-like nodule on central chest at site of previous trauma; *keloid*

(*continued*)

TABLE 18-2. Additional Primary Lesions: Pustules, Furuncles, Nodules, Cysts, Wheals, Burrows *(Continued)*

Subcutaneous Mass/Cyst: Whether mobile or fixed, cysts are encapsulated collections of fluid or semisolid

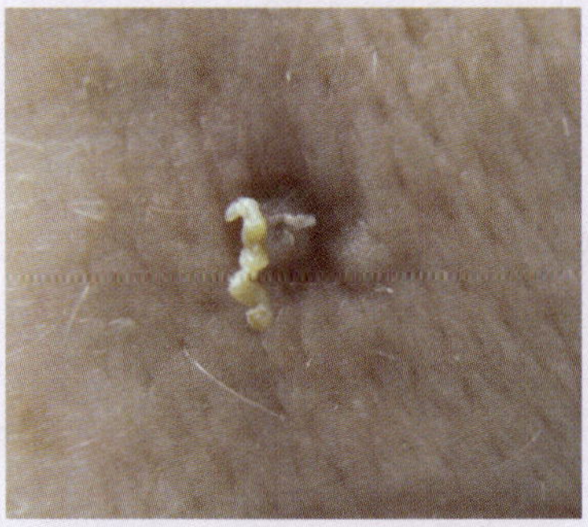

Solitary 2-cm tethered subcutaneous cyst with overlying punctum releasing caseous whitish yellow substance with foul odor; *epidermal inclusion cyst*

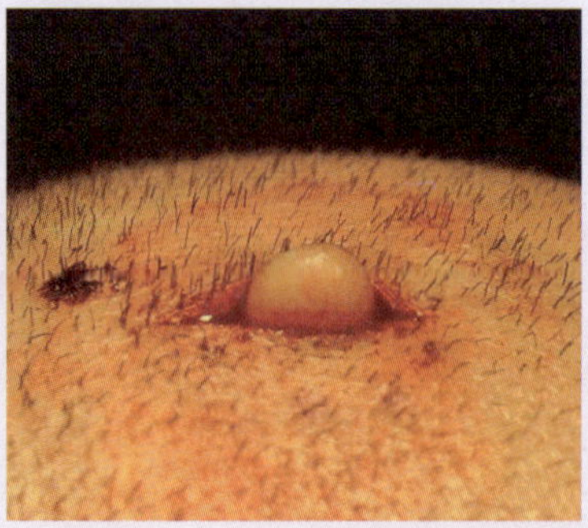

Three 6–8-mm mobile subcutaneous cysts on vertex scalp, that on excision reveal pearly white balls; *pilar cysts*

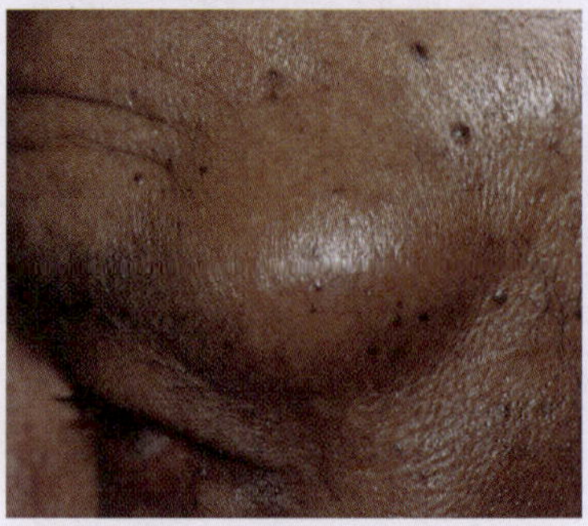

Solitary 9-cm mobile rubbery subcutaneous mass on left temple; *lipoma*

Wheal: Area of localized dermal edema that evanesces (comes and goes) within a period of 1–2 days; this is the essential primary lesion of *urticaria*

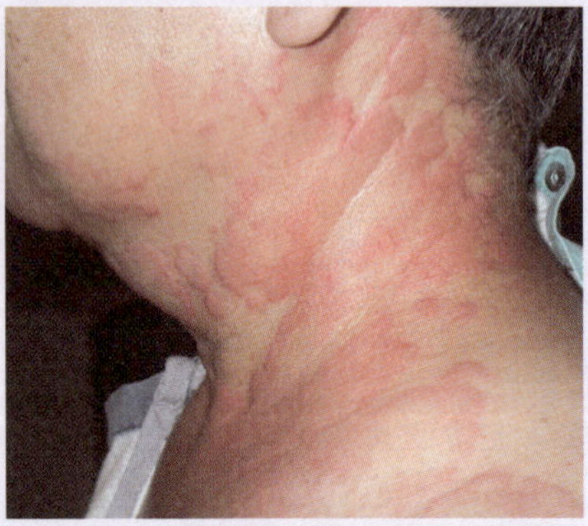

Many variably sized (1–10-cm) wheals on lateral neck, shoulders, abdomen, arms, and legs; *urticaria*

Burrow: Small linear or serpiginous pathways in the epidermis created by the scabies mite

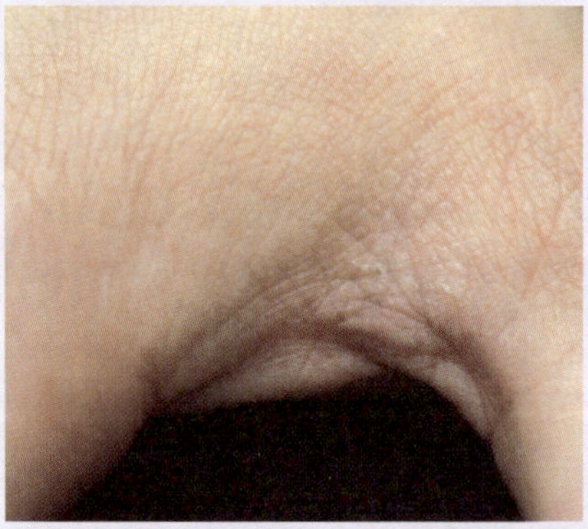

Multiple small (3–6-mm) erythematous papules on abdomen, buttocks, scrotum, and shaft and head of penis, with four *burrows* noted on interdigital web spaces; *scabies*

TABLE 18-3. Dermatology Safari: Benign Lesions

Practice makes perfect . . . Look for these common lesions during your clinical rotations. Perform a skin examination on as many patients as you can. If you are unsure about identifying the lesion, ask your instructors or supervising clinicians for help.

Cherry Angiomas

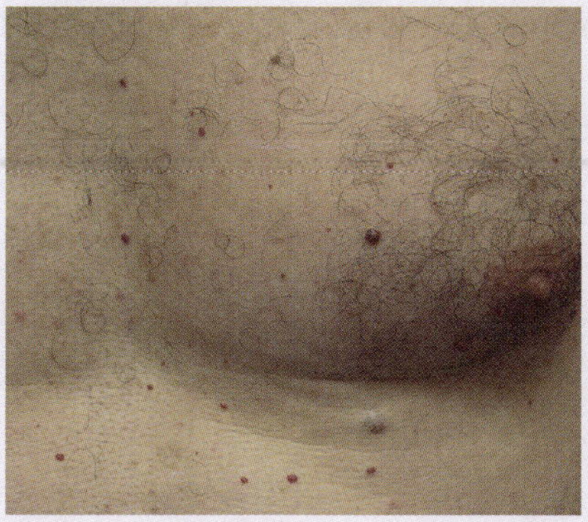

Seborrheic Keratosis

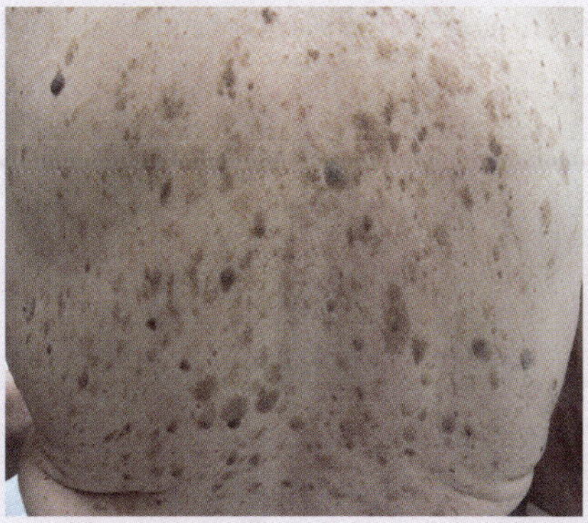

Solar Lentigines

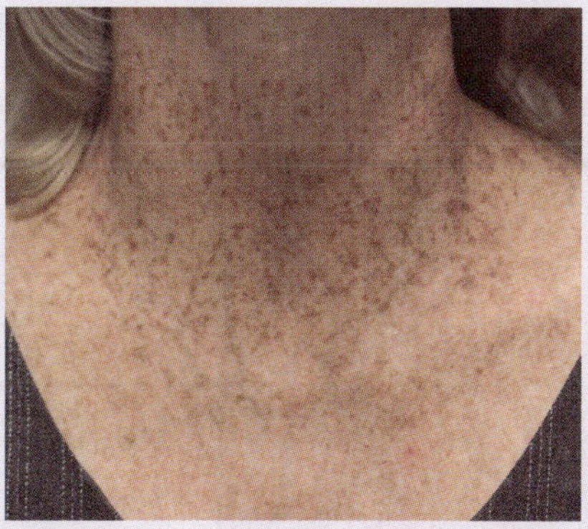

Benign Melanocytic Nevi

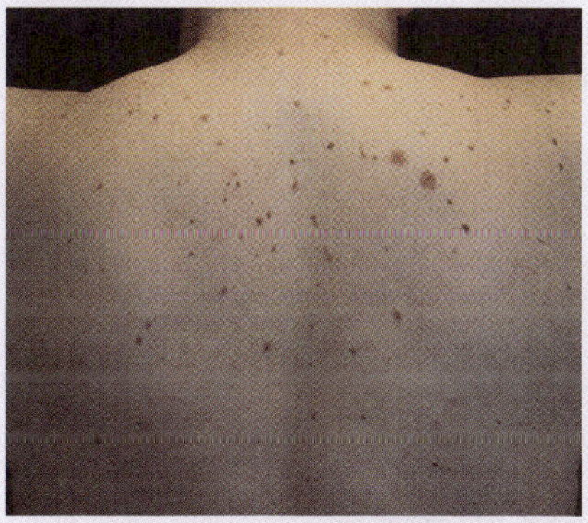

Dermatofibroma

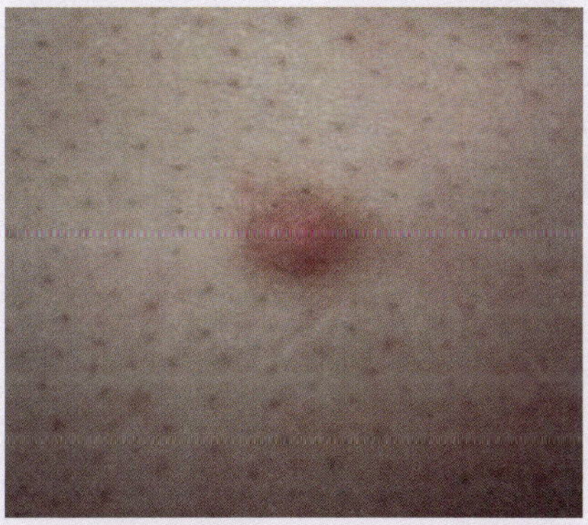

Keloids

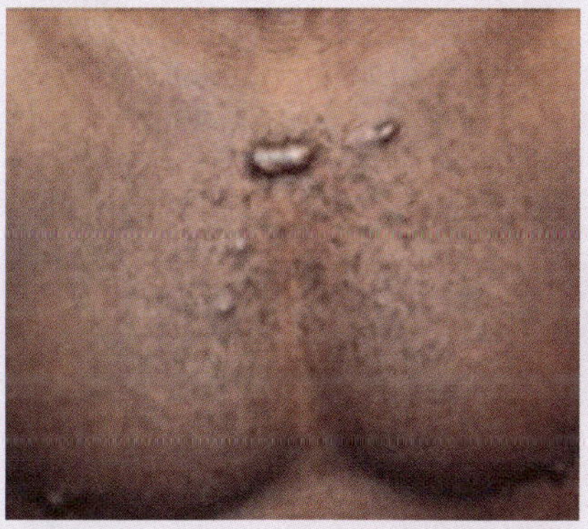

Epidermal Inclusion Cyst

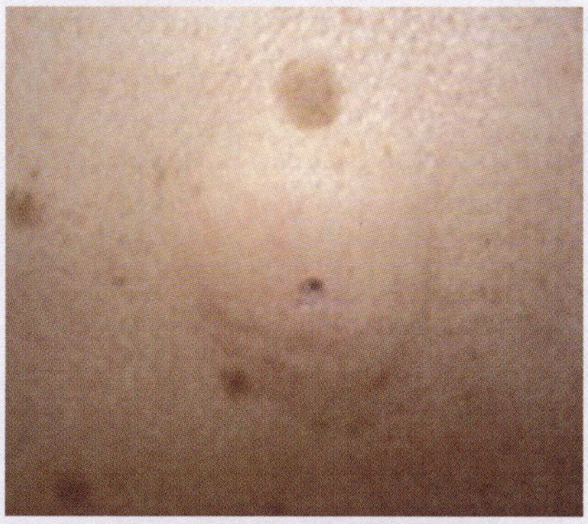

Pilar Cyst

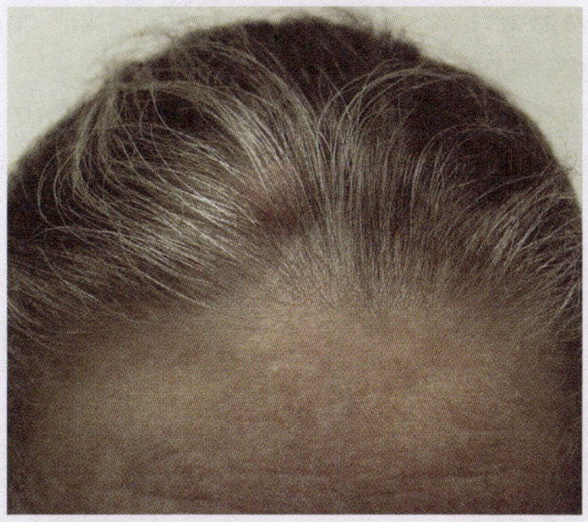

Lipoma

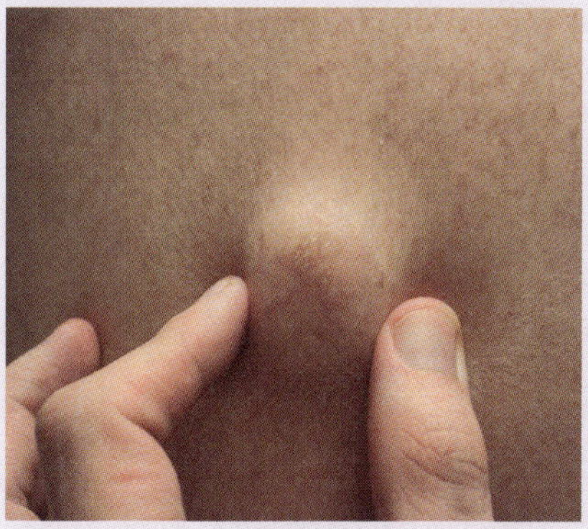

TABLE 18-4. Rough Lesions: Actinic Keratoses, Squamous Cell Carcinoma, and Their Mimics

Patients commonly report feeling rough lesions. Many are benign, like seborrheic keratoses or warts, but squamous cell carcinoma (SCC) and its precursor actinic keratosis can also feel rough or keratotic. *SCC* most commonly arises on sun-damaged skin of the head, neck, and dorsal arms and hands and can metastasize if left untreated. It consists of more mature cells usually resembling the spinous layer of the epidermis and accounts for ~16% of skin cancers. If left untreated, *actinic keratoses* progress to SCC at a rate of about 1 in 1,000 per year. Counsel affected patients about sun avoidance and use of sunscreen and offer treatment to prevent progression to SCC.

ACTINIC KERATOSIS AND SQUAMOUS CELL CARCINOMA

Actinic Keratosis

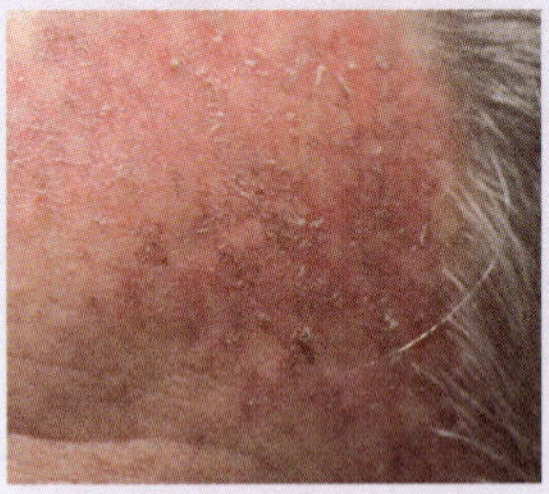

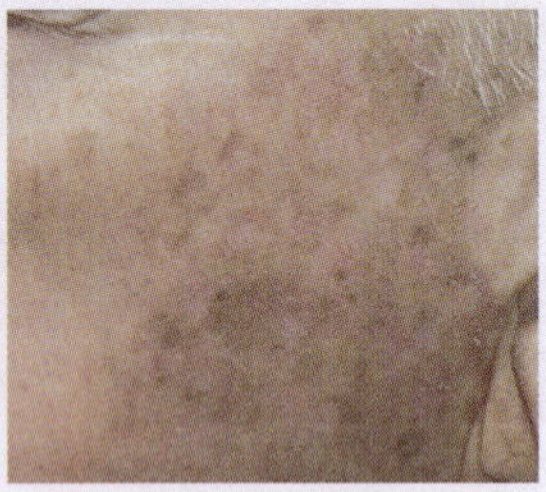

- Actinic keratosis after field therapy with 5-fluorouracil (left photo)
- Often easier to feel than to see
- Superficial keratotic papules "come and go" on sun-damaged skin

Cutaneous Horn/Keratotic Scale

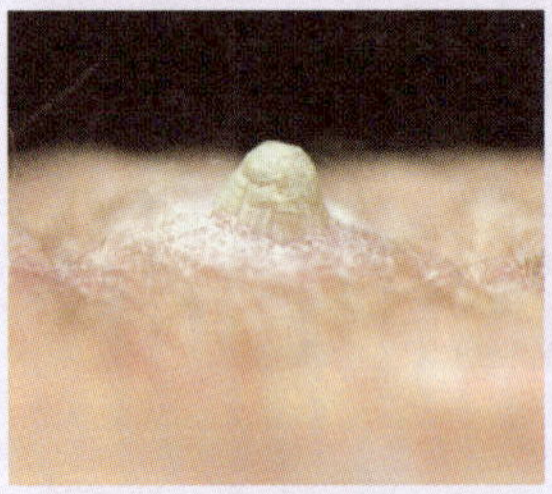

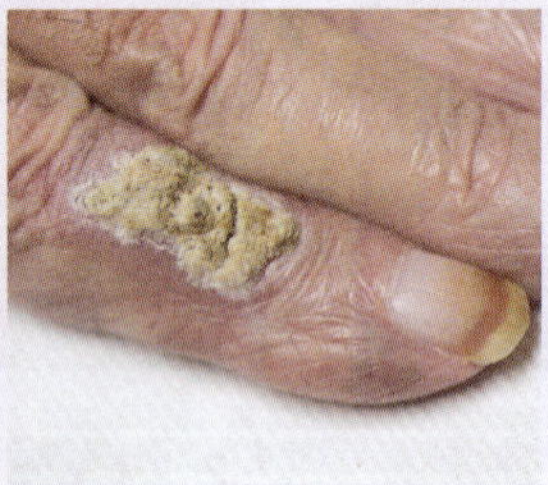

- The prototypic keratotic scale of actinic keratoses and SCC is formed by keratin and can result in a cutaneous horn
- Cutaneous horns should generally be biopsied to rule out SCC

Squamous Cell Carcinoma

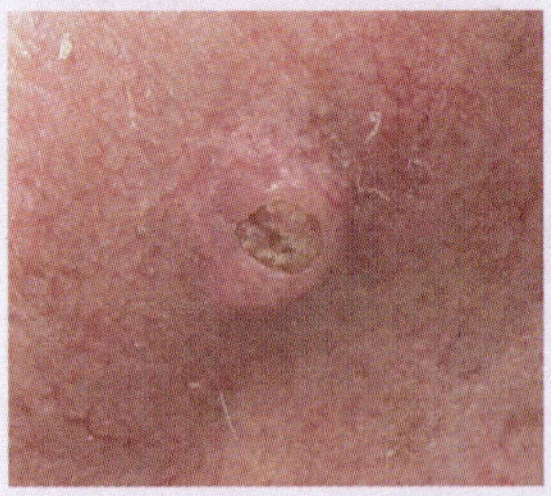

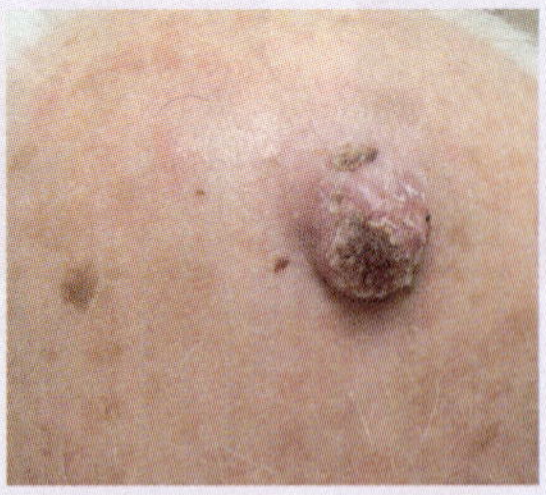

- Keratoacanthomas are SCCs that arise rapidly and have a crateriform center
- Often have a smooth but firm border
- SCCs can become quite large if left untreated (Note: highest sites of metastasis are the scalp, lips, and ears)

MIMICS

Superficial Xerosis or Seborrheic Dermatitis

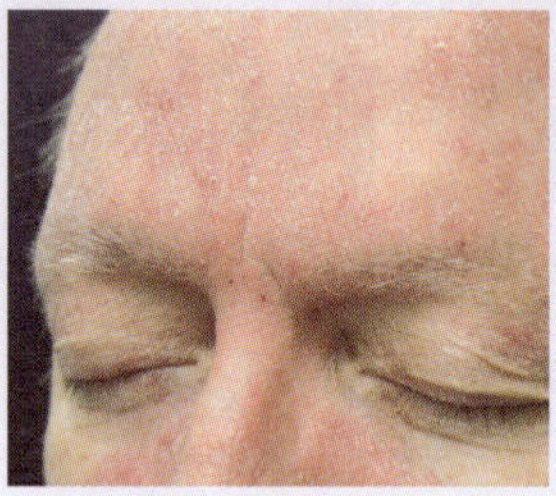

- May occur in same distribution on forehead, central face
- Scale is less keratotic and will improve with moisturizers, mild topical steroids

Warts

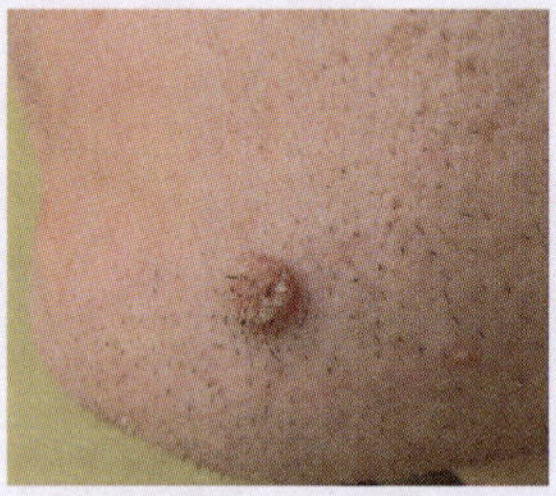

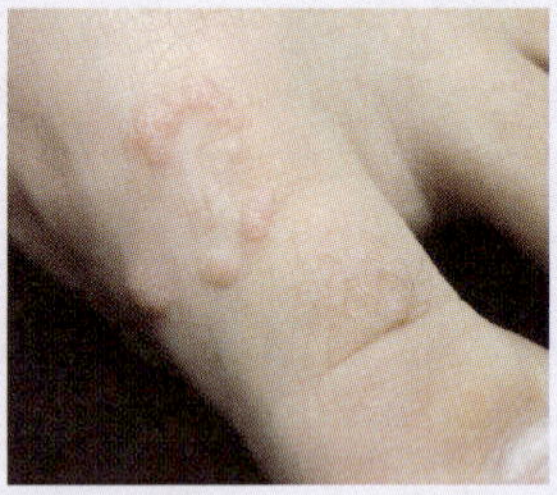

- Usually skin-colored to pink, texture more verrucous than keratotic
- May be filiform
- Often have hemorrhagic punctae that can be seen with a magnifying glass or dermatoscope

Seborrheic Keratosis

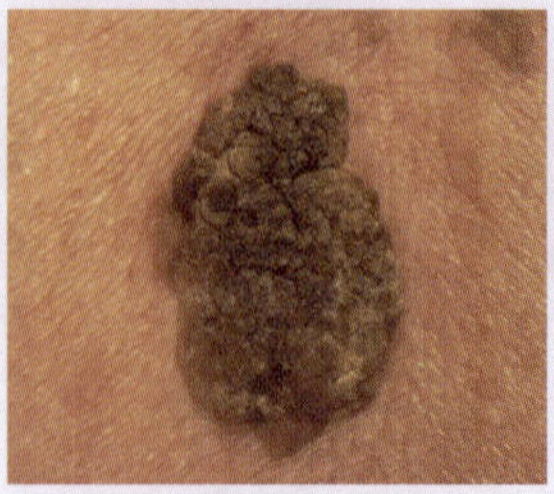

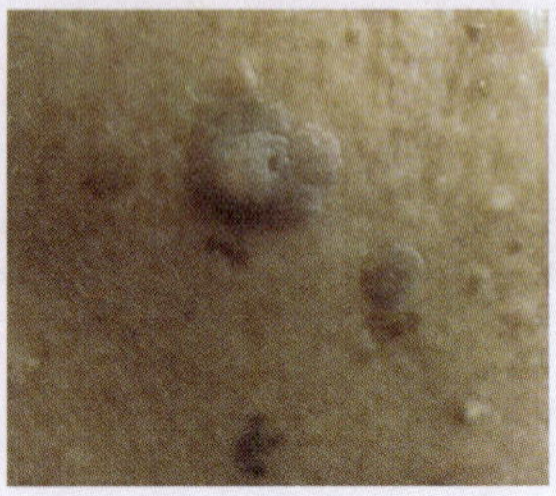

- Often have a verrucous texture
- Appear like a "stuck-on" or flattened ball of wax
- May crumble or bleed if picked
- Specific features on dermoscopy such as milia-like cysts or comedone-like openings are reassuring, if present
- May be erythematous, if inflamed

TABLE 18-5. Pink Lesions: Basal Cell Carcinoma and Its Mimics

Basal cell carcinoma (BCC) is the most common cancer in the world. Fortunately, it rarely spreads to other parts of the body. Nonetheless, it can invade and destroy local tissues, causing significant morbidity to the eye, nose, or brain. BCC consists of immature cells similar to those in the basal layer of the epidermis, and accounts for roughly 80% of all skin cancers. BCCs should be biopsied for confirmation before treatment. Review the BCC features below and how they contrast with mimics that are benign.

BASAL CELL CARCINOMAS

Superficial Basal Cell Carcinoma

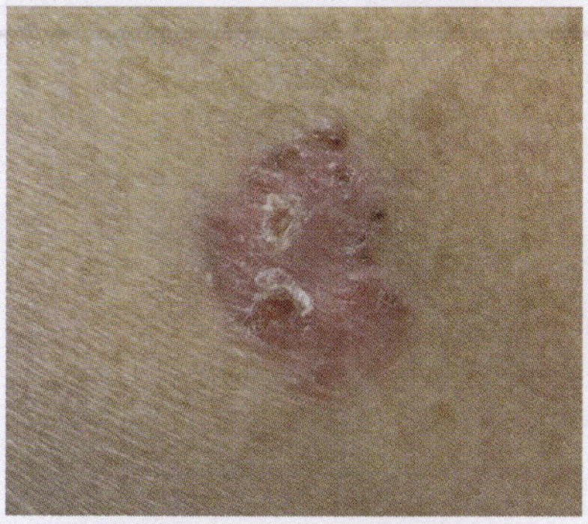

- Pink patch that does not heal
- May have focal scaling

Nodular Basal Cell Carcinoma

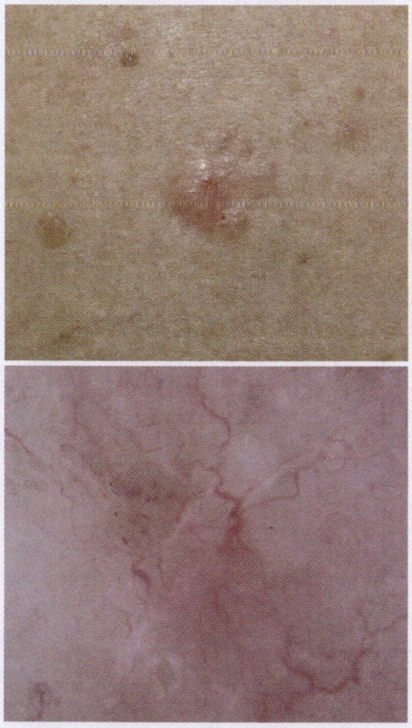

- Pink papule (top), often with translucent or pearly appearance and overlying telangiectasias
- May have focal pigmentation
- Dermoscopy (bottom) shows arborizing vessels, focal pigment globules, and other specific patterns

MIMICS

Actinic Keratosis and Squamous Cell Carcinoma In Situ

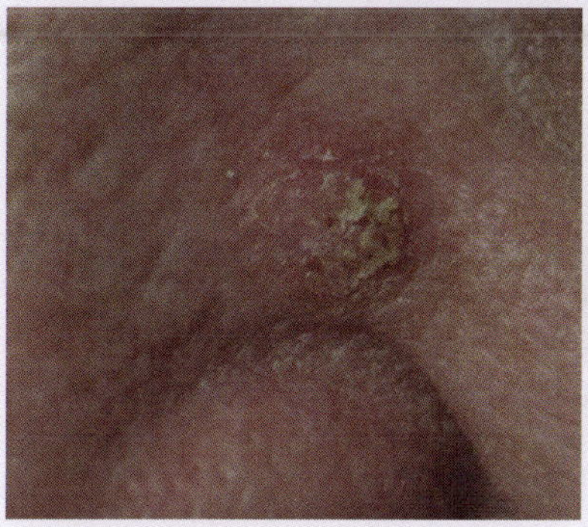

- Actinic keratosis or squamous cell carcinoma in situ usually has keratotic scaling

Sebaceous Hyperplasia

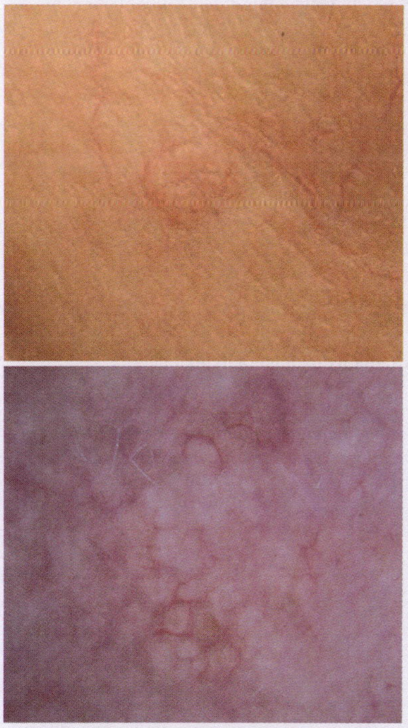

- Yellowish globular papules, often with central depression, on forehead and cheeks (top)
- Dermoscopy (bottom) shows telangiectasias that go around sebaceous glands rather than over them as in BCC

(continued)

TABLE 18-5. Pink Lesions: Basal Cell Carcinoma and Its Mimics *(Continued)*

BASAL CELL CARCINOMAS

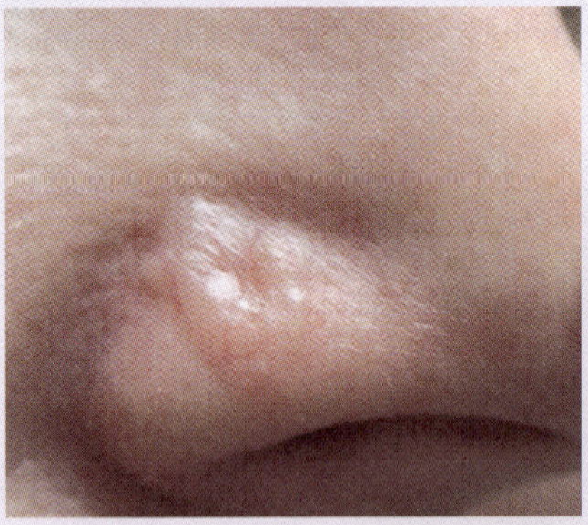

- 1-cm pearly pink plaque with central depression and overlying arborizing telangiectasias on nasal ala

Ulcerated Basal Cell Carcinoma

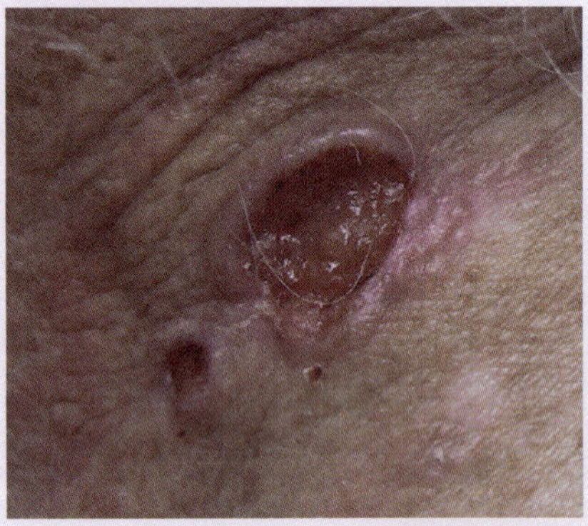

- Nonhealing ulcer, resulting in *"rolled border"*

MIMICS

Fibrous Papule

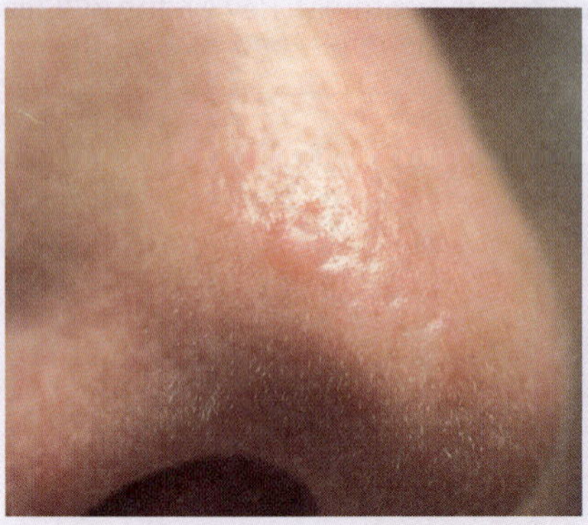

- Skin-colored to pink papule on the nose, without telangiectasias
- May become excoriated

Squamous Cell Carcinoma

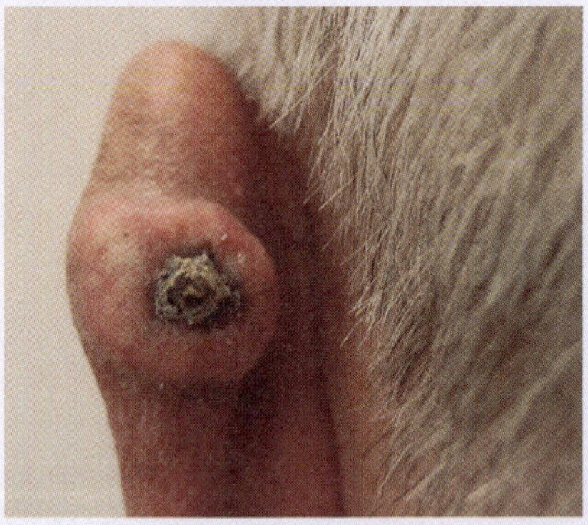

- May also be ulcerated
- Firmer at edges than BCC

TABLE 18-6. Brown Lesions: Melanoma and Its Mimics

Most patients have brown spots on their body surface if you look thoroughly. Although these are usually freckles, benign nevi, solar lentigines, or seborrheic keratoses, you and the patient must look closely for any that stand out as a possible melanoma. The best way to detect a melanoma is to do numerous skin examinations so that you recognize brown lesions that are benign. With enough practice, when you see a melanoma, it will stick out as the "ugly duckling." Review the ABCDE rule and photographs on p. 515, which provide additional helpful identifiers and comparisons.

MELANOMAS

Amelanotic Melanoma

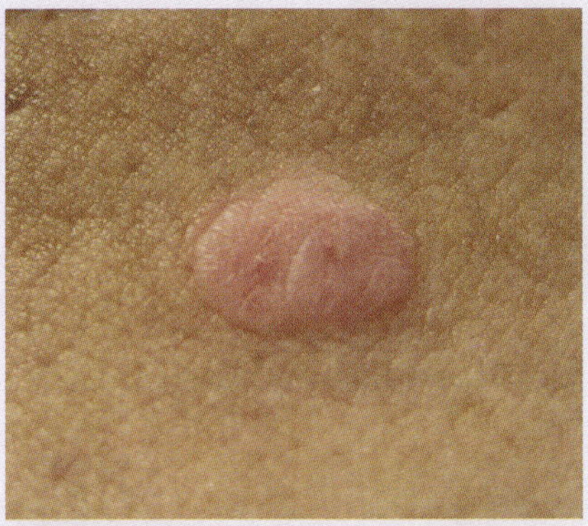

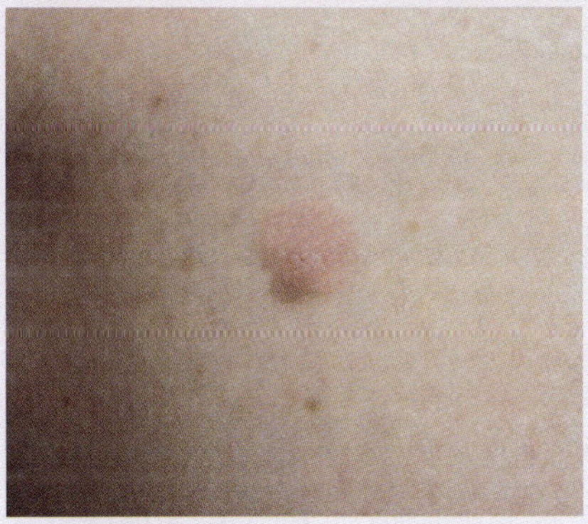

- Usually in very fair-skinned people
- *Evolution or rapid change* is the most important feature, because variegation or dark pigment is missing in this type

MIMICS

Skin Tags or Intradermal Nevi

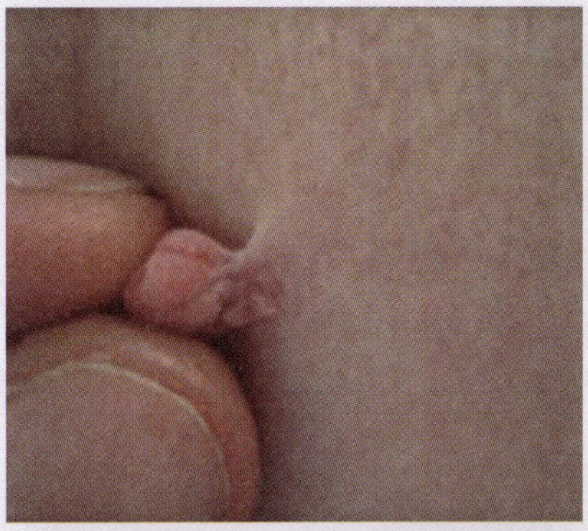

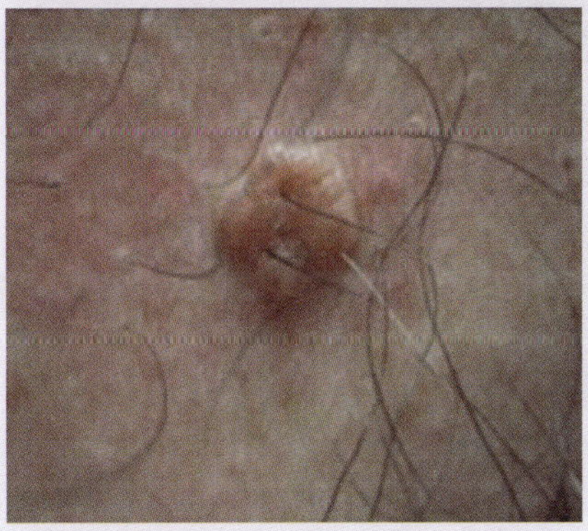

- Soft and fleshy
- Often around neck, axillae, or back
- Sessile nevi may have a hint of brown pigmentation

(continued)

TABLE 18-6. Brown Lesions: Melanoma and Its Mimics *(Continued)*

MELANOMAS	MIMICS
Melanoma *In Situ*	**Solar Lentigo**
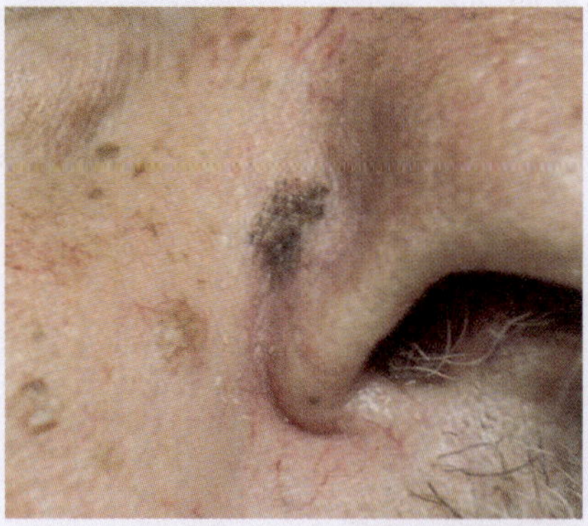	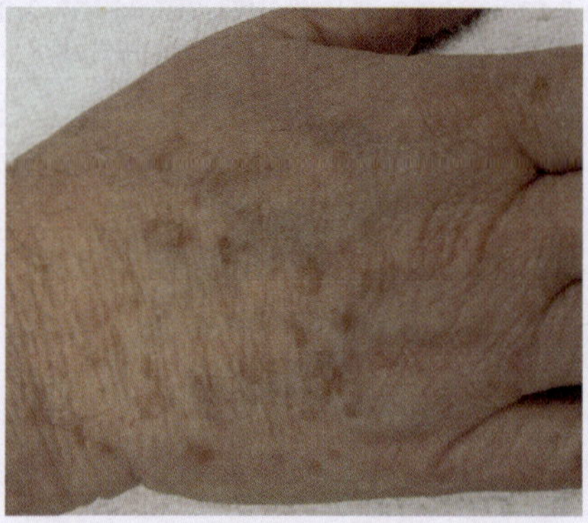
■ On sun-exposed or sun-protected skin ■ Look for ABCDE features	■ On sun-exposed skin ■ Light brown and uniform in color but may be asymmetric
Melanoma	**Dysplastic Nevus**
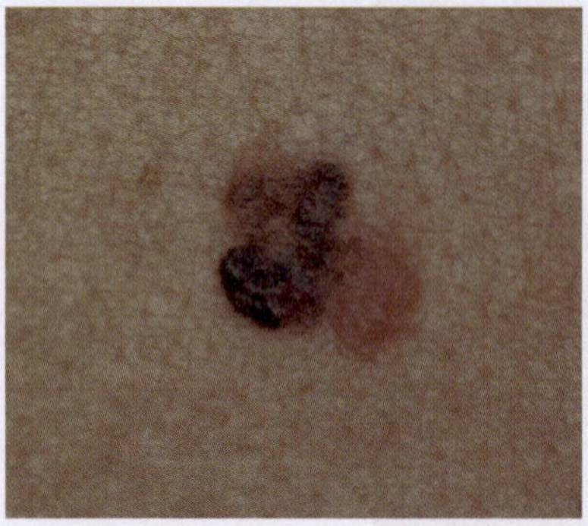	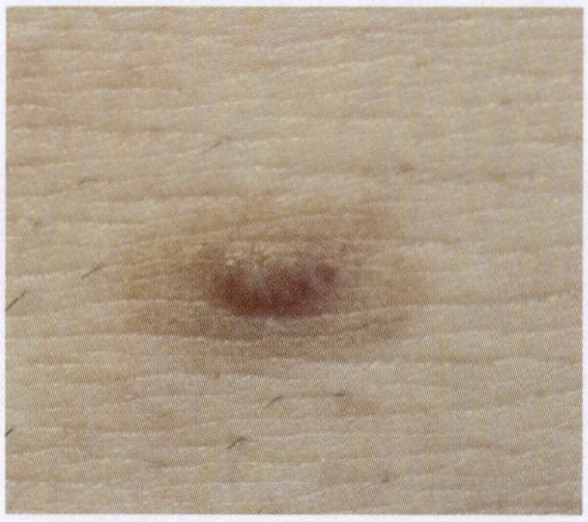
■ May arise de novo or in existing nevi and exhibits ABCDEs ■ Patients with many dysplastic nevi have increased risk of melanoma	■ May have macular base and papular central "fried egg" component ■ Compare to the patient's other nevi and monitor changes
Melanoma	**Inflamed Seborrheic Keratosis**
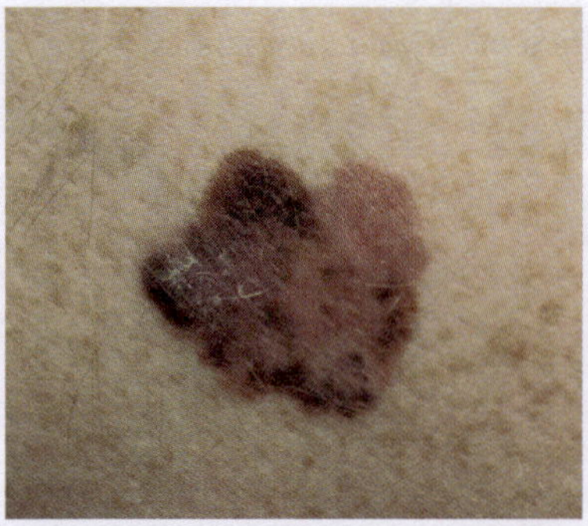	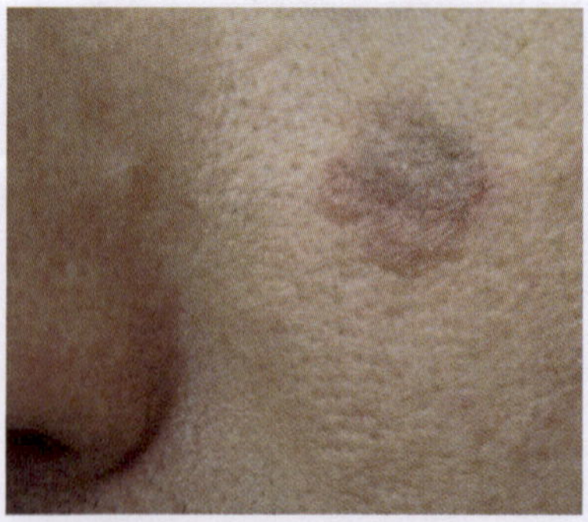
■ May have *variegated color* (browns, red) ■ Has melanocytic features on dermoscopy	■ Can sometimes mimic a melanoma if it has an erythematous base ■ Dermoscopy helps the trained eye distinguish these

(continued)

TABLE 18-6. Brown Lesions: Melanoma and Its Mimics *(Continued)*

MELANOMAS	MIMICS
Melanoma	**Seborrheic Keratosis**
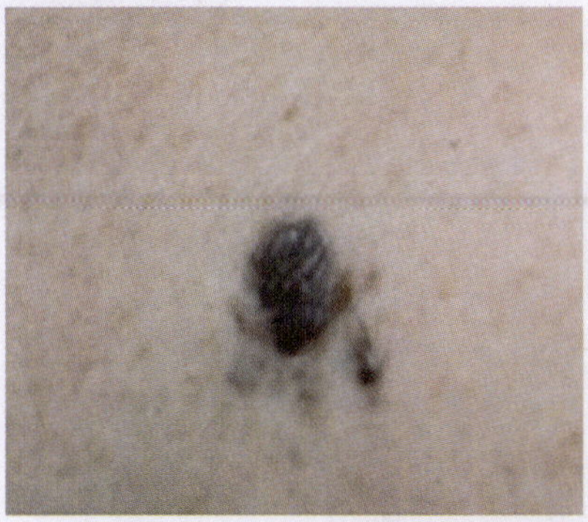	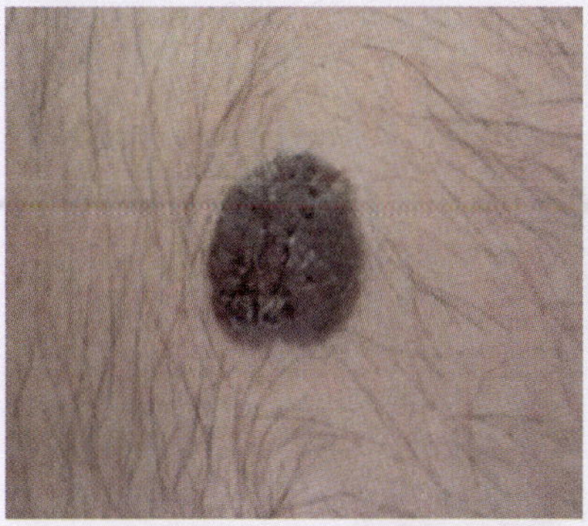
■ May be uniform in color but *asymmetric;* key feature is *rapid change or evolution*	■ Stuck-on and verrucous, may be darkly pigmented
Acral Melanoma	**Acral Nevus**
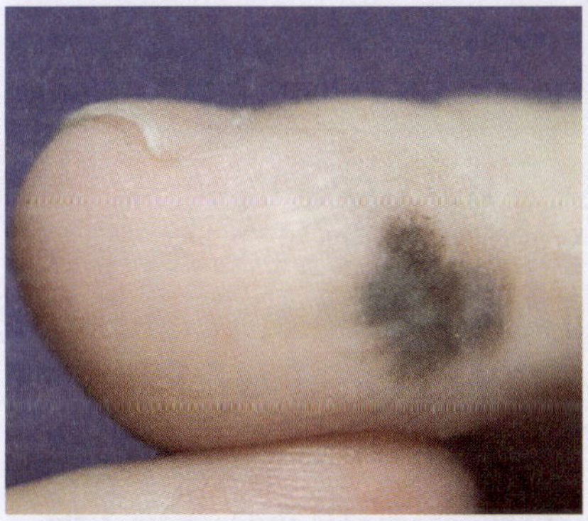	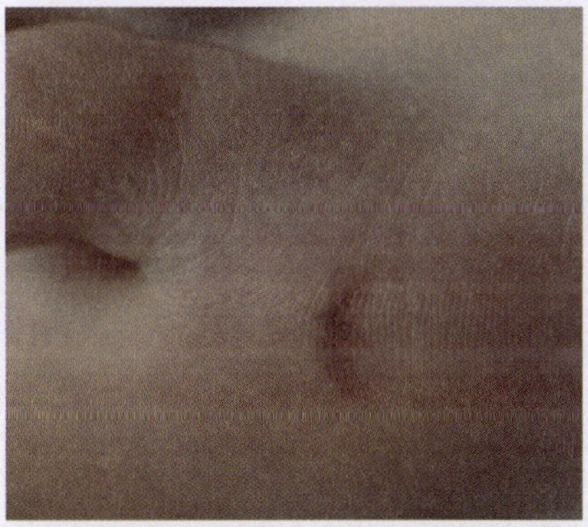
■ Rapid change or evolution helps detect acral melanoma ■ Consider biopsies if >7 mm, rapidly growing, or concerning features on dermoscopy	■ Likely benign if <7 mm and has a reassurance pattern on dermoscopy, such as the parallel furrow or lattice patterns

(continued)

TABLE 18-6. Brown Lesions: Melanoma and Its Mimics (*Continued*)

MELANOMAS

Melanoma with Blue-Black Areas

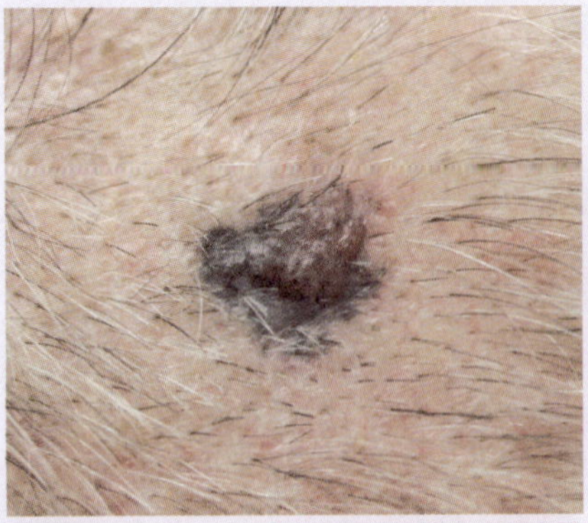

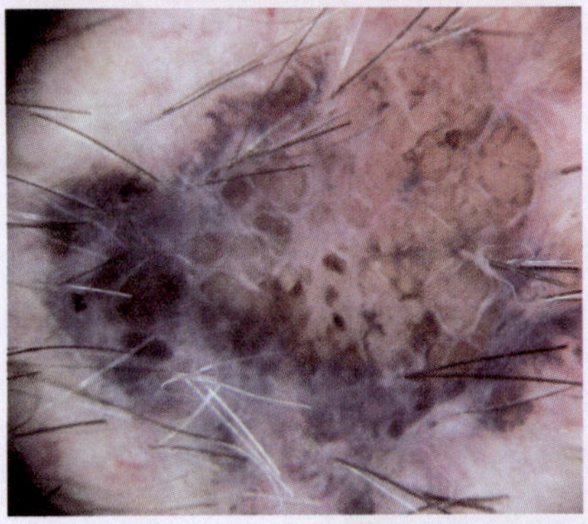

- Blue-black areas are concerning for melanoma, especially if they are asymmetric

MIMICS

Blue Nevus

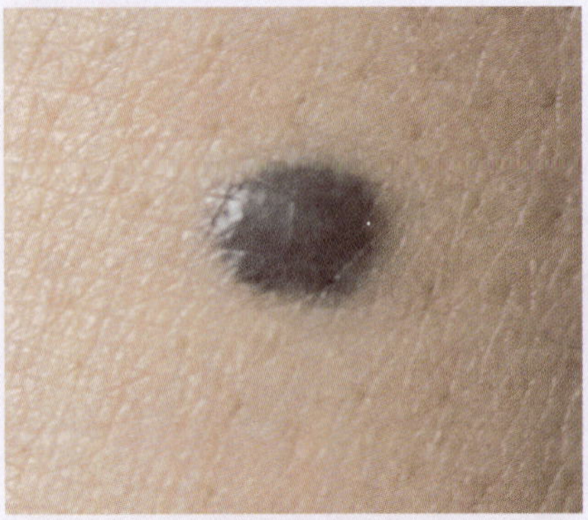

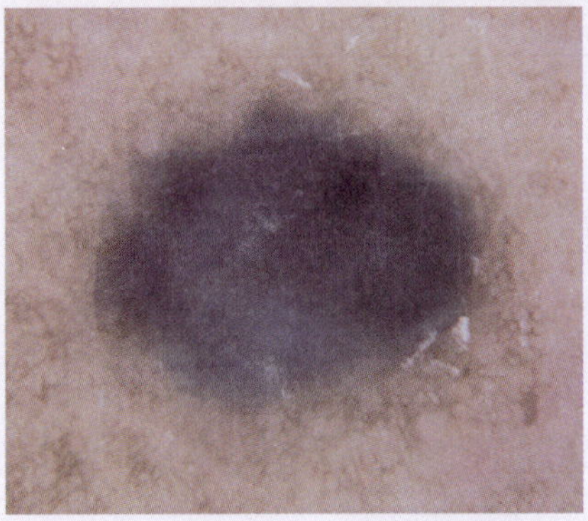

- Blue nevi have a homogenous blue-gray appearance, clinically and on dermoscopy

Finding the Ugly Duckling: As you evaluate changing brown lesions in the context of the patient's other nevi and lentigines, the "ugly duckling" is the nevus that looks different from the patient's other nevi. A patient may make many atypical nevi with surrounding macular components and central papular components, but they all look the same. Find the patient's *signature nevus,* then search for the ugly duckling that looks different from the patient's typical "signature" nevi.

Most dermatologists now rely on a dermoscope to evaluate pigmented lesions, which allows them to detect melanomas when they are thinner. With training, dermoscopy can help distinguish nevi with reassuring patterns from possible early melanomas. Even without dermoscopy, however, a keen eye actively inspecting the skin for "ugly ducklings" is likely to detect melanomas when they arise.

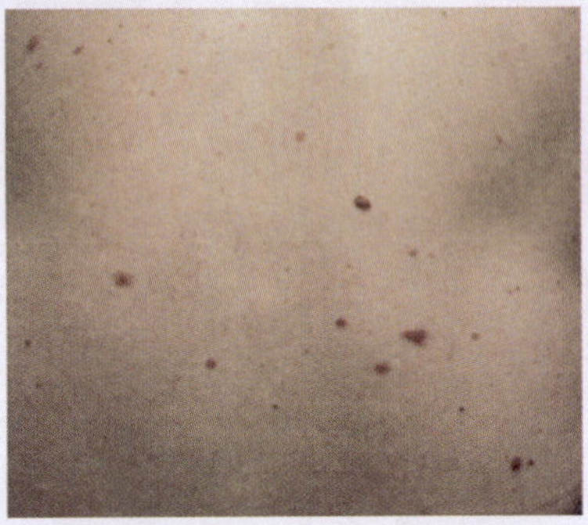

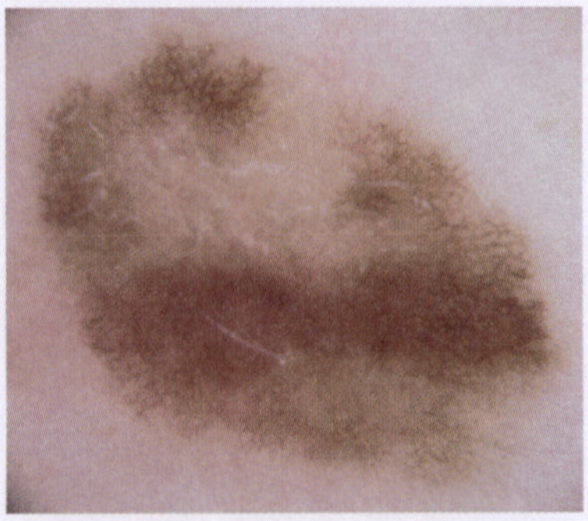

This patient has multiple atypical nevi on his back (left), but the one on his back just to the right of midline (enlarged right image) stands out as the "ugly duckling" because it has three colors; the white area showed melanoma in situ on biopsy.

TABLE 18-7. Vascular and Purpuric Lesions of the Skin

VASCULAR LESIONS

	Spider Angioma[a]	Spider Vein[a]	Cherry Angioma
	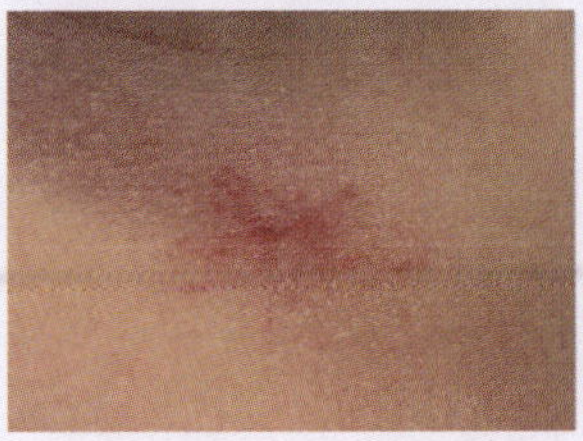	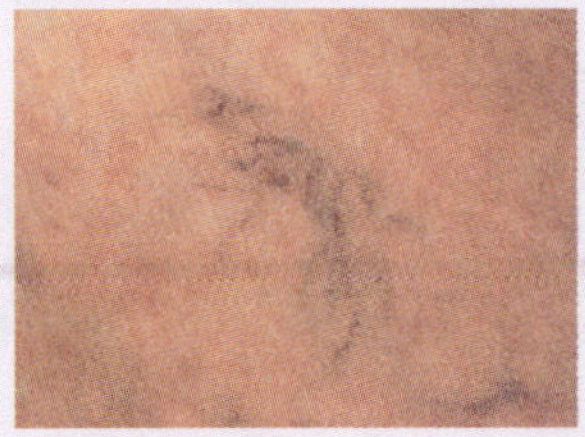	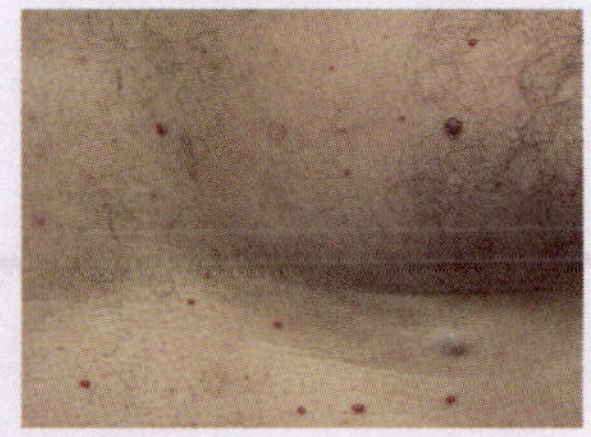
Color and Size	Fiery red; from very small to 2 cm	Bluish; size variable, from very small to several inches	Bright or ruby red; may become purplish with age; 1–3 mm
Shape	Central body, sometimes raised, surrounded by erythema and radiating legs	Variable; may resemble a spider or be linear, irregular, cascading	Round, flat, or sometimes raised; may be surrounded by a pale halo
Pulsatility and Effect of Pressure	Often seen in center of the spider when pressure with a glass slide is applied; pressure on the body causes blanching of the spider	Absent; pressure over the center does not cause blanching, but diffuse pressure blanches the veins	Absent; may show partial blanching, especially if pressure applied with edge of a pinpoint
Distribution	Face, neck, arms, and upper trunk; almost never below the waist	Most often on the legs, near veins; also on the anterior chest	Trunk; also extremities
Significance	Single spider angiomas are normal and are common on the face and chest; also seen in pregnancy and liver disease	Often accompanies increased pressure in the superficial veins, as in varicose veins	None; increases in size and numbers with aging

(continued)

TABLE 18-7. Vascular and Purpuric Lesions of the Skin *(Continued)*

	PURPURIC LESIONS	
	Petechia/Purpura	**Ecchymosis**
	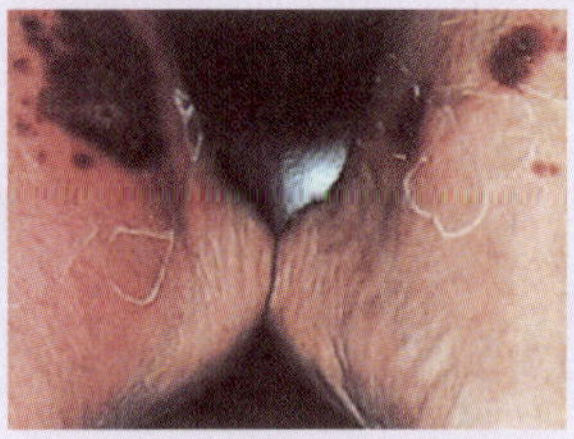	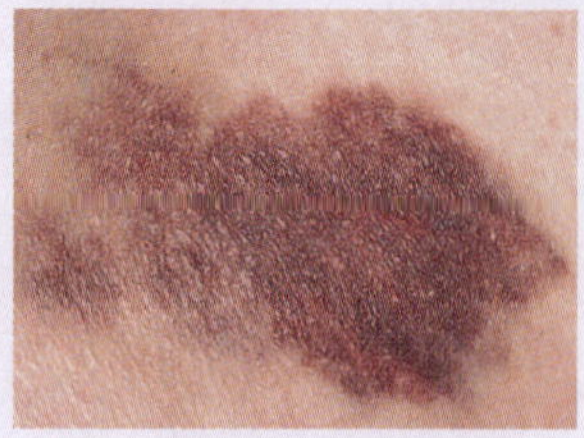
Color and Size	Deep red or reddish purple, fading away over time; petechia, 1–3 mm; purpura are larger	Purple or purplish blue, fading to green, yellow, and brown with time; variable size, larger than petechiae, >3 mm
Shape	Rounded, sometimes irregular; flat	Rounded, oval, or irregular; may have a central subcutaneous flat nodule (a hematoma)
Pulsatility and Effect of Pressure	Absent; no effect from pressure	Absent; no effect from pressure
Distribution	Variable	Variable
Significance	Blood outside the vessels; may suggest a bleeding disorder or, if petechiae, emboli to skin; palpable purpura in *vasculitis*	Blood outside the vessels; often secondary to bruising or trauma; also seen in bleeding disorders

[a]These are telangiectasias, or dilated small vessels that look red or bluish.

Sources of photos: *Spider Angioma*—Marks R. *Skin Disease in Old Age*. JB Lippincott; 1987 and *Petechia/Purpura*—Kelley WN. *Textbook of Internal Medicine*. JB Lippincott; 1989.

TABLE 18-8. Hair Loss

When taking a complete history of hair loss, include the duration, acuity of onset, cause from decreased hair density or increased shedding, the pattern (diffuse or localized), medication history, hair care practices, and associated medical conditions or stressors. *Decrease in hair density* is usually caused by male or female pattern hair loss, but less commonly by scarring alopecias. *Hair shedding from the roots* is often caused by *telogen effluvium, alopecia areata, anagen effluvium* (insults to the hair shaft from exposure to agents like chemotherapy) or less commonly, scarring alopecias. Perform a hair pull test to look for the percentage of telogen hairs. *Hair shedding from breakage at the hair shaft* is often caused by *tinea capitis,* improper hair care, and less commonly hair shaft disorders or *anagen effluvium.* Perform a tug test to look for hair fragility. See Figures 18-27 and 18-28 for examples of the hair pull test and tug test.

GENERALIZED OR DIFFUSE HAIR LOSS

Male and female pattern hair loss affects over half of men by their 50 years of age, and over half of women by their 80 years of age. In men, look for frontal hairline regression and thinning on the posterior vertex; in women, look for thinning that spreads from the crown down without hairline regression. Severity is described by standardized classifications: Norwood–Hamilton (men) and Ludwig (women). The *hair pull test* is normal or only pulls a few hairs.

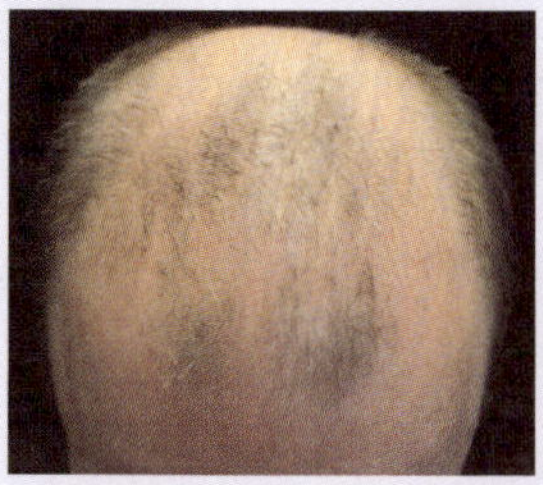

Male pattern hair loss (MPHL)

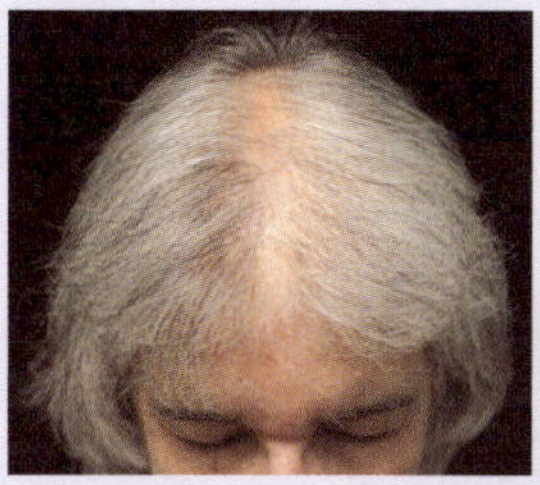

Female pattern hair loss (FPHL)

Telogen Effluvium and Anagen Effluvium

In *telogen effluvium,* overall, the patient's scalp and hair distribution appear normal, but a positive *hair pull test* reveals most hairs have telogen bulbs. In *anagen effluvium,* there is diffuse hair loss from the roots. The *hair pull test* shows few if any hairs with telogen bulbs.

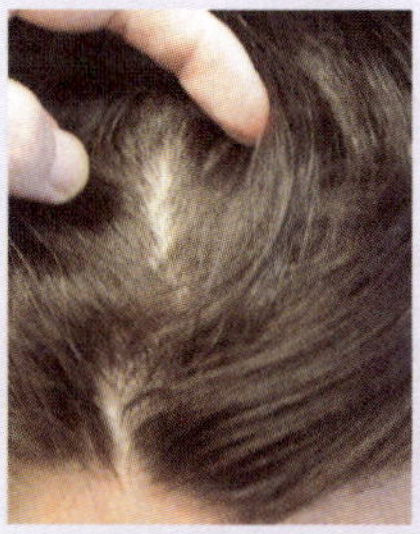

Normal hair part width in telogen effluvium

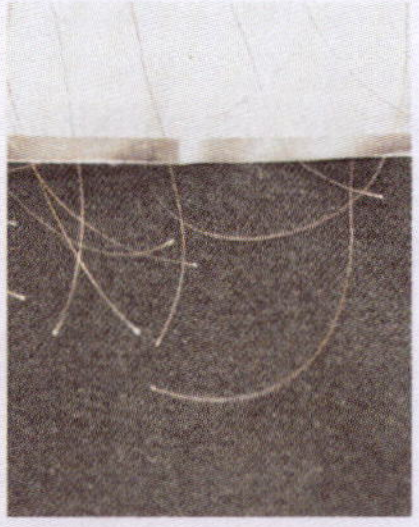

Positive hair pull test in telogen effluvium showing all hairs have telogen bulbs

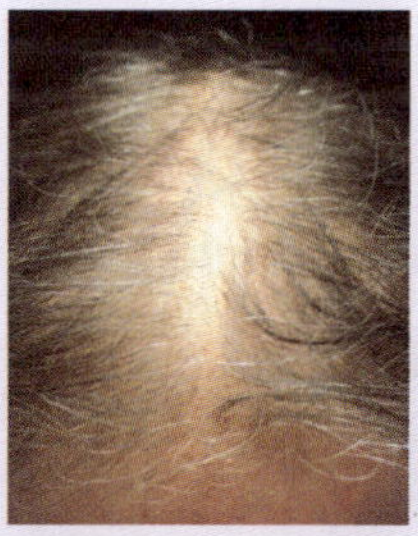

Anagen effluvium

(*continued*)

TABLE 18-8. Hair Loss *(Continued)*

FOCAL HAIR LOSS

Alopecia Areata

There is sudden onset of clearly demarcated, usually localized, round or oval patches of hair loss leaving smooth skin without hairs, in children and young adults. There is no visible scaling or erythema.

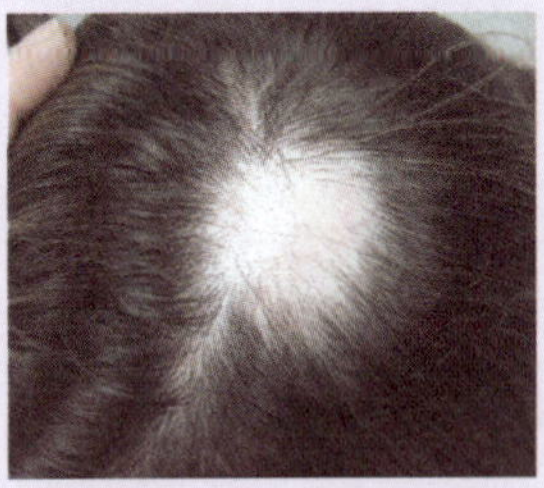

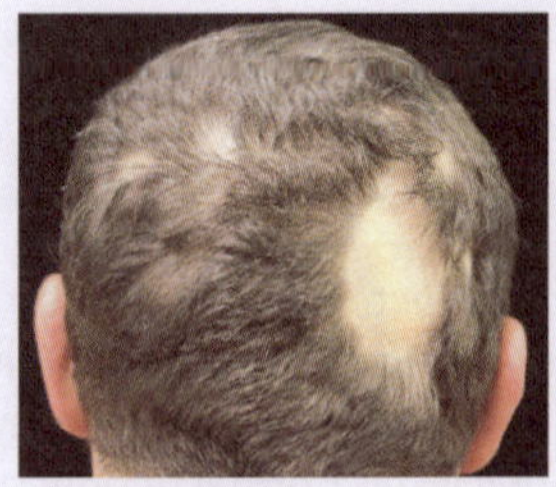

Tinea Capitis ("Ringworm")

There are round scaling patches of alopecia, mostly seen in children. There may be "black dots" of broken hairs and comma or corkscrew hairs on dermoscopy. Usually caused by *Trichophyton tonsurans* from humans, and less commonly, *Microsporum canis* from dogs or cats. Boggy plaques are called kerions.

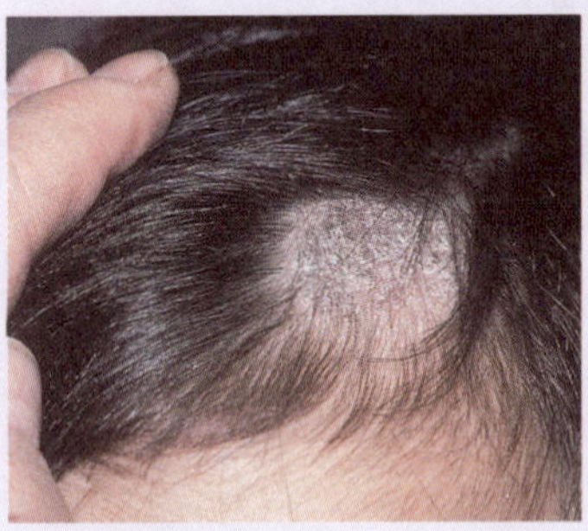

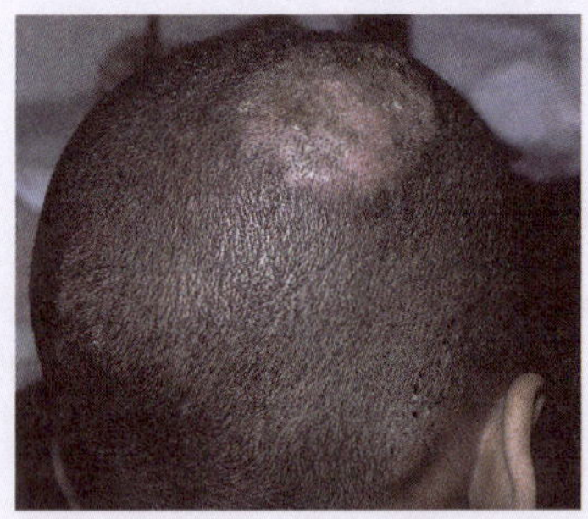

Scarring Alopecia

Scarring on the scalp is characterized by shiny skin, complete loss of hair follicles, and often, discoloration. Presence of any scarring should prompt referral to a dermatologist for possible scalp biopsy if the patient desires treatment. Examples of scarring alopecia include central centrifugal scarring alopecia and discoid lupus erythematosus, among others.

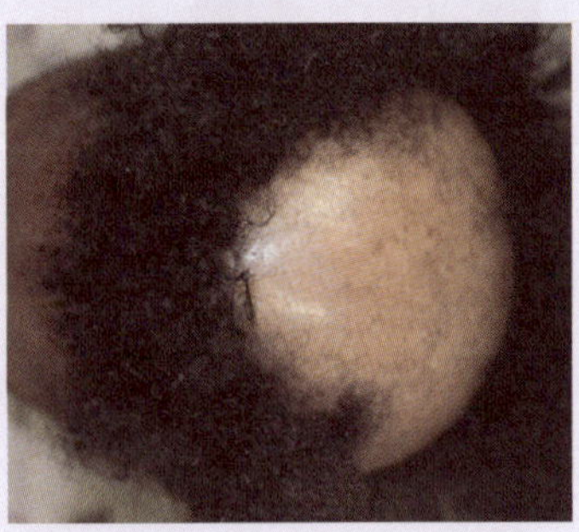

Central centrifugal scarring alopecia

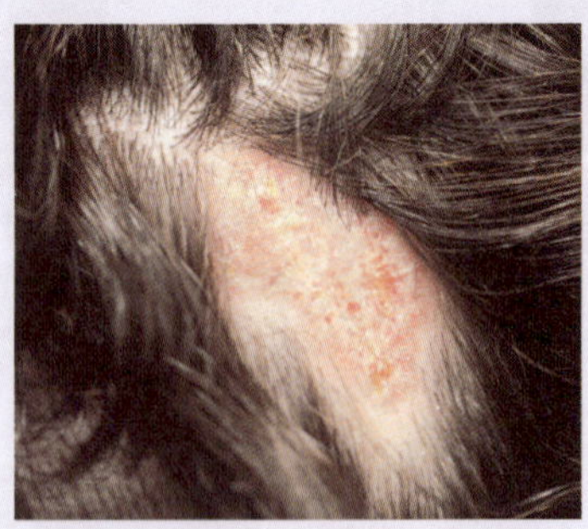

Discoid lupus scarring alopecia

(*continued*)

TABLE 18-8. Hair Loss (Continued)

Hair Shaft Disorders

Patients with abnormal hair from birth, as in this patient with a genetic condition called monilethrix, should be referred to dermatology.

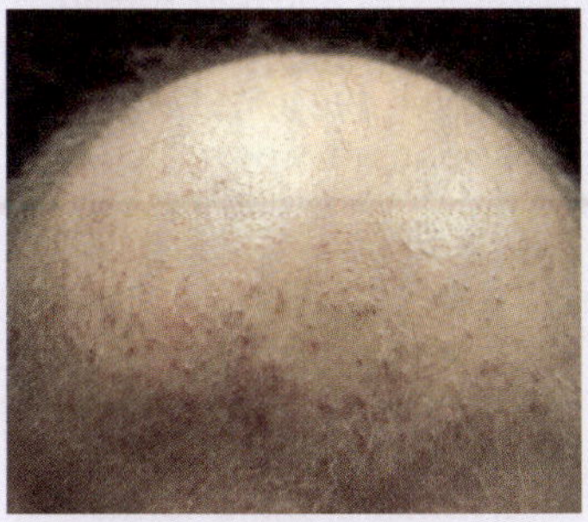

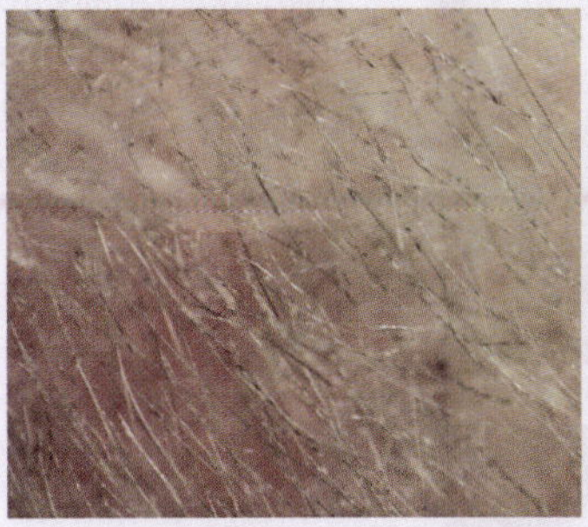

Hair shaft disorder with alternating bands

Sources of photo: Alopecia Areata [left]—Goodheart H, Gonzalez M. *Goodheart's Photoguide to Common Pediatric and Adult Skin Disorders*. 4th ed. Wolters Kluwer; 2016, Appendix Figure 10.

TABLE 18-9. Findings in or Near the Nails

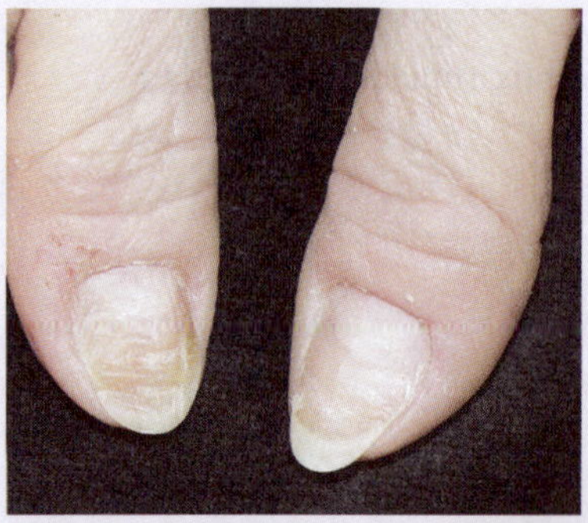

Paronychia

A superficial infection of the proximal and lateral nail folds adjacent to the nail plate. The nail folds are often red, swollen, and tender. Represents the most common infection of the hand, usually from *Staphylococcus aureus* or *Streptococcus* species, and may spread until it completely surrounds the nail plate. Creates a felon (closed-space infection) if it extends into the pulp space of the finger. Arises from local trauma due to nail biting, manicuring, or frequent hand immersion in water. Chronic infections may be related to *Candida.*

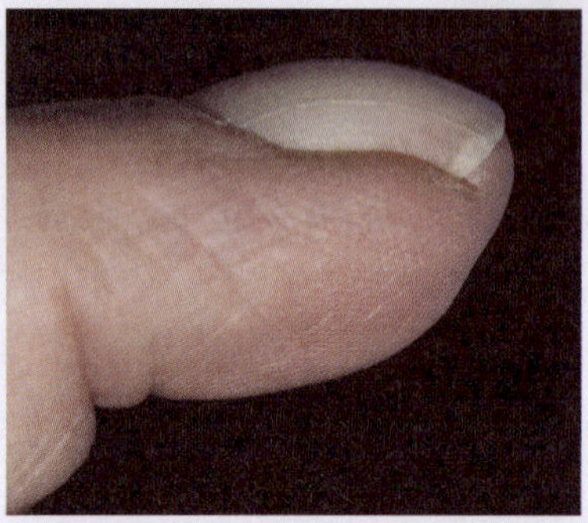

Clubbing of the Fingers

Clinically, a bulbous swelling of the soft tissue at the nail base, with loss of the normal angle between the nail and the proximal nail fold. The angle increases to 180 degrees or more, and the nail bed feels spongy or floating. The mechanism is still unknown but involves vasodilation with increased blood flow to the distal portion of the digits and changes in connective tissue, possibly from hypoxia, changes in innervation, genetics, or a platelet-derived growth factor from fragments of platelet clumps. Seen in congenital heart disease, interstitial lung disease and lung cancer, inflammatory bowel diseases, and malignancies.

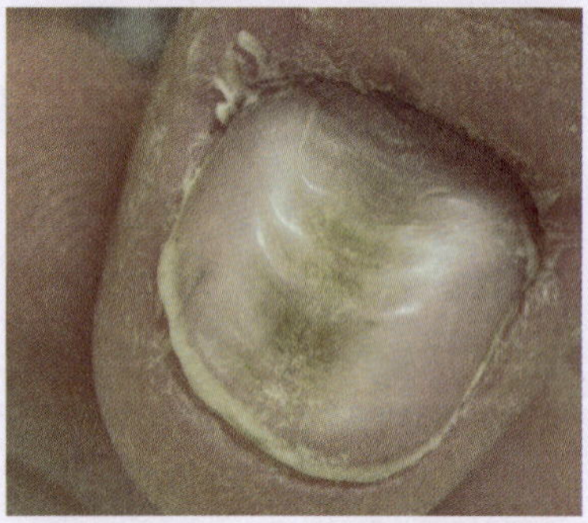

Habit Tic Deformity

There is depression of the central nail with a "Christmas tree" appearance from small horizontal depressions, resulting from repetitive trauma from rubbing the index finger over the thumb or vice versa. Pressure on the nail matrix causes the nail to grow out abnormally. Avoidance of the behavior leads to normal nail growth.

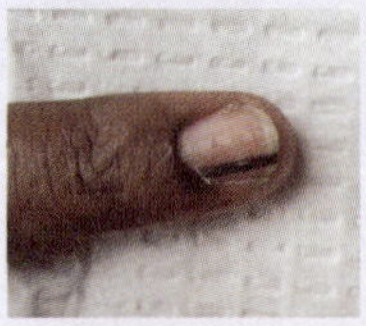

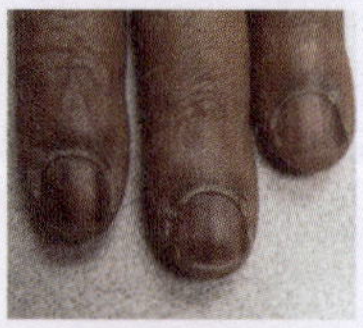

Melanonychia

Melanonychia is caused by increased pigmentation in the nail matrix, leading to a streak as the nail grows out. This may be a normal ethnic variation if found in multiple nails. A thin uniform streak may be caused by a nevus, but a wide streak, especially if growing or irregular, could represent a subungual melanoma.

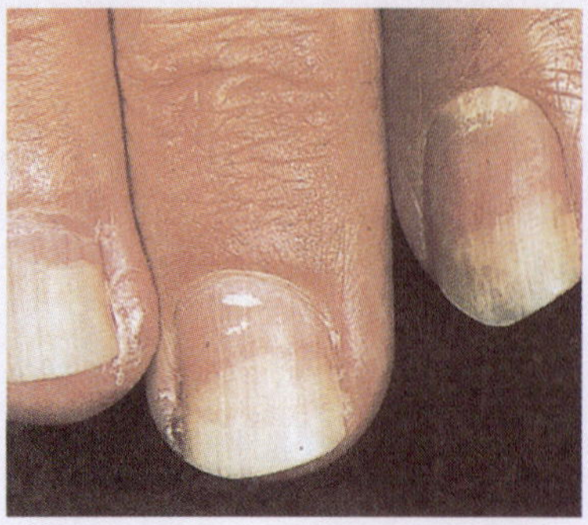

Onycholysis

A painless separation of the whitened opaque nail plate from the pinker translucent nail bed. Fingernails that extend past the fingertip are more likely to result in the traumatic shearing forces that produce onycholysis. Starts distally and progresses proximally, enlarging the free edge of the nail. Local causes include trauma from excess manicuring, psoriasis, fungal infection, and allergic reactions to nail cosmetics. Systemic causes include diabetes, anemia, photosensitive drug reactions, hyperthyroidism, peripheral ischemia, bronchiectasis, and syphilis.

(*continued*)

TABLE 18-9. Findings in or Near the Nails *(Continued)*

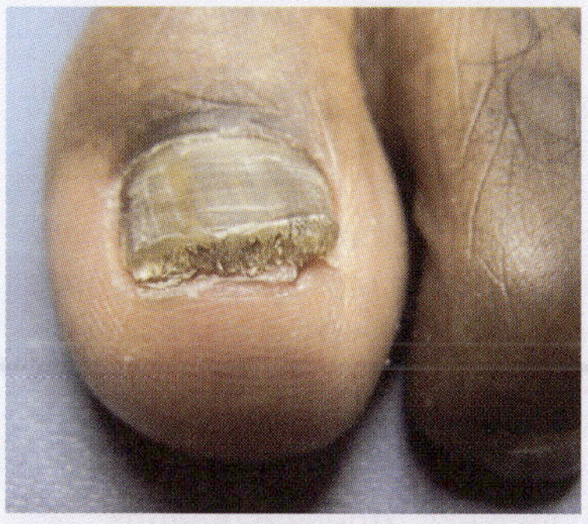

Onychomycosis

The most common cause of nail thickening and subungual debris is onychomycosis, most often from the dermatophyte *Trichophyton rubrum,* but also from other dermatophytes and some molds such as *Alternaria* and *Fusarium* species. Onychomycosis affects 1 in 5 over age 60. The best prevention is to treat and prevent tinea pedis. Only half of all nail dystrophies are caused by onychomycosis, so a positive fungal culture, potassium hydroxide examination, or pathologic evaluation of nail clippings is recommended before treating with oral antifungals.

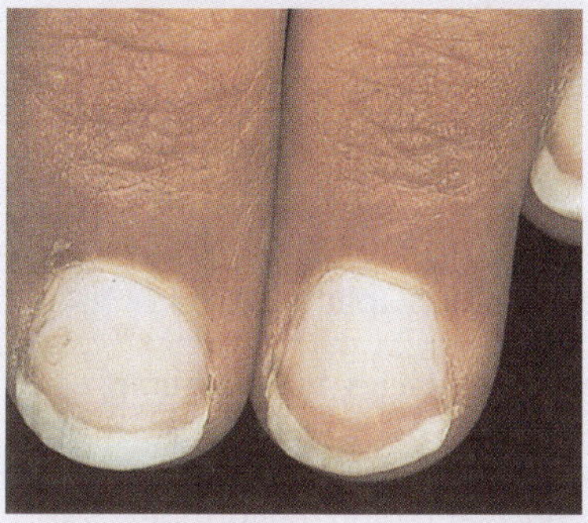

Terry Nails

Nail plate turns white with a ground-glass appearance, a distal band of reddish brown, and obliteration of the lunula. Commonly affects all fingers, although may appear in only one finger. Seen in liver disease, usually cirrhosis, heart failure, and diabetes. May arise from decreased vascularity and increased connective tissue in nail bed.

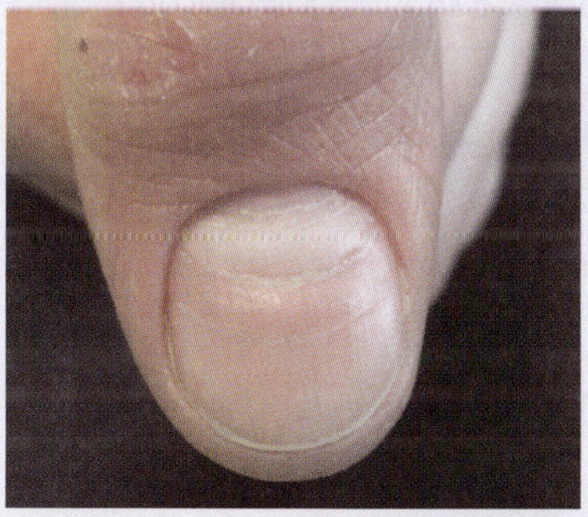

Transverse Linear Depressions (*Beau Lines*)

Transverse depressions of the nail plates, usually bilateral, resulting from temporary disruption of proximal nail growth from systemic illness. Timing of the illness may be estimated by measuring the distance from the line to the nail bed (nails grow approximately 1 mm every 6 to 10 days). Seen in severe illness, trauma, and cold exposure if Raynaud disease is present.

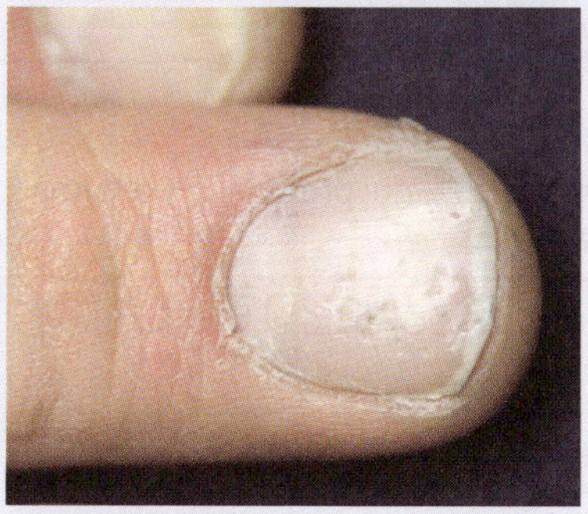

Pitting

Punctate depressions of the nail plate caused by defective layering of the superficial nail plate by the proximal nail matrix. Usually associated with psoriasis but also seen in reactive arthritis, sarcoidosis, alopecia areata, and localized atopic or chemical dermatitis.

Sources of photos: Onycholysis, Terry Nails—Reprinted from Habif TP. *Clinical Dermatology: A Color Guide to Diagnosis and Therapy*. 2nd ed. CV Mosby; 1990.

TABLE 18-10. Systemic Diseases and Associated Skin Findings

Systemic Disease	Associated Findings or Diagnoses
Addison disease	Hyperpigmentation of oral mucosa as well as sun-exposed skin, sites of trauma, and creases of palms and soles
Acquired immune deficiency syndrome	Human papillomavirus, herpes simplex virus, varicella zoster virus, cytomegalovirus, molluscum contagiosum, bacterial abscesses, mycobacterium (tuberculosis, leprae, avium) infections, candidiasis, deep fungal infections (cryptococcus, histoplasmosis), oral hairy leukoplakia, Kaposi sarcoma, oral and anal squamous cell carcinoma, acquired ichthyosis, severe psoriasis, severe seborrheic dermatitis, eosinophilic folliculitis
Chagas disease (American trypanosomiasis)	Unilateral conjunctivitis and lid edema associated with preauricular lymphadenopathy
Chronic renal disease	Pallor, xerosis, uremic frost, pruritus, "half and half" nails, calciphylaxis.
CREST syndrome	Calcinosis, Raynaud phenomenon, sclerodactyly, matted telangiectasias of face and hands (palms)
Crohn disease	Erythema nodosum, pyoderma gangrenosum, enterocutaneous fistulas, aphthous ulcers
Cushing disease	Striae, atrophy, purpura, ecchymoses, telangiectasias, acne, moon facies, buffalo hump, hypertrichosis
Dermatomyositis	Violaceous erythema as macules, patches or papules in periocular region (heliotrope), on interphalangeal joints (Gottron sign), and on upper back and shoulders (shawl sign); poikiloderma in sun-exposed areas; periungual telangiectasia, ragged cuticles (Samitz sign)
Diabetes	Pruritus, diabetic dermopathy, acanthosis nigricans, candidiasis, neuropathic ulcers, necrobiosis lipoidica, eruptive xanthomas
Disseminated intravascular coagulation	Purpura, petechiae, hemorrhagic bullae, induration, necrosis
Dyslipidemias	Xanthomas (tendon, eruptive, and tuberous), xanthelasma (may also occur in healthy people)
Gonococcemia	Purple to gray macules, papules or hemorrhagic pustules distributed over acral and periarticular surfaces
Hemochromatosis	Skin bronzing and hyperpigmentation
Hyperthyroidism	Warm, moist, soft, and velvety skin; thin and fine hair; alopecia; vitiligo; pretibial myxedema (in Graves disease); hyperpigmentation (local or generalized)
Hypothyroidism	Dry, rough, and pale skin; coarse and brittle hair; myxedema; alopecia (lateral third of the eyebrows to diffuse); skin cool to touch; thin and brittle nails
Infective endocarditis	Janeway lesions, Osler nodes, splinter hemorrhages, petechiae
Kawasaki disease	Mucosal erythema (lips, tongue, and pharynx), strawberry tongue, cherry red lips, polymorphous rash (primarily on trunk), erythema of palms and soles with later desquamation of fingertips
Leukemia/lymphoma	Pallor, exfoliative erythroderma, nodules, petechiae, ecchymoses, pruritus, vasculitis, pyoderma gangrenosum, bullous diseases

(*continued*)

TABLE 18-10. Systemic Diseases and Associated Skin Findings *(Continued)*

Systemic Disease	Associated Findings or Diagnoses
Leukocytoclastic vasculitis (postcapillary venules)	Palpable purpura, purpuric wheals, hemorrhagic bullae in dependent areas
Liver disease	Jaundice, spider angiomas and other telangiectasias, palmar erythema, Terry nails, pruritus, purpura, caput medusae
Lymphogranuloma venereum	Lymphadenopathy above and below Poupart ligament (groove sign)
Medium vessels vasculitides (e.g., polyarteritis nodosa, granulomatosis with polyangiitis, eosinophilic granulomatosis with polyangiitis, microscopic polyangiitis)	Livedo racemosa, purpuric nodules, ulcers
Meningococcemia	Angular or stellate purpuric patches and plaques with gunmetal gray center. Progresses to ecchymoses, bullae, necrosis
Neurofibromatoses 1 (von Recklinghausen syndrome)	Neurofibromas, café-au-lait spots, freckling in the axillae (Crowe sign), plexiform neurofibroma
Pancreatic carcinoma	Panniculitis, migratory thrombophlebitis (Trousseau sign)
Pancreatitis (hemorrhagic)	Bruising and induration over the costovertebral angle (Grey Turner sign), Cullen sign, panniculitis
Porphyria cutanea tarda	Photosensitivity with bullae and skin fragility on dorsal hands and forearms; bullae rupture and heal with scarring and milia; hypertrichosis of the face; bronzing of skin when associated with hemochromatosis
Pyoderma gangrenosum	Painful pustule quickly progressing to ragged ulcer with sharply marginated violaceous border and undermined edges
Rocky Mountain spotted fever	Pink or reddish papules progressing to purpuric papules; starts on wrists and ankles and spreads to palms and soles and then to trunk and face
Sarcoidosis	Red-brown plaques, often annular, typically involving the head and neck and especially the nose and ears; may show apple jelly color with dermoscopy
Systemic lupus erythematosus	Malar erythema (mid cheeks, spans bridge of nose), relative sparing of nasolabial folds, periungual erythema, interphalangeal erythema

TABLE 18-11. Acne Vulgaris—Primary and Secondary Lesions

Acne is a disorder of the pilosebaceous unit that involves proliferation of the keratinocytes at the opening of the follicle; increased production of sebum, stimulated by androgens, which combines with keratinocytes to plug the follicular opening; growth of *Propionibacterium acnes,* an anaerobic diphtheroid normally found on the skin; and inflammation from bacterial activity and release of free fatty acids and enzymes from activated neutrophils. Cosmetics, humidity, heavy sweating, and stress are contributing factors. Most recommendations for treatment of acne are divided along its morphologic subdivisions: comedonal (mild), inflammatory (moderate), and nodulocystic (severe).

Lesions appear in areas with the greatest number of sebaceous glands, namely the face, neck, chest, upper back, and upper arms. They may be primary, secondary, or mixed.

Primary Lesions

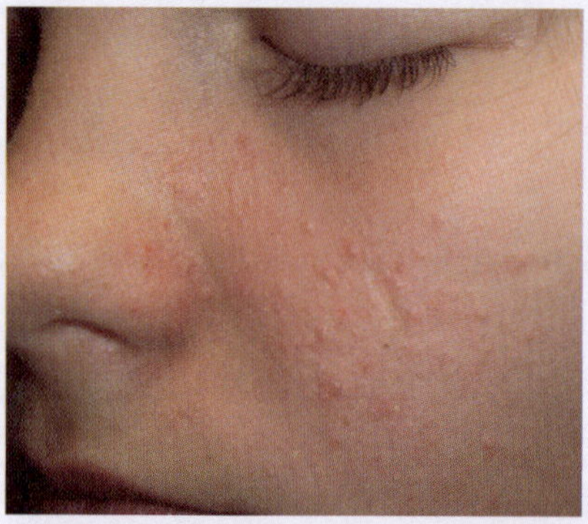

Mild Acne: Open and closed comedones, occasional papules

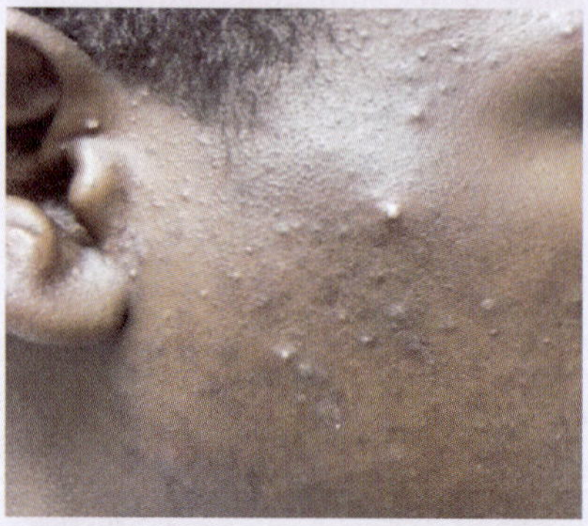

Moderate Acne: Comedones, papules, pustules

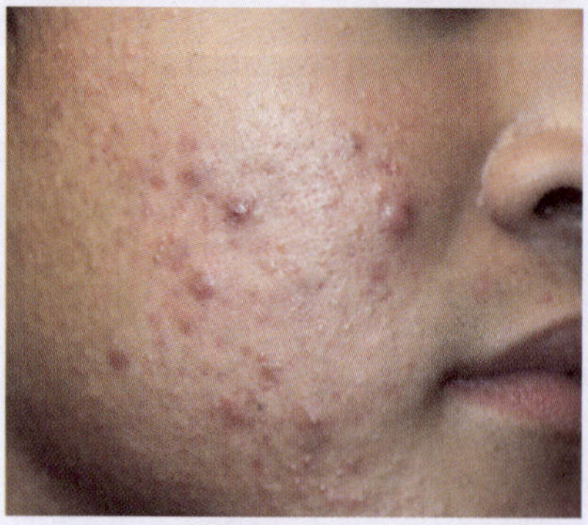

Severe Cystic Acne

Secondary Lesions

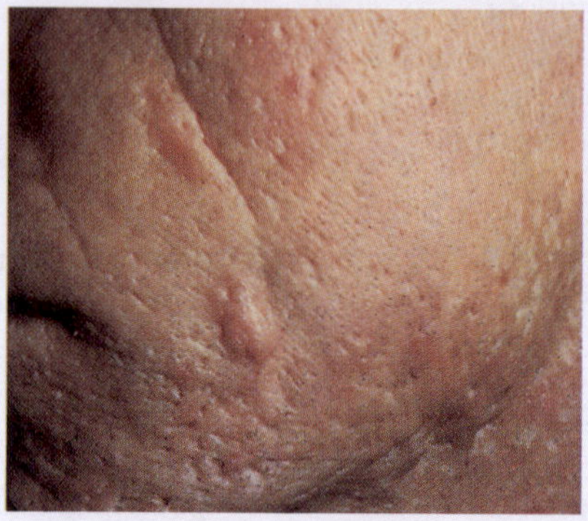

Acne with Pitting and Scars

TABLE 18-12. Signs of Sun Damage

Sun damage is one of the most important clues that a patient is at risk of skin cancer. Study carefully the following indicators of sun damage accrued throughout life. These indicators should prompt close inspection for *pink lesions* that are possible basal cell carcinomas; rough or keratotic lesions that may be actinic keratoses or squamous cell carcinomas; or asymmetric, multicolored, or changing lesions that could be melanoma. Counsel affected patients about proper sun protection, not only for themselves but for their families.

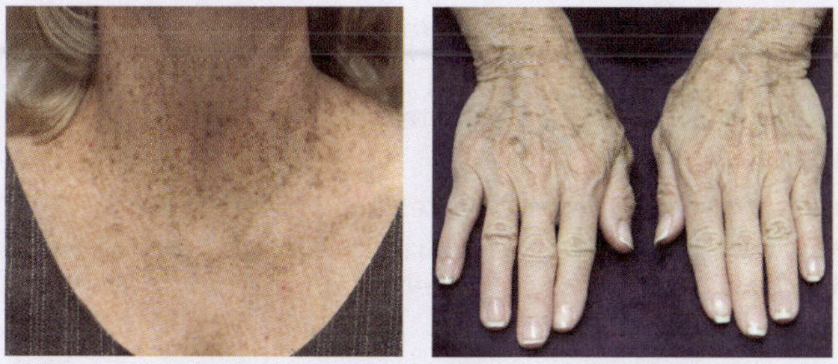

Solar Lentigo: Bilaterally symmetric brown macules located on sun-exposed skin, including the face, shoulders, and arms and hands

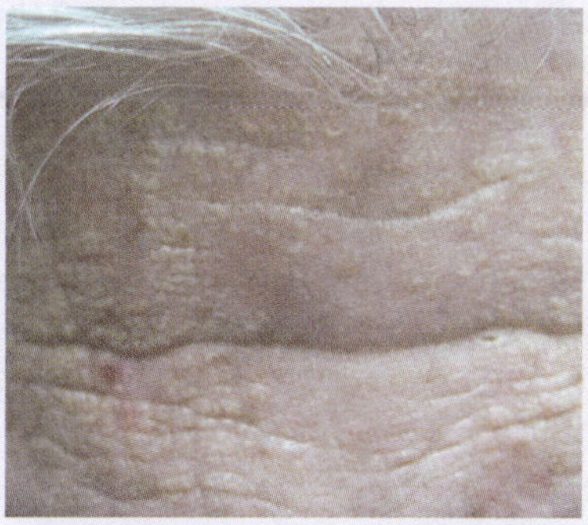

Solar Elastosis: Yellowish white macules or papules in sun-exposed skin, especially on the forehead

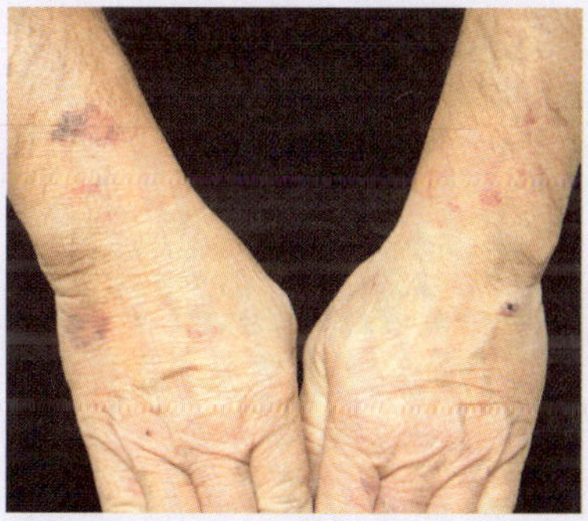

Actinic Purpura: Ecchymoses limited to the dorsal forearms and hands but not extending above the "shirt sleeve" line on the upper arm

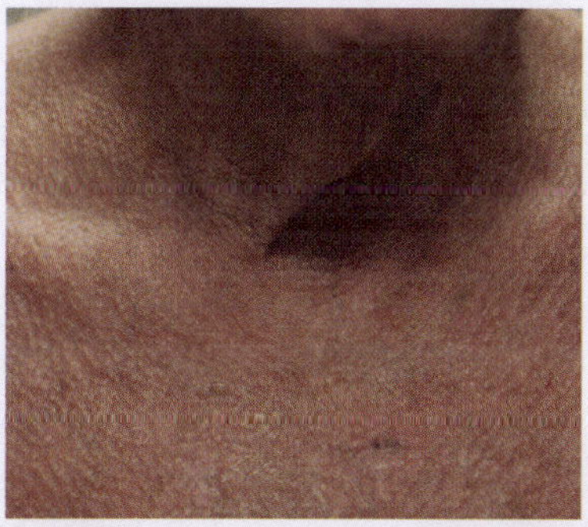

Poikiloderma: Red patches in sun-damaged areas, especially the V of the neck, and lateral neck (usually sparing the shadow inferior to the chin) with fine telangiectasias, and both hyper- and hypopigmentations

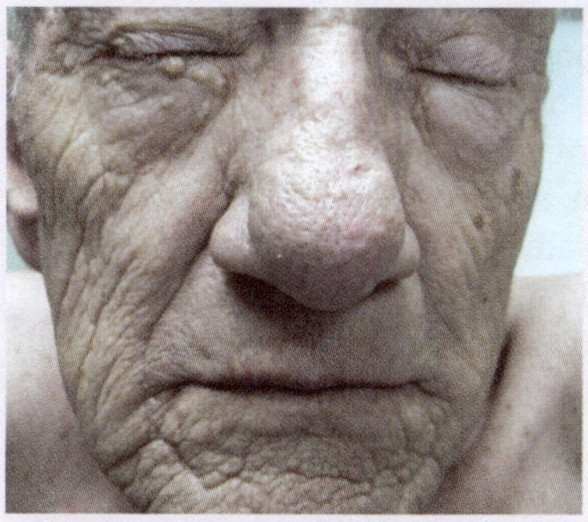

Wrinkles: Increased sun damage and tanning leads to deeper wrinkles at an earlier age

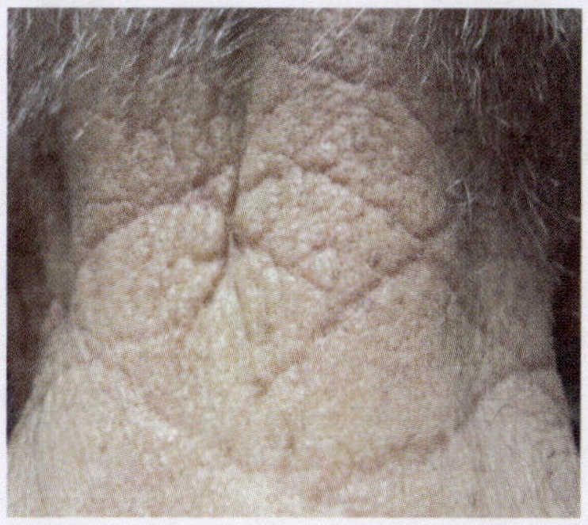

Cutis Rhomboidalis Nuchae: Deep wrinkles on the posterior neck that "crisscross"

TABLE 18-13. Pressure Injuries

A pressure injury is localized damage to the skin and underlying soft tissue usually over a bony prominence or related to a medical or other device. The injury can present as intact skin or an open ulcer and may be painful. The injury occurs as a result of intense and/or prolonged pressure or pressure in combination with shear. The tolerance of soft tissue for pressure and shear may also be affected by microclimate, nutrition, perfusion, comorbidities, and condition of the soft tissue.

Pressure injuries or ulcers usually develop over bony prominences subject to unrelieved pressure, resulting in ischemic damage to underlying tissue. Prevention is important: Inspect the skin thoroughly for early warning signs of erythema that still blanches with pressure, especially in patients with risk factors. Pressure injuries form most commonly over the sacrum, ischial tuberosities, greater trochanters, and heels.

A commonly applied staging system, based on depth of destroyed tissue, is illustrated below. Note that necrosis or eschar must be debrided before injuries can be staged. They may not progress sequentially through the four stages.

Address the patient's overall health, including comorbid conditions such as vascular disease, diabetes, immune deficiencies, collagen vascular disease, malignancy, psychosis, or depression; nutritional status; pain and level of analgesia; risk for recurrence; psychosocial factors such as learning ability, social supports, and lifestyle; and evidence of polypharmacy, overmedication, or abuse of alcohol, tobacco, or illicit drugs.

RISK FACTORS FOR PRESSURE INJURIES

- Decreased mobility, especially if accompanied by increased pressure or movement causing friction or shear stress
- Decreased sensation, from brain or spinal cord lesions or peripheral nerve disease
- Decreased blood flow from hypotension or microvascular disease such as diabetes or atherosclerosis
- Fecal or urinary incontinence
- Presence of fracture
- Poor nutritional status or low albumin

Stage 1 Pressure Injury: Nonblanchable Erythema of Intact Skin

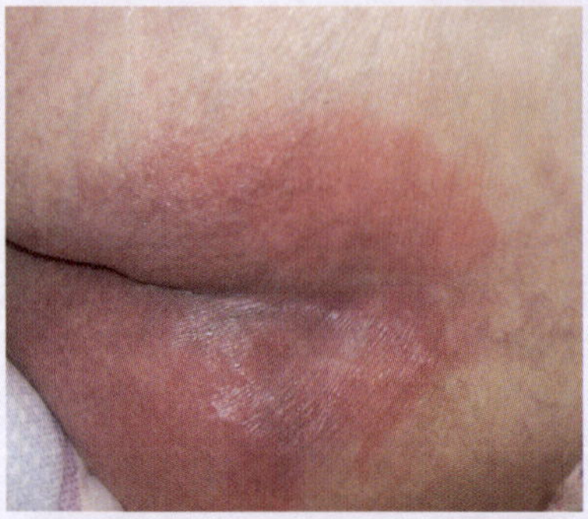

Intact skin with a localized area of nonblanchable erythema, which may appear differently in darkly pigmented skin. Presence of blanchable erythema or changes in sensation, temperature, or firmness may precede visual changes. Color changes do not include purple or maroon discoloration; these may indicate deep tissue pressure injury.

Stage 2 Pressure Injury: Partial-Thickness Skin Loss with Exposed Dermis

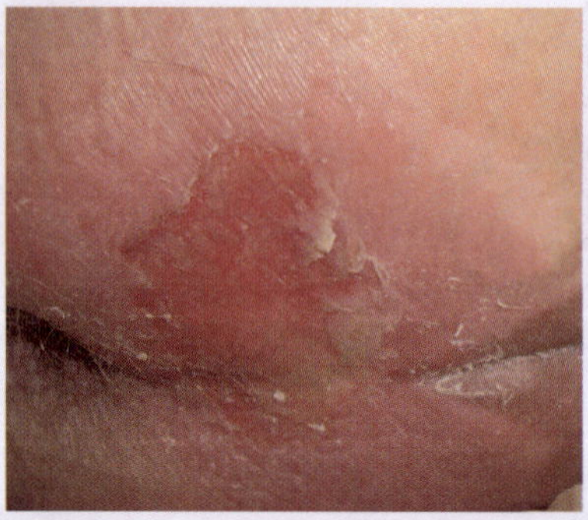

Partial-thickness loss of skin with exposed dermis. The wound bed is viable, pink or red, moist, and may also present as an intact or ruptured serum-filled blister. Adipose (fat) is not visible and deeper tissues are not visible. Granulation tissue, slough, and eschar are not present. These injuries commonly result from adverse microclimate and shear in the skin over the pelvis and shear in the heel. This stage should not be used to describe moisture-associated skin damage (MASD) including incontinence-associated dermatitis (IAD), intertriginous dermatitis (ITD), medical adhesive–related skin injury (MARSI), or traumatic wounds (skin tears, burns, abrasions).

(continued)

TABLE 18-13. Pressure Injuries *(Continued)*

RISK FACTORS FOR PRESSURE INJURIES

Stage 3 Pressure Injury: Full-Thickness Skin Loss

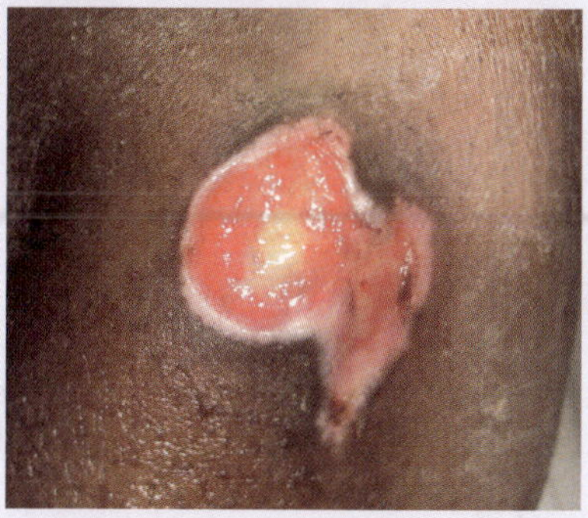

Full-thickness loss of skin, in which adipose (fat) is visible in the ulcer and granulation tissue and epibole (rolled wound edges) are often present. Slough and/or eschar may be visible. The depth of tissue damage varies by anatomical location; areas of significant adiposity can develop deep wounds. Undermining and tunneling may occur. Fascia, muscle, tendon, ligament, cartilage and/or bone are not exposed. If slough or eschar obscures the extent of tissue loss, this is an unstageable pressure injury.

Stage 4 Pressure Injury: Full-Thickness Skin and Tissue Loss

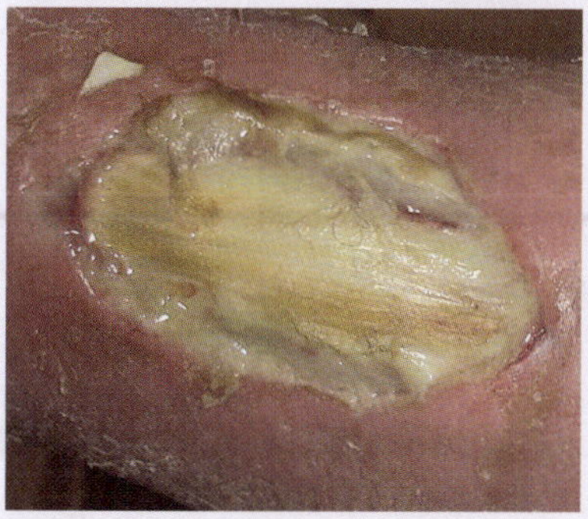

Full-thickness skin and tissue loss with exposed or directly palpable fascia, muscle, tendon, ligament, cartilage, or bone in the ulcer. Slough and/or eschar may be visible. Epibole (rolled edges), undermining and/or tunneling often occur. Depth varies by anatomical location. If slough or eschar obscures the extent of tissue loss, this is an unstageable pressure injury.

Unstageable Pressure Injury: Obscured Full-Thickness Skin and Tissue Loss

Full-thickness skin and tissue loss in which the extent of tissue damage within the ulcer cannot be confirmed because it is obscured by slough or eschar. If slough or eschar is removed, a stage 3 or stage 4 pressure injury will be revealed. Stable eschar (i.e., dry, adherent, intact without erythema or fluctuance) on the heel or ischemic limb should not be softened or removed.

Deep Tissue Pressure Injury: Persistent Nonblanchable Deep Red, Maroon, or Purple Discoloration

Intact or nonintact skin with localized area of persistent nonblanchable deep red, maroon, purple discoloration or epidermal separation revealing a dark wound bed or blood-filled blister. Pain and temperature change often precede skin color changes. Discoloration may appear differently in darkly pigmented skin. This injury results from intense and/or prolonged pressure and shear forces at the bone–muscle interface. The wound may evolve rapidly to reveal the actual extent of tissue injury or may resolve without tissue loss. If necrotic tissue, subcutaneous tissue, granulation tissue, fascia, muscle or other underlying structures are visible, this indicates a full-thickness pressure injury (unstageable, stage 3, or stage 4). Do not use DTPI to describe vascular, traumatic, neuropathic, or dermatologic conditions.

Source: Used with permission of National Pressure Injury Advisory Panel, Westford, MA.

CHAPTER 19

Head and Neck

This is the introduction to the organ systems and structures in the head and neck. This chapter, as well as the succeeding ones on the eyes, ears, nose, throat, and oral cavity, should be viewed as a unit not only due to their close anatomical proximity and interconnection but also because they have related symptoms. The physical examination of these structures is also performed sequentially. However, for this edition, these structures have been divided into separate chapters so you can learn about their distinct anatomic and physiologic structures individually. Separating the head and neck systems also helps you to understand the clinical data underlying their pathological symptoms.

ANATOMY AND PHYSIOLOGY

Head

Regions of the head take their names from the underlying bones of the skull. Knowing this anatomy helps to locate and describe physical findings (see Figs. 19-1 to 19-3).

Two paired salivary glands lie near the mandible: the *parotid gland*, superficial to and behind the mandible (both visible and palpable when enlarged), and the *submandibular gland*, located deep to the mandible. Feel for the latter as you press your tongue against your lower incisors. Its lobular surface can often be felt against the tightened muscle. The opening of the parotid duct (*Stensen duct*) as well as the submandibular ducts are visible within the oral cavity.

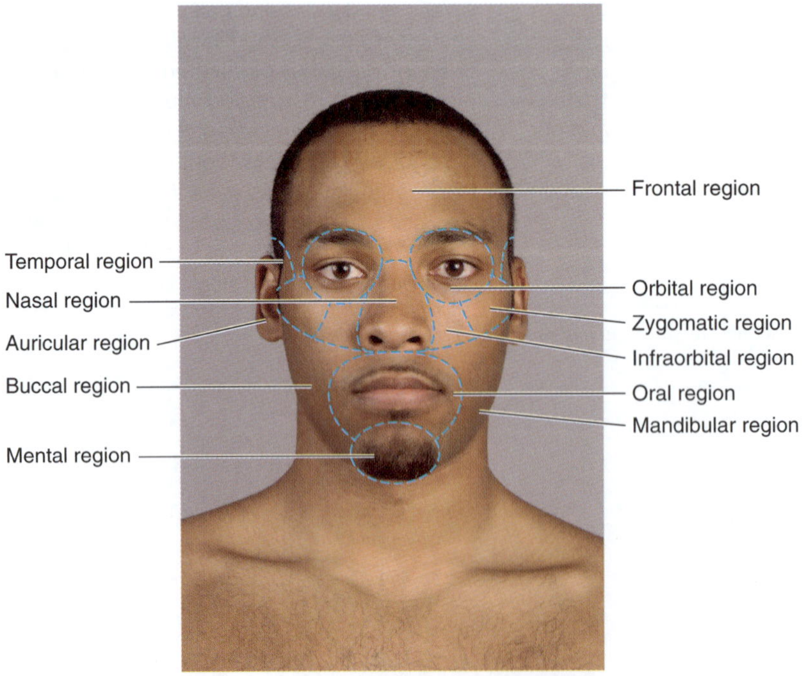

FIGURE 19-1. Surface anatomy of head, anterior view. (From Harrell KM, Dudek RW. *Lippincott® Illustrated Reviews: Anatomy*. Wolters Kluwer; 2019, Fig. 8-23.)

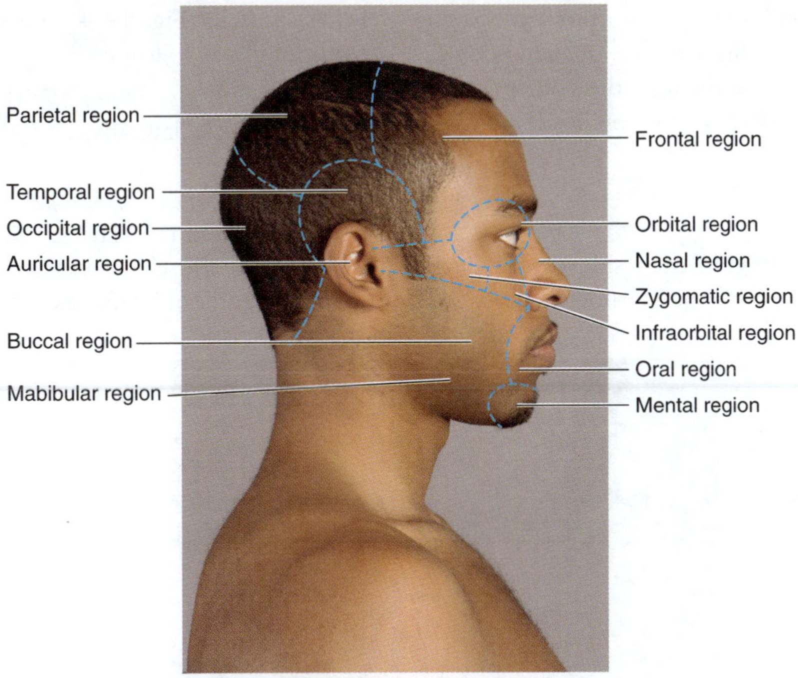

FIGURE 19-2. Surface anatomy of head, right lateral view. (From Harrell KM, Dudek RW. *Lippincott® Illustrated Reviews: Anatomy.* Wolters Kluwer; 2019, Fig. 8-6.)

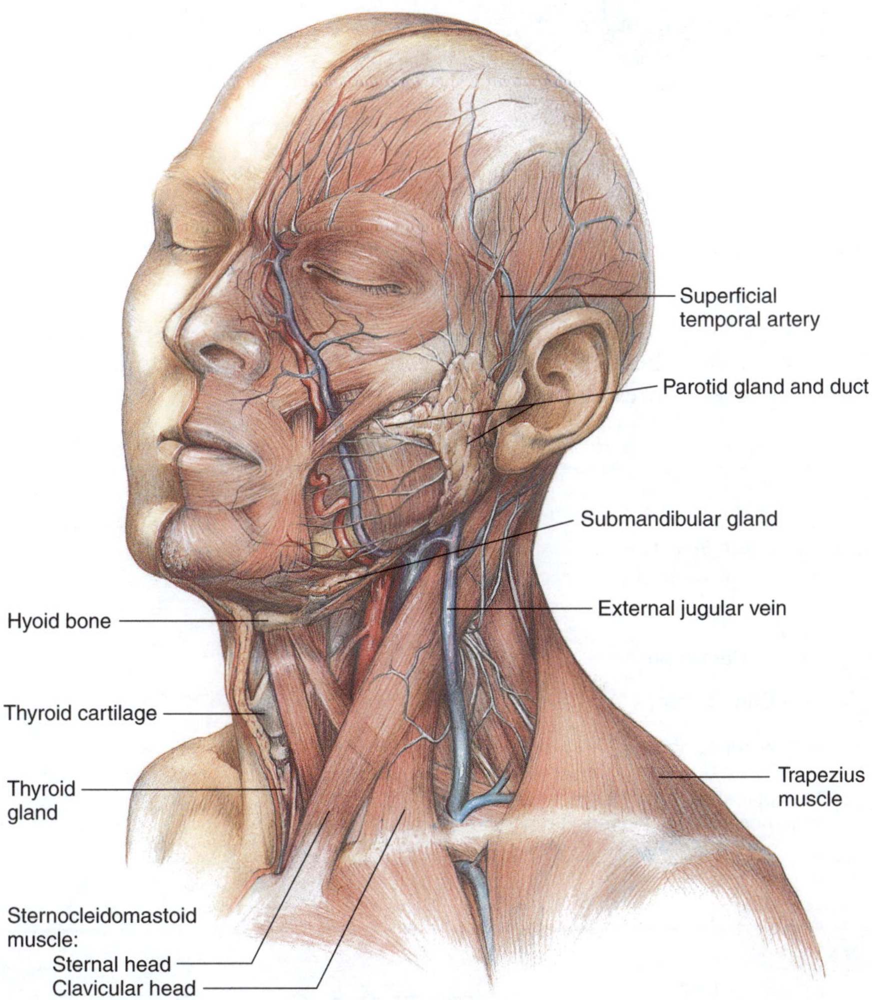

FIGURE 19-3. Anatomy of the head. (From Anatomical Chart Company: Head and Neck Anatomical Chart, 2000.)

The superficial temporal artery passes upward just in front of the ear, where it is readily palpable. In many people, especially thin and elderly ones, the tortuous course of one of its branches can be traced across the forehead.

Neck

For descriptive purposes, divide each side of the neck into two triangles bounded by the sternocleidomastoid (SCM) muscle (Fig. 19-4). Visualize the borders of the two triangles as follows:

- *Anterior cervical triangle:* the mandible above, the SCM muscle laterally, and the midline of the neck medially.
- *Posterior cervical triangle:* the SCM muscle, the trapezius, and the clavicle. Note that a portion of the omohyoid muscle crosses the lower portion of this triangle and can be mistaken for a lymph node or mass.

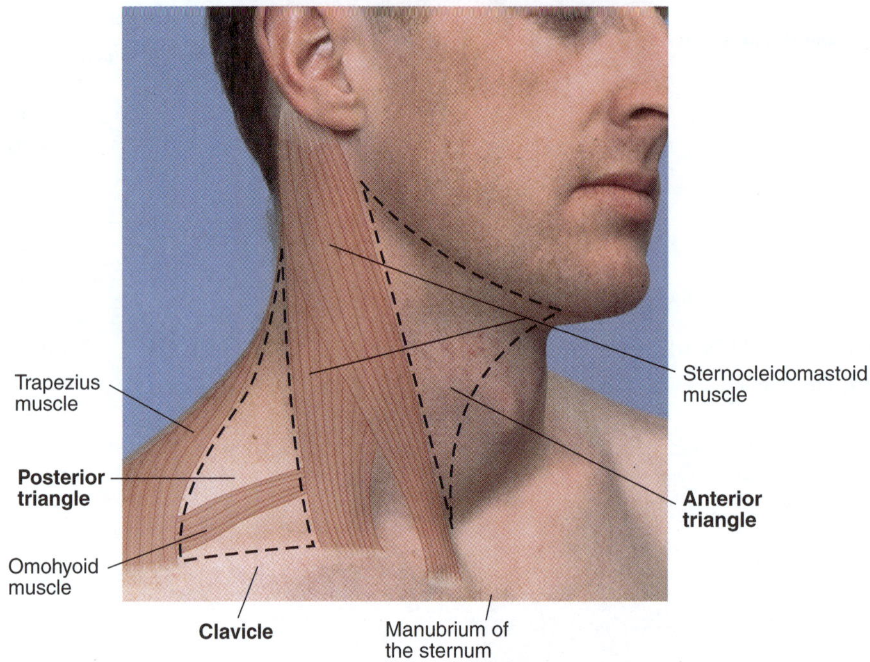

FIGURE 19-4. Anterior and posterior triangles of the neck.

Great Vessels. Deep to the SCM muscles run the great vessels of the neck: the *carotid artery* and the *internal jugular vein* (Fig. 19-5). The *external jugular vein* passes diagonally over the surface of the SCM muscle and may be helpful when trying to identify the jugular venous pressure.

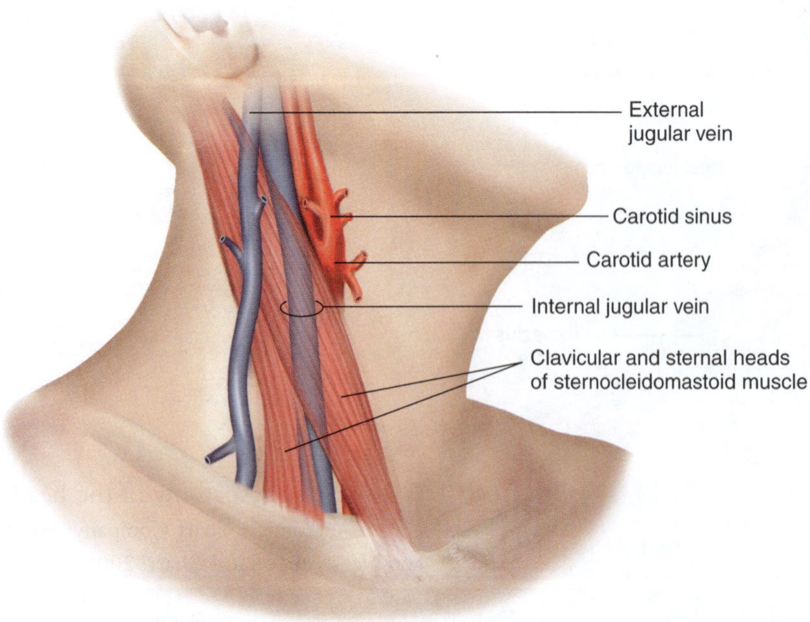

FIGURE 19-5. Great vessels of the neck.

Midline Structures and Thyroid Gland. Now identify the following midline structures: (1) the mobile hyoid bone just below the mandible; (2) the thyroid cartilage, readily identified by the notch on its superior edge; (3) the cricoid cartilage; (4) the tracheal rings; and (5) the thyroid gland (Figs. 19-6 and 19-7).

The thyroid gland is usually located above the suprasternal notch. The thyroid isthmus spans the second, third, and fourth tracheal rings just below the cricoid cartilage. The lateral lobes of the thyroid curve posteriorly around the sides of the trachea and the esophagus; each is about 4 cm to 5 cm in length. Except in the midline, the thyroid gland is covered by thin strap-like muscles anchored to the hyoid bone and more laterally by the SCM muscles, which are readily visible.

Lymph Nodes. See Chapter 8, General Examination.

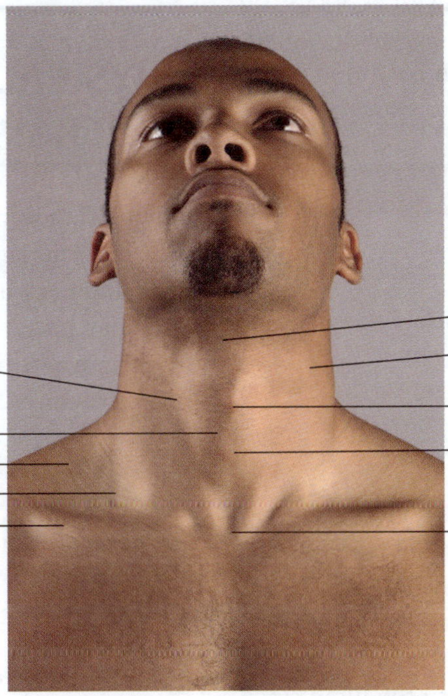

FIGURE 19-6. Surface anatomy of neck, anterior view. (From Surface Anatomy Photography Collection.)

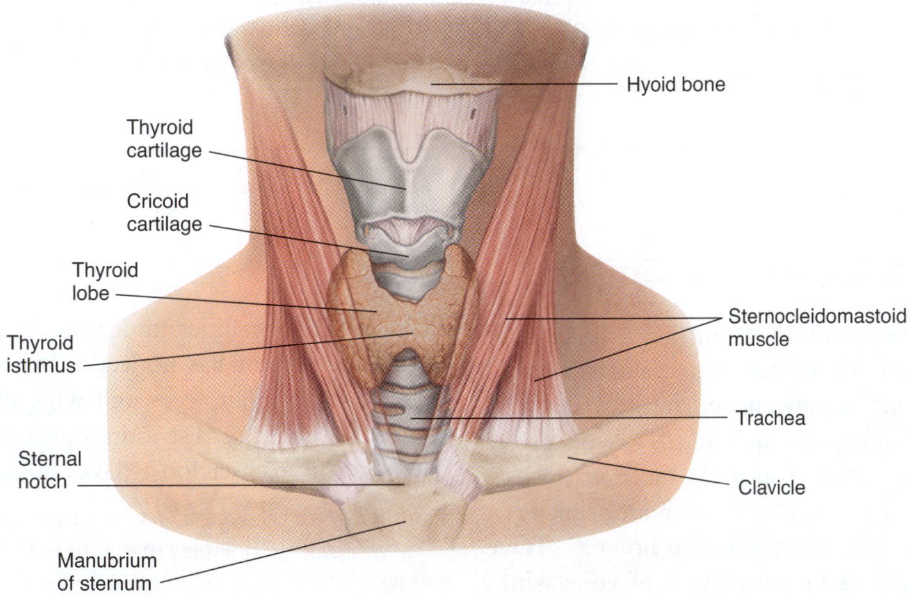

FIGURE 19-7. Midline structures of the neck.

HEALTH HISTORY: GENERAL APPROACH

Note that symptoms relating to the head and neck may involve major structures like the sensory organs, cranial nerves (CNs), and major blood vessels, which originate in these two areas. Many of these symptoms represent common benign processes, but sometimes they reflect serious underlying conditions. Careful attention to the interview and physical examination, with a focus on features and findings that do not fit a typical benign pattern, can often distinguish a common condition of the head and neck from serious underlying disease.

Common or Concerning Symptoms

- Neck mass or lump
- Thyroid mass, nodule, or goiter
- Neck pain (See Chapter 15: Musculoskeletal System)
- Headache (See Chapter 13: Nervous System)

Neck Mass or Lump

Ask "Have you noticed any lumps or swollen glands in your neck?" because patients are often more familiar with lay terms than with "lymph nodes." Other questions you may ask are: "When did you first notice the lump?" "How did you notice it?" "Was it noticed accidentally or told by others?" "Is it painful?" "Any changes to the lump since you first noticed it?" "How does the lump bother you?" "Are there any other symptoms such as discharge, pain in swallowing (dysphagia), difficulty breathing (dyspnea)?" "Have you ever had any other lumps before this?"

A persistent neck mass in an adult older than 40 years should raise a suspicion of malignancy.

Enlarged tender lymph nodes commonly accompany pharyngitis.

Thyroid Mass, Nodule, or Goiter

Assess thyroid function and ask about any enlargement of the thyroid gland, or **goiter**. To evaluate thyroid function, ask about temperature intolerance and sweating. Opening questions include: "Do you prefer hot or cold weather?" "Do you dress more warmly or less warmly than other people?" "What about blankets … do you use more or fewer than others at home?" "Have you noticed any changes in the texture of your skin?" "Do you perspire more or less than others?" "Any new palpitations or change in weight?" Recall that as people grow older, they sweat less, have less tolerance for cold, and tend to prefer warmer environments.

With goiter, thyroid function may be increased, decreased, or normal; see Table 19-1, Symptoms and Signs of Thyroid Dysfunction.

Intolerance to cold, weight gain, dry skin, and slowed heart rate point to hypothyroidism; intolerance to heat, weight loss, moist velvety skin, and palpitations point to possible hyperthyroidism. See Table 19-1, Symptoms and Signs of Thyroid Dysfunction.

PHYSICAL EXAMINATION: GENERAL APPROACH

The key in examining the head and neck is knowing and locating your landmarks. You must adequately expose the head and neck up to the clavicles for proper examination. You may have to ask patients to move or tilt their head in certain positions to properly examine the head and neck structures.

Key Components of the Head and Neck Examination

- Examine the hair (quantity, distribution, texture, any pattern of loss).
- Examine the scalp (scaliness, lumps, nevi, lesions).
- Examine the skull (size, contour, deformities, depressions, lumps, tenderness).
- Inspect the skin in the head and face (expression, contours, asymmetry, involuntary movements, edema, masses).
- Palpate the cervical lymph nodes (size, shape, delimitation, mobility, consistency, tenderness).
- Examine the trachea (deviation, breath sounds over it).
- Examine thyroid gland (size, shape, and consistency).

TECHNIQUES OF EXAMINATION

Hair

Because abnormalities under the hair are easily missed, ask if the patient has noticed anything wrong with the scalp or hair. Hairpieces and wigs should be removed. Note hair quantity, distribution, texture, and any pattern of loss. You may see loose flakes of dandruff.

Fine hair is seen in hyperthyroidism, coarse hair in hypothyroidism. Tiny white ovoid granules that adhere to hairs may be nits (lice eggs).

Scalp

Part the hair in several places and look for scaliness, lumps, nevi, and other lesions.

Look for redness and scaling that may indicate seborrheic dermatitis or psoriasis, soft lumps that may be pilar cysts (wens), and pigmented nevi that raise concern of melanoma. See Table 18-6, Brown Lesions: Melanoma and Its Mimics.

Skull

Observe the general size and contour of the skull. Inspect for any deformities, depressions, lumps, or tenderness. Learn to recognize the irregularities in a normal skull, such as those near the suture lines between the parietal and occipital bones.

An enlarged skull may signify hydrocephalus or Paget disease of bone. Palpable tenderness or bony step-offs may be present after head trauma.

Face

Note the patient's facial expression and contours. Inspect for asymmetry, involuntary movements, edema, and masses.

See Table 19-2, Selected Facies.

Skin

Inspect the skin on the face and head, noting its color, pigmentation, texture, thickness, hair distribution, and any lesions.

Acne is common in adolescents. *Hirsutism* (excessive facial hair) may appear in some women with polycystic ovary syndrome.

Cervical Lymph Nodes

See Chapter 8, General Examination.

Trachea

To orient yourself to the neck, identify the thyroid and cricoid cartilages and the trachea below them.

Physiology OSCE Video:
Palpation of Trachea

Inspection. *Inspect the trachea* for any deviation from its usual midline position. Then *palpate for any deviation.* See Chapter 10, Respiratory System. Place your finger along one side of the trachea and note the space between it and the SCM muscle. Compare it with the other side. The spaces should be symmetric.

Masses in the neck may cause tracheal deviation to one side, raising suspicion of conditions in the thorax such as a mediastinal mass, atelectasis, or a large pneumothorax.

Auscultation. *Auscultate breath sounds over the trachea.* This allows subtle counting of the respiratory rate and establishes a point of reference when assessing upper versus lower airway causes of shortness of breath. When assessing shortness of breath, always remember to listen over the trachea for stridor for upper airway etiologies in addition to examining the lungs.

Stridor is an ominous, high-pitched musical sound from severe subglottic or tracheal obstruction that signals a respiratory emergency. Causes include epiglottitis, foreign body, goiter, and stenosis from placement of an artificial airway. See also Chapter 10, Respiratory System, p. 209.

Thyroid Gland

Inspection. *Inspect the neck for the thyroid gland.* Tip the patient's head slightly back. Using tangential lighting directed downward from the tip of the patient's chin, inspect the region below the cricoid cartilage to identify the contours of the gland. The shadowed lower border of the thyroid glands shown here is outlined by arrows (Fig. 19-8).

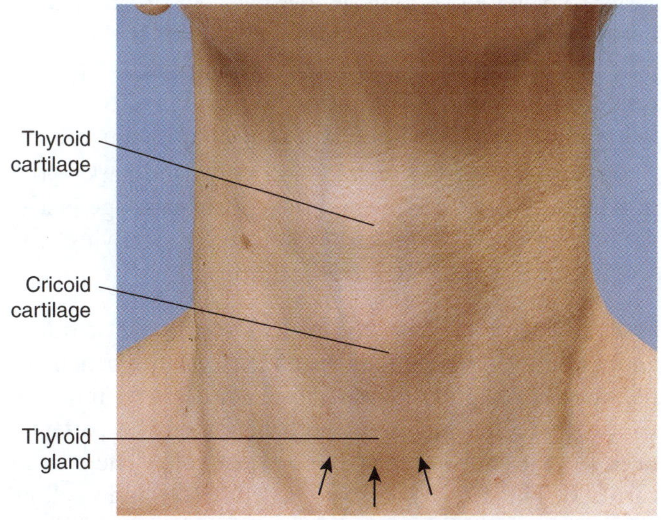

FIGURE 19-8. Thyroid gland position at rest.

The patient in Figure 19-9 has a *goiter*, defined as enlargement of the thyroid gland to twice its normal size. Goiters may be simple, without nodules, or multinodular. See Table 19-3, Thyroid Enlargement and Function.

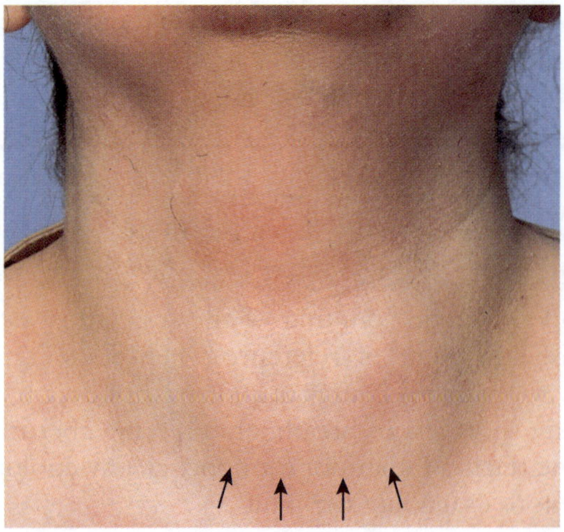

FIGURE 19-9. Thyroid gland with goiter.

Observe the patient swallowing. Ask the patient to sip some water and to extend the neck again and swallow. Watch for upward movement of the thyroid gland, noting its contour and symmetry. The thyroid cartilage, the cricoid cartilage, and the thyroid gland all rise with swallowing and then fall to their resting positions. With swallowing, the lower border of this large gland rises and looks less symmetric.

Confirm your visual observations by palpating the gland outlines as you stand facing the patient. This helps prepare you for the more systematic palpation to follow.

Palpation. This may seem difficult at first. Use the cues from visual inspection. The thyroid gland is usually easier to palpate in a long slender neck. In shorter necks, hyperextension of the neck may be helpful. If the lower pole of the thyroid gland is not palpable, suspect a retrosternal location. If the thyroid gland is retrosternal, below the suprasternal notch, it is often not palpable.

Palpate the thyroid gland. Find your landmarks—the notched thyroid cartilage and the cricoid cartilage below it. Locate the thyroid isthmus, usually overlying the second, third, and fourth tracheal rings.

Posterior Approach. With the patient seating or standing and you positioned behind the patient, ask the patient to flex the neck slightly forward to relax the SCM muscles. Gently place the fingers of both hands on the patient's neck so that your index fingers are just below the cricoid cartilage (Fig. 19-10). Ask the patient to sip and swallow water as before. Feel for the thyroid isthmus rising up under your finger pads. It is often, but not always, palpable. Find the lateral margin. In a similar fashion, examine the left lobe. The lobes are somewhat harder to feel than the isthmus, so practice is needed. The anterior surface of a lateral lobe is approximately the size of the distal phalanx of the thumb and feels somewhat rubbery. Displace the trachea to the right with the fingers of the left hand; with the right-hand fingers, palpate laterally for the right lobe of the thyroid in the space between the displaced trachea and the relaxed SCM muscle.

Retrosternal goiters can cause hoarseness, shortness of breath, stridor, or dysphagia from tracheal compression; neck hyperextension and arm elevation may cause flushing from compression of the thoracic inlet from the gland itself or from clavicular movement (**Pemberton sign**). More than 85% of goiters are benign.

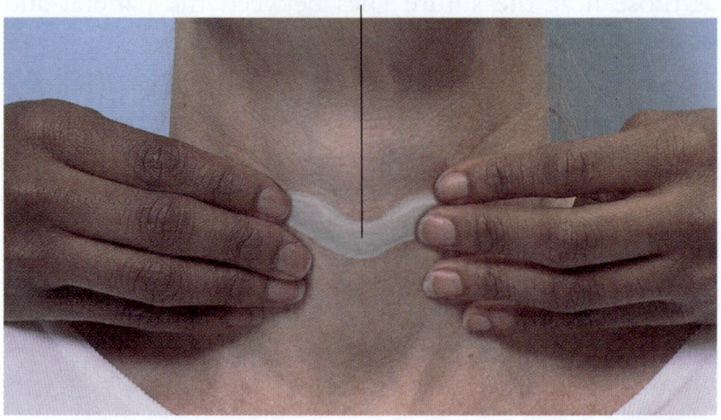

FIGURE 19-10. Palpating the thyroid gland, posterior approach.

Anterior Approach. The patient is examined in the seated or standing position. Attempt to locate the thyroid isthmus by palpating between the cricoid cartilage and the suprasternal notch. Use one hand to slightly retract the SCM muscle while using the other to palpate the thyroid. Have the patient swallow a sip of water as you palpate, feeling for the upward movement of the thyroid gland.

Note the *size, shape,* and *consistency* (soft, firm, or hard) of the gland and identify any nodules or tenderness. In general, benign (or colloid) nodules tend to be more uniform, ovoid structures and are not fixed to surrounding tissue.

The thyroid is soft in Graves disease and may be nodular; it is firm in Hashimoto thyroiditis (though not always uniformly) and malignancy.

The thyroid is tender in thyroiditis.

If the thyroid gland is enlarged, listen over the lateral lobes with a stethoscope to detect a *bruit,* a sound similar to a cardiac murmur but of not of cardiac origin.

A localized systolic or continuous bruit may be heard in hyperthyroidism from Graves disease or toxic multinodular goiter.

For palpable solitary nodules, ultrasound and possible fine-needle aspiration are advised.

Carotid Arteries and Jugular Veins

Defer a detailed examination of the neck vessels until the cardiovascular examination, when the patient is supine with the head elevated to 30 degrees. For jugular venous distention visible with the patient in the sitting position, assess the heart and lungs promptly. Also, be alert to unusually prominent arterial pulsations. See Chapter 11, Cardiovascular System, p. 219.

Jugular venous distention is a hallmark of heart failure.

RECORDING YOUR FINDINGS

Initially you may use sentences to describe your findings; later you will use phrases. The style in the next box contains phrases appropriate for most write-ups.

Recording the Head, Eyes, Ears, Nose, and Throat (HEENT) Examination

HEENT: Head*—The skull is normocephalic/atraumatic (NC/AT). Hair with average texture.** ***Eyes—Visual acuity 20/20 bilaterally. Sclera white, conjunctiva pink. Pupils are 4 mm constricting to 2 mm, equally round and reactive to light and accommodations. Disc margins sharp; no hemorrhages or exudates, no arteriolar narrowing. ***Ears*—Acuity good to** whispered voice. Tympanic membranes (TMs) with good cone of light. Weber midline. AC > BC. ***Nose***—Nasal mucosa pink, septum midline; no sinus tenderness. ***Throat (or mouth)***—Oral mucosa pink, dentition good, pharynx without exudates.

***Neck*—Trachea midline. Neck supple; thyroid isthmus palpable, lobes not felt.**

***Lymph Nodes*—No cervical, axillary, epitrochlear, inguinal adenopathy.**

OR

HEENT: Head*—The skull is normocephalic/atraumatic. Frontal balding.** ***Eyes—Visual acuity 20/100 bilaterally. Sclera white; conjunctiva injected. Pupils constrict 3 mm to 2 mm, equally round and reactive to light and accommodation. Disc margins sharp; no hemorrhages or exudates. Arteriolar-to-venous ratio (AV ratio) 2:4; no AV nicking. ***Ears***—Acuity diminished to whispered voice; intact to spoken voice. TMs clear. ***Nose***—Mucosa swollen with erythema and clear

(continued)

drainage. Septum midline. Tender over maxillary sinuses. ***Throat***—Oral mucosa pink, dental caries in lower molars, pharynx erythematous, no exudates.

***Neck*—Trachea midline. Neck supple; thyroid isthmus midline, lobes palpable but not enlarged.**

***Lymph Nodes*—Submandibular and anterior cervical lymph nodes tender, 1 cm × 1 cm, rubbery and mobile; no posterior cervical, epitrochlear, axillary, or inguinal lymphadenopathy.**

HEALTH PROMOTION AND COUNSELING: EVIDENCE AND RECOMMENDATIONS

Important Topics for Health Promotion and Counseling

- Screening for thyroid dysfunction
- Thyroid cancer screening

Screening for Thyroid Dysfunction

Epidemiology. Thyroid dysfunction is characterized as either underactive (hypothyroidism) or overactive (hyperthyroidism) and can be either subclinical or overt. Dysfunction can be defined biochemically based on levels of thyroid-stimulating hormone (TSH) and thyroid hormones (thyroxine [T_4], triiodothyronine [T_3]). Subclinical hypothyroidism is associated with increased risk for cardiovascular disease, whereas subclinical hyperthyroidism is associated with cardiovascular mortality, atrial fibrillation, and decreased bone density. Risk factors for hypothyroidism include autoimmune thyroiditis, older age, Caucasian race, type 1 diabetes, Down syndrome, goiter, external beam radiation to the head and neck area, and family history. Risk factors for hyperthyroidism include female gender, older age, African ancestry, low iodine intake, family history, and medications (amiodarone).

Screening. The American Association of Clinical Endocrinologists/American Thyroid Association guideline advises an aggressive case-finding approach for patients with risk factors and nonspecific symptoms potentially suggestive of thyroid dysfunction.

Screening for Thyroid Cancer

Epidemiology. The overall 5-year survival rate for thyroid cancer is 98.2%, ranging from 99.9% for early-stage cancers to 56.4% for cancers diagnosed at advanced stage. More than two thirds of thyroid cancers are diagnosed at an early stage. Risk factors for thyroid cancer include head and neck radiation exposure; having a first-degree relative diagnosed with thyroid cancer; and hereditary conditions such as multiple endocrine neoplasia syndrome type 2 or familial medullary thyroid cancer. Women are three times as likely to be diagnosed with thyroid cancer as men.

Screening. The head and neck examination section describes palpating the thyroid gland to characterize glandular tissue and to identify nodules. Nodules are common findings and are usually benign; however, nodules that are ≥2 cm, firm, and fixed to adjacent tissues are concerning for malignancy. Ultrasound imaging is recommended to further evaluate thyroid nodules to determine whether biopsy is indicated.

TABLE 19-1. Symptoms and Signs of Thyroid Dysfunction

	Hyperthyroidism	Hypothyroidism
Symptoms	Nervousness Weight loss despite increased appetite Excessive sweating and heat intolerance Palpitations Frequent bowel movements Tremor and proximal muscle weakness	Fatigue, lethargy Modest weight gain with anorexia Dry, coarse skin and cold intolerance Swelling of face, hands, and legs Constipation Weakness, muscle cramps, arthralgias, paresthesias, impaired memory, and hearing
Signs	Warm, smooth, moist skin With Graves disease, eye signs such as stare, lid lag, and exophthalmos Increased systolic and decreased diastolic blood pressures Tachycardia or atrial fibrillation Hyperdynamic cardiac pulsations with an accentuated S_1 Tremor and proximal muscle weakness	Dry, coarse, cool skin, sometimes yellowish from carotene, with nonpitting myxedema and loss of hair Periorbital myxedema Low-pitched speech Decreased systolic and increased diastolic blood pressures Bradycardia and, in late stages, hypothermia Sometimes decreased intensity of heart sounds Prolonged relaxation phase during ankle reflex Impaired memory, mixed hearing loss, somnolence, peripheral neuropathy, carpal tunnel syndrome

Sources: Siminoski K. *JAMA*. 1995;273:813; McDermott MT. *Ann Intern Med*. 2009;151:ITC6–1; McDermott MT. *Ann Intern Med*. 2012;157:ITC1–1; Franklyn JA. *Ann Endocrinol. 2007;68:229.*

TABLE 19-2. Selected Facies

FACIAL SWELLING

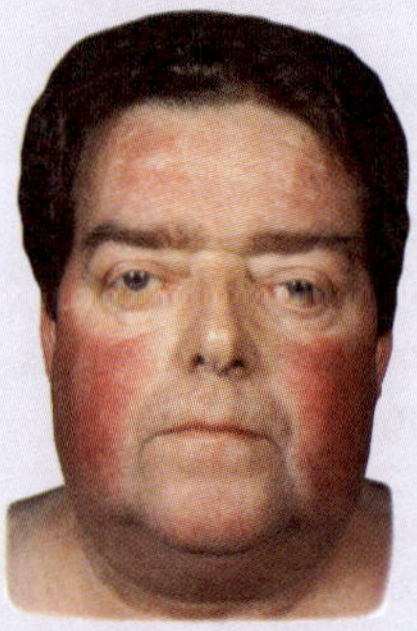

Cushing Syndrome

The increased adrenal cortisol production of Cushing syndrome produces a round or "moon" face with red cheeks. Excessive hair growth may be present in the mustache, sideburn areas, and chin (as well as the chest, abdomen, and thighs).

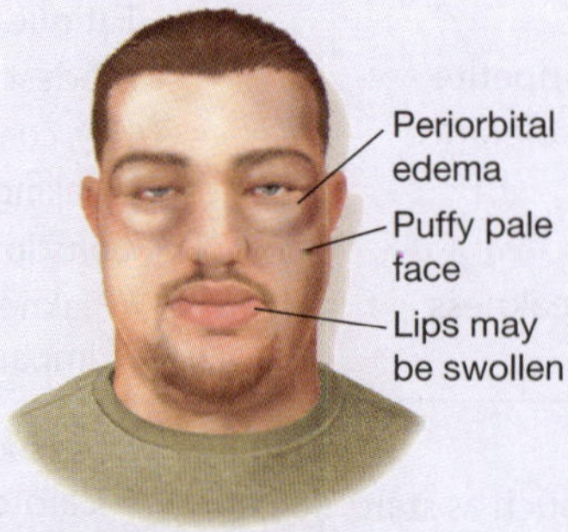

Nephrotic Syndrome

Glomerular disease causes excess albumin excretion, which reduces intravascular colloid osmotic pressure, causing hypovolemia, then sodium and water retention. The face becomes edematous and often pale. Swelling usually appears first around the eyes and in the morning. When severe, the eyes appear slit like.

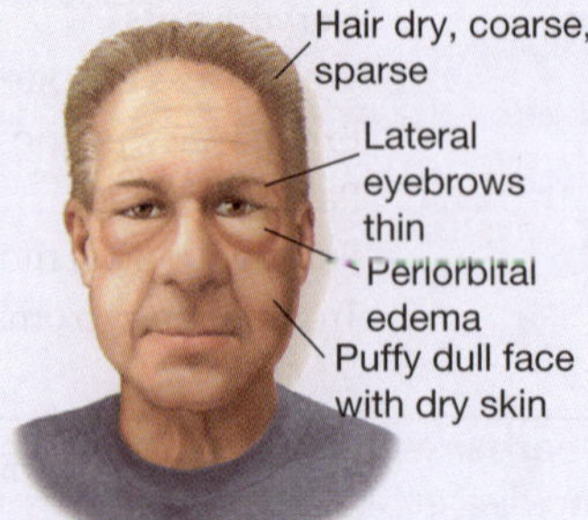

Myxedema

In severe hypothyroidism (myxedema) mucopolysaccharide deposition in the dermis leads to a dull, puffy facies. The edema, often pronounced around the eyes, does not pit with pressure. The hair and eyebrows are dry, coarse, and thinned, classically with loss of the lateral third of the eyebrows. The skin is dry.

OTHER FACIES

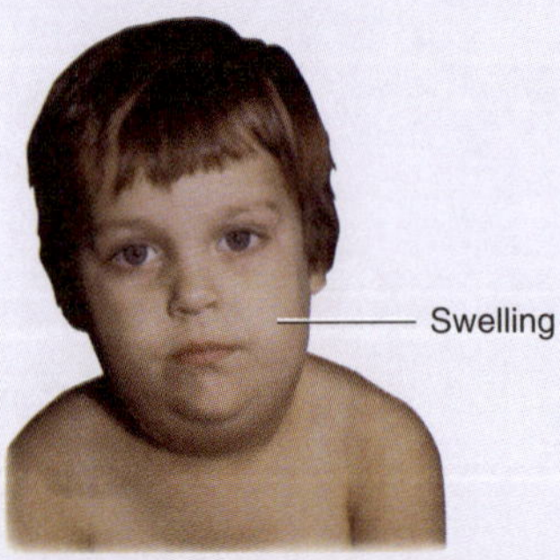

Parotid Gland Enlargement

Chronic bilateral asymptomatic parotid gland enlargement may be associated with obesity, diabetes, cirrhosis, and other conditions. Note the swellings anterior to the ear lobes and above the angles of the jaw. Gradual unilateral enlargement suggests neoplasm. Acute enlargement is seen in mumps.

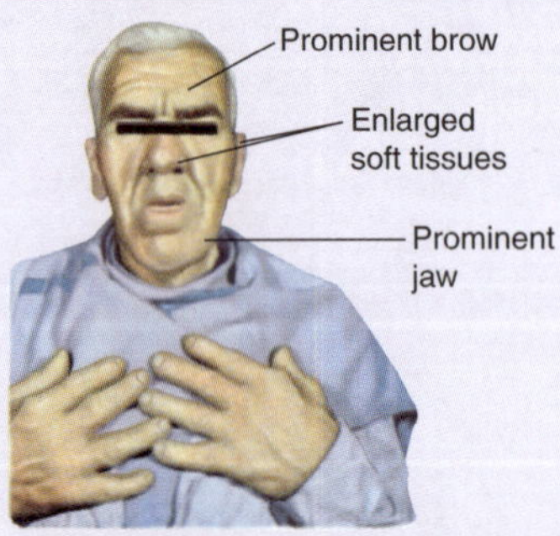

Acromegaly

The increased growth hormone of acromegaly produces enlargement of both bone and soft tissues. The head is elongated, with bony prominence of the forehead, nose, and lower jaw. Soft tissues of the nose, lips, and ears also enlarge. The facial features appear generally coarsened.

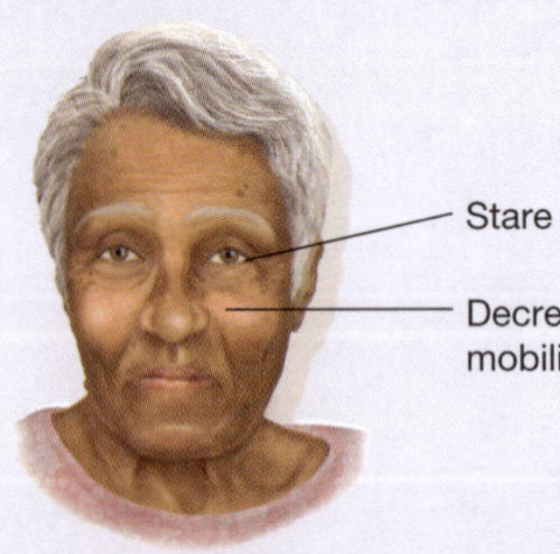

Parkinson Disease

In this neurodegenerative disorder linked to loss of the neurotransmitter dopamine, there is decreased facial mobility and masklike facies, with decreased blinking and a characteristic stare. Since the neck and upper trunk tend to flex forward, the patient seems to peer upward toward the observer. Facial skin becomes oily, and drooling may occur.

Source of photo: **Cushing Syndrome**—Courtesy of Getty Images.

TABLE 19-3. Thyroid Enlargement and Function

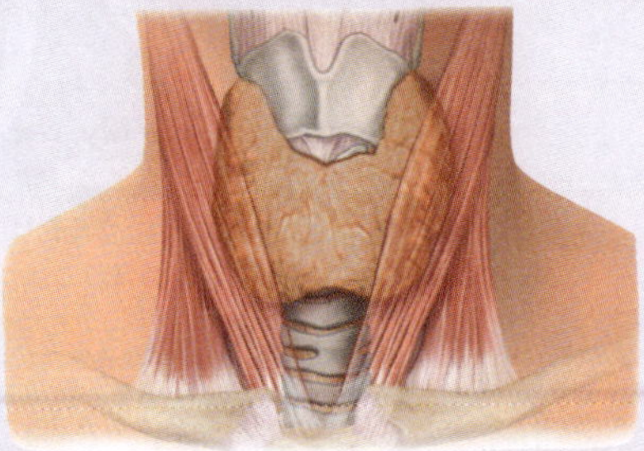

Diffuse Enlargement. Includes the isthmus and lateral lobes; there are no discretely palpable nodules. Causes include Graves disease, Hashimoto thyroiditis, and endemic goiter.

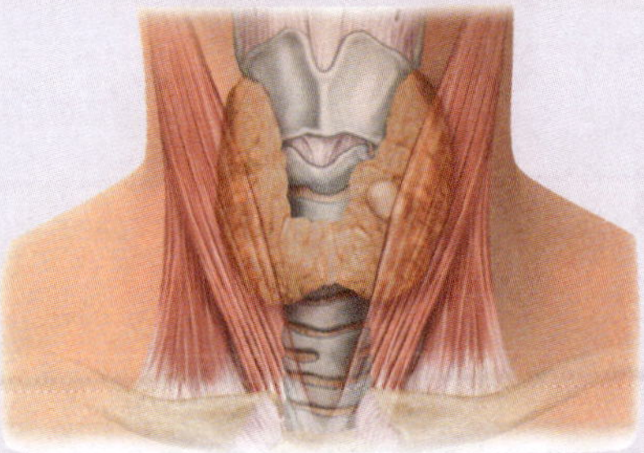

Single Nodule. May be a cyst, a benign tumor, or one nodule within a multinodular gland. It raises the question of malignancy. Risk factors are prior irradiation, hardness, rapid growth, fixation to surrounding tissues, enlarged cervical nodes, and occurrence in men.

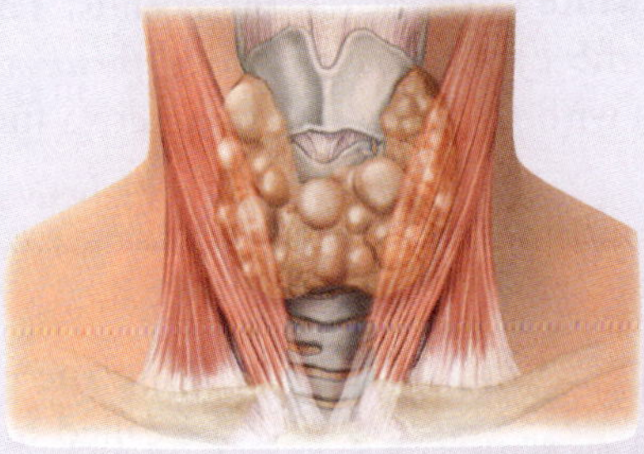

Multinodular Goiter. An enlarged thyroid gland with two or more nodules suggests a metabolic rather than a neoplastic process. Positive family history and continuing nodular enlargement are additional risk factors for malignancy.

CHAPTER 20

Eyes

ANATOMY AND PHYSIOLOGY

The eye sits in the quadrilateral-shaped bony socket called the *orbit.* In addition to protecting its contents, the orbit supports and ensures that the eye's functions are optimized. The extraocular muscles originating from the orbit attach to the relatively tough outer white covering of the eyeball called the *sclera* (white of the eye). This external covering of the eye is continuous with the dura of the central nervous system (Fig. 20-1).

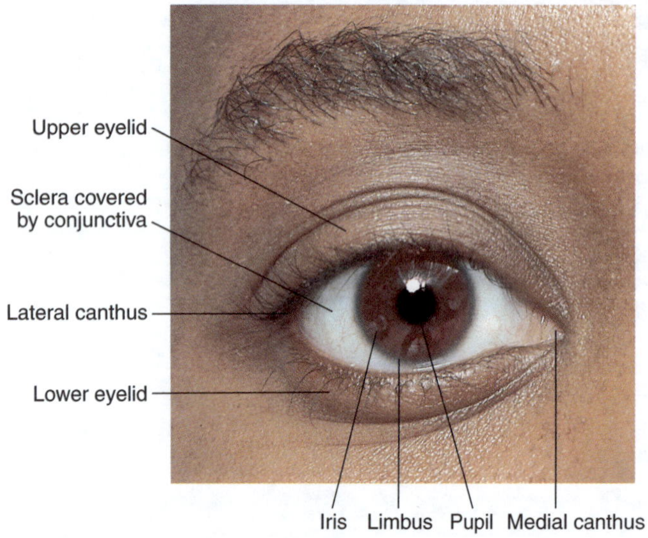

FIGURE 20-1. Surface anatomy of the eye and eyelids.

The colored circular muscle, the *iris,* gives us our eye color. The muscles of the iris dilate and constrict to control the amount of light allowed to enter the eye through its central aperture, the *pupil.* A transparent external surface, the *cornea,* covers both the pupil and the iris and is continuous with the sclera. Identify the structures illustrated in Figure 20-2. Note that the upper eyelid covers a portion of the iris but does not normally overlay the pupil. The opening between the eyelids is called the *palpebral fissure.*

The surface of the eye and the inner surfaces of the eyelids are covered with a thin, transparent membrane called the *conjunctiva.* The conjunctiva is a clear but highly vascularized mucous membrane with two components. The *bulbar conjunctiva* covers most of the anterior eyeball, adhering loosely to the underlying tissue. It meets the cornea at the *limbus.* The *palpebral conjunctiva* lines the eyelids. The two parts of the conjunctiva merge in a folded *fornix* that permits movement of the eyeball. The conjunctiva functions to lubricate and protect the eye.

The conjunctivae are usually transparent but can swell and become injected ("bloodshot") during times of infection, inflammation, or injury.

Along the eyelid margins lie firm strips of connective tissue called *tarsal plates* (Fig. 20-3). Each plate contains parallel rows of *meibomian glands* (also known as *tarsal glands*), which open on the lid margin and provide oily lubrication to the ocular surface. The *levator palpebrae superioris,* the primary muscle that raises the upper eyelid, is innervated by the *oculomotor nerve,* cranial nerve (CN) III. *Müller's muscle* is a smooth muscle innervated by the sympathetic nervous system, which also contributes to lid elevation.

The *tear film* protects the conjunctiva and cornea from drying, inhibits microbial growth, and gives a smooth optical surface to the cornea. This fluid consists of three layers: an *oily layer* from the meibomian glands, an *aqueous layer* from the lacrimal glands, and a *mucinous layer* from the conjunctival glands. The *lacrimal gland* lies in the superolateral orbit (Fig. 20-4). The tear fluid spreads across the eye and drains medially through two tiny holes on the superior and inferior medial eyelid margin called *lacrimal puncta.* The tears then pass through the canaliculi into the *lacrimal sac* and on into the nose through the *nasolacrimal duct.*

Located behind the iris is a transparent structure, the *lens,* suspended by ligaments (*zonule fibers*). The contraction or relaxation of these ligaments by muscles of the ciliary body control the thickness of the lens, allowing the eye to adjust focus on near or distant objects

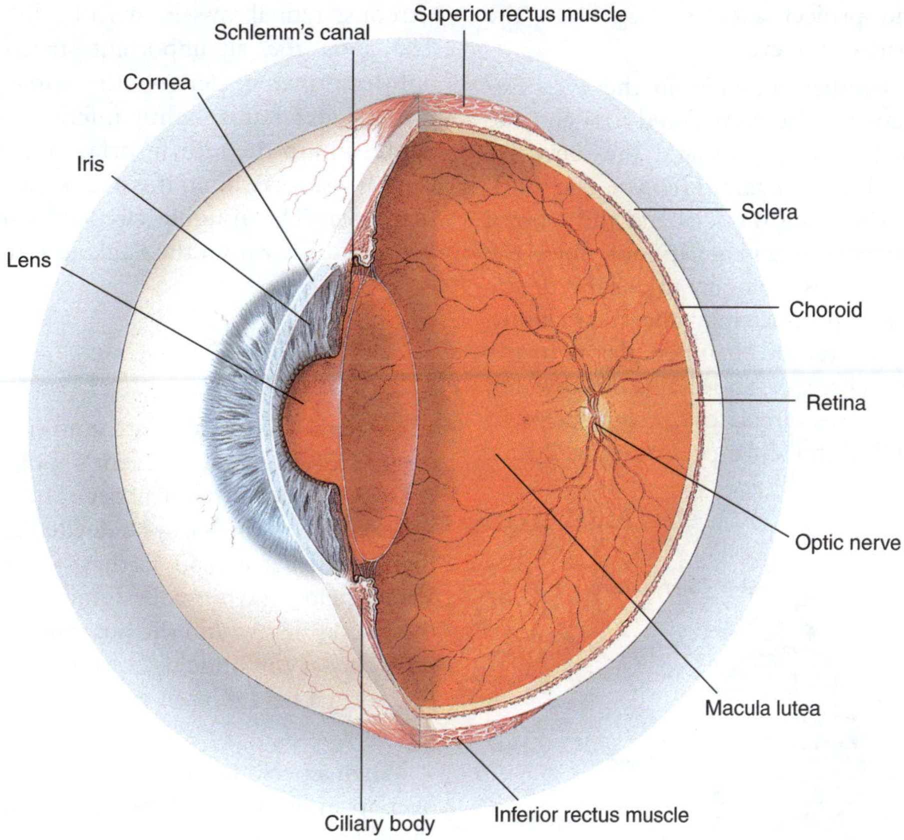

FIGURE 20-2. The normal eye, whole and cutaway views.

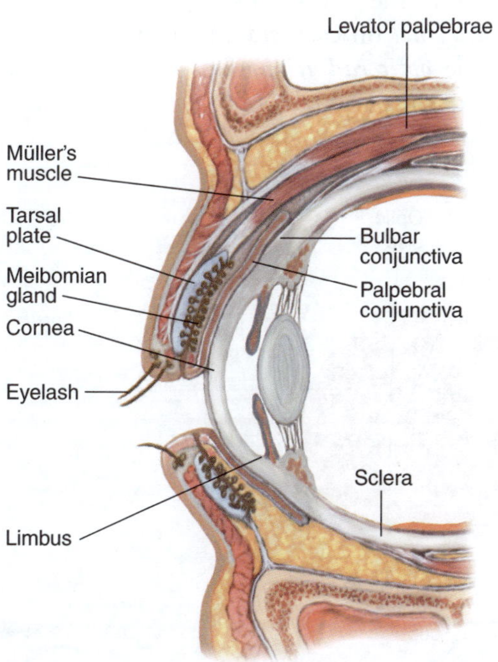

FIGURE 20-3. Sagittal section of the anterior eye.

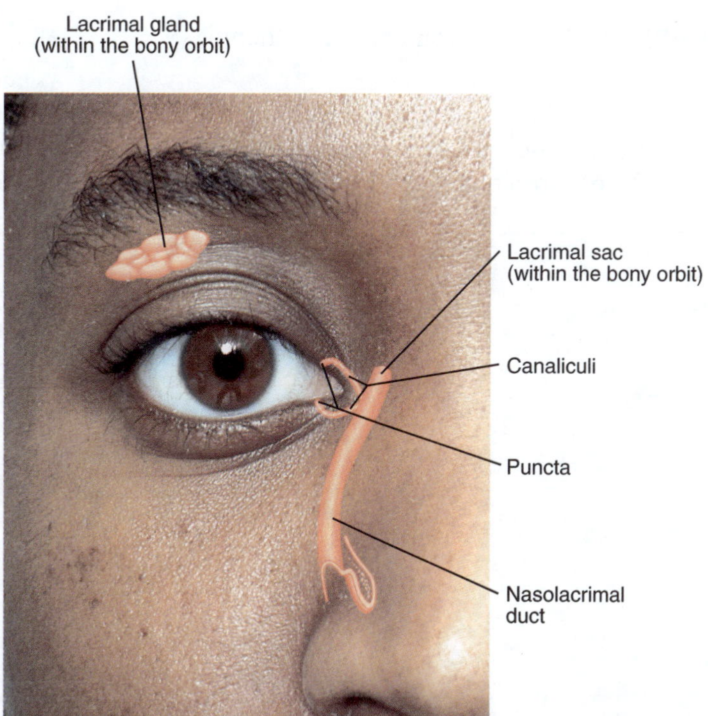

FIGURE 20-4. Lacrimal apparatus and drainage system.

(*accommodation*) and project a clear image into the *retina*, the sensory part of the eye.

There are three chambers of fluid in the eye. The *anterior chamber* (between the cornea and iris) and the *posterior chamber* (between the iris and the lens) are filled with a clear liquid called *aqueous humor*. The third, the *vitreous chamber* (between the lens and the retina), is filled with a more viscous and gelatinous fluid, the *vitreous humor*, which helps maintain the shape of the eye. Aqueous humor is produced by the ciliary body, circulates from the posterior chamber through the pupil into the anterior chamber, and drains out through the *canal of Schlemm*. This circulatory system helps to maintain and control the intraocular pressure (Fig. 20-5).

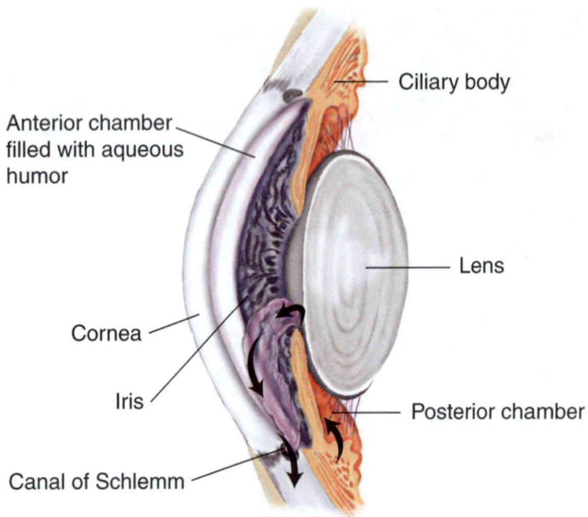

FIGURE 20-5. Circulation of aqueous humor.

The posterior portion of the eye that is seen through the ophthalmoscope is commonly called the *optic fundus* (Fig. 20-6). Structures here include the retina, choroid, vitreous, retinal vessels, macula, fovea, and optic disc. The *optic disc*, an important structure visible with an ophthalmoscope, denotes the entry point of the optic nerve. Lateral and slightly inferior to the disc is a small depression in the retinal surface that marks the point of central vision. Around it is a darkened circular area called the *fovea*. The roughly circular *macula* surrounds the fovea and lies within the flanking retinal vessels.

Visual Fields

A *visual field* is the entire area seen by an eye when it looks at a central point. Fields are conventionally diagrammed on circles from the patient's point of view looking "through" the piece of paper. The cross represents the focus of gaze, which can be divided into quadrants. Note that the fields extend farthest on the temporal sides. Visual fields are normally limited by the brows above, the cheeks below, and the nose medially. A lack of retinal receptors at the optic disc produces an oval *blind spot* in the normal field of each eye, 15 degrees temporal to the line of gaze.

When a person is using both eyes, the two visual fields overlap in an area of binocular vision—this phenomenon allows for *stereopsis*, or *3D depth perception* (Fig. 20-7).

Visual Pathways

To see an image, light reflected from the target must pass through the pupil and be focused on photoreceptors in the retina. Nerve impulses, stimulated by light, are conducted from the retina through the *optic nerve* (CN II), *optic tract* on each side, then on to a curving tract called the *optic radiation*. This ends in the *visual cortex*, a part of the occipital lobe.

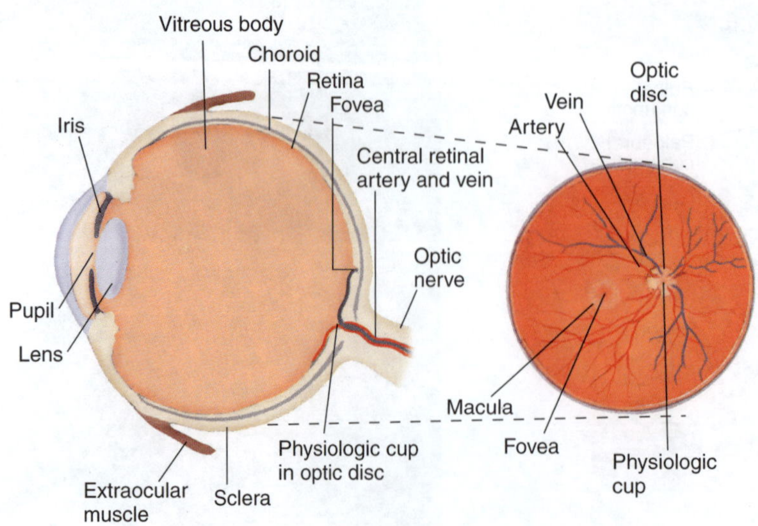

FIGURE 20-6. Cross-section of right eye showing the fundus as seen with an ophthalmoscope.

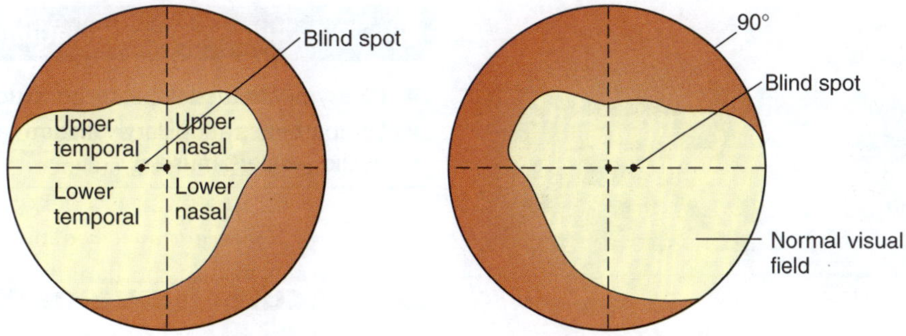

FIGURE 20-7. Visual field of left and right eyes.

Pupillary Reactions. Pupillary size changes in response to light and to the effort of focusing on a near object.

Light Reaction. A light beam shining onto one retina causes pupillary constriction in that eye, termed the *direct* reaction to light, and in the contralateral eye, the *consensual* reaction to light. The initial sensory pathways are similar to those described for vision: retina, optic nerve (CN II), and optic tract, which diverges in the midbrain. The motor impulses back to the constrictor muscles of the iris of each eye are transmitted through both oculomotor nerves (CN III) (Fig. 20-8).

Near Reaction. When a person shifts gaze from a far object to a near object, the pupils constrict (Fig. 20-9). This response, like the light reaction, is mediated by the oculomotor nerve (CN III). Coincident with this pupillary constriction, but not part of it, are (1) convergence of the eyes, a bilateral medial rectus movement; and (2) accommodation, an increased convexity of the lenses caused by contraction of the ciliary muscles. In accommodation, the change in shape of the lenses brings near objects into focus; physically, this takes place behind the iris and is not visible to the examiner.

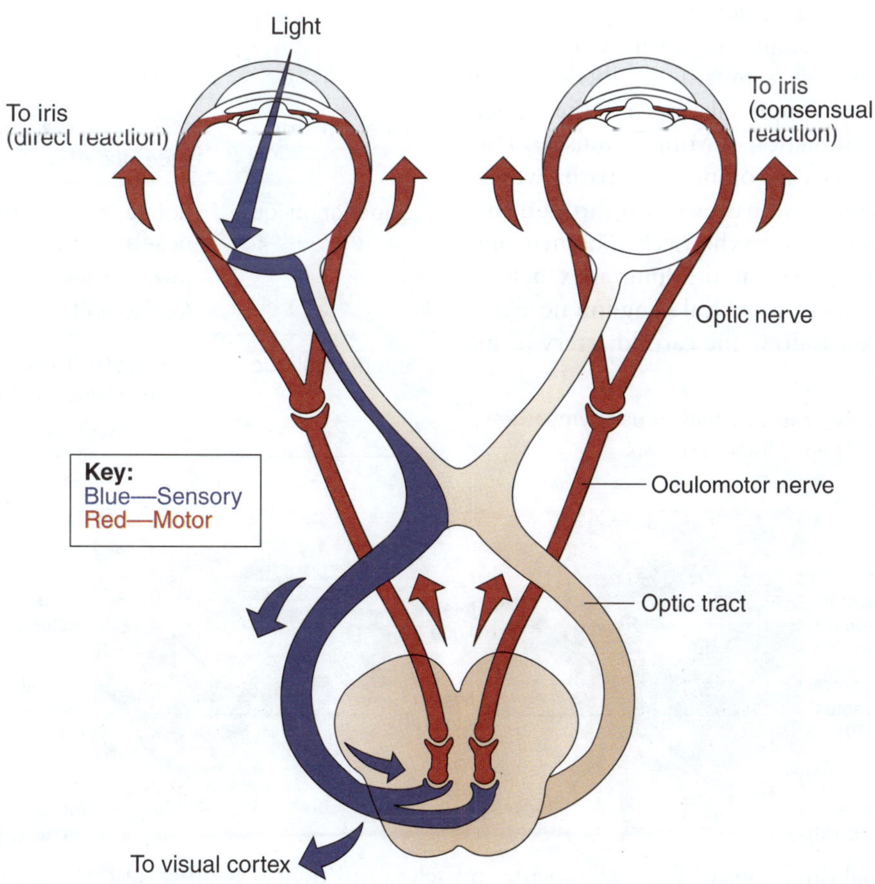

FIGURE 20-8. Pathways of the light reaction.

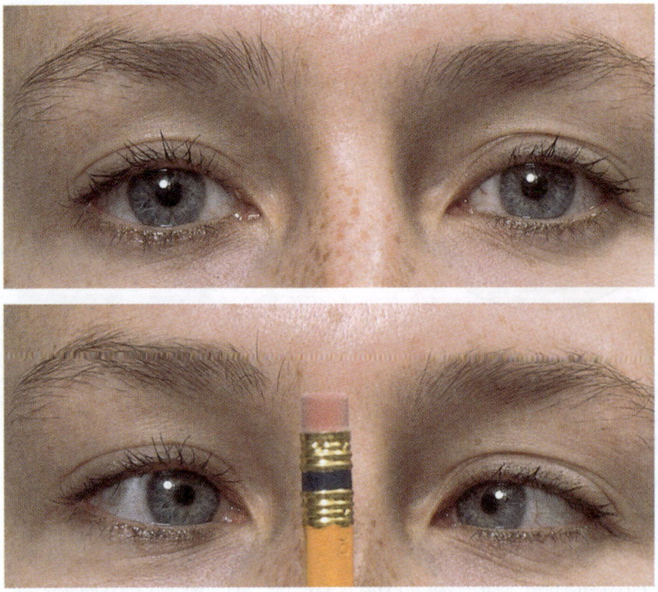

FIGURE 20-9. The pupils constrict when the focus shifts to a close object.

Autonomic Nerve Supply to the Eyes

Fibers traveling in the oculomotor nerve (CN III) and producing pupillary constriction are part of the parasympathetic nervous system, as shown in Box 20-1. The iris is also supplied by sympathetic fibers. When these are stimulated, the pupil dilates, and the upper eyelid will rise due to stimulation of Müller's muscle. The sympathetic pathway takes a complicated path, which starts in the hypothalamus and passes down through the brainstem and cervical cord into the neck. The neurons travel with the brachial plexus at the lung apex before returning back to the superior cervical ganglion near the mandible. From there, it follows the carotid artery or its branches into the orbit.

A lesion anywhere along this pathway may impair sympathetic effects that dilate the pupil and will cause **miosis**.

Box 20-1. Autonomic Stimulation

- Parasympathetics: Pupillary constriction
- Sympathetics: Pupillary dilation and raising of upper eyelid (Müller's muscle)

Extraocular Movements

The extraocular muscles that are responsible for eye movements are the *lateral* and *medial recti*, the *superior* and *inferior recti*, and the *superior* and *inferior obliques* (Box 20-2). You can test the function of each muscle and its CN innervation by asking the patient to move the eye in the direction controlled by that muscle. There are six cardinal directions, indicated by the lines in Figure 20-10.

Box 20-2. Extraocular Muscles and Actions

Extraocular Muscle	Action
Superior rectus	Moves the eye upward (*elevation*)
Inferior rectus	Moves the eye downward (*depression*)
Medial rectus	Moves the eye inward toward the nose (*adduction*)
Lateral rectus	Moves the eye outward away from the nose (*abduction*)
Superior oblique	Rotates the top of the eye toward the nose around the long axis (*intorsion*) Also moves the eye downward (*depression*)
Inferior oblique	Rotates the top of the eye away from the nose around the long axis (*extorsion*) Also moves the eye upward (*elevation*)

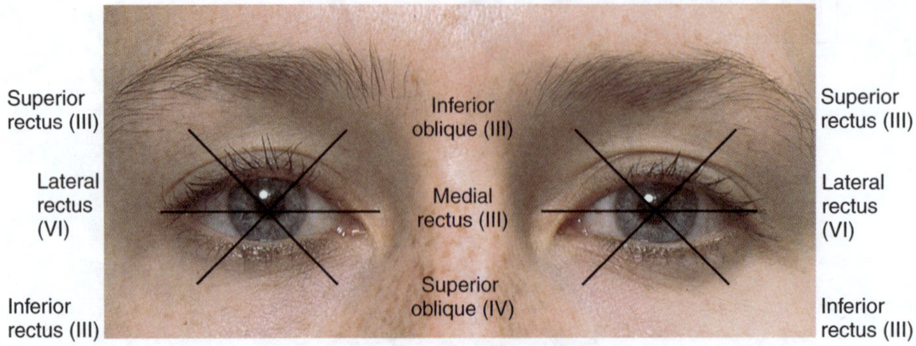

FIGURE 20-10. Cardinal directions of gaze, extraocular muscles, and their CN innervation.

In each position of gaze, a muscle of one eye is coupled (*yoked*) with a muscle of the other eye for conjugate gaze in a certain direction. If one of these muscles is paralyzed, the eye will deviate from its normal position in that direction of gaze, and the eyes will no longer appear conjugate, or parallel.

The extraocular muscles are innervated by three cranial nerves: the abducens, the trochlear, and the oculomotor. The *abducens nerve* (CN VI) innervates the lateral rectus muscle. The *trochlear nerve* (CN IV) supplies the superior oblique muscle. The *oculomotor nerve* (CN III) supplies all the rest of the extraocular muscles.

Nerve damage or injury to the muscle, due to head trauma, congenital causes, or central lesions, can cause aberrations in this yoked system and lead to *diplopia* (double vision).

HEALTH HISTORY: GENERAL APPROACH

The eyes are considered to be the "windows to the soul." Not only does our visual system allow us to interpret and interact with the outside world, but the eyes and vision can reflect the state of our current health. Careful interpretation of a thorough ocular history helps generate a comprehensive differential diagnosis. Furthermore, clues from the eye examination may prompt a more comprehensive neurologic examination or further diagnostic work-up. Careful attention to the health interview and physical examination, with a focus on features and findings that do not fit a typical benign pattern, can often distinguish a common condition from a serious underlying disease.

Start with general questions about vision and ocular function: "How is your vision?" and "How are your eyes?" Make sure to ask whether the symptoms involve one eye or both as well as the onset and duration of any symptoms. You can then hone in on the area involved with specific questions. Make sure to ask about inflammatory signs, such as pain, swelling, erythema, warmth, and/or loss of function.

In addition to previous medical history, always remember to ask about previous ocular history, including questions about surgery, eye drops, and use of glasses. When asking about eye medications, ask about over-the-counter medications, vitamins, or supplements. Family ocular history can be relevant as well.

Common or Concerning Symptoms

- Change in vision: blurred vision, loss of vision, floaters, flashing lights
- Eye pain, redness, or tearing
- Double vision (*diplopia*)

Vision Changes

Begin with open-ended questions such as "Have you had any trouble with your eyes?" If the patient reports a change in vision, pursue the related details.

- Is vision worse during close work or at distances?

Difficulty with close work suggests **hyperopia** (farsightedness) or **presbyopia** (aging vision), and, difficulty with distance vision, suggest **myopia** (nearsightedness).

- Is there blurred vision? If yes, is the onset sudden or gradual? If sudden and unilateral, is the visual loss painless or painful? Is it associated with headache?

If sudden visual loss is unilateral and painless, consider vitreous hemorrhage from diabetes or trauma, macular degeneration, retinal detachment, retinal vein occlusion, or central retinal artery occlusion.

If painful, causes are usually in the cornea and anterior chamber such as corneal ulcer, uveitis, traumatic **hyphema**, and acute angle closure glaucoma. Optic neuritis from multiple sclerosis may also be painful. Immediate referral is warranted. If associated with headache, a thorough neurologic examination is warranted.

- Is the visual loss unilateral? If so, is it painful or painless?

If it is associated with headache, jaw pain or claudication, it may be associated with giant-cell arteritis. If painless, it may be associated with a vascular occlusion, retinal detachment, or hemorrhage.

- Is the visual loss bilateral? (Sudden bilateral visual loss is rare.) If so, is it painful?

If bilateral and painless, consider vascular etiologies, stroke, or non-physiologic causes. If bilateral and painful, consider intoxication, trauma, chemical or radiation exposures.

- Is the onset of bilateral visual loss gradual?

Gradual vision loss usually arises from **cataracts**, glaucoma, or macular degeneration.

- Location of visual loss may also be helpful. Is there blurring of the entire field of vision or only parts of it?

Slow central loss may occur with nuclear cataract (p. 592) and macular degeneration (p. 777). Peripheral loss can be seen in advanced open-angle glaucoma with unilateral loss with hemianopsia and quadrantic defects. Though they may be asymmetric, these conditions are often bilateral disease processes.

- If the visual field defect is partial, is it central, peripheral, or on only one side?
- Is the visual field defect bilateral? Are there any patterns that we can help localize the lesion?
- Are there specks in the vision or areas where the patient cannot see (scotomas)? If so, do they move around in the visual field with shifts in gaze or are they fixed?

Moving specks or strands suggest vitreous floaters; fixed defects, or *scotomas*, suggest lesions in the retina, visual pathway, or brain.

- Are there lights flashing across the field of vision?

Vitreous floaters may accompany this symptom.

Flashing lights with new vitreous floaters suggest traction on the retina with detachment of the vitreous body from the retina. Prompt consultation is indicated to rule out retinal tears or detachments.

- Does the patient wear glasses? Contact lenses? Has the patient undergone refractive surgery?

Eye Pain, Redness, or Tearing

Ask about pain in or around the eyes, redness, and excessive tearing or watering.

A red painless eye is seen in **subconjunctival hemorrhage** and **episcleritis.** A red eye with a gritty sensation is seen in viral conjunctivitis and dry eye. A red painful eye is seen in corneal abrasions, foreign bodies, **corneal ulcers**, acute angle closure glaucoma, herpes keratitis, fungal keratitis, hyphema, and uveitis. See Table 20-1, Red Eyes.

Double Vision

Check for double vision, or ***diplopia***. If present, find out if the images are side by side (***horizontal diplopia***) or on top of each other (***vertical diplopia***). Does diplopia persist with one eye closed? Which eye is affected?

Diplopia is seen in lesions in the brainstem or cerebellum and with weakness or paralysis of one or more extraocular muscles, as in horizontal diplopia from palsy of CN III or VI or vertical diplopia from palsy of CN III or IV. Diplopia in one eye, with the other closed, suggests a problem in the ocular surface, cornea, lens, or macula.

One kind of horizontal diplopia is physiologic. Hold one finger upright approximately 6 inches in front of your face, a second at arm's length. When you focus on either finger, the image of the other is double. A patient who notices this phenomenon can be reassured.

PHYSICAL EXAMINATION: GENERAL APPROACH

After the patient interview, a thorough physical examination should follow. Keen observation complements a thoughtful understanding of normal physiology while performing and interpreting the ophthalmologic examination. The eye examination can often provide useful clues to diagnose and monitor systemic diseases. Furthermore, in the nonverbal patient, valuable information regarding the neurologic system, occult intoxications, metabolic derangements, or life-threatening infections can be uncovered. It is important, especially as you begin learning the examination, to follow a systematic approach. Visual acuity is a must in any ophthalmologic examination. Pupillary examination, ocular motility, confrontational visual fields, and color vision should also be tested. The best ophthalmologic examinations require keen observation and detailed reporting. Remember to look at the eye as a whole before focusing on the individual components of the eyeball.

Key Components of the Ophthalmologic Examination

- Test visual acuity using a Snellen eye chart.
- Test visual fields by confrontation.
- Test color vision and contrast sensitivity.
- Assess position and alignment of the eyes (protrusion, deviation).
- Inspect eyebrows (fullness, distribution, scaliness).
- Inspect eyelids and eyelashes (width, edema, color, lesions, eyelid closure).
- Assess the lacrimal apparatus (lumps, swelling, tearing, dryness).
- Inspect the conjunctivae and sclerae (vascular pattern, color, nodules, swelling).
- Inspect the cornea, iris, and lens (opacity, anterior chamber depth).
- Inspect the pupils (size, shape, symmetry).
- Test for pupillary reaction to light (direct and consensual light reactions).
- Inspect the light reflection in the corneas.
- Test the extraocular muscle movements.
- Perform ophthalmoscopic (funduscopic) examination including optic disc and cup, retina, and retinal vessels.

TECHNIQUES OF EXAMINATION

Visual Acuity

Test the acuity of central vision by using a *Snellen eye chart* in a well-lit area, if possible. Position the patient 20 ft from the chart. Patients who wear glasses other than for reading should put them on. Ask the patient to cover one eye with a card (to prevent looking through the fingers) and to read the smallest line of print possible. Coaxing to attempt the next line may improve performance. A patient who cannot read the largest letter can be positioned closer to the chart; note the intervening distance. Identify the smallest line of print where the patient can identify more than half the letters. Record the visual acuity designated at the side of this line, along with use of glasses, if any. For patients who cannot identify the English alphabet, there are other options to test vision. *Tumbling "E's"* can be used, in which the patient points to the direction of the open face of the letter "E." *Allen cards* display standardized pictures that can be recognized by children over the age of 2 years.

Visual acuity is expressed as two numbers (e.g., 20/30): the first indicates the distance of the patient from the chart, and the second, the distance at which a normal eye can read the line of letters. Vision of 20/200 means that, at 20 ft, the patient can read print that a person with normal vision could read at 200 ft. The larger the second number, the worse the vision. "20/40 corrected" means the patient could read the 20/40 line with glasses (a correction).

Myopia (nearsightedness) causes focusing problems for distance vision, whereas *hyperopia* (farsightedness) describes eyesight that is blurry on objects nearby. *Astigmatism* is an imperfection of the cornea or lens causing distortion while looking at near and far objects (Fig. 20-11).

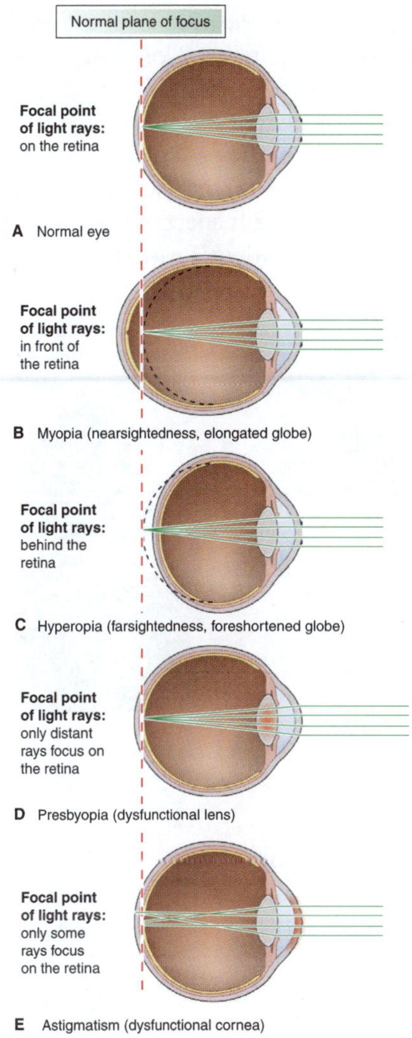

FIGURE 20-11. Refractive disorders. (From McConnell TH. *The Nature of Disease: Pathology for the Health Professions.* 2nd ed. Wolters Kluwer Health/Lippincott Williams & Wilkins; 2014, Fig. 20-6.)

Testing near vision with a handheld card can help identify the need for reading glasses (bifocals or progressive lenses) in patients older than 45 years. You can also use this card to test visual acuity at the bedside. Held 14 inches from the patient's eyes, the card simulates a Snellen chart.

Physiology OSCE Video: **Assessment of Vision**

Presbyopia causes focusing problems for near vision, found in middle-aged and older adults. A person with presbyopia often sees better when the card is farther away.

If you have no charts, screen visual acuity with any available print. If patients cannot read even the largest letters, test their ability to count your raised fingers, detect direction of hand motion, and distinguish light (such as a penlight) from dark.

Visual Fields

Confrontation visual field testing is a valuable screening technique for detection of lesions in the anterior and posterior visual pathway. Nevertheless, even relatively dense quadrantic or hemianopic visual field defects can be missed by confrontation screening tests. A formalized automated perimetry test such as the Humphrey visual field performed by an ophthalmologist is needed to make a definitive diagnosis of a visual field defect.

Refer patients with suspected visual field defects for dedicated ophthalmology evaluation. Causes of anterior pathway defects include glaucoma, optic neuropathy, optic neuritis, and compressive lesions. Posterior pathway defects include stroke and chiasmal tumors.

Static Finger Wiggle Test. Position yourself about an arm's length away from the patient. Close one eye and have the patient cover the opposite eye while staring at your open eye. So, for example, when the patient covers the left eye, to test the visual field of the patient's right eye, you should cover your right eye to mirror the patient's field of view. Place your hands about 2 ft apart out of the patient's view, roughly lateral to the patient's ears (Fig. 20-12).

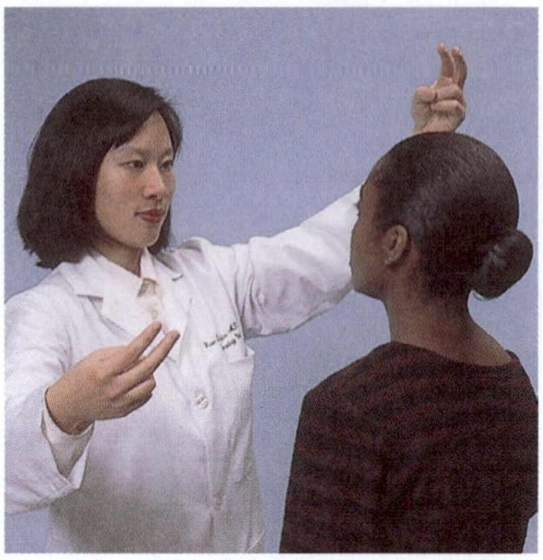

FIGURE 20-12. Starting to test visual fields using static finger wiggle technique.

While in this position, wiggle your fingers and slowly bring your moving fingers forward into the patient's center of view. Ask the patient to tell you as soon as he or she sees your finger movement. Test each clock hour, or at least each quadrant. Test each eye individually and record the extent of visits in each area. Note any abnormal "field cuts" (Figs. 20-13 and 20-14).

Physiology OSCE Video:
Field of Vision

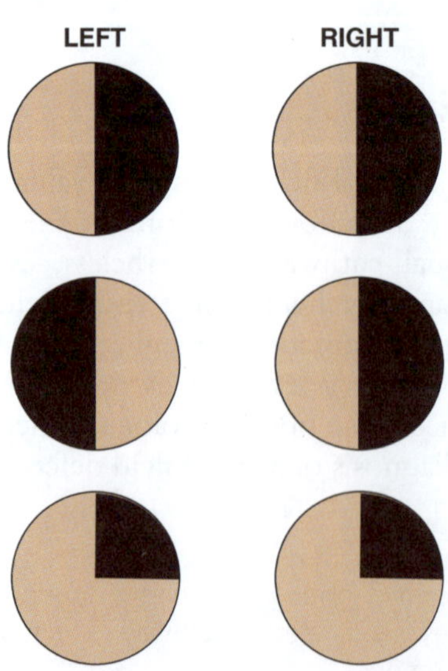

FIGURE 20-13. Visual field defects. Note that visual fields are diagrammed from the patient's viewpoint.

Review these patterns in Table 20-2, Visual Field Defects.

For example, when the patient's left eye repeatedly does not see your fingers until they have crossed the line of gaze, a left *homonymous hemianopsia* is present.

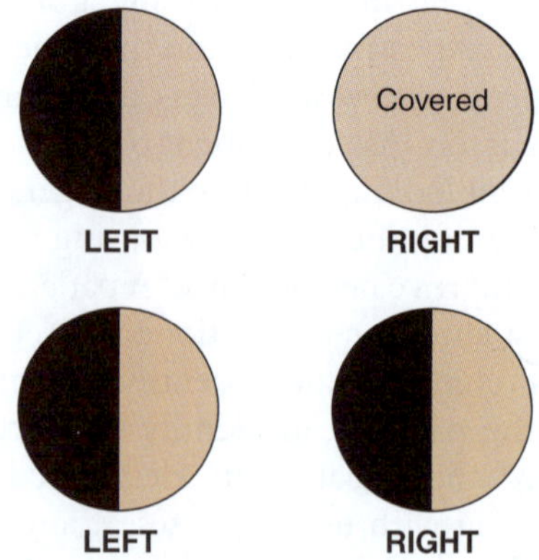

FIGURE 20-14. Visual field defects in a patient with left homonymous hemianopsia.

Color Vision

Testing for color vision can be particularly helpful in ruling out damage to the optic nerve, which often exhibits red-green color deficits and red color desaturation. Generally, pseudoisochromatic color plates can be used to screen for color vision defects (Fig. 20-15). Ask the patient to identify the colored figure embedded in a background of the plate. With normal color vision, the patient will be able to detect the hue difference between figure and background and, as a result, can easily read the figure.

Physiology OSCE Video:
Assessment of Vision

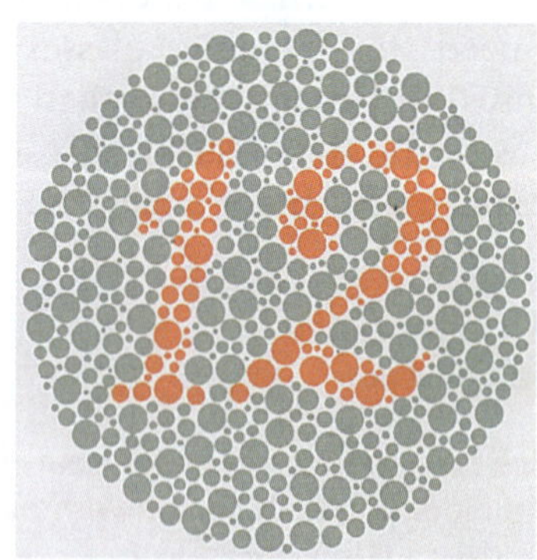

FIGURE 20-15. A pseudoisochromatic color plate for assessing color vision. (From Savino PJ, Danesh-Meyer HV. *Color Atlas and Synopsis of Clinical Ophthalmology—Wills Eye Hospital—Neuro-Ophthalmology*. 3rd ed. Wolters Kluwer; 2019, Fig. 1–3b.)

Persons with defective color vision may fail to distinguish between figure and background colors in a pseudoisochromatic test and hence fail to read the figures.

Contrast Sensitivity

A method for testing contrast sensitivity is to have the patient observe a bright red object (a pen cap or a bottle cap). After alternating cover of the right and left eye, you can ask the patient if the color saturation is equal in both eyes. If the color is less saturated in one of the eyes, you can ask the patient to describe what percent brightness the less saturated color would be in comparison to the full color saturation observed in the contralateral eye.

Though the most commonly recognized color vision abnormalities are *sex-linked congenital red-green deficiencies*, other color vision and contrast sensitivity anomalies can reflect acute or chronic optic nerve or retinal disease.

Eye Position and Alignment

Stand in front of the patient and survey the eyes for position and alignment. If one or both eyes seem to protrude, have the patients look up and assess the axial projection of the eyes from below, looking from the nostrils in a "worm's eye view" using other facial landmarks as a guide.

Abnormalities in eye movements include *esotropia* (inward deviation), *exotropia* (outward deviation), *hypertropia* (upward deviation), and *hypotropia* (downward deviation) of the eyes.

Hyper- or hypoglobus may refer to deviation in the globe position, which may result from congenital abnormalities, lacrimal gland enlargement, mucocele, or ocular tumors.

Abnormal protrusion or *proptosis* may be due to thyroid eye disease, congenital abnormalities, orbital infections, or ocular tumors.

Eyebrows

Inspect the eyebrows, noting their fullness, hair distribution, and any scaliness of the underlying skin.

Scaliness occurs in seborrheic dermatitis, lateral sparseness in hypothyroidism.

Eyelids

Note the position of the eyelids in relation to the eyeballs. Inspect for the following:

See Table 20-3, Variations and Abnormalities of the Eyelids.

- Width of the palpebral fissures

  Upslanting palpebral fissures are noted in Down syndrome.

- Edema of the lids
- Color of the lids

  Red inflamed lid margins occur in blepharitis, often with crusting.

- Lesions
- Condition and direction of the eyelashes
- Adequacy of eyelid closure. Look for this especially when the eyes are unusually prominent, when there is facial paralysis, or when the patient is unconscious.

  Lagophthalmos, or failure of the eyelids to close, which can happen after neuromuscular palsy, trauma, and thyroid eye disease, exposes the corneas to serious damage. These patients should be referred to ophthalmology for urgent evaluation and possible treatment.

Lacrimal Apparatus

Briefly and gently *inspect the regions of the lacrimal gland and lacrimal sac* for swelling.

See Table 20-4, Lumps and Swellings in and Around the Eyes.

Look for excessive tearing or dryness of the eyes. Assessment of dryness or nasolacrimal duct obstruction may require special testing by an ophthalmologist.

Excessive tearing may be from increased production, caused by conjunctival inflammation or corneal irritation, or impaired drainage, caused by *ectropion* (p. 590) and/or nasolacrimal duct obstruction. Dryness from impaired secretion is seen in Sjögren syndrome.

See Table 20-1, Red Eyes.

Conjunctiva and Sclera

Ask the patient to look up as you depress the lower lid with your thumbs, exposing the sclera and conjunctiva (Fig. 20-16). Inspect for color and the vascular pattern

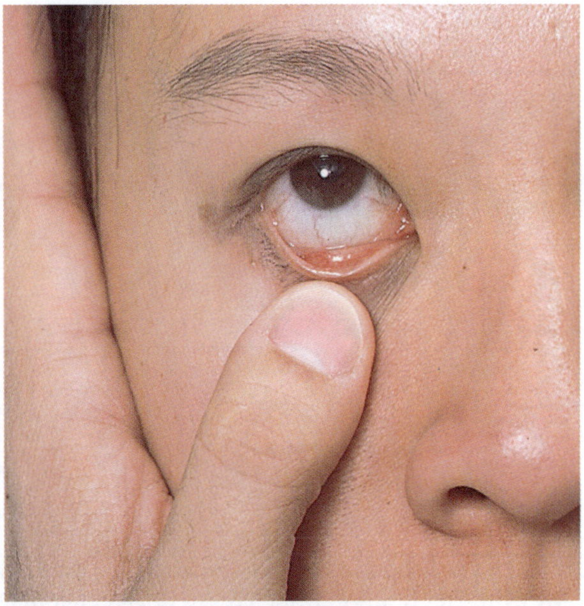

FIGURE 20-16. Inspecting the sclera and conjunctiva.

against the white scleral background. The slight vascularity of the sclera in Figure 20-16 is normal and present in most people. Look for any nodules or swelling (**chemosis**). If you need a fuller view of the eye, rest your thumb and finger on the bones of the cheek and brow, respectively, and spread the lids. Ask the patient to look to each side and down. This technique gives you a good view of the sclera and bulbar conjunctiva, but not of the palpebral conjunctiva of the upper lid. For this, you need to evert the lid. Jaundice is shown in Figure 20-17.

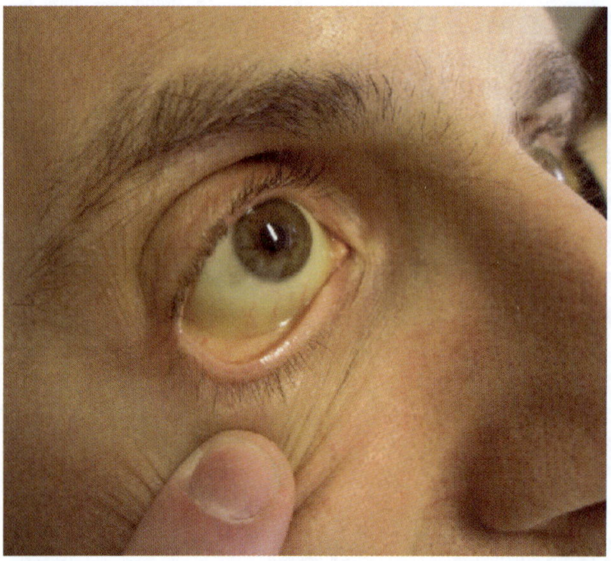

FIGURE 20-17. A yellowish discoloration of the sclera indicating jaundice. (From Weksler BB et al. *Wintrobe's Atlas of Clinical Hematology*. 2nd ed. Wolters Kluwer; 2018, Fig. 3-61a.)

Cornea and Lens

With oblique lighting, *inspect the cornea* of each eye for opacities. Note any opacities in the lens that may be visible through the pupil.

See Table 20-5, Opacities of the Cornea and Lens.

Iris

At the same time, *inspect each iris*, which is the colored ring of the eye underneath the cornea. The markings should be clearly defined. With your light shining directly from the temporal side, look for a crescentic shadow on the medial side of the iris (Fig. 20-18). Because the iris is normally fairly flat and forms a relatively open angle with the cornea, this lighting casts no shadow.

Pupils

In dim light, *inspect* the size, shape, and symmetry of *both pupils*. Measure the pupils with a card showing black circles of varying sizes, and test the light reaction. Note if the pupils are large (>5 mm), small (<3 mm), or unequal (Fig. 20-19). **Miosis** refers to constriction of the pupils, **mydriasis** to dilation.

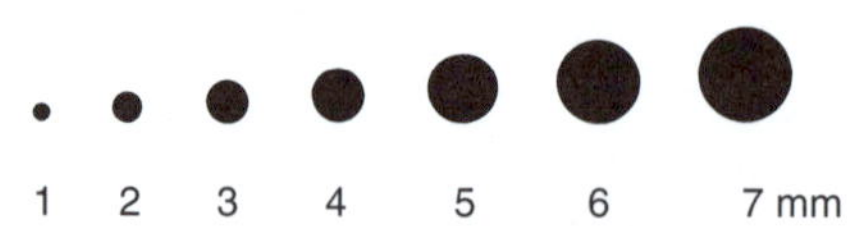

FIGURE 20-19. Pupillary sizes.

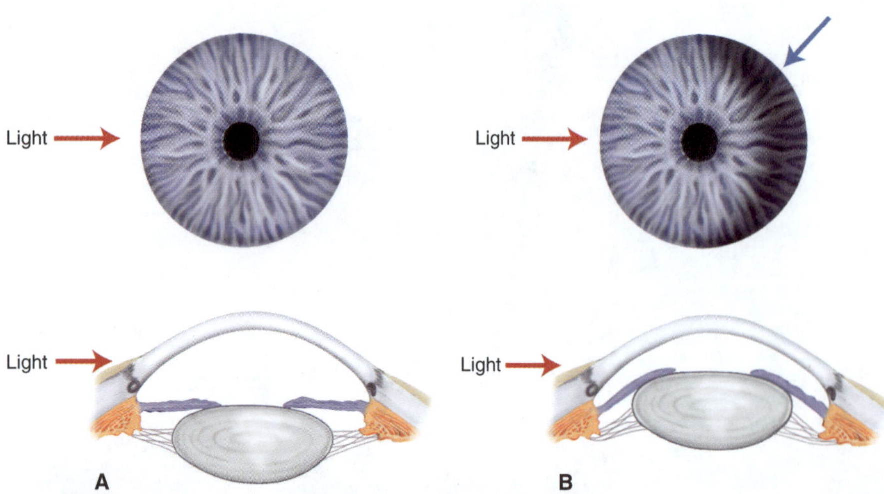

Occasionally, the iris bows abnormally far forward, forming a very narrow angle with the cornea. The light then casts a crescentic shadow (Fig. 20-18). This narrow angle increases the risk for acute *narrow-angle glaucoma,* a sudden increase in intraocular pressure when drainage of the aqueous humor is blocked.

In *open-angle glaucoma*, the common form of glaucoma, the normal spatial relation between iris and cornea is preserved and the iris is fully lit.

FIGURE 20-18. Oblique light illumination for estimating depth of the anterior chamber. **A:** A light source illuminates the iris from the temporal side. With a deep chamber, nearly the entire iris is illuminated. **B:** When the iris is bowed forward, only the proximal portion is illuminated, and a shadow is seen in the distal half on the nasal side (blue arrow).

Simple **anisocoria**, or a difference in pupillary diameter ≥0.4 mm without a known pathologic cause, can be visible in approximately 20% of healthy people, though rarely exceeds 1 mm. Simple anisocoria is considered benign if it is equal in dim and bright light, and there is brisk pupillary constriction to light (the light reaction).

Compare benign anisocoria with Horner syndrome, oculomotor nerve paralysis, and tonic pupil. See Table 20-6, Pupillary Abnormalities.

Light Reaction. In dim light, test the pupillary reaction to light. Ask the patient to look into the distance, and shine a bright light obliquely into each pupil in turn. Both the distant gaze and the oblique lighting help to prevent a near reaction. Look for:

- The *direct reaction* (pupillary constriction in the same eye)
- The *consensual reaction* (pupillary constriction in the opposite eye)

Always darken the room and use a bright light before deciding that a light reaction is abnormal or absent.

Near Reaction. If the reaction to light is impaired or questionable, test the near reaction in both dim and normal light. Testing one eye at a time makes it easier to concentrate on pupillary responses, without the distraction of extraocular muscles (EOMs). Hold your finger or pencil about 10 cm from the patient's eye. Ask the patient to look alternately at it and into the distance directly behind it. Watch for pupillary constriction with near effort and convergence of the eyes. The third component of the near reaction, accommodation of the lens that brings the near object into focus, is not visible.

Testing the near reaction is helpful in diagnosing Argyll Robertson, tonic (Adie) pupils, and other neurologic syndromes (see p. 593).

See Table 20-6, Pupillary Abnormalities.

Extraocular Muscles

Standing about 2 ft directly in front of the patient, shine a light into the patient's eyes and ask the patient to look at it. *Inspect the light reflection in the corneas.* They should be visible slightly nasal to the center of the pupils (Fig. 20-20).

Asymmetry of the corneal reflections indicates a deviation from normal ocular alignment. A temporal light reflection on one cornea, for example, indicates a nasal deviation of that eye.

A cover–uncover test may reveal a slight or latent muscle imbalance not otherwise seen; this is particularly useful in examining children (see p. 594).

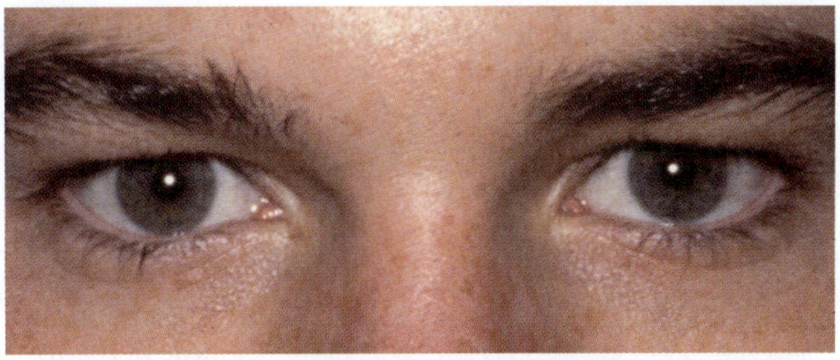

FIGURE 20-20. Inspecting light reflection in the corneas.

Now assess the EOMs, looking for:

- The normal *conjugate* movements of the eyes in each direction. Note any deviation from normal (**strabismus**), or *dysconjugate* gaze.

See Table 20-7, Dysconjugate Gaze.

- *Nystagmus*, a fine rhythmic oscillation of the eyes. A few beats of nystagmus on extreme lateral gaze are normal. If you see this, bring your finger in to within the field of binocular vision and look again.

Sustained nystagmus within the binocular field of gaze is seen in congenital disorders, labyrinthitis, cerebellar disorders, and drug toxicity. See Table 13-9, Nystagmus.

- *Lid lag* as the eyes move from up to down.

In the lid lag of hyperthyroidism, a rim of sclera is visible above the iris with downward gaze (Fig. 20-23).

Test the Six EOMs. Ask the patient to follow your finger or pencil as you sweep through the six cardinal directions of gaze. Making a wide H in the air, lead the patient's gaze (Fig. 20-21):

Review Box 20-2, Extraocular Muscles and Actions.

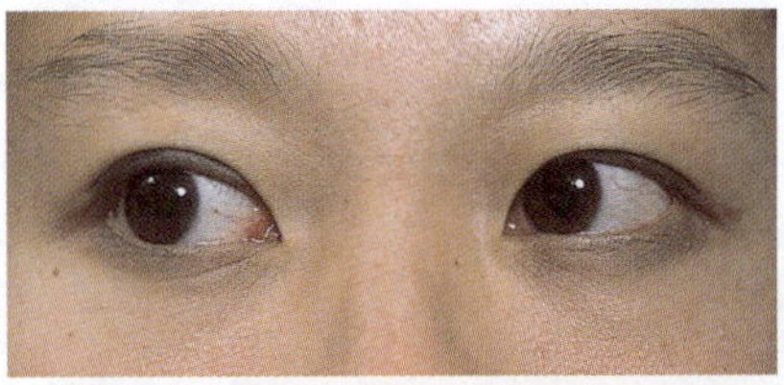

1

1. to the patient's extreme right,

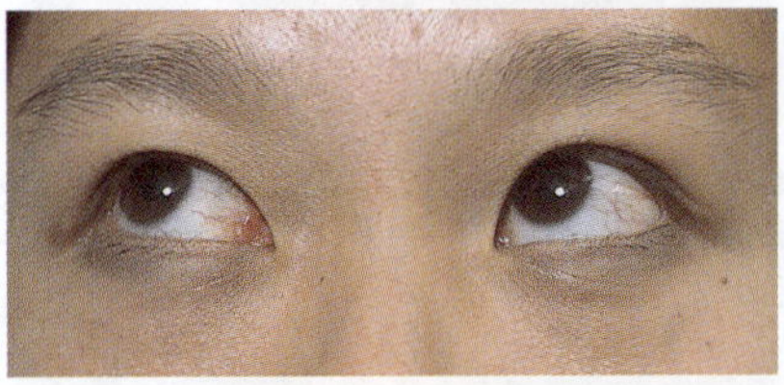

2

2. to the right and upward, and

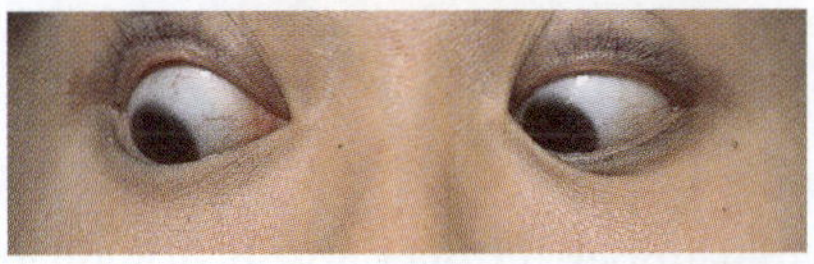

3

3. down on the right; then

FIGURE 20-21. (*continued*)

4 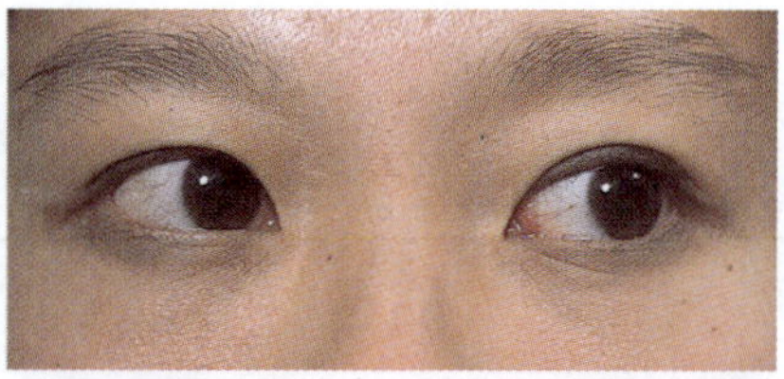

4. without pausing in the middle, to the extreme left,

5 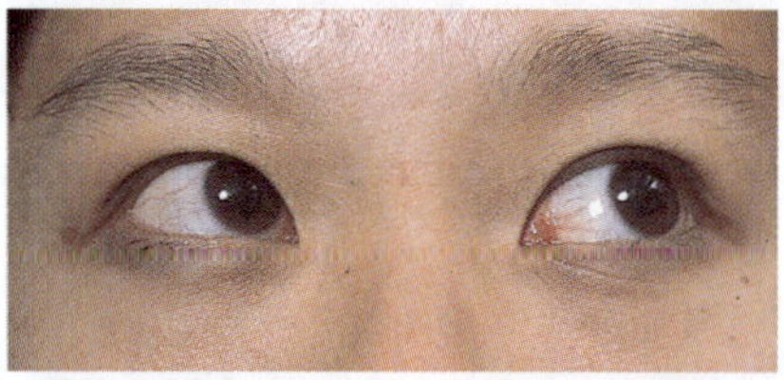

5. to the left and upward, and

6 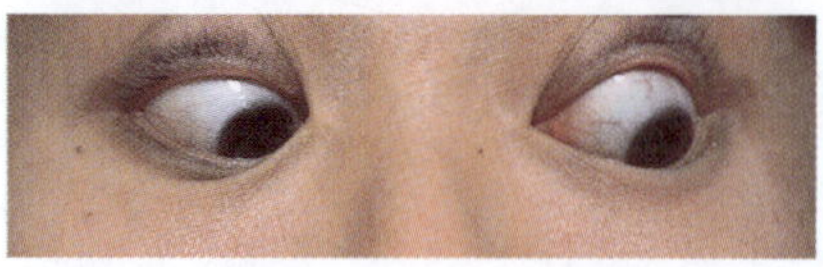

6. down on the left.

FIGURE 20-21. Test extraocular movements.

Pause during vertical and lateral gaze to detect nystagmus. Move your finger or pencil at a comfortable distance from the patient. Because middle-aged or older adults may have difficulty focusing on near objects, increase this distance. Some patients move their heads to follow your finger. If necessary, hold the head in the proper midline position.

Note the rim of sclera from *proptosis*, an abnormal protrusion of the eyeballs in hyperthyroidism, leading to a characteristic "stare" on frontal gaze. If unilateral, consider an *orbital tumor* or *retrobulbar hemorrhage* from trauma.

If you suspect lid lag or hyperthyroidism, ask the patient to follow your finger again as you move it slowly from up to down in the midline. The upper eyelid should overlap the iris slightly throughout this movement as shown in Figure 20-22. Figure 20-23 shows *proptosis*.

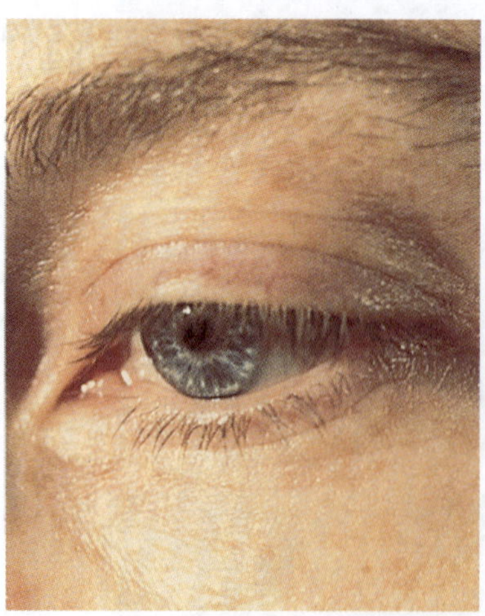

FIGURE 20-22. Normal upper lid overlap on downward gaze.

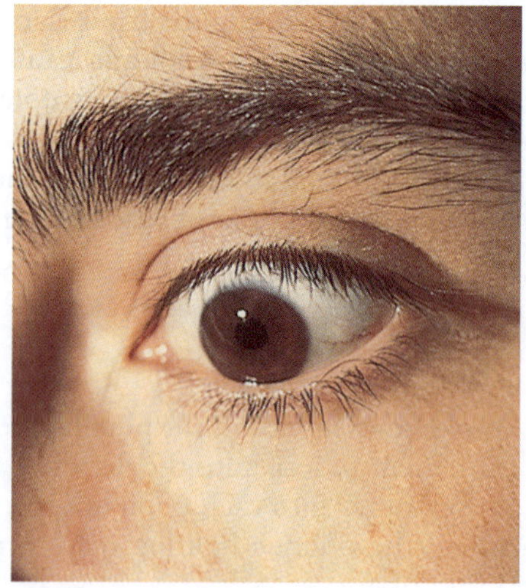

FIGURE 20-23. Lid lag. Note visible rim of sclera on downward gaze caused by proptosis.

Finally, if the near reaction has not already been tested, *test for convergence*. Ask the patient to follow your finger or pencil as you move it in toward the bridge of the nose. The converging eyes normally follow the object to within 5 cm to 8 cm of the nose (Fig. 20-24).

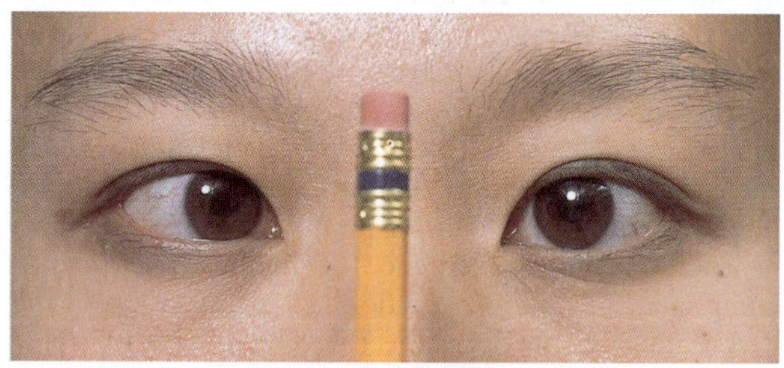

FIGURE 20-24. Testing for convergence.

Ophthalmoscopic (Funduscopic) Examination

In general health care, examine your patients' eyes without dilating their pupils. Therefore, your view is limited to the posterior structures of the retina, which can obscure important neurologic findings. To see more peripheral structures, to evaluate the macula well, or to investigate unexplained visual loss, consider referral to ophthalmologists for pupillary dilatation with mydriatic drops.

Contraindications for mydriatic drops include (1) head injury and coma, since continuing observations of pupillary reactions are essential, and (2) any suspicion of narrow-angle glaucoma. Pregnancy and breastfeeding are relative contraindications for administration of mydriatic drops.

This section describes how to use the traditional direct ophthalmoscope. Of note, some medical offices may use a PanOptic direct ophthalmoscope. The PanOptic direct ophthalmoscope allows clinicians to view the retina, even when the pupils are not dilated. It provides a five-fold greater view of the fundus than the traditional direct ophthalmoscope, enables a 25-degree field of view, and increases the examining distance between the patient and the clinician. Since most clinical settings still use the traditional direct ophthalmoscope, it is emphasized in Box 20-3.

Box 20-3. Steps for Using the Ophthalmoscope

- Darken the room. Switch on the ophthalmoscope light and turn the lens disc until you see the large round beam of white light. Shine the light on the back of your hand to check the type of light, its desired brightness, and the electrical charge of the ophthalmoscope.
- Turn the focusing wheel to the 0 diopter. (A *diopter* is a unit that measures the power of a lens to converge or diverge light.) At this diopter, the lens neither converges nor diverges light. Keep your finger on the edge of the lens disc so that you can turn the focusing wheel to focus the lens when you examine the fundus.
- Hold the ophthalmoscope in your right hand and *use your right eye to examine the patient's right eye*; hold it in your left hand and *use your left eye to examine the patient's left eye*. This keeps you from bumping the patient's nose and gives you more mobility and closer range for visualizing the fundus. With practice, you will become accustomed to using your nondominant eye.
- Hold the ophthalmoscope firmly braced against the medial aspect of your bony orbit, with the handle tilted laterally at about 20 degrees slant from the vertical. Check to make sure you can see clearly through the aperture. *Instruct the patient to look slightly up and over your shoulder at a point directly ahead on the wall.*
- Place yourself about 15 inches away from the patient and at an angle *15° lateral to the patient's line of vision.* Shine the light beam on the pupil and look for the orange glow in the pupil—the *red reflex*. Note any opacities interrupting the red reflex. If you are nearsighted and have taken off your glasses, you may need to adjust the focusing wheel toward the minus/red diopters until the structures you see at a distance is in focus.

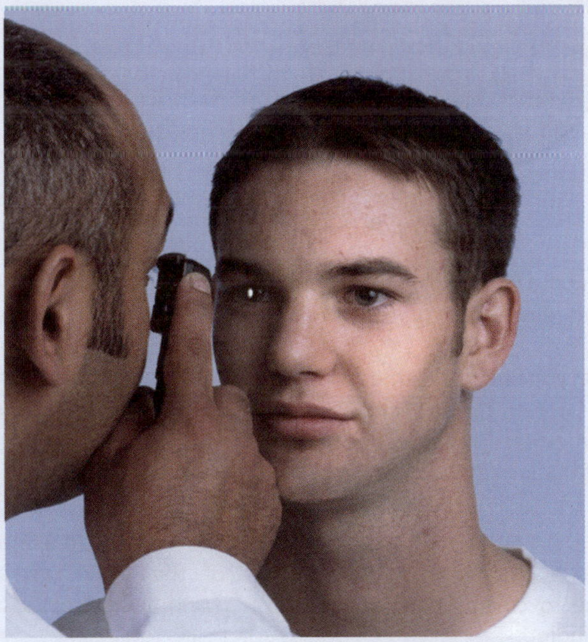

Examiner at 15° angle from patient's line of vision, eliciting red reflex.

Absence of a red reflex suggests an opacity of the lens (*cataract*) or, possibly, the vitreous (or even an artificial eye). Less commonly, a detached retina; mass; or; in children, a retinoblastoma may obscure this reflex.

- Now *place the thumb of your other hand across the patient's eyebrow*, which steadies your examining hand. Keeping the light beam focused on the red reflex, move in with the ophthalmoscope on the 15-degree angle toward the pupil until you are very close to it, almost touching the patient's eyelashes and the thumb of your other hand.
- Try to keep both eyes open and relaxed, as if gazing into the distance, to help minimize any fluctuating blurriness as your eyes attempt to accommodate.
- You may need to lower the brightness of the light beam to make the examination more comfortable for the patient, avoid *hippus* (spasm of the pupil), and improve your observations.

Using the ophthalmoscope to visualize the fundus is one of the most challenging skills of physical examination. With feedback and dedicated practice of proper technique, the fundus, optic disc, and retinal vessels will come into focus. Remove your glasses unless you have marked nearsightedness or severe astigmatism, or your refractive error makes it difficult to see the fundi.

Now you are ready to inspect the optic disc and the retina. The *optic disc* is a round, yellow-orange to creamy pink structure with a pink neuroretinal rim and central depression that often takes practice to locate. The ophthalmoscope magnifies the normal disc and retina about 15 times and the normal iris about 4 times. The optic disc actually measures about 1.5 mm. Follow the next steps shown in Box 20-4 for this important segment of the physical examination.

When the lens has been removed surgically, its magnifying effect is lost.

Retinal structures then look much smaller than usual, and you can see a much larger expanse of the fundus.

Box 20-4. Steps for Examining the Optic Disc and Retina

Optic Disc

- First, locate the optic disc. Look for the round yellowish-orange structure described above, or follow a blood vessel centrally until it enters the disc. The vessel size will help you. The vessel size becomes progressively larger at each branch point as you approach the disc. If you follow each of the branch points back, you will find the nerve.

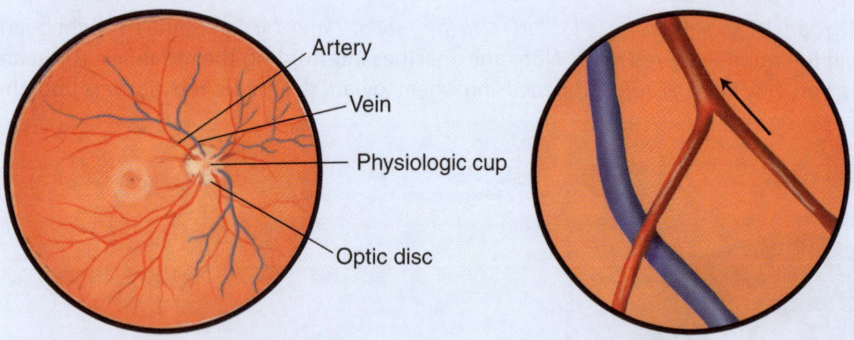

The optic disc and fundus.

- Now, bring the optic disc into sharp focus by adjusting the focusing wheel of your ophthalmoscope. If both you and the patient have no refractive errors, the retina should be in focus at 0 diopters.
- If structures are blurred, rotate the focusing wheel until you find the sharpest focus. For example, if the patient is myopic (nearsighted), rotate the focusing wheel counterclockwise to the minus/red diopters; in a hyperopic (farsighted) patient, move the focusing wheel clockwise to the plus/green diopters. You can correct your own refractive error in the same way.
- Inspect the optic disc. Note the following features:
  - The sharpness or clarity of the disc outline.
  - The color of the disc, normally yellowish-orange to creamy pink. White or pigmented crescents may ring the disc, a normal finding.
  - The size of the central physiologic *cup*, if present. It is usually yellowish-white. The horizontal diameter is usually less than half the horizontal diameter of the disc.
  - The comparative symmetry of the eyes and findings in the fundi.

(continued)

In a *refractive error*, light rays from a distance do not focus on the retina. In *myopia*, they focus anterior to the retina, in *hyperopia*, posterior to it. Retinal structures in a myopic eye look larger than normal.

See Table 20-8, Normal Variations of the Optic Disc, and Table 20-9, Abnormalities of the Optic Disc.

An enlarged cup suggests chronic open-angle glaucoma.

Box 20-4. Steps for Examining the Optic Disc and Retina (*continued*)

Importance of Detecting Papilledema

Swelling of the optic disc and anterior bulging of the physiologic cup suggest *papilledema* (Fig. 20-25), which is optic nerve head swelling associated with increased intracranial pressure. This pressure is transmitted to the optic nerve, causing stasis of axoplasmic flow, intra-axonal edema, and swelling of the optic nerve head. Papilledema signals serious disorders of the brain, such as meningitis, subarachnoid hemorrhage, trauma, and mass lesions, so searching for this important disorder is a priority during all your funduscopic examinations (see technique as described on prior page).

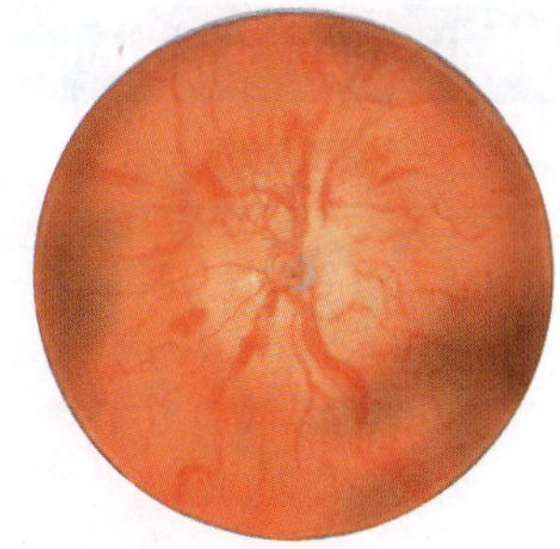

FIGURE 20-25. Papilledema.

Inspect the fundus for *spontaneous venous pulsations* (SVPs), rhythmic variations in the caliber of the retinal veins as they cross the fundus (narrower in systole; wider in diastole), present in 90% of normal patients.

Loss of SVPs occurs with high intracranial pressures (above 190 mm H_2O) that change the pressure gradient between cerebral spinal fluid pressure and intraocular pulse pressure in the optic disc. Other causes include glaucoma and retinal vein occlusion.

Retina—Arteries, Veins, Fovea, and Macula

- *Inspect the retina,* including arteries and veins as they extend to the periphery, arteriovenous crossings, the fovea, and the macula. Distinguish arteries from veins based on the features listed below.

See Tables 20-10 to 20-12 for information on retinal arteries and AV crossings, spots and streaks in the fundi, and light-colored spots in the fundi.

	Arteries	**Veins**
Color	Light red	Dark red
Size	Smaller (2/3 to 3/4 the diameter of veins)	Larger
Light reflex (*reflection*)	Bright	Inconspicuous or absent

- Follow the vessels peripherally in each direction, noting their relative sizes and the character of the arteriovenous crossings.

  Identify any lesions of the surrounding retina and note their size, shape, color, and distribution. As you search the retina, move your head and instrument as a unit, using the patient's pupil as an imaginary fulcrum. At first, you may lose your view of the retina because your light falls out of the pupil, but you will improve with practice. Lesions of the retina can be measured in terms of "disc diameters" from the optic disc.

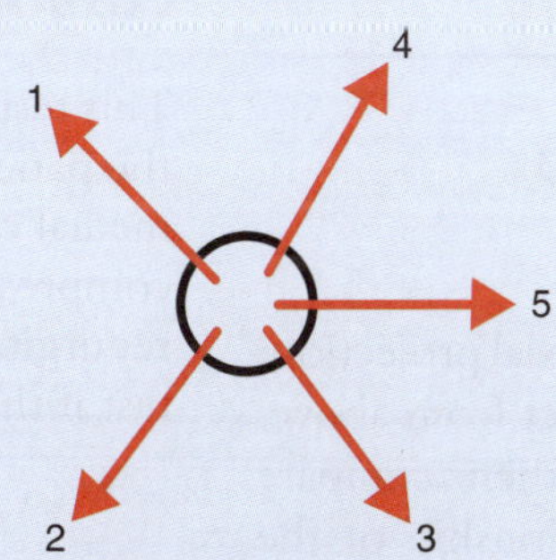

Sequence of inspection from disc to macula (left eye)

- *Inspect the fovea and surrounding macula.* Direct your light beam laterally or ask the patient to look directly into the light. In younger people, the tiny bright reflection at the center of the fovea helps to orient you; shimmering light reflections in the macular area are common.

Macular degeneration is an important cause of poor central vision in older adults. Types include dry atrophic (more common but less severe) and wet exudative, or neovascular. Cellular debris, called *drusen*, may be "hard" and sharply defined, as seen in Figure 20-26, or "soft" and confluent with altered pigmentation (see p. 777).

(continued)

Box 20-4. Steps for Examining the Optic Disc and Retina (*continued*)

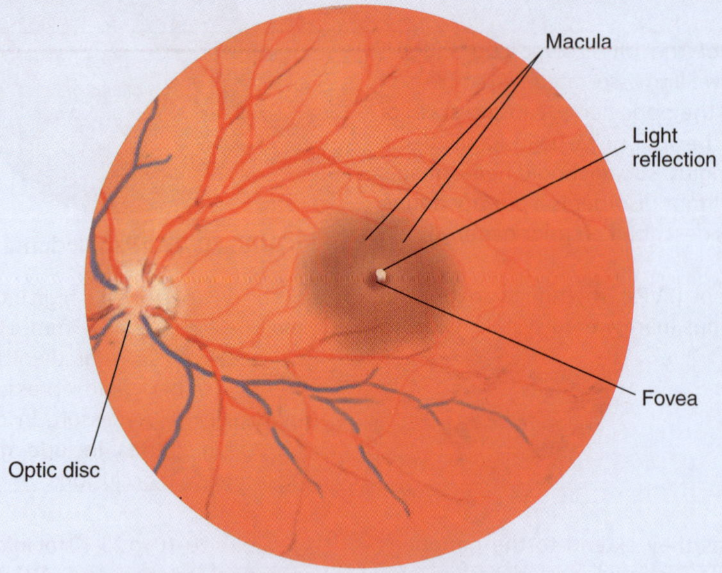

Structures of the left fundus.

- *Inspect the anterior structures.* Look for opacities in the vitreous or lens. Rotate the focusing wheel progressively to diopters of around +10 or +12, so you can focus on the more anterior structures in the eye.

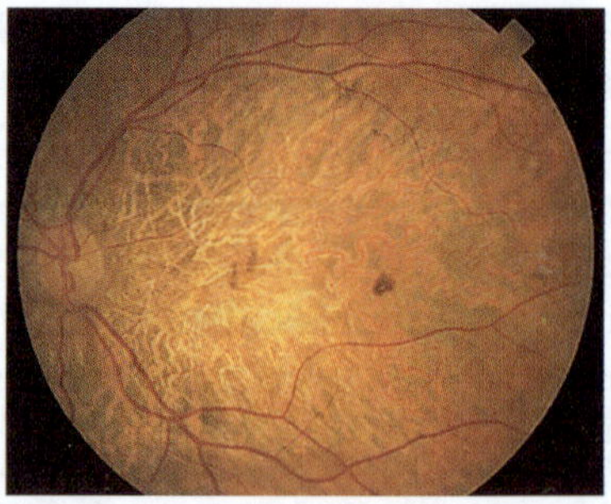

FIGURE 20-26. Hard drusen. (From Tasman W, Jaeger E, eds. *The Wills Eye Hospital Atlas of Clinical Ophthalmology.* 2nd ed. Lippincott Williams & Wilkins; 2001.)

Vitreous floaters are dark specks or strands seen between the fundus and the lens. *Cataracts* are densities in the lens (see p. 592).

SPECIAL TECHNIQUES

Eye Protrusion (Proptosis or Exophthalmos)

For eyes with **exophthalmos** or increased axial projection, stand behind the seated patient and inspect from above. Draw the upper lids gently upward, then compare the protrusion of the eyes and the relationship of the corneas to the lower lids. For objective measurement, ophthalmologists use a Hertel exophthalmometer. This instrument measures the distance between the lateral angle of the orbit and an imaginary line across the most anterior point of the cornea. The upper limits of normal are 20 to 22 mm.

Exophthalmos is a common finding in thyroid eye disease and is found in approximately 60% of patients. Other common symptoms of thyroid disease include eyelid retraction (91%), restricted ocular motility (43%), ocular pain (30%), lacrimation (23%), and dry eye (85%). See also Table 19-1, Symptoms and Signs of Thyroid Dysfunction.

When protrusion exceeds normal, further evaluation by CT or MRI often follows.

Nasolacrimal Duct Obstruction

This test helps identify the cause of excessive tearing. Ask the patient to look up. Press on the lower lid close to the medial canthus, just inside the rim of the bony orbit; this compresses the lacrimal sac (Fig. 20-27). Look for fluid regurgitated out of the puncta into the eye. Avoid this test if the area is inflamed and tender.

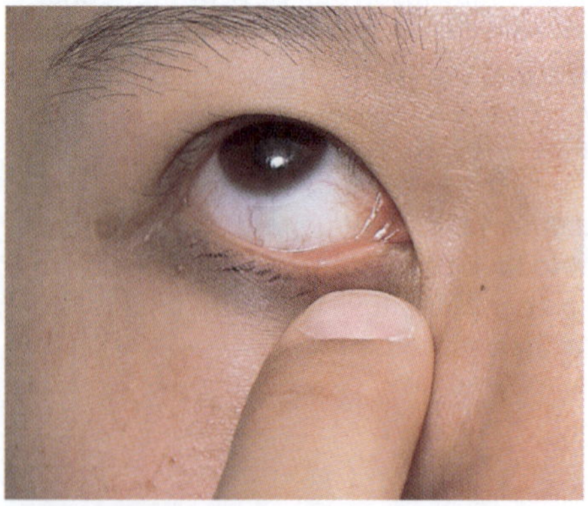

FIGURE 20-27. Expressing tears from the lacrimal sac by compressing the lower lid close to the medial canthus.

Discharge of mucopurulent fluid from the puncta suggests an obstructed nasolacrimal duct or a canaliculitis.

Everting Upper Eyelid to Search for Foreign Body

A foreign body in the eye often involves dust, a speck of sand, a paint chip, an insect, or a dislodged eyelash trapped underneath the lid, causing patients to sense something in their eye. Foreign bodies can be superficial, sticking to the eye surface or beneath the lid, or penetrating—usually a piece of metal that pierces the outer cornea or sclera.

To search thoroughly for a foreign body in the eye, evert the upper lid following the steps below.

- Ask the patient to look down and relax the eyes. Be reassuring and use gentle deliberate movements. Raise the upper eyelid slightly so that the lashes protrude, then grasp the upper eyelashes and pull them gently down and forward (Fig. 20-28).

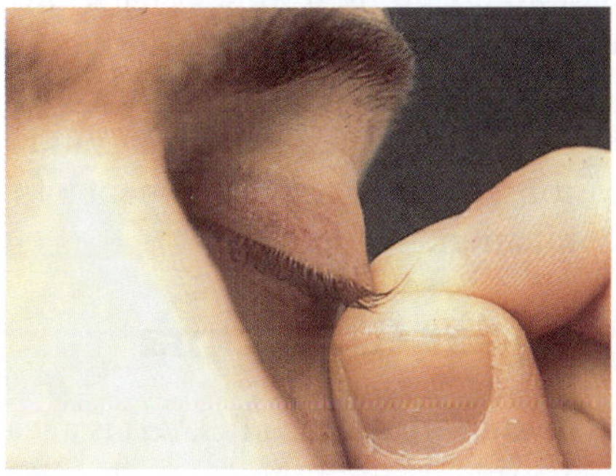

FIGURE 20-28. Start by pulling down on the upper eyelashes.

- Then place a small stick such as a tongue blade or an applicator at least 1 cm above the lid margin at the upper border of the tarsal plate. Push down on the tongue blade as you raise the edge of the lid, thus everting the eyelid or turning it "inside out." Do not press on the eyeball itself (Fig. 20-29).

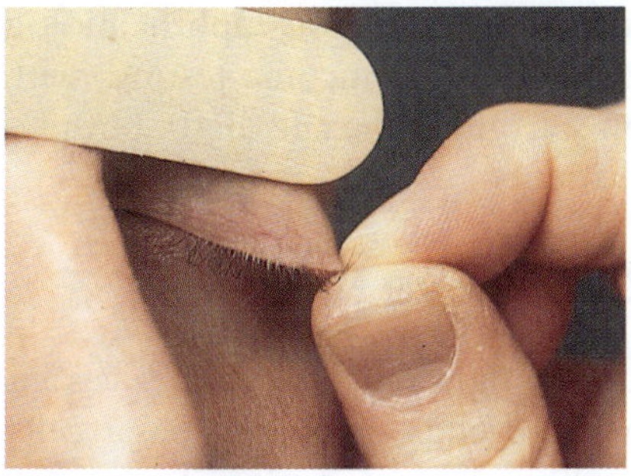

FIGURE 20-29. Everting the eyelid with the use of a tongue blade.

- Secure the upper lashes against the eyebrow with your thumb and inspect the palpebral conjunctiva (Fig. 20-30). After your inspection, grasp the upper eyelashes and pull them gently forward. Ask the patient to look up. The eyelid will return to its normal position.

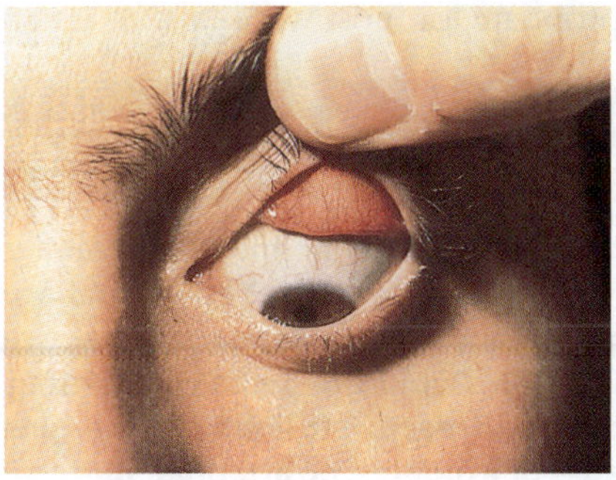

FIGURE 20-30. Securing the everted lid and inspecting the palpebral conjunctiva.

This view allows you to see the upper palpebral conjunctiva and look for a foreign body that might be lodged there.

Swinging Flashlight Test

The swinging flashlight test is a clinical test for functional impairment of the optic nerves (Fig. 20-31). In dim light, note the size of the pupils. After asking the patient to gaze into the distance, swing the beam of a penlight for 1 to 2 seconds first into one pupil, then into the other. Normally, each illuminated eye constricts promptly. The opposite eye also constricts consensually.

In left-sided optic nerve damage, the pupils usually react as follows: When the light beam shines into the normal right eye, there is brisk constriction of both pupils (direct response on the right and consensual response on the left). When the light swings over to the abnormal left eye, partial dilation of both pupils will occur. The afferent stimulus on the left is reduced, so the efferent signals to both pupils are also reduced and a net dilation occurs. This demonstrates an **afferent pupillary defect**, sometimes termed a *Marcus Gunn pupil.*

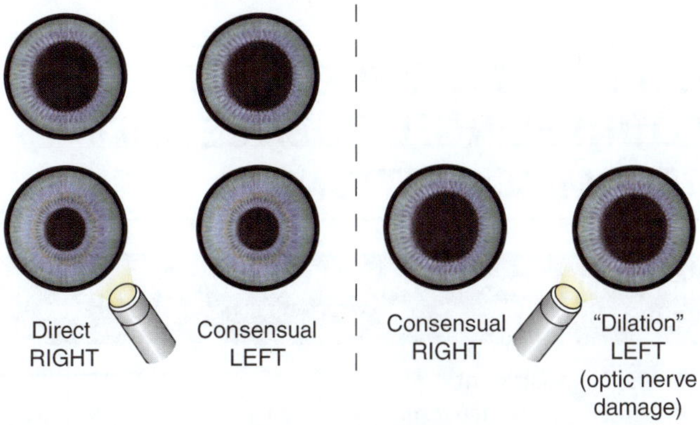

FIGURE 20-31. Swinging flashlight test.

RECORDING YOUR FINDINGS

Initially you may use sentences to describe your findings; later you will use phrases. The style in the next box contains phrases appropriate for most write-ups.

Recording the Head, Eyes, Ears, Nose, and Throat (HEENT) Examination

HEENT: Head—The skull is normocephalic/atraumatic (NC/AT). Hair with average texture. ***Eyes*—Visual acuity 20/20 bilaterally. Lids and adnexa appear normal. Sclera white, conjunctiva pink. Pupils are 5 mm constricting to 4 mm, equally round and reactive to light. Disc margins sharp; no hemorrhages or exudates, no arteriolar narrowing.** ***Ears***—Acuity good to whispered voice. Tympanic membranes (TMs) with good cone of light. Weber midline. AC > BC. ***Nose***—Nasal mucosa pink, septum midline; no sinus tenderness. ***Throat (or Mouth)***—Oral mucosa pink, dentition good, pharynx without exudates.

Neck—Trachea midline. Neck supple; thyroid isthmus palpable, lobes not felt.

Lymph Nodes—No cervical, axillary, epitrochlear, inguinal adenopathy.

OR

Head—The skull is normocephalic/atraumatic. Frontal balding. ***Eyes****—**Visual acuity 20/100 bilaterally. Eyelashes with scurf. Sclera white; conjunctiva injected. Pupils constrict 3 mm to 2 mm, equally round and reactive to light. Disc margins sharp; no hemorrhages or exudates. Arteriolar-to-venous ratio (AV ratio) 2:4; no AV nicking.** ***Ears***—Acuity diminished to whispered voice; intact to spoken voice. TMs clear. ***Nose***—Mucosa swollen with erythema and clear drainage. Septum midline. Tender over maxillary sinuses. ***Throat***—Oral mucosa pink, dental caries in lower molars, pharynx erythematous, no exudates.

Neck—Trachea midline. Neck supple; thyroid isthmus midline, lobes palpable but not enlarged.

Lymph Nodes—Submandibular and anterior cervical lymph nodes tender, 1 cm × 1 cm, rubbery and mobile; no posterior cervical, epitrochlear, axillary, or inguinal lymphadenopathy.

*These findings suggest myopia and mild arteriolar narrowing.

HEALTH PROMOTION AND COUNSELING: EVIDENCE AND RECOMMENDATIONS

Important Topics for Health Promotion and Counseling

- Visual impairment
- Screening for glaucoma
- UV-related eye injuries

Visual Impairment

Visual impairment is defined as having corrected visual acuity of only 20/40 or worse in the better eye, whereas corrected visual acuity of only 20/200 or worse in the better eye defines legal blindness. Non-Hispanic whites, women, and older adults are most affected by visual impairment and blindness. The major causes of visual impairment are *cataracts*, *age-related macular degeneration*, glaucoma, and *diabetic retinopathy*. Visual impairment is associated with decreased functional capacity, poor quality of life, loss of independent living, falls, cognitive decline, family stress, and increased risk for premature death and experiencing other medical comorbidities. Because onset can be gradual, those affected may not recognize their visual decline. The American Academy of Ophthalmology strongly recommends a comprehensive screening medical eye examination, including testing visual acuity and visual fields, funduscopic examination, and intraocular pressure measurement, for all adults. The recommended frequency for these examinations depends upon age and risk factors. Assessing vision is a standard component of a thorough physical examination.

Screening for Glaucoma

Primary open-angle glaucoma (POAG) is a leading cause of visual impairment and blindness. In POAG, there is gradual loss of vision in the peripheral visual fields, resulting from loss of retinal ganglion cell axons. Retinal examination reveals pallor and increasing size of the optic cup, which can enlarge to more than half the diameter of the optic disc. Risk factors include age ≥65 years, diabetes, myopia, and ocular hypertension (intraocular pressure [IOP] is ≥21 mm Hg). Not all people with POAG have elevated IOP, and those with elevated IOP may not develop visual impairment. Further, diagnosis of optic disc enlargement is variable, even among experts. The American Academy of Ophthalmology strongly recommends periodic glaucoma testing, with a baseline examination starting at the age of 40, but possibly earlier for at-risk patients.

UV-Related Eye Injuries

Ultraviolet (UV) light can damage the eyes and cause skin cancers on the eyelids, including basal cell carcinoma, squamous cell carcinoma, and melanoma. In addition, there is some evidence that UV light is associated with the development of cataracts. Furthermore, directly staring at the sun can cause solar retinopathy. Recommended preventive actions include use of sunscreen on the face and eyelids and wearing sunglasses during exposure to direct sunlight.

TABLE 20-1. Red Eyes

	Conjunctivitis	Subconjunctival Hemorrhage
	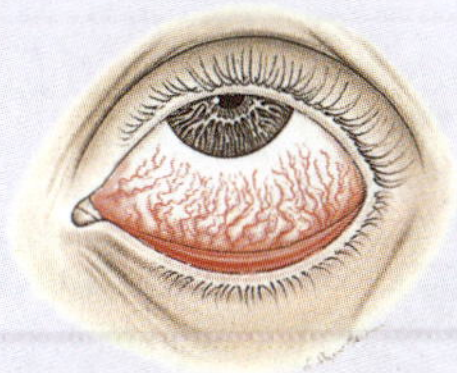	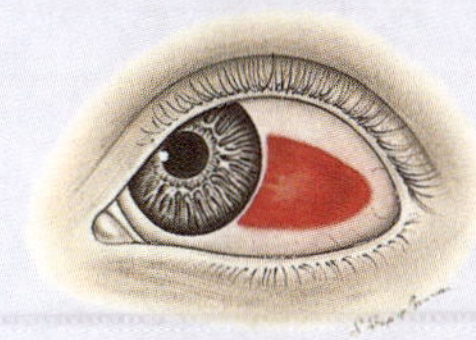
Pattern of Redness	Conjunctival injection: diffuse dilatation of conjunctival vessels with redness that tends to be maximal peripherally	Leakage of blood outside of the vessels, producing a homogeneous, sharply demarcated, red area that resolves over 2 wks
Pain	Mild discomfort rather than pain	Absent
Vision	Not affected except for temporary mild blurring due to discharge	Not affected
Ocular Discharge	Watery, mucoid, or mucopurulent	Absent
Pupil	Not affected	Not affected
Cornea	Clear	Clear
Significance	Bacterial, viral, and other infections; highly contagious; allergy; irritation	Often none. May result from trauma, bleeding disorders, or sudden increase in venous pressure, as from cough

(continued)

TABLE 20-1. Red Eyes *(Continued)*

	Corneal Injury or Infection	Acute Iritis	Acute Angle Closure Glaucoma
	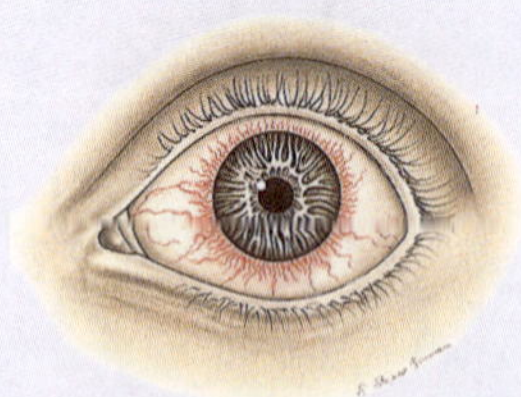	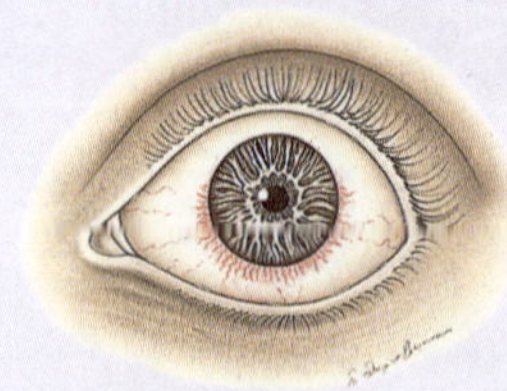	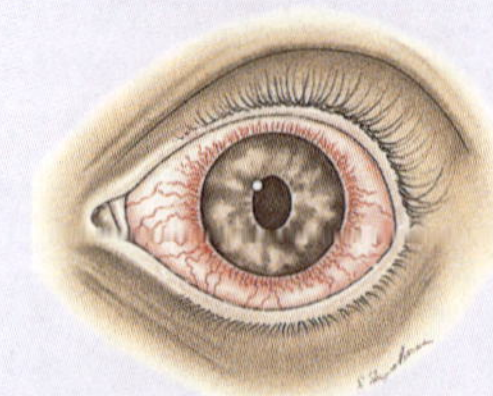
Pattern of Redness	Ciliary injection: The deeper vessels radiating from the limbus are dilated, creating a reddish violet flush. Ciliary injection is an important sign of these three conditions but is not always visible. The eye may be diffusely red instead. Other signs of these serious disorders are pain, decreased vision, unequal pupils, and a clouded cornea.		
Pain	Moderate to severe, superficial	Moderate, aching, deep, photophobia	Severe, aching, deep, severe photophobia
Vision	Usually decreased	Decreased	Decreased
Ocular Discharge	Watery or purulent	Absent	Absent
Pupil	Not affected unless iritis develops	Small and irregular	Dilated, fixed
Cornea	Changes depending on cause, often with epithelial defect. May have corneal opacity if infection involved.	Clear or slightly clouded; injection confined to corneal limbus	Steamy, cloudy
Significance	Abrasions, and other injuries; viral and bacterial infections	Associated with systemic infection, herpes zoster, tuberculosis, or autoimmune diseases; refer promptly	Acute increase in intraocular pressure constitutes an emergency

TABLE 20-2. Visual Field Defects

Visual Field Defects

1. *Horizontal Defect* Occlusion of a branch of the central retinal artery may cause a horizontal (altitudinal) defect. Ischemia of the optic nerve can produce a similar defect.

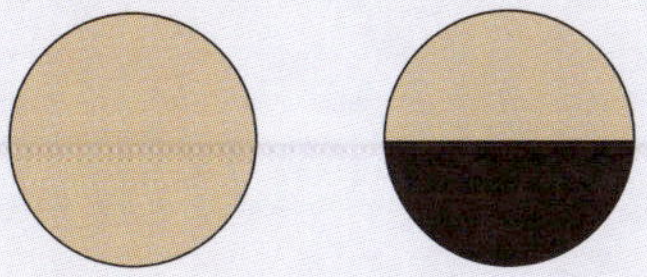

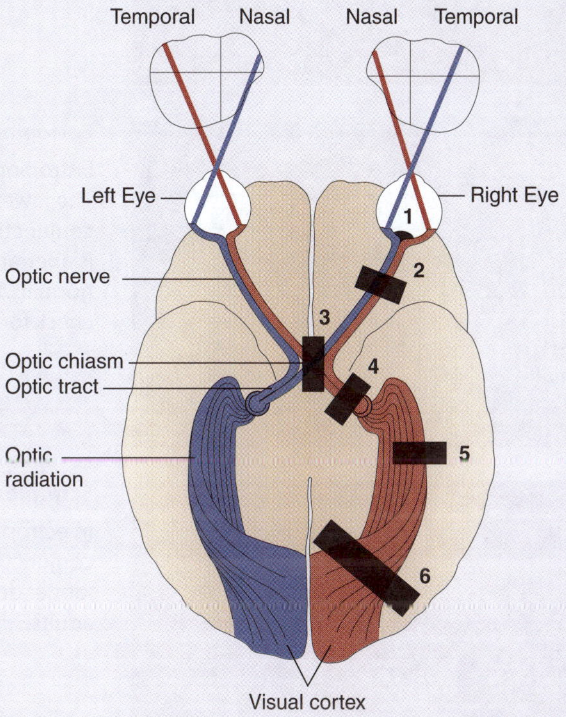

2. *Blind Right Eye (Right Optic Nerve)* A lesion of the optic nerve and, of course, of the eye itself, produces unilateral monocular blindness.

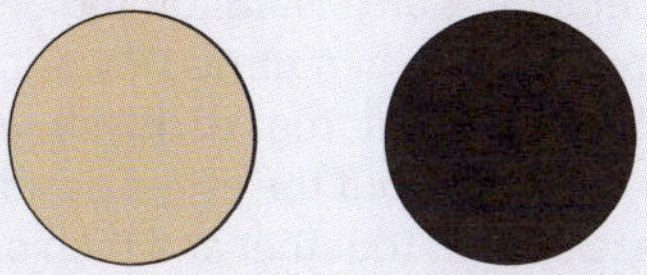

3. *Bitemporal Hemianopsia (Optic Chiasm)* A lesion at the optic chiasm (such as a pituitary tumor), may involve only fibers crossing over to the opposite side. Since these fibers originate in the nasal half of each retina, visual loss involves the temporal half of each field.

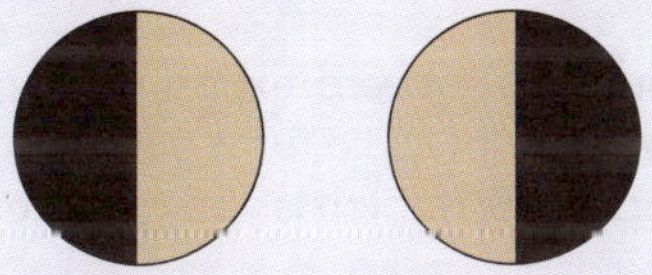

4. *Left Homonymous Hemianopsia (Right Optic Tract)* A lesion of the optic tract, interrupts fibers originating on the same side of both eyes. Visual loss in the eyes is, therefore, similar (homonymous) and involves half of each field (hemianopsia).

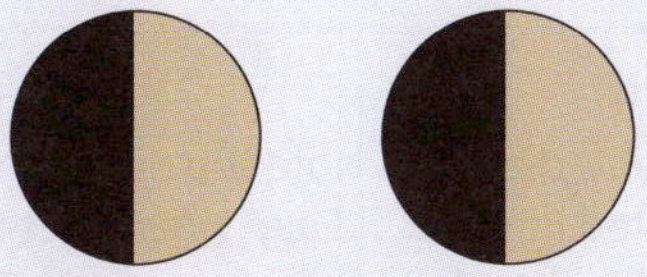

5. *Homonymous Left Superior Quadrantic Defect (Right Optic Radiation, Partial)* A partial lesion of the optic radiation in the temporal lobe, may involve only a portion of the nerve fibers, producing, for example, a homonymous quadrantic ("pie in the sky") defect.

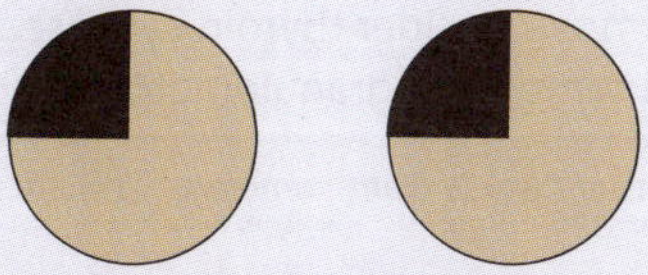

6. *Left Homonymous Hemianopsia (Right Optic Radiation)* A complete interruption of fibers in the optic radiation, produces a visual defect similar to that produced by a lesion of the optic tract.

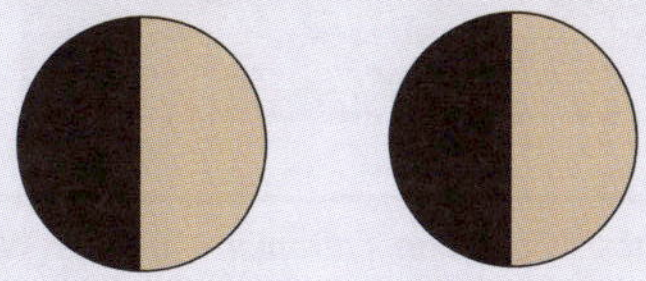

TABLE 20-3. Variations and Abnormalities of the Eyelids

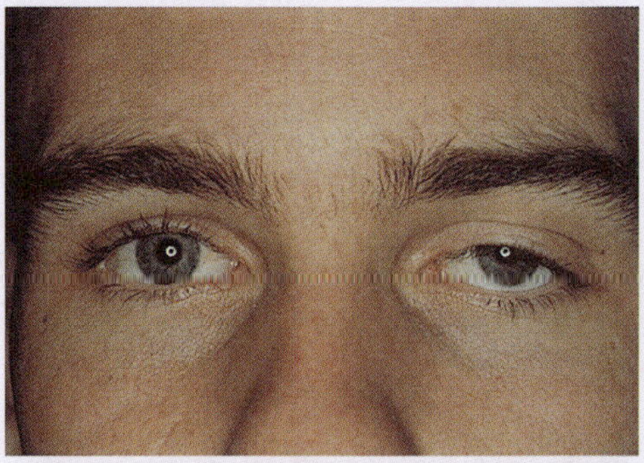

Ptosis

Ptosis is a drooping of the upper lid. Causes include senescence, myasthenia gravis, damage to the oculomotor nerve (CN III), and damage to the sympathetic nerve supply (Horner syndrome). A weakened muscle, relaxed tissues, and the weight of herniated fat may cause senile ptosis. Ptosis may also be congenital.

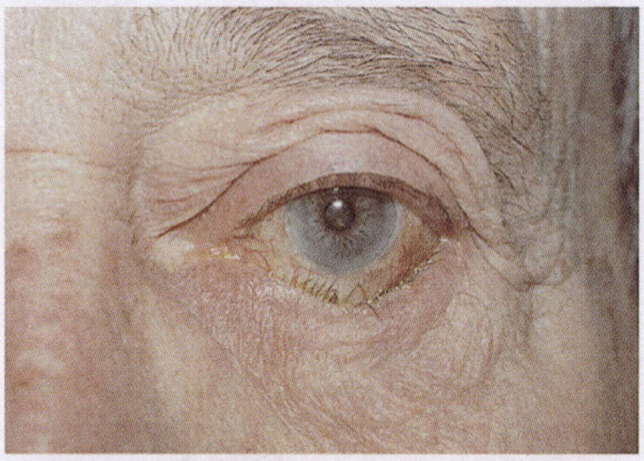

Entropion

Entropion, more common in the elderly, is an inward turning of the lid margin. The lower lashes, which are often invisible when turned inward, irritate the conjunctiva and lower cornea. This is different from **trichiasis** where there is aberrant inward growth of the eyelashes, but the eyelid position remains normal. Ask the patient to squeeze the lids together and then open them; then check for an entropion that is less obvious.

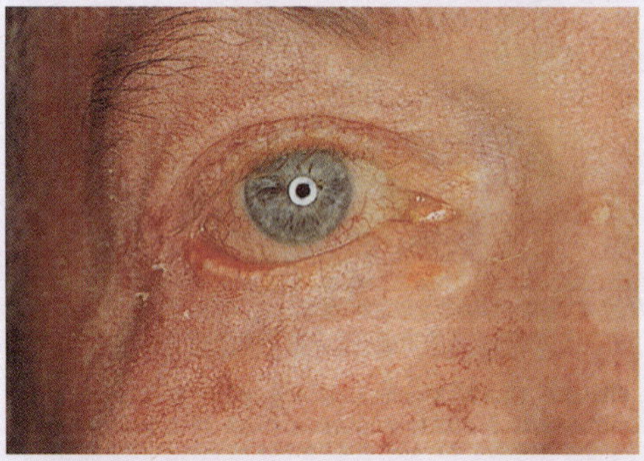

Ectropion

In ectropion, the lower lid margin turns outward, exposing the palpebral conjunctiva. When the punctum of the lower lid turns outward, the eye no longer drains well, and tearing occurs. Ectropion is also more common in older adults.

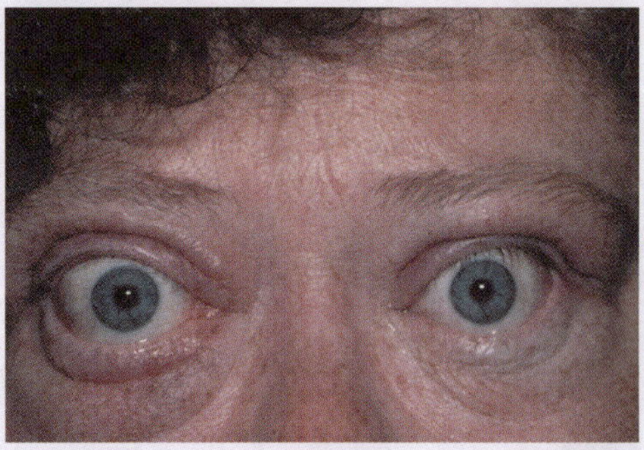

Lid Retraction and Exophthalmos

A wide-eyed stare suggests retracted eyelids. Note the rim of sclera between the upper lid and the iris. Retracted lids and "lid lag" when eyes move from up to down markedly increase the likelihood of hyperthyroidism, especially when accompanied by a fine tremor, moist skin, and heart rate >90 beats/min.

Exophthalmos describes protrusion of the eyeball, a common feature of thyroid eye disease, triggered by autoreactive T lymphocytes. In this disorder, there is a spectrum of eye changes, ranging from lid retraction to extraocular muscle dysfunction, dry eyes, ocular pain, and lacrimation. Changes do not always progress. In unilateral exophthalmos, consider thyroid eye disease (though usually bilateral), trauma, orbital tumor, and granulomatous disorders.

Source of photos: *Ptosis, Ectropion, Entropion*—Tasman W, Jaeger E, eds. *The Wills Eye Hospital Atlas of Clinical Ophthalmology*. 2nd ed. Lippincott Williams & Wilkins; 2001.

TABLE 20-4. Lumps and Swellings In and Around the Eyes

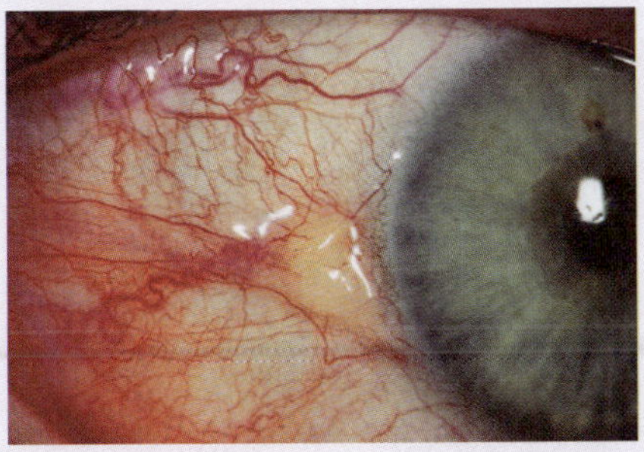

Pinguecula

A harmless yellowish triangular nodule in the bulbar conjunctiva on either side of the iris. Appears frequently with aging, first on the nasal and then on the temporal side.

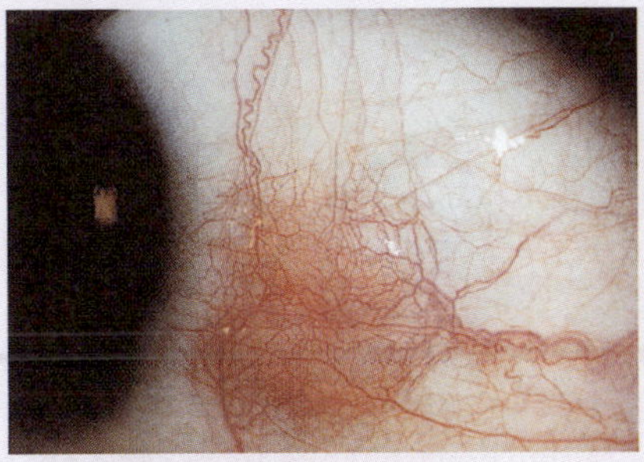

Episcleritis

A benign, usually painless localized ocular inflammation of the episcleral vessels. Vessels appear movable over the scleral surface. May be nodular or show only redness and dilated vessels.

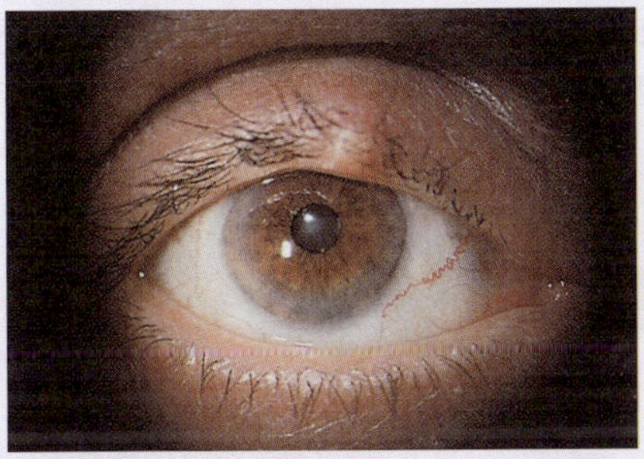

Stye (Hordeolum)

A painful, tender, red infection at the inner or outer margin of the eyelid, usually from *Staphylococcus aureus* (at the inner margin—from an obstructed meibomian gland; at the outer margin—from an obstructed eyelash follicle or tear gland).

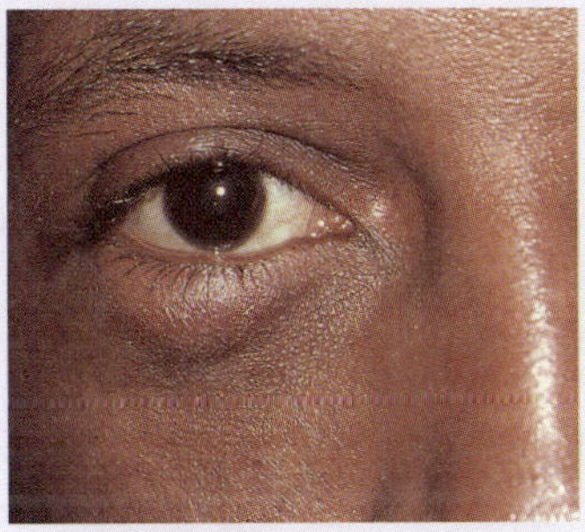

Chalazion

A subacute nontender, usually painless nodule caused by a blocked meibomian gland. May become acutely inflamed but, unlike a stye, usually points inside the lid rather than on the lid margin.

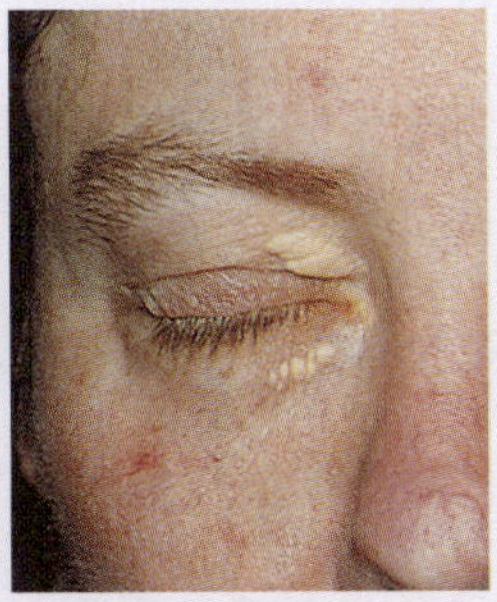

Xanthelasma

Slightly raised, yellowish, well-circumscribed cholesterol-filled plaques that appear along the nasal portions of one or both eyelids. Half of affected patients have hyperlipidemia; it is also common in primary biliary cirrhosis.

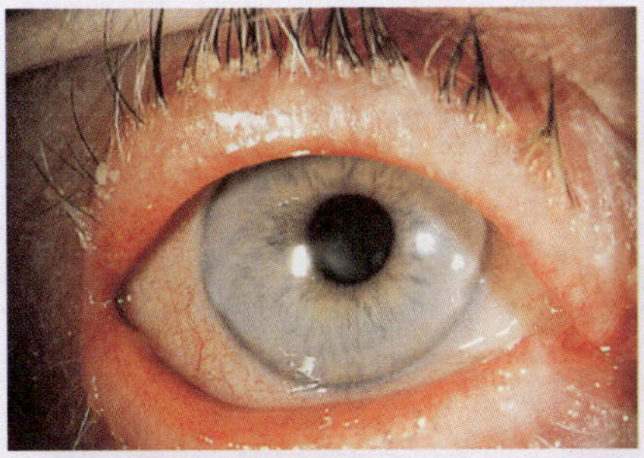

Blepharitis

A chronic inflammation of the eyelids at the base of the hair follicles, often from *S. aureus*. There is also a scaling seborrheic variant.

Source of photos: Tasman W, Jaeger E, eds. *The Wills Eye Hospital Atlas of Clinical Ophthalmology.* 2nd ed. Lippincott Williams & Wilkins; 2001.

TABLE 20-5. Opacities of the Cornea and Lens

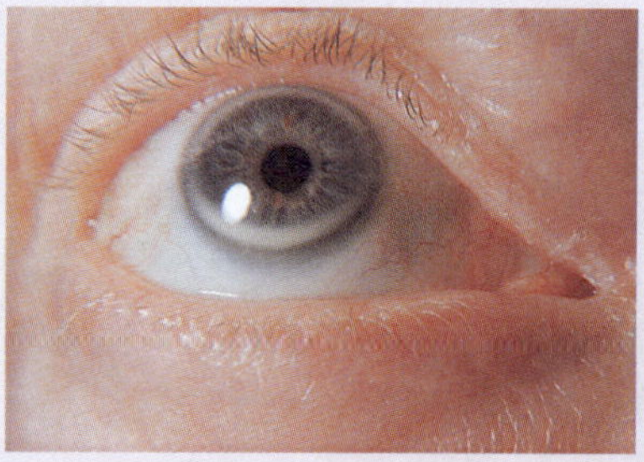

Corneal Arcus. A thin grayish-white arc or circle not quite at the edge of the cornea. Accompanies normal aging but also seen in younger adults, especially African Americans. In young adults, suggests possible hyperlipoproteinemia. Usually benign.

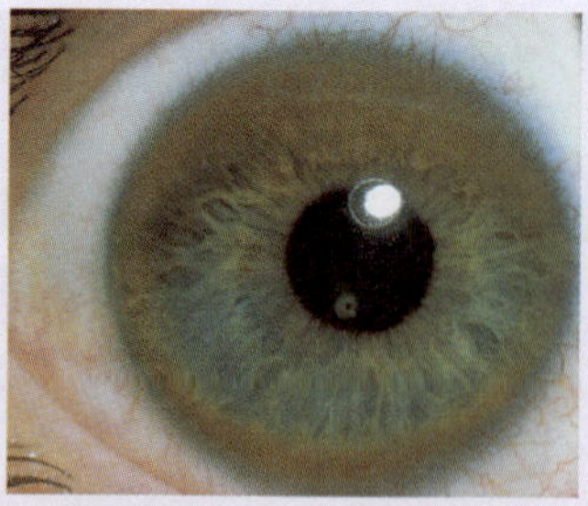

Kayser–Fleischer Ring. A golden to red brown ring, sometimes shading to green or blue, from copper deposition in the periphery of the cornea found in Wilson disease. Due to a rare autosomal recessive mutation of the ATO7B gene on chromosome 13 causing abnormal copper transport, reduced biliary copper excretion, and abnormal accumulation of copper in the liver and tissues throughout the body. Patients present with liver disease, renal failure, and neurologic symptoms of tremor, dystonia, and a variety of psychiatric disorders.

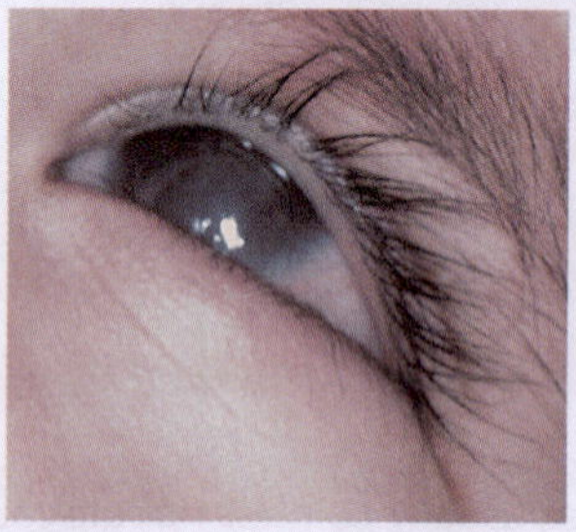

Corneal Scar. A superficial grayish-white opacity in the cornea, secondary to an old injury or to inflammation. Size and shape are variable. Do not confuse with the opaque lens of a cataract, visible on a deeper plane and only through the pupil.

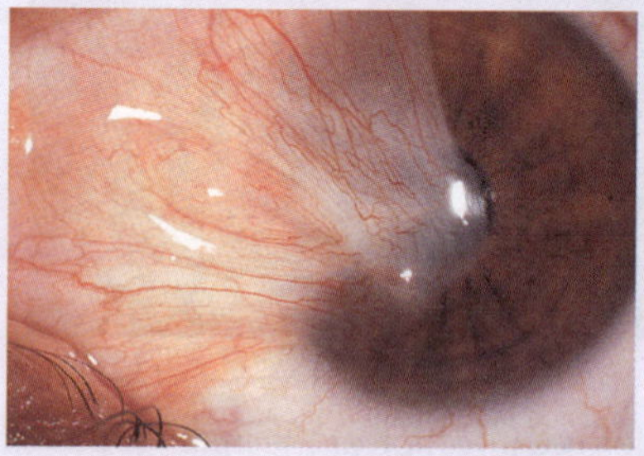

Pterygium. A triangular thickening of the bulbar conjunctiva that grows slowly across the outer surface of the cornea, usually from the nasal side. Reddening and irritation may occur. May interfere with vision as it encroaches on the pupil.

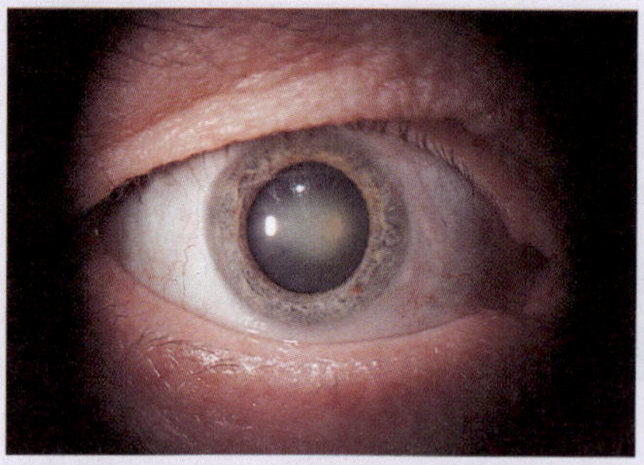

Cataracts. Opacity of the lenses visible through the pupil. Risk factors are older age, smoking, diabetes, corticosteroid use.

Nuclear Cataract. A nuclear cataract looks gray when seen by a flashlight. If the pupil is widely dilated, the gray opacity is surrounded by a black rim.

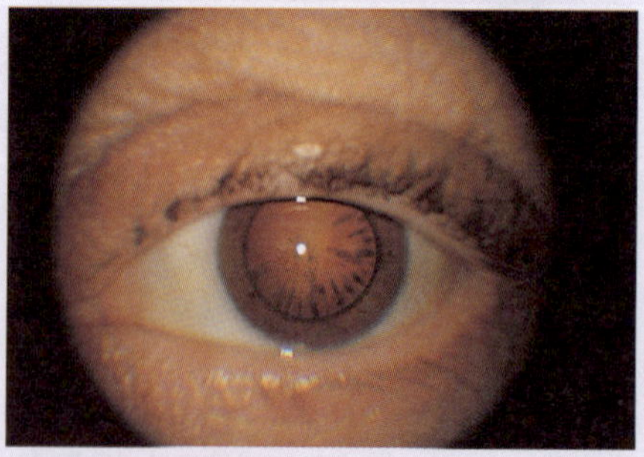

Peripheral Cataract. Produces spoke-like shadows that point—gray against black, as seen with a flashlight, or black against red with an ophthalmoscope. A dilated pupil, as shown here, facilitates this observation.

TABLE 20-6. Pupillary Abnormalities

Unequal Pupils (Anisocoria)—Anisocoria represents a defect in the constriction or dilatation of one pupil. Constriction to light and near effort is mediated by parasympathetic pathways, and pupillary dilatation by sympathetic pathways. The light reaction in bright and dim light identifies the abnormal pupil. When anisocoria is greater in bright light than in dim light, the larger pupil cannot constrict properly. Causes include blunt trauma to the eye, open-angle glaucoma, and impaired parasympathetic innervation to the iris, as in tonic pupil and oculomotor nerve (CN III) paralysis. When anisocoria is greater in dim light, the smaller pupil cannot dilate properly, as in Horner syndrome, caused by an interruption of the sympathetic innervation. Assessing the near reaction is also important in determining the cause. See also Table 13-15, Pupils in Comatose Patients.

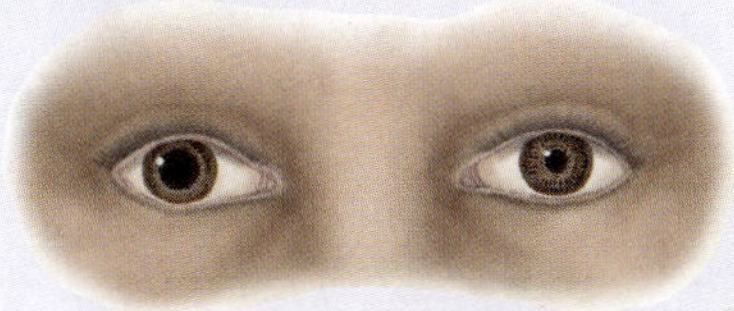

Tonic Pupil *(Adie Pupil)*. Pupil is large (dilated), regular, and usually unilateral. Reaction to light is severely reduced and slowed, or even absent. Constriction during the near vision is present, although very slow (tonic). These changes reflect parasympathetic denervation. Slow accommodation causes blurred vision.

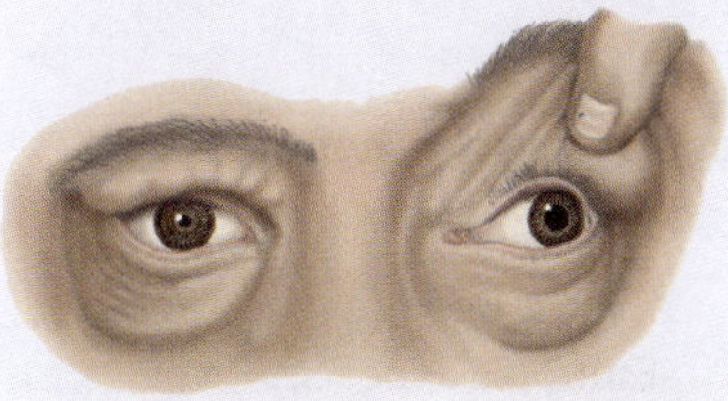

Oculomotor Nerve (CN III) Paralysis. The pupil is large and fixed to light and near effort. Ptosis of the upper eyelid (due to impaired CN III innervation of the levator palpebrae muscle) and lateral deviation of the eye downward and outward are almost always present.

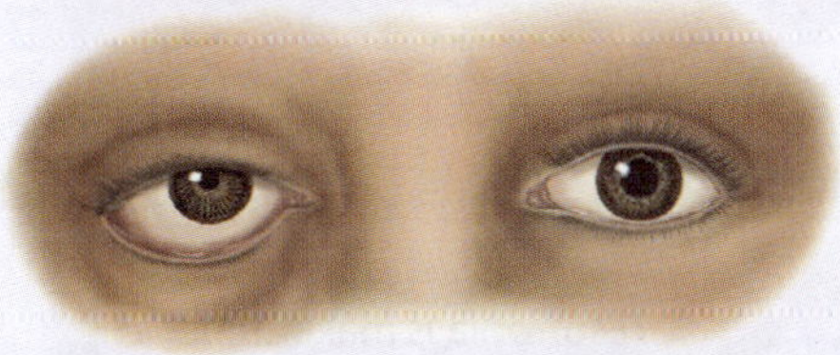

Horner Syndrome. The affected pupil is small, unilateral, reacts briskly to light and near effort, but dilates slowly, especially in dim light. Anisocoria is >1 mm, with ipsilateral ptosis of the eyelid and often loss of sweating on the forehead. These findings reflect the classic triad of Horner syndrome—miosis, ptosis and anhydrosis, due to a lesion in the sympathetic pathways anywhere from the hypothalamus through the brachial plexus and cervical ganglia into the sympathetic fibers of the eye. Causes include ipsilateral brainstem lesions, neck and chest tumors affecting the ipsilateral sympathetic ganglia, orbital trauma, or migraines. In congenital Horner syndrome, the involved iris is lighter in color than its fellow (heterochromia).

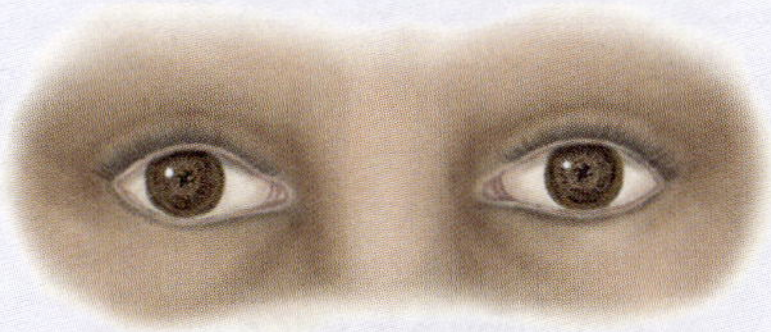

Small, Irregular Pupils (Argyll Robertson Pupils). The pupils are small, irregular and usually bilateral. They constrict with near vision and dilate with far vision (a normal near reaction) but do not react to light, seen in neurosyphilis and rarely in diabetes.

Equal Pupils and One Blind Eye. Unilateral blindness does not cause anisocoria as long as the sympathetic and parasympathetic innervation to both irises is normal. A light directed into the seeing eye produces a direct reaction in that eye and a consensual reaction in the blind eye. A light directed into the blind eye, however, causes no response in either eye.

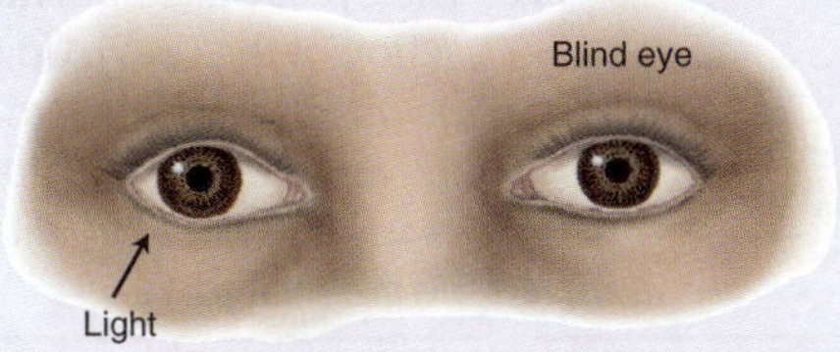

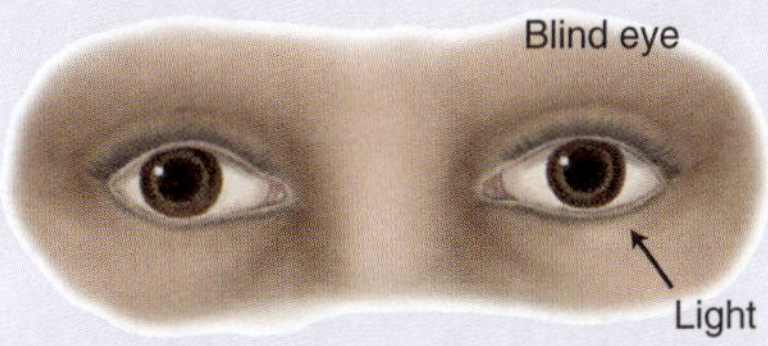

TABLE 20-7. Dysconjugate Gaze

There are a number of abnormal patterns of gaze related to developmental disorders and cranial nerve abnormalities.

Developmental Disorders

Developmental dysconjugate gaze is caused by an imbalance in ocular muscle tone. This imbalance has many causes, may be hereditary, and usually appears in early childhood. These gaze deviations are classified according to direction:

Esotropia

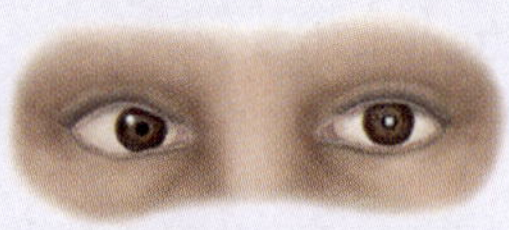

Exotropia

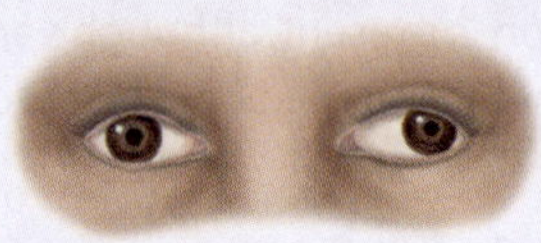

Cover–Uncover Test

A cover–uncover test may be helpful. Here is what you would see in the right monocular esotropia illustrated above.

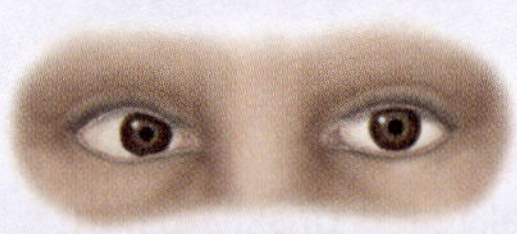

Corneal reflections are asymmetric.

COVER

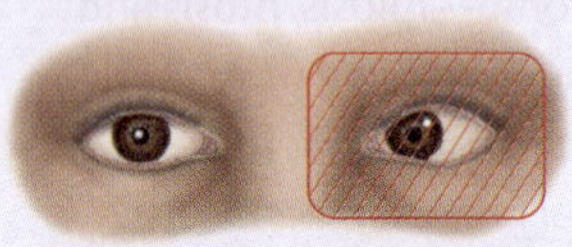

The right eye moves outward to fix on the light. (The left eye is not seen but moves inward to the same degree.)

UNCOVER

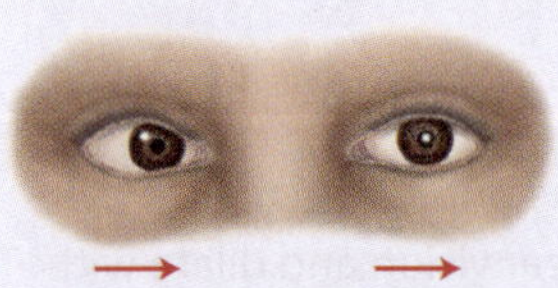

The left eye moves outward to fix on the light. The right eye deviates inward again.

Disorders of Cranial Nerves

New onset of dysconjugate gaze in adults usually results from cranial nerve injuries, lesions, or abnormalities from causes such as trauma, multiple sclerosis, syphilis, and others.

A Left Cranial Nerve VI Paralysis

LOOKING TO THE RIGHT

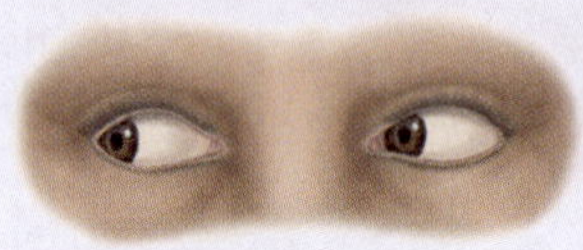

Eyes are conjugate.

LOOKING STRAIGHT AHEAD

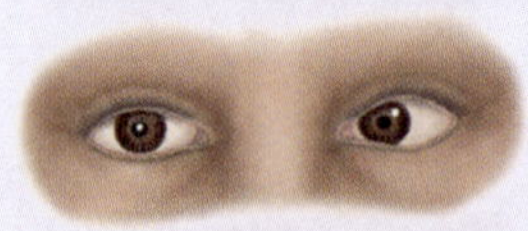

Esotropia appears.

LOOKING TO THE RIGHT

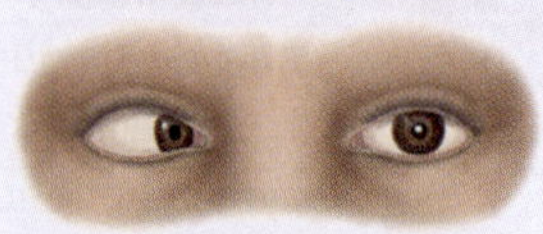

Esotropia is maximum.

A Left Cranial Nerve IV Paralysis

LOOKING DOWN AND TO THE RIGHT

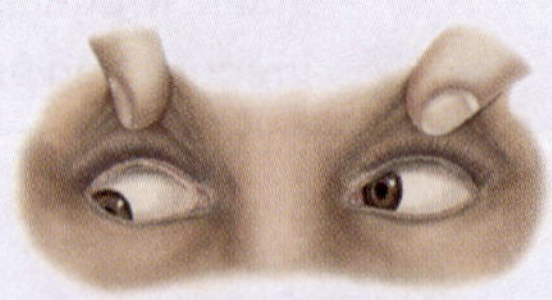

The left eye cannot look down when turned inward. Deviation is maximum in this direction.

A Left Cranial Nerve III Paralysis

LOOKING STRAIGHT AHEAD

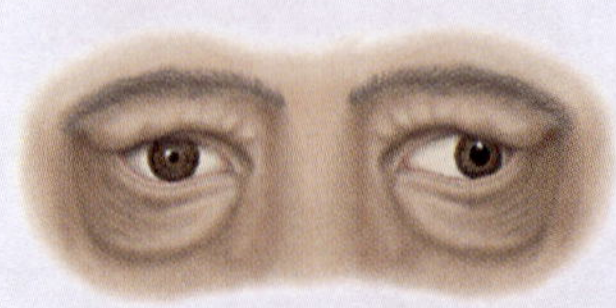

The eye is pulled outward by action of the CN VI. Upward, downward, and inward movements are impaired or lost. Ptosis and pupillary dilation may be associated.

TABLE 20-8. Normal Variations of the Optic Disc

Physiologic Cupping

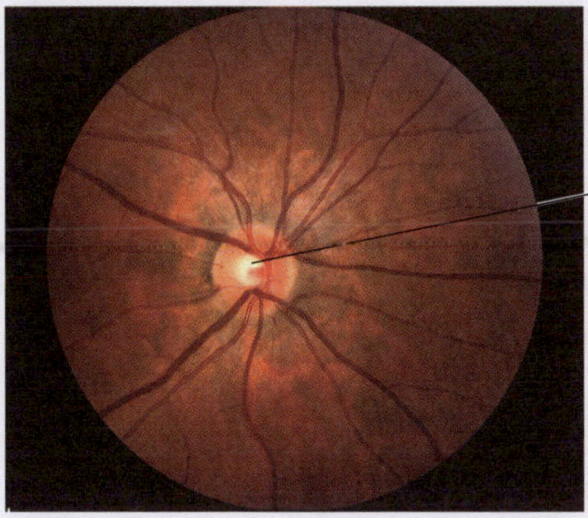

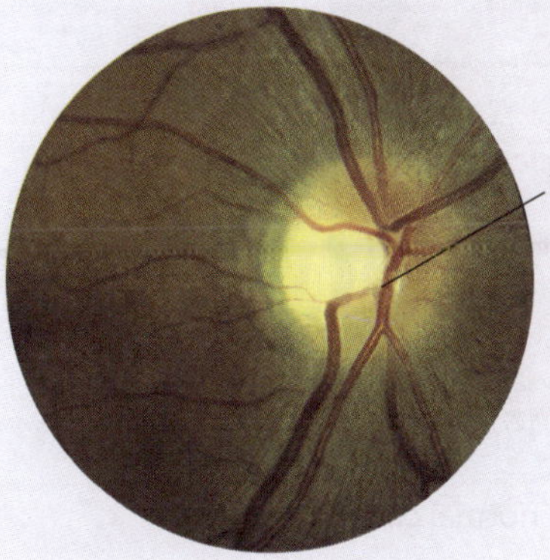

The physiologic cup is a small whitish depression in the optic disc, the entry point for the retinal vessels. Although sometimes absent, the cup is usually visible either centrally or toward the temporal side of the disc. Grayish spots are often seen at its base.

Medullated Nerve Fibers

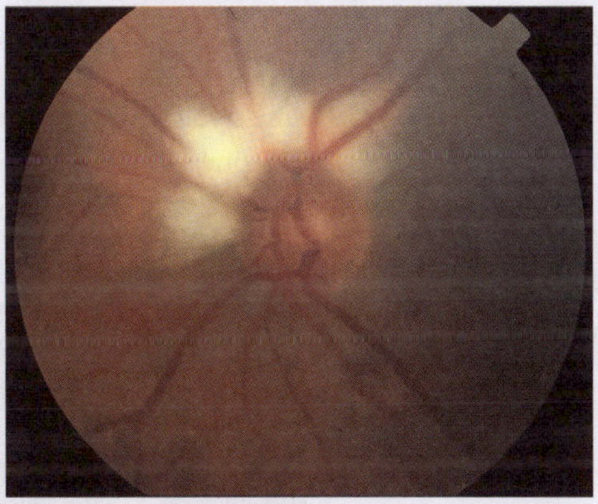

Medullated or myelinated nerve fibers are a much less common but dramatic finding. Appearing as irregular white patches with feathered margins, they obscure the disc edge and retinal vessels. They have no pathologic significance.

TABLE 20-9. Abnormalities of the Optic Disc

Normal

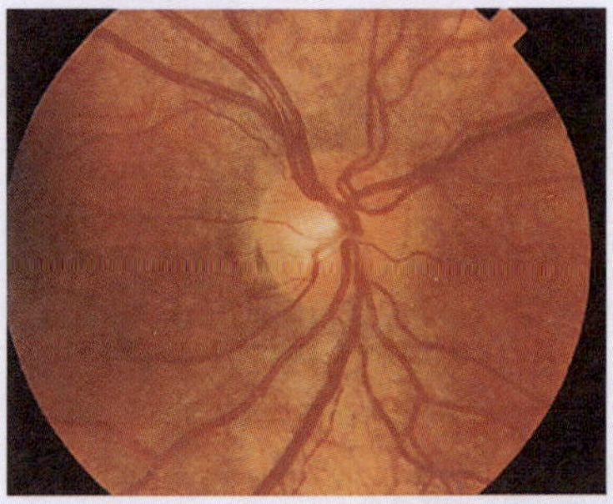

Process

Tiny disc vessels give normal color to the disc.

Appearance

Color yellowish orange to creamy pink

Disc vessels tiny

Disc margins sharp (except perhaps nasally) The physiologic cup is located centrally or somewhat temporally. It may be conspicuous or absent. Its diameter from side to side is usually less than half that of the disc.

Papilledema

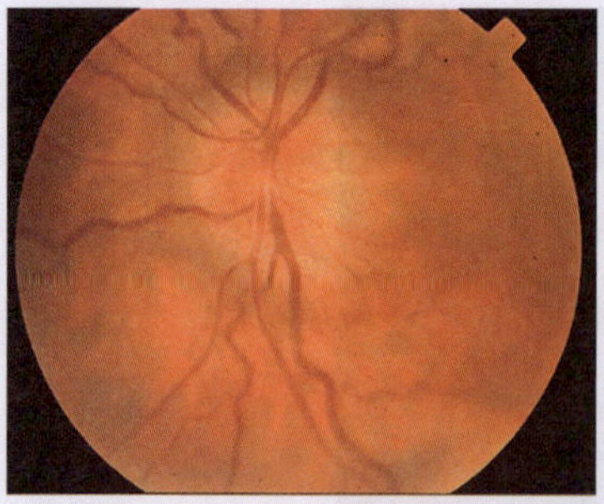

Process

Elevated intracranial pressure causes intra-axonal edema along the optic nerve, leading to engorgement and swelling of the optic disc.

Appearance

Color pink, hyperemic

Often with loss of venous pulsations

Disc vessels more visible, more numerous, curve over the borders of the disc

Disc swollen with margins blurred

The physiologic cup is not visible

Seen in intracranial mass, lesion, or hemorrhage, meningitis

Glaucomatous Cupping

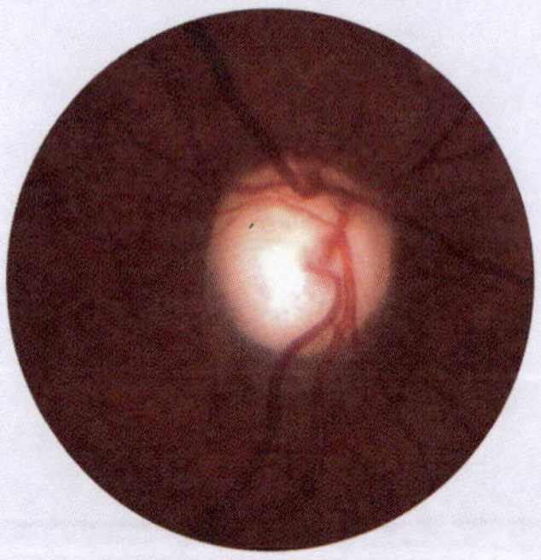

Process

Increased intraocular pressure within the eye leads to increased cupping (backward depression of the disc) and atrophy. The base of the enlarged cup is pale.

Appearance

Death of optic nerve fibers leads to loss of the tiny disc vessels.

Optic Atrophy

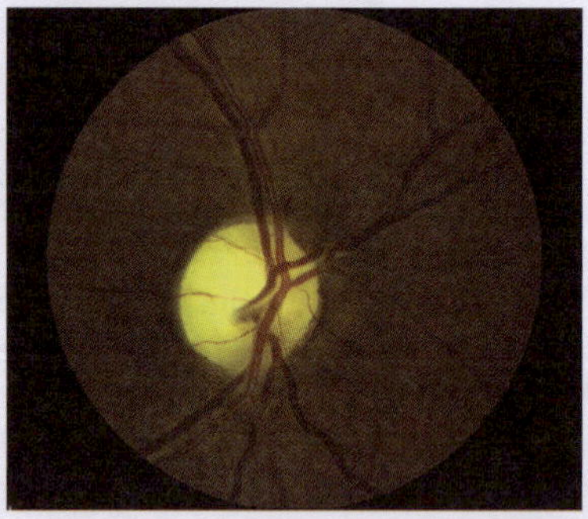

Process

The physiologic cup is enlarged, occupying more than half of the disc's diameter, at times extending to the edge of the disc. Retinal vessels sink in and under the cup, and may be displaced nasally.

Appearance

Color white

Tiny disc vessels absent

Seen in optic neuritis, multiple sclerosis, temporal arteritis

Sources of photos for *Normal*—Tasman W, Jaeger E, eds. *The Wills Eye Hospital Atlas of Clinical Ophthalmology.* 2nd ed. Lippincott Williams & Wilkins; 2001; *Papilledema, Glaucomatous Cupping, Optic Atrophy*—Courtesy of Kenn Freedman, MD.

TABLE 20-10. Retinal Arteries and Arteriovenous Crossings: Normal and Hypertensive

Normal Retinal Artery and Arteriovenous (AV) Crossing

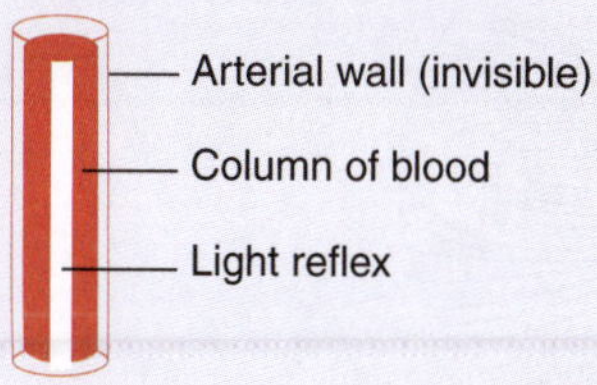

The normal arterial wall is transparent; usually only the column of blood is visible. The normal light reflex is narrow—about one-fourth the diameter of the blood column. Because the arterial wall is transparent, a vein crossing beneath the artery appears right up to the column of blood on either side.

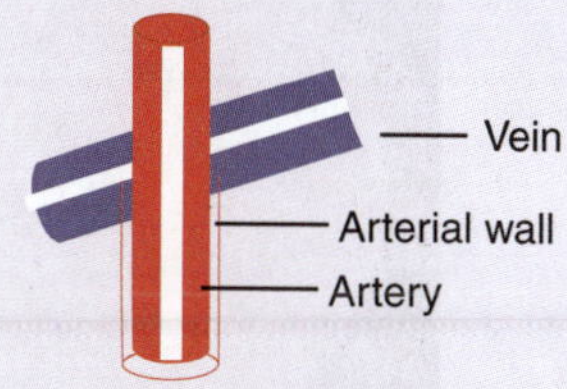

Retinal Arteries in Hypertension

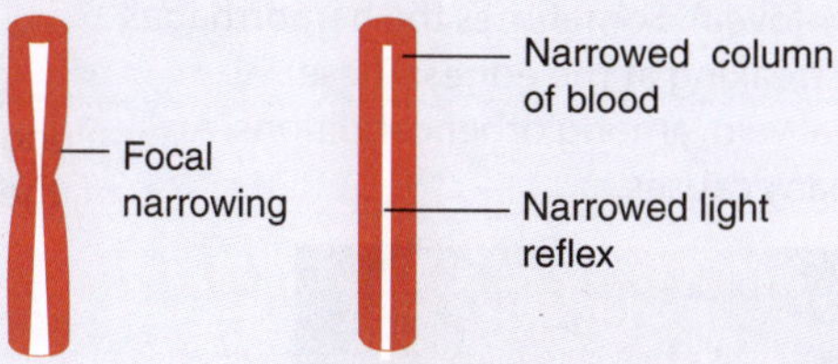

In hypertension, increased pressure damages the vascular endothelium, leading to deposition of plasma macromolecules and thickening of the arterial wall, causing focal or generalized narrowing of the lumen and the light reflex.

Copper Wiring

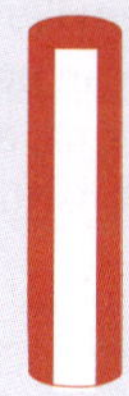

Sometimes the arteries, especially those close to the disc, become full and somewhat tortuous and develop an increased light reflex with a bright coppery luster, called copper wiring.

Silver Wiring

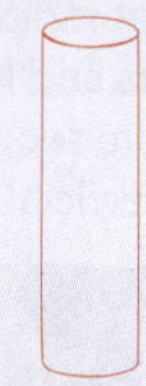

Occasionally the wall of a narrowed artery becomes opaque so there is no visible blood, called silver wiring.

AV Crossing

When the arterial walls lose their transparency, changes appear in the arteriovenous crossings. Decreased transparency of the retina probably also contributes to the first two changes shown below.

Concealment or AV Nicking. The vein appears to stop abruptly on either side of the artery.

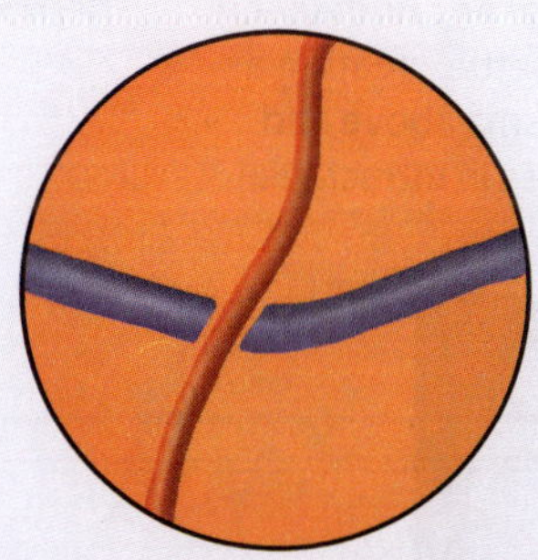

TABLE 20-11. Red Spots and Streaks in the Fundi

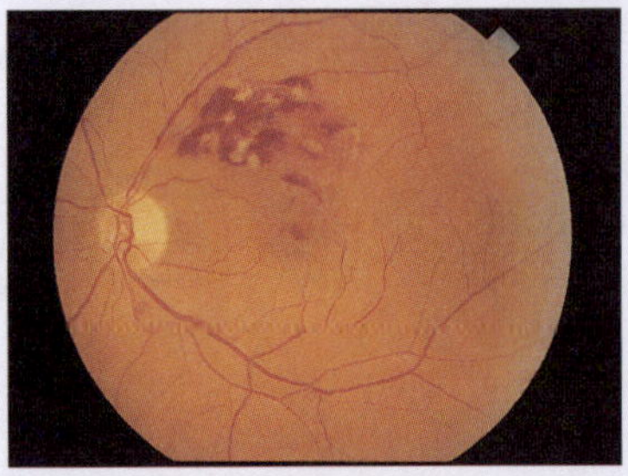

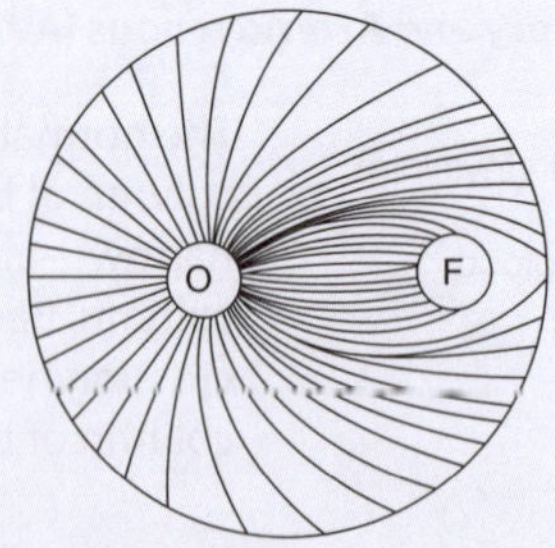

Superficial Retinal Hemorrhages. Small, linear, flame-shaped, red streaks in the fundi, shaped by the superficial bundles of nerve fibers that radiate from the optic disc in the pattern illustrated (O = optic disc; F = fovea). Sometimes the hemorrhages occur in clusters and look like a larger hemorrhage but can be identified by the linear streaking at the edges. These hemorrhages are seen in severe hypertension, papilledema, and occlusion of the retinal vein, among other conditions. An occasional superficial hemorrhage has a white center consisting of fibrin, which has many causes.

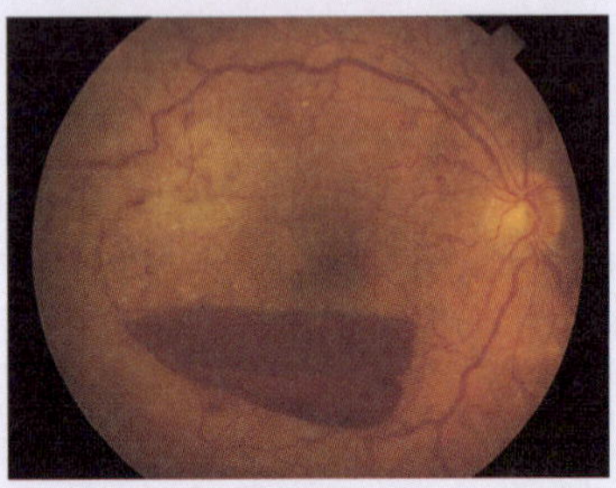

Preretinal Hemorrhage. Develops when blood escapes into the potential space between the retina and vitreous. This hemorrhage is typically larger than retinal hemorrhages. Because it is anterior to the retina, it obscures any underlying retinal vessels. In an erect patient, red cells settle, creating a horizontal line of demarcation between plasma above and cells below. Causes include a sudden increase in intracranial pressure.

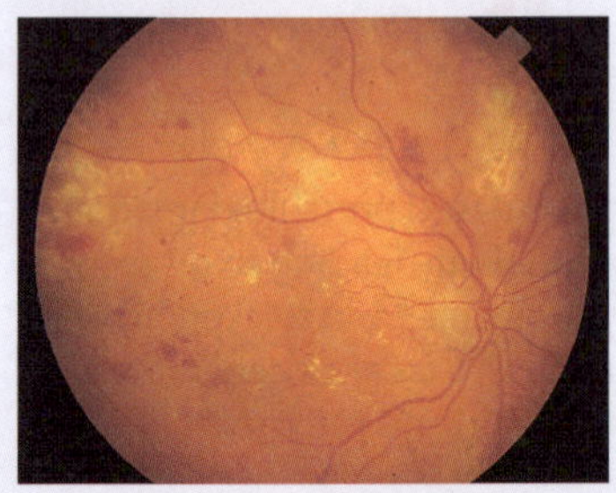

Deep Retinal Hemorrhages. Small, rounded, slightly irregular red spots that are sometimes called dot or blot hemorrhages. They occur in a deeper layer of the retina than flame-shaped hemorrhages. Diabetes is a common cause.

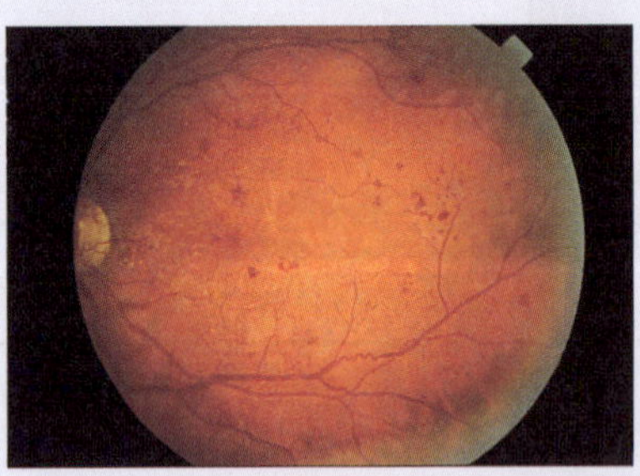

Microaneurysms. Tiny, round, red spots commonly seen in and around the macular area. They are minute dilatations of very small retinal vessels; the vascular connections are too small to be seen with an ophthalmoscope. A hallmark of diabetic retinopathy.

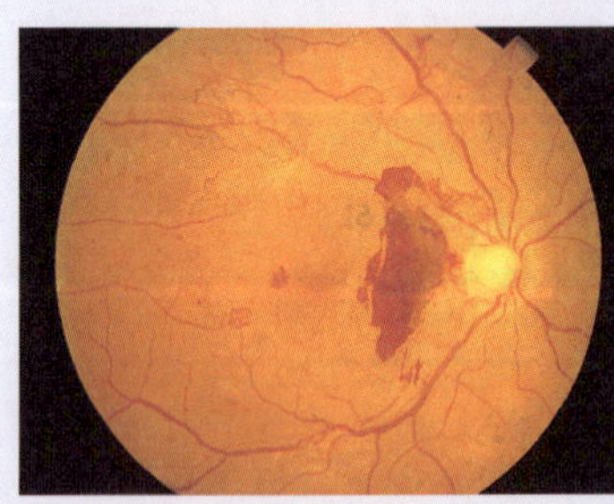

Neovascularization. Refers to the formation of new blood vessels. They are more numerous, more tortuous, and narrower than neighboring blood vessels in the area and form disorderly looking red arcades. A common feature of the proliferative stage of diabetic retinopathy. The vessels may grow into the vitreous, where retinal detachment or hemorrhage may cause loss of vision.

Source of photos: Tasman W, Jaeger E, eds. *The Wills Eye Hospital Atlas of Clinical Ophthalmology.* 2nd ed. Lippincott Williams & Wilkins; 2001.

TABLE 20-12. Light-Colored Spots in the Fundi

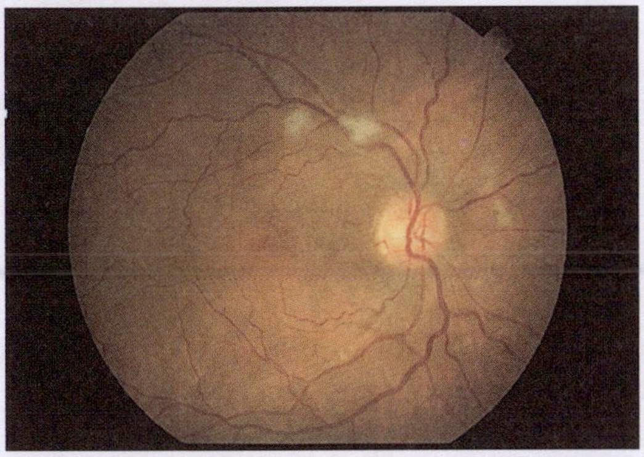

Soft Exudates: Cotton-Wool Spots

Cotton-wool spots are white or grayish, ovoid lesions with irregular "soft" borders. They are moderate in size but usually smaller than the disc. They result from extruded axoplasm from retinal ganglion cells caused by microinfarcts of the retinal nerve fiber layer. Seen in hypertension, diabetes, HIV and other viruses, and numerous other conditions.

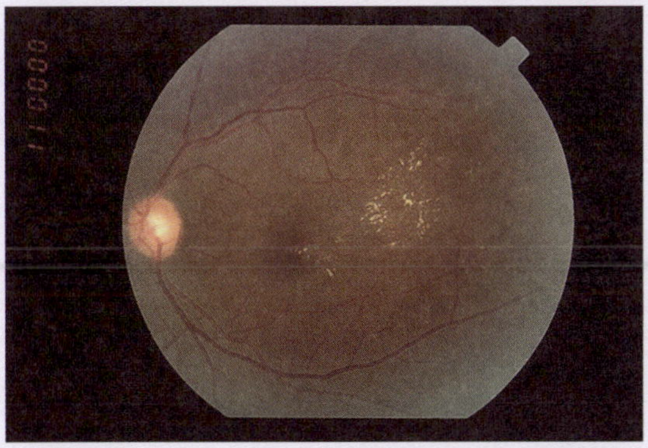

Hard Exudates

Hard exudates are creamy or yellowish, often bright, lesions with well-defined "hard" borders. They are small and round but may coalesce into larger irregular spots. They often occur in clusters or in circular, linear, or star-shaped patterns. They are lipid residues of serous leakage from damaged capillaries. Causes include diabetes and vascular dysplasias.

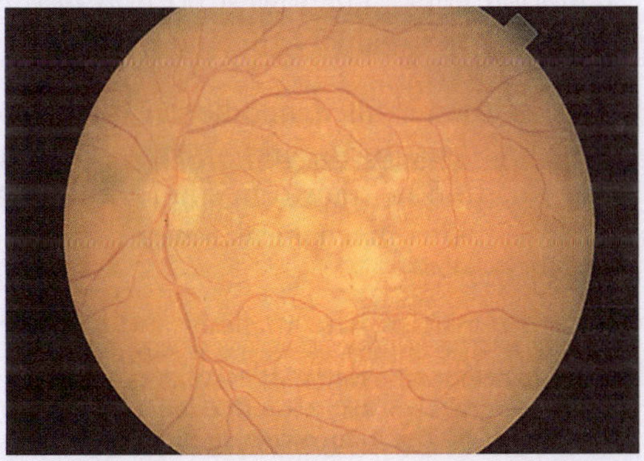

Drusen

Drusen are yellowish round spots that vary from tiny to small. The edges may be soft, as here, or hard. They are haphazardly distributed but may concentrate at the posterior pole between the optic disc and the macula. Drusen consist of dead retinal pigment epithelial cells. Seen in normal aging and age-related macular degeneration.

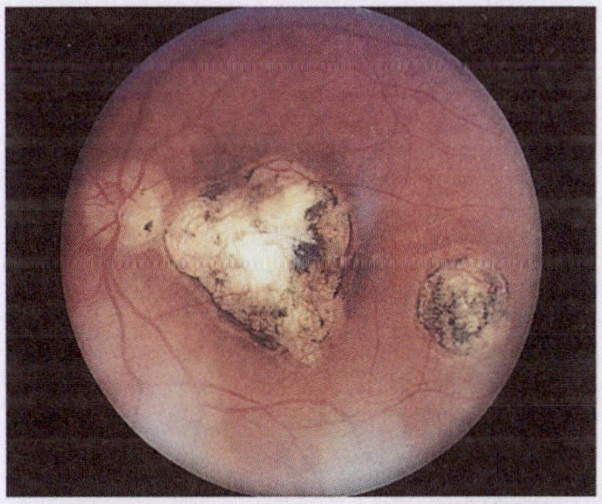

Healed Chorioretinitis

Here inflammation has destroyed the superficial tissues to reveal a well-defined, irregular patch of white sclera marked with dark pigment. Size varies from small to very large. Toxoplasmosis is illustrated. Multiple, small, somewhat similar-looking areas may be due to laser treatments. Here there is also a temporal scar near the macula.

Source of photos: *Cotton-Wool Patches, Drusen, Healed Chorioretinitis*—Tasman W, Jaeger E, eds. *The Wills Eye Hospital Atlas of Clinical Ophthalmology.* 2nd ed. Lippincott Williams & Wilkins; 2001; *Hard Exudates*—Courtesy of Kenn Freedman, MD. American Academy of Ophthalmology. Optic fundus signs. At http://www.aao.org/theeyeshaveit/optic-fundus/index.cfm. Accessed March 23, 2015.

CHAPTER 21

Ears and Nose

ANATOMY AND PHYSIOLOGY

Ear

The ear has three compartments: the external ear, the middle ear, and the inner ear.

External Ear. The *external ear* comprises the auricle and ear canal. The *auricle* consists chiefly of cartilage covered by skin and has a firm elastic consistency. Its prominent curved outer ridge is the *helix*. Parallel and anterior to the helix is another curved prominence, the *antihelix*. Inferiorly is the fleshy projection of the earlobe, or *lobule*. The ear canal opens behind the *tragus*, a nodular protrusion that points backward over the entrance to the canal (Fig. 21-1).

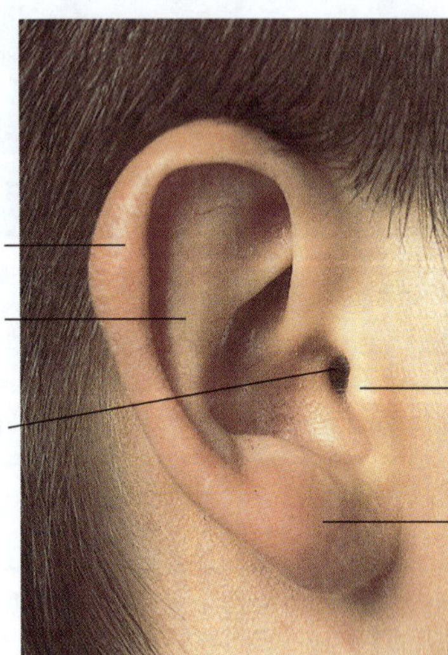

FIGURE 21-1. Anatomy of the external ear.

The ear canal is approximately 24 mm long, starting laterally at the external auditory meatus and traveling inward to end at the eardrum. It has an S shape and travels anteriorly and inferiorly as it moves medially toward the eardrum. Cartilage encases its outer one-third. This segment is covered by hair-bearing skin and contains glands that produce *cerumen* (wax). The inner two-thirds of the canal are surrounded by bone and lined by thin, hairless skin. Pressure on this inner two-thirds of the canal area causes pain—a point to remember during your examination. At the end of the ear canal lies the lateral *tympanic membrane*, or eardrum, marking the medial limit of the external ear. The external ear captures sound waves for transmission into the middle and inner ear (Fig. 21-2).

Behind and below the ear canal is the mastoid portion of the temporal bone. The lowest portion of this bone, the *mastoid process*, is palpable behind the lobule.

Middle Ear. In the air-filled middle ear, there are three *ossicles*—the *malleus, incus,* and *stapes*—which are tiny bones that function to transform sound vibrations from the external ear into mechanical waves that then travel through the inner ear.

Two of the ossicles, the malleus and the incus, are visible through the tympanic membrane and are angled obliquely. The ossicles are attached to the center of the tympanic membrane by the *malleus* (Fig. 21-3). Find the *handle* and the *short process* of the malleus, the two chief landmarks. From the *umbo*, where the eardrum meets the tip of the malleus, a light reflection called the *cone of light* fans downward and anteriorly. Above the short process lies a small portion of the eardrum called the *pars flaccida*. The remainder of the drum is the *pars tensa*. Anterior and posterior malleolar folds, which extend obliquely upward from the short process of the malleus, separate the pars flaccida from the pars tensa, but are usually invisible unless the eardrum is retracted. A second ossicle, the *incus*, can sometimes be seen through the drum in the area posterior and superior to the umbo.

The middle ear connects to the nasopharynx via the proximal end of the eustachian tube. The *eustachian tube* acts to ventilate the middle ear space and allows for pressure regulation between the middle ear and surrounding environment. It also functions to drain mucus from the middle ear into the nasopharynx.

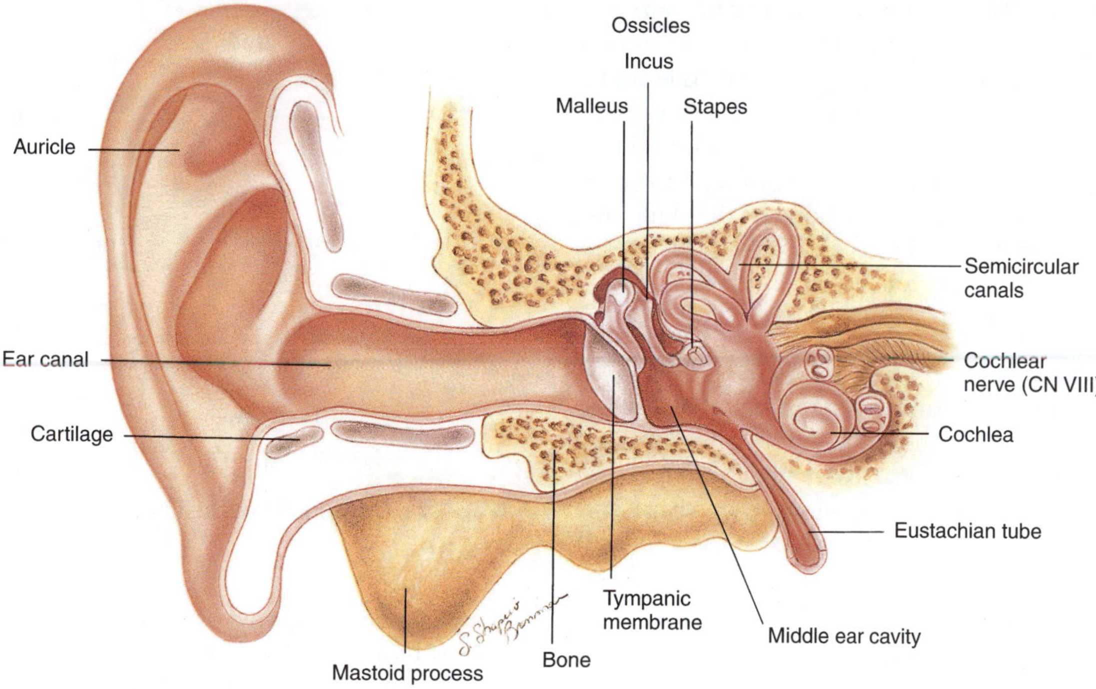

FIGURE 21-2. Anatomy of the external, middle, and inner ear.

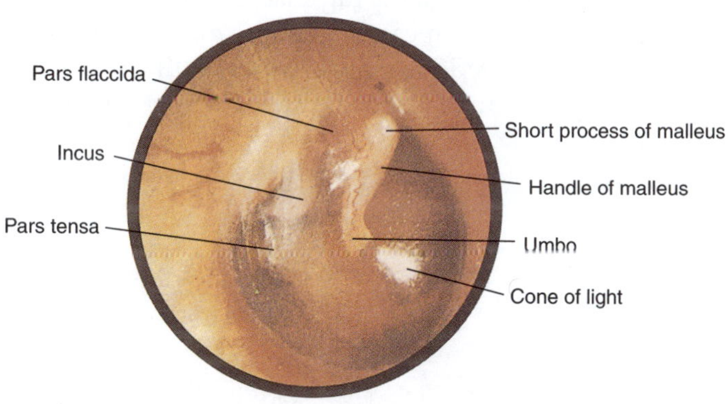

FIGURE 21-3. Right tympanic membrane.

Inner Ear. The inner ear includes the cochlea; the semicircular canals; the otolith organs housed in the *vestibule*; and the distal end of the auditory nerve, also known as the *vestibulocochlear nerve*, or *CN VIII*. The *cochlea* is dedicated to hearing, whereas the *semicircular canals* and *otolith organs* are dedicated to balance. Together these three structures form the *labyrinth*. The stapes bone in the middle ear connects to the inner ear through the oval window. Movements of the stapes vibrate the *perilymph* (liquid of the inner ear) in the labyrinth, which then causes movement of the *hair cells* and *endolymph* in the ducts of the cochlea. These vibrations are converted in the hair cells of the cochlea into electrical nerve impulses transmitted by the auditory nerve to the brain to be interpreted.

Much of the middle ear and all of the inner ear are inaccessible to direct examination. Assess their condition by testing auditory function.

Hearing Pathways. The first part of the hearing pathway, from the external ear through the middle ear, is known as the *conductive phase*. The second part of the pathway, involving the cochlea and the cochlear branch of CN VIII, is the *sensorineural phase* (Fig. 21-4).

Hearing disorders of the external and middle ear cause *conductive hearing loss*. External ear causes include cerumen impaction, infection (**otitis externa**), trauma, squamous cell carcinoma, and benign bony growths such as **exostosis** or *osteoma*. Middle ear disorders include **otitis media**, congenital conditions, cholesteatomas, otosclerosis, **tympanosclerosis**, tumors, and perforations of the tympanic membrane.

Disorders of the inner ear cause *sensorineural hearing loss* from congenital and hereditary conditions, presbycusis, viral infections such as rubella or cytomegalovirus, Ménière disease, noise exposure, ototoxic drug exposure, and acoustic neuromas.

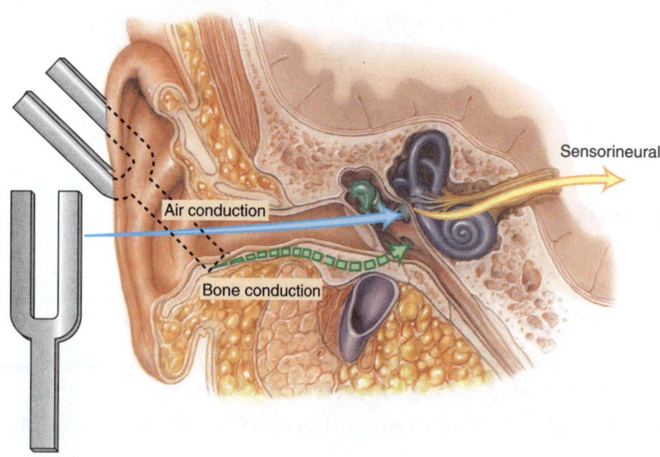

FIGURE 21-4. Hearing pathways.

Air conduction (AC) describes the normal first phase in the hearing pathway, where sound waves travel through the air and are transmitted from the external and middle ear to the cochlea. An alternative pathway, known as *bone conduction* (BC), bypasses the external and middle ear and is used for testing purposes. A vibrating tuning fork, placed on the head, sets the bone of the skull into vibration and stimulates the cochlea directly. In those with normal hearing, air conduction is more sensitive than bone conduction (AC > BC).

Equilibrium. The vestibular system senses the position and movements of the head contributing to our overall sense of balance and motion. The three semicircular canals in the inner ear sense rotational movement, whereas the otolith organs sense linear movement. Our visual and proprioceptive feedback also contribute to our overall sense of balance.

Nose and Paranasal Sinuses

Approximately the upper third of the nose is supported by bone, and the lower two-thirds by cartilage (Fig. 21-5). Air enters the nasal cavity through the *anterior naris* on either side, then passes into the widened area known as the *vestibule* and on through the narrow nasal passage to the *nasopharynx*.

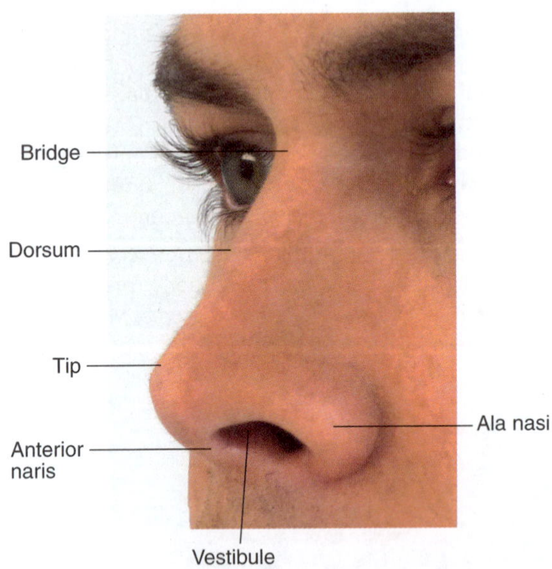

FIGURE 21-5. External anatomy of the nose.

The medial wall of each nasal cavity is formed by the *nasal septum*, which, like the external nose, is supported by both bone and cartilage (Fig. 21-6). It is covered by a highly vascular *mucous membrane*. The vestibule, unlike the rest of the nasal cavity, is lined with hair-bearing skin, not mucosa.

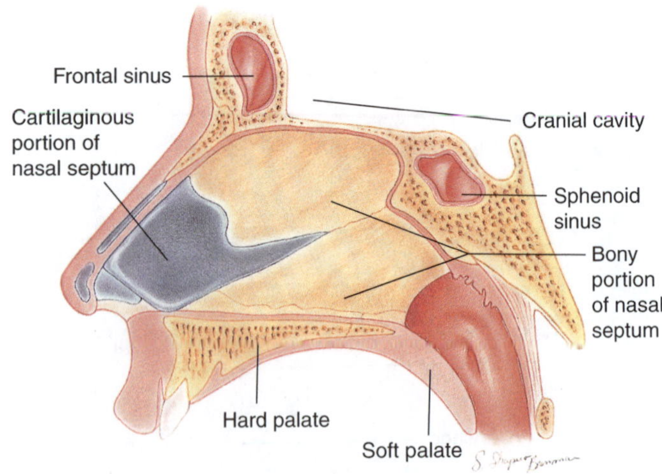

FIGURE 21-6. Medial wall—left nasal cavity (mucosa removed).

Laterally, the anatomy is more complex (Fig. 21-7). Curving bony structures, the *turbinates*, covered by a highly vascular mucous membrane, protrude into the nasal cavity. Below each turbinate is a groove, or *meatus*, each named according to the turbinate above it—*superior*, *middle*, and *inferior* meatuses. The *nasolacrimal duct* drains into the inferior meatus. Most of the paranasal sinuses drain into the middle meatus. Their openings are not usually visible.

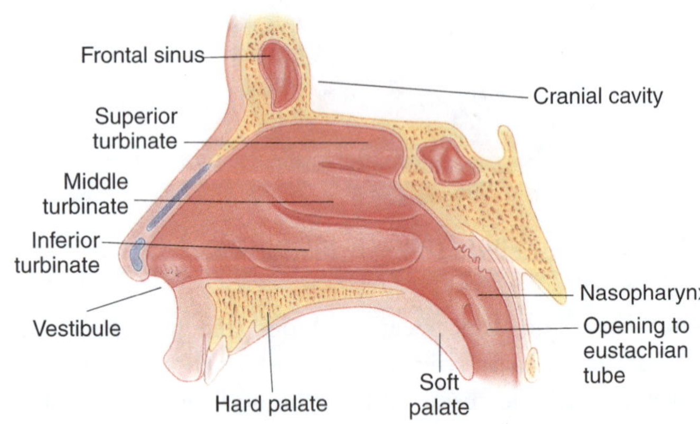

FIGURE 21-7. Lateral wall—right nasal cavity.

The additional surface area provided by the turbinates and their overlying mucosa aids the nasal cavities in their principal functions: *cleansing, humidification, and temperature control of inspired air*.

The *paranasal sinuses* consist of four paired air-filled cavities within the bones of the skull: the *maxillary*, *ethmoid*, *frontal*, and *sphenoid sinuses*. Like the nasal cavities into which they drain, they are lined with a mucous membrane. Their locations are diagrammed in Figure 21-8. Only the frontal and maxillary sinuses are readily accessible on clinical examination (Fig. 21-9).

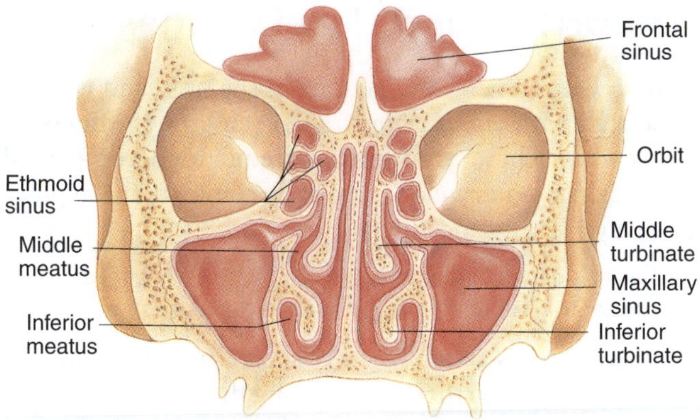

FIGURE 21-8. Cross-section of nasal cavity—anterior view.

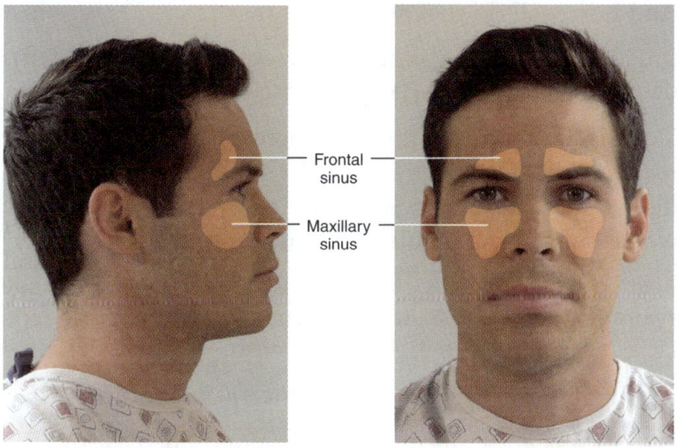

FIGURE 21-9. Frontal and maxillary sinuses.

HEALTH HISTORY: GENERAL APPROACH

Here we will review how to approach the health history interview as it relates to a patient's ears and nose.

When acquiring a patient's ear-related history, potential initial open-ended questions include, "How is your hearing?" and "Have you had any trouble with your ears?" In a comprehensive ear history, you should inquire about hearing loss, ringing in the ears (*tinnitus*), ear drainage (*otorrhea*), ear pain (*otalgia*), and *vertigo*.

For the nose-related history, opening questions include, "Do you have any complaints related to your nose?" Ask questions pertaining to any nosebleed (*epistaxis*), nasal discharge (*rhinorrhea*), nasal obstruction, and postnasal drip.

Common or Concerning Symptoms

- Hearing loss
- Earache and ear discharge
- Ringing in the ears (*tinnitus*)
- Dizziness and vertigo
- Nasal discharge (*rhinorrhea*) and nasal congestion
- Nosebleed (epistaxis)

Hearing Loss

If the patient has noticed hearing loss, does it involve one or both ears? Did it start suddenly or gradually? What are the associated symptoms, if any? It is critical to establish a timeline related to any reported hearing loss. Sudden onset hearing loss, particularly sensorineural hearing loss, without a known cause should be immediately referred to an otolaryngologist. These patients may benefit from urgent medical intervention.

Hearing loss may also be congenital, from single gene mutations.

Distinguish *conductive loss*, which results from problems in the external or middle ear, from *sensorineural loss*, resulting from problems in the inner ear, the cochlear nerve, or its central connections in the brain. People with sensorineural loss have trouble understanding speech, often complaining that others mumble; noisy environments make hearing worse. In conductive loss, noisy environments may help.

Pursue symptoms associated with hearing loss, such as earache or vertigo to help sort out likely causes.

Ask about medications that might affect hearing and about sustained exposure to loud noise.

Medications known to cause permanent hearing loss include aminoglycosides (e.g., gentamicin) and many chemotherapeutic agents (e.g., cisplatin and carboplatin). Temporary damage to hearing may be caused by aspirin, nonsteroidal anti-inflammatory agents (NSAIDs), quinine, and loop diuretics (e.g., furosemide).

Earache and Ear Discharge

Complaints of earache, or pain in the ear, are especially common. Ask about associated fever, sore throat, cough, and concurrent upper respiratory infection; if present, these heighten the likelihood of ear infection.

Pain occurs in the external canal in *otitis externa* (inflammation of the external ear canal) and deeper within the ear in *otitis media* (infection of the middle ear). Pain in the ear may also be referred from other structures in the mouth, throat, or neck.

Ask about discharge from the ear, especially if associated with earache or trauma. Wax or debris in the ear is usually normal.

Acute otitis externa and acute or chronic otitis media with perforation usually present with yellow-green discharge.

Tinnitus

Tinnitus is a perceived sound that has no external stimulus—commonly, a musical ringing or a rushing or roaring noise in one or both ears. Tinnitus may accompany hearing loss and often remains unexplained. Occasionally, popping sounds originate in the temporomandibular joint, or sounds from the vessels in the neck may be audible.

Tinnitus is a common symptom, increasing in frequency with age. When associated with fluctuating hearing loss and vertigo, suspect Ménière disease.

Dizziness and Vertigo

Complaints of *dizziness* and *lightheadedness* are challenging because they are often nonspecific and suggest a diverse set of conditions ranging from vertigo to presyncope, weakness, unsteadiness, and dysequilibrium.

See Table 21-1, Dizziness and Vertigo, for distinguishing symptoms and time course.

Clarify by asking the patient to describe how he or she is feeling without using the word "dizzy." Responses to this question often fall into one of the following categories: a sensation as if the room is spinning or tilting (*vertigo*), the sense that passing out is imminent (*presyncope*), or a sense of unsteadiness as if about to lose balance and fall (*dysequilibrium*). The question, "Do your symptoms get worse when you move your head (positional)?" may also be helpful.

Vertigo is the sensation of true rotational movement of the patient or the surroundings. These sensations point primarily to a problem in the labyrinths of the inner ear, peripheral lesions of CN VIII, or lesions in its central pathways or nuclei in the brain.

If there is true vertigo, distinguish peripheral from central neurologic causes (see Chapter 13, Nervous System, p. 612).

Establish the time course of symptoms, as well as any associated symptoms or triggers (such as loud noises, bright lights, standing from sitting). Check for nausea, vomiting, double vision, and gait disturbance. Review the patient's medications. Proceed with a careful neurologic examination focusing on the presence of **nystagmus** and focal neurologic signs.

Vertigo represents vestibular disease, usually from peripheral causes in the inner ear such as benign positional vertigo, labyrinthitis, vestibular neuritis, and Ménière disease. Ataxia, diplopia, and dysarthria signal central neurologic causes in the cerebellum or brainstem such as cerebral vascular disease or posterior fossa tumor; also consider vestibular migraine. Feeling lightheaded, weak in the legs, or about to faint points to presyncope from arrhythmia, orthostatic hypotension, or vasovagal stimulation.

Rhinorrhea and Nasal Congestion

Rhinorrhea refers to drainage from the nose and is often associated with *nasal congestion*, a sense of stuffiness or obstruction. These symptoms are frequently accompanied by sneezing; watery eyes; throat discomfort; and itching in the eyes, nose, and throat.

Causes include viral infections, allergic rhinitis ("hay fever"), and vasomotor rhinitis. Itching favors an allergic cause.

Do symptoms occur when colds are prevalent and last less than 7 days? Do they occur during the same season each year when pollens are in the air? Are symptoms triggered by specific animal or environmental exposures? Are there indoor environmental triggers such as dust or animals?

Seasonal onset or environmental triggers suggests allergic rhinitis.

What remedies has the patient used? For how long? And how well do they work?

Drug-induced rhinitis occurs with excessive use of topical decongestants or intranasal use of cocaine.

Is nasal or sinus congestion preceded by a viral upper respiratory tract infection (URI)? Is there purulent nasal discharge, loss of smell, tooth pain, facial pain made worse by bending forward, ear pressure, cough, or fever?

Acute bacterial sinusitis (*rhinosinusitis*), is unlikely until viral URI symptoms persist more than 7 days; both purulent drainage and facial pain should be present for diagnosis.

Ask about drugs that may induce nasal stuffiness.

Inquire about all medications or drugs, particularly oral contraceptives, alcohol, and cocaine.

Is the nasal congestion only on one side?

Consider a deviated nasal septum, nasal polyp, foreign body, granulomatous disease, or carcinoma.

Epistaxis

Epistaxis is bleeding from the nasal passages. Bleeding can also originate in the paranasal sinuses or nasopharynx. Note that bleeding from posterior nasal structures may pass into the throat instead of out through the nostrils. Ask the patient to pinpoint the source of the bleeding. Is it from the nose, or has the patient actually coughed up blood (*hemoptysis*) or vomited blood (*hematemesis*)? These conditions have very different causes.

Local causes of epistaxis include trauma (especially nose-picking), inflammation, drying and crusting of the nasal mucosa, tumors, and foreign bodies.

Is epistaxis a recurrent problem? Has there been easy bruising or bleeding elsewhere in the body?

Anticoagulants, NSAIDs, vascular malformations, and coagulopathies can contribute to epistaxis.

PHYSICAL EXAMINATION: GENERAL APPROACH

Both the ears and nose require external and internal examination. The examination for the ear begins externally with the inspection and palpation of the auricle and surrounding tissues. Attention is then directed to the internal structures, including the ear canal and eardrum, using an otoscope. The external nose is first examined in the nasal examination. Subsequently the anterior nasal cavity can also be inspected with an otoscope.

Key Components of the Ear Examination

- Inspect the auricle and surrounding tissue (deformities, lumps, pits, or skin lesions).
- Move the auricle and palpate the auricle, tragus and mastoid (tenderness).
- Examine ear canals and tympanic membranes with an otoscope.
  - Inspect the ear canal (cerumen, discharge, foreign bodies, redness of the skin, or swelling).
  - Inspect the tympanic membrane and malleus (color, contour, perforations, mobility).
- Test auditory acuity or gross hearing with the whispered voice test.
- If hearing loss or difficulty is present, determine sensorineural versus conductive hearing loss with tuning fork tests.
  - Test lateralization if unilateral hearing loss or difficulty (Weber) is present.
  - Compare air conduction versus bone conduction (Rinne).

TECHNIQUES OF EXAMINATION

Auricle

Inspect the auricle and surrounding tissue for deformities, lumps, pits, or skin lesions.

See Table 21-2, Lumps on or Near the Ear.

If ear pain, discharge, or inflammation is present, move the auricle up and down, press the tragus (*tug test*), and press firmly just behind the ear over the mastoid.

Movement of the auricle and tragus is painful in acute otitis externa (inflammation of the ear canal), but *not* in otitis media (inflammation of the middle ear).

Ear Canal and Tympanic Membrane

As shown in Box 21-1, to examine the ear canal and tympanic membrane, use an otoscope with the largest ear speculum that inserts easily into the canal.

Tenderness behind the ear occurs in otitis media and mastoiditis.

Otitis media can occasionally progress to acute mastoiditis, which presents with postauricular swelling, fluctuance, erythema, and significant tenderness. **Bullous myringitis** is also a common sequela presenting with painful hemorrhagic vesicles on the tympanic membrane. Both of these conditions require urgent, often surgical, management by an otolaryngologist.

Inspect the ear canal, noting any discharge, foreign bodies, redness of the skin, or swelling. Cerumen, which varies in color and consistency from yellow and flaky to

Box 21-1. Examining the Ears with the Otoscope

- Position the patient's head so that you can see comfortably through the otoscope.
- Straighten the right ear canal using the fingers of your left hand to grasp the auricle firmly but gently and pull it upward, backward, and slightly away from the head.
- Hold the otoscope handle securely with the right hand between your thumb and fingers, and brace your remaining right fingers against the patient's face. Your right hand and instrument can then follow unexpected movements by the patient.

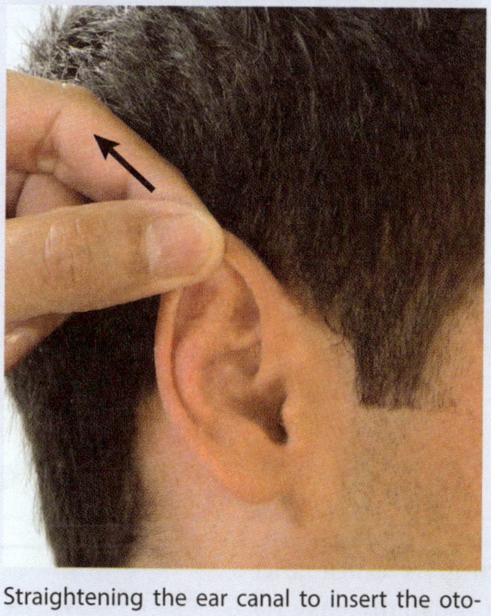

Straightening the ear canal to insert the otoscope speculum.

(continued)

Box 21-1. Examining the Ears with the Otoscope (*continued*)

- Insert the speculum gently into the ear canal, directing it somewhat down and forward and through the hairs, if any.
- Switch hands when examining the left ear by holding the otoscope with your left hand and straightening the ear canal with your right hand.
- If you are uncomfortable switching hands for the left ear, as shown in the figure below, you may reach over that ear to pull it up and back with your left hand and hold the otoscope steady with your right hand as you gently insert the speculum.

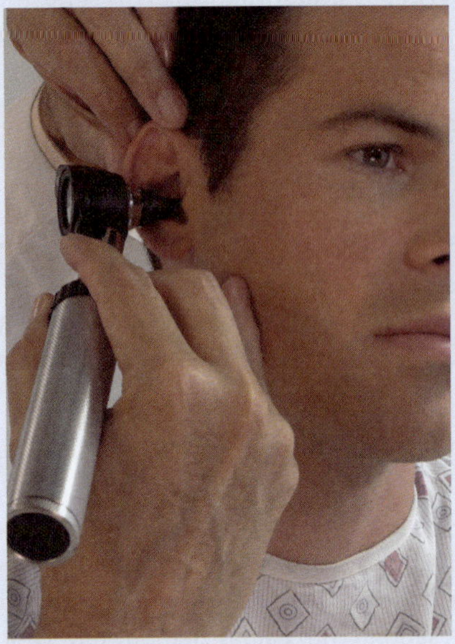

Bracing the otoscope with the right hand against the face and examining the right ear

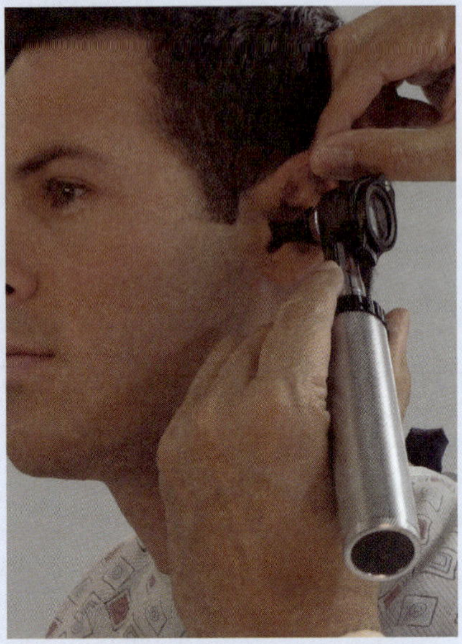

Bracing the otoscope with the left hand against the face and examining the left ear.

Nontender nodular swellings covered by normal skin deep in the ear canals suggest osteomas or exostoses (Fig. 21-10). These are nonmalignant overgrowths, which may obscure the tympanic membrane.

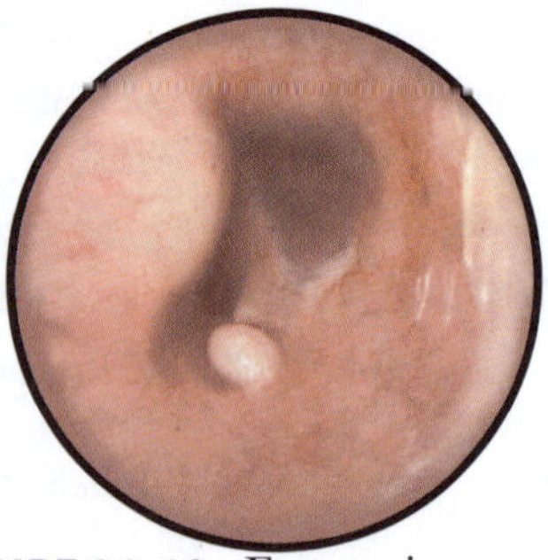

FIGURE 21-10. Exostosis.

brown and sticky or even to dark and hard, may wholly or partly obscure your view.

In acute otitis externa (Fig. 21-11), the canal is often swollen, narrowed, moist, erythematous or pale, and tender.

In chronic otitis externa, the skin of the canal is often thickened, red, and itchy.

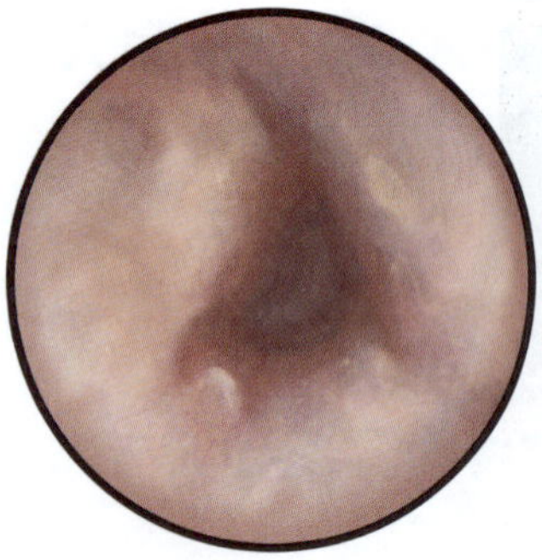

FIGURE 21-11. Acute otitis externa.

Inspect the tympanic membrane, noting its color and contour (Fig. 21-12). The cone of light—usually easy to see—helps to orient you.

Look for the red bulging tympanic membrane of acute purulent otitis media and for the amber color of a **serous effusion**.

See Table 21-3, Abnormalities of the Tympanic Membrane, and Chapter 23, Children: Infancy through Adolescence, Table 23-7, Abnormalities of the Eyes, Ears, and Mouth.

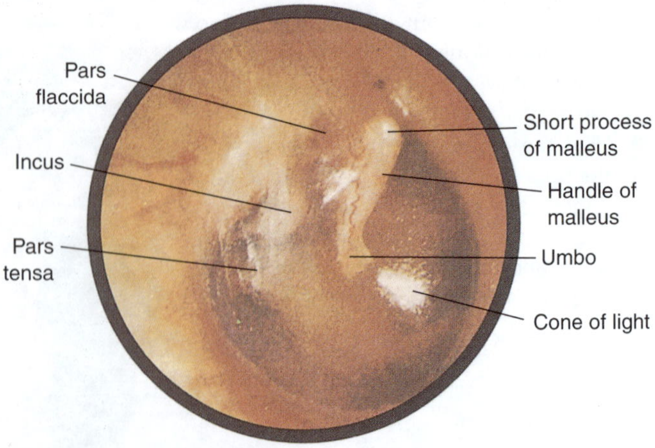

FIGURE 21-12. Anatomy of the right tympanic membrane.

Identify the handle of the malleus, noting its position, and inspect the short process of the malleus.

An unusually prominent short process and a prominent handle that looks more horizontal suggest a retracted tympanic membrane.

Gently move the speculum so that you can see as much of the tympanic membrane as possible, including the pars flaccida superiorly and the margins of the pars tensa. *Look for any perforations*. The anterior and inferior margins of the drum may be obscured by the curving wall of the ear canal. Mobility of the eardrum can be evaluated with a pneumatic otoscope (see Chapter 13, Assessing the Comatose Patient, p. 335).

A serous effusion, a thickened tympanic membrane, or purulent otitis media may decrease mobility. If there is a perforation, there will be no mobility.

Testing Auditory Acuity or Gross Hearing

To begin screening, ask the patient "Do you feel you have hearing loss or difficulty hearing?" Ask if the hearing loss or difficulty is more pronounced in one ear compared to the other.

Patients who answer "yes" are twice as likely to have a hearing deficit; for patients who report normal hearing, the likelihood of moderate to severe hearing impairment is only 0.13.

If the patient reports hearing loss, proceed to the whispered voice test (Box 21-2). The whispered voice test is a reliable screening test for hearing loss if the examiner uses a standardized and consistent method of testing. Positive likelihood ratio (LR) is 2.3 and negative LR is 0.73. This test detects significant hearing loss of greater than 30 dB. A formal hearing test is still the reference standard.

Testing for Conductive Versus Sensorineural Hearing Loss: Tuning Fork Tests

For patients failing the whispered voice test, the Weber and Rinne fork tests may help determine if the hearing loss is conductive or sensorineural in origin. However, their precision, or test–retest reproducibility, and their accuracy compared to air–bone gap reference standards have been questioned.

Note also that tuning fork tests do not distinguish normal hearing from bilateral sensorineural loss or from mixed conductive–sensorineural loss. Sensitivity of the Weber test is about 55%; specificity for sensorineural loss is about 79%, and for conductive loss, 92%. Sensitivity and specificity of the Rinne test are 60% to 90% and 95% to 98%.

To conduct these tests, make sure the room is quiet, and use a tuning fork of 512 Hz. These frequencies fall within the range of conversational speech, namely 500 to 3,000 Hz and between 45 and 60 dB.

- *Test for lateralization* **(Weber test)**. Set the fork into light vibration by briskly stroking the prongs (the "U") between the thumb and index finger or by tapping the prongs on your forearm just in front of your elbow. Place the base of the lightly vibrating tuning fork firmly on top of the patient's head or on the midforehead

Box 21-2. Whispered Voice Test for Auditory Acuity

- Inform the patient that you will be whispering a combination of numbers and letters and then asking him or her to repeat the sequence.
- Then stand at arm's length (2 ft) behind the seated patient so that the patient cannot read your lips.
- Each ear is tested individually. Occlude the non-test ear with a finger and gently rub the tragus in a circular motion to prevent transfer of sound to the non-test ear.
- Exhale a full breath before whispering to ensure a quiet voice.
- Whisper a combination of three words of numbers and letters, such as 4-K-2 or 5-B-6.
  - If the patient responds correctly, hearing is considered normal for that ear.
  - If the patient responds incorrectly or not at all, the test is repeated once more using a different three-numeral/letter combination. It is important to use a different combination each time to exclude the effect of learning.
  - If the patient repeats at least three out of a possible total of six letters or numerals correctly, he or she has passed the screening test.
  - If the patient repeats less than three words correctly, conduct further testing by audiometry.
- Using a different number/letter combination, the other ear is then tested in a similar manner.

Physiology OSCE Video: **Tests for Hearing**

Note that older adults with *presbycusis* (sensorineural hearing loss related to age-appropriate changes in the auditory system) have higher frequency hearing loss, making them more likely to miss *sibilant* consonants (producing the sound of or a sound resembling that of the *s* or the *sh*), which have higher frequency sounds than vowels. The hearing loss is typically gradual, progressive, and bilateral.

(Fig. 21-13). Ask where the patient hears the sound best: "On one side or both sides?" Normally, the vibration is heard in the midline or equally in both ears. If nothing is heard, try again, pressing the fork more firmly on the head. Restrict this test to patients with unilateral hearing loss because patients with normal hearing may lateralize, and patients with bilateral conductive or sensorineural deficits will not lateralize.

In unilateral conductive hearing loss, sound is heard in (lateralized to) the impaired ear. Explanations include otosclerosis, otitis media, perforation of the eardrum, and cerumen. See Table 21-4, Patterns of Hearing Loss.

In unilateral sensorineural hearing loss, sound is heard in the good ear.

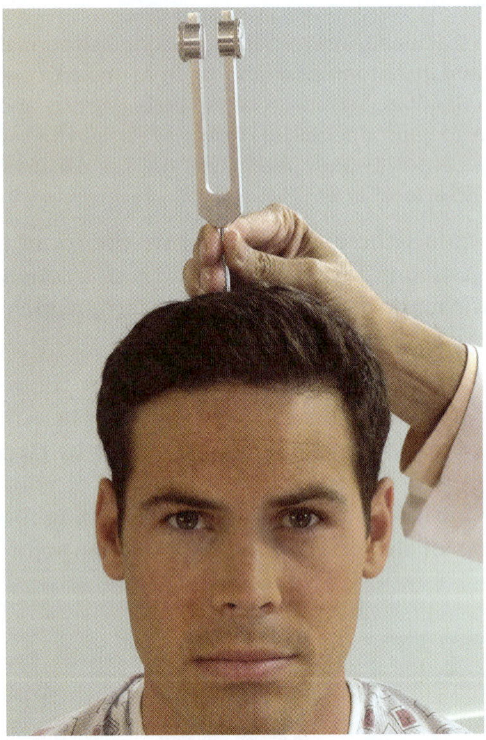

FIGURE 21-13. Lateralization (Weber) test.

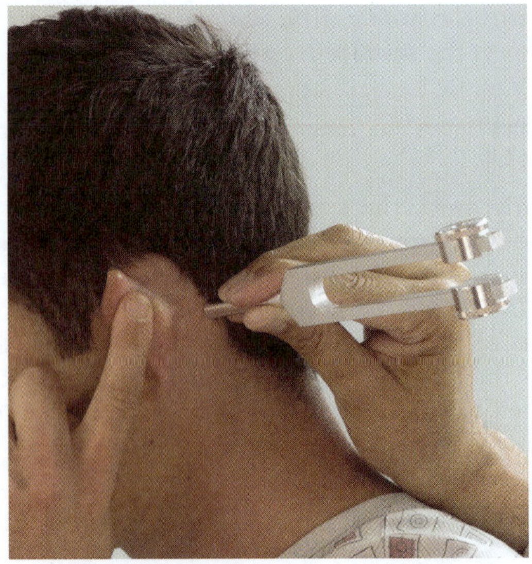

FIGURE 21-14. Rinne: Testing bone conduction.

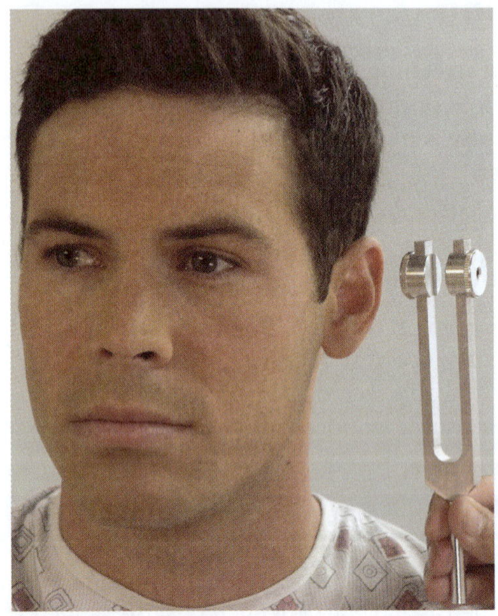

FIGURE 21-15. Rinne: Testing air conduction.

- *Compare air conduction (AC) and bone conduction (BC)* **(Rinne test)**. Place the base of a lightly vibrating tuning fork on the mastoid bone, behind the ear and level with the canal (Fig. 21-14). When the patient can no longer hear the sound, quickly place the prongs of the fork close to the ear canal and ask if the patient hears a vibration (Fig. 21-15). Here, the prongs of the fork should face forward, which maximizes sound transmission for the patient. Normally, the sound is heard longer through air than through bone (AC > BC).

In conductive hearing loss, sound is heard through bone as long as or longer than it is through air (BC = AC or BC > AC). In sensorineural hearing loss, sound is heard longer through air (AC > BC).

Key Components of the Nose and Paranasal Sinus Examination

- Inspect the anterior and inferior surfaces of the nose (asymmetry, deformities, tenderness).
- Test for nasal obstruction on each ala nasi (if indicated).
- Inspect the nasal mucosa, nasal septum, inferior and middle turbinates, and corresponding meatuses with a light source or otoscope with large speculum (deviation, marked asymmetry, polyps, ulcers).
- Palpate the frontal sinuses (tenderness, pressure, fullness).
- Palpate the maxillary sinuses (tenderness, pressure, fullness).

Surface of the Nose

Inspect the anterior and inferior surfaces of the nose. Gentle pressure on the tip of the nose with your thumb usually widens the nostrils. Use a penlight or otoscope light to obtain a partial view of each nasal vestibule. If the nasal tip is tender, be gentle and manipulate the nose as little as possible. Note any asymmetry or deformity of the nose.

Tenderness of the nasal tip or ala suggests local infection such as a furuncle, particularly if there is a small erythematous and swollen area.

Test for nasal obstruction, if indicated, by pressing on each ala nasi in turn and asking the patient to breathe in.

Nasal Cavity and Mucosa

Inspect the inside of the nares with an otoscope and the largest available ear speculum. Tilt the patient's head back a bit and insert the speculum gently into the vestibule of each nostril, avoiding contact with the sensitive nasal septum (Fig. 21-16). Hold the otoscope handle to one side to avoid the patient's chin and improve your mobility. By directing the speculum posteriorly, then upward in small steps, try to see the inferior and middle turbinates, the nasal septum, and the narrow nasal passage between them, as shown in Figure 21-17. Some asymmetry of the two sides is normal.

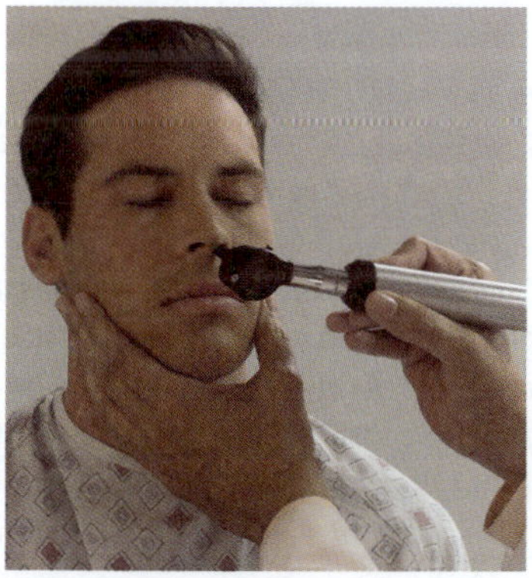

FIGURE 21-16. Inspecting inside the nares with an otoscope.

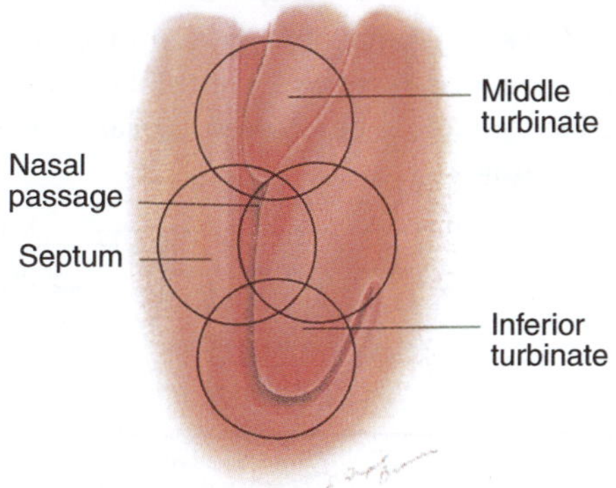

FIGURE 21-17. Inferior and middle turbinates.

Deviation of the lower septum is common and may be easily visible, as in Figure 21-18. Deviation seldom obstructs airflow.

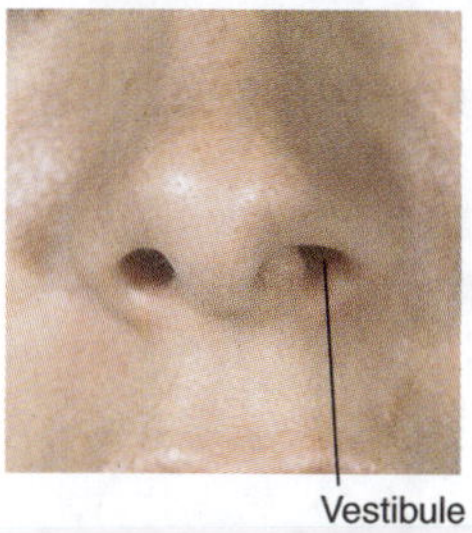

FIGURE 21-18. Deviation of the lower septum.

Inspect the nasal mucosa that covers the septum and turbinates. Note its color and any swelling, bleeding, or exudate. If exudate is present, note its character: clear, mucopurulent, or purulent. The nasal mucosa is normally somewhat redder than the oral mucosa.

In viral rhinitis, the mucosa is reddened and swollen; in allergic rhinitis, it may be pale, bluish, or red.

Nasal Septum

Inspect the nasal septum. Note any deviation, inflammation, or perforation of the septum. The lower anterior portion of the septum (where the patient's finger can reach) is a common source of *epistaxis* (nosebleed). Inspect for any abnormalities such as ulcers or polyps (Fig. 21-19).

Fresh blood or crusting may be seen. Causes of septal perforation include trauma, surgery, and intranasal use of cocaine or amphetamines, which also cause septal ulceration.

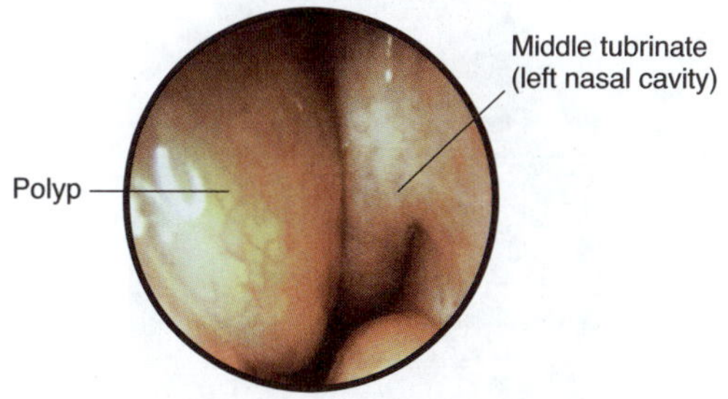

FIGURE 21-19. Nasal polyp.

Nasal polyps are pale saclike growths of inflamed tissue that can obstruct the air passage or sinuses, seen in allergic rhinitis, aspirin sensitivity, asthma, chronic sinus infections, and cystic fibrosis.

Malignant tumors of the nasal cavity occur rarely, associated with exposure to tobacco or chronically inhaled toxins.

Inspection of the nasal cavity through the anterior naris is usually limited to the vestibule, the anterior portion of the septum, and the lower and middle turbinates. Examination of posterior abnormalities requires a nasopharyngeal mirror, and its proper use is beyond the scope of this book. Remember to properly discard or clean and disinfect all nasal and ear specula after use.

Paranasal Sinuses

Palpate for sinus tenderness. Press up on the frontal sinuses from under the bony brows, avoiding pressure on the eyes (Fig. 21-20). Then press up on the maxillary sinuses (Fig. 21-21).

Local tenderness, together with symptoms such as facial pain, pressure or fullness, purulent nasal discharge, nasal obstruction, and smell disorder, especially when present for >7 days, suggest acute bacterial rhinosinusitis involving the frontal or maxillary sinuses.

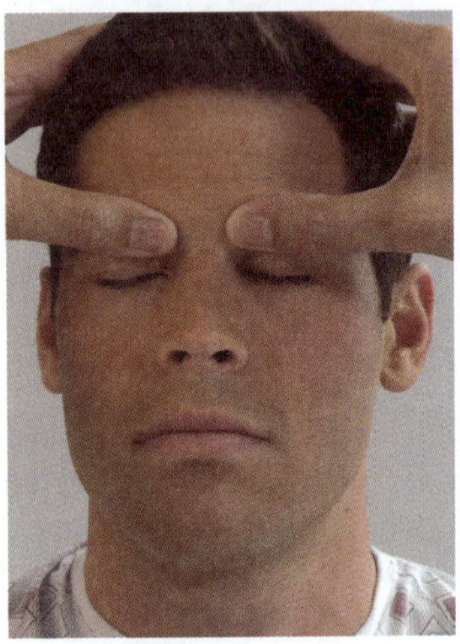

FIGURE 21-20. Palpating the frontal sinuses.

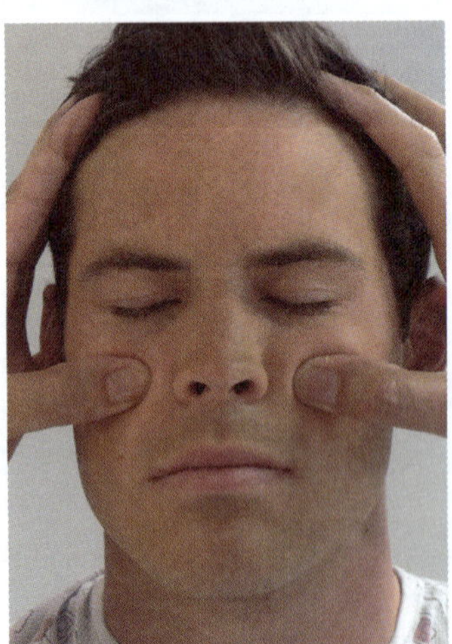

FIGURE 21-21. Palpating the maxillary sinuses.

RECORDING YOUR FINDINGS

Initially you may use sentences to describe your findings; later you will use phrases. The style in the next box contains phrases appropriate for most write-ups.

Recording the Head, Eyes, Ears, Nose, and Throat (HEENT) Examination

HEENT: Head—The skull is normocephalic/atraumatic (NC/AT). Hair with average texture. ***Eyes***—Visual acuity 20/20 bilaterally. Sclera white, conjunctiva pink. Pupils are 4 mm constricting to 2 mm, equally round and reactive to light and accommodations (PERRLA). Disc margins sharp; no hemorrhages or exudates, no arteriolar narrowing. ***Ears*—Acuity good to whispered voice. External auditory canals (EACs) intact bilaterally. Tympanic membranes (TMs) intact and mobile, with good cone of light. 512 Tuning Fork (TF): Weber midline. Rinne AC > BC bilaterally. *Nose*—Nasal mucosa pink, septum midline; no sinus tenderness.** ***Throat (or Mouth)***—Oral mucosa pink, dentition good, pharynx without exudates.

Neck—Trachea midline. Neck supple; thyroid isthmus palpable, lobes not felt.

Lymph Nodes—No cervical, axillary, epitrochlear, inguinal adenopathy.

OR

Head—The skull NC/AT. Frontal balding. ***Eyes***—Visual acuity 20/100 bilaterally. Sclera white; conjunctiva injected. Pupils constrict 3 mm to 2 mm, PERRLA. Disc margins sharp; no hemorrhages or exudates. Arteriolar-to-venous ratio (AV ratio) 2:4; no AV nicking. ***Ears***—Acuity diminished to whispered voice; intact to spoken voice. Bilateral external auditory canals and TMs clear. *Nose*—Mucosa swollen with erythema and clear drainage. Septum midline. Tender over bilateral maxillary sinuses.* Throat—Oral mucosa pink, dental caries in lower molars, pharynx erythematous, no exudates.

Neck—Trachea midline. Neck supple; thyroid isthmus midline, lobes palpable but not enlarged.

Lymph Nodes—Submandibular and anterior cervical lymph nodes tender, 1 cm × 1 cm, rubbery and mobile; no posterior cervical, epitrochlear, axillary, or inguinal lymphadenopathy.

*These findings suggest bilateral hearing loss possibly due to sinus infection and accompanying nasopharyngeal and mucosal congestion.

HEALTH PROMOTION AND COUNSELING: EVIDENCE AND RECOMMENDATIONS

Important Topic for Health Promotion and Counseling

- Screening for hearing loss

Screening for Hearing Loss

Hearing loss is frequently considered the inability to hear tones at frequencies between 500 and 4,000 Hz, the most important for speech processing. This impairment, which can adversely affect social, psychological, and cognitive functioning, often goes undetected and untreated. Hearing loss can be accurately and reliably detected by a number of screening tests, including single-item screening test (e.g., "Do you have difficulty with your hearing?"), multi-item questionnaires (such as the Hearing Handicap Inventory for the Elderly—Screening Version), handheld audiometers, the watch tick test, the whispered voice test, and the finger rub test. The most common cause of hearing loss is *presbycusis*, age-related degeneration of hair cells in the ears, which leads to gradually progressive hearing loss, particularly for high-frequency sounds. Exposure to hazardous noise levels, including from occupational and other environmental sources, is the next leading risk factor for hearing loss, particularly in younger adults. Other risk factors include history of inner ear infections, ototoxic drug exposures, and systemic illnesses such as diabetes mellitus. Hearing aids may improve hearing and quality of life for some adults with age-related hearing loss.

Noise reduction and avoidance are recommended strategies for preventing or delaying hearing loss.

TABLE 21-1. Dizziness and Vertigo

"Dizziness" is a nonspecific term used by patients encompassing several disorders that clinicians must carefully sort out. A detailed history usually identifies the primary etiology. It is important to learn the specific meanings of the following terms or conditions:

- *Vertigo*—a spinning sensation accompanied by nystagmus and ataxia; usually from peripheral vestibular dysfunction (~40% of "dizzy" patients), but may be from a central brainstem lesion (~10%; causes include atherosclerosis, multiple sclerosis, vertebrobasilar migraine, or transient ischemic attack)
- *Presyncope*—a near faint from "feeling faint or lightheaded"; causes include orthostatic hypotension, especially from medication, arrhythmias, and vasovagal attacks (~5%)
- *Disequilibrium*—unsteadiness or imbalance when walking, especially in older patients; causes include fear of walking, visual loss, weakness from musculoskeletal problems, and peripheral neuropathy (up to 15%)
- *Psychiatric*—causes include anxiety, panic disorder, hyperventilation, depression, somatization disorder, alcohol, and substance abuse (~10%)
- *Multifactorial or unknown* (up to 20%)

Peripheral and Central Vertigo

	Onset	Duration and Course	Hearing	Tinnitus	Additional Features
Peripheral Vertigo					
Benign Positional Vertigo	Sudden, often when rolling onto the affected side or tilting up the head	Onset a few seconds to <1 min Lasts a few weeks, may recur	Not affected	Absent	Sometimes nausea, vomiting, nystagmus
Vestibular Neuronitis	Sudden	Onset hours to up to 2 wks May recur over 12–18 mo	Not affected	Absent	Nausea, vomiting, nystagmus
Acute Labyrinthitis	Sudden	Onset hours to up to 2 wks May recur over 12–18 mo	Sensorineural hearing loss—unilateral	May be present	Nausea, vomiting, nystagmus
Ménière Disease	Sudden	Onset several hours to ≥1 day Recurrent	Sensorineural hearing loss—fluctuating, recurs, eventually progresses	Present, fluctuating	Pressure or fullness in affected ear; nausea, vomiting, nystagmus
Drug Toxicity	Insidious or acute—linked to loop diuretics, aminoglycosides, salicylates, alcohol	May or may not be reversible Partial adaptation occurs	May be impaired	May be present	Nausea, vomiting
Acoustic Neuroma	Insidious from CN VIII compression, vestibular branch	Variable	Impaired, one side	Present	May involve CN V and VII
Central Vertigo	Often sudden (see causes above)	Variable but rarely continuous	Not affected	Absent	Usually with other brainstem deficits—dysarthria, ataxia, crossed motor and sensory deficits

Sources: Chan Y. *Curr Opin Otolaryngol Head Neck Surg.* 2009;17:200; Kroenke K et al. *Ann Intern Med.* 1992;117:898; Tusa RJ. *Neurol Clin.* 2001;19:23; Lockwood AH et al. *N Engl J Med.* 2002;347:904.

TABLE 21-2. Lumps on or Near the Ear

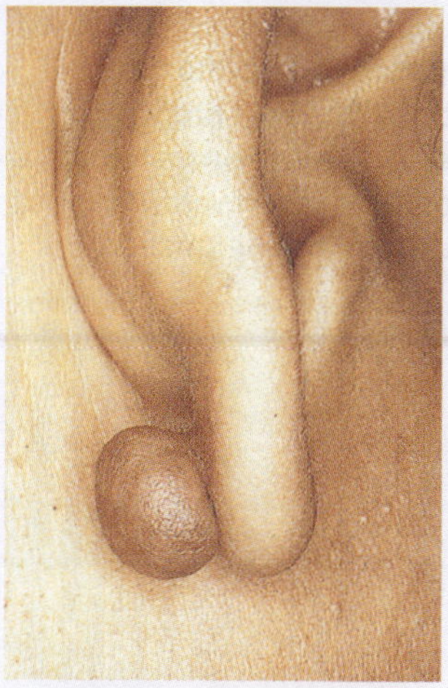

Keloid. A firm, nodular, hypertrophic mass of scar tissue extending beyond the area of injury.

It may develop in any scarred area but is most common on the shoulders and upper chest. A keloid on a pierced earlobe may have unwanted cosmetic effects.

Keloids are more common in people with darker skin and may recur following treatment.

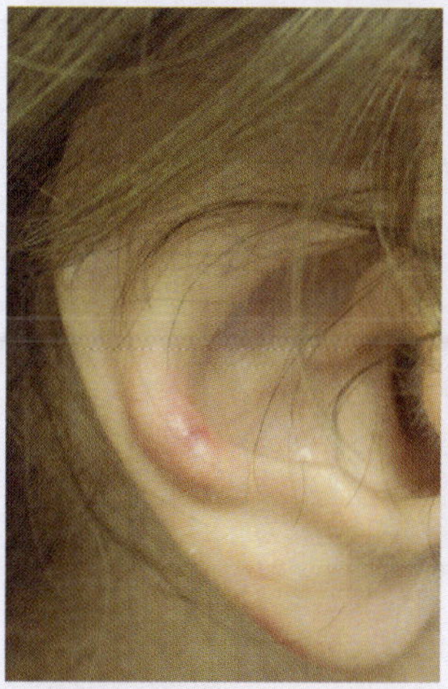

Chondrodermatitis helicis. This chronic inflammatory lesion starts as a painful, tender papule on the helix or antihelix. Reddening may occur. Biopsy is needed to rule out carcinoma.

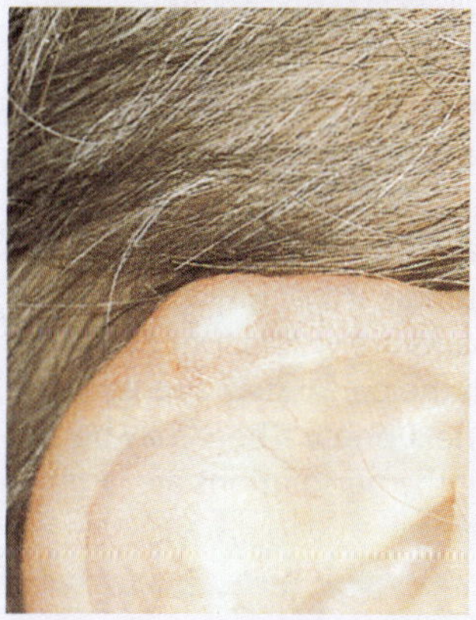

Tophi. A deposit of uric acid crystals characteristic of chronic tophaceous gout.

It appears as hard nodules in the helix or antihelix and may discharge chalky white crystals through the skin. It also may appear near the joints, hands, feet, and other areas. It usually develops after chronic sustained high blood levels of uric acid.

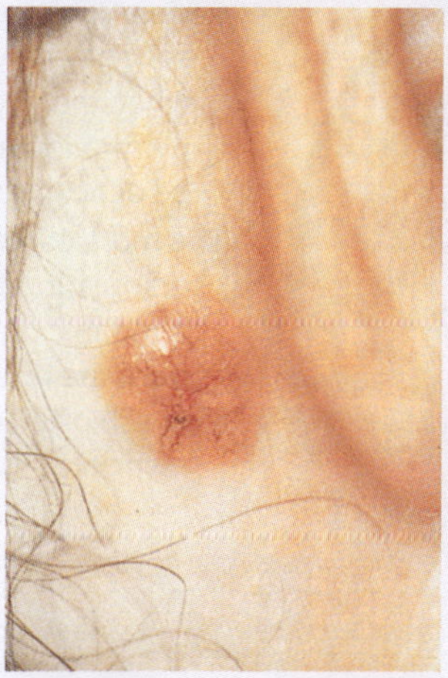

Basal Cell Carcinoma. This raised nodule shows the lustrous surface and telangiectatic vessels of basal cell carcinoma, a common slow-growing malignancy that rarely metastasizes. Growth and ulceration may occur.

These are more frequent in people with fair skin overexposed to sunlight.

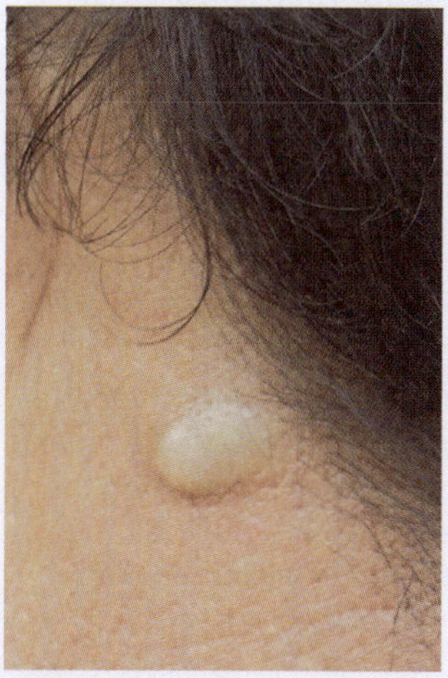

Cutaneous Cyst. Also known as a sebaceous cyst, a dome-shaped lump in the dermis forms a benign closed firm sac attached to the epidermis.

A dark dot (blackhead) may be visible on its surface. Histologically, it is usually either (1) an epidermoid cyst, common on the face and neck, or (2) a pilar (trichilemmal) cyst, common in the scalp. Both may become inflamed.

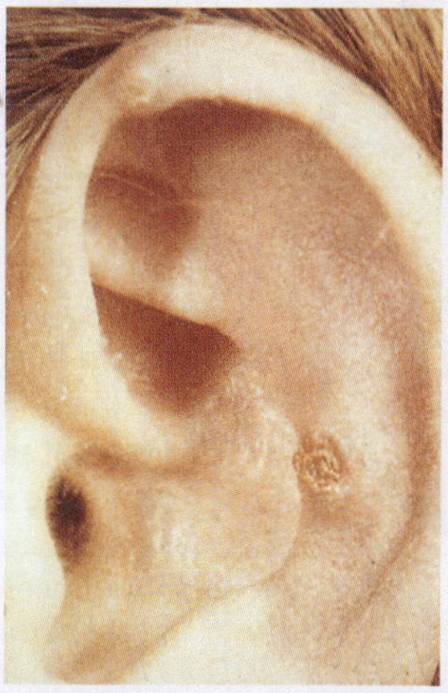

Rheumatoid Nodules. In chronic rheumatoid arthritis, look for small lumps on the helix or antihelix and additional nodules elsewhere on the hands and along the surface of the ulna distal to the elbow, and on the knees and heels. Ulceration may result from repeated injuries. These nodules may antedate the arthritis.

Sources of photos: *Keloid*—Reprinted from Sams WM Jr, Lynch PJ, eds. *Principles and Practice of Dermatology.* Churchill Livingstone; 1990. Copyright © 1990 Elsevier. With permission; *Chondrodermatitis Helicis*—Image provided by Stedman's; *Tophi*—Weber J, Kelley J. *Health Assessment in Nursing.* 2nd ed. Wolters Kluwer; 2003, Fig. 12-2; *Basal Cell Carcinoma*—Phillips T, Dover J. *N Engl J Med.* 1992;326(3):169–178. Copyright © 1992 Massachusetts Medical Society. Reprinted with permission from Massachusetts Medical Society; *Cutaneous Cyst*—Shutterstock photo by jaojormami; *Rheumatoid Nodules*—Champion RH et al., eds. *Rook/Wilkinson/Ebling Textbook of Dermatology.* 5th ed. Blackwell Scientific; 1992. Copyright © 1992 by Blackwell Scientific Publications. Reprinted by permission of John Wiley & Sons, Inc.

TABLE 21-3. Abnormalities of the Tympanic Membrane

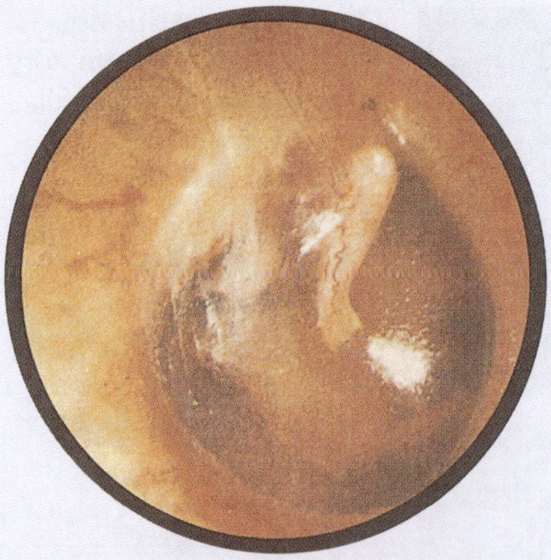

Normal Tympanic Membrane (Right)

This normal right tympanic membrane or eardrum, is pinkish gray. Note the malleus lying behind the upper part of the drum. Above the short process lies the pars flaccida. The remainder of the tympanic membrane is the pars tensa. From the umbo, the bright cone of light fans anteriorly and downward. Posterior to the malleus, part of the incus is visible behind the eardrum. The small blood vessels along the handle of the malleus are normal.

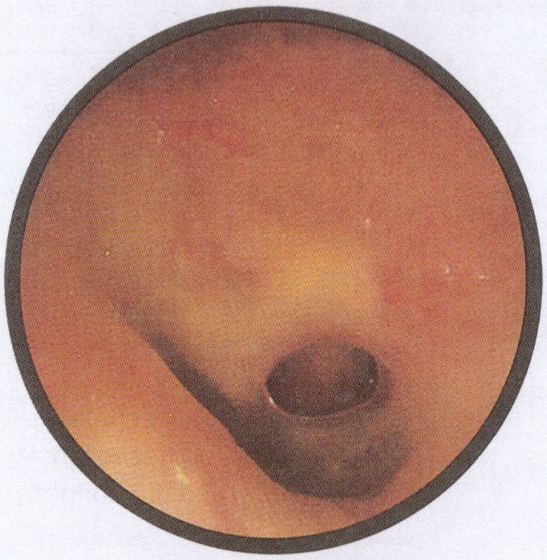

Perforation of the Tympanic Membrane

Perforations are holes in the eardrum, usually from purulent infections of the middle ear. They may be central, if not involving the edge of the drum, or marginal, when the edge is involved. When perforations heal the membrane covering the perforation may be notably thin and transparent; this is called a *monomer* and may be difficult to distinguish from a true perforation.

The more common central perforation is illustrated here. A reddened ring of granulation tissue surrounds the perforation, indicating chronic infection. The tympanic membrane itself is scarred, and no landmarks are visible. Discharge from the infected middle ear may drain out through the perforated opening, which often closes in the healing process, as in the next photo. There may be associated earache or even hearing loss, especially if the perforations are large.

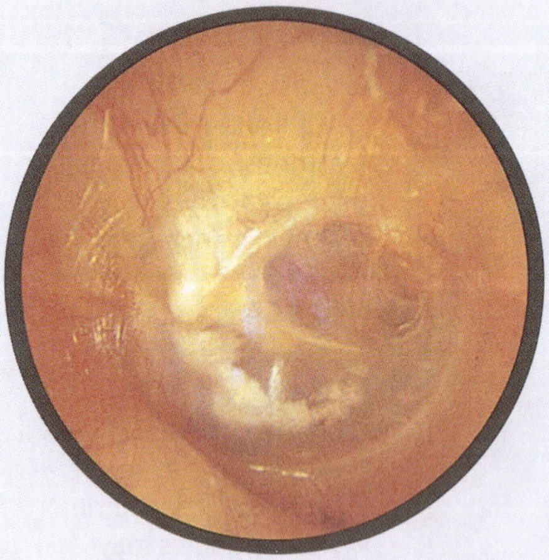

Tympanosclerosis

Tympanosclerosis is a scarring process of the middle ear from otitis media that involves deposition of hyaline and calcium and phosphate crystals in the tympanic membrane and middle ear. When severe it may entrap the ossicles and cause conductive hearing loss.

In the inferior portion of this left tympanic membrane, note the large, chalky white patch with irregular margins. It is typical of tympanosclerosis: a deposition of hyaline material within the layers of the tympanic membrane that sometimes follows a severe episode of otitis media. It does not usually impair hearing and is seldom clinically significant.

Other abnormalities in this tympanic membrane include a healed perforation (the large oval area in the upper posterior eardrum) and signs of a retracted tympanic membrane. A retracted tympanic membrane is pulled medially, away from the examiner's eye, and the malleolar folds are tightened into sharp outlines. The short process often protrudes sharply, and the handle of the malleus, pulled inward at the umbo, looks foreshortened and more horizontal.

(continued)

TABLE 21-3. Abnormalities of the Tympanic Membrane *(Continued)*

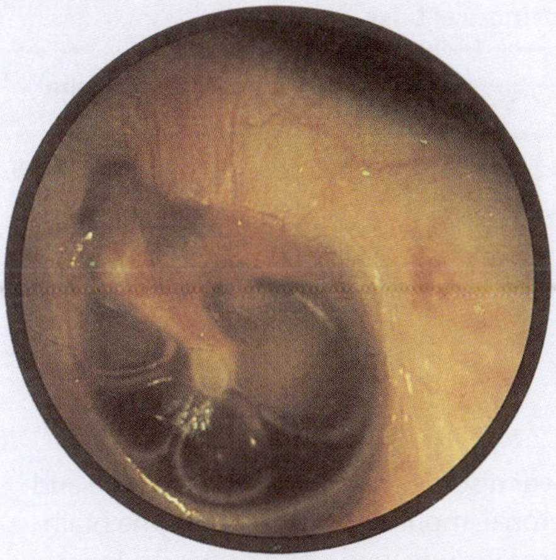

Serous Effusion

Serous effusions are usually caused by viral upper respiratory infections (otitis media with serous effusion) or by sudden changes in atmospheric pressure as from flying or diving (*otitic barotrauma*). The eustachian tube cannot equalize the air pressure in the middle ear and outside air. Air is absorbed from the middle ear into the bloodstream, and serous fluid accumulates in the middle ear instead. Symptoms include fullness and popping sensations in the ear, mild conduction hearing loss, and, sometimes, pain.

Amber fluid behind the eardrum is characteristic, as in this patient with otitic barotrauma. A fluid level, a line between air above and amber fluid below, can be seen on either side of the short process. Air bubbles (not always present) can be seen here within the amber fluid.

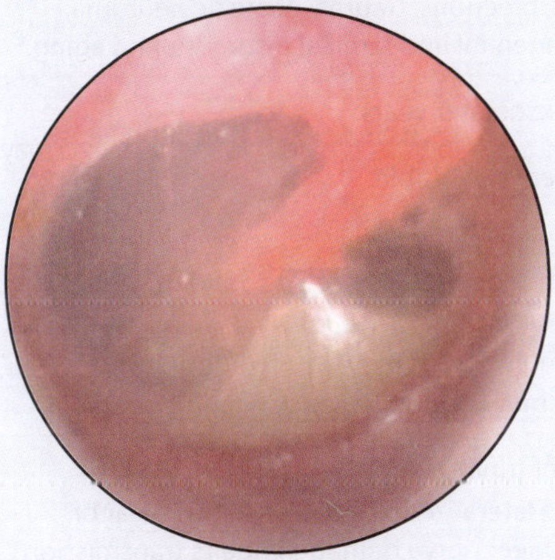

Acute Otitis Media with Purulent Effusion

Acute otitis media with purulent effusion is commonly caused by bacterial infection from *S. pneumoniae* or *H. influenzae*. Symptoms include earache, fever, and hearing loss. The tympanic membrane reddens, loses its landmarks, and bulges laterally, toward the examiner's eye.

Here the tympanic membrane is bulging with fluid level. A diffuse redness of the entire tympanic membrane often develops. Spontaneous rupture (perforation) of the tympanic membrane may follow, with discharge of purulent material into the ear canal.

Hearing loss is the conductive type. Acute purulent otitis media is much more common in children than in adults.

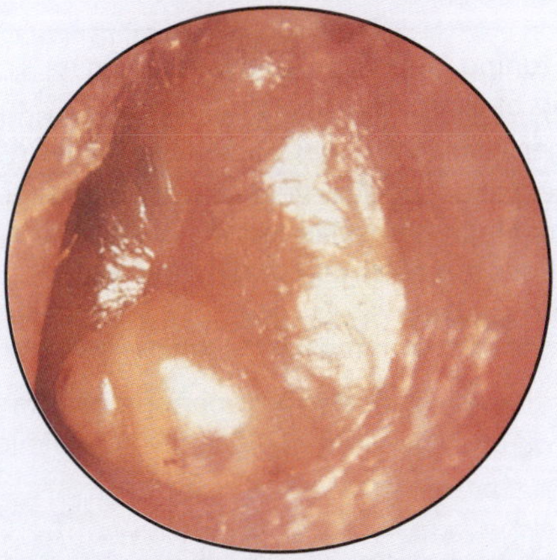

Bullous Myringitis

In bullous myringitis, painful hemorrhagic vesicles appear on the tympanic membrane, the ear canal, or both. Symptoms include earache, blood-tinged discharge from the ear, and conductive hearing loss.

In this image, a large vesicle (bulla) is discernible on the tympanic membrane. The eardrum is reddened, and its landmarks are obscured.

This condition is caused by *Mycoplasma*, viral, and bacterial otitis media.

Sources of photos: *Normal Eardrum*—Reprinted from Hawke M et al. *Clinical Otoscopy: A Text and Colour Atlas.* Churchill Livingstone; 1984. Copyright © 1984 Elsevier. With permission; *Perforation of the Tympanic membrane, Tympanosclerosis*—Courtesy of Michael Hawke, MD, Toronto, Canada; *Serous Effusion*—Reprinted from Hawke M et al. *Clinical Otoscopy: A Text and Colour Atlas.* Churchill Livingstone; 1984. Copyright © 1984 Elsevier. With permission; *Acute Otitis Media*—Johnson J. *Bailey's Head and Neck Surgery.* 5th ed. Wolters Kluwer; 2014, Figure 99-1; *Bullous Myringitis*—Jensen S. *Nursing Health Assessment: A Best Practice Approach.* 2nd ed. Wolters Kluwer Health/Lippincott Williams & Wilkins; 2011:406.

TABLE 21-4. Patterns of Hearing Loss

	Conductive Loss	Sensorineural Loss
	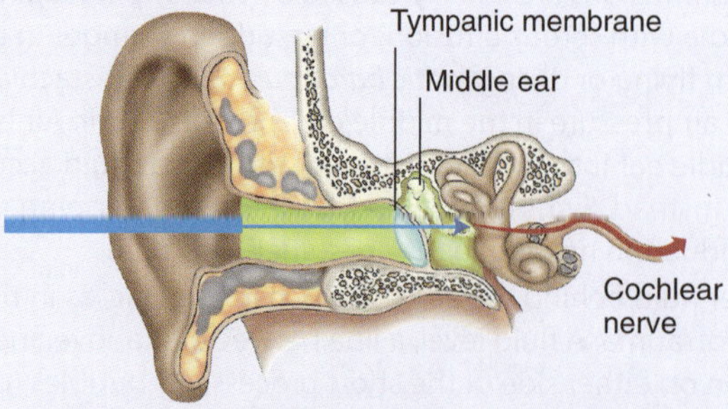	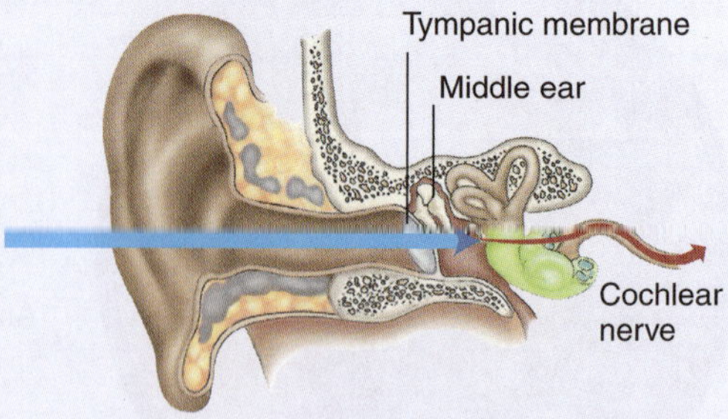
Pathophysiology	External or middle ear disorder impairs sound conduction to inner ear. Causes include foreign body, otitis media, perforated eardrum, and otosclerosis of ossicles.	Inner ear disorder involves cochlear nerve and neuronal impulse transmission to the brain. Causes include loud noise exposure, inner ear infections, trauma, acoustic neuroma, congenital and familial disorders, and aging.
Usual Age of Onset	Childhood and young adulthood, up to age 40 yrs	Middle or later years
Ear Canal and Tympanic Membrane	Abnormality usually visible, except in otosclerosis	Problem not visible
Effects	Little effect on sound Hearing seems to improve in noisy environment Voice remains soft because inner ear and cochlear nerve are intact	Higher registers are lost, so sound may be distorted Hearing worsens in noisy environment Voice may be loud because hearing is difficult
Weber Test (in Unilateral Hearing Loss)	Base of tuning fork at vertex Sound lateralizes to impaired ear—room noise not well heard, so detection of vibrations improves	Base of tuning fork at vertex Sound lateralizes to good ear—inner ear or cochlear nerve damage impairs transmission to affected ear
Rinne Test	Base of tuning fork on mastoid bone; then prongs at external auditory meatus BC longer than or equal to AC (BC ≥ AC) While air conduction through the external or middle ear is impaired, vibrations through bone bypass the problem to reach the cochlea.	Base of tuning fork on mastoid bone; then prongs at external auditory meatus AC longer than BC (AC > BC) The inner ear or cochlear nerve is less able to transmit impulses regardless of how the vibrations reach the cochlea. The normal pattern prevails.

CHAPTER 22

Throat and Oral Cavity

ANATOMY AND PHYSIOLOGY

Mouth, Gingiva, and Teeth

The *lips* are muscular folds that surround the entrance to the mouth. When opened, the gums (*gingiva*) and *teeth* are visible (Fig. 22-1). Note the scalloped shape of the *gingival margins* and the pointed *interdental papillae.*

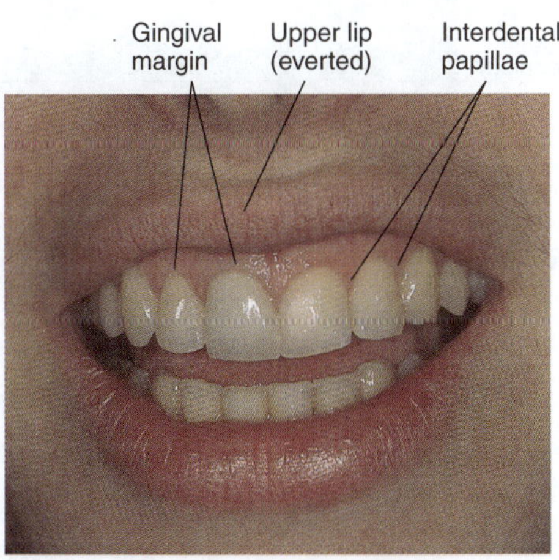

FIGURE 22-1. The mouth, gingiva, and teeth.

The *gingiva* is firmly attached to the teeth and to the maxilla and mandible in which they are seated. In people with lighter skin, the gingiva is pale or coral pink and lightly stippled. In people with darker skin, it may be diffusely or partly brown (Fig. 22-2). A midline mucosal fold, called a *labial frenulum*, connects each lip with the gingiva. A shallow *gingival sulcus* between the gum's thin margin and each tooth is not readily visible (but is probed and measured by dentists and oral health professionals). Adjacent to the gingiva is the *alveolar mucosa*, which merges with the *labial mucosa* of the lip (Fig. 22-2).

Each tooth, composed chiefly of *dentin*, lies rooted in a bony socket with only its enamel-covered *crown* exposed. Small blood vessels and nerves enter the tooth through its apex and pass into the *pulp canal* and *pulp chamber* (Fig. 22-3).

Note that there are 32 adult teeth, numbered 1 to 16 right to left on the upper jaw and 17 to 32 left to right on the lower jaw (Fig. 22-4).

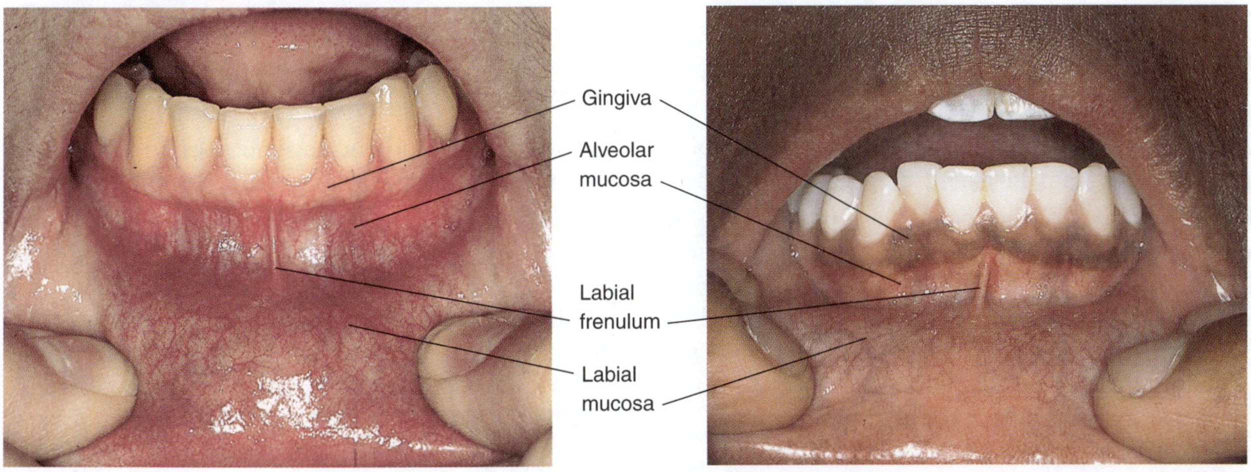

FIGURE 22-2. Alveolar and labial mucosa, labial frenulum.

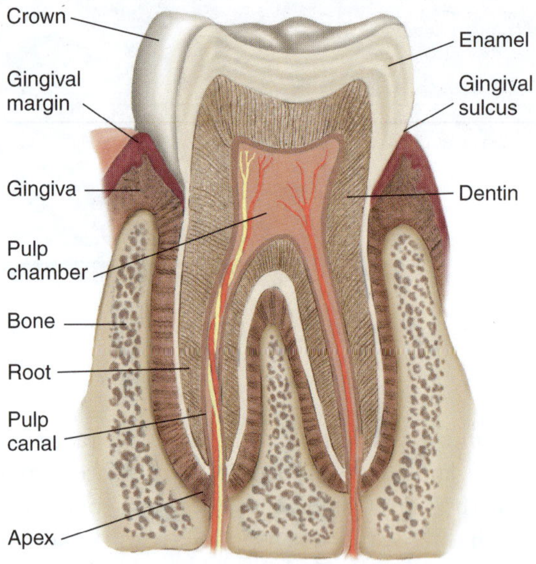

FIGURE 22-3. Anatomy of a tooth.

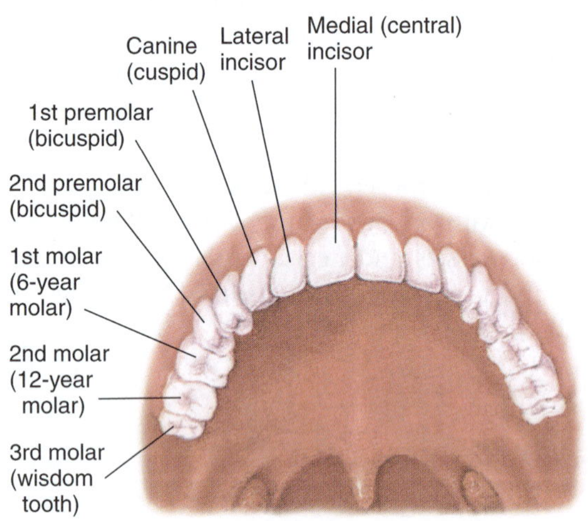

FIGURE 22-4. Adult teeth (upper jaw).

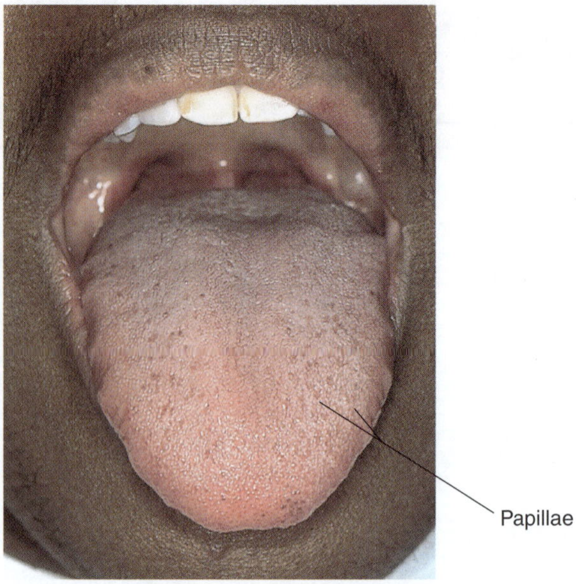

FIGURE 22-5. Dorsal papillae of the tongue.

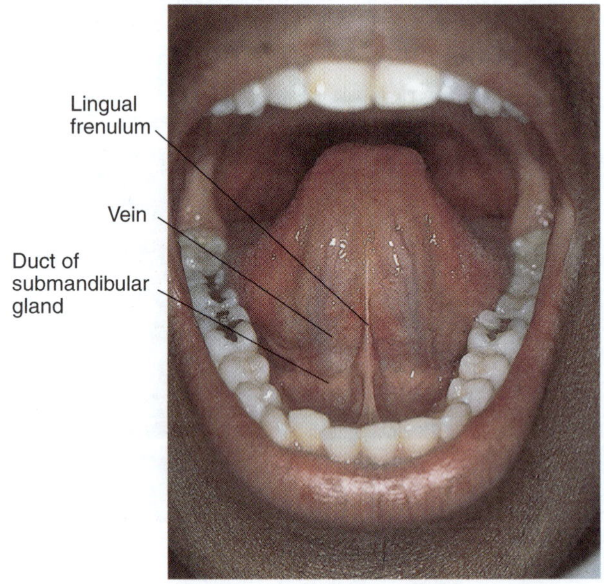

FIGURE 22-6. Undersurface of the tongue.

Tongue

The dorsum of the tongue is covered with *papillae*, giving it a rough surface. Some of these papillae look like red dots, which contrast with the thin white coat that often covers the tongue (Fig. 22-5).

The undersurface of the tongue has no papillae. Note the midline *lingual frenulum* that connects the tongue to the floor of the mouth and the ducts of the *submandibular gland* (*Wharton ducts*), which pass forward and medially (Fig. 22-6). They open on papillae that lie on each side of the lingual frenulum. The paired *sublingual salivary glands* lie just under the floor of the mouth mucosa.

Pharynx

Above and behind the tongue rises an arch formed by the anterior and posterior pillars, the *soft palate*, and the *uvula* (Fig. 22-7). A meshwork of small blood vessels may web the soft palate. The *posterior pharynx* is visible in the recess behind the soft palate and tongue.

In Figure 22-7, note the right *tonsil* protruding from the hollowed *tonsillar fossa*, or cavity, between the anterior and posterior pillars. In adults, tonsils are often small or absent, as in the empty left tonsillar fossa.

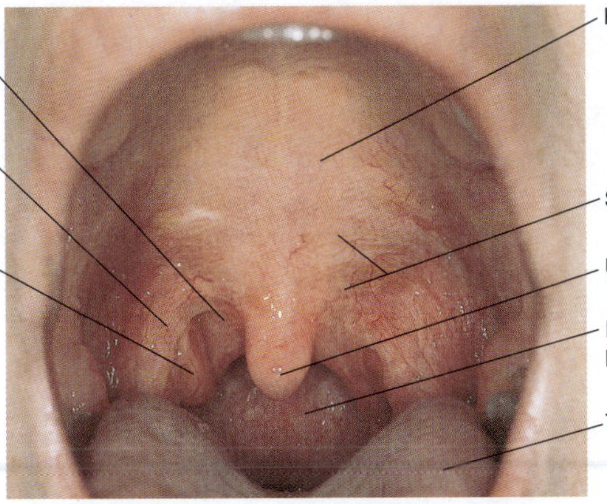

FIGURE 22-7. Anatomy of the posterior pharynx.

The *buccal mucosa* lines the cheeks. Each *parotid duct* (*Stensen duct*) opens onto the buccal mucosa near the upper second molar. Its location is frequently marked by its own small papilla (Fig. 22-8).

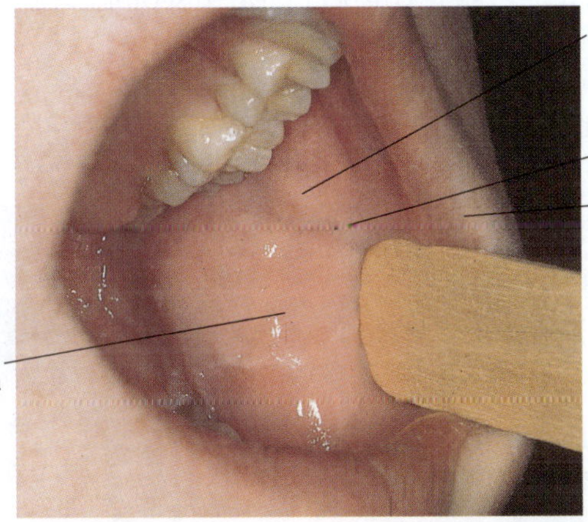

FIGURE 22-8. Buccal mucosa and opening of the parotid duct.

HEALTH HISTORY: GENERAL APPROACH

Many symptoms of the throat and oral cavity represent common benign processes, but sometimes these symptoms reflect a serious underlying condition. Careful attention to the interview and physical examination can often distinguish a common condition from a more worrisome underlying disease. Here we will review how to conduct a medical interview as it relates to conditions of the throat and oral cavity. These aspects will be useful in the context of performing the larger "HEENT" history, as head and neck symptoms are often interrelated.

Common or Concerning Symptoms

- Sore throat
- Gum swelling/bleeding gums
- Hoarseness
- Malodorous breath (*halitosis*)

Sore Throat

Sore throat or *pharyngitis* is a frequent complaint, usually associated with an acute upper respiratory illness (URI). However, sometimes a sore throat is the only symptom.

A *sore tongue* may result from local lesions such as *oral candidiasis*, as well as from systemic illness.

Abnormalities include **aphthous ulcers** and the sore smooth tongue of nutritional deficiency. See Table 22-4, Findings in or under the Tongue.

Bleeding or Swollen Gums

Bleeding from the gums, especially when brushing teeth, is a common symptom. Ask about local lesions and any tendency to bleed or bruise elsewhere.

Bleeding gums are usually caused by **gingivitis**. See Table 22-3, Findings in the Gums and Teeth.

Hoarseness

Hoarseness refers to a change in voice quality, often described as husky, rough, harsh, or lower pitched than usual.

Causes range from diseases of the larynx to extralaryngeal lesions that press on the laryngeal nerves.

Ask the patient about environmental allergies, acid reflux, smoking, alcohol use, and inhalation of fumes or other irritants. Also ask if the patient talks a great deal at work.

If hoarseness is acute, consider voice overuse, acute viral laryngitis, and possible neck trauma.

Is the problem chronic, lasting more than 2 weeks? Is there prolonged tobacco or alcohol use, cough or hemoptysis, weight loss, or unilateral throat pain?

If hoarseness lasts over 2 weeks, refer for laryngoscopy and consider causes such as reflux; vocal cord nodules; hypothyroidism; head and neck cancers including thyroid masses; and neurologic disorders like Parkinson disease, amyotrophic lateral sclerosis, or myasthenia gravis.

Malodorous Breath

Malodorous breath (*halitosis*) is an unpleasant or offensive odor emanating from the breath. Not all persons with malodorous breath are aware of it. Questions may include "Have you noticed any bad breath when you talk?" or "Has anyone mentioned to you that you have bad breath?" One thing to note is that even for a healthy mouth, there is often malodor upon waking from sleep, probably due to putrefaction of debris not cleared by low level salivation during sleep.

Common oral causes of breath malodor include poor oral hygiene, tobacco smoking, plaque retention on teeth and mouth appliances such as retainers and dentures, periodontal diseases (gingivitis, ulcers, periodontitis).

Causes of breath malodor may also be systemic. The most common ones are respiratory causes such as sinusitis, **tonsillitis**, pharyngitis, foreign bodies, neoplasms, abscesses, and bronchiectasis. Other systemic causes are uncommon such as gastric acid reflux, hepatic cirrhosis, poorly controlled diabetes mellitus, impaired fat digestion, and inborn errors of metabolism such as trimethylaminuria.

PHYSICAL EXAMINATION: GENERAL APPROACH

Examination of the mouth and pharynx requires appropriate lighting and thorough visual inspection and often palpation. The general integrity of the oral mucosa, lips, teeth and gingiva, palate, oral tongue, and pharynx, including the tonsils, should all be noted. Here we review key aspects of the examination which can then be interpreted in the greater context of the head and neck examination. If the patient wears dentures, offer a paper towel and ask the patient to remove them so that you can inspect the underlying mucosa.

Key Components of the Mouth and Pharynx Examination

- Inspect the lips (color, moisture, lumps, ulcers, cracking, or scaliness).
- Inspect the oral mucosa (discoloration, ulcers, white patches, nodules).
- Palpate the oral mucosa (if indicated for any lesions, thickening).
- Inspect the gingiva (erythema, discoloration, ulceration, swelling).
- Inspect the gum margins and interdental papillae (swelling, ulceration).
- Inspect the teeth (missing, discolored, misshapen, or abnormally positioned).
- Inspect the roof (hard palate) and floor of the mouth (erythema, discoloration, nodules, ulcerations, or deformities).

(continued)

- Test the hypoglossal nerve, or CN XII (symmetry of tongue protrusion).
- Inspect the tongue (color, texture, lesions).
- Palpate the tongue (if indicated for any lesions, thickening).
- Inspect the soft palate, anterior and posterior pillars, uvula, tonsils, and pharynx (color, symmetry, exudate, swelling, ulceration, or tonsillar enlargement).
- Test the vagus nerve, or CN X (symmetry of uvula).

TECHNIQUES OF EXAMINATION

Lips and Oral Mucosa

Inspect the lips. Observe their color and moisture, and note any lumps, ulcers, cracking, or scaliness.

Inspect the oral mucosa. Look inside the patient's mouth with a good light source and the help of a tongue blade (Fig. 22-9). Inspect for discoloration, ulcers (Fig. 22-10), white patches, and nodules.

Watch for central cyanosis or pallor from anemia. See Table 22-1, Abnormalities of the Lips.

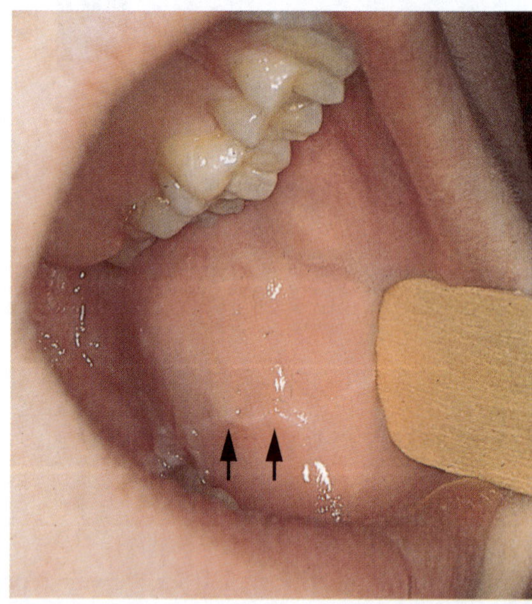

FIGURE 22-9. Inspecting the oral mucosa with a tongue blade.

If you detect any suspicious ulcers or nodules, put on a glove and palpate any lesions, noting any thickening or infiltration of the tissues that might suggest malignancy.

In the patient shown in Figure 22-9, the wavy white line indicated by the arrows on the adjacent buccal mucosa developed where the upper and lower teeth meet, related to irritation from sucking or chewing.

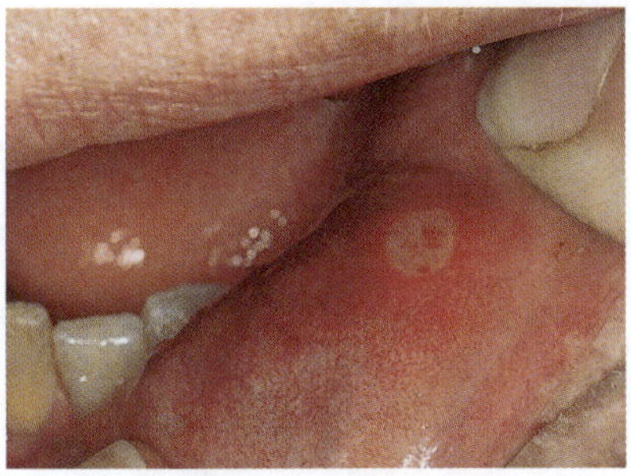

FIGURE 22-10. Aphthous ulcer on the labial mucosa of the lip.

See Table 22-2, Findings in the Pharynx, Palate, and Oral Mucosa.

Bright red edematous mucosa underneath a denture suggests *denture stomatitis* (denture sore mouth). There may be ulcers or papillary granulation tissue.

Gums and Teeth

Inspect the gingiva. Note the color of the gums, which are normally pink. Brown patches may be present, especially but not exclusively in dark-skinned individuals.

Redness of the gingiva suggests gingivitis; a black line might indicate lead poisoning.

Inspect the gum margins and the interdental papillae for swelling or ulceration.

The interdental papillae are swollen in *gingivitis.* See Table 22-3, Findings in the Gums and Teeth.

Inspect the teeth. Are any of them missing, discolored, misshapen, or abnormally positioned? To assess tooth, jaw, or facial pain, carefully palpate the teeth for looseness and the gums with your gloved thumb and index finger.

Roof and Floor of the Mouth and the Tongue

Inspect the roof of the mouth (hard palate). Note for any erythema, discoloration, nodules, ulcerations, or deformities.

Torus palatinus is a startling but benign midline lump (Fig. 22-11).

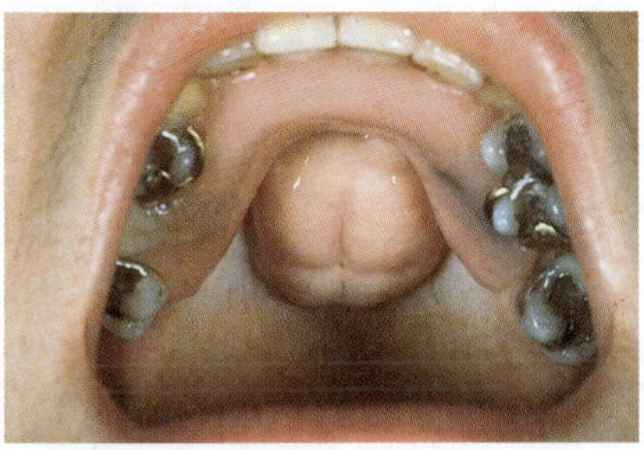

FIGURE 22-11. Torus palatinus.

Inspect the floor of the mouth. Note any white or reddened areas, nodules, or ulcerations.

Test the hypoglossal nerve (CN XII). Ask the patient to put out his or her tongue (Fig. 22-12). Inspect it for symmetry (Fig. 22-13).

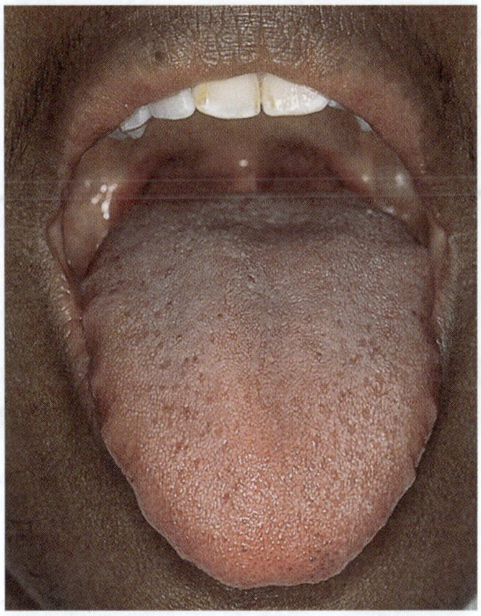

FIGURE 22-12. Inspecting the dorsum of the tongue.

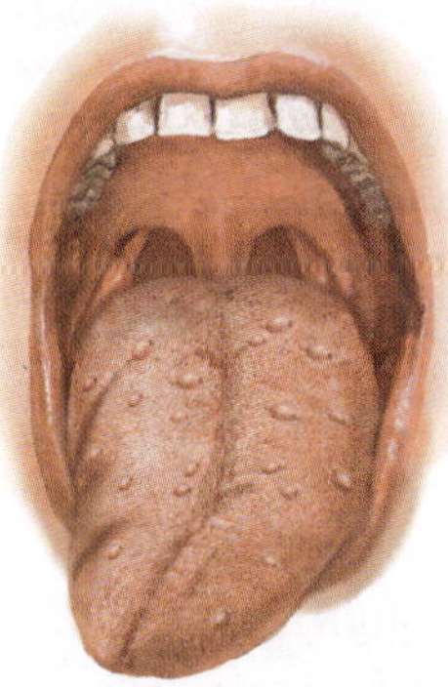

FIGURE 22-13. Asymmetric protrusion suggests a lesion of CN XII (tongue points toward the side of the lesion).

Inspect the tongue. Look especially at the sides and undersurface of the tongue, areas where cancer often develops. Note the color and texture of the dorsum of the tongue.

Men age >50 years, smokers, and heavy users of chewing tobacco and alcohol are at highest risk for cancers of the tongue and oral cavity, usually squamous cell carcinomas on the side or base of the tongue. Any persistent nodule or ulcer, red or white, is suspect, especially if indurated. These discolored lesions represent **erythroplakia** and **leukoplakia**, respectively, and should be biopsied.

Palpate any lesions with gloved hands. Ask the patient to protrude the tongue. With your right hand, grasp the tip of the tongue with a gauze and gently pull it toward the patient's left. Inspect the side of the tongue, and then palpate it with your gloved left hand, feeling for any induration (Figs. 22-14 and 22-15). Reverse the procedure for the other side.

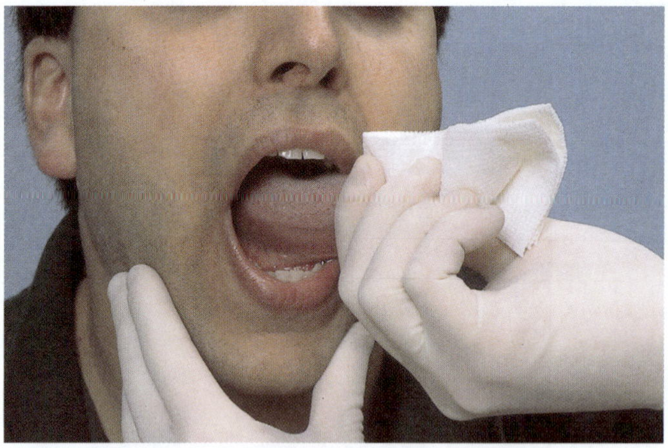

FIGURE 22-14. Grasping the tongue and inspecting its lateral margins.

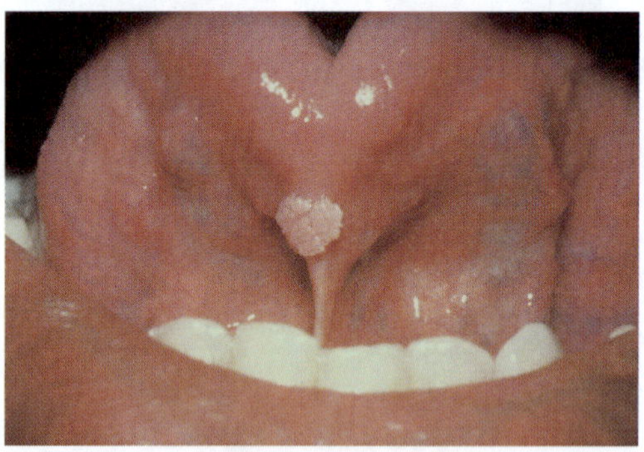

FIGURE 22-15. Carcinoma on the tongue. (Courtesy of the U.S. Department of Veteran's Affairs.)

Note the carcinoma on the left side of the tongue in Figure 22-15. Inspection and palpation remain the standard for detection of oral cancers.

See Table 22-4, Findings in or under the Tongue.

Pharynx

Visualize the pharynx. With the patient's mouth open but the tongue not protruded, ask the patient to say "ah" or yawn. This action helps you see the posterior pharynx well. Alternatively, you can press a tongue blade firmly down on the midpoint of the arched tongue—back far enough to visualize the pharynx but not so far that you cause gagging. Note the rise of the soft palate—a test of CN X (vagus nerve).

In CN X paralysis, the soft palate fails to rise and the uvula deviates to the opposite side and "points away from the lesion" (Fig. 22-16).

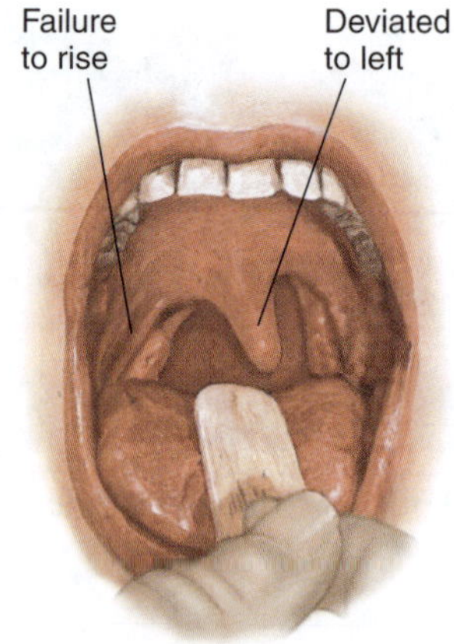

FIGURE 22-16. CN X paralysis with the uvula pointing away from the lesion.

Inspect the soft palate, anterior and posterior pillars, uvula, tonsils, and pharynx. Note their color and symmetry and look for exudate, swelling, ulceration, or tonsillar enlargement.

Asymmetric tonsils, particularly when associated with other symptoms, may signify an underlying pathology such as lymphoma.

If possible, palpate any suspicious area for induration or tenderness. Tonsils have crypts, or deep infoldings of squamous epithelium, where whitish spots of normal exfoliating epithelium may sometimes be seen. The size of the tonsils and any asymmetry should be noted.

Tonsillar exudates with a beefy red uvula are common in streptococcal pharyngitis but warrant rapid antigen-detection testing or throat culture for diagnosis.

Discard your tongue blade after use.

RECORDING YOUR FINDINGS

Initially you may use sentences to describe your findings; later you will use phrases. The style in the box contains phrases appropriate for most write-ups.

Recording the Head, Eyes, Ears, Nose, and Throat (HEENT) Examination

HEENT: Head—The skull is normocephalic/atraumatic (NC/AT). Hair with average texture. ***Eyes***—Visual acuity 20/20 bilaterally. Sclera white, conjunctiva pink. Pupils are 4 mm constricting to 2 mm, equally round and reactive to light and accommodations. Disc margins sharp; no hemorrhages or exudates, no arteriolar narrowing. ***Ears***—Acuity good to whispered voice. Tympanic membranes (TMs) with good cone of light. Weber midline. AC > BC. ***Nose***—Nasal mucosa pink,

(continued)

Recording the Head, Eyes, Ears, Nose, and Throat (HEENT) Examination (*continued*)

septum midline; no sinus tenderness. ***Throat (or Mouth)*—Oral mucosa pink, dentition good, tongue midline, tonsils absent bilaterally, pharynx without exudates or erythema.**

Neck—Trachea midline. Neck supple; thyroid isthmus palpable, lobes not felt.

Lymph Nodes—No cervical, axillary, epitrochlear, inguinal adenopathy.

OR

Head—The skull is normocephalic/atraumatic. Frontal balding. ***Eyes***—Visual acuity 20/100 bilaterally. Sclera white; conjunctiva injected. Pupils constrict 3 mm to 2 mm, equally round and reactive to light and accommodation. Disc margins sharp; no hemorrhages or exudates. Arteriolar-to-venous ratio (AV ratio) 2:4; no AV nicking. ***Ears***—Acuity diminished to whispered voice; intact to spoken voice. TMs clear. ***Nose***—Mucosa swollen with erythema and clear drainage. Septum midline. Tender over maxillary sinuses. ***Throat*—Oral mucosa pink, dental caries in lower molars, tongue midline, pharynx erythematous, bilateral tonsils enlarged, no exudates.**

Neck—Trachea midline. Neck supple; thyroid isthmus midline, lobes palpable but not enlarged.

Lymph Nodes—Submandibular and anterior cervical lymph nodes tender, 1 cm × 1 cm, rubbery and mobile; no posterior cervical, epitrochlear, axillary, or inguinal lymphadenopathy.

*These findings suggest pharyngitis or mild tonsillitis.

HEALTH PROMOTION AND COUNSELING: EVIDENCE AND RECOMMENDATIONS

Important Topics for Health Promotion and Counseling

- Oral health
- Oral and pharyngeal cancer

Oral Health

Clinicians should play an active role in promoting oral health because it is integral to an individual's overall health and well-being. Up to 19% of children aged 5 to 19 years have untreated caries, as do about 91% of adults aged 20 to 64 years. Dental caries among adults aged 35 to 64 years were higher (94% to 97%) compared with adults aged 20 to 34 years (82%). Nearly 19% of those older than age 60 years have no teeth at all (*edentulous*).

Nearly 50% of dentate adults aged 30 years and above have some form of periodontal disease, including 8.9% with severe disease. Risk factors for periodontal disease include low income, male sex at birth, smoking, diabetes, and poor oral hygiene.

To improve oral health, counsel patients to adopt daily hygiene measures. Use of fluoride-containing toothpastes reduces tooth decay, and brushing and flossing retard periodontal disease by removing bacterial plaques. Urge patients to seek dental care at least annually to receive the benefits of more specialized preventive care such as scaling, planing of roots, and topical fluorides.

Address diet and tobacco use. As with children, adults should avoid excessive intake of foods high in starches and refined sugars such as sucrose, which enhance attachment and colonization of cariogenic bacteria. Urge patients to avoid use of all tobacco products and to limit alcohol consumption to reduce risk of oral cancer.

Saliva cleanses and lubricates the mouth. Many medications reduce salivary flow, increasing risk for tooth decay, mucositis, and gum disease from xerostomia, especially for older adults. If medications cannot be changed, recommend drinking higher amounts of water and chewing sugarless gum. For those wearing dentures, recommend removal and cleaning each night to reduce bacterial plaque and risk of malodor. Regular massage of the gums relieves soreness and pressure from dentures on the underlying soft tissue.

Oral and Pharyngeal Cancer

Men are two to three times more likely than women to be diagnosed with and die from these cancers. Tobacco and alcohol account for about 75% of oral cavity cancers. Sexually transmitted human papillomavirus (HPV) infection is an increasingly important cause of oropharyngeal cancers (lesions of the tonsils, oropharynx, and base of tongue), accounting for about 70% of cases. Risk for oropharyngeal HPV infection is associated with age (highest prevalence among those 35 to 39 years, 50 to 54 years); male gender; a higher number of sexual partners; sexual behaviors (oral sex); and tobacco and marijuana smoking. The primary screening test for these cancers is a thorough examination of the oral cavity.

TABLE 22-1. Abnormalities of the Lips

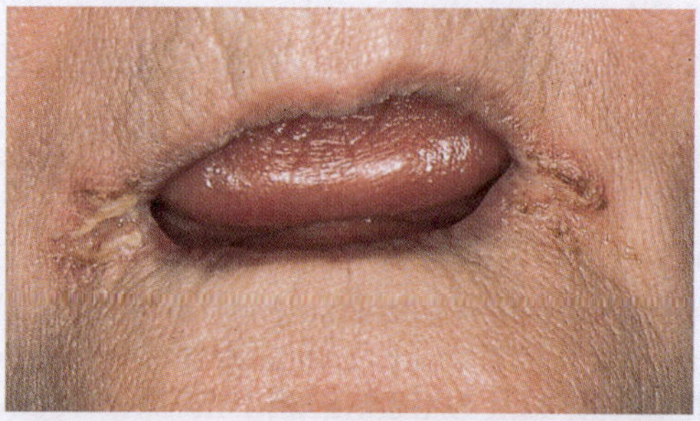

Angular Cheilitis

Angular cheilitis starts with softening of the skin at the angles of the mouth, followed by fissuring. It may be due to nutritional deficiency or, more commonly, overclosure of the mouth, seen in people with no teeth or with ill-fitting dentures. Saliva wets and macerates the infolded skin, often leading to secondary infection with *Candida*, as seen here.

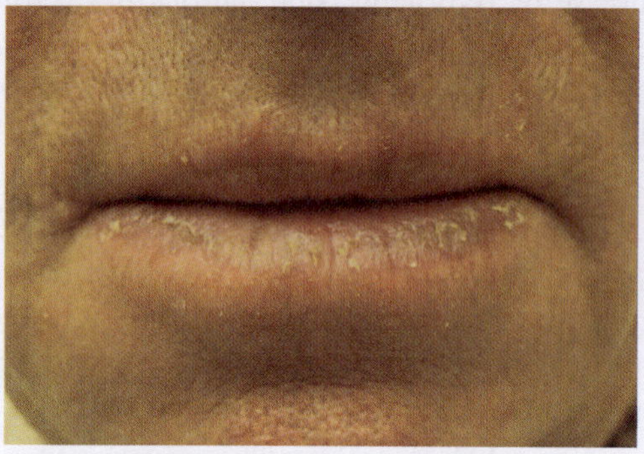

Actinic Cheilitis

Actinic cheilitis is a precancerous condition that results from excessive exposure to sunlight and affects primarily the lower lip. Fair-skinned men who work outdoors are most often affected. The lip loses its normal redness and may become scaly, somewhat thickened, and slightly everted. Solar damage predisposes to squamous cell carcinoma of the lip, so examine these skin lesions carefully.

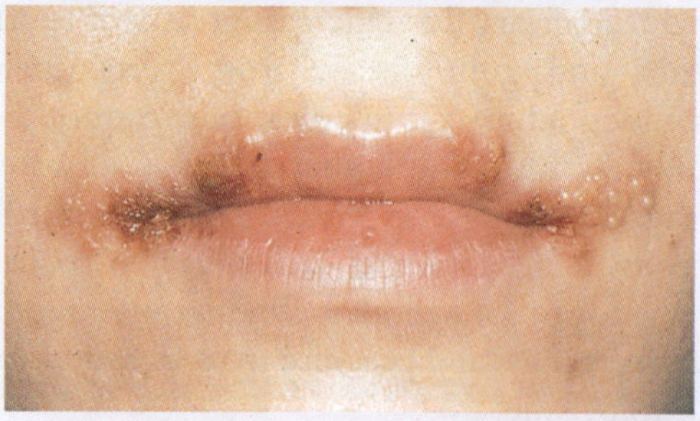

Herpes Simplex (*Cold Sore, Fever Blister*)

Herpes simplex virus (HSV) produces recurrent and painful vesicular eruptions of the lips and surrounding skin. A small cluster of vesicles first develops. As these break, yellow-brown crusts form. Healing takes 10–14 days. Both new and erupted vesicles are visible here.

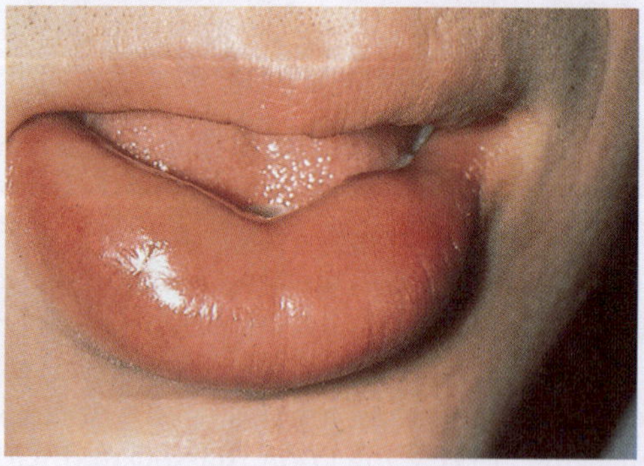

Angioedema

Angioedema is a localized subcutaneous or submucosal swelling caused by leakage of intravascular fluid into interstitial tissue. Two types are common. When vascular permeability is triggered by mast cells in allergic and NSAID reactions, look for associated urticaria and pruritus. These are uncommon in angioedema from bradykinin and complement-derived mediators, the mechanism in ACE-inhibitor reactions. Angioedema is usually benign and resolves within 24–48 hrs. It can be life threatening when it involves the larynx, tongue, or upper airway or develops into anaphylaxis.

(continued)

TABLE 22-1. Abnormalities of the Lips *(Continued)*

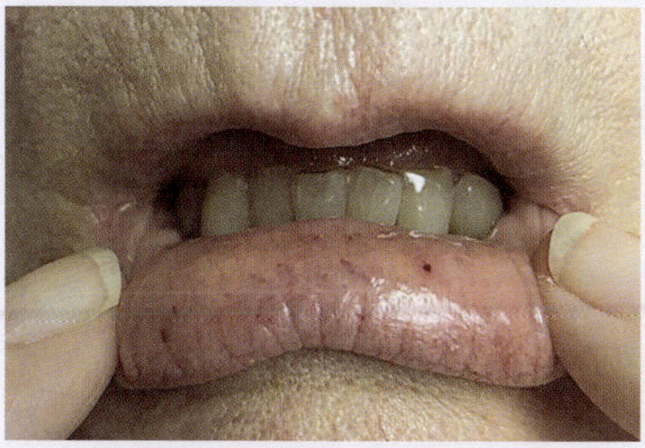

Hereditary Hemorrhagic Telangiectasia (Osler–Weber–Rendu syndrome)

Multiple small red spots on the lips strongly suggest hereditary hemorrhagic telangiectasia, an autosomal dominant endothelial disorder causing vascular fragility and arteriovenous malformations (AVMs). Telangiectasias are also visible on the oral mucosa, nasal septal mucosa, and fingertips. Nosebleeds, gastrointestinal bleeding, and iron deficiency anemia are common. AVMs in the lungs and brain can cause life-threatening hemorrhage and embolic disease.

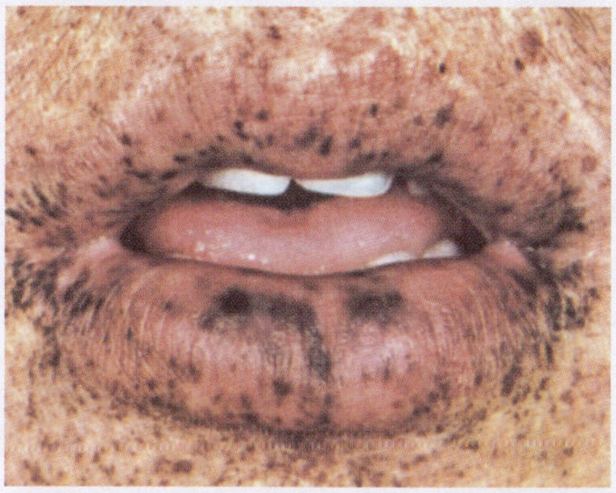

Peutz–Jeghers Syndrome

Look for prominent small brown pigmented spots in the dermal layer of the lips, buccal mucosa, and perioral area. These spots may also appear on the hands and feet. In this autosomal dominant syndrome, these characteristic skin changes accompany numerous intestinal polyps. The risk of gastrointestinal and other cancers ranges from 40–90%. Note that these spots rarely appear around the nose and mouth.

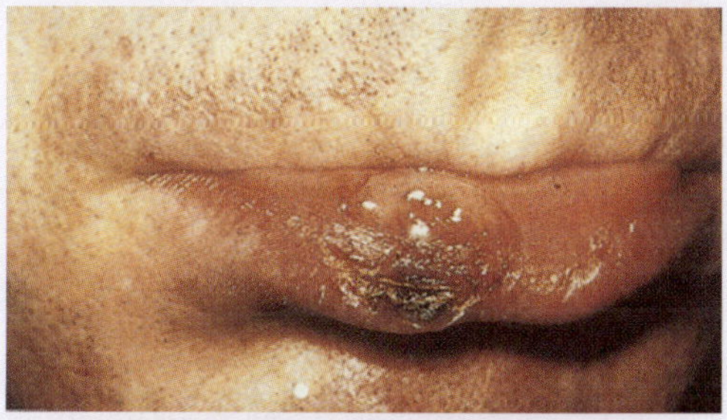

Chancre of Primary Syphilis

This ulcerated papule with an indurated edge usually appears after 3–6 wks of incubating infection from the spirochete *Treponema pallidum*. These lesions may resemble a carcinoma or crusted cold sore. Similar primary lesions are common in the pharynx, anus, and vagina but may escape detection since they are painless, nonsuppurative, and usually heal spontaneously in 3–6 wks. Wear gloves during palpation since these chancres are infectious.

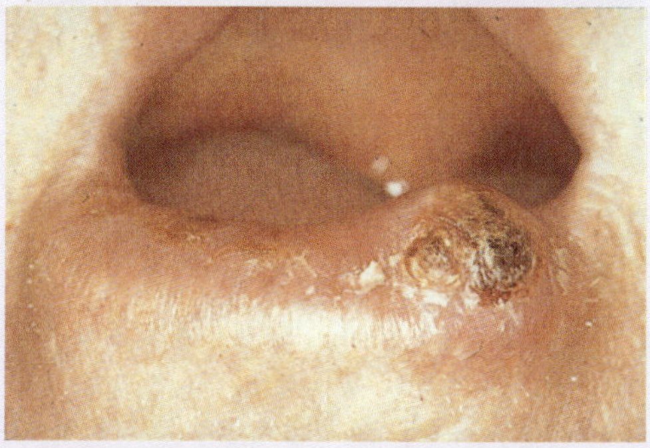

Carcinoma of the Lip

Like actinic cheilitis, squamous cell carcinoma usually affects the lower lip. It may appear as a scaly plaque, as an ulcer with or without a crust, or as a nodular lesion, as illustrated here. Fair skin and prolonged exposure to the sun are common risk factors.

Sources of photos: *Angular Cheilitis, Herpes Simplex, Angioedema*—Neville BW et al. *Color Atlas of Clinical Oral Pathology.* Lea & Febiger; 1991; *Actinic Cheilitis*—Langlais RP, Miller CS. *Color Atlas of Common Oral Diseases.* Lea & Febiger; 1992. Used with permission; *Hereditary Hemorrhagic Telangiectasia*—Mansoor N. *Frameworks for Internal Medicine.* Wolters Kluwer; 2019, Figure 40-2; *Peutz-Jeghers Syndrome*—Robinson HBG, Miller AS. *Colby, Kerr, and Robinson's Color Atlas of Oral Pathology.* 5th ed. JB Lippincott; 1990; *Chancre of Syphilis*—Reprinted from Wisdom A. *A Colour Atlas of Sexually Transmitted Diseases.* 2nd ed. Wolfe Medical Publications; 1989. Copyright © 1989 Elsevier. With permission; *Carcinoma of the Lip*—Reprinted from Tyldesley WR. *A Colour Atlas of Orofacial Diseases.* 2nd ed. Wolfe Medical Publications; 1991. Copyright © 1991 Elsevier. With permission.

TABLE 22-2. Findings in the Pharynx, Palate, and Oral Mucosa

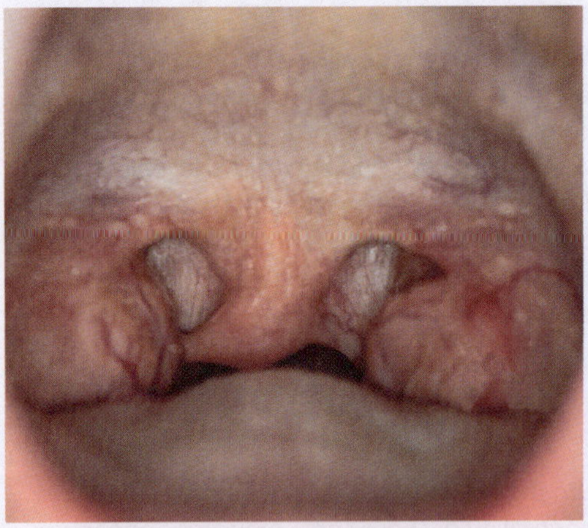

Large Normal Tonsils

Normal tonsils may be large without being infected, especially in children. They may protrude medially beyond the pillars and even to the midline. Here they slightly obscure the pharynx. Their color is pink.

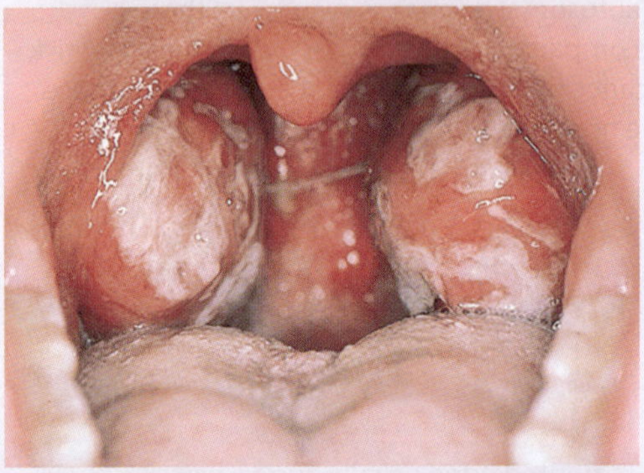

Exudative Tonsillitis

This red throat has thick white exudates on the tonsils. This, together with fever and enlarged cervical nodes, increases the probability of *group A streptococcal infection* or *infectious mononucleosis.* Anterior cervical lymph nodes are usually enlarged in the former, posterior nodes in the latter.

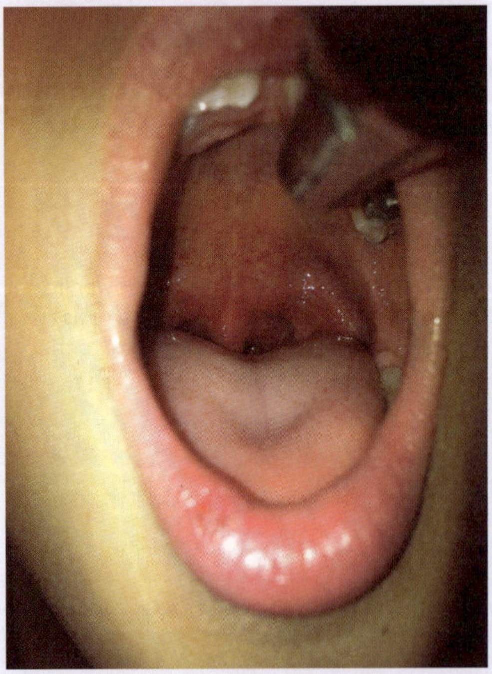

Pharyngitis

This photo shows a reddened throat without exudate. Redness and vascularity of the pillars and uvula are mild to moderate.

(continued)

TABLE 22-2. Findings in the Pharynx, Palate, and Oral Mucosa *(Continued)*

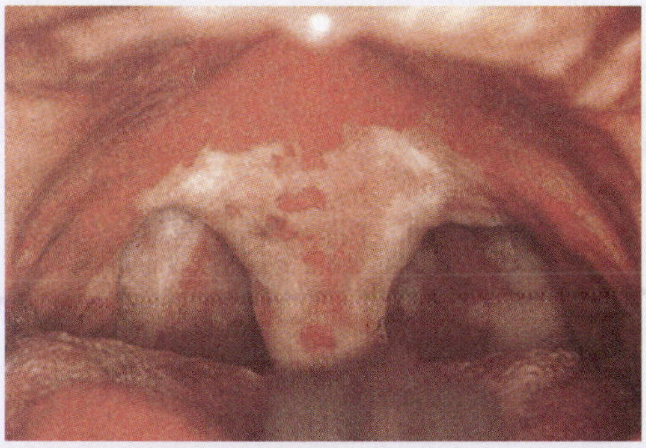

Diphtheria

Diphtheria, an acute infection caused by *Corynebacterium diphtheriae,* is now rare but still important. Prompt diagnosis may lead to life-saving treatment. The throat is dull red, and a gray exudate (pseudomembrane) is present on the uvula, pharynx, and tongue. The airway may become obstructed. Prompt diagnosis may lead to life-saving treatment.

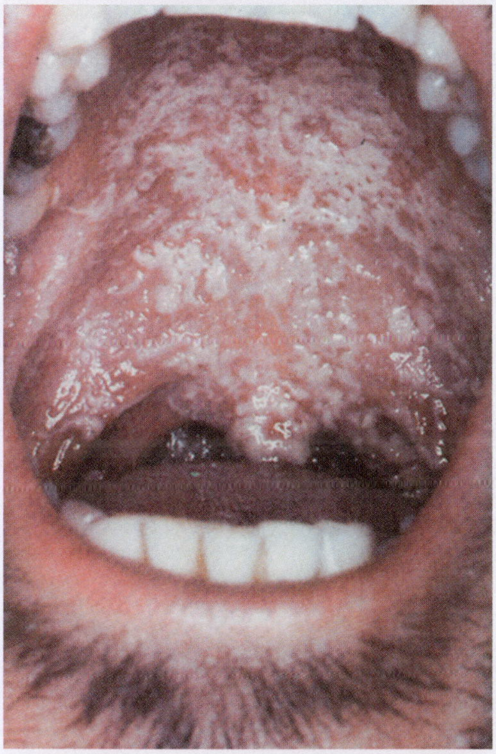

Thrush on the Palate (Candidiasis)

Thrush is a yeast infection from *Candida* species. Shown here on the palate, it may appear as cream-colored or bluish white pseudomembranous patches on the tongue, mouth, or pharynx. Thick, white plaques are somewhat adherent to the underlying mucosa. Predisposing factors include prolonged treatment with antibiotics or corticosteroids and immunocompromised status.

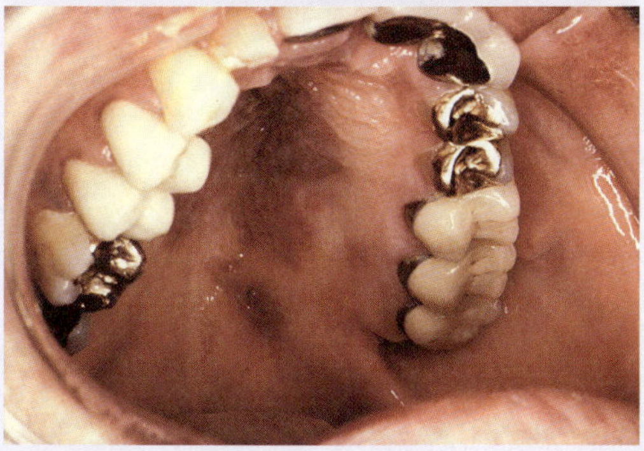

Kaposi Sarcoma in AIDS

The deep purple color of these lesions suggests Kaposi sarcoma (KS), a low-grade vascular tumor associated with human herpesvirus 8 (HHV-8). These nontender lesions may be raised or flat. About a third of patients with KS have lesions in the oral cavity; other affected sites are the gastrointestinal tract and the lungs.

(continued)

TABLE 22-2. Findings in the Pharynx, Palate, and Oral Mucosa *(Continued)*

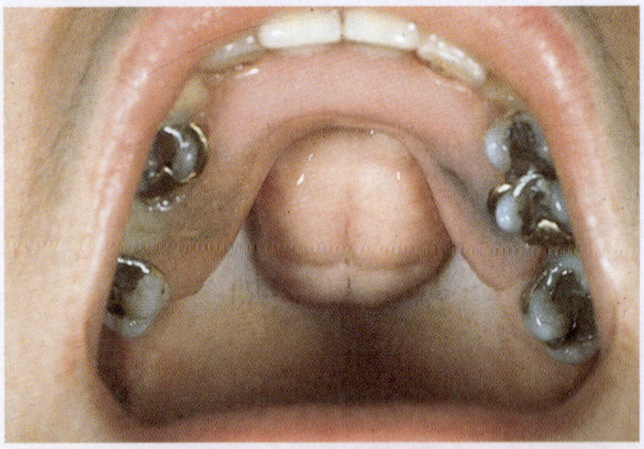

Torus Palatinus

A torus palatinus is a midline bony growth in the hard palate that is fairly common in adults. Its size and lobulation vary. Although alarming at first glance, it is harmless. In this example, an upper denture has been fitted around the torus.

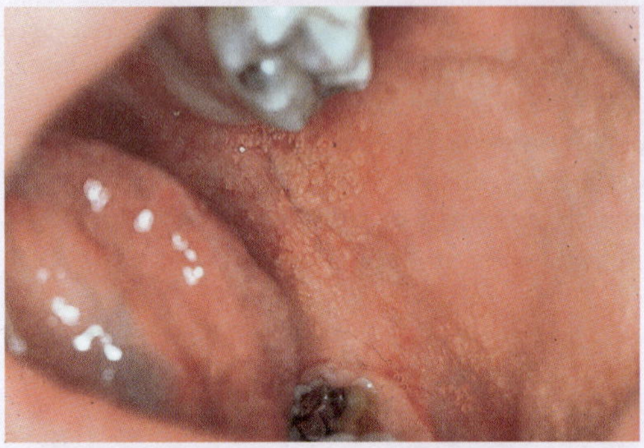

Fordyce Spots (*Fordyce Granules*)

Fordyce spots are normal sebaceous glands that appear as small yellowish spots in the buccal mucosa or on the lips. Here they are seen best anterior to the tongue and lower jaw. These spots are usually not numerous.

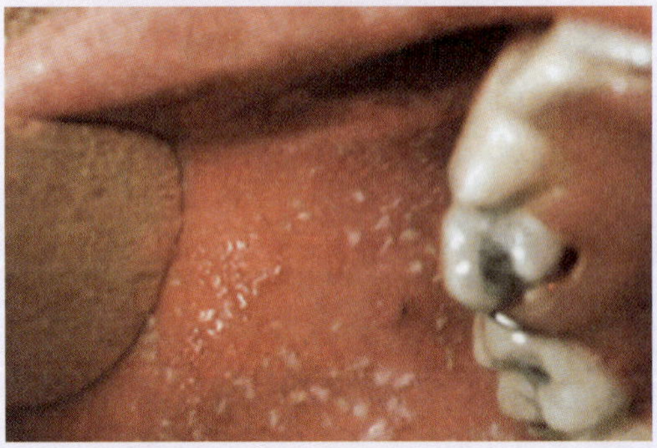

Koplik Spots

Koplik spots are an early sign of measles (*rubeola*). Search for small white specks that resemble grains of salt on a red background. They usually appear on the buccal mucosa near the first and second molars. In this photo, look also in the upper third of the mucosa. The rash of measles appears within a day.

(*continued*)

TABLE 22-2. Findings in the Pharynx, Palate, and Oral Mucosa *(Continued)*

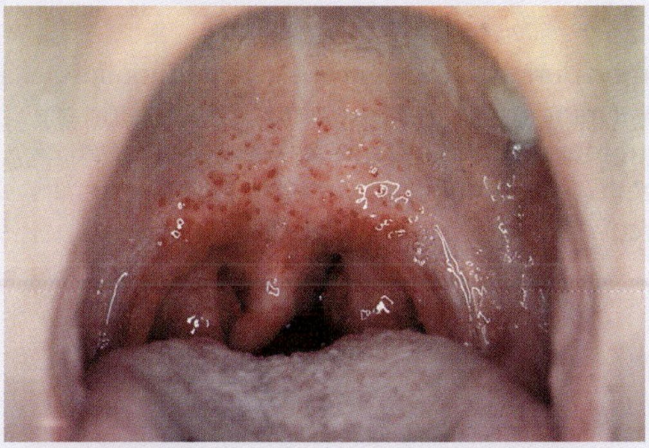

Petechiae

Petechiae are small red spots caused by blood that escapes from capillaries into the tissues. Petechiae in the buccal mucosa, as shown, are often caused by accidentally biting the cheek. Oral petechiae may be due to infection or decreased platelets, and trauma.

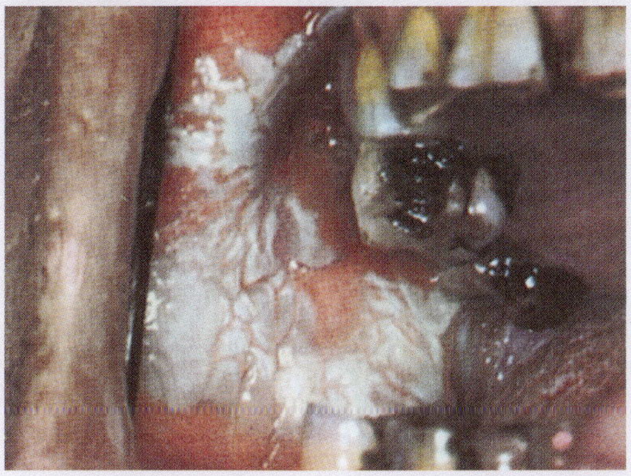

Leukoplakia

A thickened white patch (*leukoplakia*) may occur anywhere in the oral mucosa. The extensive example shown on this buccal mucosa resulted from frequent chewing of tobacco, a local irritant. This benign reactive process of the squamous epithelium may lead to cancer and should be biopsied. Another risk factor is human *papillomavirus* infection.

Sources of photos: *Large Normal Tonsils*—Moore KL et al. *Essential Clinical Anatomy.* 5th ed. Wolters Kluwer; 2015, Figure 9-23A; *Exudative Tonsillitis*—Hatfield NT, Kincheloe C. *Introductory Maternity & Pediatric Nursing.* 4th ed. Wolters Kluwer; 2018, Figure 41-12; *Pharyngitis*—Courtesy of Naline Lai, MD; *Diphtheria*—Harnisch JP et al. *Ann Intern Med.* 1989,111(1).71–82. Copyright © 1989 American College of Physicians. All Rights Reserved. Reprinted with the permission of American College of Physicians, Inc.; *Thrush on the Palate (Candidiasis)*—Engleberg NC et al. *Schaechter's Mechanisms of Microbial Disease.* 5th ed. Wolters Kluwer; 2013, Figure 48-2; *Kaposi Sarcoma in AIDS*—From the Centers for Disease Control Public Health Image Library, photo credit Sol Silverman, Jr., DDS; ID #6071; *Fordyce Spots*—Neville BW et al. *Color Atlas of Clinical Oral Pathology.* Lea & Febiger; 1991; *Koplik Spots*—Harvey RA, Cornelissen CN. *Microbiology.* 3rd ed. Wolters Kluwer Health/Lippincott Williams & Wilkins; 2013:313; *Petechiae*—From the Centers for Disease Control Public Health Image Library, photo credit Heinz F. Eichenwald, MD; ID #3185; *Leukoplakia*—Robinson HBG, Miller AS. *Colby, Kerr, and Robinson's Color Atlas of Oral Pathology.* 5th ed. JB Lippincott; 1990.

TABLE 22-3. Findings in the Gums and Teeth

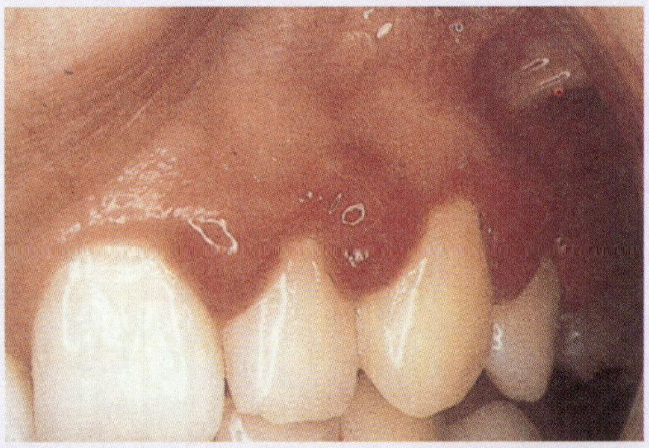

Marginal Gingivitis

Marginal gingivitis is common during adolescence, early adulthood, and pregnancy. The gingival margins are reddened and swollen, and the interdental papillae are blunted, swollen, and red. Brushing the teeth often makes the gums bleed. *Plaque*—the soft white film of salivary salts, protein, and bacteria that covers the teeth and leads to gingivitis—is not readily visible.

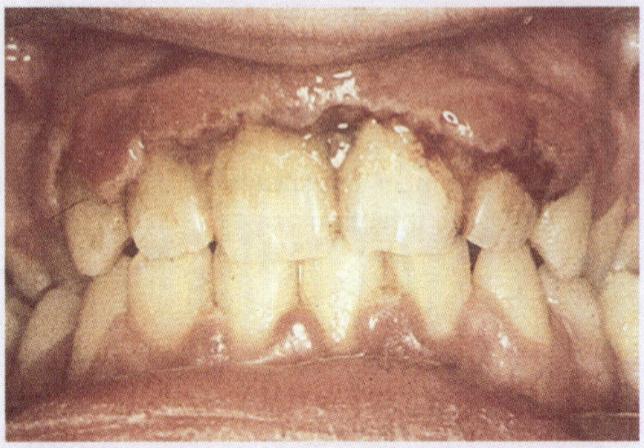

Acute Necrotizing Ulcerative Gingivitis

This uncommon form of gingivitis occurs suddenly in adolescents and young adults and is accompanied by fever, malaise, and enlarged lymph nodes. Ulcers develop in the interdental papillae. Then the destructive (necrotizing) process spreads along the gum margins, where a grayish pseudomembrane develops. The red, painful gums bleed easily; the breath is foul.

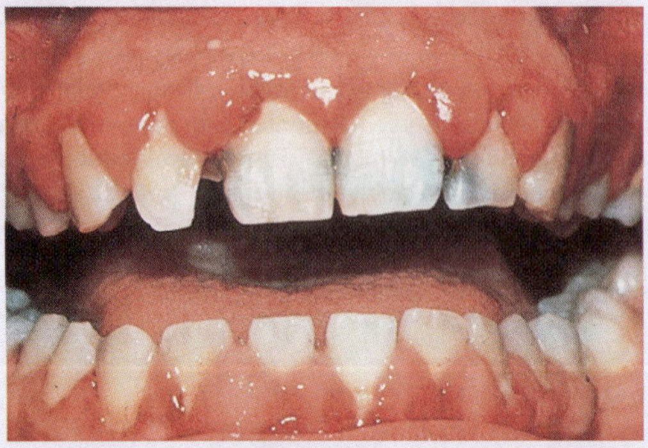

Gingival Hyperplasia

Gums enlarged by hyperplasia are swollen into heaped-up masses that may even cover the teeth. The redness of inflammation may coexist, as in this example. Causes include phenytoin therapy (as in this case), puberty, pregnancy, and leukemia.

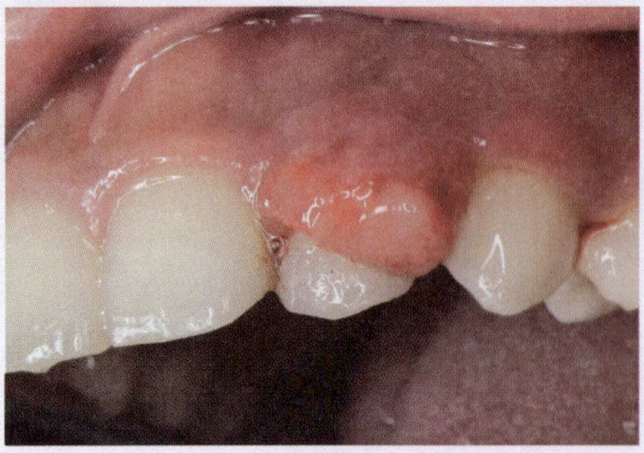

Pregnancy Tumor (Pregnancy Epulis or Pyogenic Granuloma)

Red purple papules of granulation tissue form in the gingival interdental papillae, in the nasal cavity, and sometimes on the fingers. They are red, soft, painless, and usually bleed easily. They occur in 1–5% of pregnancies and usually regress after delivery. Note the accompanying gingivitis.

(*continued*)

TABLE 22-3. Findings in the Gums and Teeth *(Continued)*

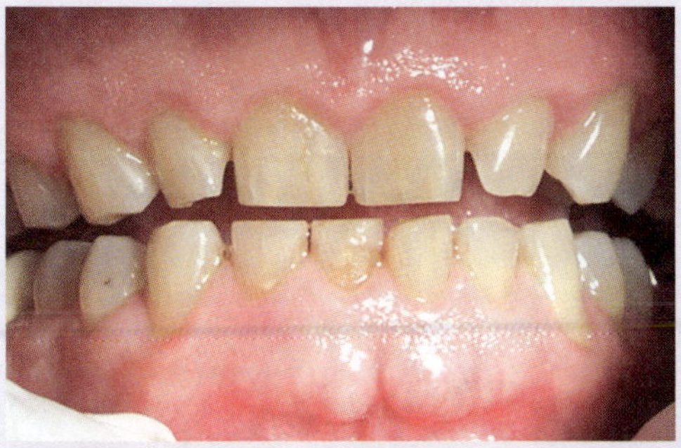

Attrition of Teeth; Recession of Gums

In many older adults, the chewing surfaces of the teeth are worn down by repetitive use so that the yellow-brown dentin becomes exposed—a process called *attrition*. *Recession of the gums,* which exposes the roots of the teeth may occur, giving a "long in the tooth" appearance.

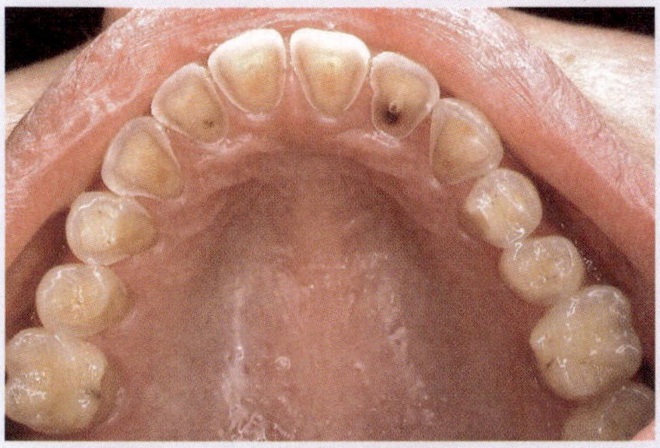

Erosion of Teeth

Severe erosion is evident on the lingual surfaces of these maxillary teeth, especially the anterior teeth exposing the yellow-brown dentin. This pattern of tooth destruction typically results from recurrent regurgitation of stomach contents as in bulimia and in persons with severe acid reflux.

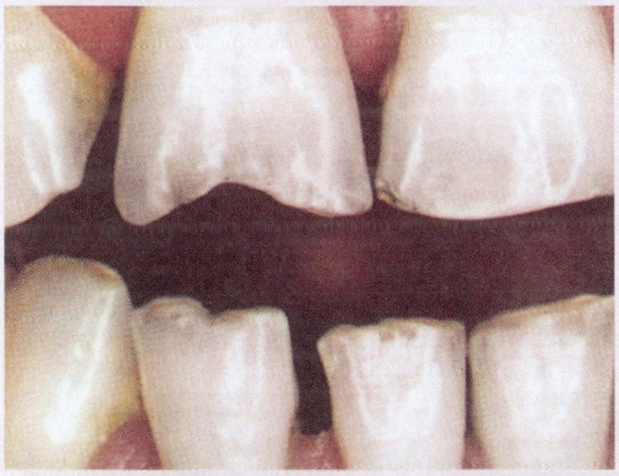

Abrasion of Teeth with Notching

The biting surface of the teeth may become abraded or notched by recurrent trauma, such as holding nails or opening bobby pins between the teeth. Unlike Hutchinson teeth, the sides of these teeth show normal contours; size and spacing of the teeth are unaffected.

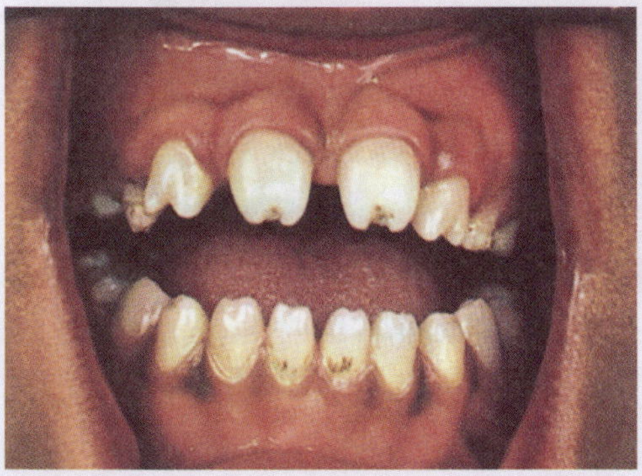

Hutchinson Teeth in Congenital Syphilis

Hutchinson teeth are smaller and more widely spaced than normal and are notched on their biting surfaces. The sides of the teeth taper toward the biting edges. The upper central incisors of the permanent (not the deciduous) teeth are most often affected. These teeth are a sign of congenital syphilis.

Sources of photos: *Marginal Gingivitis, Acute Necrotizing Ulcerative Gingivitis*—Reprinted from Tyldesley WR. *A Colour Atlas of Orofacial Diseases.* 2nd ed. Wolfe Medical Publications; 1991. Copyright © 1991 Elsevier. With permission; *Gingival Hyperplasia*—Courtesy of Dr. James Cottone; *Pregnancy Tumor*—Shutterstock photo by Kasama Kanpittaya; *Attrition of Teeth*—DeLong L, Burkhart N. *General and Oral Pathology for the Dental Hygienist.* 2nd ed. Wolters Kluwer; 2013, Figure 21-1; *Erosion of Teeth*—Timby BK, Smith NE. *Introductory Medical-Surgical Nursing.* 12th ed. Wolters Kluwer; 2018, Fig. 70-2B; *Abrasion of Teeth, Hutchinson Teeth*—Robinson HBG, Miller AS. *Colby, Kerr, and Robinson's Color Atlas of Oral Pathology.* 5th ed. JB Lippincott; 1990.

TABLE 22-4. Findings in or under the Tongue

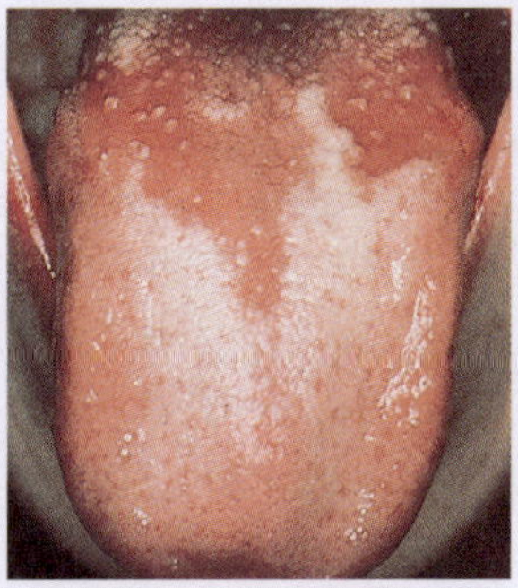

Geographic Tongue. In this benign condition, the dorsum shows scattered smooth red areas denuded of papillae. Together with the normal rough and coated areas, they give a map-like pattern that changes over time.

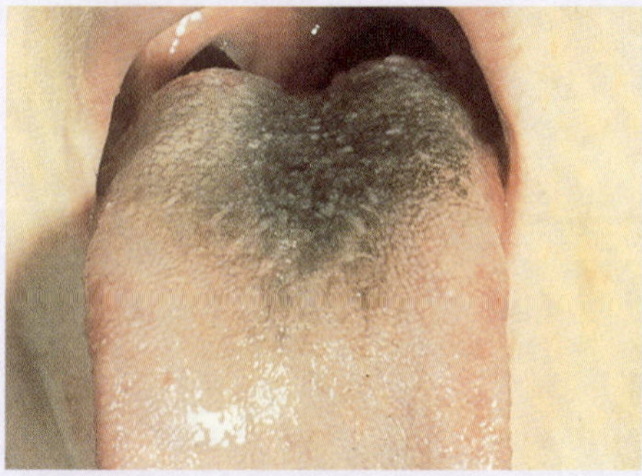

Black Hairy Tongue. Note the "hairy" yellowish to brown and black hypertrophied and elongated papillae on the tongue's dorsum. This benign condition is associated with *Candida* and bacterial overgrowth, antibiotic therapy, and poor dental hygiene. It also may occur spontaneously.

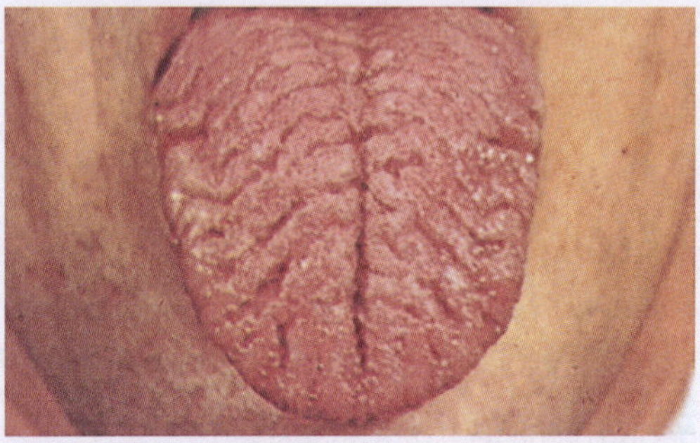

Fissured Tongue. Fissures appear with increasing age, sometimes termed *furrowed tongue.* Food debris may accumulate in the crevices and become irritating, but a fissured tongue is benign.

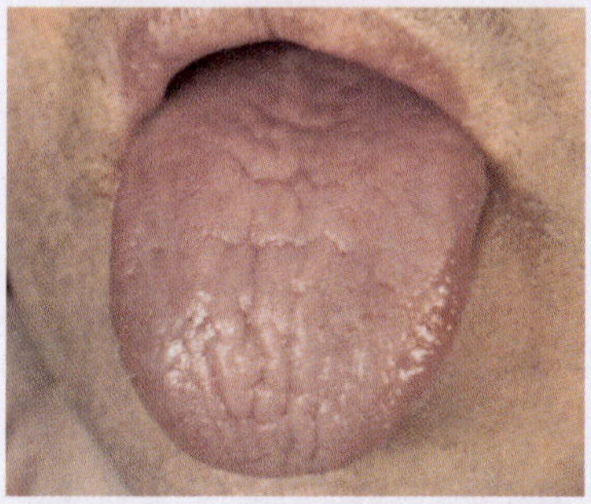

Smooth Tongue (*Atrophic Glossitis*). A smooth and often sore tongue that has lost its papillae, sometimes just in patches, suggests a deficiency in riboflavin, niacin, folic acid, vitamin B_{12}, pyridoxine, or iron, or treatment with chemotherapy.

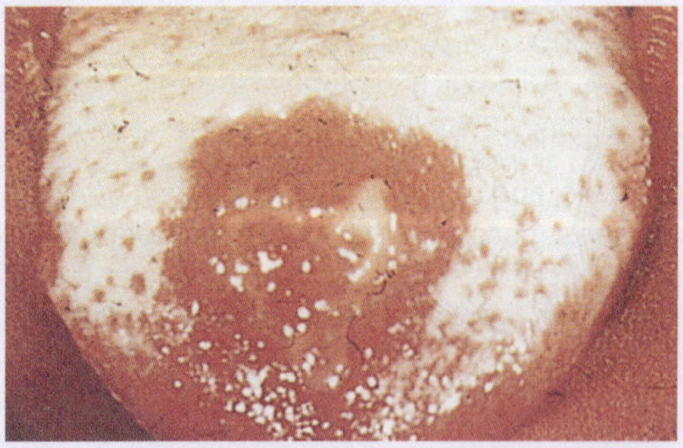

Candidiasis. Note the thick white coating from *Candida* infection. The raw red surface is where the coat was scraped off. Infection may also occur without the white coating. It is seen in immunosuppression from chemotherapy or prednisone therapy.

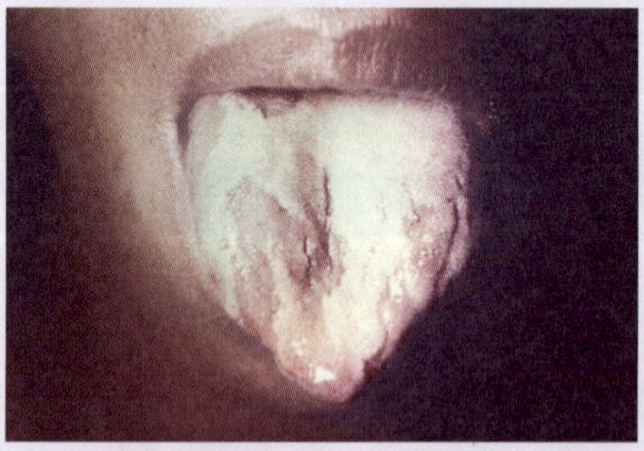

Oral Hairy Leukoplakia. These whitish raised asymptomatic plaques with a feathery or corrugated pattern occur most often on the sides of the tongue. Unlike candidiasis, these areas cannot be scraped off. This condition is caused by Epstein–Barr virus infection and is seen in HIV and AIDS infection.

(*continued*)

TABLE 22-4. Findings in or under the Tongue *(Continued)*

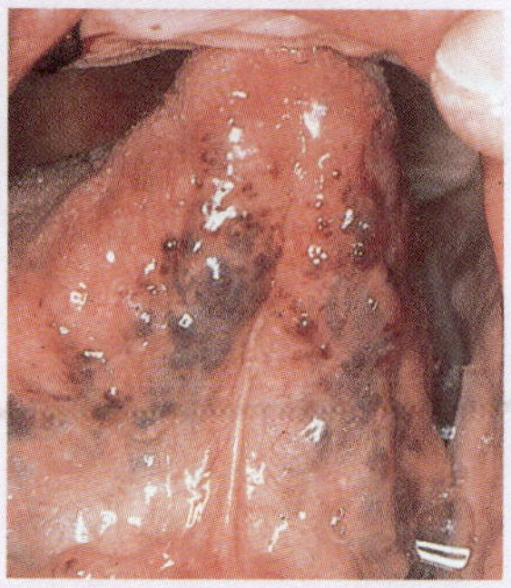

Varicose Veins. Small purplish or blue-black round swellings appear under the tongue with age. These dilatations of the lingual veins have no clinical significance.

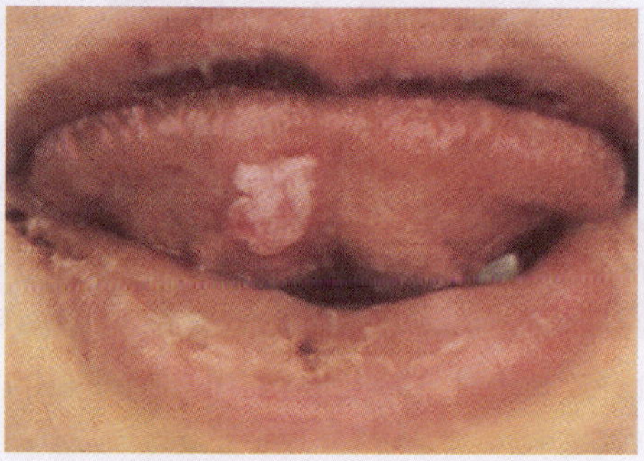

Mucous Patch of Syphilis. This painless lesion of secondary syphilis is highly infectious. It is slightly raised, oval, and covered by a grayish membrane. It may be multiple and occur elsewhere in the mouth.

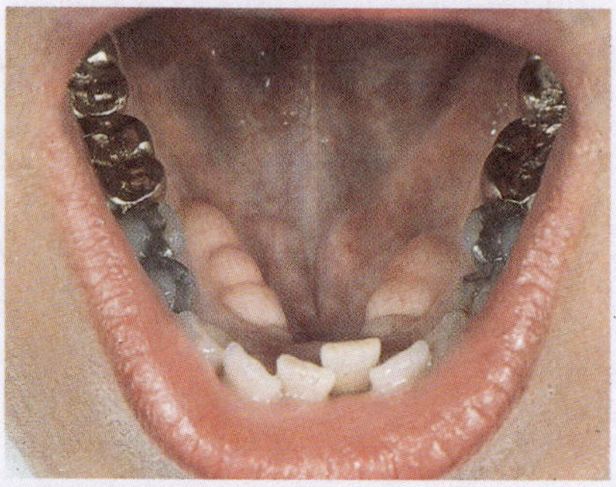

Tori Mandibularis. Rounded bony growths on the inner surfaces of the mandible are typically bilateral, asymptomatic, and harmless.

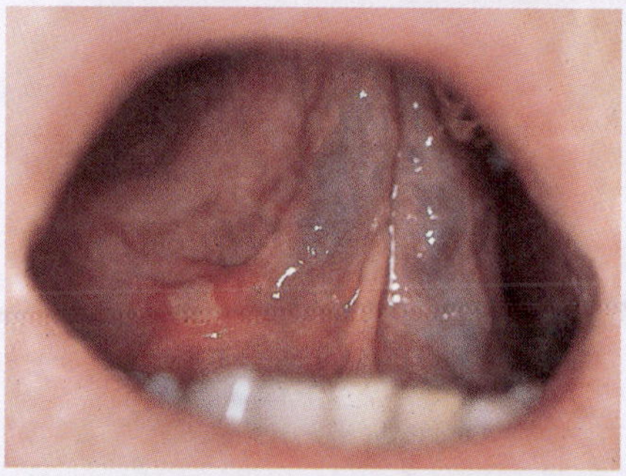

Aphthous Ulcer (*Canker Sore*). A painful, shallow whitish-gray oval ulceration surrounded by a halo of reddened mucosa. It may be single or multiple and may also occur on the gingiva and oral mucosa. It heals in 7–10 days, but may recur, as in Behçet disease.

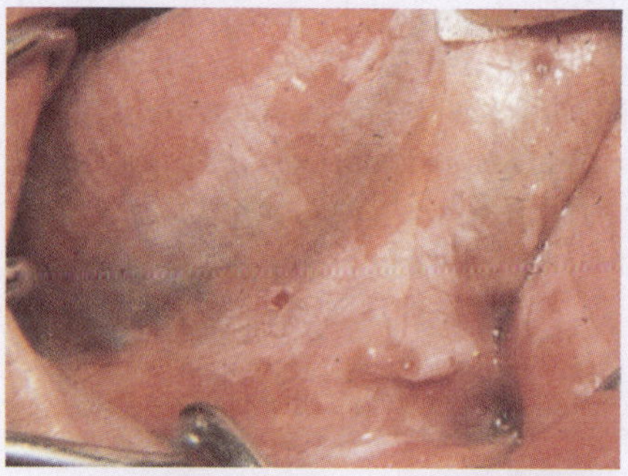

Leukoplakia. With this persisting painless white patch in the oral mucosa, the undersurface of the tongue appears painted white. Patches of any size raise the possibility of squamous cell carcinoma and require biopsy.

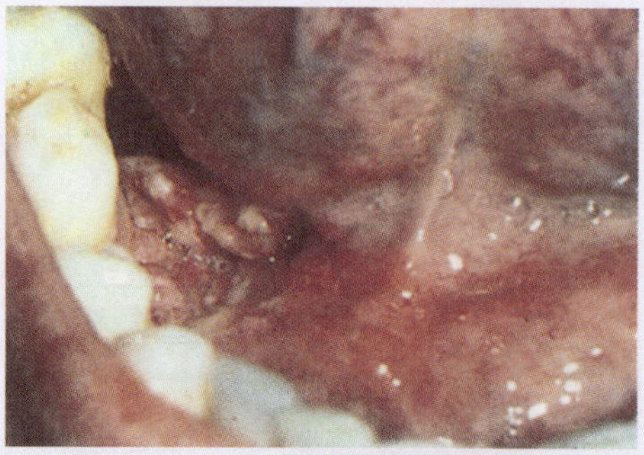

Carcinoma, Floor of the Mouth. This ulcerated lesion is in a common location for carcinoma. Medially, note the reddened area of mucosa, called *erythroplakia,* which is suspicious for malignancy and should be biopsied.

Sources of photos: *Fissured Tongue, Candidiasis, Mucous Patch, Leukoplakia, Carcinoma*—Robinson HBG, Miller AS. *Colby, Kerr, and Robinson's Color Atlas of Oral Pathology.* 5th ed. JB Lippincott; 1990; *Smooth Tongue*—*Jensen S. Nursing Health Assessment: A Best Practice Approach.* 3rd ed. Wolters Kluwer; 2019, Figure 15-25; *Geographic Tongue*—From the Centers for Disease Control Public Health Image Library; ID #16520; *Oral Hairy Leukoplakia*—From the Centers for Disease Control Public Health Image Library, photo credit Sol Silverman, Jr., DDS; ID #6061; *Varicose Veins*—Neville B et al. *Color Atlas of Clinical Oral Pathology.* Lea & Febiger; 1991.

UNIT 3 Special Populations

CHAPTER 23

Children: Infancy through Adolescence

This chapter highlights clinical assessments for each pediatric age group: newborns or neonates (0–30 days of age), infants (1 month–1 year), preschool children (1–5 years), school-aged children (6–11 years), and adolescents (12–18 years), as shown in Figures 23-1 to 23-3. It begins with general principles of development and key components of health promotion. Each age group is then covered in separate sections, with relevant discussions of history taking, development surveillance, techniques of examination, and health promotion and counseling.

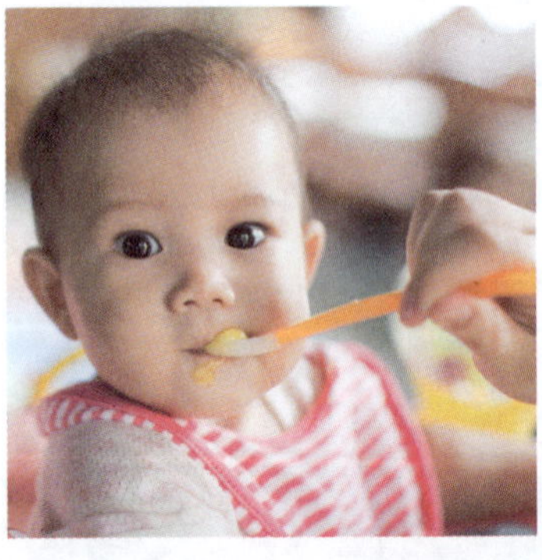

FIGURE 23-1. Infants have surprising abilities.

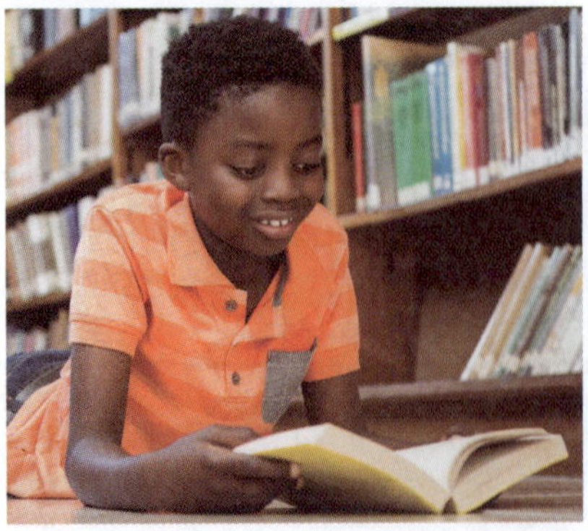

FIGURE 23-2. A drive for independence appears in school-aged children.

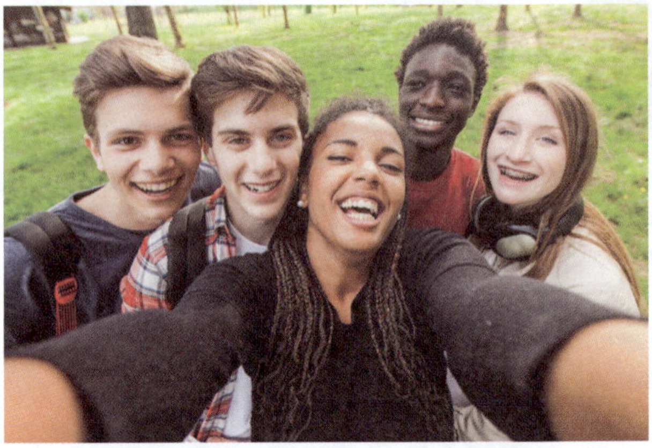

FIGURE 23-3. Social interactions become important in adolescence.

Inexperienced examiners are often intimidated when approaching a tiny baby or an upset child, especially under the watchful eyes of anxious parents. When examining infants and children, the sequence should vary according to the child's age and comfort level. *Perform less invasive maneuvers early and potentially distressing maneuvers near the end of the examination.* For example, auscultate the heart and lungs early and examine the ears and mouth and palpate the abdomen near the end. *If the child reports pain in one area, examine that area last.* Although it is initially challenging, you will come to enjoy almost all pediatric encounters.

GENERAL PRINCIPLES OF CHILD DEVELOPMENT

Childhood is a period of remarkable physical, cognitive, and social growth—by far the greatest in a person's lifetime. Within a few short years, children's weight increases 20-fold, they acquire sophisticated language and reasoning, develop complex social interactions, and progress toward mature adults (Fig. 23-4 and Box 23-1). Understanding the normal physical, cognitive, and social development of children facilitates effective interviews and physical examinations and is the basis for distinguishing normal from abnormal findings.

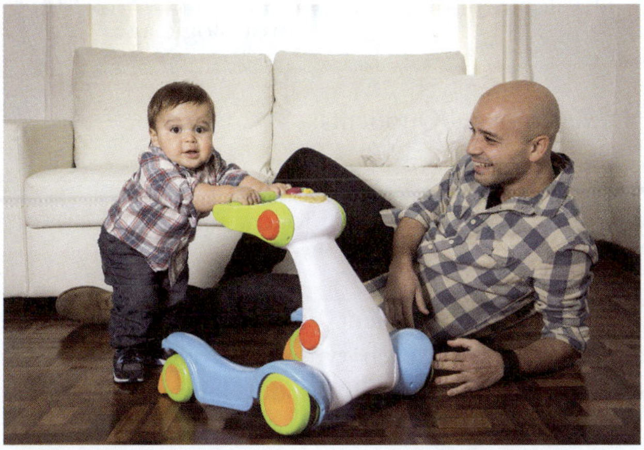

FIGURE 23-4. Parents can enhance the development of their children through play. (Used with permission from Shutterstock. By Marcos Mesa Sam Wordley.)

Box 23-1. Four Principles of Child Development

1. Child development proceeds along a predictable pathway.
2. The range of normal development is wide.
3. Various physical, social, and environmental factors, as well as diseases, can affect child development and health.
4. The child's developmental level affects how you conduct the history and physical examination.

- Principle #1: *Child development proceeds along a predictable pathway* governed by the maturing brain. You can measure age-specific milestones and use them to characterize development as normal or abnormal (i.e., typical or atypical). Because your health care visit and physical examination take place at one point in time, you need to determine where the child fits along a developmental trajectory. Milestones are achieved in a predictable order. *Loss of milestones is always concerning.*
- Principle #2: *The range of normal (typical) development is wide.* Children mature at different rates. Each child's physical, cognitive, and social development should fall within a broad developmental range.
- Principle #3: *Various physical, social, and environmental factors, as well as diseases, can affect child development and health.* For example, chronic illnesses, child abuse, and adverse childhood experiences (ACEs) can all cause detectable physical abnormalities or alter the rate and course of development. Additionally, *children with physical or cognitive disabilities may not follow the expected age-specific developmental trajectory* (Fig. 23-5).

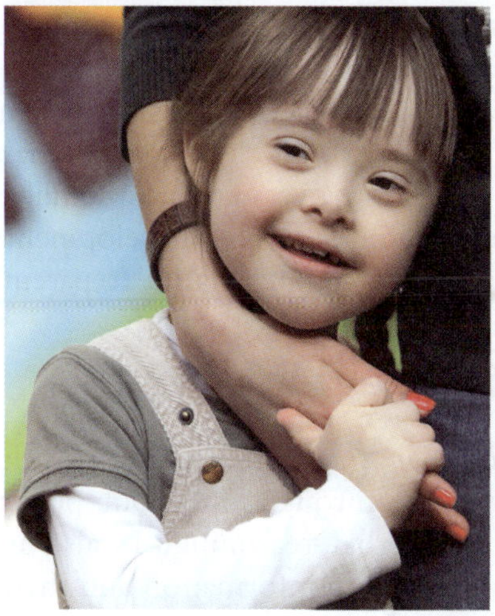

FIGURE 23-5. Child development is affected by many factors including genetics (this child has Down syndrome).

- Principle #4: *The child's developmental level affects how you conduct the clinical history and physical examination.* For example, interviewing a 5-year-old is fundamentally different than interviewing an adolescent. Both the order and style differ from the adult examination. Before performing a history and physical examination, attempt to ascertain the child's approximate developmental level and adapt your evaluation to that level. An understanding of typical child development helps you achieve these tasks.

SURVEILLANCE OF DEVELOPMENT

A child's development proceeds along a predictable pathway. They progress through milestones in an orderly fashion, attaining these functions in a clear and sequential process. Developmental assessment is the process of mapping the status of a child compared with other children of similar age. Information about the child's development and behavior are gathered from multiple sources which can involve direct observation of the child's behavior as well as expressed concerns from parents and others.

In general, pediatric clinicians assess five critical domains of development: *physical* including *gross* and *fine motor skills, cognitive (or problem-solving), language (communication),* and *social–emotional domains.*

Physical Development

Physical development encompasses both *gross* and *fine motor* abilities. Examples of gross motor skills include walking, sitting, or transferring from one position to another. Manipulation of objects with the hands in order to eat, draw, or play are examples of fine motor skills. Milestones in these two developmental domains are what most parents and caregivers are most familiar with. Any delay in achieving a physical development milestone often prompts visits to clinicians due to parental concern.

Cognitive Development

Cognitive development is a measure of the child's ability to problem solve through intuition, perception, and verbal and nonverbal reasoning. It also involves the child's ability to retain information and then to apply it when appropriate.

Language Development

Language development consists of the ability of a child to articulate, receive, and express information. It also involves nonverbal modes of communication such as waving and head nodding. A child develops these skills through their ability to put words together to express a thought which can also be influenced by their interaction with their environment.

Social and Emotional Development

Social and emotional development encompasses the child's ability to form and maintain relationships. It also measures their responsiveness to the presence of others. It involves the formation of self-help skills in various activities of daily living, such as feeding, dressing, and toileting.

Standardized screening instruments are used to assess the developmental domains. These screening instruments should be used as adjuncts to a comprehensive developmental examination. Several developmental screening instruments have been tested widely and validated in many nations and include the Ages and Stages Questionnaire (ASQ), the Early Language Milestone Scale (ELM Scale-2), the Modified Checklist for Autism in Toddlers (MCHAT), the Parents' Evaluation of Developmental Status (PEDS), and the Survey of Well-Being of Young Children (SWYC).

If a cooperative child fails items on a standardized screening instrument, evelopmental delay is possible, necessitating more precise testing and evaluation.

Developmental Quotient

A normative measure of development is the developmental quotient:

$$\text{Development quotient} = \frac{\text{Development age}}{\text{Chronologic age}} \times 100$$

Developmental Quotients:

- >85 = Normal
- 70–85 = Possibly delayed; follow-up needed
- <70 = Delayed

Assess the development of an infant or child using standard scales for each type of development. Assign to each child a gross motor developmental quotient, a fine motor developmental quotient, a cognitive developmental quotient, and so forth. Importantly, these estimates are never a perfect assessment of a child's development or potential because both can change over time (see Box 23-2 for an example of its application).

Box 23-2. Case Examples of Gross and Fine Motor Developmental Quotients

Gross Motor Development	Fine Motor Development
A 12-month-old child who is just pulling to stand (gross motor developmental age of 9 months), cruising (10 months), and walking when both hands are held (10 months) has a gross motor developmental age of 10 months. This child's gross motor developmental quotient is: $\left(\frac{10}{12} \times 100\right) = 83$ This child is in the gray zone, is likely to do well without intervention, but requires close follow-up.	A 12-month-old child can transfer objects from hand to hand (a fine motor developmental age of 6 months), rake objects into his palm (7 months), and pull things (7 months). He cannot hold blocks in each hand and does not have thumb and finger grasp (8–9 months). He has normal primitive reflexes (most absent), increased tone, scissoring of legs when held, spasticity, and delays on the gross motor part of a standardized developmental screening instrument. This child's fine motor developmental quotient is: $\left(\frac{7}{12} \times 100\right) = 58$ This child is delayed in fine motor development and has signs of *cerebral palsy.*

KEY COMPONENTS OF HEALTH PROMOTION

Prevention and health promotion at a young age can result in improved health outcomes for decades (Figs. 23-6 to 23-8).

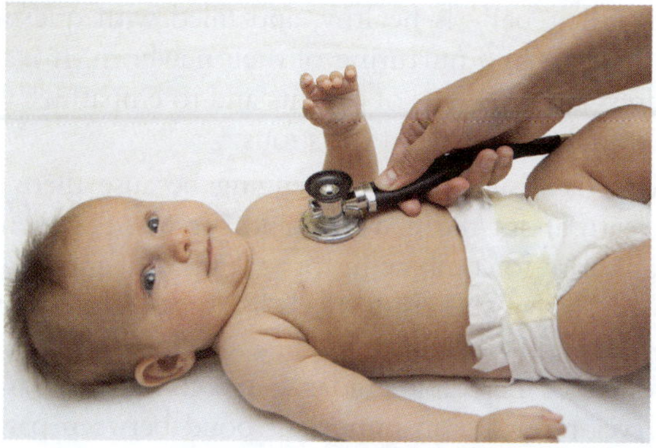

FIGURE 23-6. Clinician examining an infant. (Used with permission from Shutterstock. By Olha Birieva.)

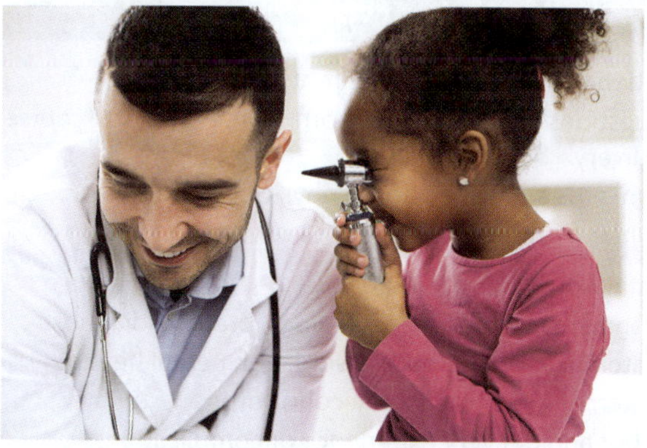

FIGURE 23-7. Clinician with a 3-year-old child. (Used with permission from Shutterstock. By didesign021.)

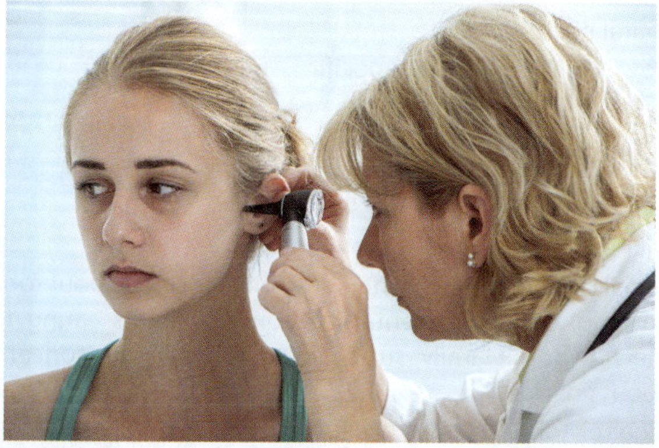

FIGURE 23-8. Clinician with an adolescent. (Used with permission from Shutterstock. By Alexander Raths.)

Current concepts of health promotion include the detection and prevention of disease as well as active promotion of the well-being of children and their families spanning physical, cognitive, emotional, and social health.

Every interaction with a child and family is an opportunity for health promotion. From the interview to the physical examination, think of your interactions as an opportunity for two important tasks: the detection of clinical problems and the promotion of health. Capitalize on the examination to offer age-appropriate guidance about the child's development. Provide suggestions about reading, conversing, playing music, and optimizing opportunities for gross and fine motor development. Advise parents about upcoming developmental stages and strategies to encourage their child's development. Parents are the major agents of health promotion for children and your advice is implemented through them.

Integrate explanations of your physical findings with health promotion. Provide advice about expected maturational changes or how health behaviors can affect physical findings (e.g., exercise may reduce blood pressure and prevent obesity). Be sure to demonstrate the relationship between healthy lifestyles and physical health

Childhood immunizations are a mainstay for health promotion and have been heralded as the most significant clinical achievement in public health worldwide. The childhood immunization schedule is updated yearly.

Age-specific screening procedures are performed at specific ages. These include newborn genetic and metabolic screening, newborn screening for hearing and critical congenital heart disease (oximetry), and (if appropriate) newborn screening for bilirubin, growth parameters and developmental screening and behavioral/mental health screening at all ages, blood pressure screening after age 3 years, BMI screening after age 2 years, and vision and hearing screening at key ages.

Anticipatory guidance is a major component of the pediatric visit. Key areas cover a broad range of topics, from clinical to developmental, social, and emotional health (Box 23-3).

NEWBORNS AND INFANTS

The first year of life, or infancy, is divided into the neonatal period (the first 28 days) and the post neonatal period (29 days to 1 year).

Box 23-3. Key Components of Pediatric Health Promotion

1. Age-appropriate developmental achievement of the child
   - Physical (maturation, growth, puberty)
   - Motor (gross and fine motor skills)
   - Cognitive (developmental milestones, language, school performance)
   - Emotional (self-regulation, mood, self-efficacy, self-esteem, independence)
   - Social (social competence, self-responsibility, integration with family and community, peer interactions)
2. Health supervision visits
   - Periodic assessment of physical, developmental, socio-emotional, and oral health
   - More frequent visits for children with special health care needs
3. Integration of physical examination findings with health promotion
4. Immunizations
5. Screening procedures
6. Oral health
7. Anticipatory guidance
   - Healthy habits
   - Nutrition and healthy eating
   - Safety and prevention of injury
   - Physical activity
   - Sexual development and sexuality
   - Self-responsibility, efficacy, and healthy self-esteem
   - Family relationships (interactions, strengths, supports)
   - Positive parenting strategies
   - Reading aloud with the child
   - Emotional and mental health
   - Oral health
   - Recognition of illness
   - Sleep
   - Screen time
   - Prevention of risky behaviors
   - School and vocation
   - Peer relationships
   - Community interactions
8. Partnership among health care provider, child/adolescent, and family

HEALTH HISTORY: GENERAL APPROACH

The newborn visit, which is generally performed within the first 12 to 24 hours after delivery, is a critical opportunity for the health care provider to engage with the family, learn about the newborn's family and environment, understand key aspects of the pregnancy, bond with the family, and observe the family's interactions with the newborn. It is also a time to demonstrate the newborns' abilities, and to role-model interactions with the newborn. Remember that although parents will be elated with the birth of their newborn, they will also be exhausted, anxious about whether their baby is healthy, and filled with questions about the care and nurturing of their newborn. It is vital to address any concerns of parents and to empathize with their natural anxieties and questions.

The initial visit can be challenging because there is a lot to learn about the newborn and parents. Experienced clinicians learn to combine history-taking with anticipatory guidance, so that the history feels like a conversation with new parents. An empathetic, calm, and helpful clinician can be a source of incredible guidance and comfort to parents and serves to create an important bond between parents and clinicians. Important parts of the health history are shown in Box 23-4.

Box 23-4. Key Components of the Health History for the Newborn Visit

Questions and concerns by parents
- Questions about the newborn, home, prenatal course or delivery
- Concerns about newborn's physical features
- Concerns and questions about newborn care

Prenatal history, labor, and delivery
- Pregnancy history, complications, prenatal diagnoses
- Maternal and paternal physical and mental health
- Maternal use of tobacco, alcohol, drugs
- Labor and delivery experience or complications
- Prior pregnancies and siblings

Neonatal course prior to the visit
- Health and well-being of mother, other family members
- Plans for breastfeeding or bottle feeding (or both)

Neonatal history
- How it is going overall, specific issues of concern
- Cultural beliefs

Family history
- Comprehensive history if time permits

Social history
- Social determinants (living situation, concerns about food, housing, utilities, parental relationship, adults caring for the newborn, family support, family violence, concerns about finances)
- Alcohol, tobacco, drug use (even if not during pregnancy)
- Any social concerns by parents
- Siblings, other family members, babysitter

(continued)

Box 23-4. Key Components of the Health History for the Newborn Visit (*continued*)

Parents' observation of their newborn's behavior and activity
- What the newborn has been able to do so far
- Level of activity, attachment

Feeding and nutrition
- Type of feeding, how feeding is going
- Details of feeding (breast or bottle)

Sleeping, stooling, urination
- Frequency and color of stools and urine
- Sleeping duration, falling asleep

Safety
- Car safety seats
- Safe sleep

Anticipatory guidance about newborn care
- Illness prevention
- Dressing, protection against heat, pets, safe home environment
- Care of newborn's body (umbilicus, penis including circumcision decision, etc.)
- Upcoming visits, when to call for advice

Source: Adapted from Bright Futures.

SURVEILLANCE OF DEVELOPMENT

Physical Development

Newborns have surprising abilities, such as fixing upon and following human faces. Neurologic development progresses centrally to peripherally. Thus, newborns learn head control before trunk control and use of arms and legs before use of hands and fingers (Fig. 23-9).

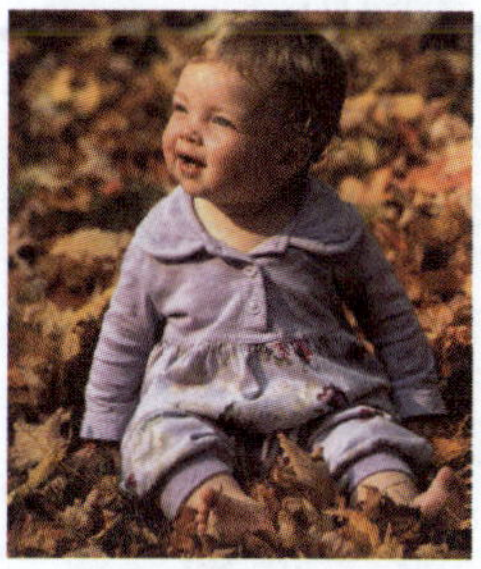

FIGURE 23-9. Sitting up is a developmental milestone among infants.

Physical growth during infancy is faster than at any other age (Box 23-5). By 1 year, the infant's birth weight

Box 23-5. Developmental Milestones: Birth to 12 Months

Age	Gross Motor	Fine Motor	Language	Social–Emotional
1 month	Lifts chin up in prone position Turns head up when prone	Hands fisted	Makes throaty noises Startles to sound	Discriminates parents' voice Follows face
4 months	Sits with support No head lag Rolls from front to back	Hands predominantly open Reaches for objects	Laughs out loud Stops crying to soothing voice	Social smile
6–7 months	Sits propped on hands Lateral protection Bounces when held	Transfers objects from hand to hand Reaches out with one hand Feeds self cracker	Babbles, consonant sounds Understands "no"	Enjoys reflection in mirror Looks from object to parent and back when wanting help
9 months	Pulls to stand Bear walks Begins creeping	Pincer grasp Bangs two cubes together	Says "mama" nonspecifically Imitates sounds Orients to name	Follows a point Enjoys peek a boo Develops stranger anxiety
12 months	Stands independently Starts taking first steps	Scribbles Hold crayon Makes tower with two cubes	Says one word with meaning Points to get objects Follows one-step commands with gestures	Shows objects to parents to share

Sources: Scharf R et al. *Pediatr Rev.* 2016;37(1); Gerber RJ et al. *Pediatr Rev.* 2010;31(7):267–277; Wilks T et al. *Pediatr Rev.* 2010;31(9):364–367; Gerber RJ et al. *Pediatr Rev.* 2011;32(12):533–536.

should have tripled and height increased by 50% from weight and height at birth.

Activity, exploration, and environmental manipulation contribute to learning. By 3 months, typical infants lift their heads and clasp their hands. By 6 months, they roll over, reach for objects, turn to voices, and possibly sit with support. With increasing peripheral coordination, infants reach for objects, transfer them from hand to hand, crawl, stand by holding on, and play with objects by banging and grabbing. At 1 year, children may be standing and even trying to walk (Fig. 23-10).

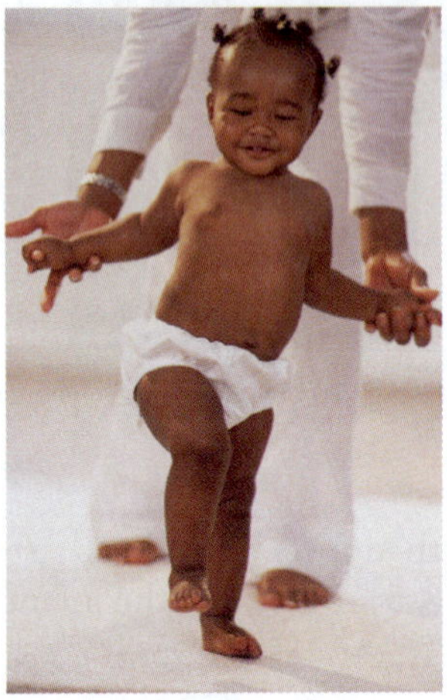

FIGURE 23-10. Children often take their first steps after 1 year.

Cognitive and Language Development

Infants reach for objects and learn cause and effect (e.g., shaking a rattle produces sound), object permanence, and use of toys. By 9 months, they imitate sounds, orient to their own name and they may recognize the examiner as a stranger deserving wary cooperation. Infants seek comfort from parents during examinations. They will actively manipulate reachable objects such as your stethoscope. Language development proceeds from cooing at 2 months, to babbling at 6 months, to saying one to three words by 1 year.

If infants are not making age-appropriate sounds and language, consider testing for a hearing deficit.

Social and Emotional Development

Understanding of self and family also matures. By a month of age infants can recognize parents' voice and follow a face, and by 4 months they smile back at you. Social tasks include bonding, attachment to caregivers, and trust that caregivers will meet their needs.

Temperaments vary. Some infants are predictable, adaptable, and respond positively to new stimuli; others are less so and respond intensely or negatively. Because environment affects social development, observe the infant's interactions with caregivers. An infant's cognitive and social–emotional development are often assessed together with the comprehensive neurologic examination.

An infant or toddler who has developmental skills that plateau or are out of sequence needs evaluation for an underlying developmental disability such as *autism* or *cerebral palsy*.

PHYSICAL EXAMINATION: GENERAL APPROACH

Newborns

Examining newborns immediately after birth is important for determining general condition, developmental status, abnormalities in gestational development, and any congenital abnormalities. A comprehensive pediatric examination is generally performed within 24 hours of birth (Fig. 23-11). This examination may reveal diseases of cardiac, respiratory, or neurologic origin. Listen to the anterior thorax with your stethoscope, palpate the abdomen, and inspect the head, face, oral cavity, extremities, genitalia, and perineum.

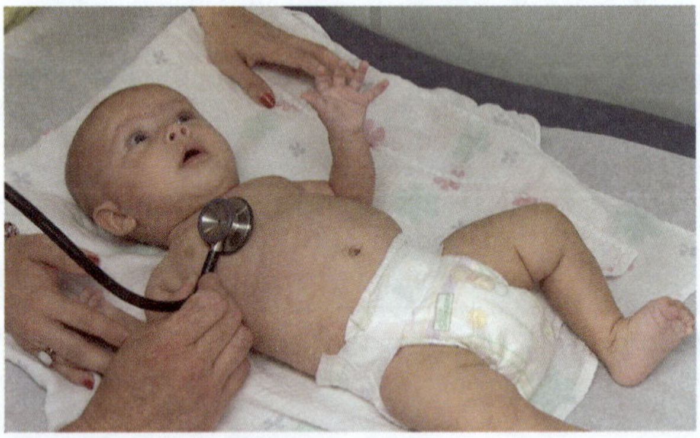

FIGURE 23-11. Physical examination starts soon after birth.

Subsequent physical examinations of newborns occur at regular intervals or when the infant is ill. If possible, do the physical examination in front of the parents so that they can interact with you and ask questions (Box 23-6). This is an excellent opportunity to educate parents about their baby and what their baby can do.

Some abnormalities on physical examination are actually identified by parents who have noted an abnormality in their infant.

Therefore, asking parents to point out any concerns or questions may help identify subtle abnormalities. Some examples include birthmarks, skin tags, asymmetries, dimples along the lower spine, or abnormal movements.

Box 23-6. Tips for Examining Newborns

- Examine the newborn in the presence of the parents.
- Swaddle and then undress the newborn as the examination proceeds.
- Dim the lights and rock the newborn to encourage the eyes to open.
- Observe feeding, if possible, particularly breastfeeding.
- Demonstrate calming maneuvers to parents (e.g., swaddling).
- Observe and teach parents about transitions as the newborn arouses.
- A typical sequence for the examination of the newborn:
    - Careful observation before (and during) the examination
    - Heart
    - Lungs
    - Head, neck, and clavicles
    - Ears and mouth
    - Hips
    - Abdomen and genitourinary system
    - Lower extremities, upper extremities, back
    - Eyes, whenever they are spontaneously open or at end of examination
    - Skin, as you go along
    - Neurologic system

Studies by Dr. T. Berry Brazelton and others have demonstrated the wide range of abilities in newborns (Box 23-7). Parents will be delighted by these abilities. You can demonstrate some of these abilities during your physical examination. For example, you can show how newborns quiet down as you speak softly to them and how they follow you with their eyes if you move your face slowly back and forth while talking to them and smiling.

Asymmetric movements of the arms or legs (if persistent and substantial) may suggest *central* or *peripheral neurologic deficits, birth injury* (such as a fractured clavicle or brachial plexus injury), or *congenital anomalies.*

Parents may have questions about their newborn's physical appearance, so stating normal findings as you go can be reassuring. Observe parents' interacting with their newborn and reinforce positive parenting behaviors. If a mother has concerns about breastfeeding technique, observe how well the newborn latches on and sucks. Breastfeeding is physiologically and psychologically ideal, but many mothers need help and support at first. Be empathetic to the normal stress of breastfeeding. Early detection of difficulties and anticipatory guidance can promote and sustain breastfeeding.

Newborns are most responsive 1 to 2 hours after a feeding, when they are neither too satiated and sleepy nor too hungry. Start with the newborn swaddled and comfortable. Then, for gradual stimulation and arousal, undress the newborn as the examination proceeds. If the newborn becomes agitated, with the parents'

Box 23-7. What a Newborn Can Do

Core Elements

Newborns use all five senses. For example, they will look at human faces and turn to a parent's voice.

Newborns are unique individuals. Marked differences exist in temperaments, personality, behavior, and learning.

Newborns interact dynamically with caregivers—a two-way street!

Examples of Complex Newborn Behavior

Habituation	Ability to selectively and progressively shut out negative stimuli (e.g., a repetitive sound)
Attachment	A reciprocal, dynamic process of interacting and bonding with the caregiver
State regulation	Ability to modulate the level of arousal in response to different degrees of stimulation (e.g., self-consoling)
Perception	Ability to regard faces, turn to voices, quiet in presence of singing, track colorful objects, respond to touch, and recognize familiar scents

Newborns who do not demonstrate these behaviors may have a neurologic condition, drug withdrawal, or a serious illness such as infection.

permission use a pacifier or a bottle of formula (if not breastfeeding) or allow the baby to suck on your gloved finger. Reswaddle the baby long enough to complete the parts of the examination that require a quiet baby.

Infants

Start with the infant sitting or lying in the parent's lap (Fig. 23-12). If the infant is tired, hungry, or ill, ask the parent to hold the baby against the parent's chest. Make sure appropriate toys, a blanket, or other familiar objects are nearby. A hungry infant may need to be fed before you initiate the examination (Box 23-8).

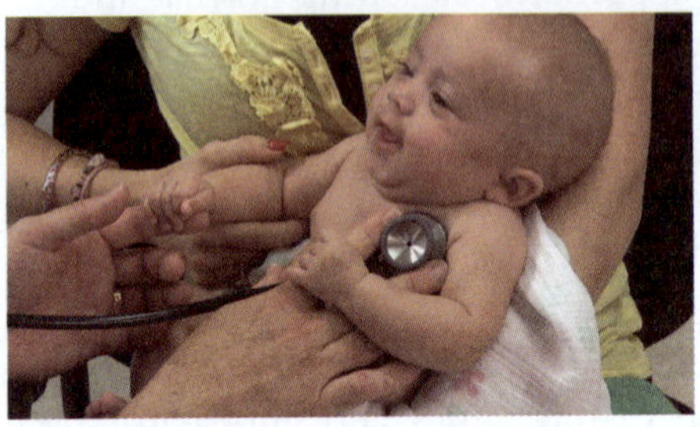

FIGURE 23-12. Start the examination while the child is still on the parent's lap.

Many neurologic conditions can be diagnosed during this general part of the examination. For example, you can detect hypotonia, conditions associated with irritability or signs of cerebral palsy (see neurologic examination below).

Box 23-8. Tips for Examining Infants

- Approach the infant gradually, using a toy or object for distraction.
- Perform as much of the examination as possible with the infant in the parent's lap.
- Speak softly to the infant or mimic the infant's sounds to attract attention.
- If the infant is cranky, make sure he or she is well fed before proceeding.
- Ask a parent about the infant's strengths to elicit useful developmental and parenting information.
- Don't expect to do a head-to-toe examination in a specific order. Work with what the infant gives you and save the mouth and ear examination for last.

Close observation of an awake infant sitting on the parent's lap can reveal potential abnormalities of tone, conditions with abnormal skin color, jaundice or cyanosis, jitteriness, or respiratory problems. Observe parent–infant interactions. Watch the parent's affect when talking about the infant. Note the parent's manner of holding, moving, dressing, and comforting the infant. Assess and comment on positive interactions, such as the obvious pride in the mother's face in Figure 23-13.

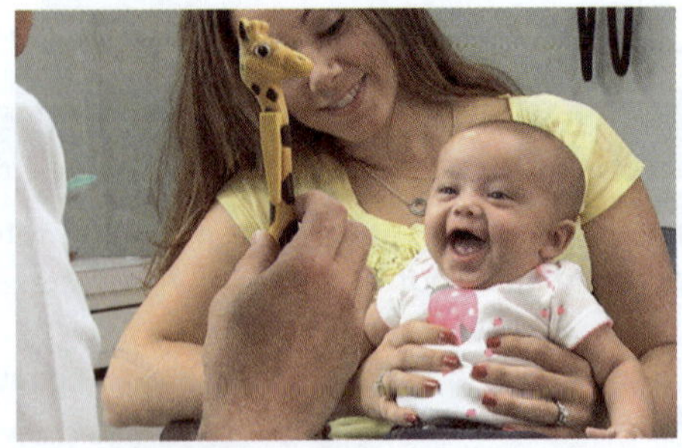

FIGURE 23-13. Children can have fun during the developmental examination.

Observation of the infant's communication with the parent can reveal abnormalities such as *developmental delay, language delay, hearing deficits,* or *inadequate parental attachment.* Likewise, such observations may identify maladaptive nurturing patterns that may stem from *maternal depression* or *inadequate social support.*

Infants do not object to having their clothing removed. To keep yourself and your surroundings dry, it is wise to leave the diaper in place throughout the examination; remove it only to examine the genitals, rectum, and hips.

Use developmentally appropriate methods such as *distraction* and *play* to examine the infant. Because infants pay attention to one thing at a time, it is relatively easy to distract the infant from the examination as it is performed. You can use a moving object, a flashing light, a toy, a game of peek-a-boo (for older infants), tickling, or any sort of noise.

If you cannot distract the infant or engage the awake infant with an object, your face, or a sound, consider a possible *visual* or *hearing deficit.*

TECHNIQUES OF EXAMINATION: INFANTS

Assessment at Birth

Apgar Score. The Apgar score is an assessment of the newborn immediately after birth. Its five components classify the newborn's neurologic recovery from the stress of birth and immediate cardiopulmonary adaptation to extrauterine life. Score each newborn at 1 and 5 minutes after birth (Box 23-9). Scoring is based on a 3-point scale (0, 1, or 2) for each component. Total scores range from 0 to 10. Scoring may continue at 5-minute intervals until the score is >7. If the 5-minute Apgar score is 8 or more, proceed to a more complete examination.

Box 23-9. Apgar Scoring System

	Assigned Score		
Clinical Sign	**0**	**1**	**2**
Heart rate	Absent	<100	>100
Respiratory effort	Absent	Slow and irregular	Good; strong
Muscle tone	Flaccid	Some flexion of the arms and legs	Active movement
Reflex irritability[a]	No responses	Grimace	Vigorous cry, sneeze, or cough
Color	Blue, pale	Pink body, blue extremities	Pink all over

1-Minute Apgar Score		**5-Minute Apgar Score**	
8–10	Normal	8–10	Normal
5–7	Some nervous system depression	0–7	High risk for subsequent central nervous system and other organ system dysfunction
0–4	Severe depression, requiring immediate resuscitation		

[a]Reaction to suction of nares with bulb syringe.

Example of Apgar score calculation for a newborn with hypoxia:

Heart rate = 110 [2]

Respiratory effort = slow, irregular [1]

Muscle tone = some flexion of arms/legs [1]

Reflex irritability = grimace [1]

Color = blue, pale [0]

Apgar score = 5

Gestational Age and Birth Weight. Classify newborns according to their gestational age of maturity and birth weight (Box 23-10). These classifications help predict clinical problems and morbidity.

Gestational age is based on specific neuromuscular signs and physical characteristics that change with gestational maturity. The Ballard Scoring System estimates gestational age to within 2 weeks, even in extremely premature infants. A complete Ballard Scoring System, with instructions for assessing neuromuscular and physical maturity, is included in Figure 23-14.

Box 23-10. Classification by Gestational Age and Birth Weight

Gestational Age Classification	**Gestational Age**
Preterm	<37 weeks
Late preterm	34–36 weeks
Term	37–41 weeks
Postterm	>42 weeks
Birth Weight Classification	**Weight**
Extremely low birth weight	<1,000 g
Very low birth weight	<1,500 g
Low birth weight	<2,500 g
Normal birth weight	≥2,500 g

Preterm infants are at risk for both short-term complications (mainly respiratory and cardiovascular) as well as long-term sequelae (e.g., neurodevelopmental).

Late preterm infants are at considerable risk for prematurity-related complications but at less risk than preterm infants.

Postterm infants are at increased risk of perinatal mortality or morbidity (relative to term infants) such as asphyxia and meconium aspiration.

The New Ballard Score for Determining Gestational Age in Weeks

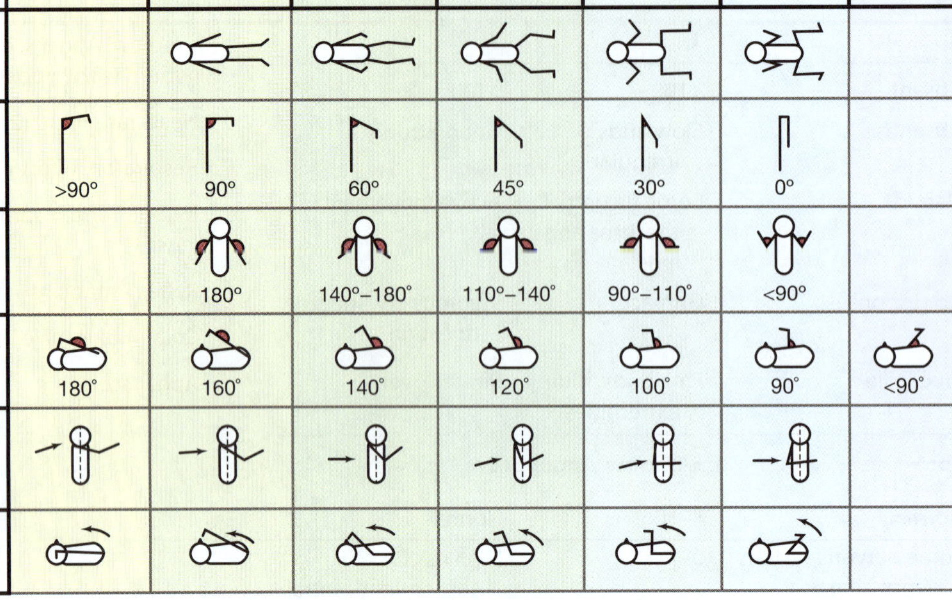

Neuromuscular Maturity

	−1	0	1	2	3	4	5
Posture							
Square window (wrist)	>90°	90°	60°	45°	30°	0°	
Arm recoil		180°	140°–180°	110°–140°	90°–110°	<90°	
Popliteal angle	180°	160°	140°	120°	100°	90°	<90°
Scarf sign							
Heel to ear							

Physical Maturity

	−1	0	1	2	3	4	5
Skin	Sticky friable transparent	Gelatinous red, translucent	Smooth pink, visible veins	Superficial peeling and/or rash, few veins	Cracking pale areas rare veins	Parchment deep cracking no vessels	Leathery cracked wrinkled
Lanugo	None	Sparse	Abundant	Thinning	Bald areas	Mostly bald	
Plantar surface	heel — toe 40–50 mm: −1 <40 mm: −2	>50 mm no crease	Faint red marks	Anterior transverse crease only	Creases anterior 2/3	Creases over entire sole	
Breast	Imperceptible	barely preceptible	flat areola no bud	Stippled areola 1–2-mm bud	Raised areola 3–4-mm bud	Full areola 5–10-mm bud	
Eye/ear	Lids fused loosely: −1 Tightly: −2	Lids open, pinna flat stays folded	Slightly curved pinna; soft, slow recoil	Well-curved pinna; soft, but ready recoil	Formed and firm instant recoil	Thick cartilage, ear stiff	
Genitals male	Scrotum flat, smooth	Scrotum empty, faint rugae	Testes in upper canal, rare rugae	Testes descending, few rugae	Testes down, good rugae	Testes pendulous, deep rugae	
Genitals female	Clitoris prominent, labia flat	Prominent clitoris, small labia minora	Prominent clitoris, enlarging minora	Majora and minora equally prominent	Majora large, minora small	Majora cover clitoris and minora	

Maturity Rating

Score	Weeks
−10	20
−5	22
0	24
5	26
10	28
15	30
20	32
25	34
30	36
35	38
40	40
45	42
50	44

FIGURE 23-14. The sum of the scores for all of the neuromuscular and physical maturity items provides an estimate of gestational age in weeks, using the maturity rating scale at the lower right potion of the figure. (Redrawn from Ballard JL et al. *J Pediatr.* 1991;119(3):417–423. Copyright © 1991 Elsevier. With permission.)

Box 23-11. Newborn Classification

Category	Abbreviation	Percentile
Small for gestational age	SGA	<10th
Appropriate for gestational age	AGA	10th–90th
Large for gestational age	LGA	>90th

LGA infants may experience difficulties during birth. Infants of mothers with diabetes are often LGA and may have metabolic abnormalities shortly after birth, as well as congenital anomalies.

A common complication among LGA newborns is hypoglycemia, which can result in jitteriness, irritability, cyanosis, or other health issues.

A useful classification (Box 23-11) is derived from the gestational age and birth weight on the intrauterine growth curve.

Figure 23-15 displays the intrauterine growth curves for the 10th and 90th percentiles and depicts the categories of maturity for newborns based on gestational age and birth weight.

While no etiology is noted for many SGA infants, known causes include fetal, placental, and maternal factors. Maternal smoking is associated with SGA newborns. SGA newborns are at risk for hypoglycemia.

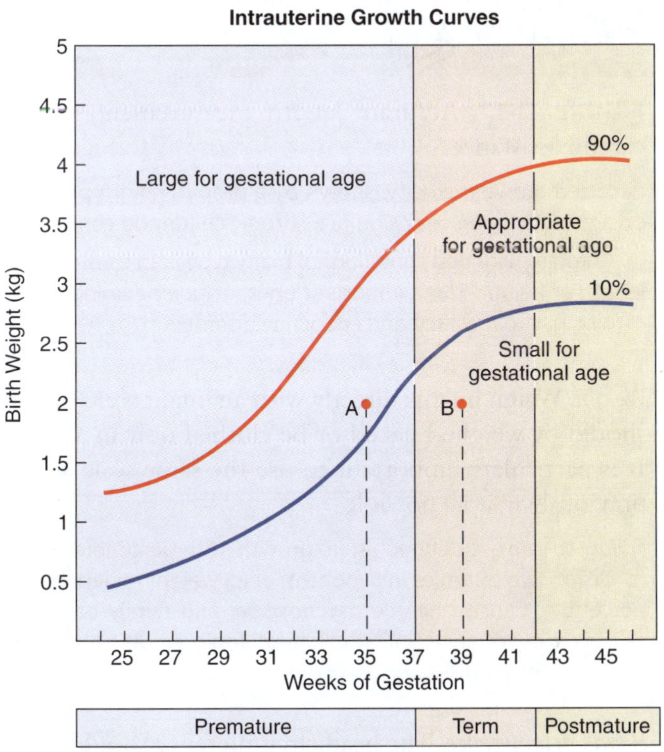

FIGURE 23-15. Level of intrauterine growth based on gestational age and birth weight of liveborn, single, white infants. Point A represents a premature infant; point B indicates an infant of similar birth weight who is mature but SGA. (Adapted from Sweet YA. Classification of the low-birth-weight infant. In: Klaus MH, Fanaroff AA, eds. *Care of the High-Risk Neonate*. 3rd ed. WB Saunders; 1986. Copyright © 1986 Elsevier. With permission.)

The three babies shown in Figure 23-16 were all born at 32 weeks' gestational age and weighed 600 g (SGA), 1,400 g (AGA), and 2,750 g (LGA). Each of these categories has a different mortality rate, highest for preterm SGA and LGA infants, and lowest for term AGA infants.

Preterm infants are more prone to respiratory distress syndrome, apnea, patent ductus arteriosus (PDA) with left-to-right shunt, and infection.

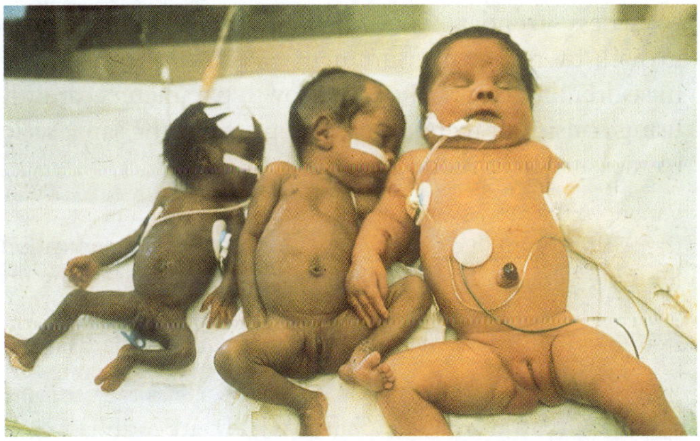

FIGURE 23-16. Infants who are small, average, and large for their gestational age. (Reprinted from Korones SB. *High-Risk Newborn Infants: The Basis for Intensive Nursing Care*. 4th ed. CV Mosby; 1986. Copyright © 1986 Elsevier. With permission.)

General Survey. During the first day of life, newborns should have a comprehensive examination. Wait until 1 or 2 hours after a feeding, when the baby is most responsive, and ask the parents to remain in the room. Follow the sequence shown in Box 23-6.

Observe the undressed newborn. Note the newborn's color, size, body proportions, nutritional status, and posture, as well as respirations and movements of the head and extremities. Most normal, full-term newborns lie in a symmetric position, with the limbs semi-flexed and the legs partially abducted at the hip.

In *breech babies* (buttock first), the knees are flexed in utero; in a *frank breech baby*, the knees are extended in utero. In both, the hips are flexed.

Note the baby's spontaneous motor activity with flexion and extension alternating between the arms and legs. The fingers are usually flexed in a tight fist but may extend in slow posturing movements. You will observe brief tremors of the body and extremities during vigorous crying, and even at rest.

By 4 days after birth, tremors at rest signal central nervous system disease from various possible causes, ranging from asphyxia to drug withdrawal.

Somatic Growth. Tables on the World Health Organization (WHO) website (https://www.who.int/childgrowth/standards) show norms for height, weight, BMI (starting age 2 years), and head circumference. Compare body proportions with age-specific norms because *they change dramatically as children grow.*

Measurement of growth is one of the most important indicators of infant health. Deviations may provide an early indication of an underlying problem. Compare growth parameters with respect to normal values for age and sex, as well as prior readings on the same child, to assess trends. Confirm abnormalities in somatic growth by repeat measurement to account for potential measurement error. Measure growth parameters carefully using consistent technique and, optimally, the same scales to measure height and weight.

Variations beyond two standard deviations for age or above the 95th percentile or below the 5th percentile are indications for more detailed evaluation. These deviations may be the first and only indicators of a variety of chronic childhood diseases (see examples in https://www.who.int/childgrowth/standards).

The most important tools for assessing somatic growth are the growth charts which are published by the National Center for Health Statistics (www.cdc.gov/nchs) and also the WHO (https://www.who.int/childgrowth/standards). All charts include height, weight, and head circumference for children up to 36 months and height and weight for children 2 to 18 years. Charts plotting weight by length as well as BMI are also available. These growth charts have percentile lines indicating the percentage of normal children above and below the child's measurement by chronologic age. Comparison with normal standards is essential because growth velocity is normally less during the second year than during the first year. Special growth charts are available for use in infants born prematurely (to correct for the level of prematurity).

Growth charts are also available for children with specific conditions such as Down syndrome or Turner syndrome.

Although many healthy infants cross percentiles on growth charts, a sudden or significant change in growth may indicate systemic disease due to various possible organ systems or inappropriate excess weight gain usually due to overfeeding.

Abnormalities that can cause deviation from normal growth patterns include chronic childhood disease or prematurity.

Length. For children younger than age 2 years, measure body length by placing the child supine on a measuring board or in a measuring tray, as shown in Figure 23-17. Direct measurement of the infant using a tape measure is inaccurate unless an assistant holds the child still with hips and knees extended. Velocity growth curves are helpful for older children, especially those who are suspected of having endocrine disorders.

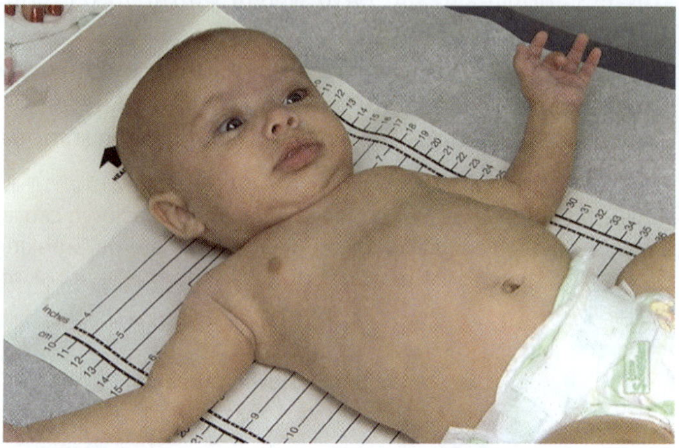

FIGURE 23-17. Accurate length measurement requires careful assistance.

Reduced growth velocity, shown by a drop in height percentile on a growth curve, may signify a chronic childhood condition.

Chronic childhood conditions of many types can cause reduced length or height. Some important ones include neurologic, renal, cardiac, gastrointestinal, and endocrine disorders.

Weight. Weigh infants directly with an infant scale. Infants should be weighed naked or be clothed only in a diaper. It is particularly important to use the same scale as used previously if at all possible.

Failure to thrive is defined as: (a) growth <5th percentile for age; (b) drop >two quartiles in 6 months; or (c) weight for length <5th percentile. Causes include psychosocial and family conditions and a variety of gastrointestinal, neurologic, cardiac, endocrine, renal, and other diseases.

Head Circumference. The head circumference should always be measured during the first 2 years of life, but measurement can be useful at any age to assess growth of the head (Fig. 23-18). The head circumference in infants reflects the rate of growth of the cranium and the brain.

A small head size is called *microcephaly*, which may be familial or due to chromosomal abnormalities, congenital infections, maternal metabolic disorders, and neurologic insults. Microcephaly may also result from premature closure of the sutures.

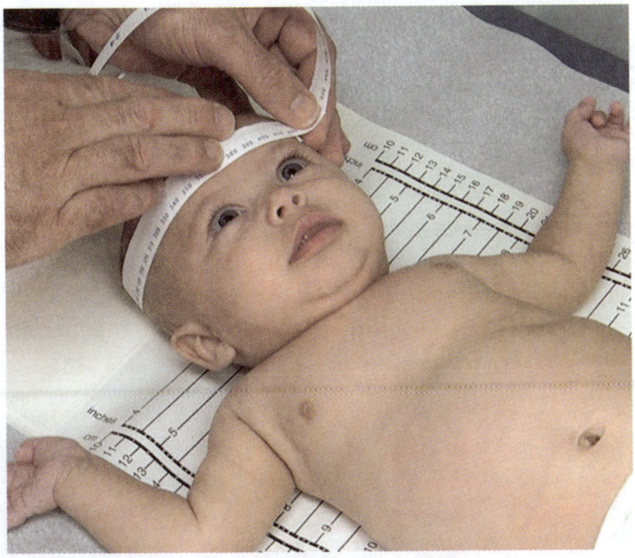

FIGURE 23-18. Head circumference is a vital metric during early childhood.

An abnormally large head size (>95th percentile or 2 standard deviations above the mean) is *macrocephaly*, which may result from hydrocephalus, intracranial hemorrhage, or rare causes like brain tumor or inherited syndromes. Familial *megaloencephaly* (large head) is a benign familial condition.

Vital Signs. Measure the infant's vital signs—blood pressure, pulse rate, respiratory rate, and temperature. Pediatric clinicians also assess pain regularly, using standardized pain scales. Another measure that can be helpful is the capillary refill time.

See pain severity assessment in Chapter 8, General Examination, p. 145.

Blood Pressure. Systolic blood pressure gradually increases throughout childhood. For example, normal systolic pressure in males is about 70 mm Hg at birth, 85 mm Hg at 1 month, and 90 mm Hg at 6 months.

Although obtaining accurate blood pressure readings in infants is challenging (Fig. 23-19), this measurement is nevertheless important for some high-risk infants. Blood pressure measurements should be routinely performed after age 3 years. An automatic cuff is an alternative to a manual blood pressure cuff. For either method, using an accurate cuff size for age and placement are critical for obtaining accurate blood pressure readings.

See page 685 for more on blood pressure cuff size and placement for children.

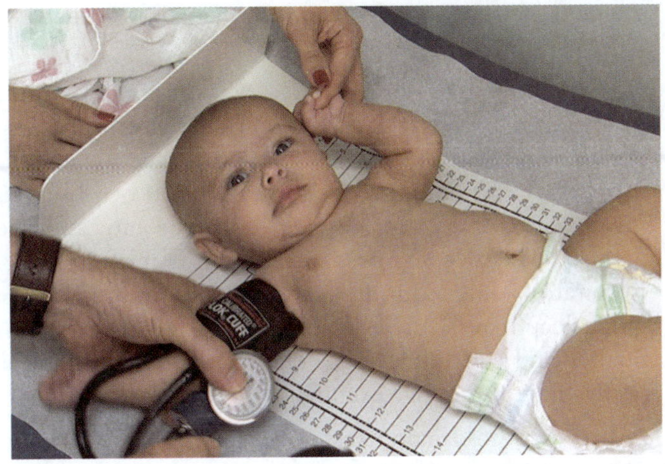

FIGURE 23-19. Practice is required to accurately measure blood pressure in early childhood.

Causes of sustained hypertension in newborns include renal artery disease (stenosis, thrombosis), congenital renal malformations, and coarctation of the aorta.

Pulse Rate. The heart rate of infants is more sensitive to the effects of illness, exercise, and emotion than that of adults (Box 23-12).

While sinus tachycardia may be extremely rapid, a pulse rate that is too rapid to count (usually >220/min in infants) may indicate paroxysmal supraventricular tachycardia (PSVT).

You may have trouble obtaining an accurate pulse rate in a squirming infant. Palpate the femoral arteries in the inguinal area or the brachial arteries in the antecubital fossa or auscultate the heart.

Respiratory Rate. As with heart rate, the respiratory rate in infants has a greater range and is more responsive to illness, exercise, and emotion than that of adults or

Box 23-12. Heart Rates of Healthy Children from Birth to 1 Year

Age	Average Heart Rate (per minute)	Range (1st to 99th percentile) per minute
Birth–1 month	140	90–165
1–6 months	130	80–175
6–12 months	115	90–170

Bradycardia may be from drug ingestion, hypoxia, intracranial or neurologic conditions, or, rarely, cardiac dysrhythmia such as heart block.

See Table 23-1, Abnormalities in Heart Rhythm and Blood Pressure.

older children. The rate of respirations per minute ranges between 30 and 68 in the newborn (1st and 99th percentiles) and between 25 and 60 per minute in infants 6 to 12 months of age.

Extremely rapid and shallow respiratory rates are seen in newborns with cyanotic cardiac disease and right-to-left shunting, metabolic acidosis, and pulmonary diseases, and can be seen in infants with neurologic diseases.

The respiratory rate may vary considerably from moment to moment in the newborn, with alternating periods of rapid and slow breathing (called "*periodic breathing*"). The respiratory pattern should be observed for at least 60 seconds to asses both the rate and the pattern. The sleeping respiratory rate is most reliable. Respiratory rates during active sleep compared with quiet sleep may be up to 10 breaths per minute faster. In infancy and early childhood, diaphragmatic breathing is predominant; thoracic excursion is minimal.

Fever can raise respiratory rates in infants by up to 10 respirations per minute for each degree centigrade of fever.

Commonly accepted cutoffs for defining *tachypnea* are >60/min from birth to 2 months, and >50/min from 2 to 12 months.

Tachypnea and increased respiratory effort in an infant can be signs of upper respiratory conditions and of lower respiratory disease such as bronchiolitis or pneumonia.

Temperature. Body temperature in infants and children is less constant than in adults. The average rectal temperature is higher in infancy and early childhood, usually above 99°F (37.2°C) until after age 3 years. Body temperature fluctuates during a single day with vigorous activity and ambient temperature. Two standard deviations above the mean for infants below 1 month is 38.0°C[31]; thus pediatric clinicians often define fever in an infant below 3 months as having a temperature above 38.0°C.

Because fever is so common in infants and children, obtain an accurate body temperature when you suspect infection. Rectal temperatures are the most accurate for infants. Axillary and thermal-tape skin temperature recordings in infants and children are inaccurate. Auditory canal temperatures are accurate.

Fever (>38°C or >100.4°F) in infants younger than age 2 to 3 months may be a sign of serious infection or disease and is an emergency. Potentially sick febrile infants under 3 months of age may have serious bacterial infection and should have temperatures assessed using a rectal thermometer.

The technique for obtaining a rectal temperature is relatively simple. One method is illustrated in Figure 23-20. Place the infant prone, separate the buttocks with the thumb and forefinger on one hand and with the other hand gently insert a well-lubricated rectal thermometer to a depth of 2 to 3 cm. Keep the thermometer in place for at least 2 minutes.

Excessive bundling of infants may elevate skin temperature but not usually core temperature, although temperature readings should be repeated in an infant who is over-bundled.

Temperature instability (either high or low temperature) in a newborn may result from sepsis, metabolic abnormality, or other serious conditions. Older infants rarely manifest temperature instability.

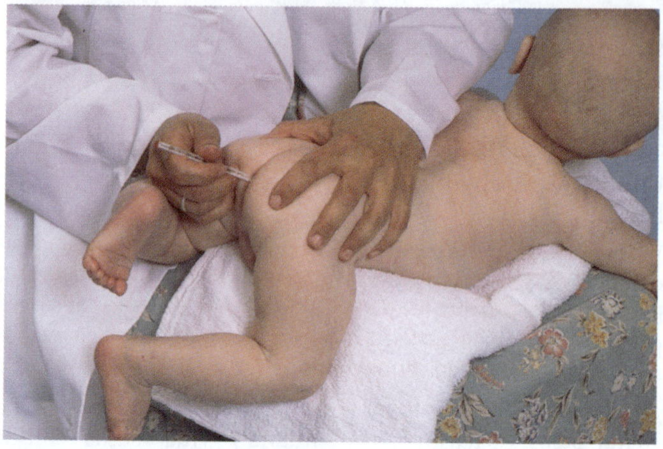

FIGURE 23-20. Rectal thermometers are the most accurate tool for infants.

Capillary Refill Time. Although it is not a vital sign, the *capillary refill time* (CRT) can be a helpful measure as a "red flag" indicator of a potentially serious condition among sick infants and young children.

Press the infant or child's finger for 5 seconds with moderate pressure and use a watch to time the number of seconds it takes for the finger to regain its original color. Normally, CRT is less than 2 seconds in children older than 1 week of age and a CRT over 3 to 4 seconds is considered prolonged.

A prolonged CRT in a sick infant or young child is a nonspecific "red flag" for potentially serious condition such as dehydration, urinary tract infection, and other serious infections.

Skin

Inspection. Examine the skin of the newborn or infant carefully to identify both normal markings and potentially abnormal ones. The photos on pp. 650–652 demonstrate normal markings. The newborn's skin has a unique characteristic *texture* and *appearance*. The texture is soft and smooth because it is thinner than the skin of older children. Within the first 10 minutes after birth a normal newborn progresses from slight *cyanosis* ("bluish") to pinkness. Some premature infants will be intensely *erythematous* (red).

Some newborns with polycythemia have a "ruddy" or purplish color.

At birth, there is a fine, downy growth of hair called *lanugo* over the entire body, especially the shoulders and back. This hair is shed within the first few weeks. Lanugo is prominent in premature infants. Hair thickness on the head varies considerably among newborns and is not predictive of later hair growth. All of the original hair is shed within months and is replaced with a new crop, sometimes of a different color.

Inspect the newborn closely for a series of common skin conditions. At birth, a cheesy white material called *vernix caseosa,* composed of water, proteins and lipids, covers the body and forms a barrier against maceration and infection and moisturizes the fetus to pass through the birth canal. Some newborns have *edema* over their hands, feet, lower legs, pubis, and sacrum; this disappears within a few days. Superficial desquamation of the skin is often noticeable 24 to 36 hours after birth, particularly in post term babies (>40 weeks' gestation), and it can last for 7 to 10 days.

Both erythema toxicum and pustular melanosis may appear similar to the pathologic vesiculopustular rash of herpes simplex or *Staphylococcus aureus* skin infection.

Note any signs of trauma from the birth process and the use of forceps or suction; these signs disappear but should prompt a careful neurologic examination.

Midline hair tufts over the lumbosacral spine region suggest a possible spinal cord defect.

Vasomotor Changes. Vasomotor changes in the dermis and subcutaneous tissue—a response to cooling or chronic exposure to radiant heat—can produce a lattice-like, bluish mottled appearance (*cutis marmorata*), particularly on the trunk, arms, and legs. This response to cold may last for months in normal infants. *Cutis marmorata* is a common, benign vascular condition, frequent among premature infants, in which the skin shows a red/blue or purplish mottled lacy blood vessel pattern that is temporary and resolves with warming.

Pigmentation. The amount of melanin in the skin of newborns varies, affecting *pigmentation*. Some infants who will eventually have dark skin may have a lighter skin color initially, except in the nail beds, genitalia, and ear folds which are dark at birth. A dark or bluish pigmentation over the buttocks and lower lumbar regions is common in newborns of African, Asian, Hispanic, and Mediterranean descent. These areas, called *congenital dermal melanocytosis,* result from pigmented cells in the deep layers of the skin; they become less noticeable with age and usually disappear during childhood. *Document these pigmented areas to avoid later concern about bruising.*

Pigmented light-brown lesions (<1 to 2 cm at birth) are *café-au-lait spots.* Isolated lesions have no significance, but multiple lesions with sharp borders may suggest neurofibromatosis.

See Table 23-2, Common Skin Rashes and Skin Findings in Newborns and Infants.

Cyanosis. Observe the infant carefully for any cyanosis. Recognizing minimal degrees of cyanosis requires care. Look inside the body (i.e., the inside of the mouth, the tongue, or the conjunctivae) in addition to assessing skin color. *Acrocyanosis,* a blue cast to the hands and feet when exposed to cold (see p. 650), is very common in newborns for the first few days and may recur throughout early infancy. *Central cyanosis* is present if in addition to the hands and feet, the lips, tongue, and sublingual tissues are also involved.

If acrocyanosis does not disappear within 8 hours or with warming, cyanotic congenital heart disease should be considered.

See discussion of central cyanosis on p. 661.

Occasionally in newborns, a remarkable color change (*harlequin dyschromia*) appears with transient cyanosis of one-half of the body or one extremity, presumably from temporary vascular instability.

Jaundice. Normal "physiologic" jaundice, which occurs in half of all newborns, appears on the second or third day, peaks at about the fifth day, and usually disappears within a week (although it may persist longer in breastfed infants). Newborn jaundice appears to progress from head to toe, with more intense jaundice on the upper body and less intense yellow color in the lower extremities.

A common and nonpathologic type of jaundice during the first couple of weeks is breastfeeding jaundice, which should completely resolve around 10 to 14 days of life. Persistent jaundice requires evaluation. A physical examination cannot reliably predict the level of bilirubin.

Jaundice within the first 24 hours of birth may be from hemolytic disease of the newborn which is always pathologic. Late-appearing jaundice or jaundice that persists beyond 2 to 3 weeks should raise suspicions of biliary obstruction or liver disease.

Carefully examine and touch the newborn's skin to assess the level of jaundice. Jaundice is best seen in natural daylight rather than artificial light. To detect jaundice, apply pressure to the skin (Fig. 23-21) to press out the normal pink or brown color. A yellowish "blanching" indicates jaundice.

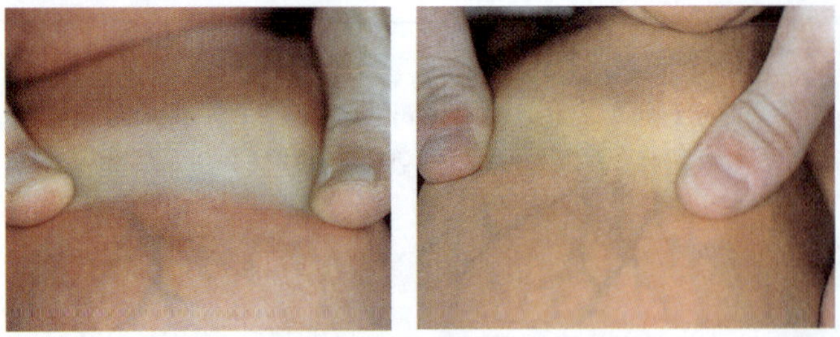

FIGURE 23-21. Pressing the red color from the skin allows better recognition of the yellow of normal skin (**left**) or jaundice (**right**). (From Fletcher M. *Physical Diagnosis in Neonatology*. Lippincott-Raven; 1998.)

Vascular Markings. A common, benign *vascular marking* is the "salmon patch" (also known as nevus simplex, "flame nevi," telangiectatic nevus, or capillary hemangioma). These flat, irregular, light pink patches (see p. 651) are most often seen on the nape of the neck ("stork bite"), upper eyelids, forehead, or upper lip ("angel kisses"). They are not true nevi but result from distended capillaries. They often disappear by 1 year of age and are covered by the hairline.

A unilateral dark, purplish lesion, or "port wine stain" over the distribution of the ophthalmic branch of the trigeminal nerve may be a sign of *Sturge–Weber syndrome,* which is associated with seizures, hemiparesis, glaucoma, and mental retardation.

Palpation. Palpate the newborn or infant's skin to assess the degree of hydration, or turgor. Roll a fold of loosely adherent skin on the abdominal wall between your thumb and forefinger to determine its consistency. The skin in well-hydrated infants returns to its normal position immediately upon release. Delay in return is a phenomenon called "tenting" and usually occurs in children with significant dehydration.

Significant edema of the hands and feet of a newborn girl may be suggestive of Turner syndrome. Other features such as a webbed neck would reinforce this diagnosis.

Dehydration is common in infants. Usual causes are insufficient intake or excess loss of fluids from diarrhea.

You should be able to identify four common dermatologic conditions in newborns—*miliaria rubra, erythema toxicum, pustular melanosis,* and *milia*—which are shown on p. 651. None of these is clinically significant (Box 23-13).

Box 23-13. Newborn Skin Findings

Finding/Description

Common Nonpathologic Conditions

Acrocyanosis

This bluish discoloration usually appears in the palms and soles. *Cyanotic congenital heart disease can present with severe acrocyanosis, which persists despite warming.*

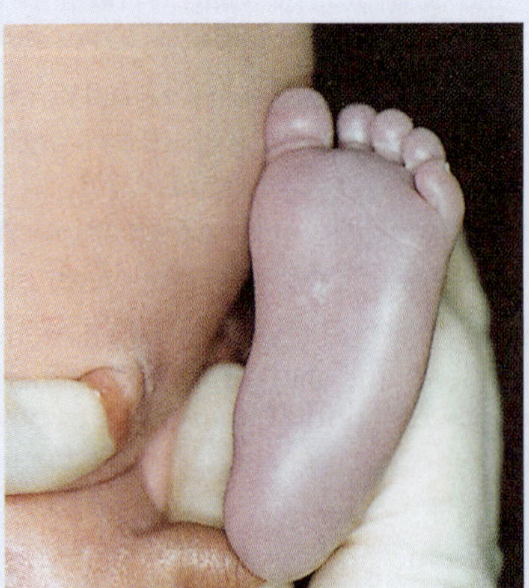

Jaundice

Physiologic jaundice occurs during days 2–5 of life and progresses from head to toe as it peaks. *Extreme jaundice may signify a hemolytic process or biliary or liver disease.*

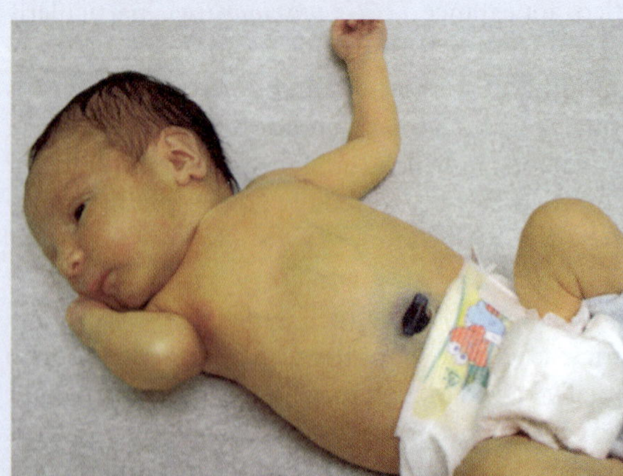

(*continued*)

Box 23-13. Newborn Skin Findings (*continued*)

Finding/Description

Common Benign Rashes

Miliaria Rubra

Scattered erythematous papules, vesicles, or pustules, usually on the face, neck and trunk, result from obstruction of the sweat gland ducts; this condition disappears spontaneously within weeks.

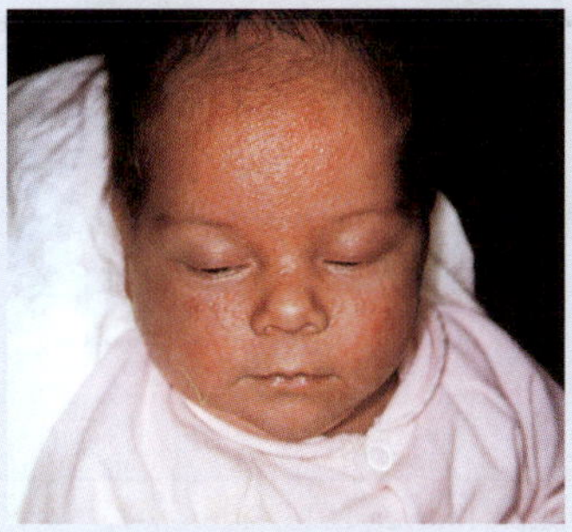

Erythema Toxicum

Usually appearing on days 2–3 of life, this rash consists of erythematous macules with central pinpoint pustules on an erythematous base, scattered diffusely over the entire body. These lesions are of unknown etiology but disappear within 1 week of birth.

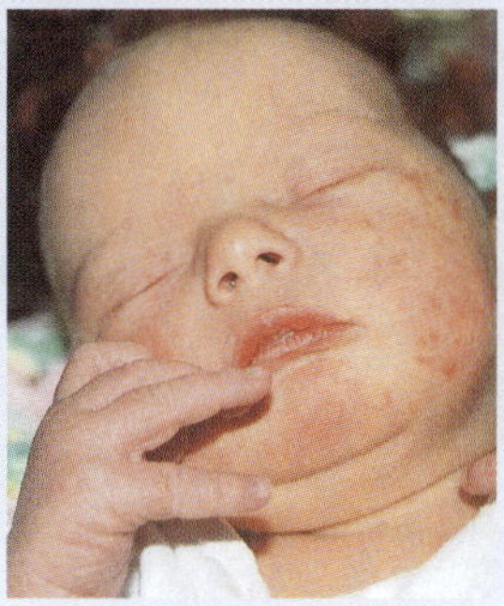

Transient Neonatal Pustular Melanosis

Seen more commonly in black infants, the rash presents at birth as some combination of pustules, scale, and hyperpigmented macules. The pustules and scale resolve by around 2 weeks, leaving behind hyperpigmented macules that resolve after several months.

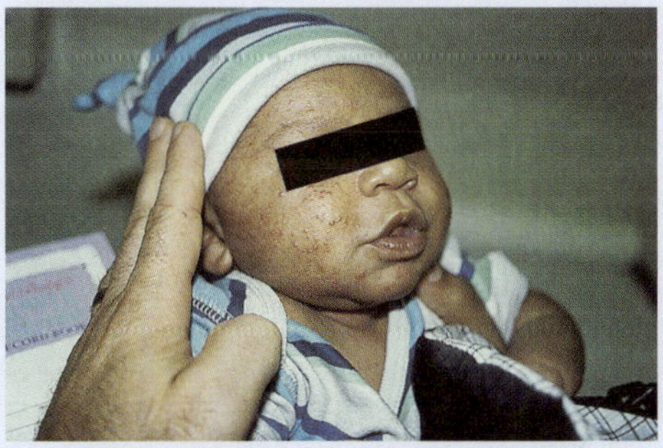

Milia

Pinhead-sized white, pearly papules, without surrounding erythema, on the nose (seen here), chin, and forehead result from retention of sebum in the openings of the sebaceous glands. Although occasionally present at birth, milia usually appear within the first few weeks and disappears over several weeks.

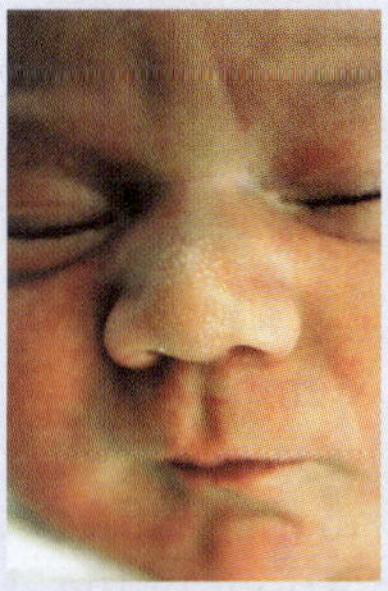

Benign Birthmarks

Eyelid Patch

This birthmark fades, usually within the first year of life.

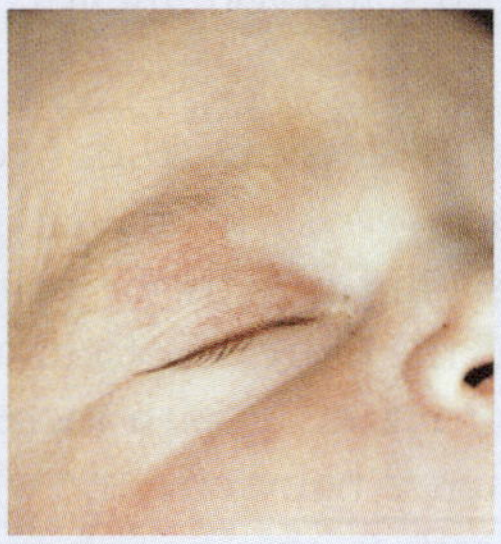

Salmon Patch

Also called the "stork bite," or "angel kiss," this splotchy pink mark fades with age.

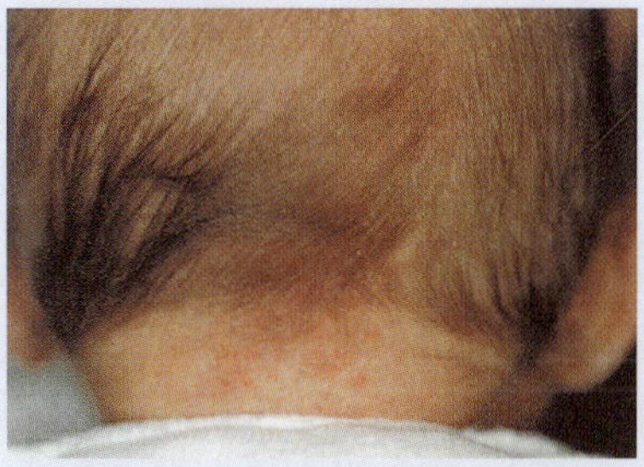

(*continued*)

Box 23-13. Newborn Skin Findings (*continued*)

Finding/Description

Benign Birthmarks (*continued*)

Café-au-lait Spots

These light-brown pigmented lesions usually have borders and are uniform. They are noted in more than 10% of black infants. *If more than five café-au-lait spots exist, consider the diagnosis of neurofibromatosis.*

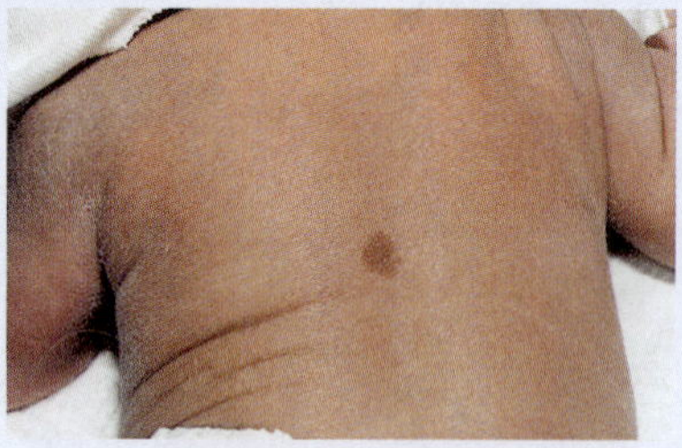

Congenital Dermal Melanocytosis

These are more common among dark-skinned babies. It is important to note them so that they are not mistaken for bruises.

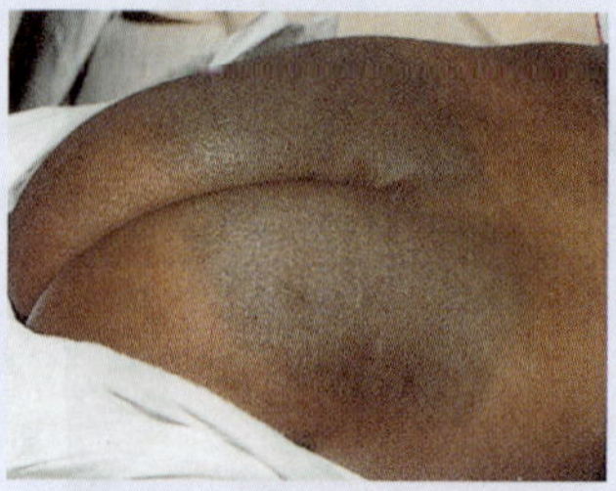

Source of photo: *Jaundice*—From Chung EK et al. *Visual Diagnosis and Treatment in Pediatrics*. 3rd ed. Wolters Kluwer; 2015, Figure 7-7.

Head. At birth, a baby's head may seem large relative to the body. A newborn's head accounts for one-fourth of the body length and one-third of the body weight; these proportions change, so that by adulthood the head accounts for one-eighth of the body length and about one-tenth of the body weight.

An enlarged posterior fontanelle may be present in congenital hypothyroidism.

Delayed closure of the fontanelles is usually a normal variant, but can be due to hypothyroidism, megalocephaly, increased intracranial pressure, or rickets.

Sutures and Fontanelles. Membranous tissue spaces called *sutures* separate the bones of the skull from one another. The areas where the major sutures intersect in the anterior and posterior portions of the skull are known as *fontanelles*. The *anterior fontanelle* at birth measures 4 to 6 cm in diameter. In about 80% of infants the anterior fontanelle will close by 18 months of age, and in about 90% by 22 months. The *posterior fontanelle* measures 1 to 2 cm at birth and usually closes by 2 months. Overlap of the cranial bones at the sutures at birth, called *molding*, results from passage of the head through the birth canal; it disappears within 2 days.

A bulging, tense fontanelle is observed in infants with *increased intracranial pressure*, which may be caused by *bleeding, central nervous system infections, neoplastic disease*, or *hydrocephalus*.

See Table 23-5, Abnormalities of the Head.

Examine the *sutures* and *fontanelles* carefully (Fig. 23-22). On palpation, the sutures feel like ridges and the fontanelles like soft concavities.

Early closure of the fontanelles can be due to developing *microcephaly* or to *craniosynostosis* or some *metabolic abnormalities*.

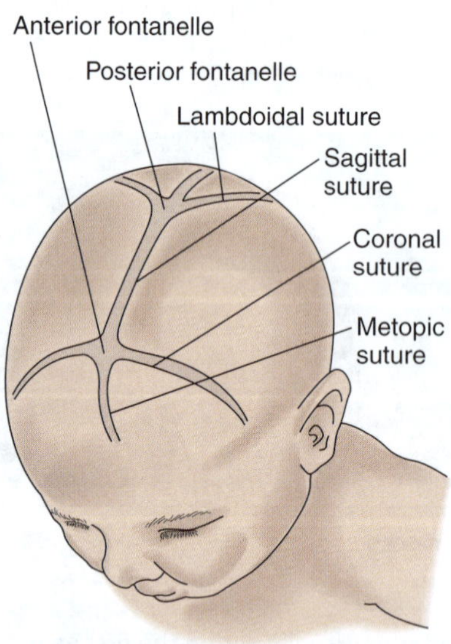

FIGURE 23-22. Sutures and fontanelles.

Carefully examine the fontanelle, because its fullness reflects *intracranial pressure*. Palpate the fontanelle while the baby is sitting quietly or being held upright. In normal infants, the anterior fontanelle is soft and flat. A full anterior fontanelle with increased intracranial pressure is seen when a baby cries or vomits. Pulsations of the fontanelle reflect the peripheral pulse and are usually completely normal (and parents often inquire about them).

Learn to palpate the fontanelle because a bulging fontanelle is concerning for increased intracranial pressure and a depressed fontanelle may suggest dehydration.

A depressed anterior fontanelle may be a sign of *dehydration.*

Inspect the scalp veins carefully to assess for dilatation.

Dilated scalp veins are indicative of long-standing *increased intracranial pressure.*

Skull Symmetry and Head Circumference. Carefully assess *skull symmetry* (Fig. 23-23). The premature infant's head at birth is relatively long in the occipitofrontal diameter and narrow in the bitemporal diameter (*dolichocephaly*). Usually, the skull shape normalizes within 1 to 2 years.

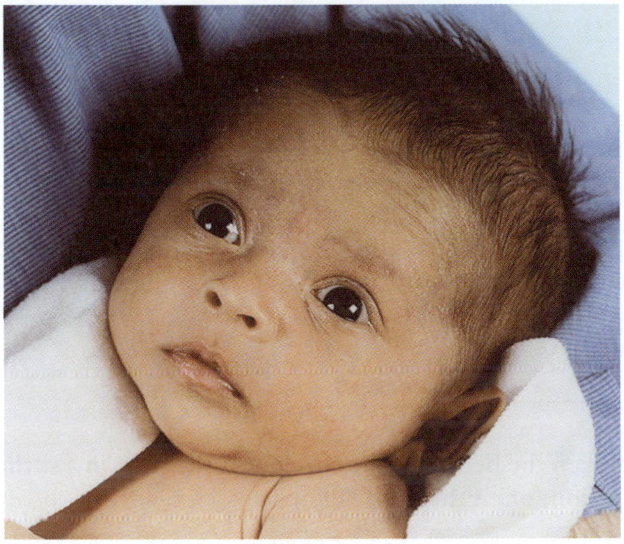

FIGURE 23-23. Skull shape and symmetry should be assessed.

A common type of localized swelling of the scalp is a *cephalohematoma,* caused by subperiosteal hemorrhage from the trauma of birth. This swelling does not cross over suture lines and resolves within 3 weeks.

See Table 23-5, Abnormalities of the Head.

Various conditions can cause asymmetry; some are benign, while others reflect underlying pathology. Look for asymmetric head swelling. A useful strategy is to inspect the baby's head from the top. Pick up the infant and examine the skull shape from behind.

A newborn's scalp may be swollen over the occipitoparietal region. This is called *caput succedaneum* and results from capillary distention and extravasation of blood and fluid resulting from the vacuum effect of rupture of the amniotic sac. This swelling *typically crosses suture lines* and resolves in 1 to 2 days.

Asymmetry of the cranial vault (*positional plagiocephaly*) occurs when an infant lies mostly on one side, resulting in a flattening of the parieto-occipital region on the dependent side and a prominence of the frontal region on the ipsilateral side. It disappears as the baby becomes more active and spends less time in one position, and symmetry is almost always restored.

Interestingly, the current trend to have newborns sleep on their backs to reduce the risk for sudden infant death syndrome (SIDS) has resulted in more cases of positional plagiocephaly (Fig. 23-24). This condition can be prevented by frequent repositioning (providing "tummy time" when the infant is awake).

Plagiocephaly may also reflect pathology such as *torticollis* from injury to the sternocleidomastoid muscle at birth or *lack of stimulation* of the infant.

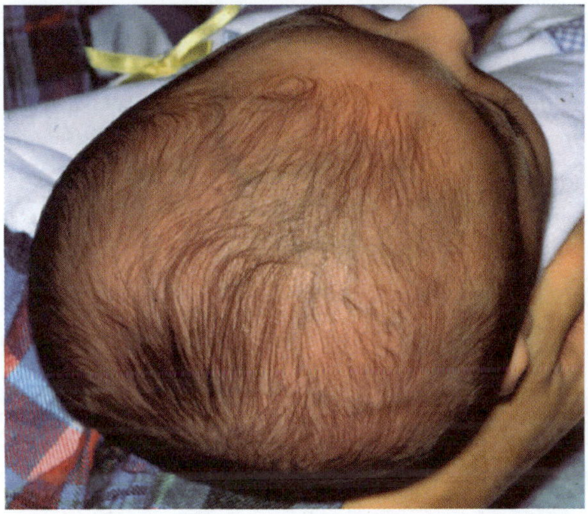

FIGURE 23-24. Careful assessment may reveal plagiocephaly.

Measure the head circumference to detect abnormally large head size (*macrocephaly*) or small head size (*microcephaly*), both of which may signify an underlying disorder affecting the brain.

Palpate along the suture lines. A raised, bony ridge at a suture suggests craniosynostosis.

Premature closure of cranial sutures causes *craniosynostosis* and an abnormally shaped skull. *Sagittal suture* synostosis causes a narrow head from lack of growth of the parietal bones.

Palpate the infant's skull with care. The cranial bones generally appear "soft" or pliable; they will normally become firmer with increasing gestational age.

In craniotabes, the cranial bones feel springy. Craniotabes can result from increased intracranial pressure, as with *hydrocephaly,* metabolic disturbances such as rickets, and infection such as congenital syphilis.

Examine the chin—an abnormally small chin is called *micrognathia or mandibular hypoplasia.*

Micrognathia may also be part of a syndrome, such as the Pierre Robin syndrome.

Box 23-14. Evaluating a Newborn or Child with Possible Abnormal Facies

Carefully review the history, especially:
- Family history
- Pregnancy
- Perinatal history

Note abnormalities on other parts of the physical examination, especially:
- Growth
- Development
- Other dysmorphic somatic features

Perform measurements (and plot percentiles), especially:
- Head circumference
- Height
- Weight

Consider the three mechanisms of facial dysmorphogenesis:
- Deformations from intrauterine constraint
- Disruptions from amniotic bands or fetal tissue
- Malformations from intrinsic abnormality in face/head or brain

Examine the parents and siblings:
- Similarity to a parent may be reassuring (e.g., large head) but may also be an indication of a familial disorder

Try to determine whether the facial features fit a recognizable syndrome, comparing with:
- References (including measurements) and pictures of syndromes
- Tables/databases of combinations of features

Most developmental and genetic syndromes with abnormal facies also have other abnormalities in other organ systems.

An infant with congenital hypothyroidism may have coarse facial features and other abnormal facial features (see Table 23-6, Diagnostic Facies in Infancy and Childhood)

A child with abnormal shape or length of palpebral fissures:

- Upslanting (*Down syndrome*)
- Downslanting (*Noonan syndrome*)
- Short (fetal alcohol effects)

See Table 23-6, Diagnostic Facies in Infancy and Childhood.

Facial Symmetry. Check the *face* of infants for symmetry.

Asymmetry of the face may reflect facial nerve palsy. If noted at birth, this may be due to congenital disorders or birth trauma; new onset in infancy may result from infection or other causes.

Examine the face for an overall impression of the facies; it is helpful to compare with the face of the parents. A systematic assessment of a child with abnormal-appearing facies can identify specific syndromes. Box 23-14 describes steps for evaluating facies.

Chvostek Sign. Percuss the cheek to check for *Chvostek sign*, which is present in some metabolic disturbances and occasionally in normal infants. Percuss at the top of the cheek just below the zygomatic bone in front of the ear, using the tip of your index or middle finger.

A positive Chvostek sign produces facial grimacing caused by repeated contractions of the facial muscles. Chvostek sign is noted in cases of *hypocalcemic tetany, tetanus, and tetany due to hyperventilation*.

Eyes

Inspection. Newborns keep their eyes closed except during brief awake periods. If you attempt to separate their eyelids, they will tighten them even more. Bright light causes infants to blink, so use subdued lighting. Awaken the baby gently and support the baby in a sitting position; often the eyes will open.

A newborn who truly cannot open an eye (even when awake and alert) may have *congenital ptosis*. Causes may include birth trauma and third cranial nerve palsy.

To examine the eyes of infants and young children, use some tricks to encourage cooperation. Small colorful toys without sounds are useful as fixation devices in examining the eyes.

Subconjunctival hemorrhages are common in neonates born via vaginal delivery.

Newborns may look at your face and follow a bright light if you catch them during an alert period. Some newborns can follow your face and turn their heads 90° to each side.

Nystagmus (wandering or shaking eye movements) persisting after a few days or persisting after the maneuver described on the left may indicate *poor vision* or *central nervous system disease*.

Examine infants for *eye movements*. Hold the baby upright, supporting the head. Rotate yourself with the baby slowly in one direction. This usually causes the baby's eyes to open, allowing you to examine the sclerae, pupils, irises, and extraocular movements (Fig. 23-25). The baby's eyes gaze in the direction you are turning.

When the rotation stops, the eyes look in the opposite direction, after a few nystagmoid movements.

If a newborn fails to gaze at you and follow your face during alert periods, pay particular attention to the rest of the ocular examination. The newborn may have *visual impairment* from congenital cataracts or other disorders.

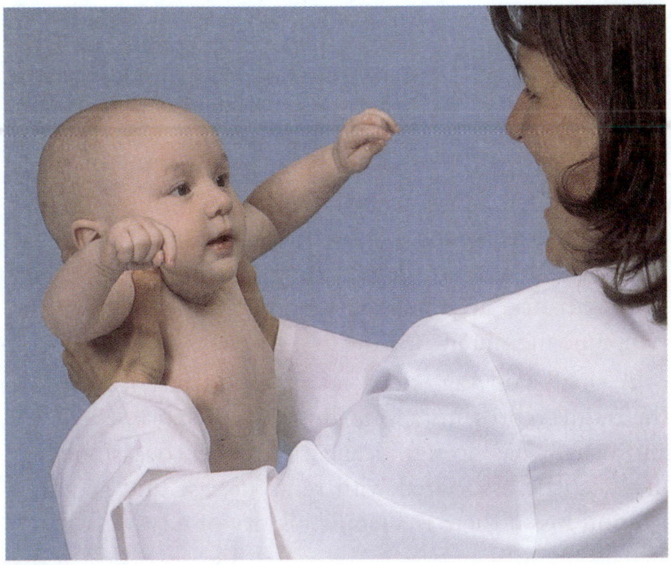

FIGURE 23-25. Carefully assess gaze and eye movements.

During the first 10 days of life, the eyes may stare in one direction if just the head is turned without moving the body (*doll's eye reflex*).

Alternating convergent or divergent *strabismus* persisting beyond 3 months, or persistent strabismus of any type, may indicate *ocular motor weakness* or another abnormality in the visual system.

During the first few months of life, some infants have intermittent crossed eyes (*intermittent alternating convergent strabismus,* or *esotropia*) or laterally deviated eyes (*intermittent alternating divergent strabismus,* or *exotropia*). These generally resolve.

Look for abnormalities or congenital problems in the *sclera* and *pupils.* Subconjunctival hemorrhages are common in newborns and resolve within a couple of weeks. The eyes of many newborns are edematous from the birth process.

Colobomas are missing sections of tissue in the eye (e.g., in the iris alone or iris plus retina). These may be seen with the naked eye and represent defects in the iris and may be associated with vision loss.

Observe pupillary reactions by response to light or by covering each eye with your hand and then uncovering it. Although there may be initial asymmetry in the size of the pupils, over time they should be equal in size and reaction to light.

Inspect the irises carefully for abnormalities.

Brushfield spots (seen with an ophthalmoscope) are a ring of white specks in the iris. Although sometimes present in normal children, these strongly suggest *Down syndrome.*

See Table 23-7, Abnormalities of the Eyes, Ears, and Mouth.

Examine the *conjunctiva* for swelling or redness. Most newborn nurseries use an antibiotic eye ointment to help prevent gonococcal eye infection. This sometimes causes temporary swelling around the eyes.

Persistent ocular discharge and tearing beginning at birth may be from *dacryocystitis* or *nasolacrimal duct obstruction.*

You will not be able to measure the *visual acuity* of newborns or infants. You can use visual reflexes to indirectly assess vision: direct and consensual pupillary constriction in response to light, blinking in response to bright light (*optic blink reflex*), and blinking in response to quick movement of an object toward the eyes.

During the first year of life, visual acuity sharpens as the ability to focus improves (Box 23-15). Infants achieve the visual milestones shown here. Failure to progress along these visual developmental milestones may indicate *delayed visual maturation.*

Box 23-15. Visual Milestones of Infancy

Age	Milestone
Birth	Blinks, may regard face
1 month	Fixes on objects
1½–2 months	Coordinated eye movements
3 months	Eyes converge, baby reaches toward a visual stimulus
12 months	Acuity around 20/60–20/80

Acoustic Blink Reflex. The *acoustic blink reflex* is a blinking of the infant's eyes in response to a sudden sharp sound. You can produce it by snapping your fingers or using a bell, beeper, or other noisemaking device approximately 1 foot from the infant's ear. Be sure you are not producing an airstream that may cause the infant to blink (Box 23-16). This reflex may be difficult to elicit during the first 2 to 3 days of life. After it is elicited several times within a brief period, the reflex disappears, a phenomenon known as *habituation.* This crude test of hearing certainly is not diagnostic.

Ophthalmoscopic Examination. A thorough ophthalmoscopic examination is difficult in young infants but may be needed if ocular or neurologic abnormalities are noted. The cornea can ordinarily be seen at +20 diopters, the lens at +15 diopters, and the fundus at 0 diopters.

Congenital glaucoma may cause cloudiness of the cornea.

Box 23-16. Signs That an Infant Can Hear

Age	Sign
0–2 months	Startle response and blink to a sudden noise Calming down with soothing voice or music
2–3 months	Change in body movements in response to sound Change in facial expression to familiar sounds Turning eyes and head to sound
3–4 months	Turning to listen to voices and conversation
6–7 months	Appropriate language development

Perinatal problems raising the risk for *hearing defects* include birth weight <1,500 g, anoxia, treatment with potentially ototoxic medications, congenital infections, severe hyperbilirubinemia, and meningitis.

In the absence of universal hearing screening, many children with *hearing deficits* are not diagnosed until 2 years. Clues to hearing deficits include parental concern about hearing, delayed speech, and lack of developmental indicators of hearing shown here.

For the ophthalmoscopic examination, with the newborn awake and eyes open, examine the *red retinal (fundus) reflex* by setting the ophthalmoscope at 0 diopters and viewing the pupil from about 10 in. Normally, a red or orange color is reflected from the fundus through the pupil.

A dark light reflex can result from cataracts, retinopathy of prematurity, or other disorders. A white retinal reflex (*leukokoria*) is abnormal, and cataract, retinal detachment, chorioretinitis, or retinoblastoma should be suspected.

Occlusion of the red reflex by the lens may represent a cataract.

Examine the optic disc area as you would for an adult. In infants, the optic disc is difficult to visualize but is lighter in color, and there is less macular pigmentation. The foveal light reflection may not be visible.

Papilledema is rare in infants because the fontanelles and open sutures accommodate any increased intracranial pressure, sparing the optic discs.

Small retinal hemorrhages may occur in normal newborns.

Extensive hemorrhages may suggest severe anoxia, subdural hematoma, subarachnoid hemorrhage, or trauma. Beyond the newborn period, retinal hemorrhages may be a sign of nonaccidental trauma (child abuse).

Ears. The physical examination of the ears of infants can detect abnormalities such as structural problems, otitis media, and hearing loss. The goals are to determine the *position*, *shape*, and *features of the ear* and to detect abnormalities. Note ear position in relation to the eyes.

An imaginary line drawn across the inner and outer canthi of the eyes should cross the pinna or auricle; if the pinna is below this line the infant has low-set ears. Draw this imaginary line across the face of the baby on p. 653; note that it crosses the pinna.

Small, deformed, or low-set auricles may indicate associated *congenital defects*, especially renal disease.

Otoscopic Examination. Otoscopic examination of the newborn's ear can detect only patency of the *ear canal* because accumulated vernix caseosa obscures the tympanic membrane for the first few days of life.

A small skin tag, cleft, or pit found just forward of the tragus represents a remnant of the *first branchial cleft* and usually has no significance. However, occasionally it may also be associated with renal disease and acquired hearing loss if there is a family history of hearing loss.

The infant's ear canal is directed downward from the outside; therefore, pull the auricle gently downward and outward, not upward, for the best view of the eardrum. Once the tympanic membrane is visible, note that the light reflex is diffuse; it does not become cone shaped for several months.

See techniques in the use of an otoscope on p. 683.

Acute otitis media can occur in infants.

Nose and Sinuses. Infants are *obligate nasal breathers* and have difficulty breathing through their mouths. The most important component of the examination of the infant nose is to *test for patency of these nasal passages.* You can do this by gently occluding each nostril alternately while holding the infant's mouth closed. This usually will not cause stress because most infants are nasal breathers. Do not occlude both nares simultaneously, as this will cause considerable distress.

The nasal passages in newborns may be obstructed in *choanal atresia.* In severe cases, nasal obstruction can be assessed by attempting to pass a no. 8 feeding tube through each nostril into the posterior pharynx. This is usually done in the delivery room to assess for choanal atresia or other sources of unilateral or bilateral obstruction. The nasal passages in newborns may be obstructed in *choanal atresia.* In severe cases, nasal obstruction can be assessed by attempting to pass a no. 8 feeding tube through each nostril into the posterior pharynx. This is usually done in the delivery room to assess for choanal atresia or other sources of unilateral or bilateral obstruction.

Inspect the nose to ensure that the nasal septum is midline.

At birth, the maxillary and the ethmoid sinuses are present but small and pneumatization occurs over time. Palpation of the sinuses of newborns is not helpful.

Mouth and Pharynx. Use both inspection with a tongue depressor and flashlight and palpation to inspect the mouth and pharynx (Fig. 23-26). A parent can help you by stabilizing the infant's head and arms. The newborn's mouth is edentulous, and the alveolar mucosa is smooth with finely serrated borders. Occasionally, pearl-like retention cysts are seen along the alveolar ridges and are easily mistaken for teeth; these disappear within 1 or 2 months. Petechiae are commonly found on the soft palate after birth.

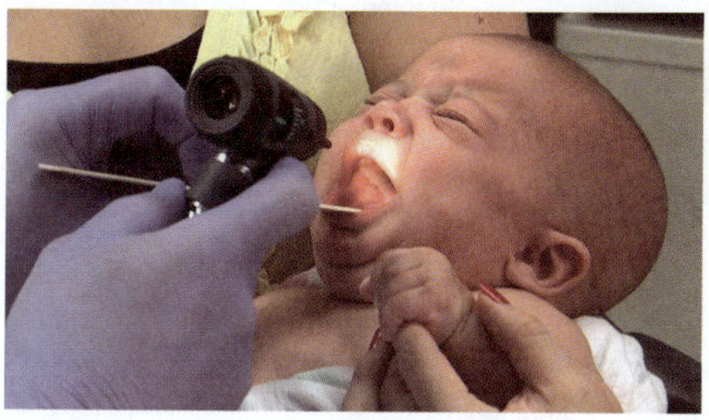

FIGURE 23-26. Parental assistance helps with oral assessment.

Rarely, supernumerary teeth are noted. These are usually dysmorphic and are shed within days but are removed to prevent aspiration.

Palpate the upper hard palate to make sure it is intact. *Epstein pearls*, tiny white or yellow, rounded mucous retention cysts, are located along the posterior midline of the hard palate. They disappear within months.

A congenital fissure of the median line of the palate is a *cleft palate*.

Infants produce little saliva during the first 3 months. Older infants produce a lot of saliva and drool frequently.

Tongue. *Inspect the tongue.* The frenulum varies in tightness; sometimes it extends almost to the tip and other times it is short, limiting protrusion of the tongue (*ankyloglossia* or *tongue tie*).

A prominent, protruding tongue may signal congenital hypothyroidism, Down syndrome, or Beckwith–Wiedemann syndrome.

If associated with hypoglycemia and omphalocele, macroglossia is likely *Beckwith–Wiedemann* syndrome.

You will often see a whitish covering on the tongue. If this coating is from milk, it can be easily removed by scraping or wiping it away. Use a tongue depressor or your gloved finger to wipe away the coating. If you do use a tongue depressor, be careful to not stick it too deep into the infant's mouth or you will elicit a gag reflex.

Oral candidiasis *(thrush)* is common in infants. The white plaques are difficult to wipe away and have an erythematous raw base. They are found on the buccal mucosa, palate, and tongue. See Table 23-7, Abnormalities of the Eyes, Ears, and Mouth.

Cysts may be noted on the tongue or mouth. Thyroglossal duct cysts may open at the posterior tongue, or more commonly in the neck.

Teeth. While there is a predictable *pattern of tooth eruption*, there is wide variation in the age at which teeth appear. A rule of thumb is that a child will have 1 tooth for each month of age between 6 and 26 months, up to a maximum of 20 primary teeth.

Natal teeth are teeth that are present at birth. They are usually simply early eruptions of normal teeth, but they can be part of syndromes.

The pharynx of the infant is best seen while the baby is crying. Do not stick a tongue depressor more than two-thirds of the way over the tongue to avoid a strong gag reflex. Infants do not have prominent lymphoid tissue so you will probably not visualize the tonsils which increase in size as children grow.

Listen to the quality of the *infant's cry*. Normal infants have a vigorous cry.

New-onset stridor that appears following birth can be due to infections such as croup, a foreign body, or gastroesophageal reflux.

Inspiratory stridor beginning at birth suggests a congenital abnormality. See Table 23-8, Abnormal Infant Cries.

Neck. Palpate the *lymph nodes of the neck* and assess for any additional masses such as *congenital cysts* (Fig. 23-27). Because the necks of infants are short, it is best to palpate the neck while infants are lying supine, whereas older children are best examined while sitting. Check the position of the thyroid cartilage and trachea.

Branchial cleft cysts appear as small dimples or openings anterior to the midportion of the sternocleidomastoid muscle. They may be associated with a sinus tract.

Preauricular cysts and sinuses are common, pinhole-size pits, usually located anterior to the helix of the ear. They are often bilateral and may be associated with hearing deficits and renal disorders.

Thyroglossal duct cysts are located at the midline of the neck, just above the thyroid cartilage. These small, firm, mobile masses move upward with tongue protrusion or with swallowing. They are usually detected after 2 years.

Congenital torticollis, or a "wry neck," is from bleeding into the sternocleidomastoid muscle during the stretching process during delivery or to in utero positioning. A firm fibrous mass is felt within the muscle 2 to 3 weeks after birth and generally disappears over months.

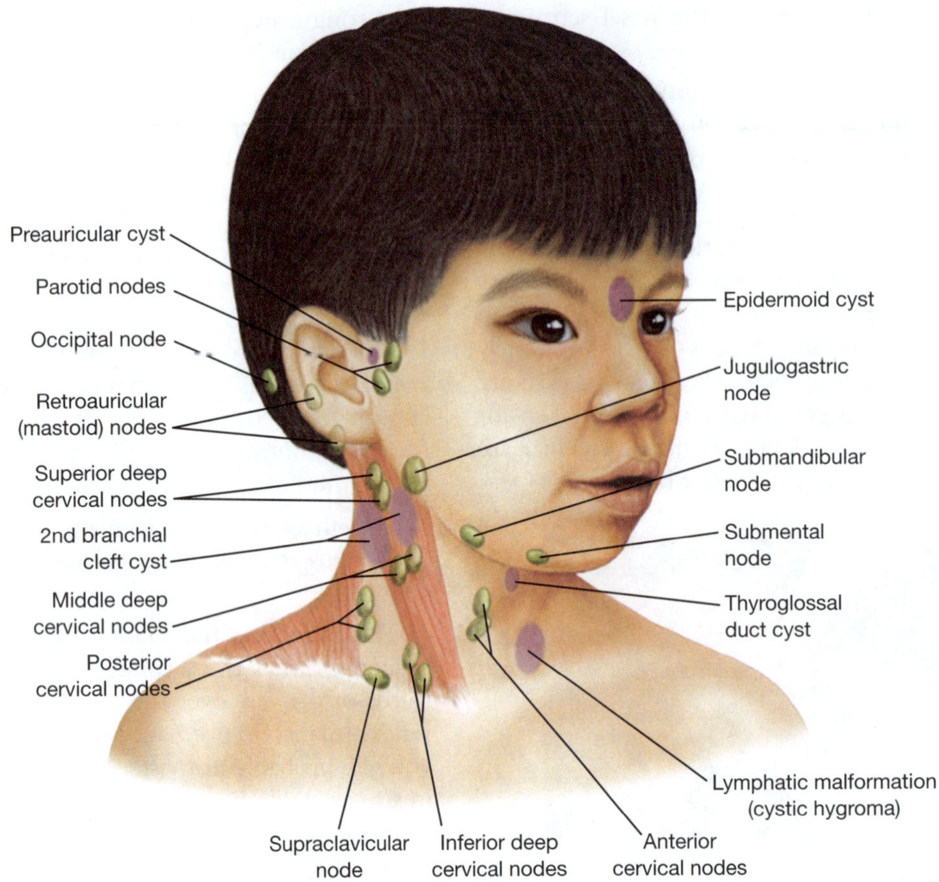

FIGURE 23-27. Nodes and cysts of the head and neck.

In newborns, palpate the *clavicles* and look for evidence of a fracture. If present, you may feel a break in the contour of the bone, tenderness, crepitus at the fracture site, and may notice limited movement of the arm on the affected side.

A fracture of the clavicle may occur during birth, particularly during delivery of a difficult arm or shoulder extraction.

Thorax and Lungs. The infant's *thorax* is more rounded than that of adults. The thin chest wall has little musculature; thus, lung and heart sounds are transmitted quite clearly. The bony and cartilaginous rib cage is soft and pliant. The tip of the xiphoid process often protrudes anteriorly, immediately beneath the skin.

Two types of chest wall abnormalities noted in childhood include pectus excavatum and pectus carinatum.

Inspection. Carefully *assess respirations* and *breathing patterns*. Newborns, especially those born prematurely, show periods of normal rate (30 to 40 per minute) alternating respirations that may even cease for 5 to 10 seconds. This alternating pattern of rapid and slow breathing is called "periodic respiration" or "periodic breathing." Periodic breathing is one reason why it is optimal to measure respiratory rate over 60 seconds.

Apnea is cessation of breathing for more than 20 seconds. It is often accompanied by bradycardia and may indicate respiratory disease, central nervous system disease, or, rarely, a cardiopulmonary condition.

Do not rush to the stethoscope. Instead, observe the infant carefully as demonstrated in Figure 23-28, which demonstrates locations for retractions among infants. Inspection is easiest when infants are not crying; thus, work with the parents to settle the child.

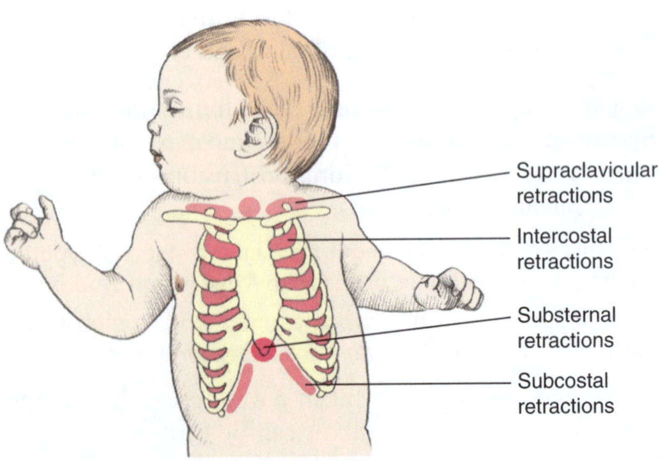

FIGURE 23-28. Anatomic locations of retractions (chest indrawing).

Box 23-17. Observing Respiration

Type of Assessment	Specific Observable Pathology
General appearance	Inability to feed or smile Lack of consolability
Respiratory rate	Tachypnea (see p. 686), apnea
Color	Pallor or cyanosis
Nasal component of breathing	Nasal flaring (enlargement of both nasal openings during inspiration)
Audible breath sounds	Grunting (repetitive, short expiratory sound) Wheezing (musical expiratory sound) Stridor (high-pitched, inspiratory noise) Obstruction (lack of breath sounds)
Work of breathing	Nasal flaring (excessive movement of nares) Grunting (expiratory noises) Retractions (chest indrawing): Supraclavicular (soft tissue above clavicles) Intercostal (indrawing of skin between ribs) Substernal (at xiphoid process) Subcostal (just below the costal margin)

Acute stridor is a potentially serious condition; causes include laryngotracheobronchitis (croup), epiglottitis, bacterial tracheitis, foreign body, hemangioma, or a vascular ring.

In infants, increased work of breathing plus abnormal findings on auscultation are the best findings for *ruling in* pneumonia. The best sign for *ruling out* pneumonia is the absence of tachypnea.

Observe for 30 to 60 seconds, note general appearance, respiratory rate, color, nasal component of breathing, audible breath sounds, and work of breathing (Box 23-17). Because infants are obligate nasal breathers, observe their nose as they breathe. Look for *nasal flaring*. Observe breathing with the infant's mouth closed or during nursing or sucking on a bottle to assess for nasal patency. Listen to the sounds of breathing; note any *grunting*, *audible wheezing*, or *lack of breath sounds (obstruction)*.

Nasal flaring, grunting, retractions, and wheezing are all signs of respiratory distress.

In newborns and young infants, nasal flaring may be the result of upper respiratory infections, with subsequent obstruction of their small nares, but it may also be caused by *pneumonia* or other serious respiratory infections.

Observe three aspects of the infant's breathing: *respiratory rate (i.e., tachypnea)*, *audible breath sounds* and *work of breathing*. These are particularly relevant in assessing both upper and lower respiratory illness. Any of the abnormalities listed in Box 23-17 should raise concern about underlying respiratory pathology.

A combination of respiratory signs such as nasal flaring plus grunting and tachypnea may indicate lower respiratory infections, defined as infections below the vocal cords. Examples include bronchiolitis and pneumonia.

In healthy infants, the ribs do not move much during quiet breathing. Any outward movement is produced by descent of the diaphragm which compresses the abdominal contents and in turn shifts the lower ribs outward.

Asymmetric chest movement may indicate a space-occupying lesion.

Chest indrawing is inward movement of the skin between the ribs during inspiration. Movement of the diaphragm primarily affects breathing with little assistance from the thoracic muscles. As mentioned in the preceding table, four types of retractions can be noted in infants: suprasternal, intercostal, substernal, and subcostal.

Pulmonary disease in young children causes increased abdominal breathing and can result in retractions.

Head bobbing may also be seen in infants with severe respiratory distress.

Thoracoabdominal paradox, or *paradoxical breathing*, is inward movement of the chest and outward movement of the abdomen during inspiration (abdominal breathing). This is a *normal finding in newborns (but not older infants)*. It persists during active, or rapid eye movement (REM), sleep even when it is no longer seen during wakefulness or quiet sleep because of the decreased muscle tone of active sleep. As muscle strength increases and chest wall compliance decreases with age, abdominal breathing should no longer be noted. If observed, it may signify respiratory disease.

Airway obstruction or lower respiratory tract disease in infants can result in the *Hoover sign*, or paradoxical (seesaw) breathing in which the abdomen moves outward while the chest moves inward during inspiration.

Children with *muscle weakness* may be noted to have paradoxical breathing at several years of age.

Palpation. Although it is challenging in infants, you can try to assess tactile fremitus by *palpation*. Place your hand on the chest when the infant cries or makes noise. Place your hand or fingertips over each side of the chest and feel for symmetry in the transmitted vibrations. Percussion is not helpful in infants except in extreme instances. The infant's chest is hyperresonant throughout, and it is difficult to detect abnormalities on palpation or percussion.

Because of the excellent transmission of sounds throughout the chest, any abnormalities of tactile fremitus or on percussion suggest severe pathology, such as a large pneumonic consolidation.

Auscultation. Infant breath sounds are louder and harsher than those of adults because the stethoscope is closer to the origin of the sounds. It is often difficult to distinguish transmitted upper airway sounds from sounds originating in the chest (Box 23-18). Upper airway sounds tend to be loud, transmitted symmetrically throughout the chest, and loudest as you move your stethoscope toward the neck. They are usually coarse inspiratory sounds. Lower airway sounds are loudest over the site of pathology, are often asymmetric, and often occur during expiration. You can also hold your stethoscope just above the infant's mouth and nose to differentiate upper airway from lower airway sounds.

Biphasic sounds imply severe obstruction from intrathoracic airway narrowing or severe obstruction from extrathoracic airway narrowing.

Expiratory sounds usually arise from an intrathoracic source, whereas inspiratory sounds can arise from an extrathoracic airway such as the trachea or from an intrathoracic source. During expiration, the diameter of the intrathoracic airways decreases because radial forces from the surrounding lung do not "tether" the airways open as occurs during inspiration. Higher flow rates during inspiration produce turbulent flow, resulting in appreciable sounds.

Upper respiratory infections are not serious in infants but can produce loud inspiratory sounds that are often transmitted to the chest.

The characteristics of the *breath sounds,* such as vesicular and bronchovesicular, and of the *adventitious* lung sounds, such as crackles, wheezes, and rhonchi, are the same as those for adults, except that they may be more difficult to distinguish in infants and often occur together.

Wheezes and rhonchi are common in infants. *Wheezes,* often audible without the stethoscope, occur more frequently than in adults because of the smaller size of the tracheobronchial tree. *Rhonchi* reflect obstruction of larger airways, or bronchi. *Crackles* (rales) are discontinuous sounds, near the end of inspiration; they are usually caused by lung disorders and are far less likely to represent cardiac failure in infants than in adults. They tend to be harsher than in adults.

Wheezes in infants occur commonly from asthma and less commonly from bronchiolitis.

Rhonchi in infants occur with upper respiratory infections.

Crackles can be heard with pneumonia and bronchiolitis.

Box 23-18. Distinguishing Upper Airway from Lower Airway Sounds in Infants

Technique	Upper Airway	Lower Airway
Compare sounds from nose/stethoscope	Same sounds	Often different sounds
Listen to harshness of sounds	Harsh and loud	Variable
Note symmetry (left/right)	Symmetric	Often asymmetric
Compare sounds at different locations (higher or lower)	Sounds are louder as stethoscope is moved up chest	Often sounds are louder lower in chest toward abdomen
Inspiratory vs. expiratory	Almost always inspiratory	Often has expiratory phase
Hold stethoscope above infant's mouth	Inspiratory sounds remain loud	Often quieter than by auscultation of the chest

Diminished breath sounds in one side of the chest of a newborn suggest unilateral lesions (e.g., congenital diaphragmatic hernia or pneumothorax).

Heart

Inspection. Before examining the heart, observe the infant carefully for any cyanosis. Check particularly for *central cyanosis* which is involvement of the lips, tongue and sublingual tissues in addition to the hands and feet (Box 23-19). The best area to look for central cyanosis is the tongue and oral mucosa, not the nail beds, lips, or the extremities. *Acrocyanosis* in the newborn, which spares the oral mucosa, is discussed on pages 650 and 733.

Central cyanosis is always abnormal because many congenital cardiac abnormalities, as well as respiratory diseases, present with cyanosis. See Table 23-10, Cyanosis in Children, and Table 23-11, Congenital Heart Murmurs.

Box 23-19. Cardiac Causes of Central Cyanosis in Infants and Children

Age of Onset	Potential Cardiac Cause
Immediately at birth or within a few days	Transposition of the great arteries Pulmonary valve atresia Severe pulmonary valve stenosis Possibly Ebstein malformation Additional conditions (often within days): Total anomalous pulmonary venous return Hypoplastic left heart syndrome Truncus arteriosus (sometimes) Single ventricle variants
Weeks, months, or years of life	All of the above plus: Pulmonary vascular disease with atrial, ventricular, or great vessel shunting (right-to-left shunting)

A true strawberry pink is normal, whereas any hint of raspberry red suggests desaturation and requires urgent evaluation. The distribution of cyanosis should be evaluated. An oximetry reading will confirm desaturation.

In general, cardiac causes of central cyanosis involve right-to-left shunting and can be caused by a variety of congenital cardiac lesions.

Observe the infant for *general signs of health*. The infant's nutritional status, responsiveness, irritability, and fatigue are all clues that may be useful in evaluating cardiac disease. Note that noncardiac findings are often present in infants with cardiac disease (Box 23-20).

Box 23-20. Noncardiac Findings Commonly Present in Infants with Cardiac Disease

Poor feeding	Tachypnea	Poor overall appearance
Failure to thrive	Hepatomegaly	Weakness
Irritability	Clubbing	Fatigue

The combination of tachypnea, tachycardia, and hepatomegaly in infants suggests *heart failure.*

Observe the respiratory rate and pattern to help distinguish the degree of illness and cardiac versus pulmonary diseases. An increase in respiratory effort is expected from pulmonary diseases, whereas in cardiac disease there may be tachypnea without increased work of breathing (called "peaceful tachypnea") until heart failure becomes significant.

Palpation. Palpation of the chest wall will allow you to assess volume changes within the heart. For example, a hyperdynamic precordium reflects a big volume change.

The *point of maximal cardiac impulse*, or *PMI*, is not always palpable in infants and is affected by respiratory patterns, a full stomach, and the infant's positioning. It is usually an interspace higher than in adults during the first few years of life because the heart lies more horizontally within the chest.

A *"rolling" heave* at the left sternal border suggests an *increase in right ventricular work,* whereas the same kind of motion closer to the apex suggests the same thing for the left ventricle.

Thrills are palpable when turbulence within the heart or great vessels is transmitted to the surface. Knowledge of the structures of the precordium helps pinpoint the origin of the thrill. Thrills are easiest to feel with your palm or the base of your fingers rather than your fingertips. Thrills have a somewhat rough, vibrating quality. Figure 23-29 shows locations of thrills that occur in infants and children from various cardiac abnormalities.

A patent ductus arteriosus (*PDA*) is associated with hyperdynamic precordium and bounding distal pulses.

Visible and palpable chest pulsations suggest a hyperdynamic state from either increased metabolic rate or inefficient pumping as a result of an underlying *cardiac defect.*

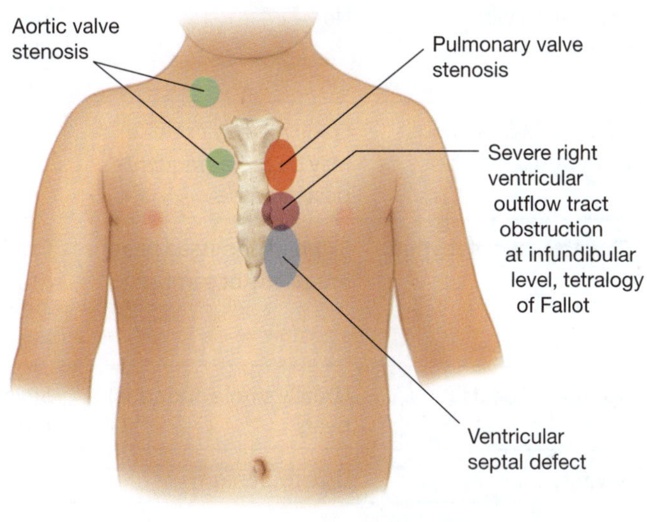

FIGURE 23-29. Location of thrills in infants and children.

Auscultation. You can evaluate the *heart rhythm* more easily in infants by listening to the heart than by feeling the peripheral pulses; in older children assess the rhythm either way (see Box 23-18).

The most common abnormal dysrhythmia in infants is supraventricular tachycardia (SVT). It can occur at any age and is sometimes found on examination. The child may look healthy, pale, or moderately ill. The heart rate is sustained and regular at around 220 beats per minute or more. SVT in older children is more likely to be truly paroxysmal, with episodes of varying duration and frequency.

Infants and children commonly have a normal sinus dysrhythmia, with the heart rate increasing on inspiration and decreasing on expiration, sometimes quite abruptly. This normal finding can be identified by its repetitive nature and its correlation with respiration (Box 23-21).

Many neonates and some older children have premature atrial or ventricular beats that are often described as "skipped" beats. You can usually eradicate them by increasing their intrinsic sinus rate through exercise such as crying in an infant or jumping in an older child, although they may also be more frequent in the postexercise period. In a completely healthy child, they are usually benign and rarely persist.

Distant heart tones suggest *pericardial effusion.*

Heart Sounds. Heart sounds are very challenging to assess in infants because they are rapid and often obscured by respiratory or other sounds. Nevertheless, attempt to evaluate the S_1 and S_2 heart sounds carefully and systematically. They are normally crisp. You can usually hear the second sounds (S_2) at the base separately, but they should fuse into a single sound in deep expiration.

Pathologic arrhythmias in children can not only be from *structural cardiac lesions* but also from other causes such as drug ingestion, metabolic abnormalities, endocrine disorders, serious infections, and postinfectious states, or conduction disturbances without structural heart disease.

Try to detect a split S_2 by examining the infant when the infant is completely quiet or asleep. This split is usually reassuring although there are exceptions as noted below.

In addition to trying to detect splitting of the S_2, listen for the intensity of A_2 and P_2. The aortic, or first component of the second sound at the base, is normally louder than the pulmonic, or second component (Fig. 23-30).

A louder-than-normal pulmonic component, particularly when louder than the aortic sound, suggests pulmonary hypertension or an atrial septal defect (ASD).

Box 23-21. Characteristics of Normal Variants of Heart Rhythms in Children

Characteristics	Atrial Premature Contractions (APCs) or Ventricular Premature Contractions (VPCs)	Normal Sinus Dysrhythmias
Most common age	Neonates (may occur at any time)	After infancy Throughout childhood
Correlation with respiration	No	Yes: Increases on inspiration, decreases on expiration
Effect of exercise on tachycardia	Eradicated by exercise May be more frequent post-exercise	Disappears
Characteristic of rhythm	Skipped or missed beat Irregularly occurring	Gradually faster with inspiration Often suddenly slower on expiration
Number of beats	Usually single abnormal beats	Several beats, usually in repetitive cycles
Severity	Usually benign	Benign (by definition)

Although ventricular premature contractions generally occur in otherwise healthy infants, they can occur with underlying cardiac disease, particularly cardiomyopathies and congenital heart disorders. Electrolyte or metabolic disturbances are also possible causes.

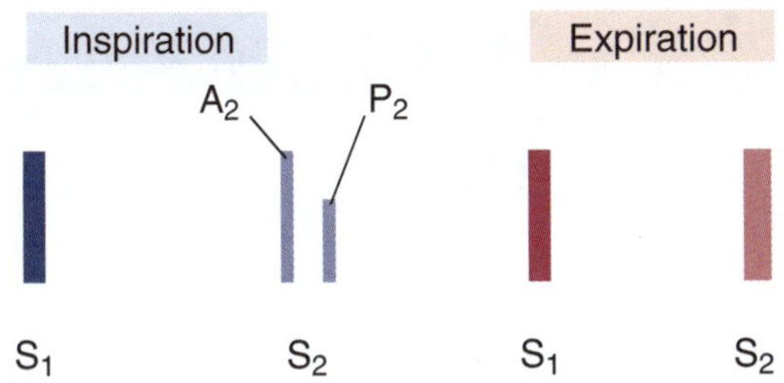

FIGURE 23-30. Healthy heart sounds in infants.

Persistent splitting of S_2 may indicate a right ventricular volume load such as atrial septal defect, or cardiac lesions associated with pulmonary hypertension.

You may detect *third heart sounds* which are low-pitched, early diastolic sounds best heard at the lower left sternal border, or apex; they reflect rapid ventricular filling. These are frequently heard in children and are normal. A fourth heart sound (S_4), not often heard in children, is a low-frequency, late diastolic sound, occurring just before the first heart sound.

A high-intensity third heart sound, or a gallop, is a sign of underlying pathology.

A *fourth heart sound* represents decreased ventricular compliance, suggesting heart failure.

You may also detect an *apparent gallop* (widely split S_2 that varies), in the presence of a normal heart rate and rhythm. This is frequently found in normal children and does not represent pathology.

A true *gallop rhythm* (in contrast to a widely split S_2 which gives an apparent gallop)—tachycardia plus a loud S_3, S_4, or both—is pathologic and indicates *heart failure* (*poor ventricular function*).

Heart Murmurs. One of the most challenging aspects of the cardiac examination in children is the evaluation of *heart murmurs.* In addition to listening to a squirming, perhaps uncooperative child, a major challenge is distinguishing common benign murmurs from unusual or pathologic ones.

Characterize heart murmurs in infants and children by noting their specific location (e.g., left upper sternal border, not just left sternal border), timing, intensity, and quality. If each murmur is delineated completely, the diagnosis is usually made clinically; laboratory tools such as ECG, chest x-ray, and echocardiography may be needed for confirmation and better characterization.

Many (but not all) children with serious cardiac malformations have signs and symptoms other than a heart murmur obtainable on careful history or examination. Many have noncardiac signs and symptoms, including evidence of genetic defects that may offer helpful diagnostic clues.

Any of the noncardiac findings that frequently accompany cardiac disease in children markedly raises the possibility that a murmur is pathologic.

Most children, if not all, will have one or more *functional,* or *benign, heart murmurs* before reaching adulthood. It is important to identify functional murmurs by their specific qualities rather than by their intensity. An important rule of thumb is that, by definition, *benign murmurs in children have no associated abnormal findings* and are growing normally.

Some *pathologic murmurs of congenital heart disease* are present at birth. Others are not apparent until later, depending on their severity, drop in pulmonary vascular resistance following birth, or changes associated with growth of the child. Table 23-11, Congenital Heart Murmurs, shows examples of pathologic murmurs of childhood.

Box 23-22 characterizes two *benign* heart murmurs in infants according to their locations and key characteristics.

In some infants, you will detect a soft, ejectile murmur heard in the axilla and back. This represents benign peripheral pulmonary stenosis, which is partly the result of inadequate pulmonary artery growth in utero (when there is little pulmonary blood flow) and the sharp angle at which the pulmonary artery curves backward. In the absence of any physical findings to suggest additional underlying diseases, this *peripheral pulmonary stenosis murmur* (which is common) can be considered benign and usually disappears by 1 year.

A pulmonary flow murmur in the newborn with other signs of disease is more likely to be pathologic. Diseases may include Williams syndrome, congenital rubella syndrome, and Alagille syndrome. These conditions have pulmonary artery stenosis and differ from the benign peripheral pulmonary stenosis.

When you detect a murmur in a child, note all of the qualities as described in Chapter 11, Cardiovascular System, to help you distinguish *pathologic murmurs* from benign murmurs. Heart murmurs that reflect underlying structural heart disease are easier to evaluate if you have a good knowledge of intrathoracic anatomy and the functional cardiac changes following birth and if you understand the physiologic basis for heart murmurs. Understanding these physiologic changes can help you distinguish pathologic murmurs from benign heart murmurs in children (Box 23-23).

A newborn with a heart murmur and central cyanosis is likely to have congenital heart disease and requires urgent cardiac evaluation.

Peripheral Vascular System. The major branches of the aorta can be assessed by evaluation of the *peripheral pulses.* All neonates should have an evaluation of all pulses at the time of their newborn examination. In neonates and

Box 23-22. Two Common Benign Murmurs in Infants

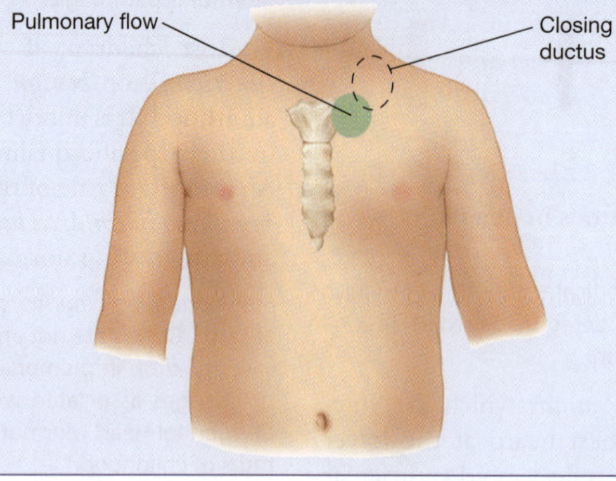

Typical Age	Name	Characteristics	Description and Location
Newborn	*Closing ductus*	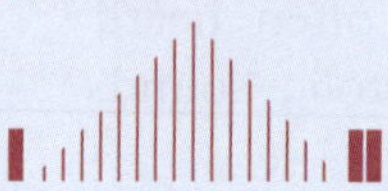	Harsh, ejectile (crescendo) systolic murmur, as PDA closes becomes continuous Upper left sternal border
Newborn to 1 yr	*Peripheral pulmonary flow murmur*	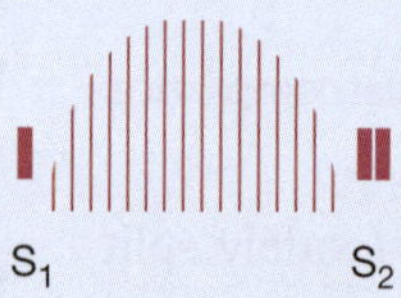	Soft, ejectile, systolic Upper left sternal border, radiating to lung fields and axillae

Box 23-23. Physiologic Basis for Selected Pathologic Heart Murmurs

Change in Pulmonary Vascular Resistance

- Heart murmurs that are dependent on a postnatal drop in pulmonary vascular resistance, allowing turbulent flow from the high-pressure systemic circuit to the lower-pressure pulmonary circuit, are not audible until such a drop has occurred. Except in premature infants, murmurs of a ventricular septal defect or PDA are sometimes not heard in the first few days of life and usually become audible after a week to 10 days.

Obstructive Lesions

- Obstructive lesions, such as pulmonic and aortic stenosis, are caused by normal blood flow through two small valves. They are not dependent on a drop in pulmonary vascular resistance. They are audible at birth.

Pressure Gradient Differences

- Murmurs of atrioventricular valve regurgitation are audible at birth because of the high-pressure gradient between the ventricle and its atrium.

Changes Associated with Growth of Children

- Some murmurs do not follow the patterns above but become audible because of alterations in normal blood flow that occur with growth. For example, even though it is an obstructive defect, aortic stenosis may not be audible until considerable growth has occurred and is frequently not heard until adulthood, although a congenitally abnormal valve is responsible. Similarly, the pulmonary flow murmur of an atrial septal defect may not be heard for a year or more because right ventricular compliance gradually increases and the shunt becomes larger, eventually producing a murmur caused by too much blood flow across a normal pulmonic valve.

infants, the *brachial artery pulse in the antecubital fossa is easier to feel than the radial artery pulse at the wrist*. Both temporal arteries should be felt just in front of the ear.

The absence or diminution of femoral pulses is indicative of *coarctation of the aorta*. If you cannot detect femoral pulses, measure blood pressures of one of the lower and both upper extremities. Normally, the blood pressure in the lower extremity is slightly higher than in the upper extremities. If they are equal or lower in the leg, coarctation is likely to be present.

Palpate the femoral pulses. They lie in the midline just below the inguinal crease, between the iliac crest and the symphysis pubis. Take your time to search for femoral pulses; they are difficult to detect in chubby, squirming infants. Use the pads of your index and middle finger together to maximize your chance of finding the pulse. If you first flex the infant's thighs on the abdomen, this may overcome the reflex flexion that occurs when you then extend the legs.

Palpate the pulses in the lower extremities using your index or middle finger. The dorsalis pedis and posterior tibial pulses (Fig. 23-31) may be difficult to feel unless there is an abnormality involving aortic run-off. Normal pulses should have a sharp rise and should be firm and well localized.

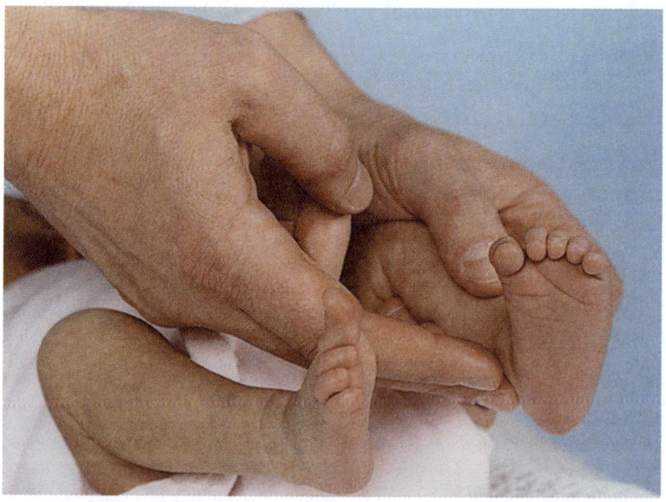

FIGURE 23-31. Palpating pulses in the lower extremity.

A weak or thready, difficult-to-feel pulse may reflect myocardial dysfunction and heart failure, particularly if associated with an unusual degree of tachycardia.

Although the pulses in the feet of neonates and infants are often faint, several conditions can cause full pulses, such as a patent ductus arteriosus or truncus arteriosus.

Carefully measure the *blood pressure* of infants and children (using an appropriate-sized infant blood pressure cuff) as part of the cardiac examination.

Breasts. The breasts of the newborn in both males and females are often enlarged from maternal estrogen effect; this may last several months. The breasts may also be engorged with a white liquid, sometimes colloquially called "witch's milk," which may last 1 or 2 weeks.

In premature thelarche, breast development occurs, most often between 6 months and 2 years. Other signs of puberty or hormonal abnormalities are not present.

Abdomen

Inspection. Inspect the abdomen with the infant lying supine (and, optimally, asleep). The infant's abdomen is protuberant as a result of poorly developed abdominal musculature. You will easily notice abdominal wall blood vessels and intestinal peristalsis.

Inspect the newborn's *umbilical cord* to detect abnormalities. Normally, there are two thick-walled umbilical arteries and one larger but thin-walled umbilical vein which is usually located at the 12 o'clock position.

A single umbilical artery may be associated with congenital anomalies or be an isolated anomaly.

The umbilicus in the newborn may have a long cutaneous portion (*umbilicus cutis*) which is covered with skin, and an amniotic portion (*umbilicus amnioticus*) which is covered by a firm gelatinous substance. The amniotic portion dries up and falls off within 2 weeks, whereas the cutaneous portion retracts to be flush with the abdominal wall.

An umbilical granuloma at the base of the navel is the development of pink granulation tissue formed during the healing process.

Inspect the area around the umbilicus for redness or swelling. The normal healing process of the umbilical stump produces a sometimes foul-smelling, moist exterior at the point of healing. However, the abdominal skin around the umbilicus should be the same color as the baby's abdomen.

Infection of the umbilical stump (*omphalitis*) is characterized by periumbilical edema and erythema.

Umbilical hernias are detectable by a few weeks of age. Most disappear by 1 year, nearly all by 5 years. Umbilical hernias in infants are caused by a defect in the abdominal wall and can be quite protuberant with increased intra-abdominal pressure (e.g., during crying).

In some infants, you will notice a *diastasis recti*. This involves separation of the two rectus abdominis muscles, causing a midline ridge most apparent when the infant contracts the abdominal muscles. A benign condition in most cases, it resolves during early childhood.

Auscultation. Auscultation of a quiet infant's abdomen is easy. You may hear an orchestra of musical tinkling bowel sounds upon placement of your stethoscope on the infant's abdomen.

An increase in pitch or frequency of bowel sounds is heard with gastroenteritis. Intestinal obstruction often produces a silent abdomen.

Percussion and Palpation. You can percuss an infant's abdomen as you would an adult's but you may note greater tympanitic sounds because of the infant's propensity to swallow air. Percussion is useful for determining the size of organs and abdominal masses.

A silent, tympanic, distended, and tender abdomen suggests peritonitis.

It is easy to palpate an infant's abdomen because infants like being touched. A useful technique to relax the infant is to hold the legs flexed at the knees and hips with one hand and palpate the abdomen with the other.

A pacifier may quiet the infant in this position.

When palpating the liver, start gently low in the abdomen, moving upward with your fingers. This technique helps to identify an extremely enlarged liver that extends down into the pelvis. With a careful examination, you can feel the liver edge in most infants, 1 to 3 cm below the right costal margin.

Among newborns, causes of hepatomegaly include hepatitis, storage diseases, vascular congestion, and late presentation of biliary obstruction.

One technique for assessing liver size in infants is simultaneous percussion and auscultation. Percuss and simultaneously auscultate, noting a change in sound as you percuss over the liver or beyond it (Box 23-24).

Box 23-24. Liver Size in Healthy Term Newborns

By palpation and percussion	Mean, 5.9 ± 0.7 cm
Projection below right costal margin	Mean, 2.5 ± 1.0 cm

The *spleen*, like the liver, is felt easily in most infants. It is soft with a sharp edge and it projects downward like a tongue from under the left costal margin. The spleen is moveable and rarely extends more than 1 to 2 cm below the left costal margin.

Splenomegaly can be due to infections, hemolytic anemias, infiltrative disorders, inflammatory or autoimmune diseases, and portal hypertension.

Palpate the *other abdominal structures*. You will commonly note pulsations in the epigastrium caused by the aorta. This is felt on deep palpation to the left of the midline. Rarely, you may be able to palpate the kidneys of infants by carefully placing the fingers of one hand in front of and those of the other behind each kidney. The descending colon is a sausage-like mass in the left lower quadrant.

Abnormal abdominal masses in infants can be associated with the kidney (e.g., hydronephrosis), bladder (e.g., urethral obstruction), bowel (e.g., stool from Hirschsprung disease, or intussusception), and tumors.

Once you have identified the normal structures in the infant's abdomen, use palpation to identify abnormal masses.

In pyloric stenosis, deep palpation in the right upper quadrant or midline can reveal an "olive," or a 2-cm firm pyloric mass. While the infant is feeding you might see peristaltic waves pass across the abdomen. Infants present at about 4 to 6 weeks of age.

Male Genitalia. *Inspect* the male genitalia with the infant supine noting the appearance of the penis, testes, and scrotum.

The *foreskin (prepuce)* completely covers the *glans penis*. It is nonretractable at birth though you may be able to retract it enough to visualize the external urethral meatus.

The foreskin gradually loosens over months to years and becomes retractable.

Hypospadias refers to an abnormal location of the urethral orifice to some point along the ventral surface of the glans or shaft of the penis The foreskin is incompletely formed ventrally.

Inspect the *shaft of the penis*, noting any abnormalities on the ventral surface. Make sure the penis appears straight.

A fixed, downward bowing of the penis is a *chordee;* this may accompany a hypospadias. *Micropenis* is a normally structured penis with length <1.9 cm.

Inspect the *scrotum* noting rugae, which should be present by 40 weeks' gestation. Scrotal edema may be present for several days following birth because of the effect of maternal estrogen.

Palpate the testes in the scrotal sacs, proceeding downward from the external inguinal ring to the scrotum. If you feel a testis up in the inguinal canal, gently milk it downward into the scrotum. The newborn's testes should be about 10 mm in width and 15 mm in length and should lie in the scrotal sacs most of the time.

In newborns with an undescended testicle, the scrotum often appears underdeveloped and tight; palpation reveals an absence of scrotal contents (see Table 23-13, Common Abnormalities in the Male Genitourinary System).

Examine the testes for swelling within the scrotal sac and over the inguinal ring. If you detect swelling in the scrotal sac try to differentiate it from the testis. Note whether the size changes when the infant increases abdominal pressure by crying. See if your fingers can get above the mass, trapping it in the scrotal sac. Apply gentle pressure to try to reduce the size of the mass and note any tenderness. Note whether it transilluminates (Fig. 23-32).

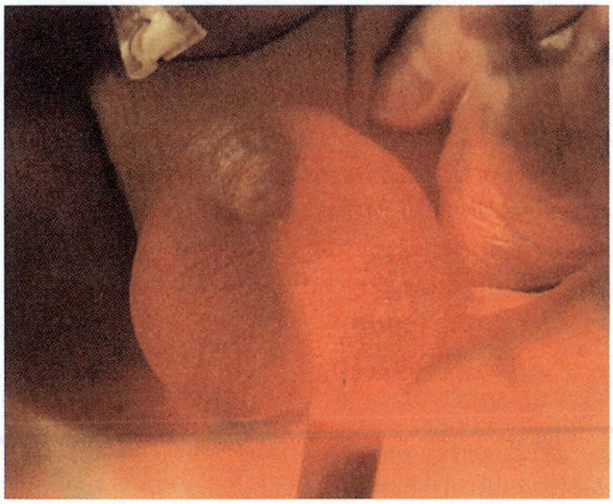

FIGURE 23-32. Transillumination of a hydrocele. (From Fletcher M. *Physical Diagnosis in Neonatology*. Lippincott-Raven; 1998.)

Two common scrotal masses in newborns are hydroceles and inguinal hernias; frequently both coexist, and both are more common on the right side. Hydroceles overlie the testes and the spermatic cord, and can be communicating (i.e., reducible) or noncommunicating (i.e., nonreducible). They can be transilluminated (Fig. 23-32). Most resolve by 18 months. Hernias are separate from the testes, are usually reducible, and often do not transilluminate. They do not resolve. Sometimes a thickened spermatic cord (called the *silk sign*) is noted.

Female Genitalia. Become familiar with the anatomy of an infant's female genitalia. Examine the female genitalia with the infant supine.

In the newborn female, the genitalia on inspection are prominent due to the effects of maternal estrogen (this decreases during the first year).

The *labia majora* and *minora* have a dull pink color in light-skinned infants and may be hyperpigmented in dark-skinned infants. During the first few weeks of life there is often a milky white vaginal discharge that may be blood tinged and is a result of the effects of hormonal withdrawal; this is not a cause for concern.

Ambiguous genitalia, involving masculinization of the female external genitalia, is a rare condition caused by endocrine disorders such as *congenital adrenal hyperplasia.*

Examine the different structures systematically, including the size of the *clitoris*, the color and size of the labia majora, and any rashes, bruises, or external lesions (Fig. 23-33).

Labial adhesions occur frequently, tend to be paper thin, and often disappear without treatment. The adhesions attach the labial minora to each other at the midline.

Next, separate the labia majora at their midpoint with the thumb of each hand, or as shown in Figures 23-85 and 23-86. Inspect the *urethral orifice* and the labia minora. Assess the *hymen*, which in newborns and infants is a thickened, avascular structure with a central orifice, covering the vaginal opening. You should note a *vaginal opening*, although the hymen will be thickened and redundant. Note any discharge.

An imperforate hymen may be noted at birth.

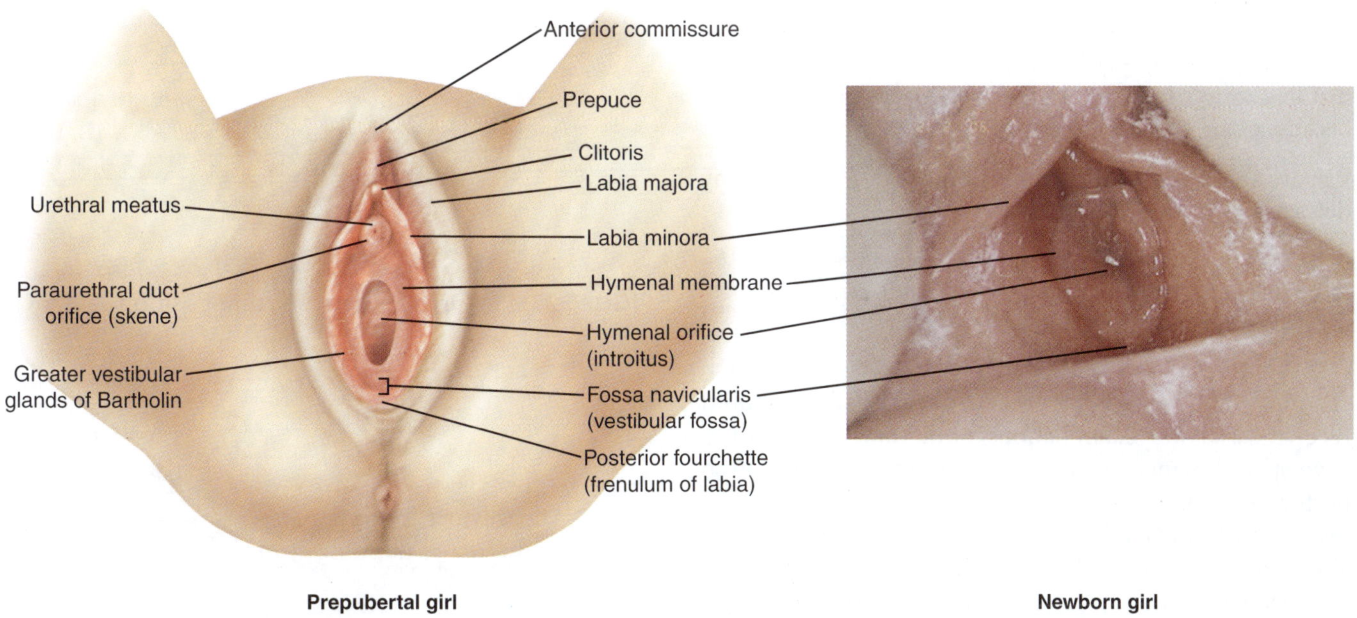

FIGURE 23-33. Highly estrogenized hymen of a newborn with thickening and hypertrophy of hymenal tissue.

Rectum and Anus. In general, a digital rectal examination is not performed on infants or children unless there is question of patency of the anus or an abdominal mass. In such cases, flex the infant's hips and fold the legs to the head. Use your lubricated and gloved pinky to perform the examination.

A common cause of blood in the stool of infants is an *anal fissure* which is a superficial break in the surface of the anus and observable with the naked eye.

Musculoskeletal System. Significant changes in the musculoskeletal system occur during infancy. Much of the examination of the infant focuses on detection of congenital abnormalities, particularly in the hands, spine, hips, legs, and feet.

Combine the musculoskeletal examination with the neurologic and developmental examination.

Inspection can reveal gross deformities such as dwarfism, congenital abnormalities of extremities or digits, and amniotic bands that constrict an extremity.

The *newborn's hands* are clenched. Because of the palmar grasp reflex, you will need to help the infant extend the fingers. Inspect the fingers carefully, noting any defects.

Skin tags, remnants of digits, *polydactyly* (extra fingers), or *syndactyly* (webbed fingers) are congenital defects noted at birth.

Palpate along the *clavicle* noting any lumps, tenderness, or crepitus; these may indicate a fracture which can occur during a difficult birth.

Inspect the *spine* carefully especially for major defects. Note any subtle abnormalities including pigmented spots, hairy patches, or deep pits.

Major defects of the spine such as meningomyeloceles are often detected by ultrasound before birth and if present within 1 cm or so of the midline, may overlie external penings of sinus tracts that extend to the spinal canal. Do not probe any sinus tracts because of the risk of infection.

Palpate the spine in the lumbosacral region, noting any deformities of the vertebrae.

Spina bifida occulta (a defect of the vertebral bodies) may be associated with defects of the spinal cord, which can cause severe neurologic dysfunction.

Examine the newborn and infant's hips carefully at each examination for signs of dislocation. All babies should receive serial hip examinations until they are walking. Two special maneuvers to detect hip instability are often performed. One tests for the presence of a posteriorly dislocated hip (*Ortolani test*), and another tests for the ability to sublux or dislocate an intact but unstable hip (*Barlow test*). The Ortolani and Barlow tests are usually performed together in either sequence.

Developmental dysplasia of the hip is important to detect as early treatment has excellent outcomes.

A soft audible "click" heard with these maneuvers does not prove a *dislocated hip* but should prompt a careful examination.

Ortolani Test. Make sure the baby is relaxed for these techniques. For the *Ortolani test*, place the baby supine with the legs pointing toward you (Fig. 23-34). Flex the legs to form right angles at the hips and knees, placing your index fingers over the greater trochanter of each femur and your thumbs over the lesser trochanters (Fig. 23-35). Abduct both hips simultaneously until the lateral aspect of each knee touches the examining table (Fig. 23-36).

With a developmental dysplasia of the hip, you feel a "clunk" as the femoral head, which lies posterior to the acetabulum, enters the acetabulum. A palpable movement of the femoral head back into place constitutes a *positive Ortolani sign*.

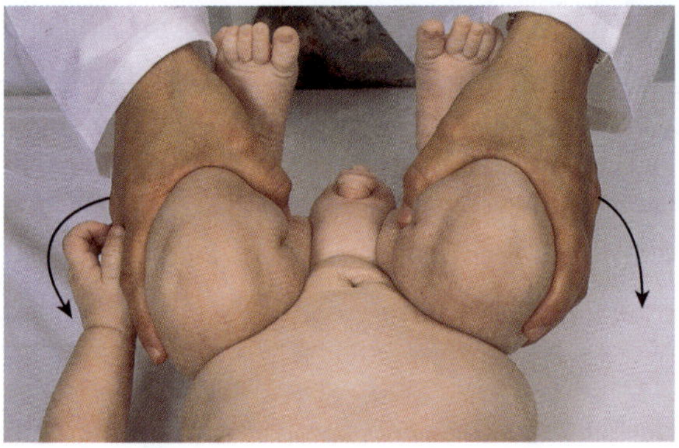

FIGURE 23-34. Ortolani test, overhead view.

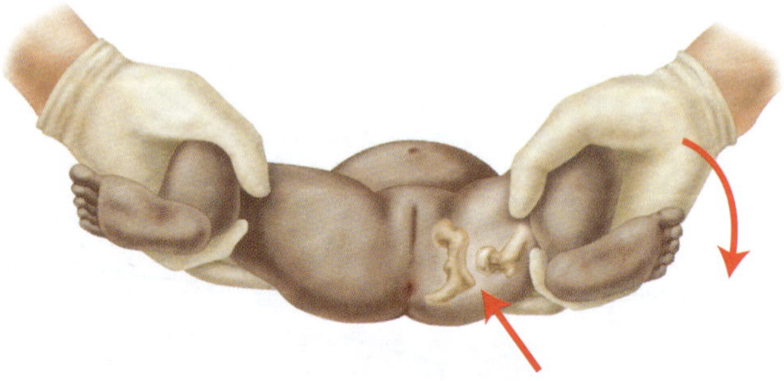

FIGURE 23-35. Ortolani test, starting position.

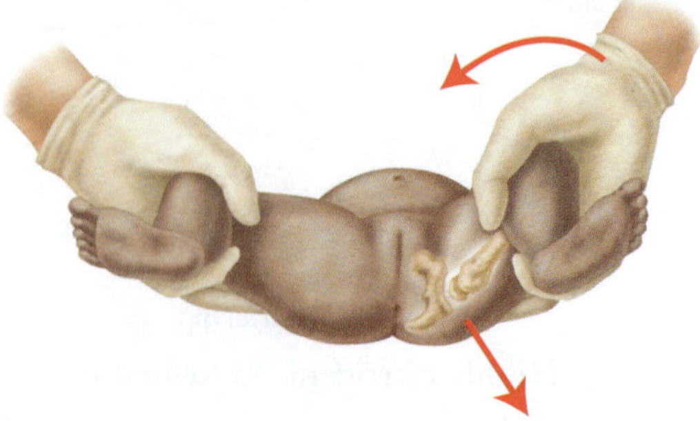

FIGURE 23-36. Ortolani test, ending position.

Barlow Test. For the *Barlow test,* place your hands in the same position as for the Ortolani test. Pull the leg forward (Fig. 23-37) and adduct with posterior force; that is, press in the opposite direction with your thumbs moving down toward the table and outward, applying pressure posteriorly (Fig. 23-38). Feel for any movement of the head of the femur laterally. Normally, there is no movement and the hips feel "stable."

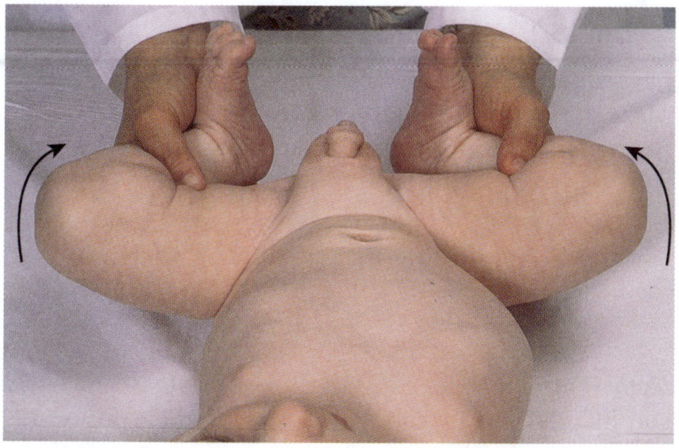

FIGURE 23-37. Barlow test, overhead view.

A positive Barlow sign is not diagnostic of a dysplastic hip but indicates laxity and a potentially dislocatable hip; the baby needs to be followed closely or obtain an ultrasound or refer to a specialist. If you feel the head of the femur slipping out onto the posterior lip of the acetabulum, this constitutes a *positive Barlow sign.* If you feel this dislocation movement, abduct the hip by pressing with your index and middle fingers back inward and feel for the movement of the femoral head as it returns to the hip socket.

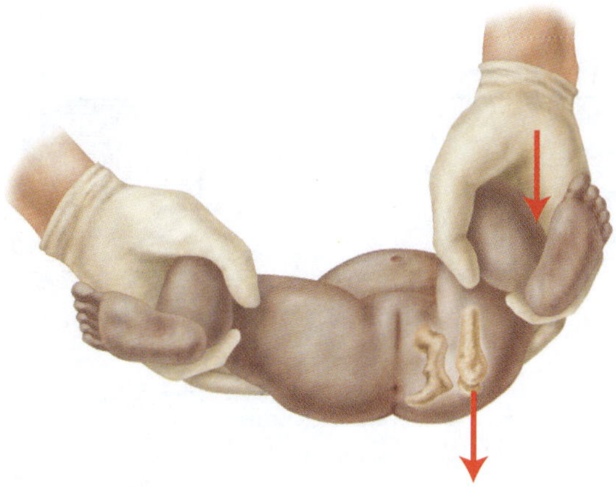

FIGURE 23-38. Barlow test, direction of force.

Children older than age 3 months may have a negative Ortolani or Barlow sign and still have a *dislocated hip* due to tightening of the hip muscles and ligaments.; in these children limited abduction is concerning for developmental dysplasia of the hip.

Test for femoral shortening using the *Galeazzi* or *Allis sign.* Place the feet (with knee flexed and sacrum flat on the table) together and note any difference in knee heights.

Examine a newborn or infant's *legs and feet* to detect developmental abnormalities. Assess symmetry, bowing, and torsion of the legs. There should be no discrepancy in leg length. It is common for normal infants to have asymmetric thigh skin folds, but if you do detect asymmetry, make sure you perform the instability tests because dislocated hips are commonly associated with this finding.

Severe bowing of the knees can be normal, but it can also be due to *rickets* or *Blount disease.* The most common cause of bowing is tibial torsion (see below).

Most newborns are *bowlegged,* reflecting their curled-up intrauterine position.

Some normal infants exhibit twisting or *torsion of the tibia* inwardly or outwardly on its longitudinal axis. Parents may be concerned about a toeing in or toeing out of the foot and an awkward gait, all of which are usually normal. *Tibial torsion usually corrects itself during the second or third year of life after months of weight bearing.*

Pathologic tibial torsion occurs only in association with *deformities of the feet or hips.*

Examine the feet of newborns and infants. *At birth, the feet may appear deformed from retaining their intrauterine positioning,* often turned inward (Fig. 23-39). You should be able to correct the feet to the neutral and even to an overcorrected position (Fig. 23-40). Scratch or stroke along the outer edge to see if the foot assumes a normal position.

True *deformities of the feet* do not return to the neutral position even with manipulation.

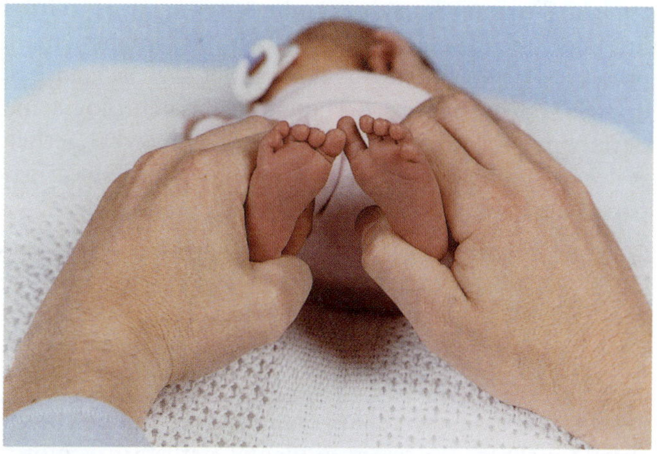

FIGURE 23-39. Assess alignment of the feet.

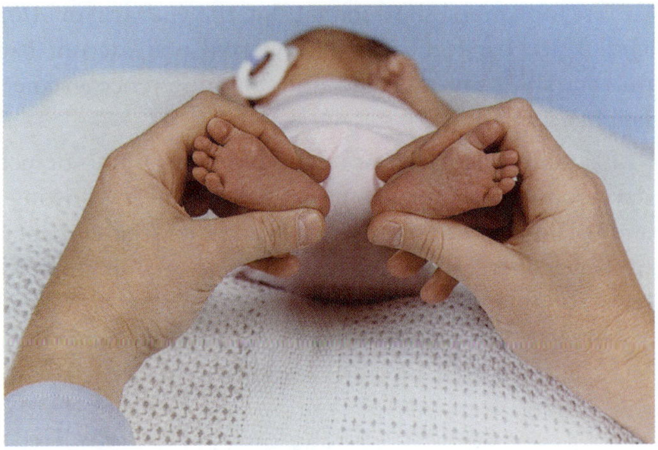

FIGURE 23-40. Assess alignment by turning to an overcorrected position.

The normal newborn's foot has several benign features that may initially cause concern. The newborn's foot appears flat because of a plantar fat pad. There is often inversion of the foot, elevating the outer margin. Other babies will have adduction of the forefoot without inversion, called *metatarsus adductus* which requires close follow-up. Still others will have adduction of the entire foot. Finally, most toddlers have some pronation during early stages of weightbearing with eversion of the foot.

In all of these normal variants the abnormal position can be easily overcorrected past midline. They all tend to resolve within 1 or 2 years.

The most common severe congenital foot deformity is talipes equinovarus or *clubfoot*.

See Table 23-14, Common Musculoskeletal Findings in Young Children.

Nervous System. The examination of the nervous system in infants includes techniques that are highly specific to this particular age group. Unlike many neurologic abnormalities in adults that produce asymmetric localized findings, neurologic abnormalities in infants often present as developmental abnormalities such as failure to do age-appropriate tasks. Therefore, the neurologic and developmental examinations need to proceed together. A developmental abnormality should prompt you to pay particular attention to the neurologic examination.

Signs of severe neurologic disease in infants include extreme irritability, persistent asymmetry of posture, persistent extension of extremities, constant turning of the head to one side, marked extension of the head, neck, and extremities (*opisthotonus*), severe flaccidity, limited response to pain, and sometimes seizures.

The neurologic screening examination of all newborns should include assessment of mental status, gross motor function, tone, cry, deep tendon reflexes, and primitive reflexes. More detailed examination of cranial nerve function and sensory function are indicated if you suspect any abnormalities from the history or screening.

Subtle neonatal behaviors such as fine tremors, irritability, and poor self-regulation may indicate *withdrawal from nicotine or opioids.*

The neurologic examination can reveal extensive disease but will not pinpoint specific functional deficits or minute lesions.

Mental Status. Assess the *mental status* of newborns by observing the newborn activities discussed in Box 23-7. Make sure you test the newborn during alert periods. A detailed description of the assessment of development follows.

Persistent irritability in the newborn may be a sign of *neurologic insult* or may reflect a variety of *metabolic, infectious,* or other *constitutional abnormalities,* or environmental conditions such as *drug withdrawal.*

Motor Function and Tone. Assess the *motor tone* of newborns and infants, first by carefully observing their position at rest and testing their resistance to passive movement.

Further, assess *tone* as you move each major joint through its range of motion, noting any spasticity or flaccidity. Hold the baby in your hands (Fig. 23-41) to determine whether the tone is normal, increased, or decreased. A baby with normal tone has normal response to vertical suspension, as in the figure, and won't "slip through the hands" without the examiner grasping the back of the infant. *Either increased or decreased tone may indicate intracranial disease* although such disease is usually accompanied by a number of other signs.

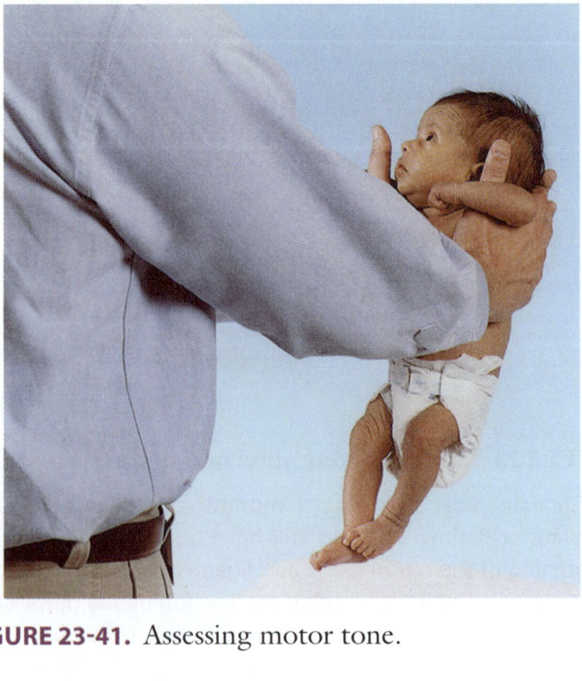

FIGURE 23-41. Assessing motor tone.

Newborns with hypotonia often lie in a frog-leg position, with arms flexed and hands near the ears. A hypotonic infant would almost slip through the examiner's hands in Figure 23-41. Hypotonia can be caused by a variety of central nervous system abnormalities and disorders of the motor unit.

Sensory Function. You can test for *sensory function* of the newborn in only a limited way. Test for pain sensation by flicking the infant's palm or sole with your finger. Observe for withdrawal, arousal, and change in facial expression. Do not use a pin to test for pain.

If changes in facial expression or cry follow a painful stimulus but no withdrawal occurs, weakness or *paralysis* may be present.

Cranial Nerves. The *cranial nerves* of the newborn or infant can be tested. Box 23-25 provides useful strategies.

Abnormalities in the cranial nerves can suggest an intracranial lesion such as hemorrhage or a congenital malformation (or alternatively peripheral nervous system problems).

Deep Tendon Reflexes. The *deep tendon reflexes* are present in newborns but may be difficult to elicit and may vary in their intensity because the corticospinal pathways are immature. Their exaggerated presence or their absence has little diagnostic significance, unless this response is different from results of previous testing or extreme responses are observed or they are very asymmetric.

A progressive increase in deep tendon reflexes during the first year of life may indicate central nervous system disease such as cerebral palsy, especially if it is coupled with increased tone. Another common pattern of presentation is central hypotonia followed by progressively increased tone.

Box 23-25. Strategies to Assess Cranial Nerves in Newborns and Infants

Cranial Nerve		Strategy
I	Olfactory	Very difficult to test
II	Visual acuity	Have infant regard your face and look for facial response and tracking.
II, III	Response to light	Darken room, raise infant to sitting position to open eyes. Use light and test for *optic blink reflex* (blink in response to light). Use the otoscope's light (without speculum) to assess pupillary responses.
III, IV, VI	Extraocular movements	Observe how well the infant tracks your smiling face (or a bright light) and whether the eyes move together.
V	Motor	Test rooting reflex. Test sucking reflex (watch infant suck breast, bottle, or pacifier) and strength of suck.
VII	Facial	Observe infant crying and smiling; note symmetry of face.
VIII	Acoustic	Test acoustic blink reflex (blinking of both eyes in response to a loud noise). Observe tracking in response to sound.
IX, X	Swallow	Observe coordination during swallowing.
	Gag	Test for gag reflex.
XI	Spinal accessory	Observe symmetry of shoulders.
XII	Hypoglossal	Observe coordination of sucking, swallowing, and tongue thrusting. Pinch nostrils; observe reflex opening of mouth with tip of tongue to midline.

Congenital facial nerve palsy can result from birth trauma or developmental defects.

Dysphagia, or difficulty in swallowing, can occasionally be due to injury to cranial nerve IX, X, and XII.

Use the same techniques to elicit deep tendon reflexes as you would for an adult. You can substitute your index or middle finger for the reflex hammer as shown in Figure 23-42.

As in adults, asymmetric reflexes suggest a lesion of the peripheral nerves or spinal segment or can be due to an intracranial lesion.

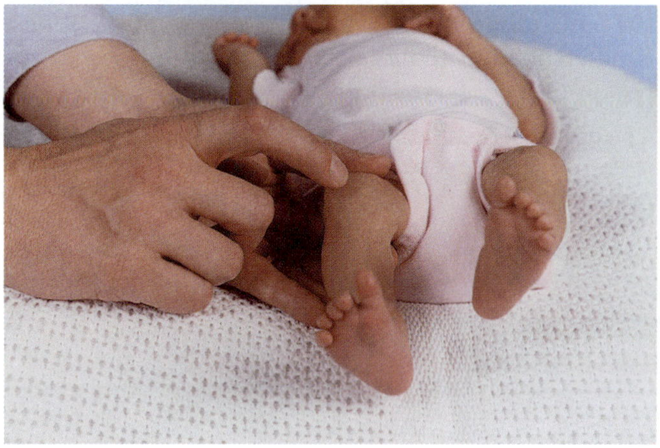

FIGURE 23-42. Assessing deep tendon reflexes with finger.

The triceps, brachioradialis, and abdominal reflexes are difficult to elicit before 6 months of age. The *anal reflex* or *"anal wink"* is present at birth and important to elicit if a spinal cord lesion is suspected. This reflex is a contraction of the external anal sphincter when the examiner touches the skin near the anus.

An absent anal reflex suggests loss of innervation of the external sphincter muscle caused by a spinal cord abnormality such as a congenital anomaly (e.g., spina bifida), tumor, or injury.

In newborns, a *positive Babinski response* to plantar stimulation (dorsiflexion of big toe and fanning of other toes) can be elicited and may persist for several months.

In order to best elicit the ankle reflex of an infant, grasp the infant's malleolus with one hand and abruptly dorsiflex the ankle (Fig. 23-43). You may note rapid, rhythmic plantar flexion of the newborn's foot (*ankle clonus*) in response to this maneuver. Up to 10 beats are normal in newborns and young infants; this is *unsustained ankle clonus.*

When the contractions are continuous (*sustained* ankle clonus), central nervous system disease should be suspected.

A newborn who is irritable, jittery and has tremors, hypertonicity, and hyperactive reflexes may have drug withdrawal from maternal substance use during pregnancy. *Neonatal abstinence syndrome* results from the use of opioids by the mother while pregnant. In addition to the signs listed above, the newborn may also have autonomic signs, as well as poor feeding and seizures.

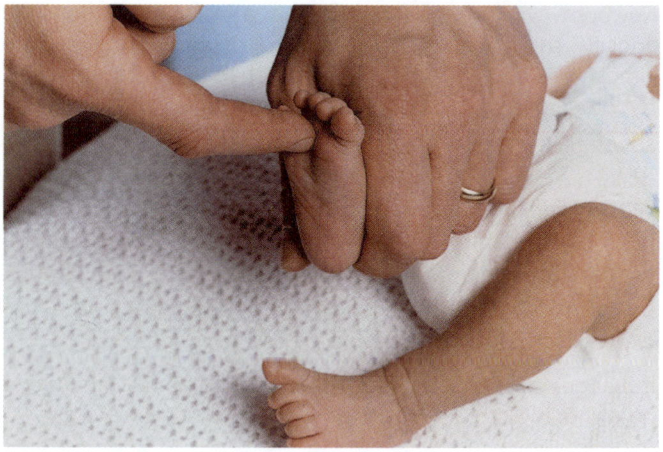

FIGURE 23-43. Assessing ankle reflexes.

Primitive Reflexes. Evaluate the newborn's and infant's developing central nervous system by assessing *infantile automatisms*, called *primitive reflexes.* These develop during gestation, are generally demonstrable at birth, and disappear at defined ages. Abnormalities in these primitive reflexes suggest neurologic disease and merit more intensive investigation.

A *neurologic* or *developmental abnormality* is suspected if primitive reflexes are:

- Absent at appropriate age
- Present longer than normal
- Asymmetric
- Associated with posturing or twitching

The most important primitive reflexes are illustrated in Box 23-26.

Developmental Assessment. By observation and play with the infant, you can both do a developmental screening examination and an assessment for gross motor and (for older infants) fine motor achievement (Box 23-27). Infants who have developmental delay may have abnormalities on the neurologic examination because much of the examination is based on age-specific norms.

Specifically, look for *weakness* by observing sitting, standing, and transitions. Note *station*, or the posture of sitting or standing. Assess fine motor development in older infants in a similar way, combining the neurologic and developmental examination. Key milestones include the development of the pincer grasp, ability to manipulate objects with the hands, and more precise tasks, such as building a tower of cubes or scribbling. Fine and gross motor development progresses in a proximal to distal direction.

Many causes of developmental delay exist but often no cause is identified. Etiologies include *prenatal* (genetic, central nervous system, congenital hypothyroidism), *perinatal* (preterm, asphyxia, infection, trauma), and *postnatal* (trauma, infection, toxin, abuse).

Box 23-26. Primitive Reflexes

Primitive Reflex		Maneuver	Ages
Palmar Grasp Reflex	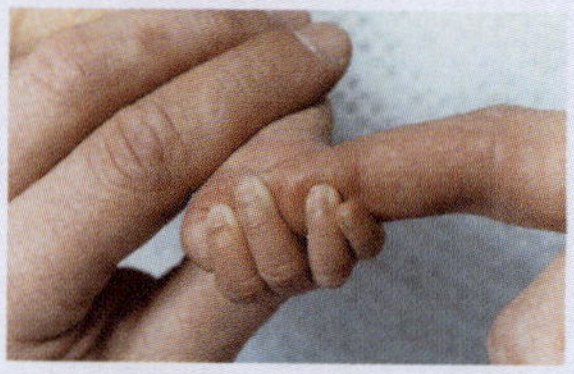	Place your fingers into the infant's hands and press against the palmar surfaces. The infant will flex all fingers to grasp your fingers.	Birth to 3–4 months
Plantar Grasp Reflex	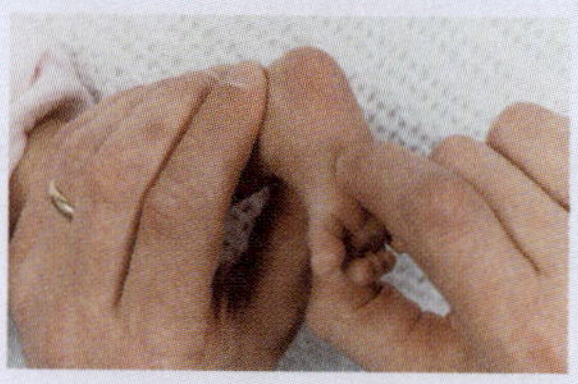	Touch the sole at the base of the toes. The toes will curl.	Birth to 6–8 months
Rooting Reflex	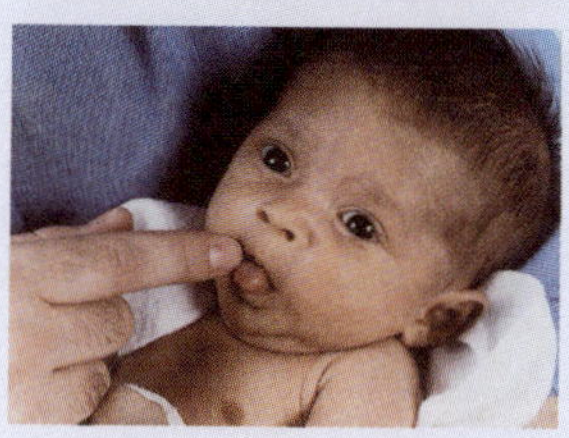	Stroke the perioral skin at the corners of the mouth. The mouth will open and the infant will turn the head toward the stimulated side and suck.	Birth to 3–4 months
Moro Reflex (Startle Reflex)	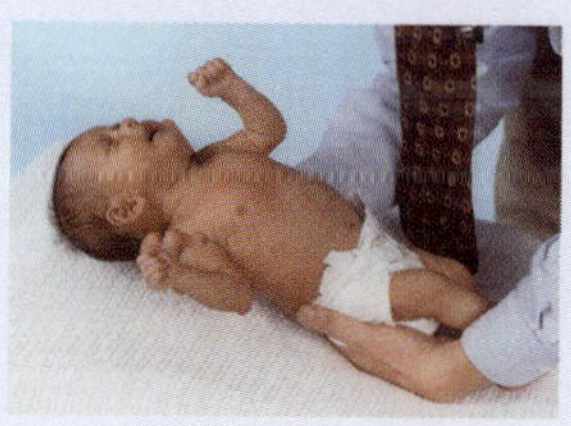	Hold the infant supine, supporting the head, back, and legs. Abruptly lower the entire body about 1 foot. The arms will abduct and extend, hands will open, and legs will flex. The infant may cry.	Birth to 4 months
Asymmetric Tonic Neck Reflex	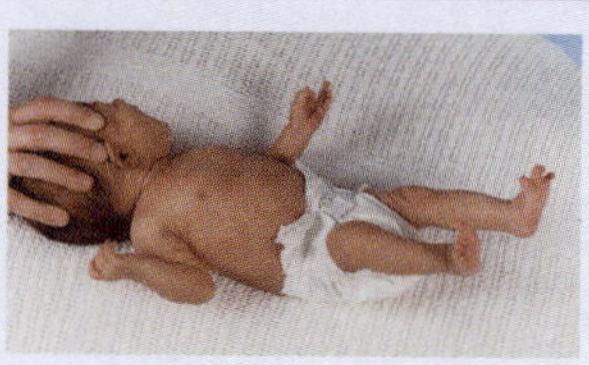	With the infant supine, turn head to one side, holding jaw over shoulder. The arms/legs on side to which head is turned will extend while the opposite arm/leg will flex. Repeat on other side.	Birth to 2–3 months

Persistence of palmar grasp reflex beyond 4 to 6 months suggests pyramidal tract dysfunction.

Persistence of clenched hand beyond 2 months suggests central nervous system damage, especially if fingers overlap the thumb.

Persistence of plantar grasp reflex beyond 8 months suggests pyramidal tract dysfunction.

Absence of rooting indicates severe generalized or central nervous system disease.

Persistence beyond 4 months suggests neurologic disease (e.g., cerebral palsy); persistence beyond 6 months strongly suggests it.

Asymmetric response suggests fracture of clavicle or humerus or brachial plexus injury.

Persistence beyond 3 months suggests asymmetric central nervous system development and sometimes predicts the development of cerebral palsy.

(*continued*)

Box 23-26. Primitive Reflexes (*continued*)

Primitive Reflex		Maneuver	Ages	
Trunk Incurvation (Galant) Reflex	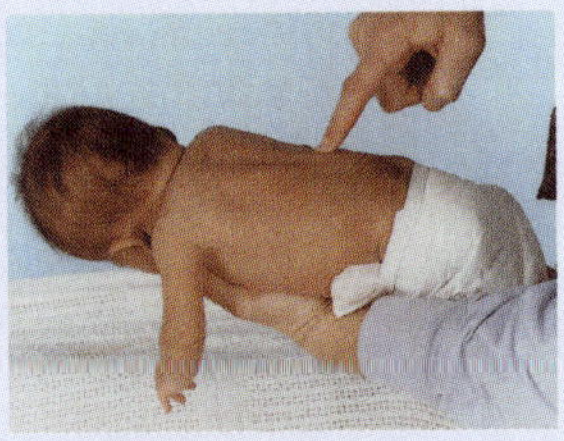	Support the infant prone with one hand and stroke one side of the back 1 cm from midline, from shoulder to buttocks. The spine will curve toward the stimulated side.	Birth to 3–4 months	Absence suggests a transverse spinal cord lesion or injury. Persistence may indicate delayed development.
Landau Reflex	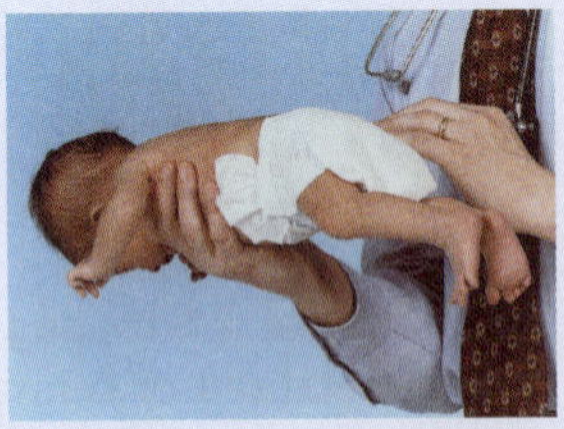	Suspend the infant prone with one hand. The head will lift up, and the spine will straighten.	Birth to 6 months	Persistence may indicate delayed development.
Parachute Reflex	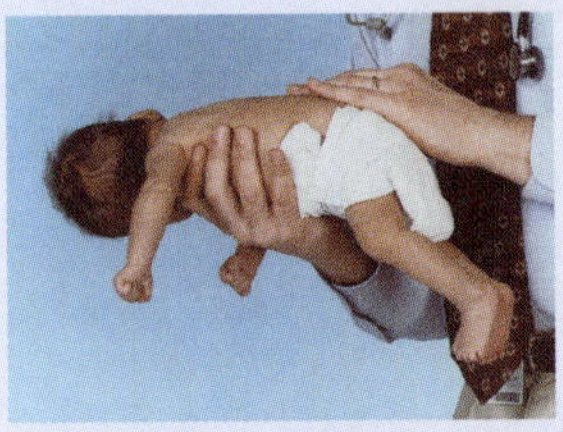	Suspend the infant prone and slowly lower the head toward a surface. The arms and legs will extend in a protective fashion.	8 months and does not disappear	Delay in appearance may predict future delays in voluntary motor development.
Positive Support Reflex	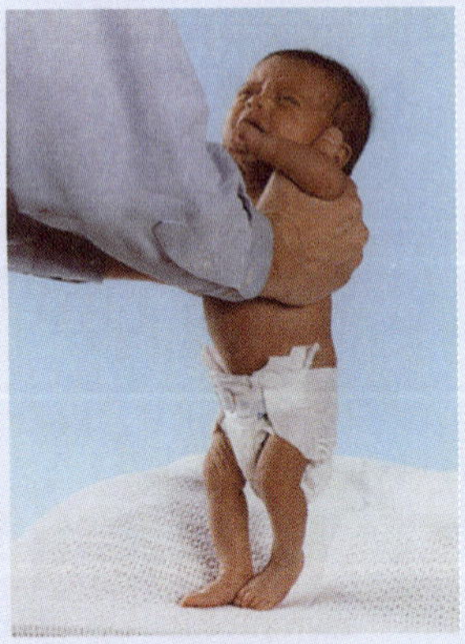	Hold the infant around the trunk and lower until the feet touch a flat surface. The hips, knees, and ankles will extend, the infant will stand up, partially bearing weight, sagging after 20–30 seconds.	Birth or 2 months until 6 months	Lack of reflex suggests hypotonia or flaccidity. Fixed extension and adduction of legs (scissoring) suggests spasticity from neurologic disease, such as cerebral palsy.
Placing and Stepping Reflexes	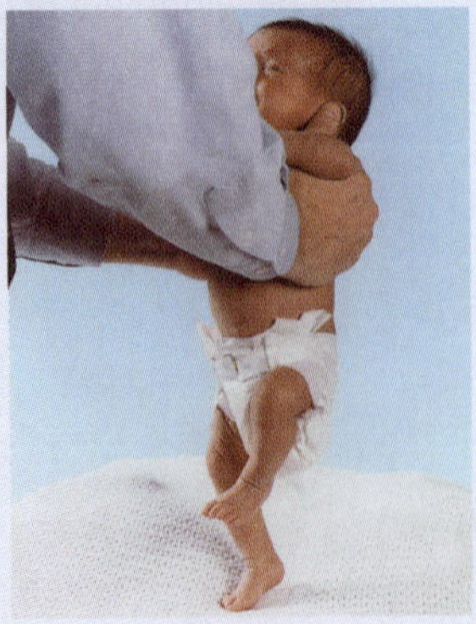	Hold the infant upright as in positive support reflex. Have one sole touch the tabletop. The hip and knee of that foot will flex and the other foot will step forward. Alternate stepping will occur.	Birth (best after 4 days; variable age to disappear)	Absence of placing may indicate paralysis. Newborns born by breech delivery may not have a placing reflex

Box 23-27. Abnormalities Detected while Observing Play

Behavioral*	Social or Environmental
Poor parent–child interactions	Parental stress, depression
Sibling rivalry	Risk for abuse or neglect
Inappropriate parental discipline	**Neurologic**
"Difficult temperament"	Weakness
Developmental	Abnormal posture
Gross motor delay	Spasticity
Fine motor delay	Clumsiness
Language delay (expressive or receptive)	Attentional problems, hyperactivity
Delay in social or emotional tasks	Autistic features
	Musculoskeletal abnormalities

*Note: The child's behavior during the visit may not represent typical behavior but your observations may serve as a springboard for discussion with parents.

In addition, since some neurologic abnormalities produce deficits or slowing in cognitive and social development, one can assess the infant's cognitive and social–emotional developmental domains as you proceed with the comprehensive neurologic and developmental examination.

Developmental delay across more than one domain (e.g., motor plus cognitive) suggests more severe disease.

RECORDING YOUR FINDINGS

The format of the clinical record is the same for both children and adults. Although the sequence of the physical examination may vary, convert your clinical findings into the same order of the traditional written or electronic format.

Initially, you may use sentences to describe your findings; later you will use phrases. The style here contains phrases appropriate for most write-ups. As you read through this write-up, you will note some atypical findings. Try to test yourself. See if you can interpret these findings. You will also note the modifications necessary to accommodate reports from the parent.

Since the structure and sequence of the write-up for the newborn or infant history and physical examination mirrors the write-up for young children, use the example shown on page 705. The key elements of the history shown in Box 23-4 could be used as a guide for the write-up of the history.

HEALTH PROMOTION AND COUNSELING: EVIDENCE AND RECOMMENDATIONS

Health supervision visits are recommended for infants below 1 year of age at the following ages: at birth, at 3 to 5 days, by 1 month, and at 2, 4, 6, 9, and 12 months (Fig. 23-44). This is called the *Infant Periodicity Schedule*. Health supervision visits provide opportunities to answer questions for parents, assess the infant's growth and development, perform a comprehensive physical examination, and provide anticipatory guidance. Age-appropriate anticipatory guidance includes healthy habits and behaviors, social competence of caregivers, parenting techniques, family relationships, and community interactions.

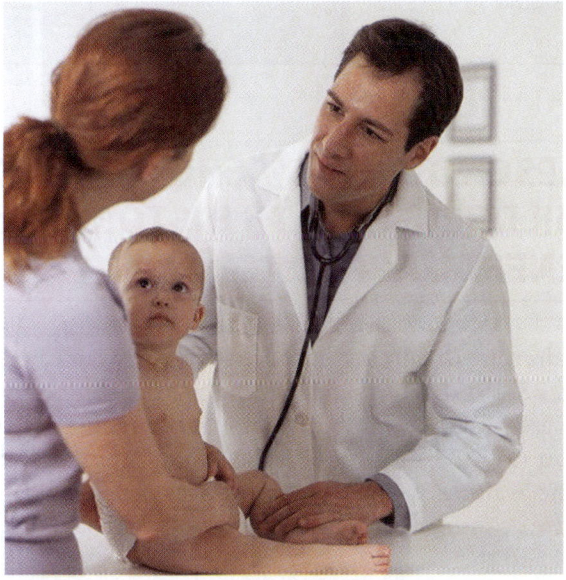

FIGURE 23-44. Regular health supervision serves many purposes.

Regular visits provide an opportunity to plot a course for healthy and successful development. Infants generally are well during these visits, enhancing the quality of the experience. Parents are usually receptive to suggestions about health promotion which can have major, long-term influences on the child and family. Strong interviewing skills are necessary as you discuss strategies to optimize the health and well-being of their infants. Adjust the content to the appropriate developmental level of the infant. As an exercise, review the critical components of a health supervision visit for a 6-month-old in Box 23-28.

Box 23-28. Components of a Health Supervision Visit for a 6-Month-Old

Discussions with Parents
- Address parents' concerns/questions
- Provide advice
- Obtain social history
- Assess development, nutrition, sleep, elimination, safety, oral health, family relationships, stressors, parenting beliefs, community factors

Developmental Assessment
- Use a standardized developmental instrument to measure milestones
- Assess milestones by history
- Assess milestones by examination

Physical Examination
- Perform a careful examination, including growth parameters with percentiles for age

Screening Tests
- Vision and hearing (by examination)
- Screen for social risk factors

Immunizations
- See schedule (AAP or CDC website)

Anticipatory Guidance

Healthy Habits and Behaviors
- Injury and illness prevention
  Use infant seat, watch for rolling, caution on walkers, poisons, tobacco exposure
- Nutrition
  Breastfeeding or bottle, iron supplementation with Vitamin D if needed, solids, no juice, prevent choking, overfeeding
- Oral health
  No bottle in bed, fluoride, brushing teeth

Parent–Infant Interaction
- Promoting development (talk, read, sing, music, play)

Family Relationships
- Time for self; babysitters

Community Interaction
- Childcare, resources

PRESCHOOL AND SCHOOL-AGED CHILDREN–HEALTH HISTORY: GENERAL APPROACH

Children are usually accompanied by a parent or caregiver (Fig. 23-45). Even when alone in the examination room, they are often seeking health care at the request of their parent (Fig. 23-46). Indeed, the parent is usually sitting in the waiting room. When interviewing a child, you need to consider the needs and perspectives of both the child and the caregivers.

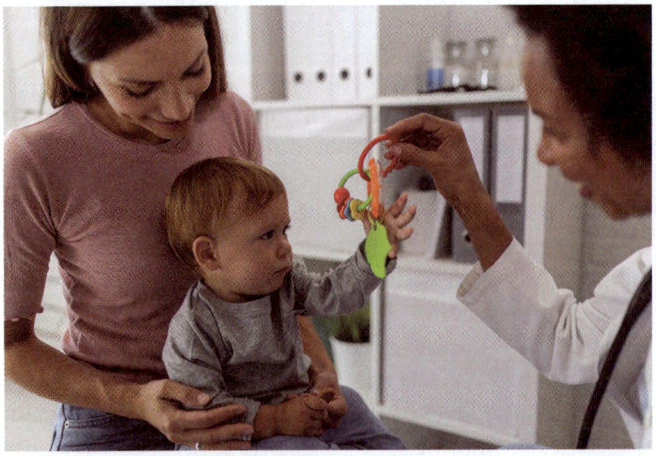

FIGURE 23-45. Pediatrician examining baby boy who is accompanied by his mother. (Used with permission from Shutterstock. By Lordn.)

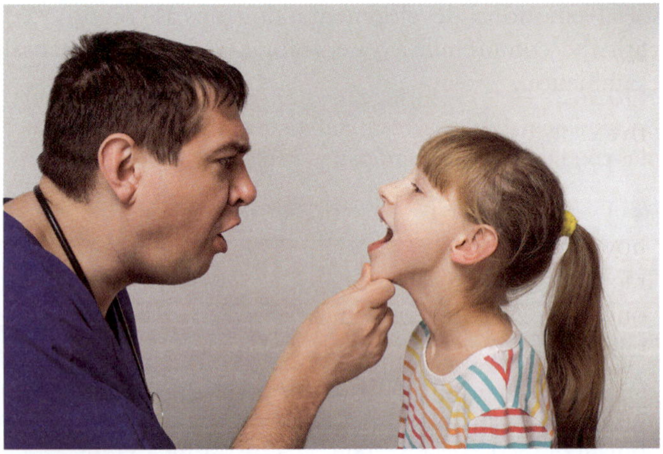

FIGURE 23-46. Examining a child's throat. (Used with permission from Shutterstock. By Business plus.)

Establishing Rapport

Begin the interview by greeting and establishing rapport with each person present (Fig. 23-47). Refer to the child by name rather than by "him" or "her." Families come in many varieties—these include traditional families, single parents, separated/divorced parents, blended, same-sex parents, kinship families, foster families, and adoptive families so clarify the role or relationship of all of the adults and children. "Now, are you Jimmy's grandmother?" "Please help me by telling me Jimmy's relationship to everyone here." Address the parents as "Mr. Smith" or "Ms. Smith" rather than by their first names or "Mom" or "Dad." When the family structure is not immediately clear, you may avoid embarrassment by asking directly about other members. "Who else lives in the home?" "Who is Jimmy's father?" "Do you live together?" Do not assume that just because parents are separated, only one parent is actively involved in the child's life.

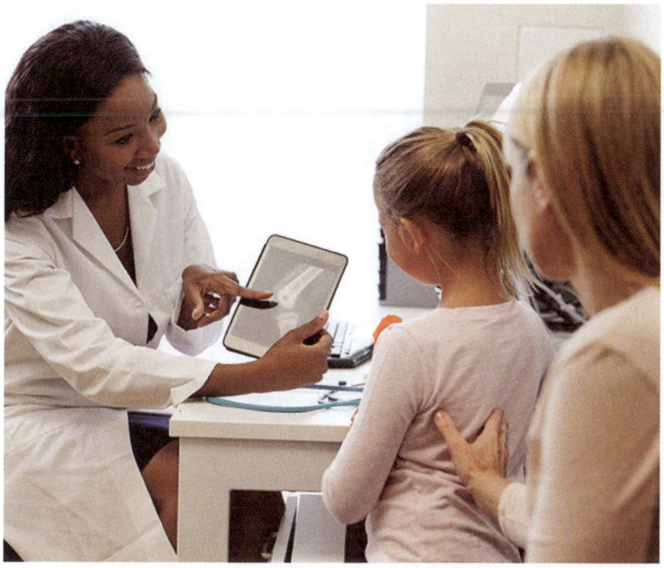

FIGURE 23-47. Establishing rapport enables more effective evaluation.

Use your personal experiences with children to guide how you interact in a health care setting. To establish rapport, meet children on their own level. Eye contact on their level, participating in playful engagement, and talking about what interests them are good strategies. Ask children about their clothes, toys, favorite book or TV show, or their adult companion in an enthusiastic but gentle style. Spending time at the beginning of the interview to calm and connect with an anxious child can put both the child and the caregiver at ease.

Working with Families

One challenge when several people are present is deciding to whom to direct your questions. While eventually you need to get information from both the child and the parent, it is useful to start with the child.

Asking simple open-ended questions like "Are you sick?... Tell me about it," followed by more specific questions, often provides much of the clinical data. The parents can then verify the information, add details that give you the larger context, and identify other issues you need to address. Sometimes children are embarrassed to begin, but once the parent has started the conversation, direct questions back to the child. Characterize symptom attributes as for adults.

"Your mom tells me that you get stomachaches. Tell me about them."
"Show me where you get the pain. What does it feel like?"
"Is it sharp like a pinprick, or does it ache?"
"Does it stay in the same spot, or does it move around?"
"What helps make it go away? What makes it worse?"
"What do you think causes it?"

The presence of family members allows you to observe how they interact with the child. A child may be able to sit still or may get restless and start fidgeting. Watch how the parents set, or fail to set, limits when needed.

Multiple Agendas

Each individual in the room, including the clinician, may have a different idea about the nature of the problem and what needs to be done about it (Fig. 23-48).

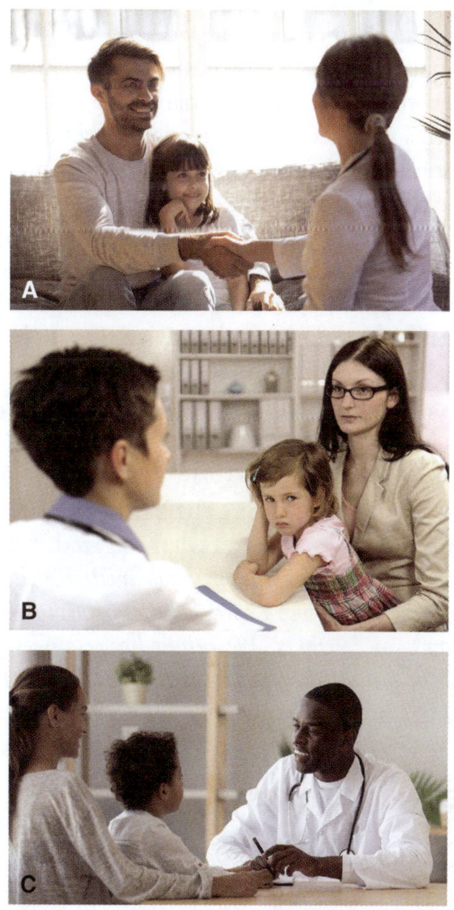

FIGURE 23-48. Pediatrician, parent, and patient sometimes have differing agendas. (Used with permission from Shutterstock. **A.** By fizkes. **B.** By mangostock. **C.** By fizkes.)

Discover as many of these perspectives and agendas as possible. Family members who are not present (e.g., the absent parent or grandparent) may also have concerns. Ask about those concerns, too. *"If Sangeeta's father were here today, what questions or concerns would he have?" "Have you, Mrs. Rana, discussed this with your mother or anyone else?" "What does she think?"*

For example, Mrs. Anurag brings Durga in for abdominal pain because she is worried that Durga may have an ulcer and also poor eating habits. Durga is not worried about the belly pain but is uneasy about the changes in her body and about getting fat. Mr. Anurag thinks that Durga's schoolwork is not getting enough attention. You, as the clinician, need to balance these concerns with what you see as a healthy 12-year-old girl in early puberty with some mild functional abdominal pain and concern for possible emerging obesity.

Your goals need to include uncovering the concerns of each person and helping the family to be realistic about the range of "normal."

Family as a Resource

In general, family members provide most of the care and are your natural allies in promoting the child's health. Being open to a wide range of parenting behaviors helps to make this alliance. Raising a child reflects cultural, socioeconomic, and family practices. It is important to respect the tremendous variation in these practices. A good strategy is to *view the parents as experts in the care of their child and yourself as their consultant.* This demonstrates respect for the parents' care and minimizes their likelihood of discounting or ignoring your advice. Parents face many challenges raising children, so practitioners need to be supportive, not judgmental. Comments like, *"Why didn't you bring him in sooner?"* or *"What did you do that for?"* do not improve your rapport with the parent.

Statements acknowledging the hard work of parenting and praising successes are always appreciated. *"Mr. Rahul, you are doing such a wonderful job with Rohit. Being a parent takes so much work and Rohit's behavior here today clearly shows your efforts. We might have some suggestions for you at the end of the visit."* Or to the child, *"Rohit you are so lucky to have such a wonderful dad."*

Hidden Agendas

As with adults, the chief complaint may not relate to the real reason the parent has brought the child to see you (Fig. 23-49). The complaint may be a bridge to concerns that may not seem like a legitimate reason to go to the clinician. Create a trusting atmosphere that allows parents to be open about all their concerns by asking facilitating questions such as:

"Do you have any other concerns about Ravi?"
"Was there anything else that you wanted to tell/ask me today?"

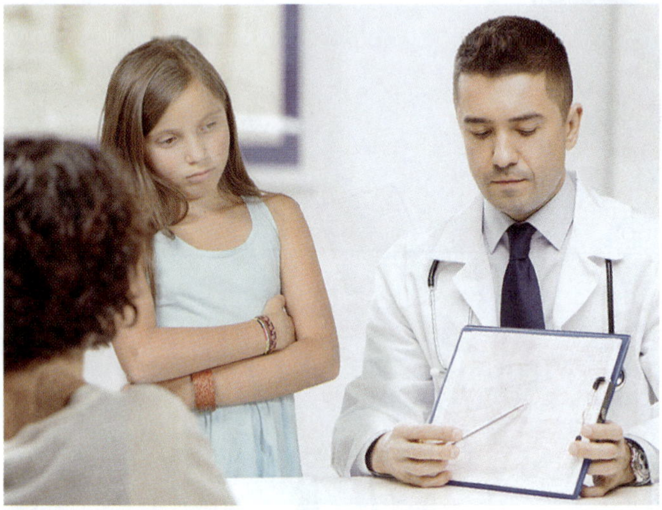

FIGURE 23-49. Engaging parents can reveal hidden agendas.

SURVEILLANCE OF DEVELOPMENT: EARLY CHILDHOOD: 1 TO 4 YEARS

Physical Development

After infancy, the rate of physical growth slows by approximately half. *After 2 years, toddlers gain about 2 to 3 kg and grow 5 cm per year.* Physical changes are impressive characterized by leaner but a more muscular bulk.

Gross and fine motor skills also develop quickly. Almost all children walk by 15 months, run well by 2 years, and pedal a tricycle and jump by 4 years. Fine motor skills develop through neurologic maturation and play (Fig. 23-50). The 18-month-old who scribbles becomes a 2-year-old who draws lines and then a 3-year-old who copies a circle; 4-year-olds can draw a simple person with a couple of body parts and can start to copy simple capital letters.

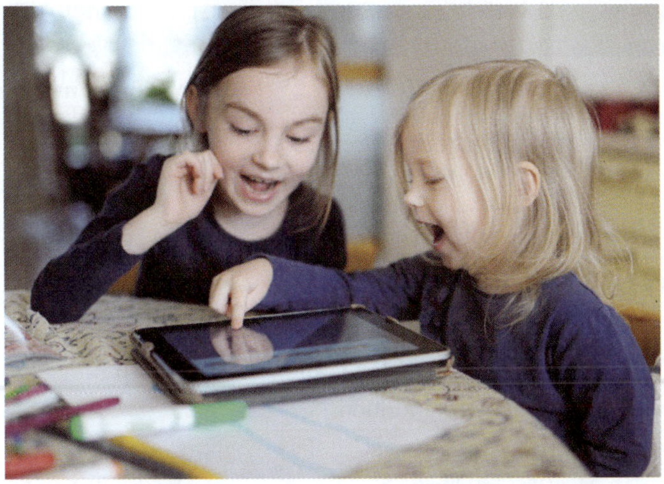

FIGURE 23-50. Fine motor skills develop along with cognition.

Cognitive and Language Development

Toddlers move from sensorimotor learning (through touching and looking) to symbolic thinking, solving simple problems, remembering songs, and engaging in imitative play. Language develops with extraordinary speed. An 18-month-old with 10 to 20 words becomes a 2-year-old with two to three word sentences, and a 3-year-old who converses well. By 4 years, preschoolers form complex sentences. They remain preoperational, however—that is, without sustained logical thought processes. You can ask children older than 3 years to draw a picture or copy objects and then discuss their pictures to test simultaneously for fine motor coordination, cognition, and language.

Distinguish between isolated delays in one aspect of development (e.g., coordination or language) and more generalized delays that occur in several components. The latter is more likely to reflect global neurologic disorders such as *cognitive disability* that can have many etiologies.

Social and Emotional Development. Toddlers develop rapidly from beginning to pretend play, to mostly parallel play, to imitating adult actions and really pretending and imagining. New intellectual pursuits are surpassed only by an emerging drive for independence (Fig. 23-51). Because toddlers are impulsive and have poor self-regulation, temper tantrums are common. Self-regulation is an important developmental task with a wide range of normal (Box 23-29).

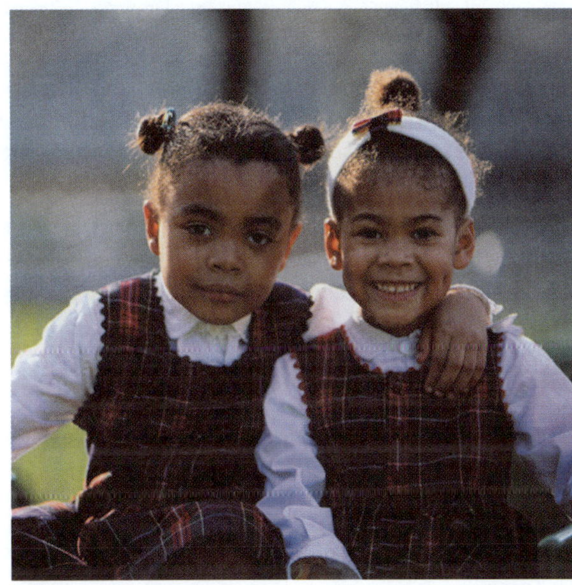

FIGURE 23-51. Individual personalities emerge as the intellect grows.

Box 23-29. Developmental Milestones: 1 to 5 Years

Age	Gross Motor	Fine Motor	Language	Social–Emotional
12 months	Stands independently Starts taking first steps	Scribbles Hold crayon Makes tower with 2 cubes	Says one word with meaning Points to get objects Follows one-step commands with gestures	Shows objects to parents to share
15 months	Stoops to pick up toys Climbs on furniture Runs stiff legged	Uses spoon with some spilling Places 10 cubes in cup Turns pages in book	Uses 3–5 words Mature jargon speech Points to one body part	Shows empathy Gives hugs on request
18 months	Creeps down stairs Runs well	Makes 4-cube tower Imitates vertical stroke	Uses 10–25 words Points to three body parts Points to self, familiar people	Engages in pretend play

(*continued*)

Box 23-29. Developmental Milestones: 1 to 5 Years (*continued*)

Age	Gross Motor	Fine Motor	Language	Social–Emotional
24 months	Walks downstairs holding rail, with both feet on one step Kicks ball	Imitates horizontal line Opens door knob Sucks through straw	Uses 2-word sentences Uses 50+ words Has 50% intelligibility Refers to self by name	Parallel play
30 months	Walks up stairs, holding on, alternating feet Jumps in place	Makes tower with 8 cubes Can wash hands, brush teeth with help	Refers to self with correct pronoun Understands action words (sleeping, eating, playing) Understands prepositions	Imitates adult actions (cooking, talking on phone, cleaning)
3 years	Goes up stairs without holding on, alternating feet Pedals tricycle	Copies circle Strings small beads Draws a 2–3 part person	Uses 3-word sentences, Has 75% intelligibility Understands negatives Knows own gender	Starts to share Imaginative play Fears imaginary things
4 years	Balances on one foot for 8 seconds Throws ball overhand Catches bounced ball	Copies square Goes to the toilet alone Draws a 4–6 part person	Speaks with 100% intelligibility Follows three-step commands Understands adjectives	Has a preferred friend Labels feelings Group play
5 years	Walks down stairs, alternating feet Hops on one foot Skips	Copies triangle Cuts with scissors Writes first name	Speaks in 6–8 word sentences, can count to 10, knows colors Knows telephone number Retells story with clear beginning, middle, end Enjoys rhyming words	Has a group of friends Apologizes for mistakes

Sources: Scharf R et al. *Pediatr Rev*. 2016;37(1); Gerber RJ et al. *Pediatr Rev*. 2010;31(7):267–277; Wilks T et al. *Pediatr Rev*. 2010;31(9):364–367; Gerber RJ et al. *Pediatr Rev*. 2011;32(12):533–536.

SURVEILLANCE OF DEVELOPMENT: MIDDLE CHILDHOOD, 5 TO 10 YEARS

Middle childhood is an active period of growth and development (Box 23-30). *Goal-directed exploration increased physical and cognitive abilities,* and *achievements by trial and error* mark this stage.

Box 23-30. Developmental Tasks during Middle Childhood

Task	Characteristic	Healthcare Needs
Physical	Enhanced strength and coordination Competence in various tasks and activities	Screening for strengths, assessing problems Involving parents Support for disabilities Anticipatory guidance: safety, exercise, nutrition, sleep
Cognitive	"Concrete operational": focus on the present	Emphasis on short-term consequences
	Achievement of knowledge and skills, self-efficacy	Support; screening for skills and school performance
Social	Achieving good "fit" with family, friends, school	Assessment, support, advice about interactions including peer relationships
	Sustained self-esteem	Support, emphasis on strengths
	Evolving self-identity	Understanding, advice, support

(continued)

Physical Development

Children grow steadily but more slowly. Strength and coordination improve dramatically with more participation in activities (Fig. 23-52). This is also when children with physical disabilities or chronic illnesses become more aware of their limitations.

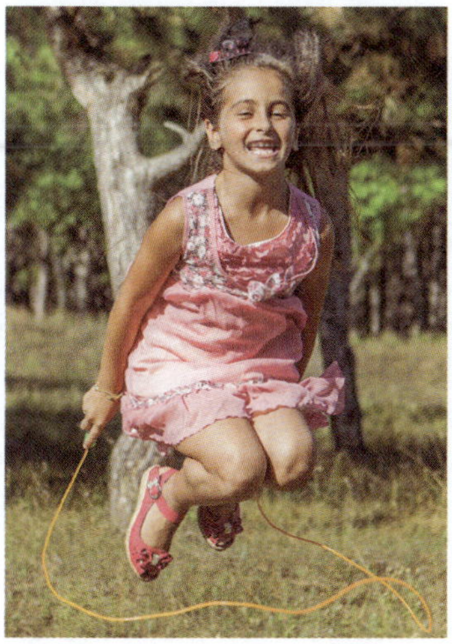

FIGURE 23-52. Physical abilities rapidly progress in early childhood.

Cognitive and Language Development

Children become "*concrete operational*"—capable of limited logic and more complex learning. They remain rooted in the present with little ability to understand consequences or abstractions. School, family, and environment greatly influence learning (Fig. 23-53). A major developmental task is *self-efficacy*, or the child's belief in their ability to thrive in different situations. Language becomes increasingly complex.

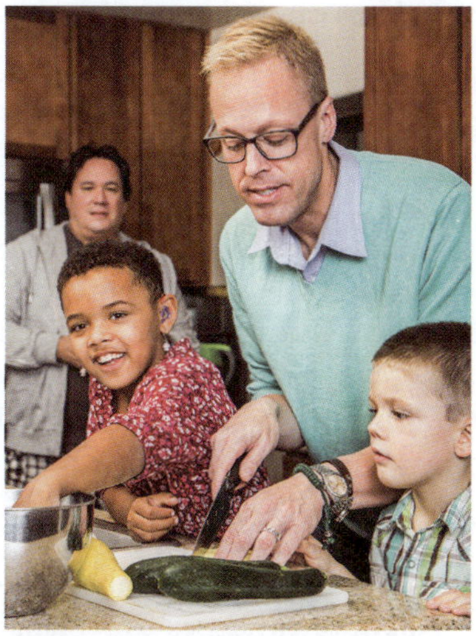

FIGURE 23-53. A child's cognitive development is shaped by family relationships.

Among school-aged children, the best test for development is their school performance. You can obtain school records or psychological testing results, obviating the need for the clinician to formally test an older child's development. Delayed or disordered development in early childhood can lead to early school failure as well as social, behavioral, and emotional problems.

Social and Emotional Development

Children become progressively more independent, initiating activities and enjoying accomplishments. Achievements are critical for self-esteem and developing a "fit" within major social structures—family, school, and peer activity groups. Guilt and poor self-esteem also may emerge. Family and environment contribute enormously to the child's self-image. Moral development remains simple and concrete with a clear sense of "right and wrong."

PHYSICAL EXAMINATION: GENERAL APPROACH

An important aspect of examining children is that parents are usually watching and taking part in the interaction, providing you the opportunity to observe the parent–child interaction. Note whether the child displays age-appropriate behaviors.

Assess the "goodness of fit" between parents and child. Although some abnormal interactions may result from the unnatural setting of the examination room, others may be a consequence of interactional problems. Careful observation of the child's interactions with parents and the child's unstructured play in the examination room can reveal *abnormalities in physical, cognitive, and social development or issues with parent–child relationship*, and also provide opportunities for gentle education and anticipatory guidance.

Normal toddlers are occasionally alarmed at the examiner. Some will be uncooperative but most eventually warm up to you. If this behavior continues or is not developmentally appropriate, there may be an *underlying behavioral or developmental abnormality.* Older, school-aged children have more self-control and prior experience with clinicians and are generally cooperative with the examination.

Assessing Younger Children

One challenge in examining children in this age group is avoiding a physical struggle, a crying child, or a distraught parent. Accomplishing this successfully is one aspect of the "art of medicine" in the practice of pediatrics.

Gain the child's confidence and allay the child's fears from the start of the encounter. Your approach will vary with the circumstances of the visit. As an example, you can start a visit with a preschooler by having a cleaned toy to play with or giving the child a book as a gift. A health supervision visit allows greater rapport than a visit when the child is ill.

The child should remain dressed during the interview to minimize the child's apprehension. It also allows you to interact more naturally and observe the child playing, interacting with the parents, and undressing and dressing.

Toddlers who are of 9 to 15 months may have *stranger anxiety*, a fear of strangers that is developmentally normal. It signals the toddler's growing awareness that the stranger is new. You should not approach these toddlers quickly, and you might want to avoid direct eye contact initially with the toddler. Play can help the child warm up to you. Make sure they remain solidly in their parent's lap throughout much of the examination and that the parent remains close when the child is on the examination table.

Engage children in age-appropriate conversation. Ask simple questions about their illness or toys. Compliment their appearance or behavior, tell a story, or play a simple game (Fig. 23-54). If a child is shy, turn your attention to the parent to allow the child to warm up gradually. Also, sometimes the parent is anxious. Helping the parent relax or asking them to help by reading to the child or playing with the child can help relax everyone in the examination room.

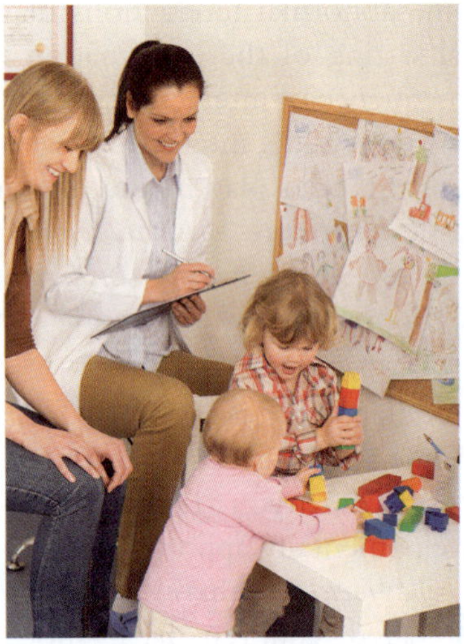

FIGURE 23-54. Engaging children in play is sometimes part of the assessment.

With certain exceptions, physical examination does not require use of the examining table; it can be done with the child in a parent's lap. The key is to engage the child's cooperation. For young children who resist undressing, expose only the body part being examined. When examining siblings, begin with the oldest child who is more likely to cooperate and set a good example. Approach the child pleasantly. Explain each step as you perform it. Continue conversing with the family to provide distraction.

Plan the examination to start with the least distressing procedures and end with the most distressing ones, usually involving the throat and ears. Begin with parts that can be done with the child sitting such as examining the eyes or palpating the neck. Lying down may make a child feel vulnerable, so change positions with care. Once a child is supine, begin with the abdomen, saving throat and ears or genitalia for last. You may need a parent's help to restrain the child for examination of the ears or throat; however, use of formal restraints is inappropriate. *Patience, distraction, play, flexibility in the order of the examination, and a caring but firm and gentle approach, are all key to successfully examining the young child* (Fig. 23-55).

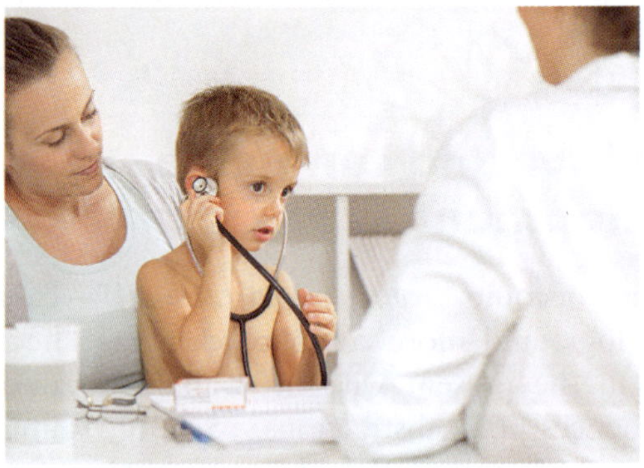

FIGURE 23-55. Familiarizing the child with the equipment and procedures can reduce anxiety in children.

Assessing Older Children

Examining children after they reach school age usually poses few difficulties. Although some have unpleasant memories of previous clinical encounters, most children respond well when the examiner is attuned to their developmental level.

Many children at this age are modest (Fig. 23-56). Providing gowns and leaving underwear in place as long as possible are wise approaches. Consider leaving the room while they change with their parents' help. Some children may prefer opposite-sex siblings to leave, but most prefer a parent of either sex to remain in the room. *Parents of children younger than 11 years should stay with them.* Adhere to your setting's chaperone policy.

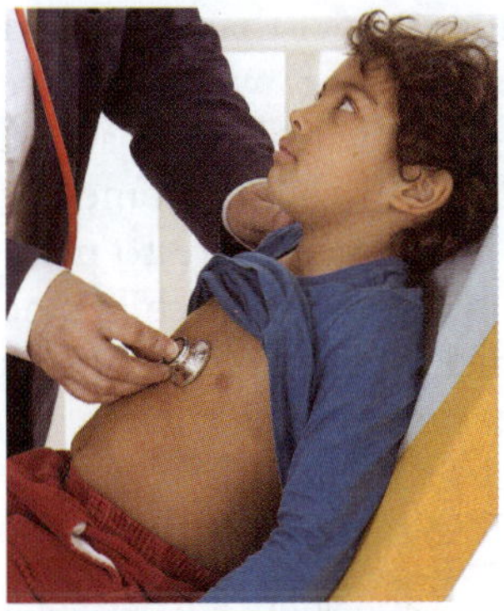

FIGURE 23-56. Clinicians need to be aware of older children's developing modesty.

TECHNIQUES OF EXAMINATION

The order of the examination now begins to follow that used for adults (Box 23-31). Examine painful areas last and forewarn children about areas you are going to examine. If a child resists part of the examination, you can return to it at the end.

Reassure parents that resistance to examination is developmentally appropriate. Some embarrassed parents scold the child, compounding the problem. Involve parents in the examination. Learn which techniques and approaches work best and are most comfortable for you.

Box 23-31. Tips for Examining Young Children (1- to 4-Year-Olds)

Useful Strategies for Examination

- Have the parent help you facilitate the examination (e.g., removing clothing, holding child on lap). Try to be at the child's eye level.
- Use a reassuring voice throughout the examination.
- Let the child see and touch the examination tools you will be using.
- First examine the child's toy or teddy bear, or even the parent, then the child (Fig. A).
- Let the child do some of the examination (e.g., move the stethoscope). Then go back and *"get the places we missed"* (Fig. B).
- Ask the toddler who keeps pushing you away to *"hold your hand."* Then have the toddler "help you" with the examination.
- *Avoid asking permission to examine a body part because you will do the examination anyway.* Instead, ask the child which ear or which part of the body he or she would like you to examine first.
- Make a game out of the examination! For example, *"Let's see how big your tongue is!"* or *"Is Elmo in your ear? Let's see!"*
- Some toddlers believe that if they can't see you, then you aren't there. Perform the examination while the child stands on the parent's lap, facing the parent.
- Hand the child an age-appropriate book and engage the child in reading.
- If 2-year-olds are holding something in each hand (such as tongue depressors), it is more difficult for them to fight or resist.
- If unable to console the child, give the child a short break.

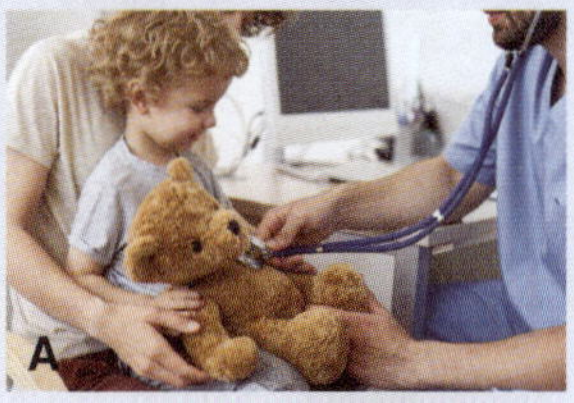

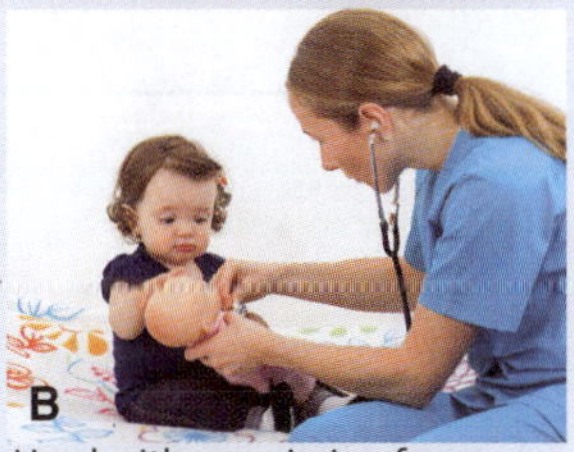

Used with permission from Shutterstock. **A.** By Seventy-Four. **B.** By Ocskay Bence.

Useful Toys and Aids

- "Blow out" the otoscope light.
- "Beep" the stethoscope on your nose.
- Make tongue-depressor puppets.
- Use the child's own toys for play.
- Jingle your keys to test for hearing.
- Shine the otoscope through the tip of your finger (or the child's finger) to show it doesn't hurt, "lighting it up," and then examine the child's ears with it.
- Use age-appropriate toys and books.
- Use a fun toy attached to the stethoscope to make it less scary.

Note: Make sure to clean toys and your stethoscope in between patients.

Somatic Growth

Figures 23-57 and 23-58 demonstrate somatic growth patterns in children.

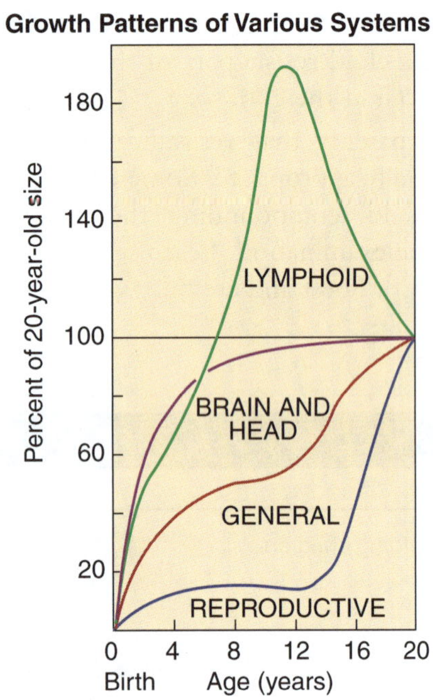

FIGURE 23-57. Growth patterns of various systems.

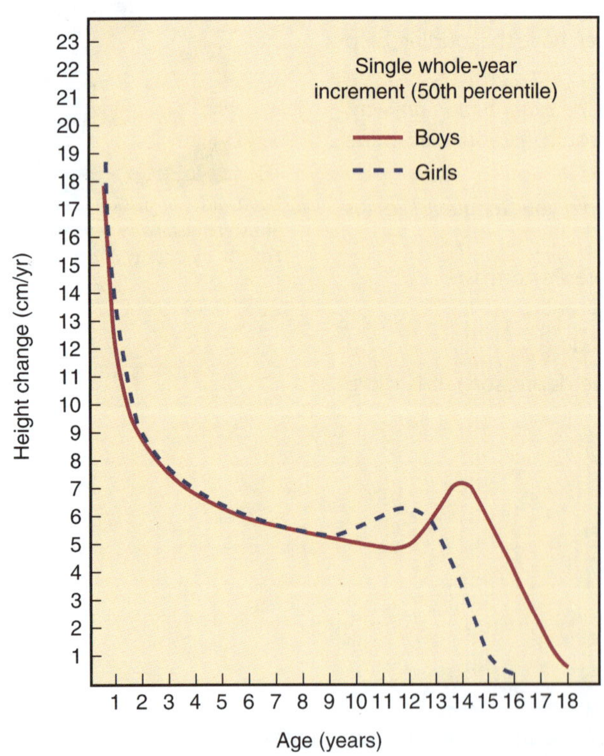

FIGURE 23-58. Velocity curves for length and height for boys and girls based on intervals of 1 year. (Reprinted from Lowrey GH. *Growth and Development of Children*. 8th ed. Year Book Medical; 1986. Copyright © 1986 Elsevier. With permission.)

Height. For children older than 2 years measure standing height, optimally using wall-mounted stadiometers. Have the child stand with heels, back, and head against a wall or the back of the stadiometer. If using a wall with a marked ruler, make sure to place a flat board or surface against the top of the child's head and at right angles to the ruler. Stand-up weight scales with a height attachment are not very accurate. After age 2 years children should grow at least 5 cm per year. During puberty, growth velocity increases.

Short stature, defined as height <5th percentile, can be a normal variant or caused by endocrine or other diseases. Normal variants include familial short stature and constitutional delay. Chronic diseases include growth hormone deficiency, other endocrine diseases, gastrointestinal disease, renal or metabolic disease, and genetic syndromes.

Weight. Children who can stand should be weighed in a gown (or in clothing without shoes) on a stand-up scale. Use the same scales across successive visits to optimize comparability.

Etiologies for insufficient caloric intake causing poor growth include psychosocial, gastrointestinal, and endocrine disorders. These conditions often cause poor growth in both height and weight.

Head Circumference. In general, head circumference is measured until the child reaches 24 months. Afterward, head circumference measurement may be helpful if you suspect a genetic or a central nervous system disorder.

Body Mass Index for Age. Age- and sex-specific charts are now available to assess BMI in children (Box 23-32). BMI in children is associated with body fat, related to subsequent health risks for obesity.

Box 23-32. Interpreting BMI in Children

Group	BMI-for-Age
Underweight	<5th percentile
Healthy weight	5th–85th percentile
Overweight	85th–95th percentile
Obese	≥95th percentile

Most children with exogenous obesity are also tall for their age. Children with endocrine causes of obesity tend to be short.

BMI measurements are helpful for early detection of obesity in children older than 2 years. BMI growth charts for children take into account differences by sex and age. Obesity is now a major childhood epidemic and it often begins before age 6 to 8 years. Consequences of childhood obesity include hypertension, diabetes, metabolic syndrome, and poor self-esteem. Childhood obesity *often leads to adult obesity* and *shortened lifespan*. It is helpful to give parents their child's BMI results (or show them the graph) together with information about the impact of healthy eating and physical activity.

Long-term morbidity from childhood obesity spans many organ systems, including cardiovascular, endocrine, renal, musculoskeletal, gastrointestinal, and psychological. Prevention, early detection, and aggressive management are needed.

Vital Signs

Blood Pressure. Hypertension during childhood is more common than previously thought and it is important to recognize, confirm, and appropriately manage it.

Children have elevated blood pressure during exercise, crying, and anxiety. Most children are cooperative with blood pressure measurement. If the blood pressure is initially elevated, you can perform blood pressure readings again at the end of the examination. Leave the cuff on the arm (deflated) and repeat the reading later. Elevated readings must always be confirmed by subsequent measurements.

A very common cause of apparent hypertension is anxiety or "white-coat hypertension." The most frequent "cause" of an elevated blood pressure in children is probably an *improperly performed examination,* often due to an incorrect cuff size.

A proper cuff size is essential for accurate determinations of blood pressure in children. Select the blood pressure cuff as you would for adults. The bladder length of the cuff should encircle 80% to 100% of the circumference of the child's arm. The cuff's width-to-arm circumference ratio should be 0.45 to 0.55 (Fig. 23-59). *A narrower cuff falsely elevates the blood pressure reading,* whereas *a wider cuff lowers it* and may interfere with proper placement of the stethoscope diaphragm over the artery.

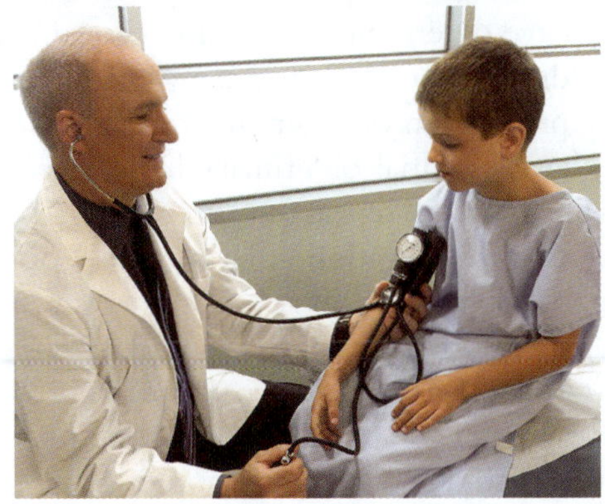

FIGURE 23-59. Blood pressure monitoring in childhood can be challenging.

With children, as with adults, the *first Korotkoff sound* indicates systolic pressure and the point at which the *Korotkoff sounds disappear* constitutes the *diastolic pressure*. At times, especially among young children with increased body fat, the Korotkoff sounds are not easily heard. Keep trying in a quiet room. If needed, you can use palpation to determine the systolic blood pressure, remembering that the systolic pressure obtained is approximately 10 mm Hg lower by palpation than by auscultation.

In children, as in adults, blood pressure readings from the thigh are approximately 10 mm Hg higher than those from the upper arm. If they are the same or lower, *coarctation of the aorta* should be suspected.

Transient hypertension in children can be caused by some common childhood medications, including those to treat asthma (e.g., prednisone) and ADHD (e.g., methylphenidate).

See Box 23-33 for updated definitions of BP categories and stages.

Box 23-33. Updated Definitions of BP Categories and Stages

	For Children Age 1 to <13 years	For Children Age ≥13 years
Normal BP	<90th percentile	<120/<80 mm Hg
Elevated BP	≥90th percentile to <95th percentile or 120/80 mm Hg to <95th percentile (whichever is lower)	120/<80 to 129/<80 mm Hg
Stage 1 HTN	≥95th percentile to <95th percentile + 12 mm Hg, or 130/80 to 139/89 mm Hg (whichever is lower)	130/80 to 139/89 mm Hg
Stage 2 HTN	≥95th percentile + 12 mm Hg, or ≥140/90 mm Hg (whichever is lower)	≥140/90 mm Hg

BP, blood pressure; *HTN*, hypertension.

Causes of *sustained hypertension* in childhood include primary hypertension (with no underlying etiology) and secondary hypertension (which has an underlying etiology). Causes of secondary hypertension include obesity, renal, endocrine, and neurologic disease, vascular causes, drugs or medications, and psychological causes.

The epidemic of childhood obesity has also resulted in a rising prevalence of childhood hypertension.

Children who have hypertension should be evaluated extensively to determine the cause. For infants and young children, a specific cause can often be found. An increasing proportion of older children and adolescents, however, have essential or primary hypertension. In all cases it is important to repeat measurements to reduce the possibility that the elevation reflects anxiety. Sometimes, repeating measurements in school is a way to obtain readings in a more relaxed environment. *Hypertension and obesity often coexist in children.* It is important not to *falsely label* a child or adolescent as having hypertension because of the stigma of labeling, potential limitations to activities, and possible side effects of treatment.

Pulse Rate. Average heart rates and normal ranges are shown in Box 23-34. Measure the heart rate over a 60-second interval.

Box 23-34. Average Heart Rate of Children at Rest

Age (Years)	Average Rate (Median)	Range (1st to 99th percentile)
1–2	110–120	88–155
2–6	100–110	65–140
6–10	75–90	52–130

Sinus bradycardia is a heart rate <100 beats per minute in infants and toddlers and <60 beats per minute in children >3 years.

Respiratory Rate. The rate of respirations per minute ranges from 20 to 40 during early childhood and 15 to 25 during late childhood, reaching adult levels at around 15 years of age.

For young children, observe the movements of the chest wall for two 30-second intervals or over 1 minute, preferably before stimulating them. Direct auscultation of the chest or placing the stethoscope in front of the mouth is also useful for counting respirations, but the measurement may be falsely elevated if the child becomes agitated. For older children use the same technique as that used for adults.

The commonly accepted standard for tachypnea in children older than age 1 year is a respiratory rate >40 breaths per minute.

The best single physical finding for *ruling out pneumonia* is an absence of tachypnea.

Temperature. In children, auditory canal temperature recordings are preferable because they can be obtained quickly with essentially no discomfort.

Children younger than 3 years, who appear very ill with a fever, should be evaluated for sepsis, urinary tract infection, pneumonia, or other serious infection.

Skin

After a child's first year of life, the techniques of examination are the same as those for the adult.

See Chapter 18, Skin, Hair, and Nails. Also see Table 23-4, Common Skin Lesions during Childhood.

Head

In examining the head and neck, tailor your examination to the child's stage of growth and development.

Even before touching the child, carefully observe the shape of the head, its symmetry, and the presence of abnormal facies. Abnormal facies may not be apparent until later in childhood; therefore, carefully examine the face as well as the head of all children.

See Table 23-6, Diagnostic Facies in Infancy and Childhood, which shows several diagnostic facies in childhood that reflect chromosomal abnormalities, endocrine defects, chronic illness, and other disorders.

Fetal alcohol syndrome can cause abnormal facies (p. 728), microcephaly, and developmental delay.

Eyes

The two most important components of the eye examination for young children are to determine whether the gaze is conjugate or symmetric and to test visual acuity in each eye.

Conjugate Gaze. Use the methods described in Chapter 7 for adults to assess conjugate gaze, or the position and alignment of the eyes, and the function of the extraocular muscles. The corneal light reflex test and the cover–uncover test are particularly useful in young children (Figs. 23-60 and 23-61).

Anisometropia (eyes with significantly different refractive errors) can result in *amblyopia,* or reduced vision in an otherwise normal eye. *Amblyopia* can lead to a "lazy eye," with permanently reduced visual acuity if not corrected early.

Strabismus (see Table 23-7, Abnormalities of the Eyes, Ears, and Mouth) in children requires treatment by an ophthalmologist because it can also lead to amblyopia. The common forms of strabismus in children involve horizontal deviation: nasal ("eso") or temporal ("exo"). A *latent strabismus* ("phoria") occurs when you disrupt fixation, whereas *manifest strabismus* ("tropia") is present without interruption.

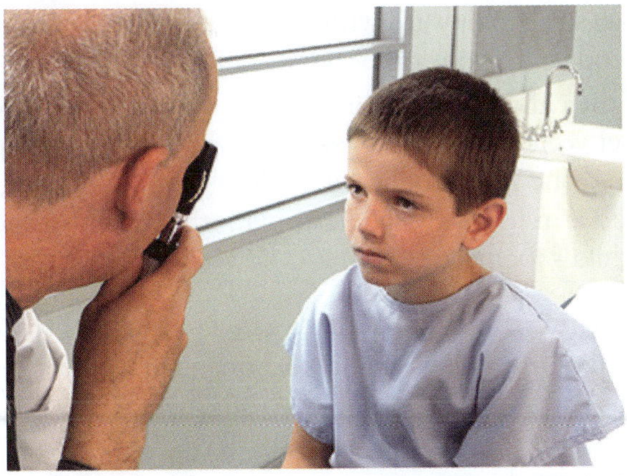

FIGURE 23-60. Corneal light reflex test.

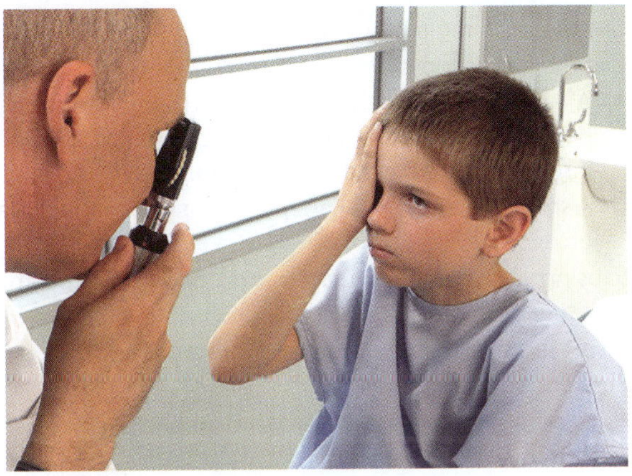

FIGURE 23-61. Cover–uncover test.

Perform the cover–uncover test as a game by having the young child watch your nose or tell you if you are smiling or not while you cover one of the child's eyes. When you uncover the eye, watch for any deviation of that eye. Repeat for the other eye. Latent strabismus is indicated by movement of either eye when uncovered.

Visual Acuity. It may not be possible to measure the *visual acuity* of children younger than 3 years who cannot identify pictures on an eye chart. For these children, the simplest examination is to assess for fixation preference by alternately covering one eye; the child with normal vision will not object, but a child with poor vision in one eye will object to having the good eye covered. Importantly, if you or the parent have any doubts about visual acuity, it is wise to refer to an optometrist or ophthalmologist because this aspect of the physical examination is insensitive (Box 23-35). In all tests of visual acuity, it is important that both eyes show the same result because of the risk for amblyopia.

Reduced visual acuity is more likely among children who were born prematurely and among those with other neurologic or developmental disorders.

Box 23-35. Visual Acuity

Age	Acuity
3 months	Eyes converge, baby reaches
12 months	~20/200
Younger than 4 years	20/40
4 years and older	20/30

Any difference in visual acuity between the eyes (e.g., 20/20 on the left and 20/30 on the right) is abnormal by age 5 years (Figs. 23-62 and 23-63).

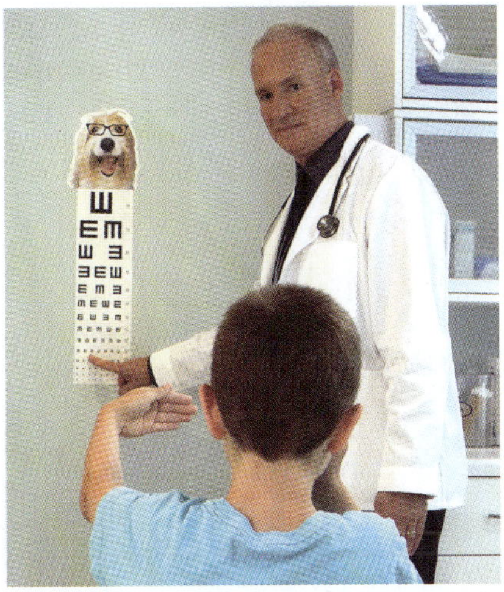

FIGURE 23-62. Testing visual acuity with a simple chart.

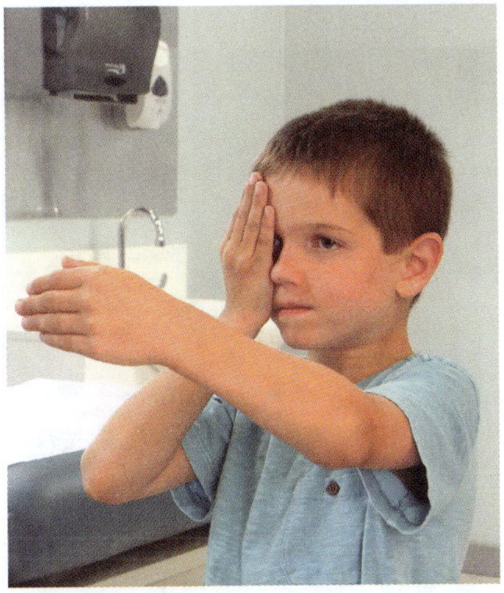

FIGURE 23-63. Test each eye and note the difference in acuity.

Some children develop *abnormalities in near vision,* which can lead to reading difficulties, headaches, and school problems, as well as double vision.

Visual acuity in children 4 years and older can usually be formally tested using an eye chart with one of a variety of optotypes (characters or symbols). A child who does not know letters or numbers reliably can be tested using pictures, symbols, or the "E" chart. Using the "E" chart, most children will cooperate by telling you in which direction the "E" is pointing.

The most common visual disorder of childhood is *myopia,* which can be easily detected using this examination technique.

Visual Fields. While it is often challenging, the *visual fields* can be examined in infants and young children with the child sitting on the parent's lap. One eye should be tested at a time with the other eye covered. Hold the child's head in the midline while bringing an object such as a toy into the field of vision from behind the child. The overall method is the same as that for adults, except that you will have to make this into a game for your patient.

Ears

Examining the *ear canal* and *tympanic membrane* can be difficult in young children who are sensitive and fearful because they cannot observe the procedure. With a little practice though, you can master this technique. Unfortunately, *many young children need to be briefly restrained during this examination, which is why you may want to leave it for the end.*

Ask the parent for a preference regarding the positioning of the child for the examination. There are two common positions: the child lying down and restrained, and if the child is not too fearful, you may examine the ears with the child sitting on a parent's lap.

If the child is held supine, have the parent hold the arms either extended (Figs. 23-64 and 23-65) or close to the sides to limit motion. Hold the head and pull the pinna (auricle) upward with one hand while you hold the otoscope with your other hand.

If the child is on the parent's lap, the child's legs should be between the parent's legs. The parent could help by placing one arm around the child's body and using the second arm to steady the head (with the parent's hand on the child's forehead).

Otoscopic Examination. Make a game out of the otoscopic examination, such as finding an imaginary object in the child's ear or talking playfully to allay fears (Box 23-36).

Box 23-36. Tips for Conducting the Otoscopic Examination

- Use the best angle of the otoscope.
- Use the largest possible speculum.
  - A larger speculum allows you to better visualize the tympanic membrane and is less painful since it is not inserted as far as a smaller speculum.
  - A small speculum may not provide a seal for pneumatic otoscopy.
- If using a pneumatic otoscope, do not apply too much pressure or the child may cry.
- Insert the speculum ¼–½ in into the canal.
- First find the landmarks.
  - Careful—sometimes the ear canal resembles the tympanic membrane.
- Note whether the tympanic membrane is abnormal.
- Remove cerumen if it is blocking your view, using one of the following:
  - Flushing of ears
  - Special plastic curettes
  - Moistened microtipped cotton swab if not totally occluded
  - Special instruments that can also be purchased.

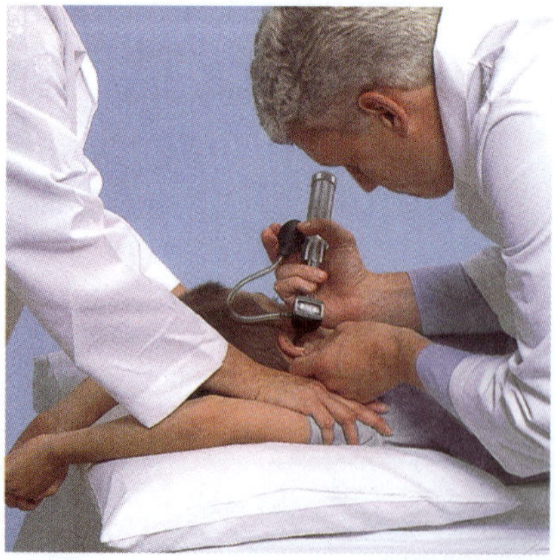

FIGURE 23-64. Gently holding the child's arms reduces reactions to the otoscope.

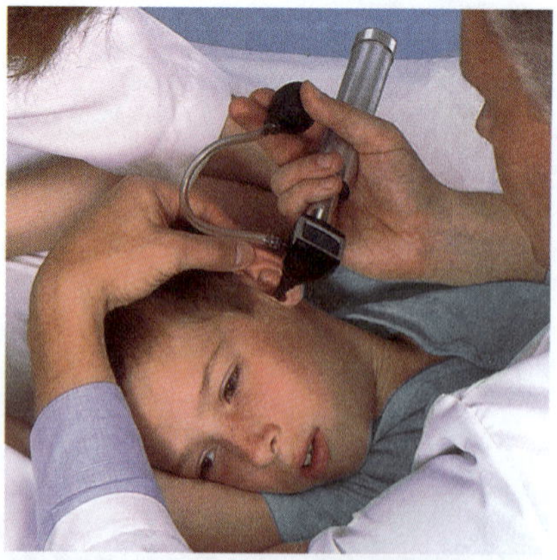

FIGURE 23-65. Hand positions for standard otoscope approach.

With otitis externa (but not otitis media), movement of the pinna elicits pain.

It may help to place the otoscopic speculum gently into the external auditory canal of one ear and then withdraw it so that the child gets used to the procedure before the actual examination. It is also helpful to show the child that the speculum does not hurt by letting the child touch it and shine a light through your finger.

Gently move and pull on the *pinna* before or during your otoscopic examination. Carefully inspect the area behind the pinna, over the mastoid bone. Many offices now use a tympanometer, which measures the compliance of the tympanic membrane and helps to diagnose a middle ear effusion.

With acute mastoiditis, the auricle may protrude forward and outward, and the area over the mastoid bone is red, swollen, and tender.

Many students have difficulty visualizing a child's tympanic membrane. In young children, the external auditory canal is directed upward and backward from the outside, and *the auricle must be pulled upward, outward, and backward to afford the best view.* Press the child's head with one hand, and with that same hand pull up on the auricle. Position the otoscope with your other hand.

There are two ways to hold the otoscope:

The first is the method generally used in adults, with the otoscope handle pointing upward or laterally while you pull up on the auricle. While holding the otoscope with the handle pointing down, pull up on the auricle. Steady your hand against the child's head and pull up on the auricle with that hand, while you hold the otoscope with the other hand (see Figs. 23-64 and 23-65).

The second method, with the handle of the otoscope pointing down toward the child's feet, is preferred by many pediatricians because of the angle of the auditory canal in children (Figs. 23-66 and 23-67).

Pneumatic Otoscopy. You can use a *pneumatic otoscope* to improve the accuracy of diagnosis of otitis media in children (Fig. 23-68). This allows you to assess the mobility of the tympanic membrane as you increase and decrease the pressure in the external auditory canal by squeezing the rubber bulb of the pneumatic otoscope.

Sometimes acute otitis media causes a ruptured tympanic membrane, leading to pus in the auditory canal. In these cases, you will generally not be able to visualize the tympanic membrane.

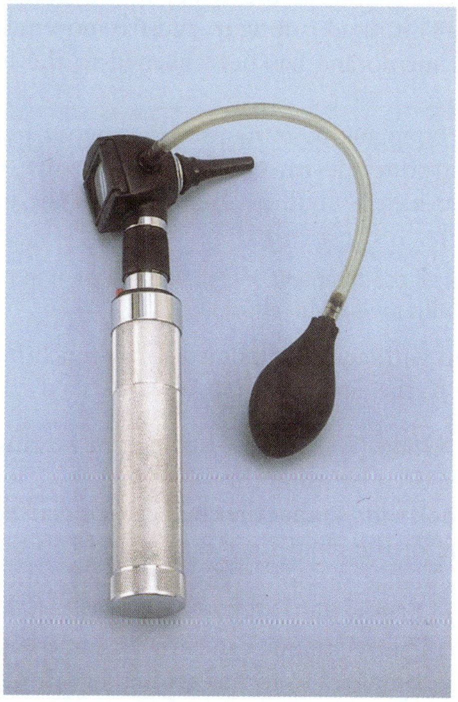

FIGURE 23-68. Pneumatic otoscope.

First, check the pneumatic otoscope for leaks by placing your finger over the tip of the speculum and

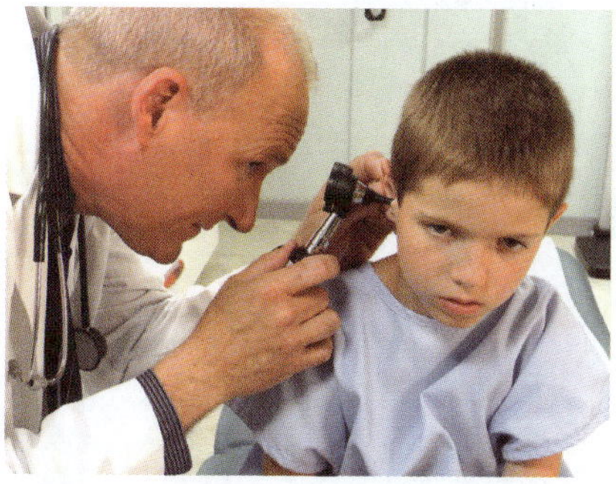

FIGURE 23-66. Gently pulling up on the auricle gives a better otoscope view with many children.

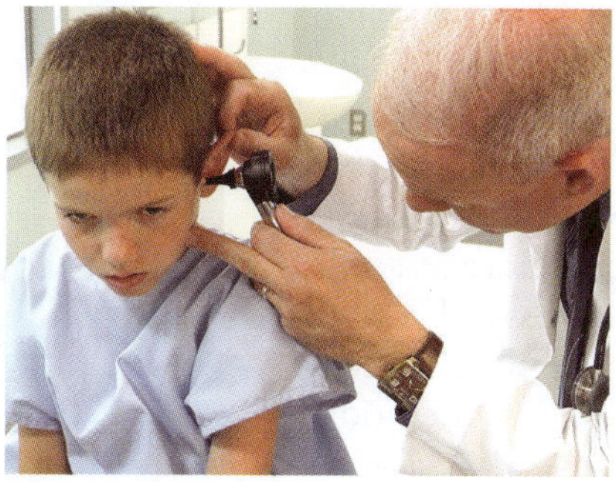

FIGURE 23-67. Auricle pulled up, handle pointed down, assessing left ear.

Acute otitis media is a common condition of childhood. A symptomatic child typically has a red, bulging tympanic membrane with a dull or absent light reflex and diminished movement on pneumatic otoscopy. Purulent material may also be seen behind the tympanic membrane. See Table 23-7, Abnormalities of the Eyes, Ears, and Mouth. The most useful symptom in making the diagnosis is ear pain, if combined with the above signs.

squeezing the bulb. Note the pressure on the bulb. Then insert the speculum, obtaining a proper seal; this is critical because failure to obtain a seal can produce a false-positive finding (lack of movement of the tympanic membrane). Of note, this process requires a patient who is not moving.

Significantly, *temporary hearing loss* for several months can accompany otitis media with effusion.

When air is introduced into the normal ear canal, the tympanic membrane and its light reflex move inward. When air is removed, the tympanic membrane moves outward. This rapid, subtle to-and-fro movement of the tympanic membrane has been likened to the luffing of a sail.

If the tympanic membrane fails to move perceptibly as you introduce positive or negative pressure, the child is likely to have a middle ear effusion (or the technique was poor).

Movement of the tympanic membrane is absent in middle ear effusion (otitis media with effusion).

A child with acute otitis media may flinch because of pain due to the air pressure.

Hearing Testing. You can grossly test for hearing in very young children by using the whispered voice test. Stand behind the child (so that the child cannot read your lips), cover one of the child's ear canals, and rub the tragus, using a circular motion. Whisper letters, numbers, or a word and have the child repeat it, and then test the other ear. This technique can have similar sensitivity and specificity compared to formal testing, but this technique is highly variable depending on the examiner.

Younger children who fail these screening maneuvers or who have speech delay should have audiometric testing. These children may have *hearing deficits* or central auditory processing disorders.

Up to 15% of school-aged children have at least *mild hearing loss*, emphasizing the importance of screening for hearing prior to school age.

The types of hearing loss seen in children are *conductive, sensorineural*, and *mixed conductive/sensorineural* hearing loss.

Causes of *conductive hearing loss* include congenital abnormalities, ossicular abnormalities, cerumen impaction, trauma, otitis media, and tympanic membrane perforation.

Formal hearing testing is necessary for accurate detection of hearing deficits in young children, and nowadays children as young as 6 months old may undergo behavioral hearing tests. Once the child is old enough to cooperate, use a formal hearing test method (Box 23-37).

Causes of *sensorineural hearing loss* include genetic, hereditary congenital infections, ototopic drugs, trauma, and some infections such as meningitis.

Box 23-37. Hearing Ranges on Formal Acoustic Screening Tests

Normal hearing	0–20 dB
Mild hearing loss	21–40 dB
Moderate hearing loss	41–60 dB
Severe hearing loss	61–90 dB
Profound hearing loss	>90 dB

All children older than 4 years should have a full-scale acoustic screening test using standardized equipment (Figs. 23-69 and 23-70). Even though a normal hearing screen at birth is reassuring, some hearing loss can be acquired as children age and hearing loss can dramatically affect a child's language and development. If you do use an acoustic screening test, be sure to test the entire acoustic range, including the speaking range (500 to 8,000 Hz). Box 23-37 shows one classification of hearing ranges.

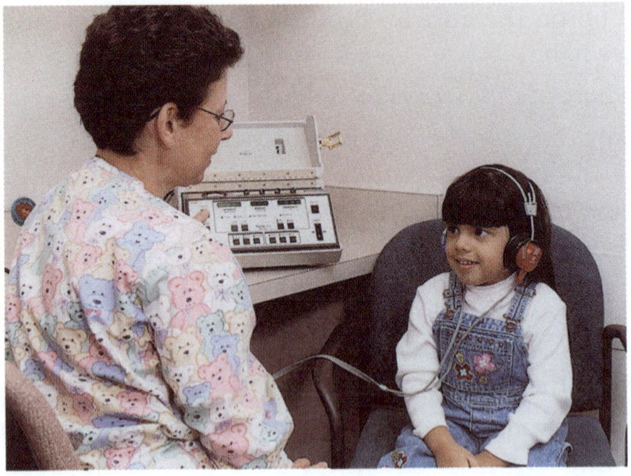

FIGURE 23-69. Standardized testing equipment provides more precise metrics.

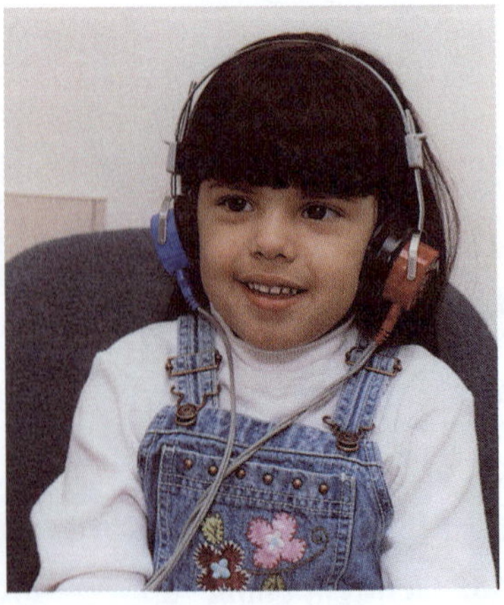

FIGURE 23-70. Children often enjoy a full-scale acoustic screening test.

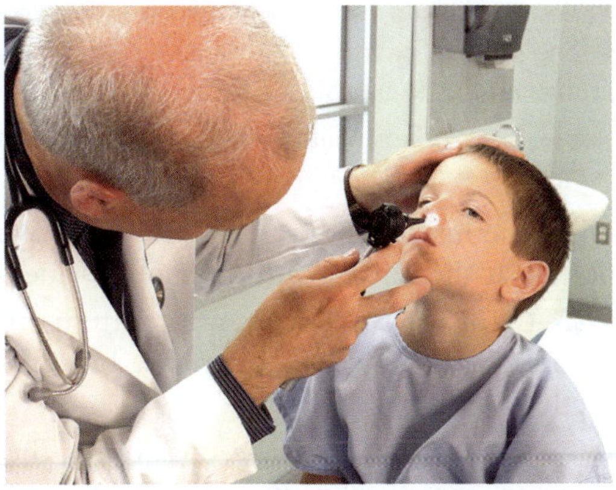

FIGURE 23-71. Nasal inspection of children.

Nose and Sinuses

Inspect the anterior portion of the nose by using a large speculum on your otoscope. Inspect the nasal mucous membranes, noting their color and condition. Look for nasal septal deviation and the presence of polyps (Fig. 23-71).

Pale, boggy nasal mucous membranes are found in children with *allergic rhinitis*.

Purulent rhinitis is common in viral infections.

Foul-smelling, purulent, unilateral discharge from the nose may be due to a foreign body. Young preschool children tend to stick objects into body orifices.

Nasal polyps are gray/yellow-colored growths inside the nares.

Sinuses develop at varying ages (Box 23-38). The sinuses of older children can be palpated or percussed as in adults, looking for tenderness. Transillumination of the paranasal sinuses of younger children has poor sensitivity and specificity for diagnosing sinusitis or fluid in the sinuses.

Children with (1) purulent rhinorrhea for more than 10 days, (2) worsening course, or (3) severe symptoms, high fever, and purulent rhinorrhea >3 days may have *sinusitis*. These children also have headache and sore throat, and you might note tenderness over the sinuses on percussion or palpation.

Box 23-38. Age of Pneumatization of Sinuses in Children

Sinus	Age of Pneumatization
Ethmoid	Birth
Maxillary	Birth to several years
Sphenoid	5–6 years
Frontal	7–8 years (continues until adolescence)

Mouth and Pharynx

For anxious or young children, it is wise to leave the examination of the mouth and pharynx until near the end because it may require parental restraint. It is often practical to examine the ears, and then the mouth. The young, cooperative child may be more comfortable sitting in the parent's lap. Healthy children are more likely to cooperate with this examination than sick children, especially if the sick child sees the tongue depressor or has had previous experience with throat cultures.

Figure 23-72 demonstrates how to get children to open their mouths. The child who can say "ahhh" will usually offer a sufficient (albeit brief) view of the posterior pharynx so that a tongue depressor is unnecessary (Box 23-39).

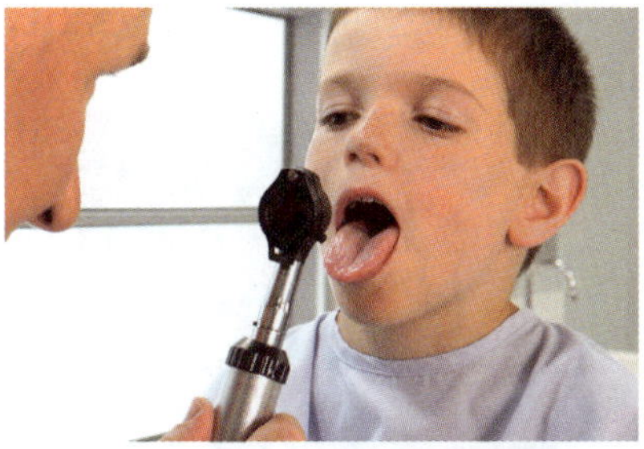

FIGURE 23-72. Children generally imitate well enough to allow you to inspect the back of their mouths.

Box 23-39. How to Get Children to Open Their Mouths (a.k.a., "Would You Please Say 'Ahhh'?")

- Turn it into a game.
  - *"Now let's see what's in your mouth."*
  - *"Can you stick out your whole tongue?"*
  - *"I bet you can't open your mouth really wide!"*
  - *"Let me see the inside of your teeth."*
  - *"Can you pant like a dog on a hot day?"*
- Don't show a tongue depressor unless really necessary.
- Demonstrate first on an older sibling (or even the parent).
- Offer enthusiastic praise for opening their mouths a little and encourage them to open even wider.

Pharynx. If you need to use a tongue depressor, push down and pull slightly forward toward yourself while the child says "ahhh," being careful not to place the depressor too far posteriorly, eliciting a gag reflex. Sometimes, young and anxious children will need to be restrained and will clamp their teeth and purse their lips. In these cases, carefully slip the tongue depressor between the teeth and the cheek in the vertical plane to the back of the gum line. Then turn the tongue depressor horizontally toward the tongue and push down. These techniques will either allow you to push down on the tongue or elicit a gag reflex, which should permit a brief look at the posterior pharynx and tonsils. Careful planning and parental help are needed.

Teeth. Examine the *teeth* for the timing and sequence of eruption, number, character, condition, and position. Abnormalities of the enamel may reflect local or general disease.

Dental caries are the most common health problem in children. They are particularly prevalent in populations living in impoverished areas and can cause both short-term and long-term problems. Caries are highly preventable and can be treated with dental visits.

Carefully inspect the upper teeth as shown in Figure 23-73. This is a common location for *early childhood caries.* The technique shown in Figure 23-73 is called "lift the lip," and it can help visualize dental caries.

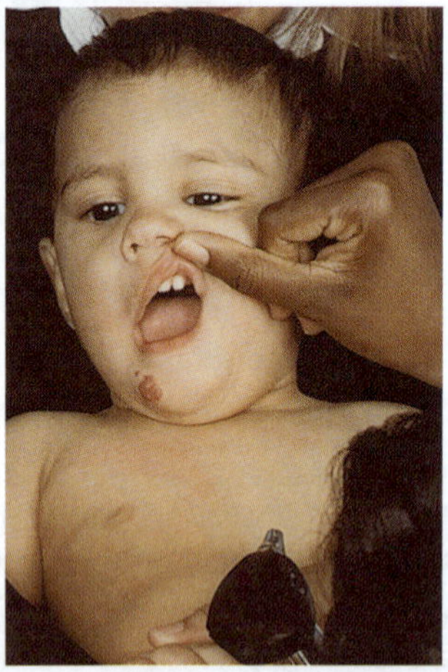

FIGURE 23-73. Lift the lip to check for dental caries.

Dental caries are caused by bacterial activity. Caries are more likely among young children who have prolonged bottle-feeding ("nursing-bottle caries").

See Table 23-9, Abnormalities of the Teeth, Pharynx, and Neck, for different stages of caries.

Visualize the inside of the upper teeth by having the child look up at the ceiling with the mouth wide open.

Box 23-40 displays the common pattern of tooth eruption. In general, lower teeth erupt a bit earlier than upper teeth.

Look for abnormalities of the position of the teeth. These include malocclusion, maxillary protrusion (*overbite*), and mandibular protrusion (*underbite*). You can demonstrate the latter two by asking the child to bite down hard while either you or the child parts the lips. Normally, the lower teeth are contained within the arch formed by the upper teeth.

Malocclusion and misalignment of teeth can be from thumb sucking, excess pacifier use, a hereditary condition, or premature loss of primary teeth.

Tongue. Carefully inspect the *tongue*, including the underside (Fig. 23-74). Most children will happily stick their tongue out at you and move it from side to side.

A *geographic tongue* is a benign but chronic condition in which a portion of the tongue has a rough, unusual appearance (looking like a map). The abnormal-appearing portion can vary over time and is thought to be a benign inflammatory process. Some children with geographic tongue also have fissured tongue, which is usually benign, and notable for small fissures.

Common abnormalities include *coated tongue* in viral infections, and *strawberry tongue,* from strep (see below) or scarlet fever.

Box 23-40. Tooth Types and Age of Eruption

	Approximate Age of Eruption	
Tooth Type	**Primary (months)**	**Permanent (years)**
Central incisor	5–8	6–8
Lateral incisor	5–11	7–9
Cuspids	24–30	11–12
First bicuspids	—	10–12
Second bicuspids	—	10–12
First molars	16–20	6–7
Second molars	24–30	11–13
Third molars	—	17–22

Staining of the teeth may be intrinsic or extrinsic. Intrinsic stains may be from tetracycline use before 8 years (yellow, gray, or brown stain). Other examples of intrinsic stains that we see are the "green stain" in teeth of children with liver disease, and fluorosis (white stain) caused by the excess of ingested fluoride during early childhood. Iron preparation (black stain) and fluoride (white stain) is an example of extrinsic stain. Extrinsic stains can be polished off; intrinsic stains cannot.

Delayed tooth eruption can be due to a variety of conditions such as *genetic disorders involving an altered craniofacial complex, or systemic diseases.*

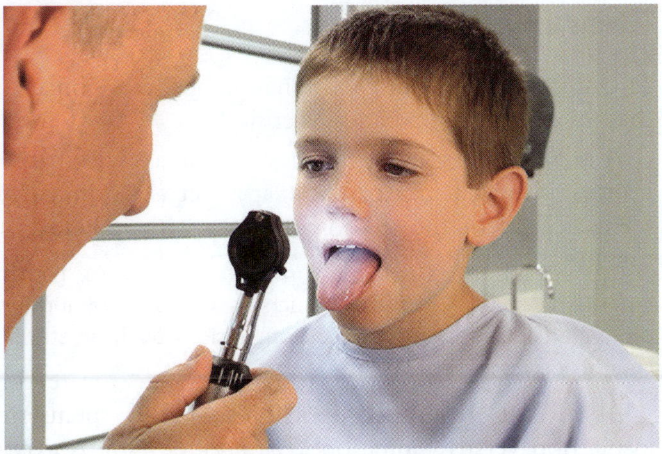

FIGURE 23-74. Inspect all parts of the tongue.

Some young children have a tight frenulum. Have the child touch the tongue to the roof of the mouth to diagnose this condition which often does not require treatment unless it interferes with eating or speech.

Children who are severely "tongue-tied" might have a speech impediment.

Tonsils. Note the size, position, symmetry, and appearance of the *tonsils*. The peak growth of tonsillar tissue is between 2 and 10 years (see Fig. 23-57). The size of the tonsils varies considerably in children and is often categorized by the percent of the width of the posterior oropharynx (e.g., reduce the opening by <25% of opening, by 50%, etc.). The tonsils in children often appear more obstructive than they really are.

Streptococcal pharyngitis typically produces white or yellow exudates on the tonsils or posterior pharynx, a beefy-red uvula, and palatal petechiae.

Tonsils in children usually have deep crypts on their surfaces, which often have white concretions or food particles protruding from their depths. This does not indicate disease.

A *peritonsillar abscess* is suggested by erythema and asymmetric protrusion of one tonsil, pain, difficulty opening the mouth (trismus), and lateral displacement of the uvula.

Look for clues of a submucosal cleft palate such as notching of the posterior margin of the hard palate or a bifid *uvula*. Because the mucosa is intact, the underlying defect is easily missed, but needs referral to otolaryngology.

Extremely rarely, you may encounter a child who has a sore throat and has difficulty swallowing saliva and who is sitting up stiffly in a "tripod" position because of throat obstruction. Do not open this child's mouth because he may have acute epiglottitis, or obstruction from another cause, and examination of the throat may induce gagging and laryngeal obstruction.

Bacterial tracheitis can cause airway obstruction.

Note the quality of the child's voice. Certain abnormalities can change the pitch and quality of the voice (Box 23-41).

Tonsillitis can be caused by bacteria, such as *Streptococcus* or *Staphylococcus*, or viruses. The "hot potato" voice is accompanied by enlarged tonsils with exudates.

The epidemic of childhood obesity has resulted in many children who snore and have *obstructive sleep apnea*.

Box 23-41. Voice Changes—Clues to Underlying Abnormalities

Voice Change	Possible Abnormality
Hypernasal speech	Submucosal cleft palate
Nasal voice plus snoring	Adenoidal hypertrophy
Hoarseness plus cough	Viral infection (croup)
"Hot potato speech"	Tonsillitis

You may note an abnormal breath odor which may help lead to a specific diagnosis.

Halitosis (bad breath) in a child can be caused by upper respiratory, pharyngeal, or mouth infection, foreign body in the nose, sinusitis, dental disease, and gastroesophageal reflux.

Neck. Beyond infancy, the techniques for examining the neck are the same as for adults. Lymphadenopathy is unusual during infancy but very common during childhood. The child's lymphatic system reaches its zenith of growth at 12 years, and cervical or tonsillar lymph nodes reach their peak size between 8 and 16 years (see Fig. 23-57).

Lymphadenopathy is usually from viral or bacterial infections.

The vast majority of enlarged lymph nodes in children are due to infections (mostly viral, but sometimes bacterial) and not due to malignant disease, even though the latter is a concern for many parents. It is important to differentiate normal lymph nodes from abnormal ones or from congenital cysts of the neck.

Malignancy is more likely if the node is *>2 cm, is hard, or is fixed to the skin or underlying tissues* (i.e., not mobile) and is *accompanied by serious systemic signs* such as weight loss.

Check for *neck mobility*. It is important to ensure that the neck of all children is supple and easily mobile in all directions. This is particularly important when the patient is holding the head in an asymmetric manner and when central nervous system disease such as meningitis is suspected.

In young children, it may be difficult to differentiate low posterior cervical lymph nodes from *supraclavicular lymph nodes (which are always abnormal and raise suspicion for an abdominal malignancy).*

In children, the presence of *nuchal rigidity* is a more reliable indicator of meningeal irritation than *Brudzinski sign* or *Kernig sign*. To detect nuchal rigidity in older children, ask the child to sit with legs extended on the examining table. Normally, children should be able to sit upright and touch their chins to their chests. Younger children can be persuaded to flex their necks by having them follow a small toy or light beam. You also can test for nuchal rigidity with the child lying on the examining table, as shown in Figure 23-75. Nearly all children with nuchal rigidity will be extremely sick, irritable, and difficult to examine.

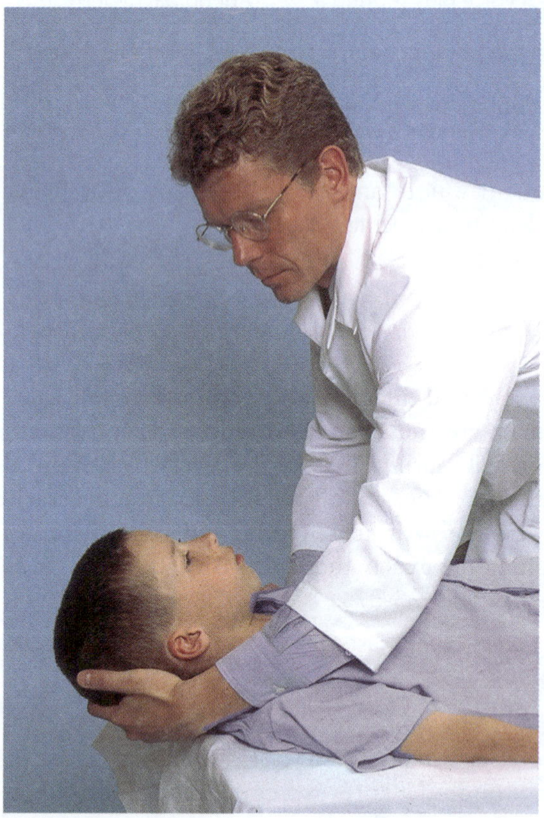

FIGURE 23-75. Inspect the neck for nuchal rigidity.

Nuchal rigidity is marked resistance to movement of the head in any direction. It suggests meningeal irritation due to meningitis, bleeding, tumor, or other causes. These children are extremely irritable and difficult to console and may have *"paradoxical irritability"*—increased irritability when being held.

When meningeal irritation is present, the child may assume the *tripod position* and is unable to assume a full upright position to perform the chin-to-chest maneuver.

Thorax and Lungs

As children age, the lung examination becomes similar to that for adults. Cooperation is critical.

Auscultation is usually easiest when a child barely notices (as when in a parent's lap). Let a toddler who seems fearful of the stethoscope play with it before it touches the child's chest.

With *upper airway obstruction* such as croup, inspiration is prolonged and accompanied by other signs such as stridor, cough, or rhonchi.

Assess the relative proportion of time spent on inspiration versus expiration. *The normal ratio is about 1:2.* Prolonged inspirations or expirations are a clue to disease location. Degree of prolongation and effort or "work of breathing" are related to disease severity.

With *lower airway obstruction* such as asthma, expiration is prolonged and often accompanied by wheezing (as well as coughing).

Young children asked to *"take deep breaths"* often hold their breath, further complicating auscultation. It is easier to let preschoolers breathe normally. Demonstrate to older children how to take nice, quiet, deep breaths. Make it a game. To accomplish a forced expiratory maneuver, ask the child to blow out candles on an imaginary birthday cake or use pinwheels (Fig. 23-76).

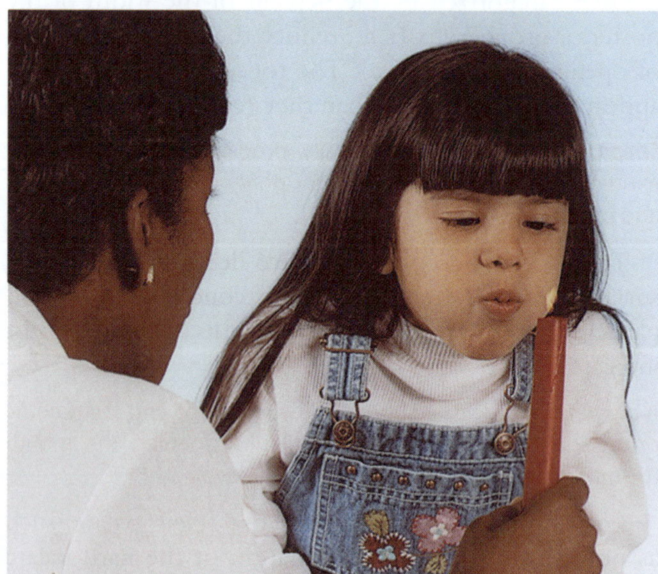

FIGURE 23-76. Getting a child to perform a forced expiration.

Pneumonia in young children is generally manifested by fever, tachypnea, dyspnea, and increased work of breathing.

Upper respiratory infections due to viruses in young children present with the same signs as in adults; children generally appear well without lower respiratory signs.

Childhood asthma is an extremely common condition throughout the world. Children with acute asthma present with varying severity and often have increased work of breathing. Expiratory wheezing and a prolonged expiratory phase, caused by reversible bronchospasm, may be heard without the stethoscope and are apparent on auscultation. Wheezes are often accompanied by inspiratory rhonchi caused by upper respiratory congestion. Asthma flares often occur with viral infections.

Older children will usually be cooperative for the respiratory examination and can even go through the maneuvers of assessing fremitus or listening to "E to A" changes Palpation, percussion, and auscultation achieve greater importance in a careful examination of the thorax and lungs.

Children in respiratory distress may assume a "*tripod position*" in which they lean forward to optimize airway patency (Fig. 23-77). This same position can also be caused by pharyngeal obstruction.

Children exhibiting these signs of respiratory distress must be managed emergently. Possible causes include upper airway obstruction (such as epiglottitis or bacterial tracheitis), bacterial or viral lower respiratory infections, and foreign-body obstruction.

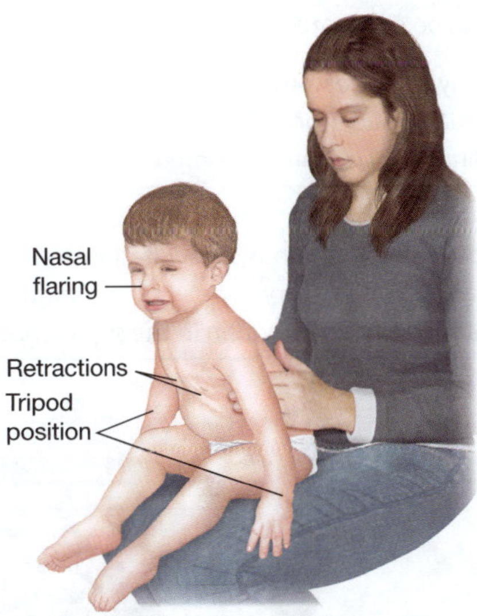

FIGURE 23-77. A child in respiratory distress.

Heart

The examination of the heart and vascular systems in infants and children is similar to that in adults. However, a child's fearfulness or inability to cooperate may make the examination difficult while the desire to play will make the examination easier and more productive (Fig. 23-78). Use your knowledge of the developmental stage of each child with some helpful techniques for cardiac examination (Box 23-42).

General abnormalities detected on examination may suggest increased likelihood of congenital cardiac disease as exemplified by Down syndrome or Turner syndrome.

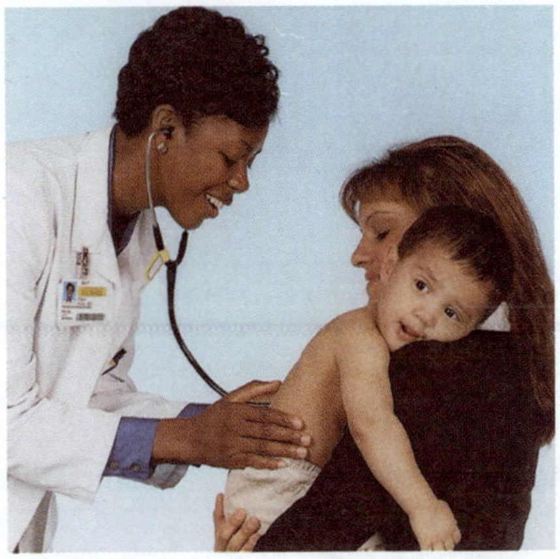

FIGURE 23-78. Young children are easiest to examine when held by a parent. You can even sneak your stethoscope around to the anterior chest.

Box 23-42. Techniques to Enhance Your Cardiac Examination in Young Children

- Young children (2–4 years)
  - Examine the child's arm or parent's arm first with your stethoscope
  - Have the child touch your stethoscope and play with it a bit
  - Examine the child while he/she is on their parent's lap, and have the parent turn them to face you
  - Give the child something to hold in each hand making it more challenging for the child to push you away
  - Have the child watch a video on a smartphone or tablet (with the volume on low)
  - Use endless chatter to hold the child's attention, pausing briefly to listen (they may forget you are listening)
- Older children (5–10 years)
  - Explain what you plan to do
  - Remind the child that the stethoscope might be cold
  - Say *"shhh"* very gently with a smile, asking the child to be quiet
  - Ask the child to just breathe normally

Benign Murmurs. Preschool and school-aged children often have benign murmurs (Box 23-43). The most common (*Still's murmur*) is a grade I–II/VI, musical, vibratory, early and midsystolic murmur with multiple overtones located over the mid or lower left sternal border; it may also be heard over the carotid arteries. Carotid artery compression will usually cause the precordial murmur to disappear. This murmur may be extremely variable and may be accentuated when cardiac

Box 23-43. Location and Characteristics of Benign Heart Murmurs in Children

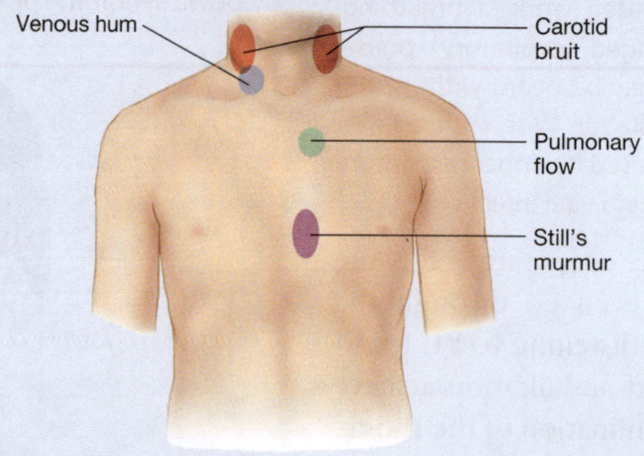

Typical Age	Name	Characteristics	Description and Location
Preschool or early school age	*Still's murmur*	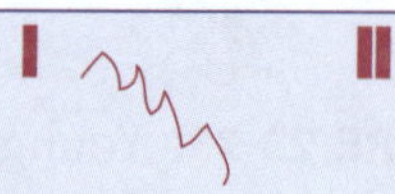	Grade I–II/VI, musical, vibratory Multiple overtones Early and midsystolic Mid/lower left sternal border Frequently also a carotid bruit
Preschool or early school age	*Venous hum*	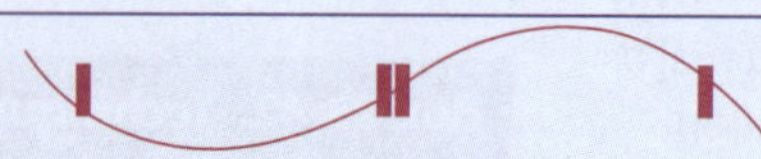	Soft, hollow, continuous Louder in diastole Just above or below the clavicle Can be eliminated by maneuvers
Preschool and later	*Carotid bruit*	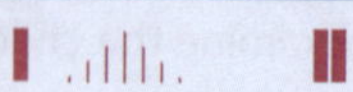	Early and midsystolic Usually louder on left Eliminated by carotid compression
Preschool and school age	*Pulmonary flow murmur*	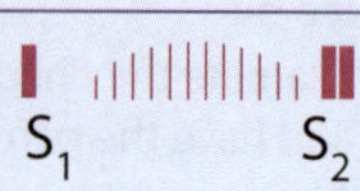	Grade 2–3 systolic crescendo–decrescendo Loudest at pulmonary auscultation area Harsh, nonvibratory Intensity increases when in the supine position

output is increased, as occurs with fever or exercise. The murmur will diminish as the child goes from supine to sitting to standing, conversely it will often sound louder as the child lies down if you started the examination while the child was sitting.

See Box 23-43, Location and Characteristics of Benign Heart Murmurs in Children.

In preschool or school-aged children, you may detect a *venous hum*. This is a soft, hollow, continuous sound, louder in diastole, heard just above or below the clavicle (Fig. 23-79). It can be completely eliminated by maneuvers that affect venous return, such as lying supine, changing head position, or jugular venous compression. It has the same quality as breath sounds and is therefore frequently overlooked.

Among young children, murmurs without the recognizable features of the common benign murmurs may signify underlying heart disease and should be evaluated thoroughly by a pediatric cardiologist.

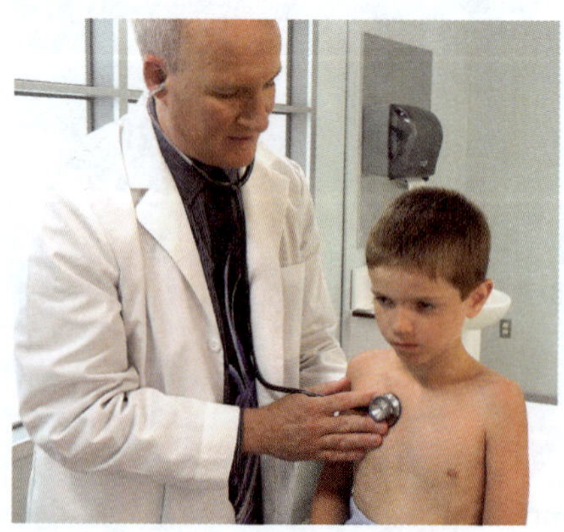

FIGURE 23-79. Listening for venous hum.

Pathologic murmurs that signify cardiac disease can first appear after infancy and during childhood. Examples include *aortic stenosis and mitral valve disease.*

The murmur heard in the carotid area or just above the clavicles is known as a *carotid bruit*. It is early and midsystolic with a slightly harsh quality. It is usually louder on the left and may be heard alone or in combination with the Still's murmur. It may be completely eradicated by carotid artery compression (Fig. 23-80).

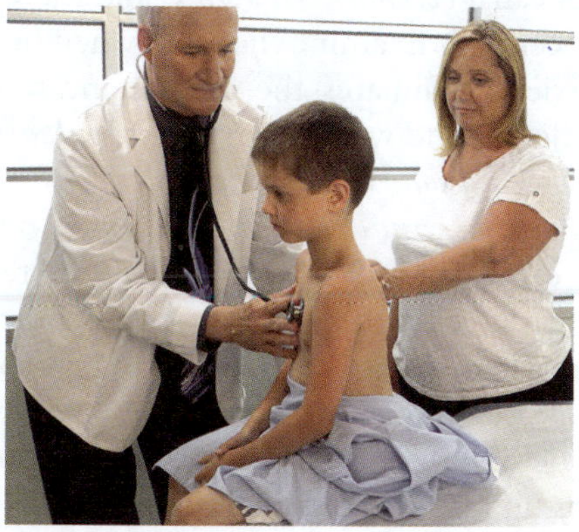

FIGURE 23-80. Carotid artery compression while listening to murmur.

A *pulmonary flow murmur* is typically located in the left upper sternal border. It is a grade I–II/VI, soft systolic crescendo–decrescendo murmur. The second heart sound is normal (i.e., not unusually loud). Like the Still's murmur, it also is louder when the child lies down. It is quieter when the patient sits or stands or holds his/her breath.

Blood Pressure in Extremities. Measure the blood pressure in both arms and one leg one time to check for possible *coarctation of the aorta*. Thereafter, only the right arm blood pressure needs to be measured after a coarctation has been ruled out.

In *coarctation of the aorta* the blood pressure is lower in the legs than in the arms.

Abdomen

Toddlers and young children commonly have protuberant abdomens, most apparent when they are upright. The examination can follow the same order as for adults except that you may need to distract the child during the examination.

An exaggerated "pot-belly appearance" may indicate *malabsorption* from celiac disease, cystic fibrosis, or constipation; in developing countries it can be a sign of kwashiorkor or intestinal parasites.

Most children are ticklish when you first place your hand on their abdomens for *palpation*. This reaction tends to disappear, particularly if you distract the child with conversation and place your whole hand flush on the abdominal surface for a few moments without probing. For children who are particularly sensitive and who tighten their abdominal muscles you can start by placing the child's hand under yours. Eventually, you will be able to remove the child's hand and palpate the abdomen freely. Palpate the *liver* edge and measure its span as you would in an adult using percussion techniques. Expected liver spans by percussion are shown in Box 23-44.

A common condition of childhood that can occasionally cause a protuberant abdomen is *constipation*. The abdomen is often tympanitic on percussion, and stool is sometimes felt on palpation.

Box 23-44. Expected Liver Span of Children by Percussion

	Mean Estimated Liver Span (cm)	
Age in Years	**Males**	**Females**
2	3.5	3.6
3	4.0	4.0
4	4.4	4.3
5	4.8	4.5
6	5.1	4.8
8	5.6	5.1
10	6.1	5.4

Try flexing the knees and hips to relax the child's abdominal wall, as shown in Figure 23-81. Palpate lightly in all areas, then deeply, leaving the site of potential pathology to the end.

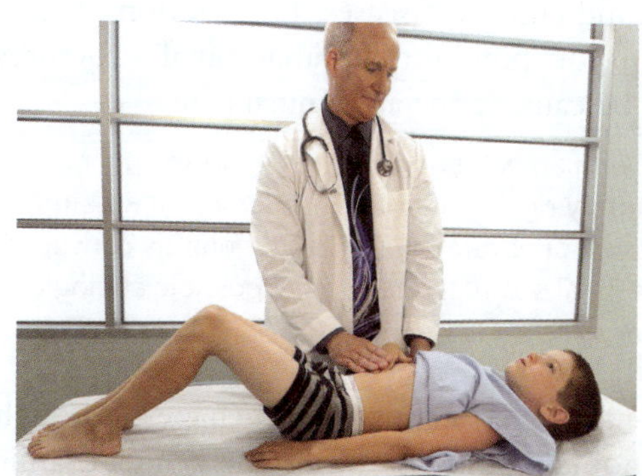

FIGURE 23-81. Position child as shown to palpate abdomen.

Chronic or recurrent abdominal pain is relatively common in children. Some functional disorders causing abdominal pain include irritable bowel syndrome, functional dyspepsia, and childhood functional abdominal pain syndrome. Other causes in children include gastritis or ulcer, gastroesophageal reflux, constipation, and inflammatory bowel disease.

Many children present with abdominal pain from *acute gastroenteritis.* Despite pain, their physical examination is relatively normal except for increased bowel sounds on auscultation and mild tenderness on palpation.

The childhood obesity epidemic has resulted in many children who have extremely obese abdomens. This makes the examination more challenging but the steps for examining the abdomen are the same.

Hepatomegaly in young children is unusual. It can be caused by cystic fibrosis, parasites, fatty liver, hepatitis, and tumors.

The *spleen,* like the liver, may be palpable in some children. It too is soft with a sharp edge, and it projects downward like a tongue from under the left costal margin. The spleen is moveable and rarely extends more than 1 to 2 cm below the costal margin.

If hepatomegaly is accompanied by splenomegaly, portal hypertension, storage diseases, chronic infections, and malignancy should be considered.

Various diseases can cause *splenomegaly,* including infections, hematologic disorders such as hemolytic anemias, infiltrative disorders, and inflammatory or autoimmune diseases, as well as congestion from portal hypertension.

Palpate the *other abdominal structures.* You will commonly note pulsations in the epigastrium caused by the aorta. This is felt most easily to the left of the midline, on deep palpation.

An *abdominal mass* felt on palpation may represent stool from constipation, a distended bladder, or a serious condition such as a tumor.

Palpating for abdominal tenderness in an older child is the same as for the adult; however, the causes of abdominal pain are often different, encompassing a wide spectrum of acute and chronic diseases. Localization of tenderness may help you pinpoint the abdominal structures most likely to be causing the abdominal pain.

In a child with an *acute abdomen,* as in acute appendicitis, check for involuntary rigidity, rebound tenderness, a Rovsing sign, or a positive psoas or obturator sign. Gastroenteritis, constipation, and gastrointestinal obstruction are other possible etiologies of acute abdominal pain.

Male Genitalia. An appropriate chaperone such as a parent should be present during the genital examination. Inspect the penis. The size in prepubertal children has little significance unless it is abnormally large or small. In boys who are obese, the fat pad over the symphysis pubis may obscure the penis.

In *precocious puberty,* the penis and testes are enlarged with signs of pubertal changes. Other pubertal changes also occur. It is due to excess androgens and can be caused by multiple conditions including adrenal or pituitary tumors.

Examination by *palpation* of the scrotum and testes of a young boy may cause the testis to retract upward into the inguinal canal (*cremasteric reflex*) and thereby appear to be undescended. Examine the child when he is relaxed because anxiety stimulates the cremasteric reflex. Have the boy lie down, and with warm hands, *palpate the lower abdomen, working your way downward toward the scrotum along the inguinal canal. This will minimize retraction of the testes* into the canal. If you can detect the testis in the scrotum it is descended, even if it spends much time in the inguinal canal. A retractile testis can be brought into the scrotum and remains there, while an undescended testis may be able to be brought into the scrotum but readily pops up into the inguinal canal.

Cryptorchidism may be noted at this age. It requires surgical correction. It should be differentiated from a retractile testis.

A *painless scrotal mass* in a young boy is usually due to a hydrocele or a nonincarcerated inguinal hernia. Other rare causes include a varicocele or tumor.

A painful testicle requires urgent consultation and treatment.

Possible causes of a *painful testicle* include infection such as epididymitis or orchitis, torsion of the testicle, or torsion of the appendix testis.

The cremasteric reflex can be elicited by gently stroking upward or downward along the medial aspect of the thigh. The testis on the side being stroked will move upward.

Examine the inguinal canal as you would for adults noting any swelling that may reflect an inguinal hernia. If desired, have the boy increase abdominal pressure by pretending to blow a balloon or fill up his cheeks by pursing his lips and blowing; note whether a bulge in the inguinal canal increases with Valsalva.

Inguinal hernias in older boys present as they do in adult men with swelling in the inguinal canal, particularly following a Valsalva maneuver.

Female Genitalia

An appropriate chaperone such as a parent should be present during the examination. The genital examination can be anxiety provoking for the older child and for parents. Nevertheless, it is important to perform it to detect abnormalities and to reassure parents in the case of normal examination findings. Depending on the child's developmental stage, explain what parts of the body you will check and that this is part of the routine examination.

The appearance of pubic hair before age 7 years should be considered *precocious adrenarche* and requires evaluation to determine the cause.

After infancy, the labia majora and minora flatten out and the hymenal membrane becomes thin, translucent, and vascular, with the edges easily identified.

Rashes on the external genitals can be from physical irritation, sweating, and candidal or bacterial infections including streptococcal infection.

The genital examination is the same for all ages of children, from late infancy until adolescence. Use a calm, gentle approach including a developmentally appropriate explanation as you do the examination. A bright light source is essential. Most children can be examined in the supine, frog-leg position.

If the child seems reluctant, it may be helpful to have the parent sit on the examination table with the child; alternatively, the examination may be performed while the child sits in the parent's lap. Do not use stirrups as these may frighten the child. Figure 23-82 demonstrates a 5-year-old girl sitting on her parent's lap with the parent holding her knees outstretched.

Vulvovaginal pruritis and erythema can be caused by external irritants, bubble baths, masturbatory activity, pinworms, or other infections such as *Candida* or sexually transmitted infections.

Examine the genitalia in an efficient and systematic manner. Inspect the external genitalia for pubic hair, the size of the clitoris, the color and size of the labia majora, and the presence of rashes, bruises, or other lesions.

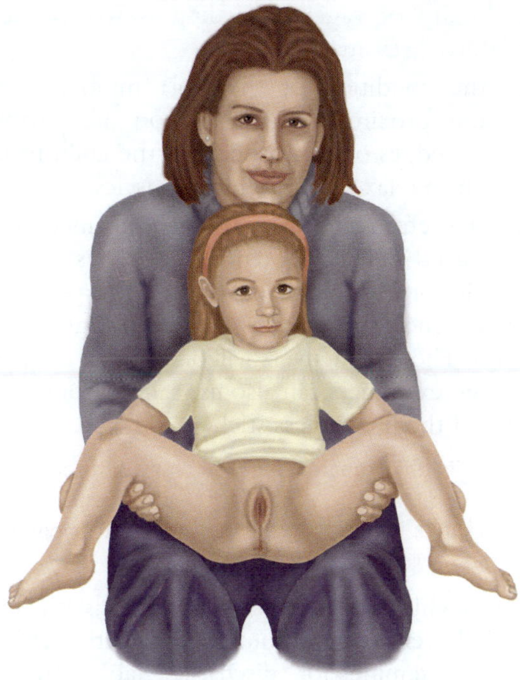

FIGURE 23-82. Positioning the mother behind her child has a calming effect.

Next, visualize the structures by separating the labia with your fingers, as shown in Figure 23-83. You can also grasp the labia between your thumb and index finger of each hand, separating the labia majora with gentle traction laterally and toward the examiner in order to the inner structures as shown in Figure 23-84. *Labial adhesions,* or fusion of the labia minora, may be noted in prepubertal children. They are normal findings. They may be a normal variant.

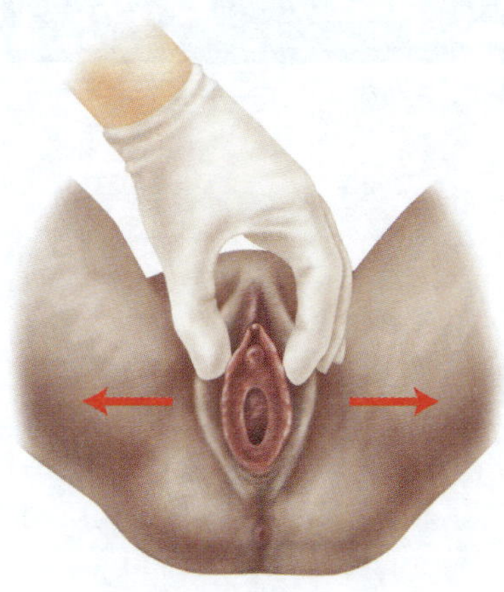

FIGURE 23-83. Separate labia to assess genital structures.

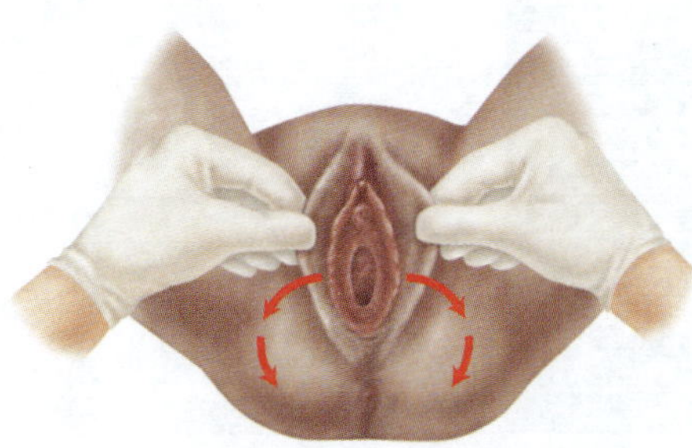

FIGURE 23-84. Using thumb and forefinger to examine inner structures.

A *vaginal discharge* in early childhood can be from *perineal irritation* (e.g., bubble baths or soaps), *foreign body, nonspecific vulvovaginitis, Candida, pinworms,* or a *sexually transmitted infection* from sexual abuse.

Precocious puberty can induce menses in a young girl.

Purulent, profuse, malodorous, and blood-tinged discharge should be evaluated for the presence of *infection, foreign body,* or *trauma.*

The finding of vaginal bleeding is worrisome and warrants further evaluation.

Note the condition of the labia minora, urethra, hymen, and proximal vagina. If you are unable to visualize the edges of the hymen, ask the child to take a deep breath to relax the abdominal muscles.

Another useful technique (to be performed only by an experienced pediatric examiner, such as during an examination for possible sexual abuse) is to position her in the knee–chest position, as shown in Figures 23-85 and 23-86. These maneuvers will often open the hymen. Experienced examiners can also use saline drops to make the edges of the hymen less sticky.

Sexual abuse is unfortunately far too common throughout the world. Up to one fifth of women report some history of sexual abuse as a child; while many of these do not involve severe physical trauma, some do.

Avoid touching the hymenal edges because the hymen is exquisitely sensitive without the protective effects of hormones. Examine for discharge, labial adhesions, lesions, estrogenization (indicating onset of puberty), hymenal variations (such as imperforate or septate hymen, which are rare), and hygiene. A thin, white discharge (leukorrhea) can be present. A speculum examination of the vagina and cervix is contraindicated in a prepubertal child unless there is suspicion of severe trauma or foreign body; it should be performed by an expert.

Abrasions or signs of trauma of the external genitalia can be from benign causes such as masturbation, irritants, or accidental trauma, but should also raise the possibility of sexual abuse. See Table 23-12, Physical Signs of Sexual Abuse.

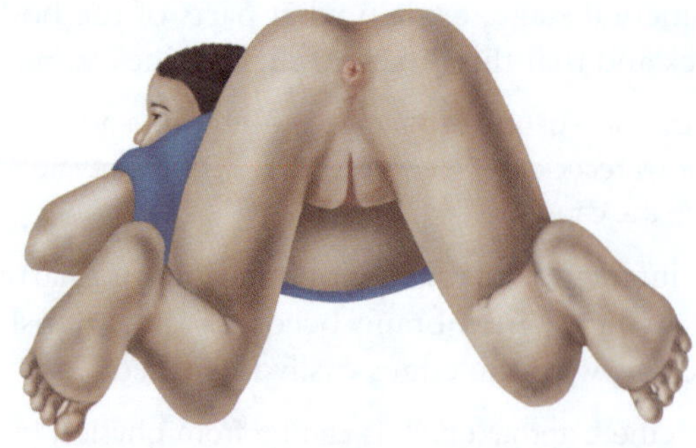

FIGURE 23-85. Position for more advanced technique to visualize hymen.

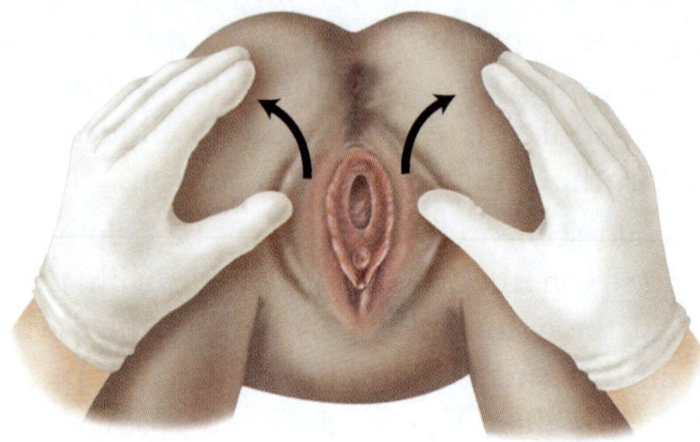

FIGURE 23-86. Using thumbs to separate labia to open the hymen.

The normal hymen in infants and young girls can have various configurations, as shown in Box 23-45. The physical examination may reveal mounds, notches, and tags on the hymen which may all be normal variants. The size of the vaginal orifice can vary with age and with examination technique. Therefore, there is no correlation between the size of the vaginal orifice and whether or not the patient has been sexually assaulted.

Box 23-45. Normal Configurations of the Hymen in Prepubertal and Adolescent Females

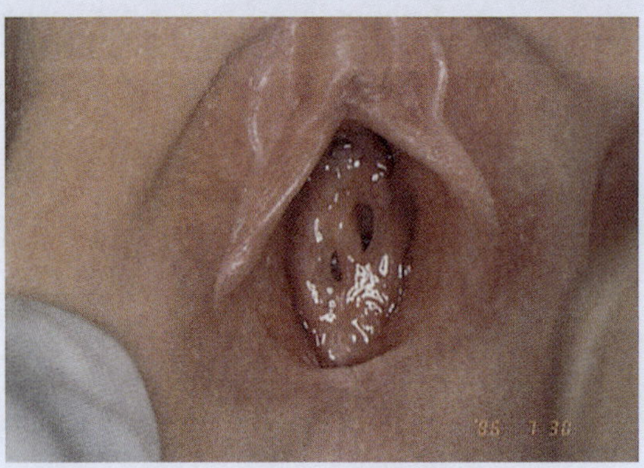

6-year-old girl with a septate hymen causing two orifices. Traction is needed to visualize the two openings.

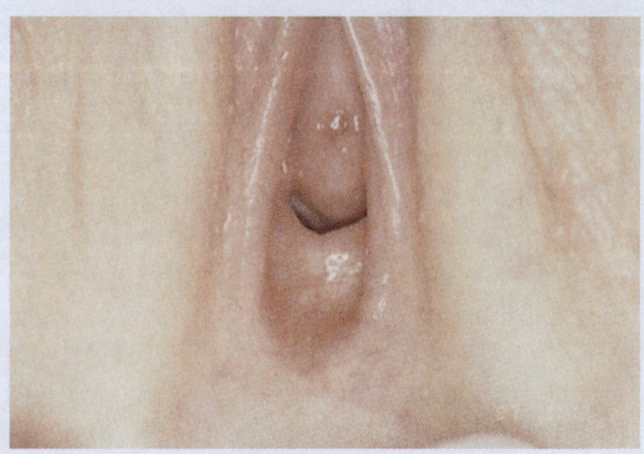

7-year-old girl with a crescent-shaped hymen. Crescentic hymens do not encircle the vaginal orifice but rather border the lower part of the vaginal orifice and extend to the posterior and lateral margins of the hymenal ring.

(*continued*)

Box 23-45. Normal Configurations of the Hymen in Prepubertal and Adolescent Females (*continued*)

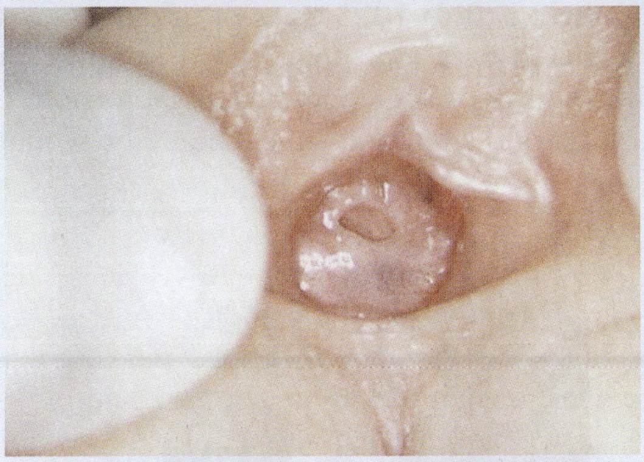

2-year-old girl with an annular hymen, visible with labial traction. Annular means that the hymen surrounds the orifice circumferentially.

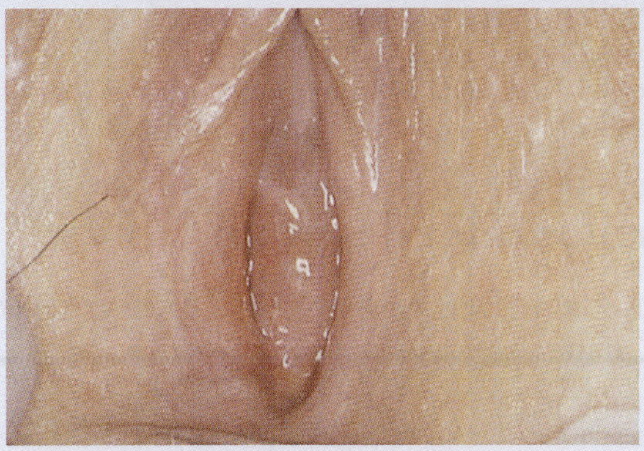

9-year-old girl with redundant labial tissue suggesting estrogen effect. Greater traction or a knee–chest position would reveal a normal orifice. If unable to locate an orifice, consider the possibility of an imperforate hymen.

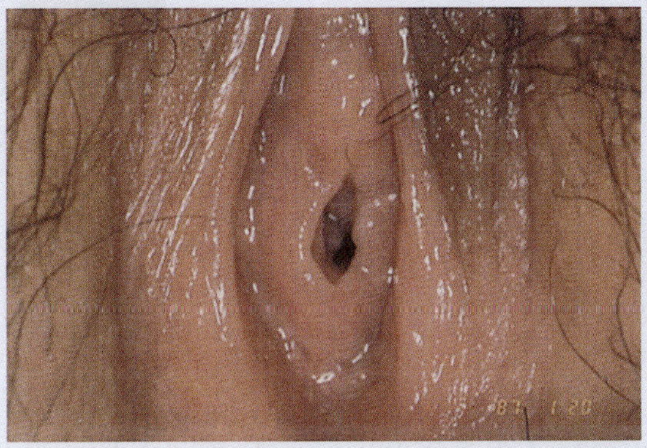

12-year-old girl with annular hymen and hormonal influence of puberty, causing thickened, pink tissue.

Source of photos: Reece R, Ludwig S, eds. *Child Abuse: Medical Diagnosis and Management*. 2nd ed. Lippincott Williams & Wilkins; 2001.

The physical examination may reveal signs that suggest *sexual abuse,* and the examination is particularly important if there are suspicious clues in the history.

As demonstrated in Table 23-12, physical signs strongly suggestive of *sexual abuse* include lacerations, ecchymoses and newly healed scars of the hymen, lack of hymenal tissue from 3 to 9 o'clock while the patient is in the supine position, and healed hymenal transections. Other signs such as purulent discharge and herpetic lesions are concerning as well.

Even with known abuse, the majority of examinations will be unremarkable; a normal genital examination does not rule out sexual abuse.

If the hymenal edges are smooth and without interruption in the inferior half, the hymen is probably normal (but does not rule out abuse since the hymen, like most other tissues, can heal over 7 to 10 days). Certain physical findings, however, suggest the possibility of sexual abuse and require more complete evaluation by an expert in the field.

Rectum and Anus

The rectal examination is not routine but should be done whenever intra-abdominal, pelvic, or perirectal disease is suspected. The examination of the young child can be performed with the child in either the side-lying or lithotomy position. For many young children, the lithotomy position is less threatening and easier to perform. Have the child lie on the back with the knees and hips flexed and the legs abducted. Drape the child from the waist down. Provide frequent reassurance during the examination and ask the child to breathe in and out through the mouth to relax. Spread the buttocks and observe the anus. You can use your lubricated gloved index finger, even in small children. Palpate the abdomen with your other hand, both to distract the child and to note the abdominal structures between your hands. The prostate gland is not palpable in young boys.

Anal skin tags are present in inflammatory bowel disease but are more often an incidental finding when located in the midline.

Tenderness noted on rectal examination of a child usually indicates an infectious or inflammatory cause, such as an *abscess or appendicitis.*

Reflex anal dilatation suggests the possibility of sexual abuse involving the rectum and requires more complete examination by an expert.

Musculoskeletal System

In older children, abnormalities of the upper extremities are rare in the absence of injury.

Toddlers may acquire *nursemaid's elbow* or subluxation of the radial head from a tugging injury. They will hold their arms slightly flexed at the elbows.

The normal young child has increased lumbar concavity and decreased thoracic convexity compared with the adult, and often has a protuberant abdomen.

Observe the child standing and walking barefoot. Ask the child to touch the toes, rise from sitting, run a short distance, and pick up objects. You will detect most abnormalities by watching carefully from both front and behind.

The cause of acute limp in childhood is usually trauma or injury, although many etiologies are possible including infection of the bone, joint, or muscle and also malignancy. In an obese child, consider *slipped capital femoral epiphysis.*

During early infancy, there is a common and normal progression from bowleggedness (Fig. 23-87) that begins to disappear at about 18 months of age, often followed by transition toward knock-knees.

The *knock-knee pattern* (Fig. 23-88) is usually maximal by age 3 years and gradually corrects by age 7 years.

The presence of tibial torsion can be assessed in several ways; one method is shown in Figure 23-89. Have the toddler lie prone on the examination table, with the knees flexed to 90 degrees. Note the thigh–foot axis. Usually there is 0 to 10 degrees of internal or external rotation noted by a foot pointing off in a direction. A negative thigh-foot angle indicates tibial torsion. Check the position of the malleoli—they should be symmetric.

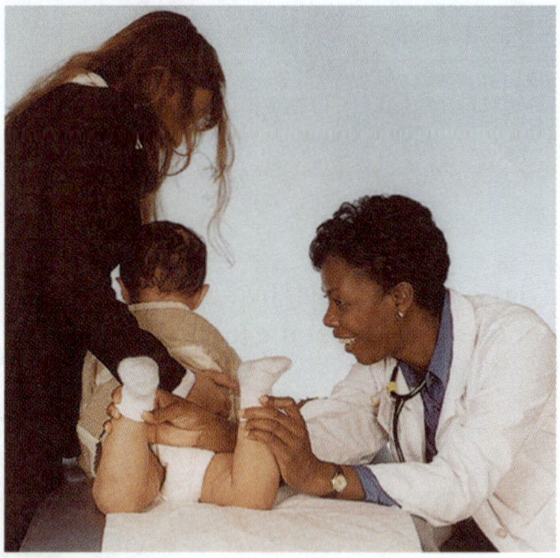

FIGURE 23-89. Checking for tibial torsion.

The most common lower extremity pathology in childhood is injury from accidents. Fractures are somewhat common in young children due to incompletely developed bones and growth plates and frequent injuries during play. Joint injuries, sprains, and strains are common in young children.

A chronic limp in childhood could be caused by *Blount disease, hip disorders* such as avascular necrosis of the hip, leg-length discrepancy, spinal disorder, or rarely a malignancy.

Medial femoral torsion (or femoral anteversion) is an inward twisting of the femur resulting in toeing in by the child after age 3 to 4 years; this tends to resolve by 8 to 10 years of age although many adults have some toeing in as well.

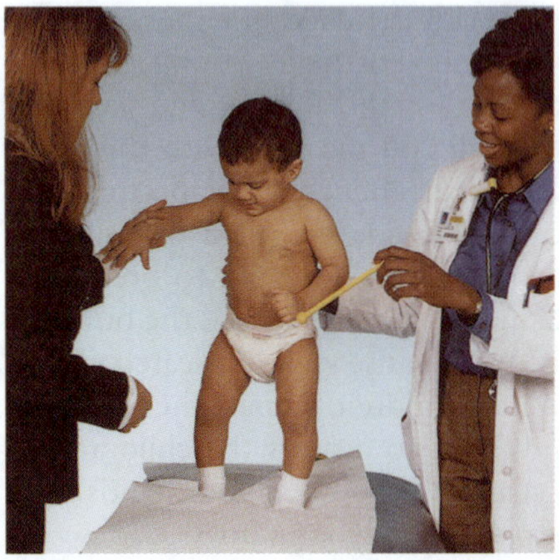

FIGURE 23-87. Bowleggedness is normal in early childhood.

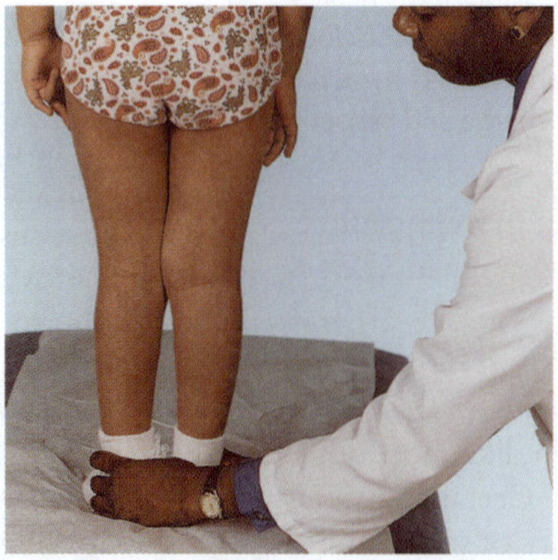

FIGURE 23-88. Knock-knee is not unusual in childhood.

Severe bowing of the legs (*genu varum*) may still be physiologic bowing that will spontaneously resolve. Extreme bowing or unilateral bowing may be from pathologic causes such as *rickets* or tibia vara (*Blount disease*).

Inspect any child who can stand for *scoliosis* using techniques described on page 1055.

Determine any *leg shortening* that may accompany hip disease by comparing the distance from the anterior superior spine of the ilium to the medial malleolus on each side. Make sure the hips are level. Straighten the child by pulling gently on the legs, and then compare the levels of the medial malleoli with each other. Put a small ink dot over the prominent malleoli and touch them together for a direct measure.

Have the child stand straight and place your hands horizontally over the iliac crests from behind. Small discrepancies can be noted. If such a discrepancy is noted and you suspect leg-length discrepancy, with one iliac crest higher than the other, place a book under the shorter leg—if this equalizes the iliac crests then a leg-length discrepancy is likely.

Test for severe hip disease with its associated weakness of the gluteus medius muscle. Observe from behind as the child shifts weight from one leg to the other (Figs. 23-90 and 23-91). A pelvis that remains level when weight is shifted from one foot to the other is a *negative Trendelenburg sign*. With an abnormal positive sign in severe hip disease, the *pelvis tilts toward the unaffected hip* (the hip muscle does not hold the hip level resulting in a drop in the nonweight-bearing leg) during weightbearing on the affected side (*positive Trendelenburg sign*).

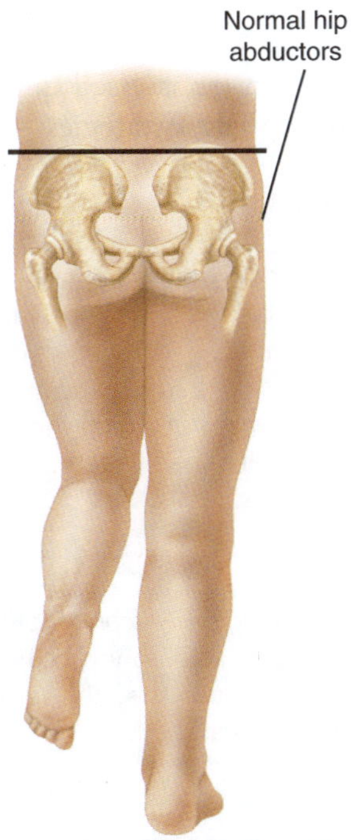

FIGURE 23-90. Negative Trendelenburg sign.

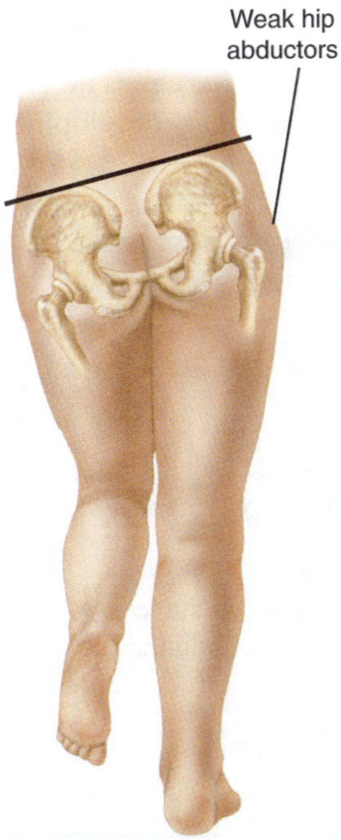

FIGURE 23-91. Positive Trendelenburg sign.

Nervous System

Beyond infancy, the neurologic examination includes the components evaluated in adults. Combine the neurologic and developmental assessment; turn this into a game with the child to assess optimal development and neurologic performance.

Children with *spastic diplegias* will often have hypotonia as infants and then excessive tone with spasticity, scissoring, and perhaps clenched fists as toddlers and young children.

Use a validated developmental screen for preschool children. Children usually enjoy this component, and you can too. Many neurologic conditions in children are accompanied by developmental abnormalities. You can ask children older than 3 years to draw a picture or copy objects and then discuss their pictures to test simultaneously for fine motor coordination, cognition, and language.

Problems with social interaction, verbal and nonverbal communication, restricted interests, and repetitive behaviors could be signs of *autism*.

Distinguish between isolated delays in one aspect of development (e.g., coordination or language) and more generalized delays several components. The latter is more likely to reflect global neurologic disorders such as *cognitive disability* that can have many etiologies.

Sensation. The sensory examination can be performed by using a cotton ball or tickling the child. This is best performed with the child's eyes closed. Do not use pin pricks.

Gait, Strength, and Coordination. Observe the child's gait while the child is walking and, optimally, running. Note any asymmetries, weakness, undue tripping, or clumsiness.

Follow developmental milestones to test for appropriate maneuvers such as heel-to-toe walking (Fig. 23-92), hopping, and jumping. Use a toy to test for coordination and strength of the upper extremities.

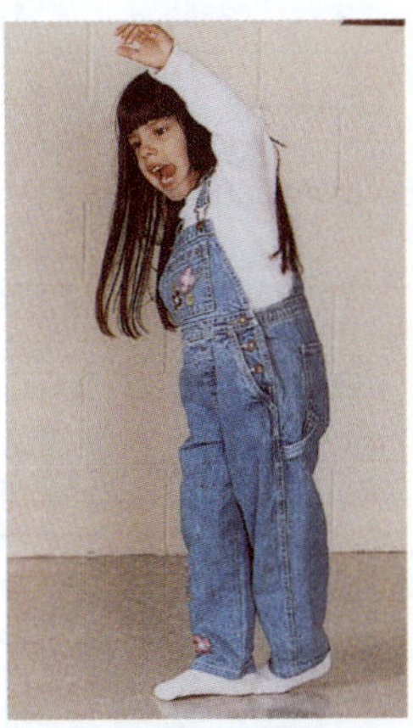

FIGURE 23-92. Heel-to-toe walking is a coordination milestone.

In children with uncoordinated gait, be sure to distinguish orthopedic causes such as positional deformities of the hip, knee, or foot from neurologic abnormalities such as *cerebral palsy, ataxia, or neuromuscular conditions.*

If you are concerned about the child's strength, have the child lie on the floor and then stand up, and closely observe the stages. Most normal children will first sit up, then flex the knees, and extend the arms to the side to push off from the floor and stand up.

In certain forms of *muscular dystrophy* with weakness of the pelvic girdle muscles, children will rise to standing by rolling over prone and pushing off the floor with the arms while the legs remain extended (*Gower sign*).

Hand preference is often demonstrated by age 2 years, although many preschool children use one hand or another preferentially for different tasks. If a younger child has clear hand preference, check for weakness in the nonpreferred upper extremity.

Deep Tendon Reflexes. Deep tendon reflexes can be tested as in adults. First, demonstrate the use of the reflex hammer on the child's hand, assuring the child that it will not hurt. Children love to feel their legs bounce when you test their patellar reflexes. Have the child keep the eyes closed during some of this examination because tensing will disrupt the results.

Children with *mild cerebral palsy* may have both slightly increased tone and hyperreflexia.

Cerebellar Function. The cerebellar examination can be tested using finger-to-nose and rapid alternating movements of the hands or fingers (Figs. 23-93 and 23-94). Children older than 5 years should be able to tell right from left so you can assign them right–left discrimination tasks as is done in the adult patient.

Some children with *attention deficit disorder with hyperactivity (ADHD)* will have difficulty cooperating with your neurologic and developmental examination because of problems focusing. These children often have high-energy levels, fidgetiness, and a history of difficulty in school or structured situations. Other conditions such as anxiety may have similar manifestations, so a complete history and physical examination is warranted.

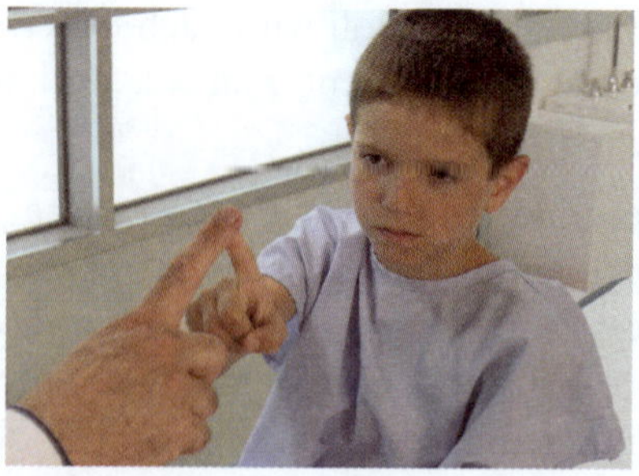

FIGURE 23-93. Finger-to-nose test—first have child touch your finger.

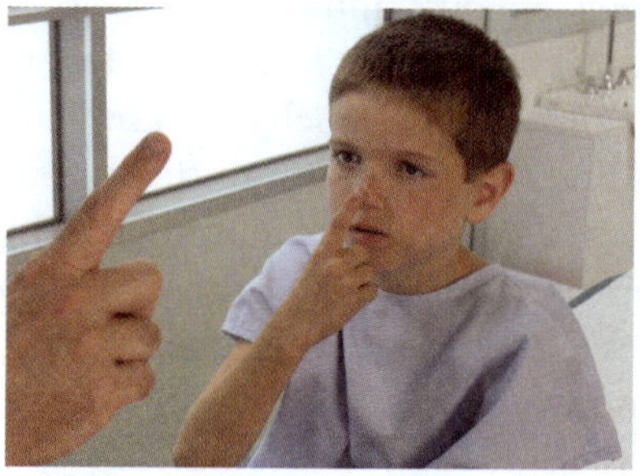

FIGURE 23-94. Then have the child touch her or his nose.

Cranial Nerves. The cranial nerves can be assessed quite well using developmentally appropriate strategies, as shown in Box 23-46.

Box 23-46. Strategies to Assess Cranial Nerves in Young Children

Cranial Nerve		Strategy
I	Olfactory	Testable in older children.
II	Visual acuity	Use Snellen chart after age 3 years. Test visual fields as for an adult. A parent may need to hold the child's head.
III, IV, VI	Extraocular movements	Have the child track a light or an object (a toy is preferable). A parent may need to hold the child's head.
V	Motor	Play a game with a soft cotton ball to test sensation. Have the child clench the teeth and chew or swallow some food.

(continued)

Localizing neurologic signs are rare in children but can be caused by *trauma, brain tumor, intracranial bleed,* or *infection.* Children with *increased intracranial pressure* can develop cranial nerve abnormalities as well as papilledema and altered mental status.

Children with *meningitis, encephalitis, or cerebral abscess* can have abnormalities of cranial nerves, although they also have altered consciousness and other signs.

Box 23-46. Strategies to Assess Cranial Nerves in Young Children (*continued*)

Cranial Nerve		Strategy
VII	Facial	Have the child "make faces" or imitate you as you make faces (including moving your eyebrows) and observe symmetry and facial movements.
VIII	Acoustic	Perform auditory testing after age 4 years. Whisper a word or command behind the child's back and have the child repeat it.
IX, X	Swallow and gag	Have the child stick the "whole tongue out" or "*say 'ah.'*" Observe movement of the uvula and soft palate. Test the gag reflex.
XI	Spinal accessory	Have the child push your hand away with his head. Have the child shrug his shoulders while you push down with your hands to *"see how strong you are."*
XII	Hypoglossal	Ask the child to *"stick out your tongue all the way."*

Although *facial nerve palsy* can be congenital, it is often caused by infection or trauma.

RECORDING YOUR FINDINGS

The format of the clinical record is the same for both children and adults. Although the sequence of the physical examination may vary, convert your clinical findings into the same order of the traditional written or electronic format.

Initially, you may use sentences to describe your findings; later you will use phrases. The style here contains phrases appropriate for most write-ups. As you read through this write-up, you will note some atypical findings. Try to test yourself. See if you can interpret these findings. You will also note the modifications necessary to accommodate reports from the small child's parent, rather than from the child.

Recording the Pediatric Examination

4/19/2020

Riyan is an active, 26-month-old boy accompanied by his father, Rajesh Das, who is concerned about his development and behavior.

Source and Reliability: Father.

Chief Complaint: Slow development and difficult behavior.

History of Present Illness: Riyan appears to be developing more slowly than his older sister did. He uses only single words and simple phrases, rarely combines words, and appears frustrated with not being able to communicate. People understand less than one-quarter of his speech. Physical development seems normal to the mother: he can throw a ball, kick, scribble, and dress himself well. He has had no head trauma, chronic illnesses, seizures, or regression in his milestones.

Riyan's dad is also concerned about his behavior. Riyan is extremely stubborn, frequently has tantrums, gets angry easily (especially with his older sister), throws objects, bites, and physically strikes others when he doesn't get his way. His behavior seems worse around his father who reports that he is "fine" at his childcare center. He moves from one activity to another with an inability to sit still to read or play a game. Of note, he is sometimes affectionate and cuddly. He does make eye contact and plays normally with toys. He has no unusual movements.

Riyan is an extremely picky eater who eats a large quantity of junk food and little else. He will not eat fruits or vegetables and drinks enormous quantities of juice and soda. His father has tried everything to get him to eat healthy food, to no avail.

The family has been under substantial stress during the past year because Riyan's father has been unemployed.

Riyan sleeps through the night.

Medications. One multivitamin daily.

Past History

Pregnancy. Uneventful. Dad reduced tobacco intake to a half-pack a day and drank alcohol at times. He denies use of other drugs or any infections.

(*continued*)

Recording the Pediatric Examination (*continued*)

Newborn Period. Born vaginally at 40 weeks; left the hospital in 2 days. Birth weight 2.5 kg. Dad does not know why Riyan was small at birth.

Illnesses. Only minor illnesses; no hospitalizations.

Accidents. Required sutures last year for a facial laceration secondary to a fall on the road. He did not lose consciousness and had no sequelae.

Preventive Care. Riyan has had regular preventive check-ups. At the last appointment 6 months ago, his regular physician said that Riyan was a bit behind on some developmental milestones and suggested a childcare center that she knew was excellent, as well as increased parental attention to reading, speaking, playing, and stimulation. Immunizations are up to date.

Family History

Strong family history of diabetes (two grandparents, none with diabetes as children) and hypertension. No family history of childhood developmental, psychiatric, or chronic illnesses.

Developmental History: Sat up at 6 months, crawled at 9 months, and walked at 13 months. First words ("mama" and "car") said at approximately 1 year.

Personal and Social History: Parents are married and live with the two children in a rented apartment. Dad has not had a steady job for 1 year but has worked intermittently in a gym. Mom works as a waitress part-time while Riyan is in childcare.

Mom had depression during Riyan's first year and attended some counseling sessions but stopped because she could not pay for them or medications. She gets support from her mother who lives 30 minutes away, and many friends, some of whom babysit occasionally.

Despite substantial family stress, Dad describes a loving and intact family. They try to eat dinner together daily, limit television, read to both children (although Riyan won't sit still), and go to the nearby park regularly to play.

Environmental Exposures. Father smokes, although generally outside the house.

Safety. Dad reports this as a major concern: he can barely leave Riyan out of his sight without him getting into something. He fears he will run under a car. Riyan sits in his car seat most of the time.

Review of Systems

General. No major illnesses.

Skin. Dry and itchy. Last year he was prescribed hydrocortisone for it.

Head, Eyes, Ears, Nose, and Throat (HEENT). Head: No trauma. *Eyes:* Vision fine. *Ears:* Multiple infections in the past year. Frequently ignores parents' requests; they can't tell if this is purposeful or if he can't hear well. *Nose:* Often runny; Dad wonders about allergies. *Mouth:* No dentist visit yet. Brushes teeth sometimes (a frequent source of dispute).

Neck. No lumps. Glands in neck seem large.

Respiratory. Frequent cough and whistle in chest. Dad cannot identify trigger; it tends to go away. He can run around all day without seeming to get tired.

Cardiovascular. No known heart disease. He had a murmur when younger, but it went away.

Gastrointestinal. Appetite and eating habits described above. Regular bowel movements. He is in the process of toilet training and wears pull-ups at night, but not at childcare.

Urinary. Good stream. No prior urinary tract infections.

Genital. Normal.

Musculoskeletal. He is "all boy" and never gets tired. Minor bumps and bruises occasionally.

Neurologic. Walks and runs well; seems coordinated for age. No stiffness, seizures, or fainting. Dad says his memory seems great, but his attention span is poor.

Psychiatric. Generally, seems happy. Cries easily; bounces back and forth from trying to be independent to needing cuddling and comforting.

Physical Examination

General Appearance: Riyan is an active and energetic toddler. He plays with the reflex hammer, pretending it is a truck. He appears closely bonded with his father, looking at him occasionally for comfort. He seems concerned that Riyan will break something. His clothes are clean.

Vital Signs. Ht 90 cm (90th percentile). Wt 16 kg (>95th percentile). BMI 19.8 (>95th percentile). Head circumference 50 cm (75th percentile). BP 108/58. Heart rate 90 beats per minute and regular. Respiratory rate 30/min; varies with activity. Temperature (ear) 37.5°C. Obviously no pain.

Skin. Normal except for bruises on the anterior aspects of his legs, and patchy, dry skin over external surface of elbows.

HEENT. Head: Normocephalic; no lesions. *Eyes:* Difficult to examine because he won't sit still. Symmetric with normal extraocular movements. Pupils 4 to 5 mm, and symmetrically reactive to light. Discs difficult to visualize; no hemorrhages noted. *Ears:* Normal pinna; no external abnormalities. Normal external canals and tympanic membranes (TMs). *Nose:* Normal nares; septum midline. *Mouth:* Several darkened teeth (inside surface of upper incisors). One clear cavity on upper right incisor. Tongue normal. Cobblestoning of posterior pharynx; no exudates. Tonsils large but adequate gap (1.5 cm) between them. No allergic shiners.

Neck. Supple, midline trachea, no thyroid palpable.

Lymph Nodes. Easily palpable (1.5 to 2 cm), firm, mobile anterior cervical lymph nodes bilaterally. Small (0.5 cm) nodes in inguinal canal bilaterally. All lymph nodes mobile and nontender.

Lungs. Good expansion. No tachypnea or dyspnea. Congestion audible but seems to be upper airway (louder near mouth, symmetric). No rhonchi, rales, or wheezes. Clear to auscultation.

Cardiovascular. PMI in 4th or 5th interspace and midsternal line. Normal S_1 and S_2. No murmurs or abnormal heart sounds. Normal femoral pulses; dorsalis pedis pulses palpable bilaterally. Capillary refill brisk.

Breasts. Normal, with some fat under both.

(*continued*)

Recording the Pediatric Examination (*continued*)

Abdomen. Protuberant but soft; no masses or tenderness. Liver span 2 cm below right costal margin (RCM) and not tender. Spleen and kidneys not palpable. Bowel sounds present.

Genitalia. Tanner I circumcised penis; no pubic hair, lesions, or discharge. Testes descended, difficult to palpate because of active cremasteric reflex. Normal scrotum both sides.

Musculoskeletal. Normal range of motion of upper and lower extremities and all joints. Spine straight. Gait normal.

Neurologic. Mental Status: Happy, cooperative, active child. *Developmental:* Gross motor—Jumps and throws objects. Fine motor—Imitates vertical line. Language—Does not combine words; single words only, three to four noted during examination. Personal–social—Washes face, brushes teeth, and puts on shirt. Overall—Normal, except for language, which appears delayed. *Cranial Nerves:* Intact, although several difficult to elicit. *Cerebellar:* Normal gait; good balance. *Deep tendon reflexes (DTRs):* Normal and symmetric throughout with downgoing toes. *Sensory:* Deferred.

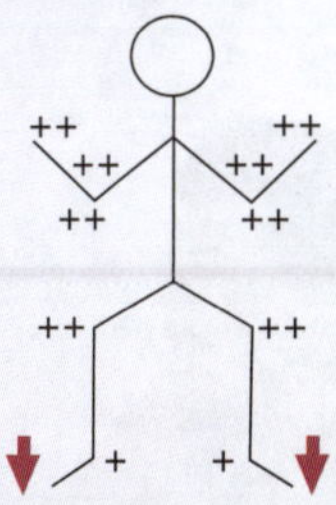

HEALTH PROMOTION AND COUNSELING: EVIDENCE AND RECOMMENDATIONS

Children 1 to 4 Years

During the health supervision visits clinicians should address concerns and questions from parents, evaluate the child's growth and development, perform a comprehensive physical examination, and provide anticipatory guidance about healthy habits and behaviors, social competence of caregivers, family relationships, and community interactions. This is a critical age for preventing childhood obesity as *many children begin their trajectory toward obesity after the age of 2 years.*

It is also important to assess the child's development. Standardized developmental screening instruments are recommended to measure the different dimensions of a child's development because clinicians often fail to identify problems in the general history and examination. Similarly, it is important to differentiate normal (but potentially challenging) childhood behavior from abnormal behavioral or mental health problems.

Box 23-47 demonstrates the major components of a health supervision visit for a 3-year-old, stressing health promotion. You do not have to wait for a health supervision visit to address many of these health promotion issues; they can be addressed during other types of visits, even when the child is mildly ill.

Box 23-47. Components of a Health Supervision Visit for a 3-Year-Old

Discussions with Parents
- Parental concerns
- Providing advice
- Childcare, school, social
- Major topic areas: development, nutrition, safety, oral health, family relationships, community

Developmental Assessment
- Assessment of milestones: gross and fine motor, personal–social, language, and cognitive; use a validated developmental screener.

Physical Examination
- Careful examination, including growth parameters with percentiles for age.

Screening Tests
- Vision (formal testing starting at age 3 years), hearing (formal testing starting at age 4 years), hematocrit and lead (if high risk), screen for social risk factors

Immunizations
- See updated AAP schedule

Anticipatory Guidance

Healthy Habits and Behaviors
- Injury and illness prevention

  Car seats, poisons, tobacco exposure, supervision
- Nutrition and exercise

  Obesity assessment; healthy meals and snacks
- Oral health

  Brushing teeth; dentist

Parent–Child Interaction
- Reading and fun times, child-directed play, limiting screen time

Family Relationships
- Activities, babysitters

Community Interaction
- Childcare, resources

Children 5 to 10 Years

As for earlier ages, these visits present opportunities to assess the child's physical, mental, and developmental health and the parent–child relationship and the child's relationships with peers and school performance (Fig. 23-95).

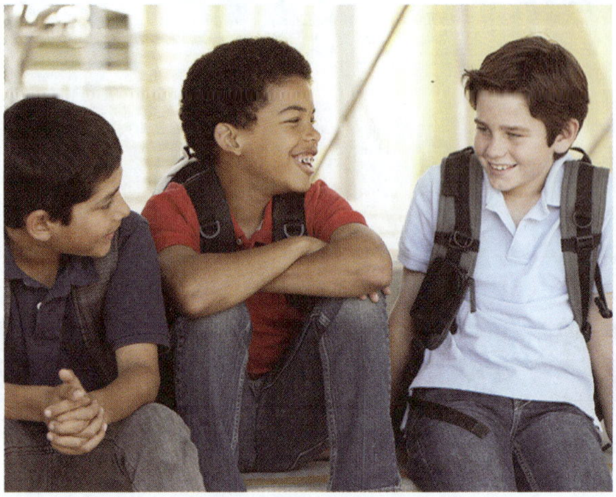

FIGURE 23-95. As children develop, mental health and peer relationships become increasingly important.

Once again, health promotion should be incorporated into all interactions with children and families. Older children enjoy talking directly with the examiner. In addition to discussing health, safety, development, and anticipatory guidance with parents, include the child in these conversations using age-appropriate language and concepts. Discuss the child's experience and perceptions of school, interactions with peers, and other cognitive and social activities.

Focus on healthy habits such as good nutrition, exercise, reading, stimulating activities, healthy sleep hygiene, screen time, and safety. About 20% of children have some type of chronic physical, developmental, or mental condition. These children should be seen more frequently for monitoring, disease management, and preventive care (Fig. 23-96). Some behaviors that become established at this age can lead to or exacerbate chronic conditions such as obesity or eating disorders. Health promotion is critical to optimize healthy habits and minimize unhealthy ones. Helping families and children with chronic diseases deal most effectively with these disorders is a key part of health promotion.

For all children, health promotion involves assessing and promoting the family's overall health.

The specific components of the health supervision visit for older children are the same as the components for younger children. Emphasize school performance and experiences as well as appropriate and safe sports and activities and healthy peer relationships.

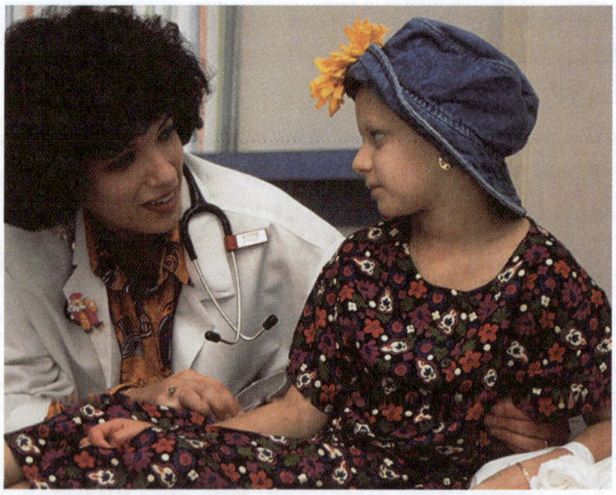

FIGURE 23-96. Connecting with children with chronic conditions can positively affect health outcomes.

ADOLESCENTS: HEALTH HISTORY

The key to successfully examining adolescents is a *comfortable, confidential environment.* This makes the examination more relaxed and informative.

Consider the teen's cognitive and social development when deciding issues of privacy, parental involvement, and confidentiality (Fig. 23-97).

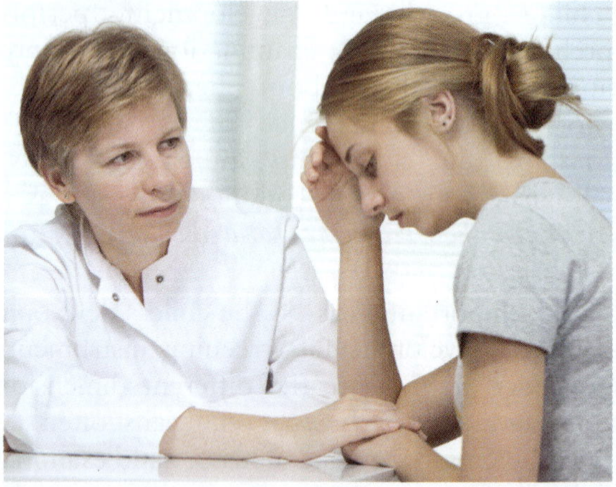

FIGURE 23-97. Trust-building is vital with the adolescent patient.

Adolescents usually respond positively to anyone demonstrating a genuine interest in them. Show such interest early and then sustain the connection for effective communication. Adolescents are more likely to open up when the interview focuses on them rather than on their problems.

In contrast to most other interviews, *start with specific questions* to build trust and rapport and get the conversation going. You may have to do more talking than usual at the beginning. Chat informally about friends, school, hobbies, and family. Using silence in an attempt to get adolescents to talk or asking about feelings directly is usually not a good idea.

It is particularly important to use summarization and transitional statements and to explain what you are going to do during the physical examination. The physical examination can also be an opportunity to engage young persons. *Once you have established rapport, return to more open-ended questions.* At that point, make sure to ask what concerns or questions the adolescent may have.

Because adolescents are often reluctant to ask their most important questions (which are sometimes about sensitive topics), ask if the adolescent has anything else to discuss. A useful phrase to use is *"tell me what other questions you have."* Another technique is to use the phrase: *"other kids your age often have questions about ..."*

Adolescents' behavior is related to their developmental stage and not necessarily to chronologic age or physical maturation. Their appearance may fool you into assuming that they are functioning on a more future-oriented and realistic level. This is particularly true regarding "early bloomers," who look older than their age. The reverse can also be true, especially in teens with delayed puberty or chronic illness.

Issues of *confidentiality* are important in adolescence. Explain to both parents and adolescents that the best health care allows adolescents some degree of independence and confidentiality. It helps if the clinician starts asking the parent to leave the room for part of the interview when the child is age 11 to 12 years. This prepares both parents and teens for future visits when the patient spends time alone with the clinician.

Before the parent leaves, obtain relevant clinical history from him or her, such as certain elements of past history, and clarify the parent's agenda for the visit. Adolescents need to know that you will hold in confidence what they discuss with you.

However, never make confidentiality unlimited. Always state explicitly that you may need to act on information that makes you concerned about safety: *"I will not tell your parents what we talk about unless you give me permission, or I am concerned about your safety. For example, if you were to talk to me about hurting yourself or someone else and I thought that you really were at risk to follow through, I would need to discuss it with others in order to help you."* Familiarize yourself with your relevant laws regarding confidentiality, reproductive care, and rights of adolescents.

An important goal is to help adolescents bring their concerns or questions to their parents. Encourage adolescents to discuss sensitive issues with their parents and offer to be present or help. Although young people may believe that their parents would *"reject them if they only knew,"* you may be able to promote more open dialogue. Occasionally, you will encounter a parent who is very rigid and punitive. It is important to carefully assess the parents' perspective prior to further discussion, and to obtain the explicit consent of the young person.

HEEADSSS Assessment

Obtaining an adequate psychosocial history from an adolescent offers you the ability to contextualize their lives. Since most adolescents have minimal clinical problems, most of their medical issues stem from risky behaviors. The HEADSS assessment is a good guide. Recently the HEADSS assessment was expanded to HEEADSSS (or HE^2ADS^3) to include questions about eating and safety. The acronym stands for **H**ome environment, **E**ducation and employment, **E**ating, peer-related **A**ctivities, **D**rugs, **S**exuality, **S**uicide/depression, and **S**afety from injury and violence. It is analogous to the "review of systems" and is a valuable tool for assessing the physical, emotional, and social well-being of adolescents (Box 23-48). The information you gather can then be used to provide appropriate support for your patient.

Box 23-48. HEEADSSS Assessment

Category	Sample Question Topics
Home environment	Who lives with you? How long have you lived there? Own room? What are relationships like at home? Recent moves or running away?
Education and employment	School/grade performance—any recent changes? Suspension, termination, dropping out? Favorite/least favorite class? Safety at school?
Eating	Likes and dislikes about one's body? Any recent changes in your weight or appetite? Any worries about weight? Worries about having food to eat?
Activities	With peers and family? Church, clubs, sports activities? Video games? History of arrests, acting out, crime?
Drugs and alcohol	Use of tobacco, vaping, alcohol, or drugs by peers, by teen, by family members?
Sexuality	Orientation? Dated anyone? Kissed anyone? Degree and types of sexual experience and acts? Number of partners? Sexually transmitted infections, contraception, pregnancy/abortion?

(continued)

Box 23-48. HEEADSSS Assessment (*continued*)

Category	Sample Question Topics
Suicide, depression, and self-harm	Have you thought about hurting yourself or someone else? Have you lost interest in things that you used to really enjoy?
Safety from injury and violence	History of accidents, physical or sexual abuse, or bullying? Concerns about online activities? Violence in home, school, or neighborhood? Access to firearms? Seatbelt use? Ridden with someone who was drunk or high? Any violence in school? Where you live? Ever been picked on or bullied? Ever felt the need to protect yourself?

Source: Republished with permission of SLACK Incorporated from Smith GL, McGuinness TM. *J Psychosoc Nurs Ment Health Serv.* 2017;55(5):24–27; permission conveyed through Copyright Clearance Center, Inc.

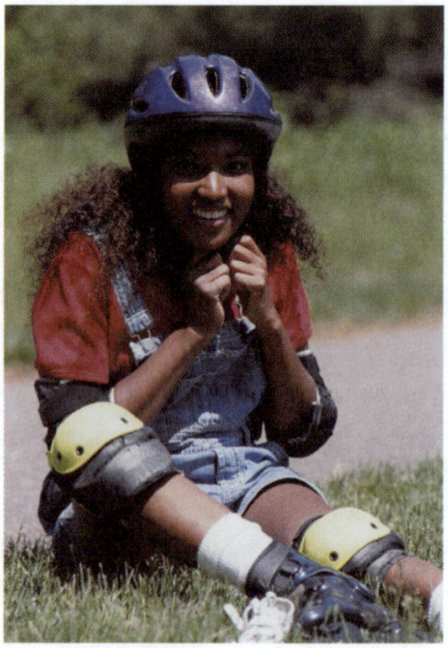

FIGURE 23-98. Rapid physical changes during adolescence provide wonderful opportunities for new activities.

SURVEILLANCE OF DEVELOPMENT: 11 TO 20 YEARS

Adolescence can be divided into three stages: early, middle, and late. Interview and examination techniques vary widely depending on the adolescent's physical, cognitive, and social–emotional levels of development.

Physical Development

Adolescence is the period of transition from childhood to adulthood. The physical transformation generally occurs over a period of years, beginning at an average age of 10 years in girls and 11 years in boys. On average, girls end pubertal development with a growth spurt by age 14 years and boys by age 16 years. The age of onset and duration of puberty vary widely, although the stages follow the same sequence in all adolescents. Early adolescents are preoccupied with these physical changes.

Cognitive Development

Although less obvious, cognitive changes during adolescence are as dramatic as changes in physique. Most adolescents progress from concrete to formal operational thinking, acquiring an ability to reason logically and abstractly and to consider future implications of current actions (Fig. 23-98).

Although the interview and examination resemble those of adults, keep in mind the wide variability in cognitive development of adolescents and their often erratic and still limited ability to see beyond simple solutions. Moral thinking becomes sophisticated with lots of time spent debating issues. Recent evidence shows that brain development (especially in the right prefrontal cortex) probably continues well into the twenties.

Social and Emotional Development

Adolescence is a tumultuous time, marked by the transition from family-dominated influences to increasing autonomy and peer influence (Fig. 23-99).

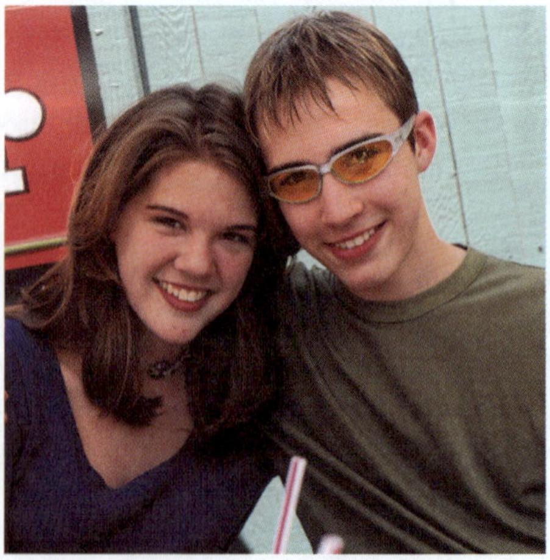

FIGURE 23-99. In adolescence, peers often become more influential than family.

The struggle for identity, independence, and eventually intimacy can lead to stress, health-related problems, and high-risk behavior. This struggle also provides an important opportunity for health promotion.

Box 23-49 demonstrates common developmental tasks or achievements of adolescence, typical characteristics you might note during the history, and helpful health care approaches. Note that there can be a wide variability of ages at which adolescents go through these stages.

Gender and Sexual Identity Formation Among Adolescents

Discussing sexuality and gender may be difficult for adolescents and young adults, and many struggle with their sexual attractions and identity formation. Clinicians must create a welcoming, supportive, confidential and nonjudgmental environment for adolescents to talk about their emerging sexual identity and concerns about their sexual activities or feelings.

Research shows lesbian, gay, bisexual, transgender, and queer (LGBTQ) youth value the opportunity to discuss their gender and sexuality with their clinician, but they often delay disclosing their sexuality until the clinician has built a trusting relationship with the patient. When initiating this conversation, it is important that the clinician emphasize and practice confidentiality to allow for a more open discussion. It is not the role of the clinician to inform parents or guardians about a teenager's sexual or gender identity, as doing so could expose the youth to harm.

It is important to understand that being LGBTQ is not abnormal and is not inherently a risk factor for high-risk behaviors or adverse health outcomes. Many LGBTQ youth experience discrimination and are negatively impacted by the presence of stigma from homophobia, transphobia, and heterosexism. This can damage the emerging self-image of an LGBTQ youth and result in psychological distress and an increase in high-risk behaviors. Ostracism, bullying, and parental rejection remain common and can lead to physical and

Box 23-49. Developmental Tasks of Adolescence

Task	Characteristic	Health Care Approaches
Early Adolescence (10- to 14-year-olds)		
Physical	Puberty (F: 10–14; M: 11–16)	Confidentiality; privacy
Cognitive	Concrete operational	Emphasis on short-term
Social identity	Am I normal? Peers increasingly important	Reassurance and positive attitude
Independence	Ambivalence (family, self, peers)	Support for growing autonomy
Middle Adolescence (15- to 16-year-olds)		
Physical	Females more comfortable, males often awkward	Support if patient varies from normal
Cognitive	Transition; many ideas, often highly emotional thinker	Problem solving; decision making, increased responsibility
Social identity	Who am I? Much introspection; global issues, sexuality	Nonjudgmental acceptance
Independence	Limit testing; experimental behaviors; dating	Consistency; limit setting
Late Adolescence (17- to 20-year-olds)		
Physical	Adult appearance	Minimal unless chronic illness
Cognitive	Formal operational (for many but not all)	Approach as an adult
Social identity	Role with respect to others; sexuality; future	Encouragement of identity to allow growth; safety and healthy decision-making
Independence	Separation from family; toward real independence	Support, anticipatory guidance

emotional abuse and the possibility of homelessness. This is often associated with health disparities and may result in poor health outcomes in the areas of mental health and suicide risk, substance abuse, and STIs. Clinicians should be aware of these disparities and appropriately screen for signs of bullying, depression and suicide risk, as well as help adolescents identify their protective factors and strengths and build upon their existing talents.

PHYSICAL EXAMINATION: GENERAL APPROACH

The sequence and content of the physical examination of the adolescent are similar to those in the adult. Keep in mind, however, issues unique to adolescents such as puberty, growth, development, family and peer relationships, sexuality, healthy decision making, and high-risk behaviors.

As in middle childhood, modesty is important. The patient should remain dressed until the examination begins (Fig. 23-100). Leave the room while the patient puts on a gown. Not all adolescents are willing to don a gown, so partially uncovering as the examination proceeds to preserve the patient's modesty is important. Most adolescents older than 13 years prefer to be examined without a parent in the room, but this depends on the patient's developmental level, familiarity with the examiner, relationship with the parent, and culture. Ask younger adolescents and their parent their preferences. In fact, it is safest to have a chaperone in the room regardless of patient gender when examining a patient's breasts or genitalia. It is best to discuss the issue of chaperones with patients/parents and record the shared decision in the clinical chart.

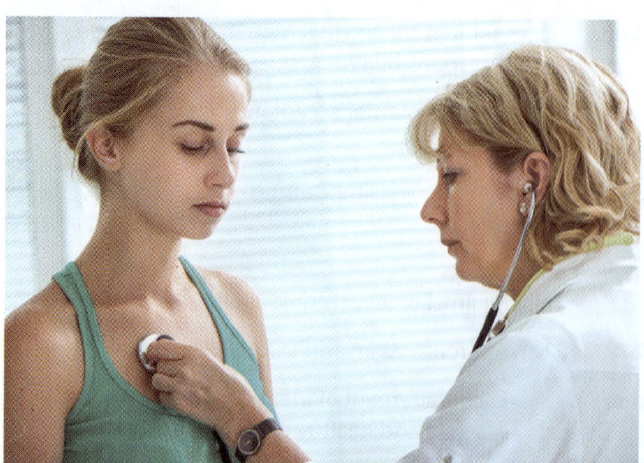

FIGURE 23-100. Some adolescents will request to remain in their clothes.

TECHNIQUES OF EXAMINATION

Somatic Growth: Height and Weight

Adolescents should wear gowns to be weighed or have them remove their shoes and heavy clothing. This is particularly important for adolescents being evaluated for underweight problems. Ideally, serial weights (and heights) should use the same scale.

Both obesity and eating disorders (*anorexia and bulimia*) are major public health problems requiring regular assessments of weight, monitoring for complications, and promoting healthy choices and self-concept.

Vital Signs

Ongoing evaluations of blood pressure are important for adolescents. The average heart rate from age 10 to 14 years is 85 beats per minute, with a range of 55 to 115 beats per minute considered normal. Average heart rate for those 15 years and older is 60 to 100 beats per minute. Percentiles for blood pressure are shown on p. 685.

Causes of sustained hypertension for this age group include *primary hypertension, renal parenchymal disease*, and *drug use.*

Skin

Examine the adolescent's skin carefully. Many adolescents will have concerns about various skin lesions, such as acne, dimples, blemishes, warts, and moles. Pay particular attention to the face and back in examining adolescents for acne. Stretch marks have become more common with the epidemic of obesity.

Adolescent acne, a common skin condition, tends to resolve eventually, but often benefits from proper treatment. It tends to begin during middle to late puberty.

Many adolescents spend considerable time in the sun and at tanning salons. You may detect this during a comprehensive health history or by noticing signs of tanning during the physical examination. This is a good opportunity to counsel adolescents about the dangers of excessive ultraviolet exposure, the need for sunscreen, and the risks of tanning salons.

See Table 23-3, "Warts, Lesions That Resemble Warts, and Other Raised Lesions". Moles or benign nevi may appear during adolescence.

Counsel older adolescents to begin performing a regular self-examination of the skin, as shown on p. 523.

Head, Eyes, Ears, Nose, Mouth, and Neck

The examination of these body parts is generally the same as for adults. The methods used to examine the eye, including testing for visual acuity, are the same as those for adults. Refractive errors become common, and it is important to test visual acuity monocularly at regular intervals, such as during the annual health supervision visit.

The ease and techniques of examining the ears and testing the hearing approach the methods used for adults. There are no ear, mouth, throat, or neck abnormalities or variations of normal unique to this age group.

An adolescent with persistent fever, sore throat, swollen tonsils, and cervical lymphadenopathy may have *streptococcal pharyngitis* or *infectious mononucleosis.*

Thorax and Lungs

The technique for examining the lungs of adolescents is the same as the technique for adults.

Breasts

Physical changes in a girl's breasts are one of the first signs of puberty. As in most developmental changes, there is a systematic progression. Generally, over a 4-year period, the breasts progress through five stages, called Tanner stages or *Tanner sex maturity rating* stages, as shown in Box 23-50. Breast buds in the preadolescent stage enlarge, changing the contour of the breasts and areola. The areola also darkens in color. These stages are accompanied by the development of pubic hair and other secondary sexual characteristics, as shown on p. 717. Menarche usually occurs when a girl is in breast stage 3 or 4. By then, she has passed her peak growth spurt (see Box 23-50).

Breast buds (pea-size firm masses inferior to the nipple) are common among both girls and boys entering puberty or during early puberty. They are benign.

For years, the normal range for onset of breast development and pubic hair was 8 to 13 years (average, 11 years), with earlier onset considered abnormal. Breast development varies by age, race, and ethnicity. Breasts develop at different rates in approximately 10% of girls, with resultant asymmetry of size or Tanner stage. Reassurance that this generally resolves is helpful to the patient.

Breast asymmetry is common in adolescents, particularly when adolescents are between Tanner stages 2 and 4. This is nearly always a benign condition.

Many adolescent boys develop *gynecomastia* (enlarged breasts) on one or both sides. Although usually slight, it can be embarrassing. It often resolves in a few years.

Box 23-50. Sexual Maturity Ratings in Girls: Breasts

Stage 1

Preadolescent: elevation of nipple only

Stage 2

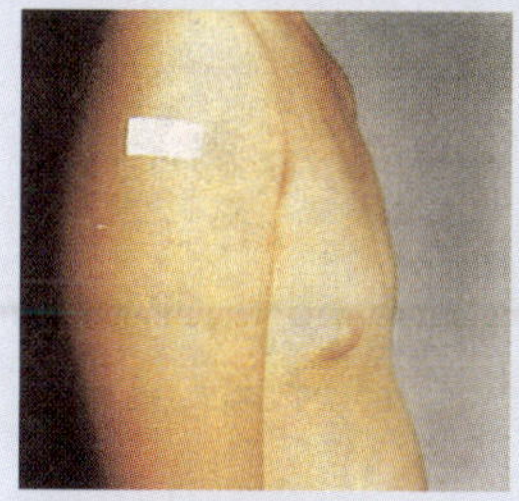

Breast bud stage: elevation of breast and nipple as a small mound; enlargement of areolar diameter

Stage 3

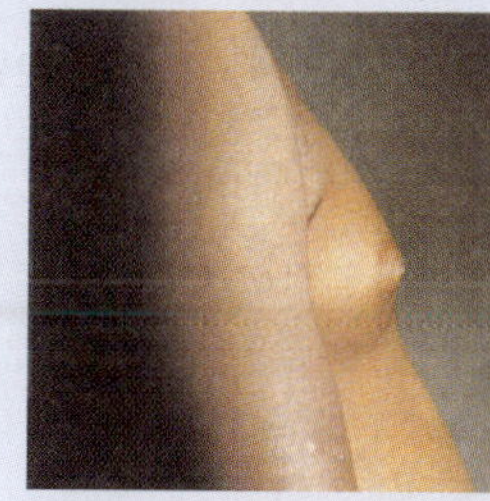

Further enlargement of elevation of breast and areola, with no separation of their contours

Stage 4

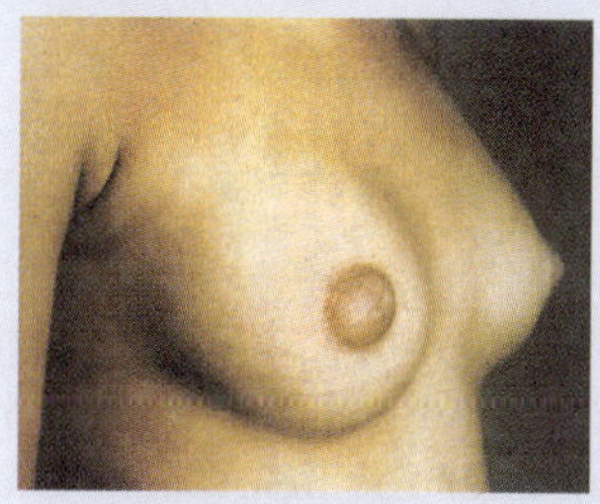

Projection of areola and nipple to form a secondary mound above the level of breast

Stage 5

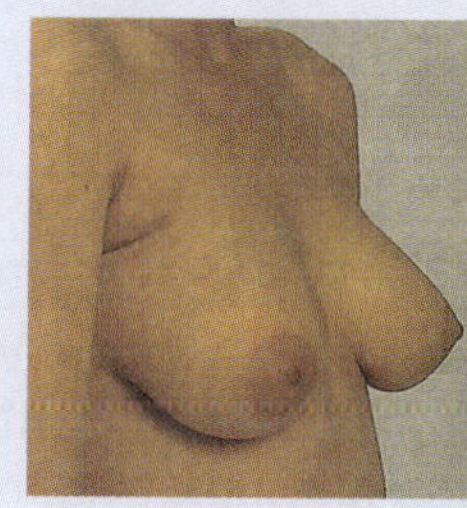

Mature stage: projection of nipple only; areola has receded to general contour of the breast (although in some normal individuals the areola continues to form a secondary mound)

Source: Photos republished with permission of American Academy of Pediatrics from Bourdony CJ et al. Assessment of Sexual Maturity Stages in Girls. Elk Grove Village: American Academy of Pediatrics, 1995; permission conveyed through Copyright Clearance Center, Inc.

Masses or nodules in the breasts of adolescent girls should be examined carefully. They are usually *benign fibroadenomas* or cysts; less likely, etiologies include abscesses or lipomas. Breast carcinoma is extremely rare in adolescence and nearly always occurs in families with a strong history of the disease.

Breasts in boys consist of a small nipple and areola. During puberty, about one-third of boys develop a breast bud 2 cm or more in diameter, usually in one breast. Boys who are obese may develop substantial breast tissue.

Heart

The technique and sequence of examination are the same as those for adults. Murmurs are a continued cardiovascular issue for evaluation.

Box 23-51. Location and Characteristics of Benign Heart Murmurs in Adolescents

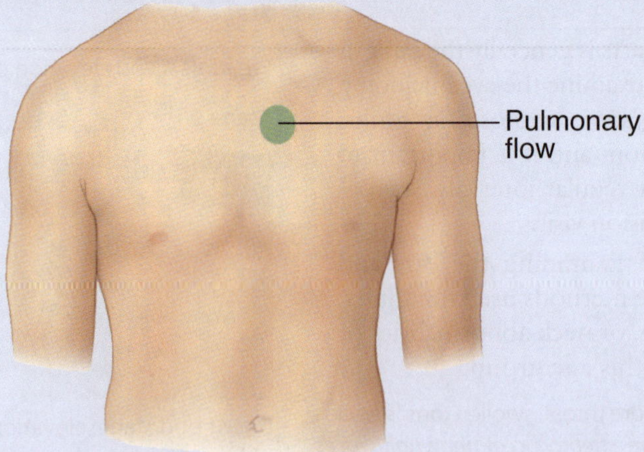

Typical Age	Name	Characteristics	Description and Location
Older child, adolescence and later	*Pulmonary flow murmur*	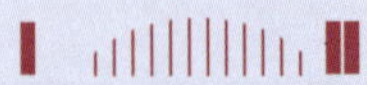 S_1 S_2	Grade I–II/VI soft, nonharsh Ejection in timing Upper left sternal border Normal P_2

The benign *pulmonary flow murmur* is a grade I–II/VI soft, non-harsh murmur with the timing characteristics of an ejection murmur, beginning after the first sound and ending before the second sound, but without the marked crescendo–decrescendo quality of an organic ejection murmur (Box 23-51). If you hear this murmur, evaluate whether the pulmonary closure sound is of normal intensity and whether splitting of the second heart sound is eliminated during expiration. An adolescent with a benign pulmonary ejection murmur will have normal intensity and normally split S_2.

A pulmonary flow murmur accompanied by a fixed split second heart sound suggests right-heart volume load such as an *atrial septal defect.*

The pulmonary flow murmur may also be heard in the presence of volume overload from any cause such as chronic anemia and following exercise. It may persist into adulthood.

Abdomen

Techniques of abdominal examination are the same as for adults. The size of the liver approaches the adult size as the teen progresses through puberty and is related to the adolescent's overall height. Although data are lacking about the usefulness of different techniques to assess liver size, it is likely that evidence from adult studies apply, particularly for older adolescents. Palpate the liver. If it is nonpalpable, hepatomegaly is highly unlikely. If you can palpate the lower edge, use light percussion to assess liver span.

Hepatomegaly in teens may be from infections such as *hepatitis* or *infectious mononucleosis, inflammatory bowel disease,* or *tumors.*

Splenomegaly in an adolescent who has had sore throat and fever may be a sign of *infectious mononucleosis.*

Male Genitalia

The genital examination of the adolescent boy proceeds like the examination of the adult male. Be aware of the embarrassment many boys experience during this aspect of the examination. Important anatomical changes in the male genitalia accompany puberty and help to define its progress. The first reliable sign of puberty (Fig. 23-101), starting between ages 9 and 13.5 years is an increase in the size of the testes. Next, pubic hair appears, along with progressive enlargement of the penis. The complete change from preadolescent to adult anatomy requires about 3 years, with a range of 1.8 to 5 years.

Delayed puberty is suspected in boys who have no signs of pubertal development by 14 years of age.

An axiom of development is that pubertal changes follow a well-established sequence. The age range for start and completion is wide, but the sequence for each boy is the same (see Fig. 23-101). This progression is helpful when counseling anxious adolescents about

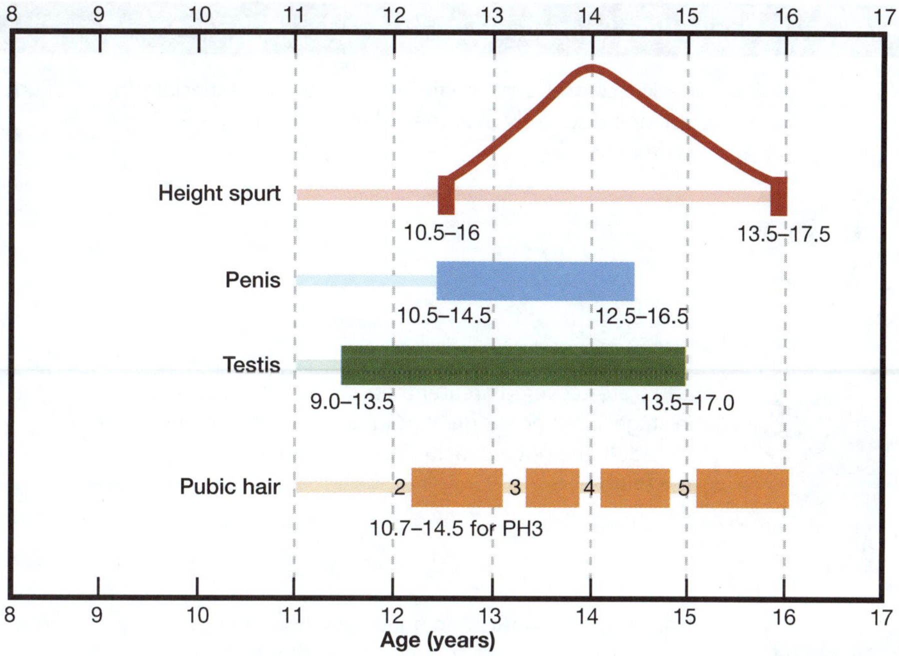

Numbers below the bars indicate the ranges in age within which the changes occur.

FIGURE 23-101. Pubertal changes in male adolescents.

current and future maturation and the wide range of normal for puberty.

When examining the adolescent male, assign a *sexual maturity rating*. The five stages of sexual development, first described by Tanner, are outlined and illustrated in Box 23-52. These involve changes in the penis, testes, and scrotum. In about 80% of men, pubic hair spreads farther up the abdomen in a triangular pattern pointing toward the umbilicus; this phase is not completed until the 20s.

The most common cause of delayed puberty in males is *constitutional delay,* frequently a familial condition involving delayed bone and physical maturation, but normal hormonal levels.

Box 23-52. Sexual Maturity Rating in Boys

In assigning sexual maturity rating in boys, observe each of the three characteristics separately because they may develop at different rates. Record two separate ratings: pubic hair and genital. If the penis and testes differ in their stages, average the two into a single figure for the genital rating. These photos demonstrate pubertal development in an uncircumcised male.

		Pubic Hair	Penis	Testes and Scrotum
Stage 1		Preadolescent—no pubic hair except for the fine body hair (vellus hair) similar to that on the abdomen	Preadolescent—same size and proportions as in childhood	Preadolescent—same size and proportions as in childhood
Stage 2	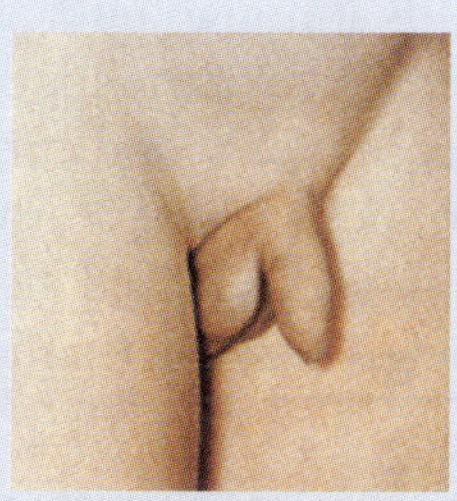	Sparse growth of long, slightly pigmented, downy hair, straight or only slightly curled, chiefly at the base of the penis	Slight or no enlargement	Testes larger; scrotum larger, somewhat reddened, and altered in texture

(*continued*)

Box 23-52. Sexual Maturity Rating in Boys (*continued*)

Stage 3	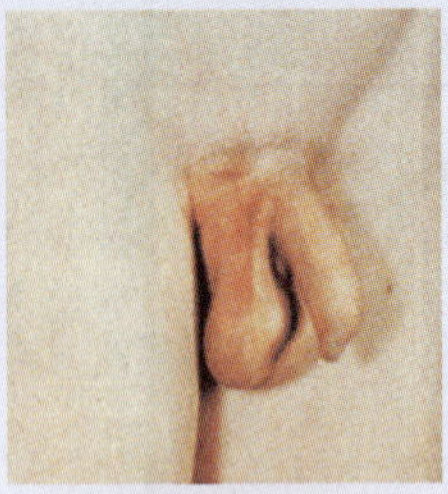	Darker, coarser, curlier hair spreading sparsely over the pubic symphysis	Larger, especially in length	Further enlarged
Stage 4	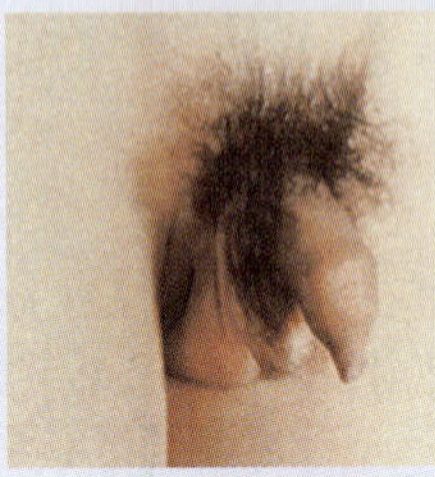	Coarse and curly hair, as in the adult; area covered greater than in stage 3, but not as great as in the adult and not yet including the thighs	Further enlarged in length and breadth, with development of the glans	Further enlarged; scrotal skin darkened
Stage 5	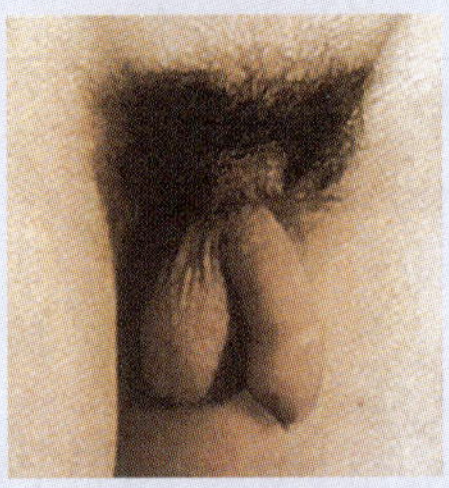	Hair adult in quantity and quality, spreads to the medial surfaces of the thighs but not up over the abdomen	Adult in size and shape	Adult in size and shape

Source: Photos reprinted from Wales JKH, Wit JM. *Pediatric Endocrinology and Growth.* 2nd ed. W.B. Saunders; 2003. Copyright © 2003 Elsevier. With permission.

Although nocturnal or daytime ejaculation tends to begin around Sexual Maturity Rating 3, a finding on either history or physical examination of penile discharge may indicate a *sexually transmitted infection.*

In addition to constitutional delay, less common causes of delayed puberty in boys include *primary* or *secondary* hypogonadism as well as congenital GnRH deficiency.

Observe the penis for sores and discharge as you would in an adult male.

In uncircumcised males, the foreskin should be easily retractable by adolescence. This is also an opportunity to discuss normal hygiene. Discuss testicular examination in older boys by age 18 years.

Female Genitalia

The external examination of adolescent female genitalia proceeds in the same manner as for school-aged children. If clinically necessary to perform a pelvic examination, the technique is the same as for an adult female. Of note, indications for performing pelvic examinations in adolescents have become much more stringent. When performing a pelvic examination, a full explanation of the steps of the examination, demonstration of the instruments, and a gentle, reassuring approach are necessary because the adolescent is usually quite anxious. A chaperone (parent or nurse) must be present.

Vaginal discharge in a young adolescent should be treated as in the adult. Causes include *physiologic leukorrhea*, sexually transmitted infections from consensual sexual activity or sexual abuse, bacterial vaginosis, foreign body, and external irritants.

An adolescent's first pelvic examination should be performed by an experienced health care provider. Routine pelvic examination is not recommended for adolescents.

A girl's initial signs of puberty are hymenal thickening and redundancy secondary to estrogen, widening of the hips, and beginning of a height spurt, although these changes are difficult to detect.

The first easily detectable sign of puberty is usually the appearance of breast buds although pubic hair sometimes appears earlier. The average age of the appearance of pubic hair has decreased in recent years, and current consensus is that the appearance of pubic hair as early as 7 years can be normal, particularly in dark-skinned girls who develop secondary sexual characteristics at an earlier age.

Pubertal development prior to the normal age range may signify *precocious puberty* which has a variety of endocrine and central nervous system causes. *Premature adrenarche* is usually

Box 23-53. Sexual Maturity Ratings in Girls: Pubic Hair

Stage 1

Preadolescent—no pubic hair except for the fine body hair (vellus hair) similar to that on the abdomen

Stage 2

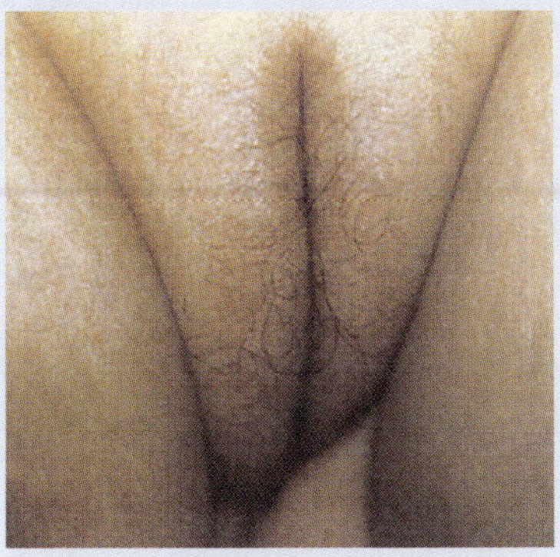

Sparse growth of long, slightly pigmented, downy hair, straight or only slightly curled, chiefly along the labia

Stage 3

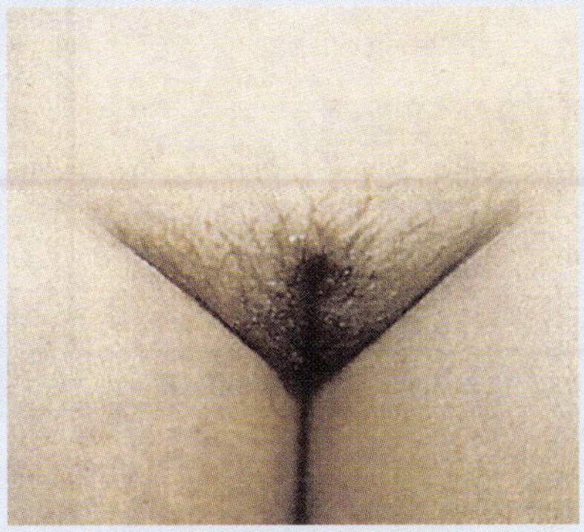

Darker, coarser, curlier hair, spreading sparsely over the pubic symphysis

Stage 4

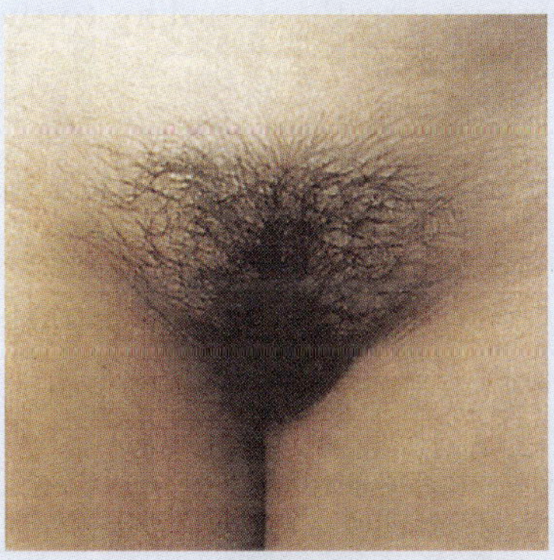

Coarse and curly hair as in adults; area covered greater than in stage 3 but not as great as in the adult and not yet including the thighs

Stage 5

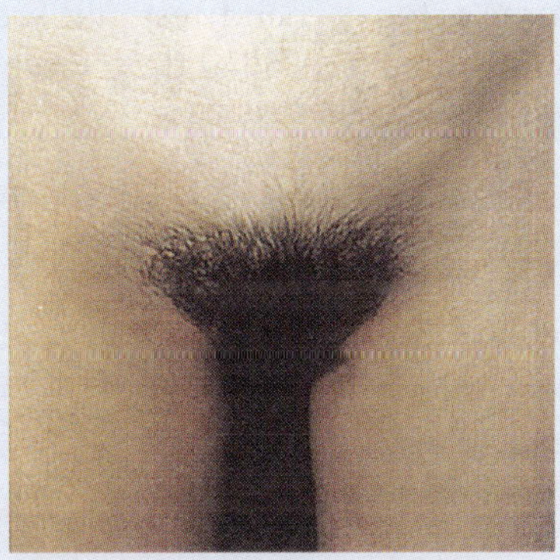

Hair adult in quantity and quality, spreads on the medial surfaces of the thighs but not up over the abdomen

Source: Photos republished with permission of American Academy of Pediatrics from Bourdony CJ et al. Assessment of Sexual Maturity Stages in Girls. Elk Grove Village: American Academy of Pediatrics, 1995; permission conveyed through Copyright Clearance Center, Inc.

Amenorrhea in adolescence can be primary (no menarche by age 16 years) or secondary (cessation of menses in an adolescent who had previously menstruated). While primary amenorrhea is usually due to anatomic or genetic causes, secondary amenorrhea can be due to a variety of etiologies such as *stress, excessive exercise, and eating disorders.*

benign, but may occasionally be associated with polycystic ovary syndrome, insulin resistance, and metabolic syndrome.

Assign a sexual maturity rating to every female, irrespective of chronologic age. The assessment of sexual maturity in girls is based on both growth of pubic hair and the development of breasts. The sexual maturity rating of pubic hair growth is shown in Box 23-53. Counsel girls about this sequence and their current stage.

Delayed puberty (no breasts or pubic hair development by age 12 years) is usually caused by inadequate gonadotropin secretion from the anterior pituitary due to defective hypothalamic GnRH production. A common cause is *anorexia nervosa.*

Although there is a wide variation in the age of onset and completion of puberty in girls, the stages occur in a predictable sequence, as shown in Figure 23-102.

Delayed puberty in an adolescent female below the third percentile in height may be from *Turner syndrome or chronic disease.* The two most common causes of delayed sexual development in an extremely thin adolescent girl are *anorexia nervosa* and *chronic disease.*

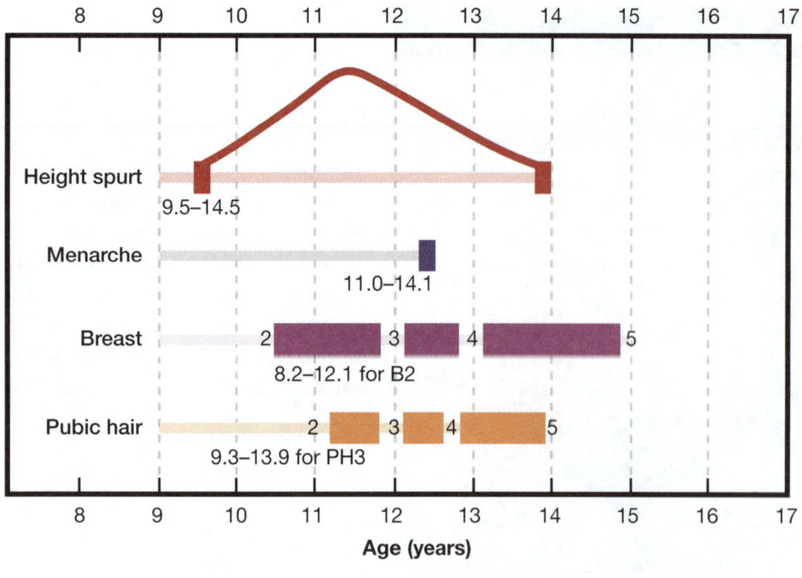

FIGURE 23-102. Pubertal changes in female adolescents.

Obesity in females can be associated with early onset of puberty.

Rectum and Anus

The examination of the rectum and anus is the same as for adults. Routine rectal examination is not recommended for adolescents unless there is a particular concern.

Musculoskeletal System

Evaluations for scoliosis and screening for participation in sports (pp. 718–721) remain common components of examination in adolescents. Other segments of the musculoskeletal examination are the same as for adults.

Assessing for Scoliosis. First, examine the patient standing assessing symmetry of shoulders, scapula, and hips. Then have the child bend forward with the knees straight and head hanging straight down between extended arms (*Adams forward bend test*). Next, evaluate any asymmetry in positioning.

Scoliosis in a young child is unusual and abnormal; mild scoliosis in an older child occurs in 2% to 4% of adolescents. Scoliosis appears as an asymmetrical rise in the thoracic region (as shown in Fig. 23-103) or lumbar region, or both.

If you detect scoliosis use a *scoliometer* to test for the degree of scoliosis. Ask the adolescent to bend forward again as previously described. Place the scoliometer over the spine at a point of maximum prominence making sure that the spine is parallel to the floor at that point, as shown in Figure 23-103. If needed, move the scoliometer up and down the spine to find the point of maximal prominence. An angle greater than 7 degrees on the scoliometer is a reason for concern and often used as a threshold for referral to a specialist. Of note, the sensitivity and specificity of both the Adams forward bend test and scoliometer vary greatly according to the skill and experience of the examiner.

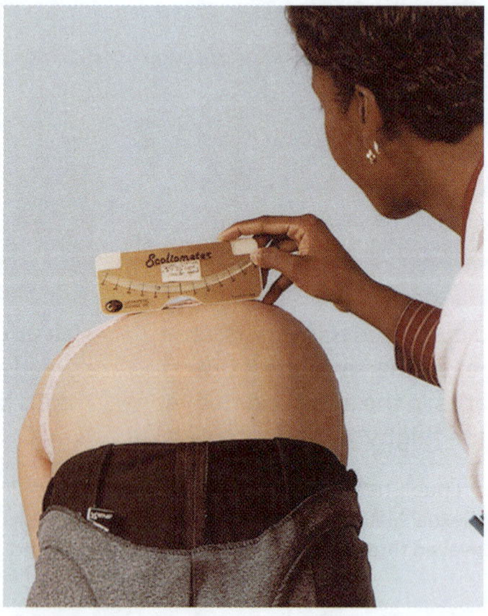

FIGURE 23-103. Measure and record scoliosis with a scoliometer.

Several types of *scoliosis* may present during childhood. *Idiopathic scoliosis* (75% of cases), seen mostly in girls, is usually detected in early adolescence. As seen in the adolescent girl in Figure 23-103, the right hemithorax is generally more prominent. Other causes include neuromuscular and congenital.

You can also use a *plumb line,* a string with a weight attached, to assess symmetry of the back (Fig. 23-104). Place the top of the plumb line at C7 and have the child stand straight. The plumb line should extend to the gluteal crease (not shown).

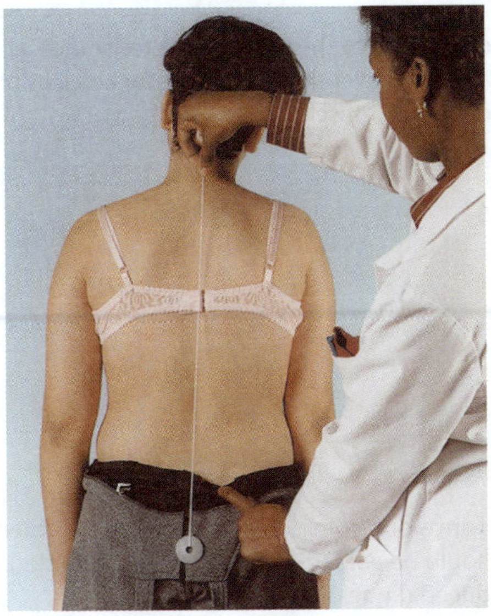

FIGURE 23-104. Measuring scoliosis with a plumb line.

Scoliosis is more common among children and adolescents with neurologic or musculoskeletal abnormalities.

Apparent scoliosis, including an abnormal plumb line test, can be caused by a *leg-length discrepancy*.

The remainder of the musculoskeletal examination is similar to that for adults, except for the sports preparticipation screening examination described below.

Sports Preparticipation Physical Evaluation. Start the evaluation with a thorough medical history focusing on cardiovascular risk factors, prior surgeries, prior injuries, other medical problems, and a family history.

In fact, a complete history is the most sensitive and specific part of the evaluation for detection of risk factors or abnormalities that would preclude participation in sports. The preparticipation physical evaluation is often one of the few times a healthy adolescent will see a clinical professional, so it is important to include some screening questions and anticipatory guidance. Finally, perform a general physical examination, with special attention to the heart and lungs and a vision and hearing screening. Include a focused, thorough musculoskeletal examination, looking for weakness, limited range of motion, and evidence of previous injury.

Important risk factors for sudden cardiovascular death during sports include episodes of dizziness or palpitations, prior syncope (particularly if associated with exercise), or family history of sudden death or cardiomyopathy in young or middle-aged relatives.

During the preparticipation sports physical examination, assess carefully for cardiac murmurs and wheezing in the lungs. Also, if the adolescent has had head injuries or a concussion, perform a careful, focused neurologic examination.

A 2-minute preparticipation screening musculoskeletal examination shown in Box 23-54 has been recommended by some experts.

Box 23-54. Screening Musculoskeletal Examination for Sports

Position and Instruction to Patient

Step 1: Stand straight, facing forward. Note for any asymmetry or swelling of joints.

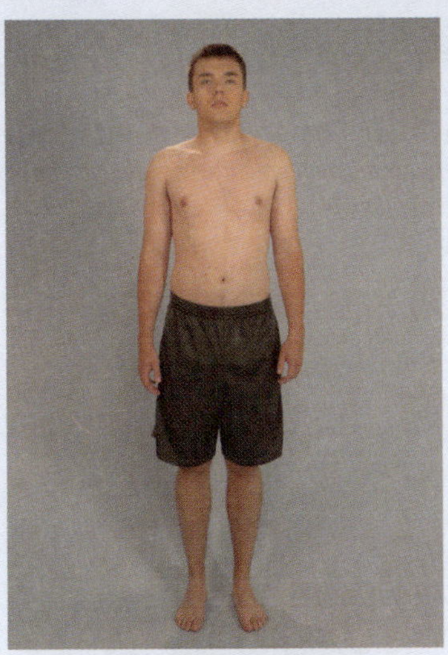

Step 2: Move neck in all directions. Note for any loss of range of motion.

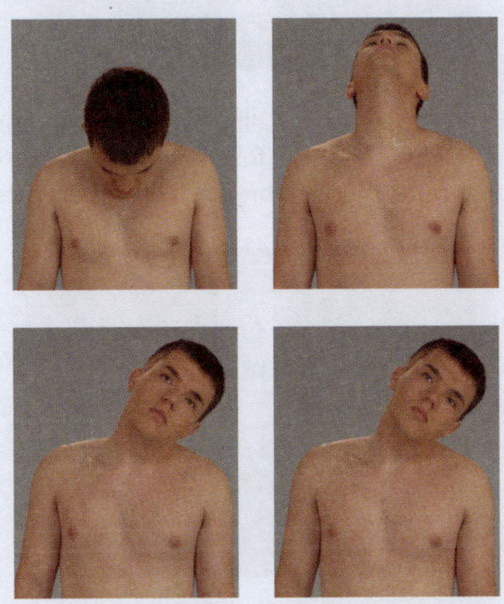

(*continued*)

Box 23-54. Screening Musculoskeletal Examination for Sports (*continued*)

Position and Instruction to Patient

Step 3: Shrug shoulders against resistance. Note for any weakness of shoulder, neck, or trapezius muscles.

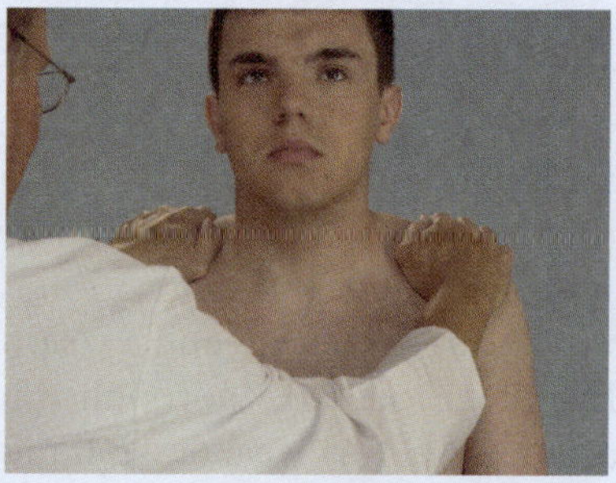

Step 4: Hold arms out to the side against resistance, and actively raise arms over the head. Note for any loss of strength of deltoid muscle.

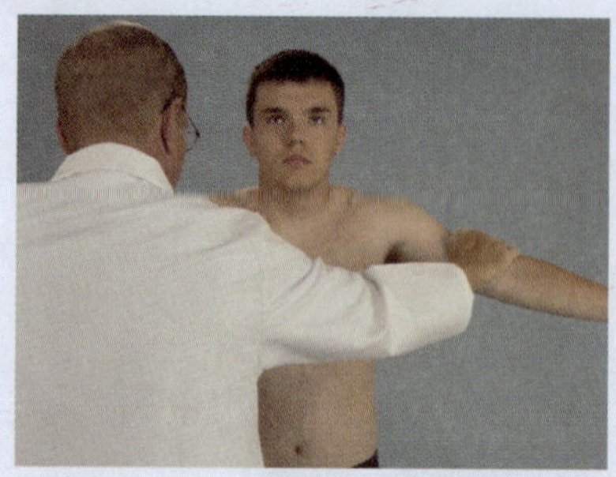

Step 5: Hold arms out to side with elbows bent 90 degrees; raise and lower arms. Note for any loss of external rotation and injury of glenohumeral joint.

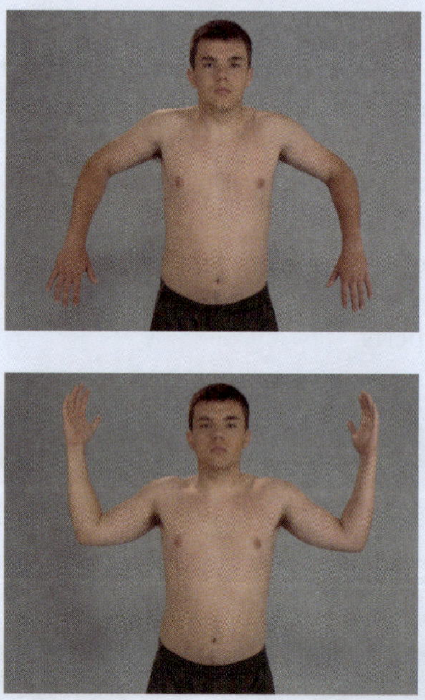

Step 6: Hold arms out, completely bend, and straighten elbows (should be able to easily touch the shoulder). Note for any reduced range of motion of elbow.

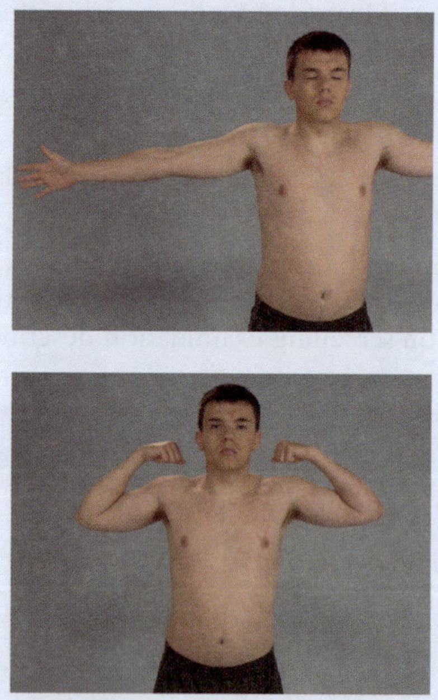

Step 7: Hold arms down, bend elbows 90 degrees, and pronate and supinate forearms. Note for any reduced range of motion from prior injury to forearm, elbow, or wrist.

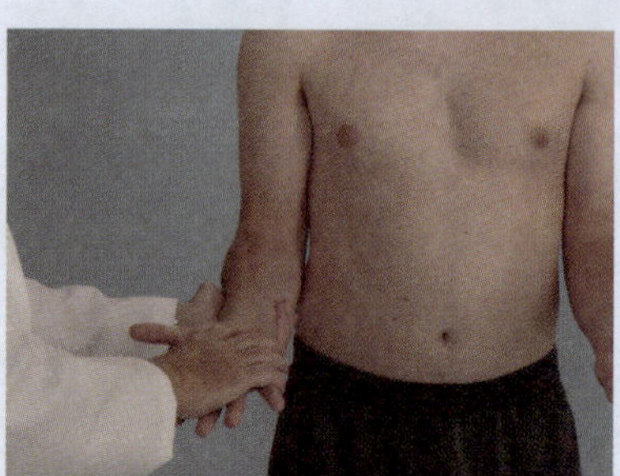

Step 8: Make a fist, clench, and then spread fingers. Note for protruding knuckle, reduced range of motion of fingers from prior sprain or fracture.

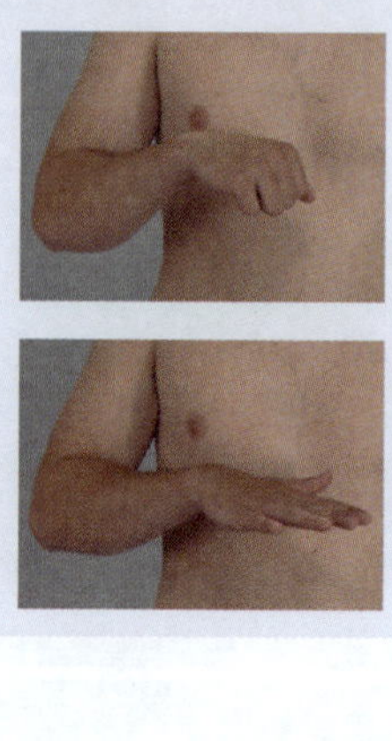

(*continued*)

Box 23-54. Screening Musculoskeletal Examination for Sports (*continued*)

Position and Instruction to Patient

Step 9: Squat and duck-walk for four steps forward. Note for inability to fully flex knees and difficulty standing up from prior knee or ankle injury.

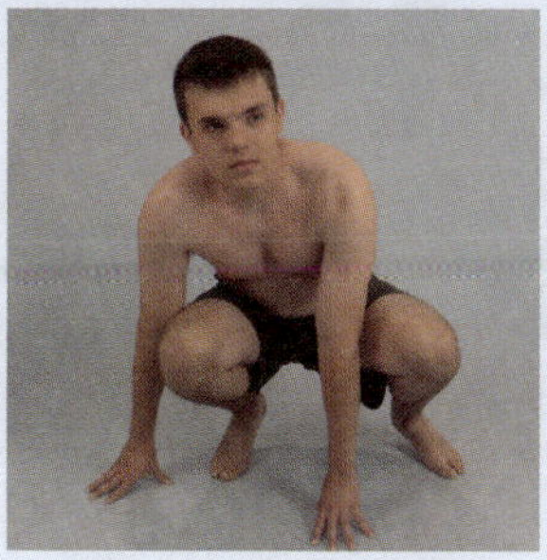

Step 10: Stand straight with arms at sides, facing back. Check whether shoulders, scapula, and hips are even. Note for asymmetry from scoliosis, leg-length discrepancy, or weakness from prior injury.

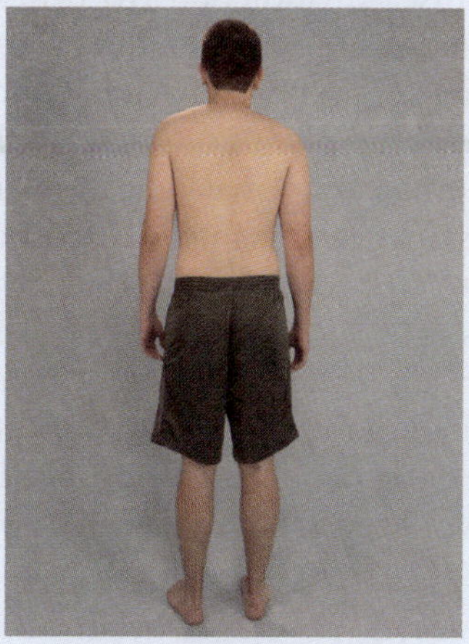

Step 11: Bend forward with knees straight and touch toes. Note any asymmetry from scoliosis and twisting of back from low back pain.

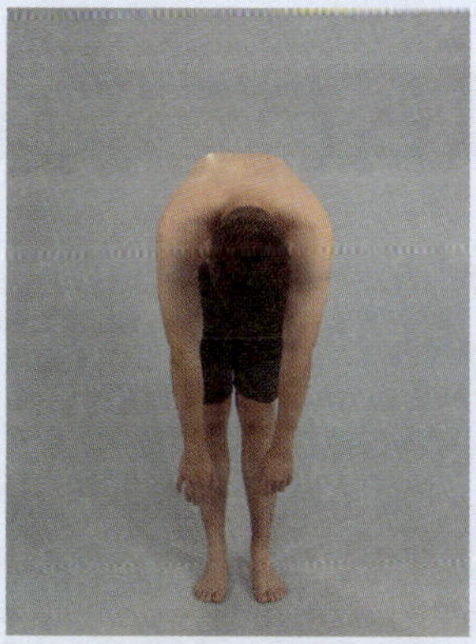

Step 12: Stand on heels and rise to the toes. Note any wasting of calf muscles from prior ankle or Achilles tendon injury.

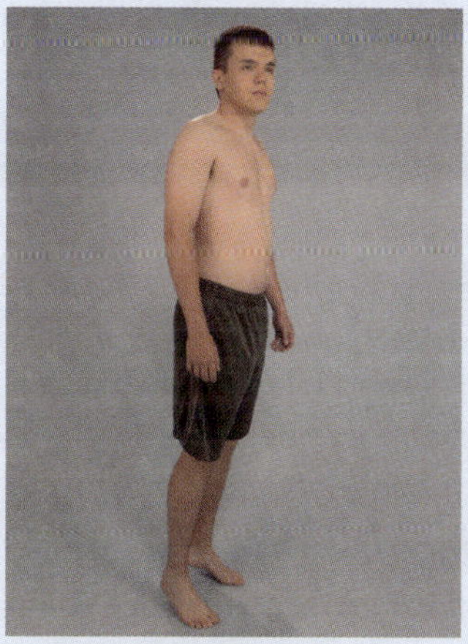

Nervous System

The neurologic examination of the adolescent and the adult is the same. Assess the adolescent's developmental achievement according to age-specific milestones.

RECORDING YOUR FINDINGS

The format of the clinical record is the same for both children and adults. Although the sequence of the physical examination may vary, convert your clinical findings into the same order of the traditional written or electronic format.

Initially, you may use sentences to describe your findings; later you will use phrases. The style here contains phrases appropriate for most write-ups. As you read through this write-up, you will note some atypical findings. Try to test yourself. See if you can interpret these findings. You will also note the modifications necessary to accommodate reports from the small child's parent, rather than from the child.

The write-up of the note for the history and physical examination of the adolescent mirrors that of the adult or younger child (p. 705). Remember to include the key elements of the HEEADSSS evaluation in the history section of the write-up.

HEALTH PROMOTION AND COUNSELING: EVIDENCE AND RECOMMENDATIONS

Most chronic diseases of adults have their antecedents in childhood or adolescence. For example, obesity, cardiovascular disease, addiction (to drugs, tobacco, or alcohol), and depression are all influenced by childhood and teen experiences and by behaviors established during adolescence. For example, most obese adults were obese as adolescents or had abnormal indicators such as elevated BMI scores. As a second example, almost all adults who are addicted to tobacco began their tobacco habits before 18 years. Therefore, a major component of health promotion for adolescents includes discussions about health behaviors or habits (Fig. 23-105). Effective health promotion can help patients develop healthy habits and lifestyles and avoid several chronic health problems.

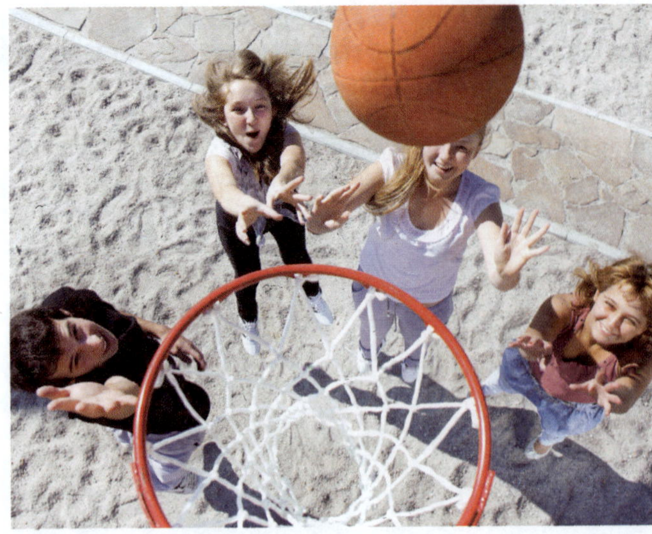

FIGURE 23-105. Inquire about and encourage adolescents to participate in healthy activities.

Because some health promotion topics involve confidential issues such as mental health, addiction, sexual behavior, and eating disorders, speak to adolescents (particularly older youth) privately during part of a visit that involves health supervision. Self-completed screening questionnaires can be completed before the visit to facilitate comprehensive assessment of youth risk behaviors. This approach saves time so that you can better address the specific risk behaviors the adolescent endorses during the visit. The AAP's Bright Futures has guidelines for preventive services for adolescents (Box 23-55).

Box 23-55. Components of a Health Supervision Visit for Adolescents Ages 11 to 18 Years

Discussions with Parents

- Address parent concerns
- Provide advice about supervision, encouraging progressively responsible decision making
- Ask about school, activities, social interactions
- Assess youth's behaviors and habits, mental health

Discussions with Adolescent

- *Social and Emotional:* mental health, friends, family, gender identity
- *Physical Development:* puberty, self-concept
- *Behaviors and Habits:* nutrition, exercise, TV or computer screen time, drugs, alcohol, tobacco, e-cigarettes, sleep
- *Relationships and Sexuality:* dating, sexual activity, sexual orientation, forced sex
- *Family Functioning:* relations with parents and siblings
- *School Performance:* activities, strengths, goals

Physical Examination

- Perform a careful examination; note growth parameters, sexual maturity ratings

Screening Tests

- Vision and hearing, blood pressure; consider hematocrit (in females); assess emotional health and risk factors (using a validated instrument)

Immunizations

- See schedule from the AAP

Anticipatory Guidance—Teen

- *Promote Healthy Habits and Behaviors:*
  - Injury and illness prevention
    - Seat belts, drunk driving, helmets, sun, weapons
  - Nutrition
    - Healthy meals/snacks, obesity prevention
  - Oral health: dentist, brushing
    - Physical activity and screen time
- *Sexuality:*
  - Confidentiality, sexual behaviors, safer sex, contraception if needed
- *High-Risk Behaviors:*
  - Prevention strategies
  - Parent–teen interaction, peer interactions
  - Communication, rules
- *Social Achievement:*
  - Activities, school, future
  - Community interaction
  - Resources, involvement

Anticipatory Guidance—Parent

- Positive interactions, support, safety, limit setting, family values, modeling behaviors, increased responsibility

TABLE 23-1. Abnormalities in Heart Rhythm and Blood Pressure

Supraventricular Tachycardia

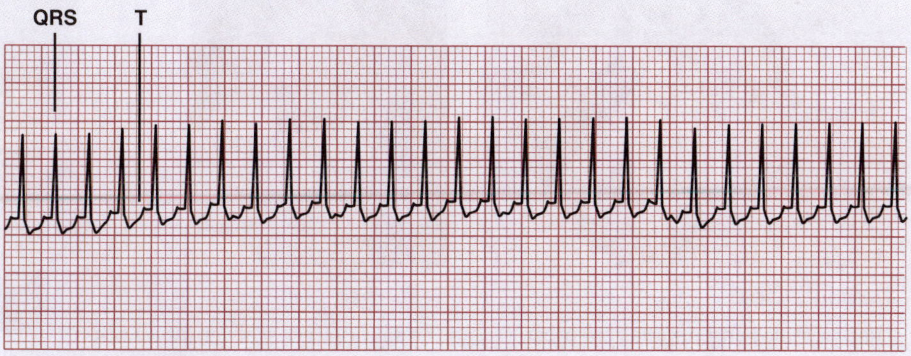

Paroxysmal supraventricular tachycardia (PSVT) is the most common dysrhythmia in children. Some infants with SVT look well or may be somewhat pale with tachypnea but have a heart rate of ≥220 beats per minute. Others are ill and in cardiovascular collapse. P waves have different morphology or are not seen.

SVT in infants is usually sustained and treated. In older children, it is more likely to be truly paroxysmal, with episodes of varying duration and frequency.

Hypertension in Childhood—A Typical Example

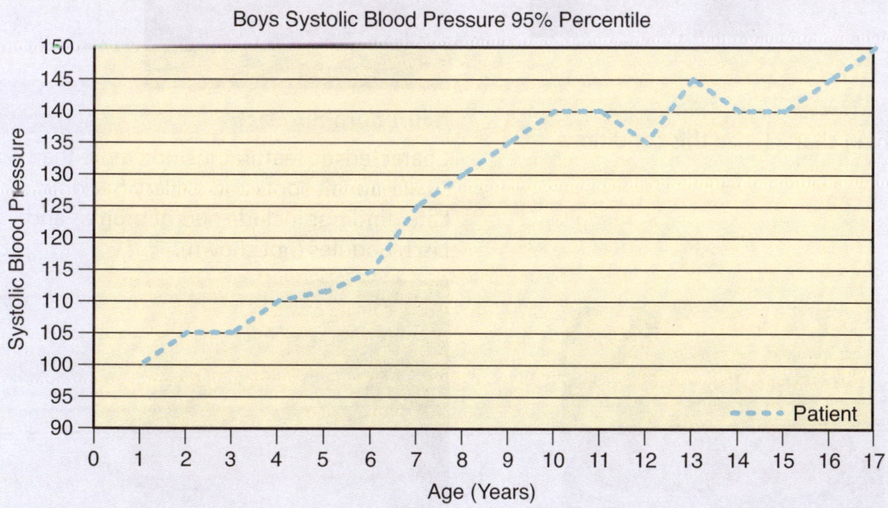

Hypertension can start in childhood. In young children it is more likely to have a renal, cardiac, or endocrine cause, whereas in older children and adolescents it is most likely to be primary or essential hypertension.

This child developed hypertension, and it "tracked" into adulthood. Children tend to remain in the same percentile for blood pressure as they grow. This tracking of blood pressure continues into adulthood, supporting the concept that adult essential hypertension often begins during childhood.

The consequences of untreated hypertension can be severe and include cardiac, renal, and visual sequelae.

TABLE 23-2. Common Skin Rashes and Skin Findings in Newborns and Infants

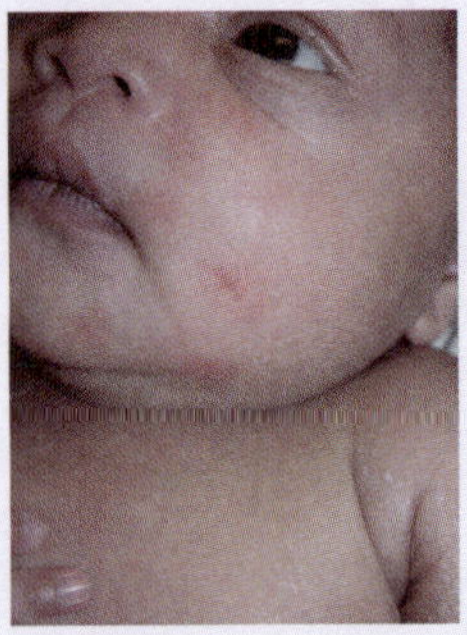

Erythema Toxicum

These common yellow or white pustules are surrounded by a red base.

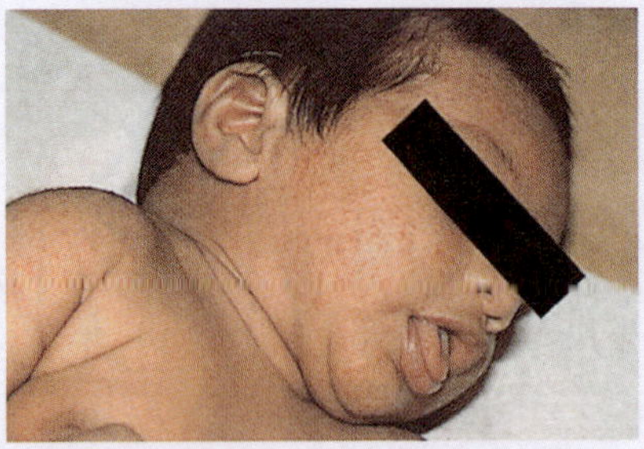

Neonatal Acne

Red pustules and papules are most prominent over the cheeks and nose of some normal newborns.

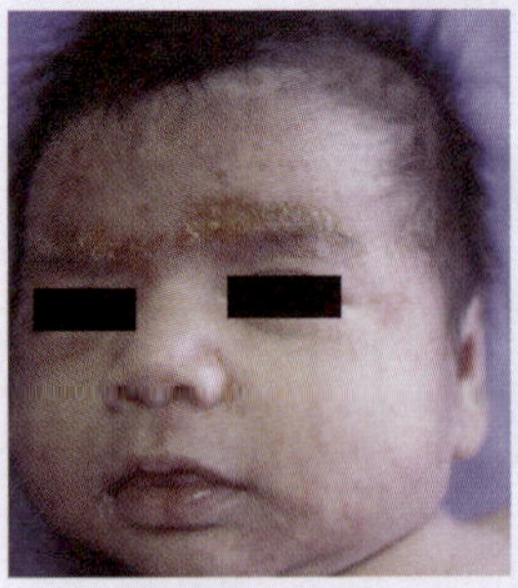

Seborrhea

The salmon red, scaly eruption often involves the face, neck, axilla, diaper area, and behind the ears.

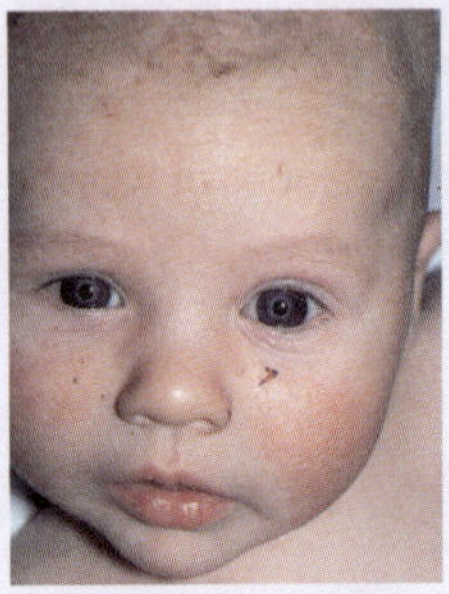

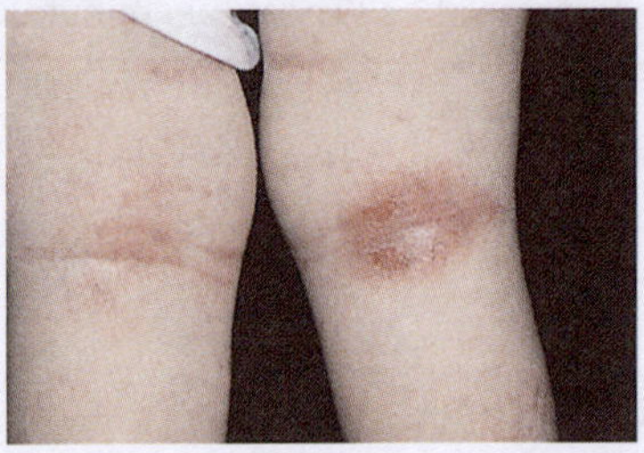

Atopic Dermatitis (Eczema)

Erythema, scaling, dry skin, and intense itching characterize this condition.

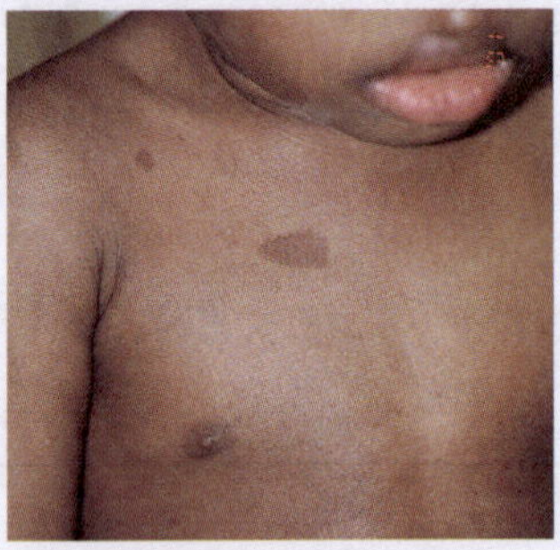

Neurofibromatosis

Characteristic features include more than 5 café-au-lait spots and axillary freckling. Later findings include neurofibromas and Lisch nodules (not shown).

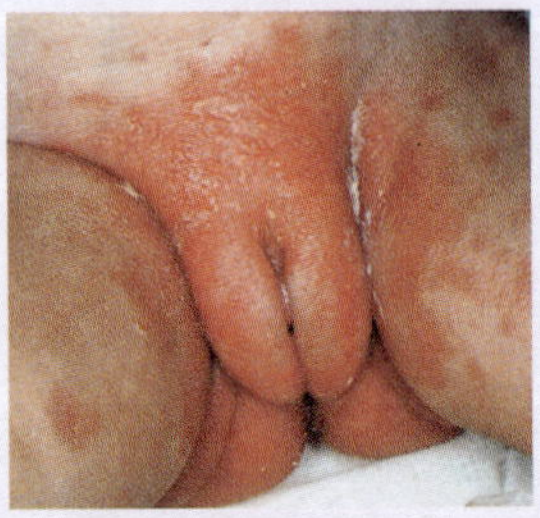

Candidal Diaper Dermatitis

This bright red rash involves the intertriginous folds, with small "satellite lesions" along the edges.

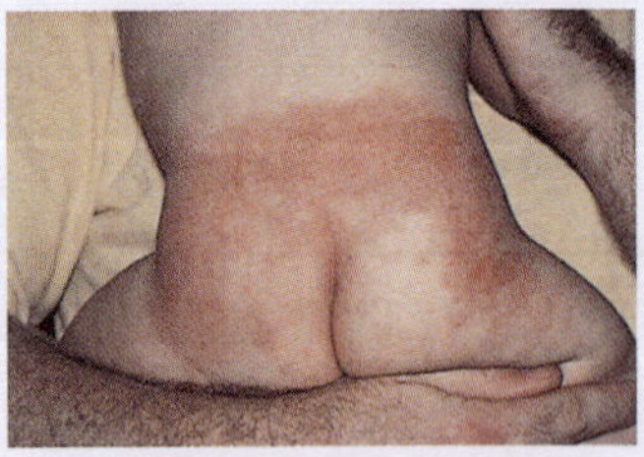

Contact Diaper Dermatitis

This irritant rash is secondary to diarrhea or irritation and is noted along contact areas (here, the area touching the diaper).

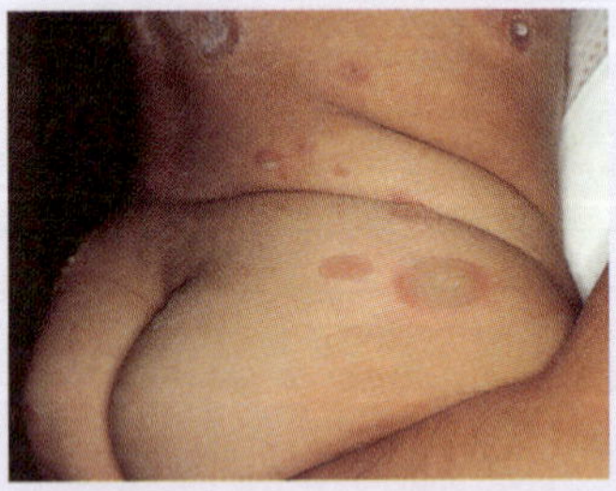

Impetigo

This infection is due to bacteria and can appear bullous or crusty and yellowed with some pus.

Source of photos: *Erythema Toxicum*—White AJ. *The Washington Manual of Pediatrics,* 2nd ed. Wolters Kluwer; 2017, Fig. 15-1; *Seborrhea*—Salimpour RR et al. *Photographic Atlas of Pediatric Disorders and Diagnosis.* Wolters Kluwer; 2014, Fig. 5-8a; *Atopic Dermatitis—Lippincott's Nursing Advisor 2011.* Wolters Kluwer; 2011, Fig. 48-1; and Goodheart HP, Gonzalez M. *Goodheart's Photoguide of Common Skin Disorders*, 2nd ed. Wolters Kluwer; 2003, Fig. 2-11.

TABLE 23-3. Warts, Lesions That Resemble Warts, and Other Raised Lesions

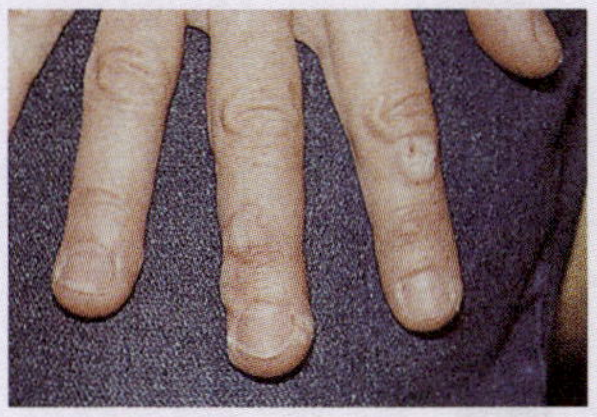

Verruca Vulgaris

Dry, rough warts on hands

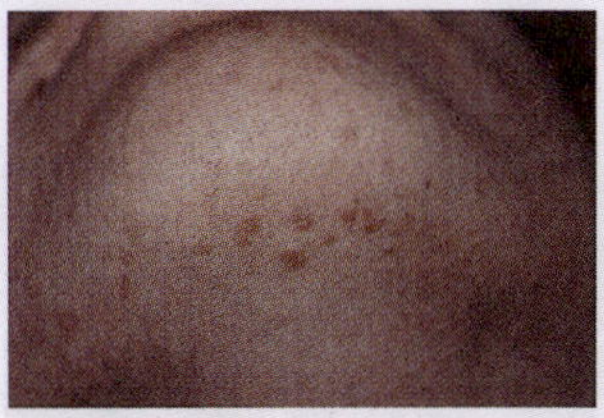

Verruca Plana

Small, flat warts

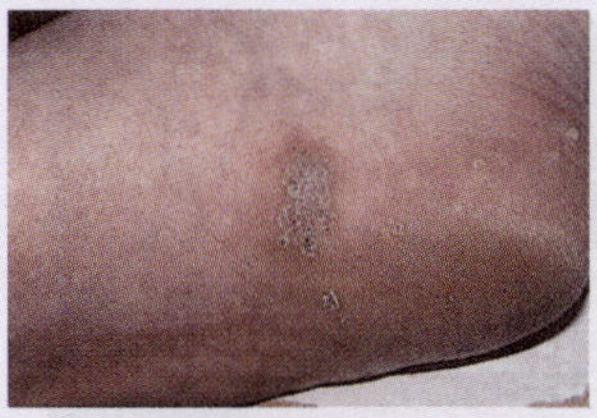

Plantar Warts

Tender warts on feet

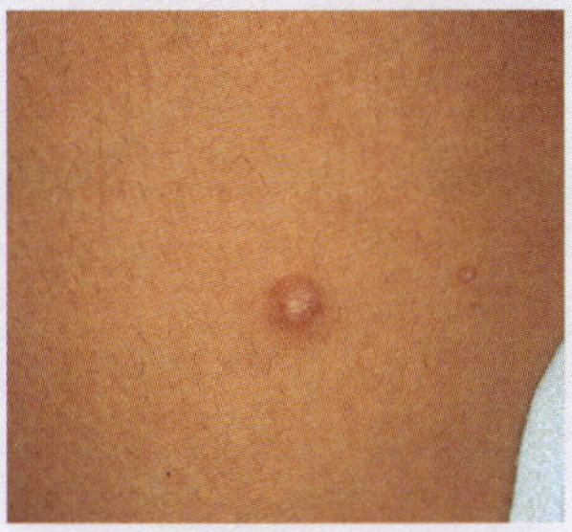

Molluscum Contagiosum

Dome-shaped, fleshy lesions with central umbilication.

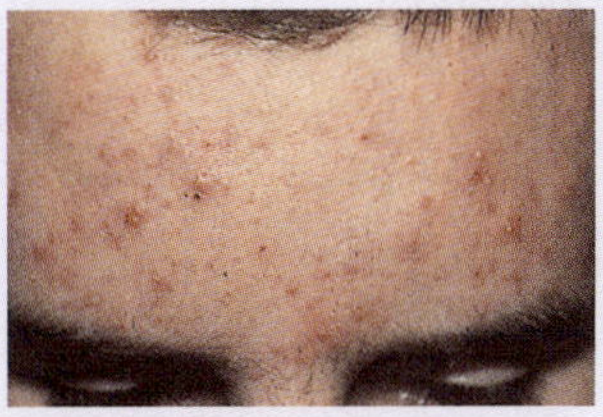

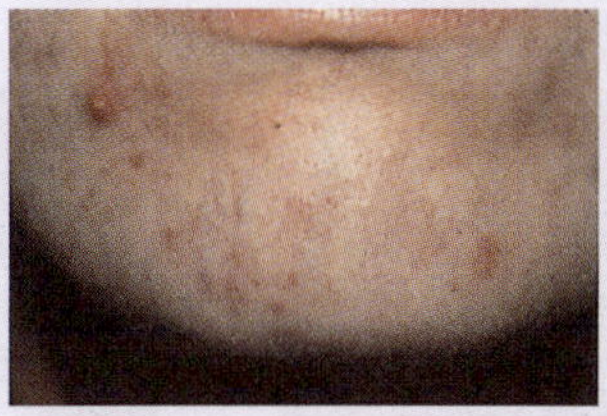

Adolescent Acne

Acne in adolescents involves open comedones (blackheads) and closed comedones (whiteheads) shown at the left, and inflamed pustules (right).

Source of photos: Molluscum Contagiosum—Fleisher GR et al. *Atlas of Pediatric Emergency Medicine.* Lippincott Williams & Wilkins; 2004, Fig. 6-25.

TABLE 23-4. Common Skin Lesions during Childhood

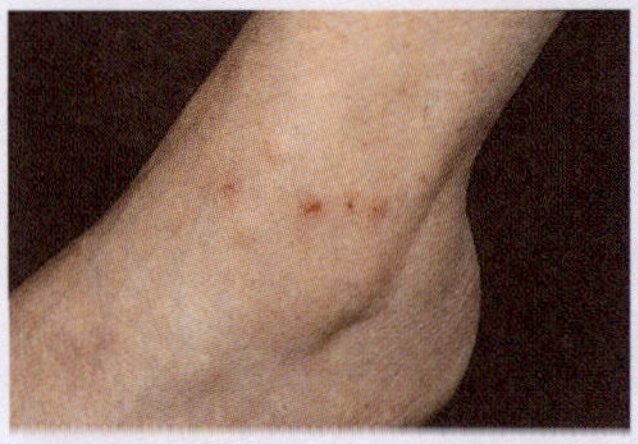

Insect Bites

Intensely pruritic, red, distinct papules characterize these lesions.

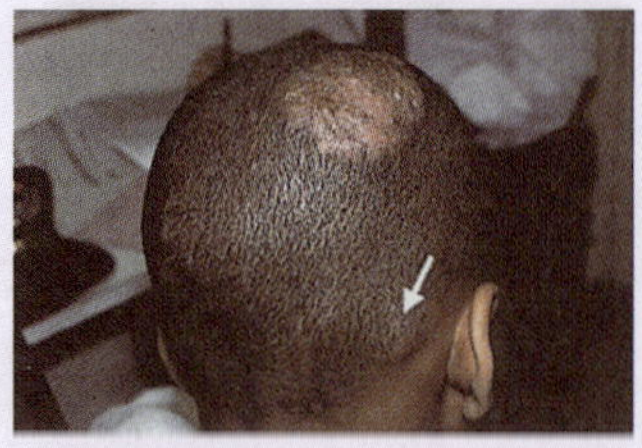

Tinea Capitis

Scaling, crusting, and hair loss are seen in the scalp, along with a painful plaque (kerion) and occipital lymph node (*arrow*).

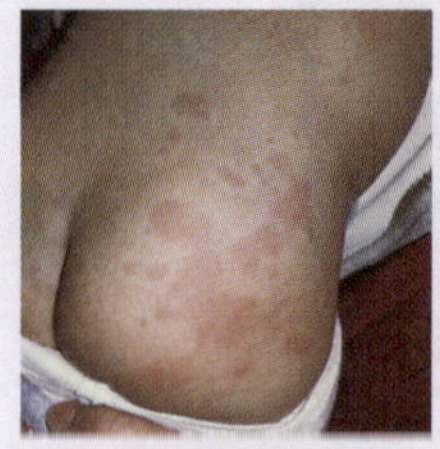

Urticaria (Hives)

This pruritic, allergic sensitivity reaction changes shape quickly.

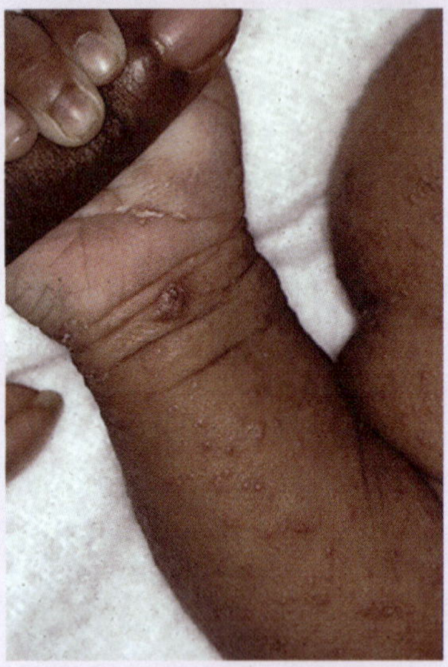

Scabies

Intensely itchy papules and vesicles, sometimes burrows, most often on extremities.

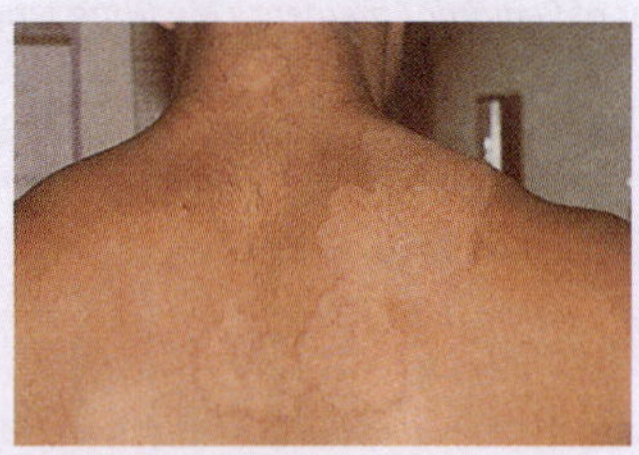

Tinea Corporis

This annular lesion has central clearing and papules along the border.

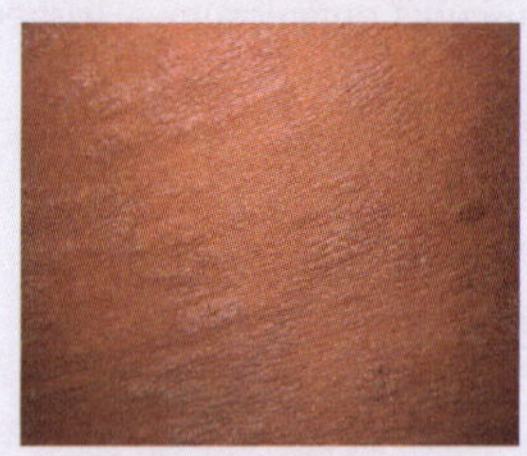

Pityriasis Rosea

Oval lesions on trunk, in older children, often in a Christmas tree pattern, sometimes a herald patch (a large patch that appears first).

Source of *Bites, Tinea Capitis, and Tinea Corporis* photos—Goodheart HP, Gonzalez ME. *Goodheart's Photoguide to Common Pediatric and Adult Skin Disorders*. 4th ed. Wolters Kluwer; 2016, Figs. 9-11, 18-8, and 29-2; *Urticaria*—Chung EK et al. *Visual Diagnosis and Treatment in Pediatrics.* 3rd ed. Wolters Kluwer; 2015, Fig. 64-1; *Scabies*—Courtesy of Ronald W. Cotliar, MD; *Pityriasis Rosea*—Fleisher GR et al. *Atlas of Pediatric Emergency Medicine.* Lippincott Williams & Wilkins; 2004, Fig. 6-23b.

TABLE 23-5. Abnormalities of the Head

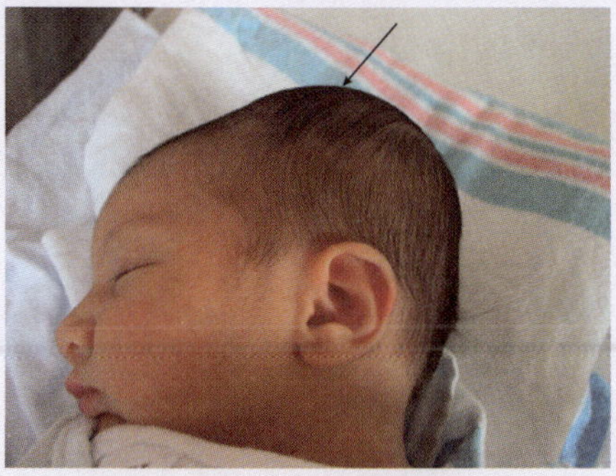

Cephalohematoma

Although not present at birth, cephalohematomas appear within the first 24 hours from subperiosteal hemorrhage involving the outer table of one of the cranial bones. The swelling, shown at the *arrow,* does not extend across a suture though it is occasionally bilateral following a difficult birth. The swelling is initially soft, then develops a raised bony margin within a few days from calcium deposits at the edge of the periosteum. It tends to resolve within several weeks.

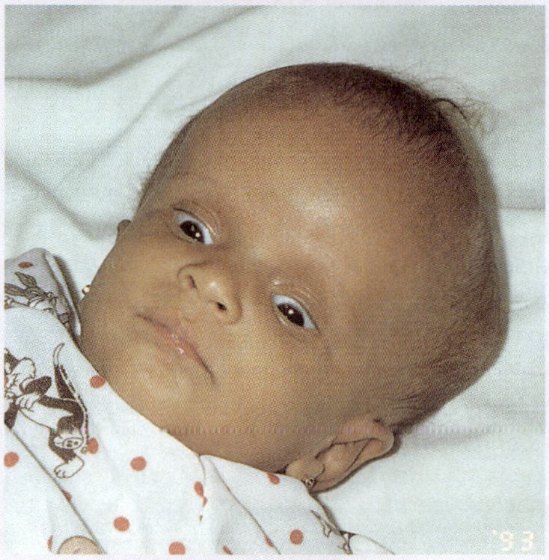

Hydrocephalus

In hydrocephaly, the anterior fontanelle is bulging, and the eyes may be deviated downward revealing the upper sclerae and creating the *setting sun* sign, as shown on the left.

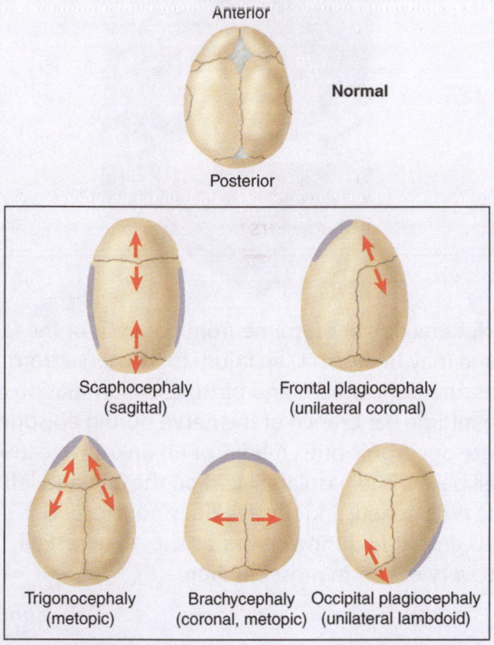

Craniosynostosis

Craniosynostosis is a condition of premature closure of one or more sutures of the skull. This results in an abnormal growth and shape of the skull because growth will occur across sutures that are not affected but not across sutures that are affected.

The figures demonstrate different skull shapes associated with the various types of craniosynostosis. The prematurely closed suture line is noted by the absence of a suture line in each figure. Scaphocephaly and frontal plagiocephaly are the most common forms of craniosynostosis. The *blue shading* shows areas of maximal flattening. The *red arrows* show the direction of continued growth across the sutures, which is normal.

Source of photos: *Cephalohematoma*—Chung EK et al. *Visual Diagnosis and Treatment in Pediatrics.* 3rd ed. Wolters Kluwer; 2015, Fig. 2-6; *Hydrocephalus*—Fleisher GR et al. *Atlas of Pediatric Emergency Medicine*. Lippincott Williams & Wilkins; 2004, Fig. 14.4.

TABLE 23-6. Diagnostic Facies in Infancy and Childhood

Fetal Alcohol Syndrome

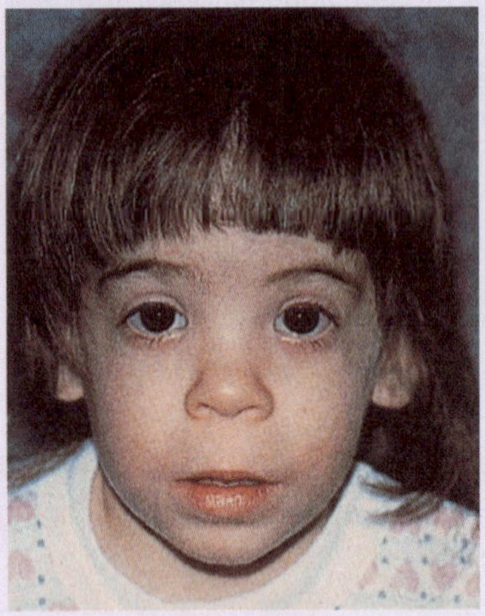

Babies born to women with chronic alcoholism are at increased risk for growth deficiency, microcephaly, and intellectual disability. Facial characteristics include short palpebral fissures, a wide and flattened philtrum (the vertical groove in the midline of the upper lip), and thin lips.

Congenital Hypothyroidism

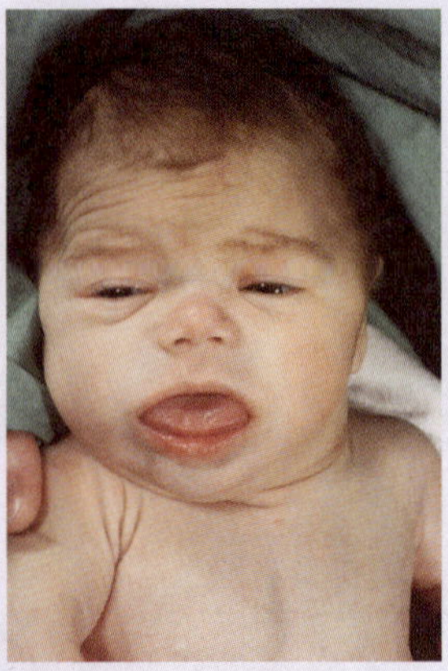

The child with congenital hypothyroidism has coarse facial features, a low-set hair line, sparse eyebrows, and an enlarged tongue. Associated features include a hoarse cry, umbilical hernia, dry and cold extremities, myxedema, mottled skin, and intellectual disability. Since most infants with congenital hypothyroidism have no physical stigmata, the United States and many other nations screen all newborns for congenital hypothyroidism.

Congenital Syphilis

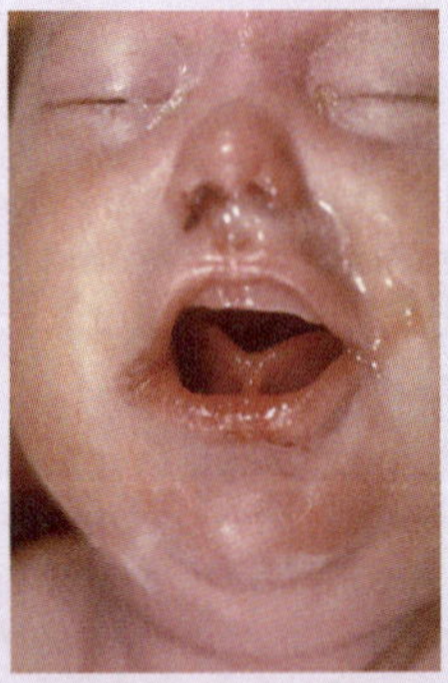

In utero infection by *Treponema pallidum* usually occurs after the 16th week of gestation and affects virtually all fetal organs. Signs of illness appear in survivors within the first month of life. Facial stigmata often include bulging of the frontal bones and nasal bridge depression (*saddle nose*), both from periostitis; rhinitis from weeping nasal mucosal lesions (*snuffles*); and a circumoral rash. Mucocutaneous inflammation and fissuring of the mouth and lips (*rhagades*), not shown here, may also occur as stigmata of congenital syphilis, as may craniotabes tibial periostitis (*saber shins*) and dental dysplasia (*Hutchinson teeth*).

Facial Nerve Palsy

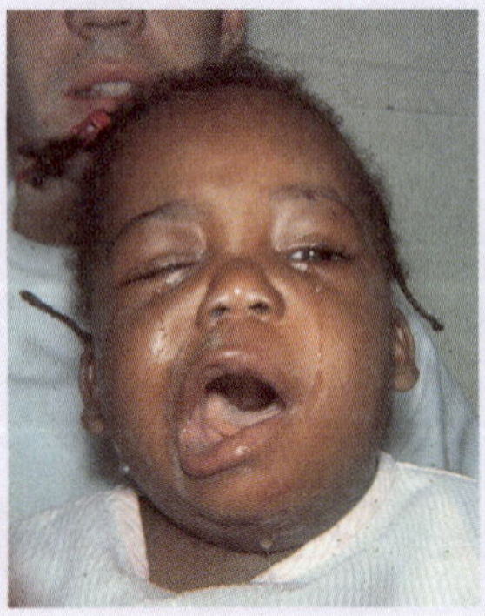

Peripheral (lower motor neuron) paralysis of the facial nerve may be from (1) an injury to the nerve from pressure during labor and birth, (2) inflammation of the middle ear branch of the nerve during episodes of acute or chronic otitis media, or (3) unknown causes (Bell palsy). The nasolabial fold on the affected left side is flattened, and the eye does not close. This is accentuated during crying, as shown here. Full recovery occurs in most children.

(*continued*)

TABLE 23-6. Diagnostic Facies in Infancy and Childhood *(Continued)*

Down Syndrome

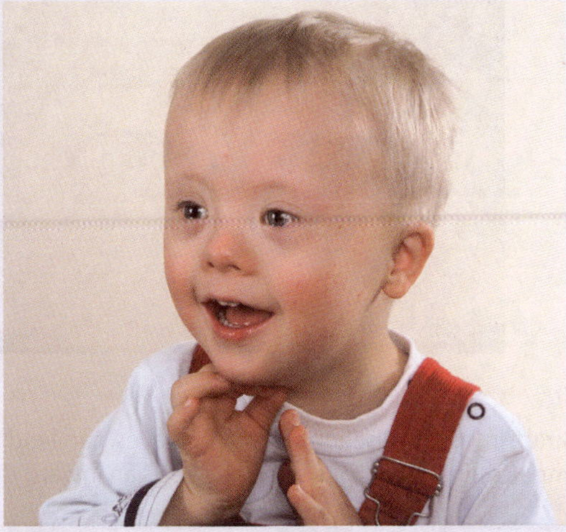

The child with Down syndrome (trisomy 21) usually has a small, rounded head, a flattened nasal bridge, oblique palpebral fissures, prominent epicanthal folds, small, low-set, shell-like ears, and a relatively large tongue. Associated features include generalized hypotonia, transverse palmar creases, shortening and incurving of the fifth fingers (*clinodactyly*), Brushfield spots, and mild to moderate cognitive impairment.

Nonaccidental Trauma

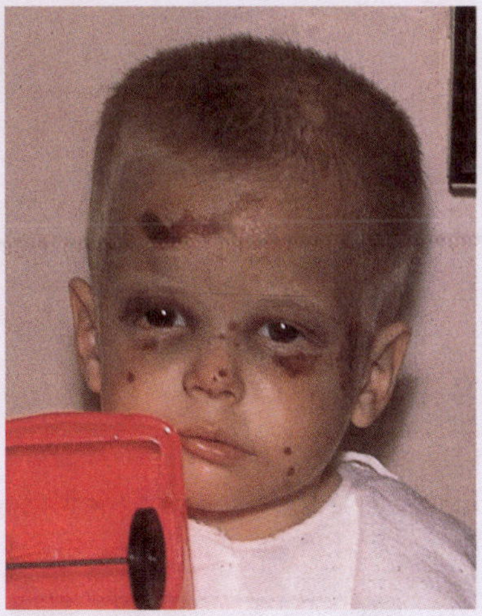

The child who has been physically abused may have *old and fresh bruises* on the head and face. Other stigmata include bruises in areas (axilla and groin) not usually subject to injury rather than the bony prominences; x-ray evidence of fractures of the skull, ribs, and long bones in various stages of healing; and skin lesions that are morphologically similar to implements used to inflict trauma (hand, belt buckle, strap, rope, coat hanger, or lighted cigarette).

Perennial Allergic Rhinitis

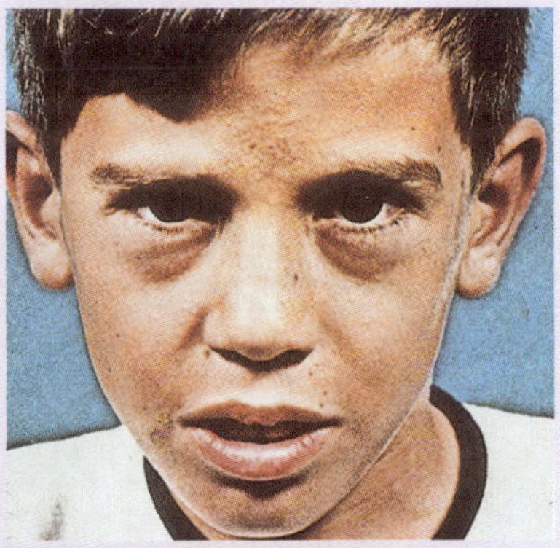

The child suffering from perennial allergic rhinitis has an open mouth (cannot breathe through the nose) and edema and discoloration of the lower orbitopalpebral grooves ("allergic shiners"). Such a child is often seen to push the nose upward and backward with a hand ("allergic salute") and to grimace (wrinkle the nose and mouth) to relieve nasal itching and obstruction.

Hyperthyroidism

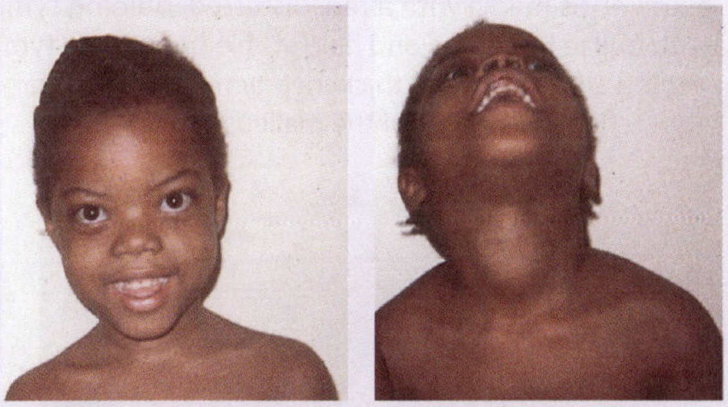

Thyrotoxicosis (*Graves disease*) causes tachycardia, hypermetabolism, and accelerated linear growth. Facial characteristics shown in this 6-year-old girl are "staring" eyes (not true exophthalmos, which is rare in children) and an enlarged thyroid gland (*goiter*).

TABLE 23-7. Abnormalities of the Eyes, Ears, and Mouth

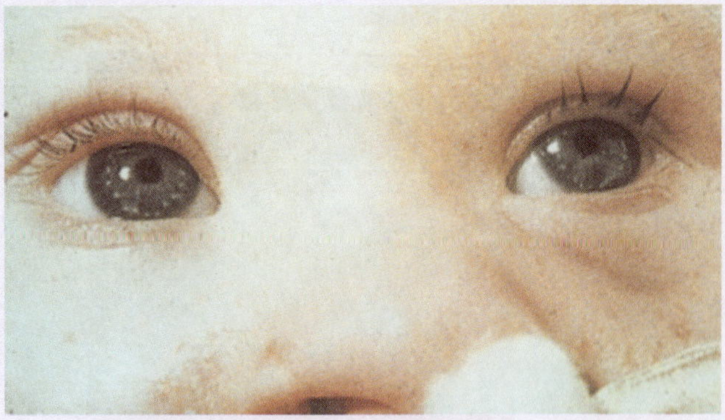

Brushfield Spots

These abnormal speckling spots on the iris suggest Down syndrome.

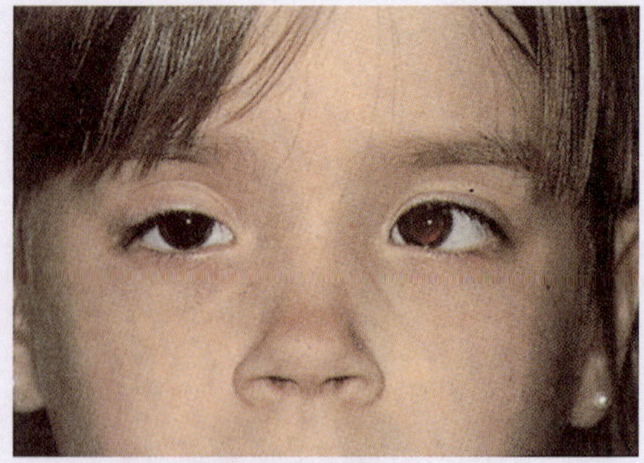

Strabismus

Strabismus, or misalignment of the eyes, can lead to visual impairment. Esotropia, shown here, is an inward deviation.

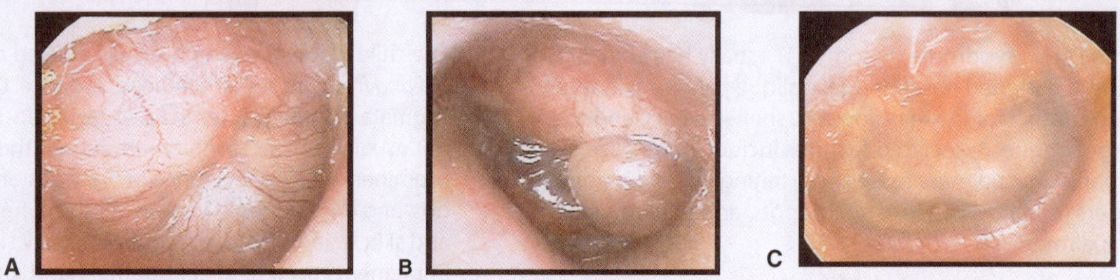

Otitis Media

Otitis media is one of the most common conditions in young children. The spectrum of otitis media is shown here. **A:** Typical acute otitis media with a red, distorted, bulging tympanic membrane in a highly symptomatic child. **B:** Acute otitis media with bullae formation and fluid visible behind the tympanic membrane. **C:** Otitis media with effusion, showing a yellowish fluid behind a retracted and thickened tympanic membrane. Often you can no longer visualize the normal landmarks such as the light reflex and handle of the malleus.

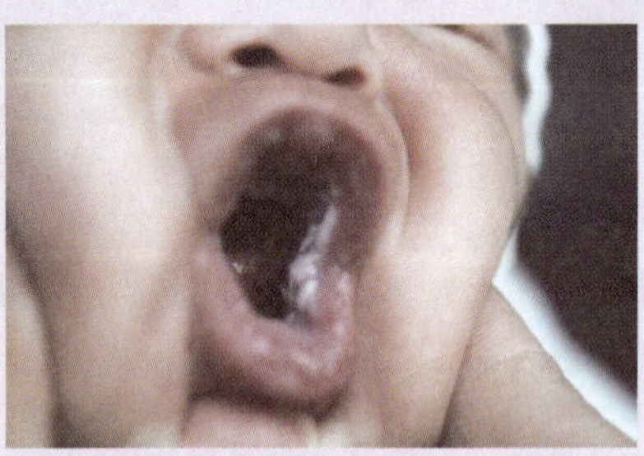

Oral Candidiasis ("Thrush")

This infection is common in infants. The white plaques do not rub off.

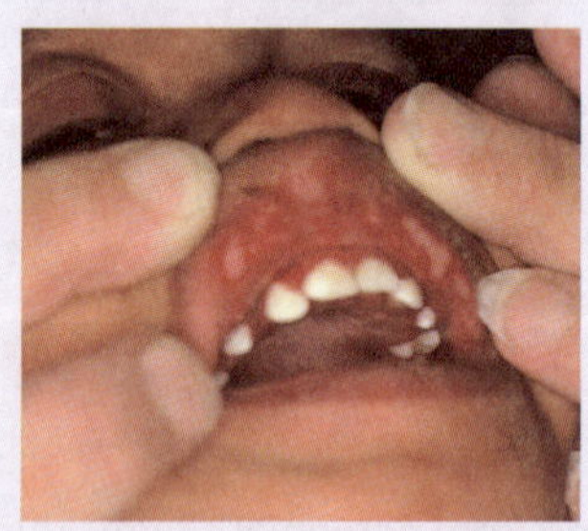

Herpetic Stomatitis

Tender ulcerations on the oral mucosa are surrounded by erythema.

Source of photos: *Otitis Media*—Courtesy of Alejandro Hoberman, Children's Hospital of Pittsburgh, University of Pittsburgh; *Thrush*—Salimpour RR et al. *Photographic Atlas of Pediatric Disorders and Diagnosis.* Wolters Kluwer; 2014, UNImage13C; *Herpetic Stomatitis*—Fleisher GR et al. *Atlas of Pediatric Emergency Medicine.* Lippincott Williams & Wilkins; 2004, Fig. 11-7b.

TABLE 23-8. Abnormal Infant Cries (If Persistent)

Type	Possible Abnormality
Shrill or high-pitched	Increased intracranial pressure. Also, in a newborn born to a mother with an addiction to narcotics.
Hoarse	Hypocalcemic tetany, congenital hypothyroidism, or unilateral vocal cord weakness.
Continuous inspiratory and expiratory stridor	Upper airway obstruction from various lesions (e.g., a polyp or hemangioma), a relatively small larynx (*infantile laryngeal stridor*), a delay in the development of the cartilage in the tracheal rings (*tracheomalacia*), or bilateral vocal cord paralysis.
Absence of cry	Severe illness, or glottis web.

TABLE 23-9. Abnormalities of the Teeth, Pharynx, and Neck

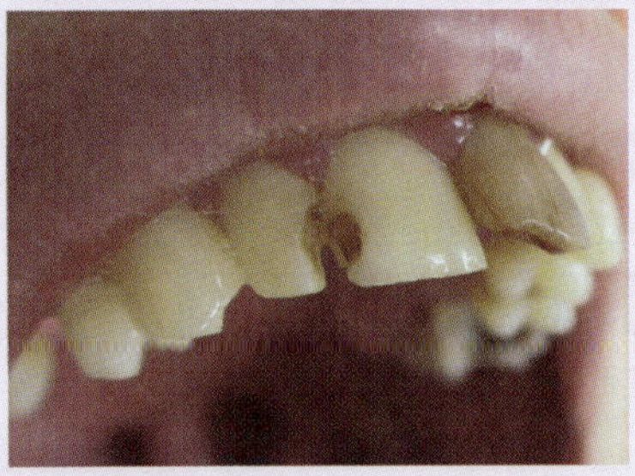

Dental Caries (Early Childhood Caries, or ECC)

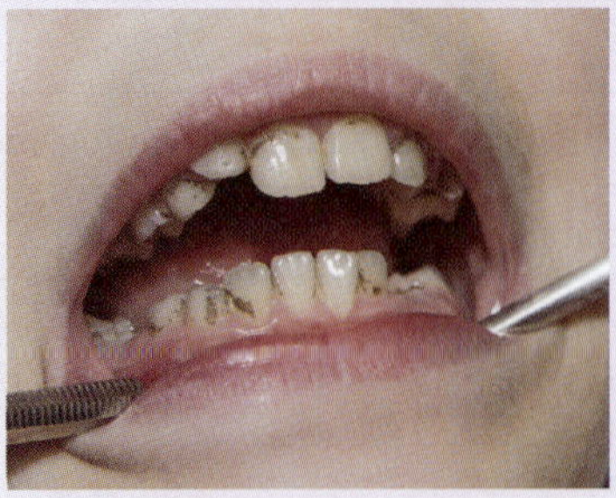

Severe early childhood caries

Dental Caries

Dental caries is a major global health and pediatric problem. White spots on the teeth often reflect early caries. The photographs to the left show different characteristics of caries.

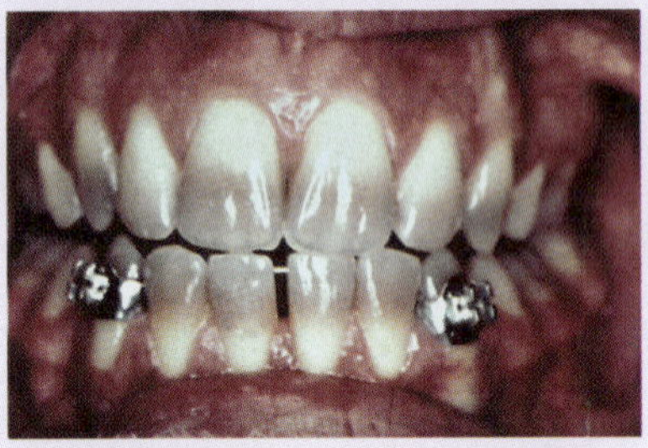

Staining of the Teeth

Various causes can lead to staining of the teeth of children, including intrinsic stains such as tetracycline (*left*) or extrinsic stains such as poor oral hygiene (carious lesions shown in previous figures). Extrinsic stains can be removed.

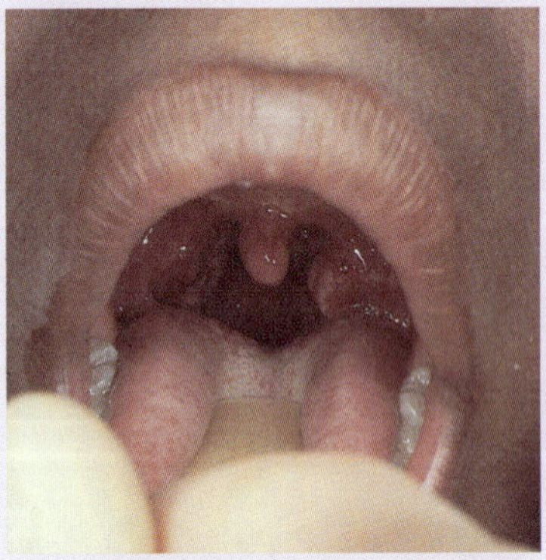

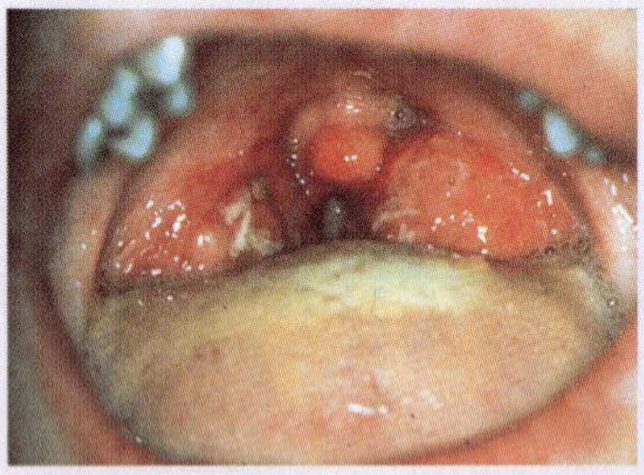

Streptococcal Pharyngitis ("Strep Throat")

This common childhood infection has a classic presentation of erythema of the posterior pharynx and palatal petechiae. A foul-smelling exudate is also commonly noted.

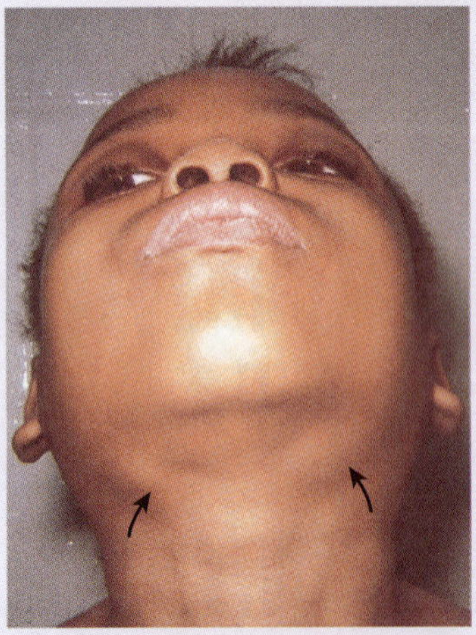

Lymphadenopathy

Enlarged and tender cervical lymph nodes are common in children. The most likely causes are viral and bacterial infections. Lymph node enlargement can be bilateral, as shown in the figure to the left.

Source of photos: *Dental Caries*—From Sherman S et al. *Atlas of Clinical Emergency Medicine.* Wolters Kluwer; 2016, Fig. 5-6; *Staining of the Teeth*—Used with permission from Shutterstock. By Maliutina Anna.

TABLE 23-10. Cyanosis in Children

Cyanosis is a "raspberry" color, whereas normal mucous membranes should have a "strawberry" color. Try to identify the cyanosis in these photographs before reading the captions.

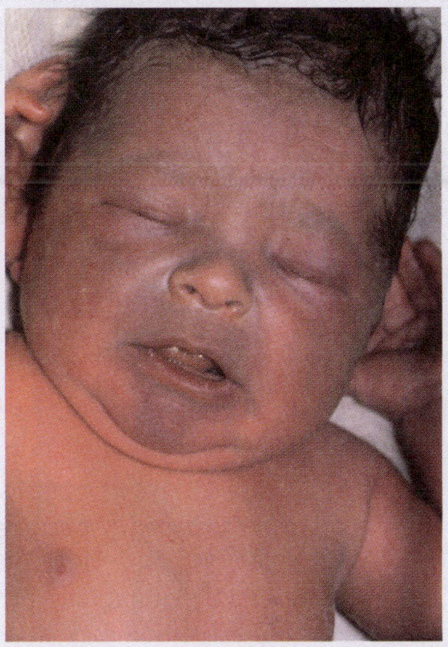

Generalized Cyanosis

This baby has total anomalous pulmonary venous return and an oxygen saturation level of 80%.

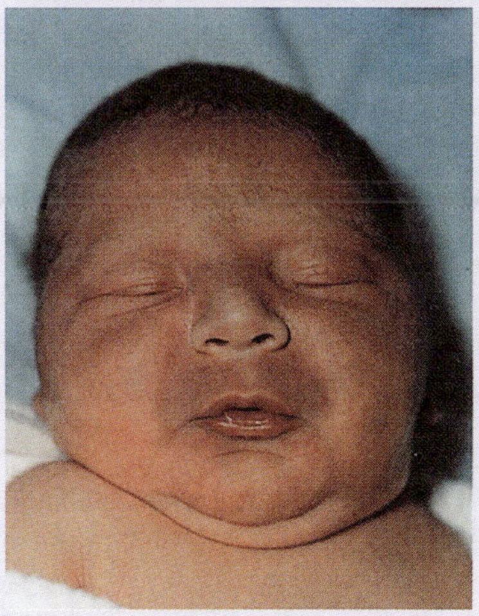

Perioral Cyanosis

This baby has mild cyanosis above the lips, but the mucous membranes remain pink.

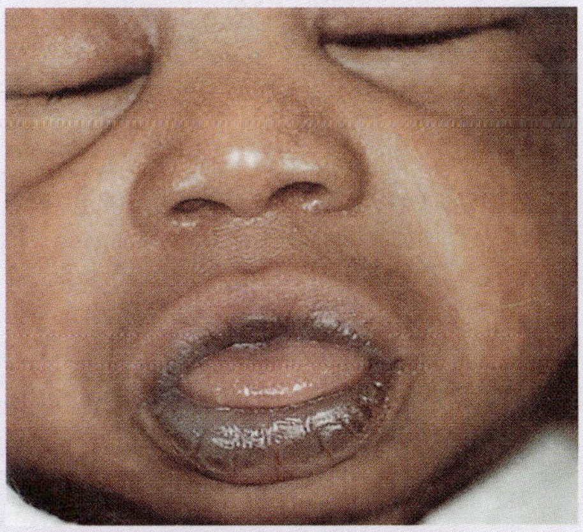

Bluish Lips, Giving Appearance of Cyanosis

Normal pigment deposition in the vermilion border of the lips gives them a bluish hue, but the mucous membranes are pink.

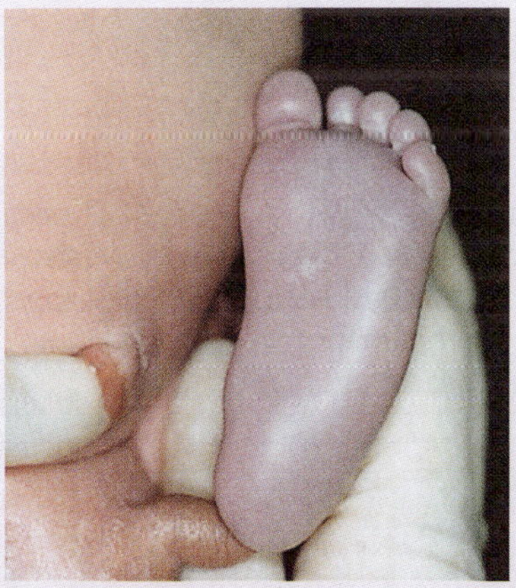

Acrocyanosis

This commonly appears on the feet and hands of babies shortly after birth. This infant is a 32-week-old newborn. Acrocyanosis does not reflect cardiac disease.

Source of photos (except *Generalized Cyanosis*): Fletcher M. *Physical Diagnosis in Neonatology*. Lippincott-Raven; 1998.

TABLE 23-11. Congenital Heart Murmurs

Some heart murmurs reflect underlying heart disease. If you understand their physiologic causes, you will more readily be able to identify and distinguish them from innocent heart murmurs. Obstructive lesions result when blood flows through under-sized valves or narrowed vessels. Because this problem does not depend on the drop in pulmonary vascular resistance following birth, these murmurs are audible at birth. Defects with left-to-right shunts, on the other hand, depend on the drop in pulmonary vascular resistance that occurs shortly after birth. High-pressured shunts such as ventricular septal defect, patent ductus arteriosus, and persistent truncus arteriosus may not be heard until 1 week or more after birth; the murmur gets louder as peripheral vascular resistance drops. Low-pressured left-to-right shunts, such as atrial septal defects, may not be heard until age 1 year or more. Many children with congenital cardiac defects have combinations of defects or variations of abnormalities, so findings on cardiac examination may not follow these classic patterns. This table shows a limited selection of the more common murmurs, starting with murmurs that appear in the newborn period.

Congenital Defect and Mechanism	Characteristics of the Murmur	Associated Findings
Pulmonary Valve Stenosis		
Usually a normal valve annulus with fusion of some or most of the valve leaflets, restricting flow across the valve *Mild* 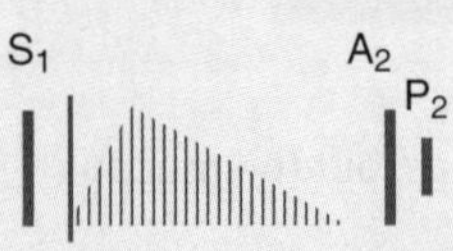 *Severe* 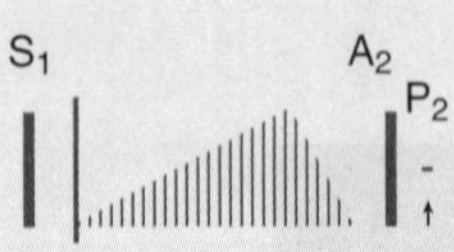	*Location.* Upper left sternal border *Radiation.* In mild degrees of stenosis, the murmur may be heard over the course of the pulmonary arteries in the lung fields *Intensity.* Increases in intensity and duration as the degree of obstruction increases *Quality.* Ejection, peaking later in systole as the obstruction increases	Usually a prominent ejection click in early systole Pulmonary component of the second sound at the base (P_2) becomes delayed and softer, disappearing as obstruction increases. Inspiration may increase murmur; expiration may increase click. Growth is usually normal. Newborns with severe stenosis may be cyanotic from right-to-left atrial shunting and rapidly develop heart failure as the ductus arteriosus closes.
Aortic Valve Stenosis		
Usually a bicuspid valve with progressive obstruction, but may occur as a result of a dysplastic valve or damage from rheumatic fever or degenerative disease 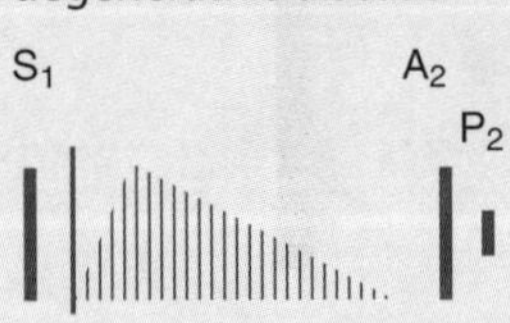	*Location.* Midsternum, upper right sternal border *Radiation.* To the carotid arteries and suprasternal notch; may also be a thrill *Intensity.* Varies, louder with increasingly severe obstruction *Quality.* An ejection, often harsh, systolic murmur	May be an associated ejection click The aortic closure sound may be increased in intensity. There may be a diastolic murmur of aortic valve regurgitation (not shown in the diagram). Newborns with severe stenosis may have weak or absent pulses and severe heart failure. May not be audible until adulthood even though the valve is congenitally abnormal

(continued)

TABLE 23-11. Congenital Heart Murmurs *(Continued)*

(continued)

Congenital Defect and Mechanism	Characteristics of the Murmur	Associated Findings
Tetralogy of Fallot Complex defect with ventricular septal defect, infundibular and usually valvular right ventricular outflow obstruction, malrotation of the aorta, and right-to-left shunting at ventricular septal level *With Pulmonic Stenosis* 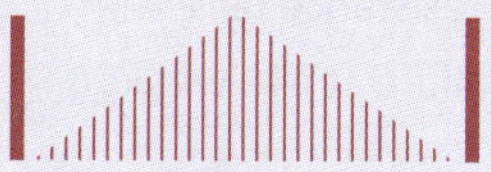 *With Pulmonic Atresia* 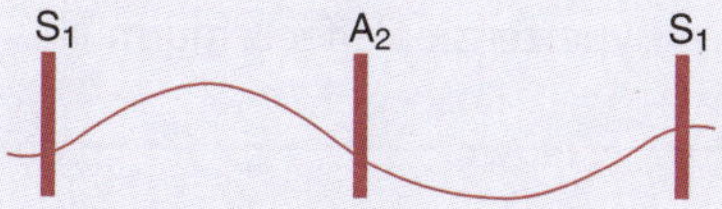	*General.* Variable cyanosis, increasing with activity *Location.* Mid-to-upper left sternal border. If pulmonary atresia, the continuous murmur of ductus arteriosus flow at upper left sternal border or in the back. *Radiation.* Little, to upper left sternal border, occasionally to lung fields *Intensity.* Usually grade III–IV *Quality.* Systolic ejection murmur	Normal pulses The pulmonary closure sound is usually not heard. May have abrupt hypercyanotic spells with sudden increase in cyanosis, air hunger, altered level of awareness Failure to gain weight with persistent and increasingly severe cyanosis Long-term persistence of cyanosis accompanied by clubbing of fingers and toes Persistent hypoxemia leads to polycythemia, which will accentuate the cyanosis.
Transposition of the Great Arteries A severe defect with failure of rotation of the great vessels, leaving the aorta to arise from the right ventricle and the pulmonary artery from the left ventricle	*General.* Intense generalized cyanosis *Location.* No characteristic murmur. If present, it may reflect an associated defect such as ventricular septal defect (VSD). *Radiation and Quality.* Depends on associated abnormalities	Single loud second sound of the anterior aortic valve Frequent rapid development of heart failure Frequent associated defects as described at the left
Ventricular Septal Defect Blood going from a high-pressure left ventricle through a defect in the septum to the lower-pressure right ventricle creates turbulence, usually throughout systole. *Small to Moderate* 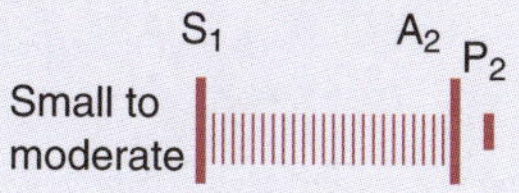	*Location.* Lower left sternal border *Radiation.* Little *Intensity.* Variable, only partially determined by the size of the shunt. Small shunts with a high-pressure gradient may have very loud murmurs. Large defects with elevated pulmonary vascular resistance may have no murmur. Grade II–IV/VI with a thrill if grade IV/VI or higher. *Quality.* Pansystolic, usually harsh, may obscure S_1 and S_2 if loud enough	With large shunts, there may be a low-pitched middiastolic murmur of relative mitral stenosis at the apex. As pulmonary artery pressure increases, the pulmonic component of the second sounds at the base increases in intensity. When pulmonary artery pressure equals aortic pressure there may be no murmur and P_2 will be very loud. In low-volume shunts, growth is normal. In larger shunts, heart failure may occur by 6–8 weeks; poor weight gain, poor feeding. Associated defects are frequent.

(continued)

TABLE 23-11. Congenital Heart Murmurs *(Continued)*

Congenital Defect and Mechanism	Characteristics of the Murmur	Associated Findings
Patent Ductus Arteriosus		
Continuous flow from aorta to pulmonary artery throughout the cardiac cycle when ductus arteriosus does not close after birth *Small to Moderate* 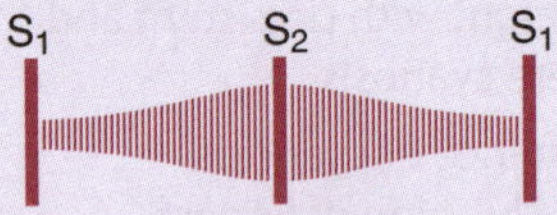	*Location.* Upper left sternal border and to left *Radiation.* Sometimes to the back *Intensity.* Varies depending on size of the shunt, usually grade II–III/VI. *Quality.* A rather hollow, sometimes machinery-like murmur that is continuous throughout the cardiac cycle, although occasionally almost inaudible in late diastole, uninterrupted by the heart sounds, louder in systole	Full to bounding pulses Noticed at birth in the premature infant who may have bounding pulses, a hyperdynamic precordium, and an atypical murmur Noticed later in the full-term infant as pulmonary vascular resistance falls May develop heart failure at 4–6 weeks if large shunt Poor weight gain related to size of shunt Pulmonary hypertension affects murmur as above.
Atrial Septal Defect		
Left-to-right shunt through an opening in the atrial septum, possible at various levels 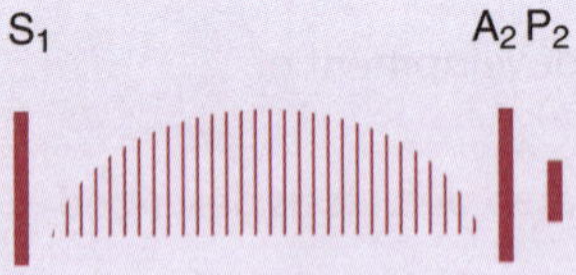	*Location.* Upper left sternal border *Radiation.* To the back *Intensity.* Variable, usually grade II–III/VI *Quality.* Ejection but without the harsh quality	Widely split second sounds throughout all phases of respiration, normal intensity Usually not heard until after age of 1 year Gradual decrease in weight gain as shunt increases Decreased exercise tolerance, subtle, not dramatic Heart failure is rare.

TABLE 23-12. Physical Signs of Sexual Abuse

Possible Indications

1. Marked and immediate dilatation of the anus in knee–chest position, with no constipation, stool in the vault, or neurologic disorders
2. Hymenal notch or cleft that extends >50% of the inferior hymenal rim (confirmed in knee–chest position)
3. Condyloma acuminata in a child older than 3 years
4. Bruising, abrasions, lacerations, or bite marks of labia or perihymenal tissue
5. Herpes of the anogenital area beyond the neonatal period
6. Purulent or malodorous vaginal discharge in a young girl (culture and view all discharges under a microscope for evidence of a sexually transmitted infection)

Strong Indications

1. Lacerations, ecchymoses, and newly healed scars of the hymen or the posterior fourchette
2. No hymenal tissue from 3 o'clock to 9 o'clock (confirmed in various positions)
3. Healed hymenal transections especially between 3 and 9 o'clock (complete cleft)
4. Perianal lacerations extending to external sphincter

A child with concerning physical signs must be evaluated by a sexual abuse expert for a complete history and sexual abuse examination.

Any physical sign must be evaluated in light of the entire history, other parts of the physical examination, and laboratory data.

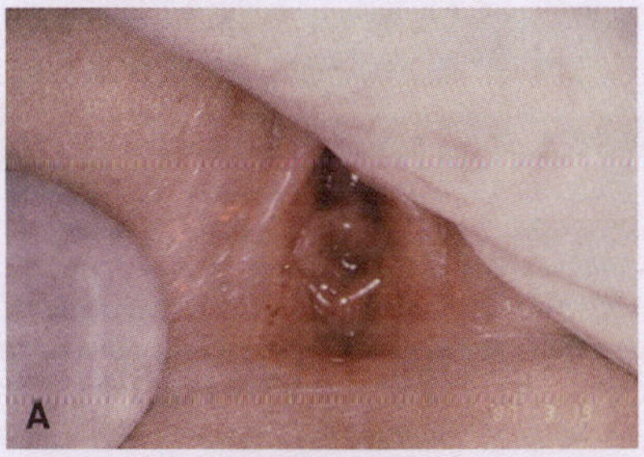

Acute hemorrhage and ecchymoses of tissues (10-month-old)

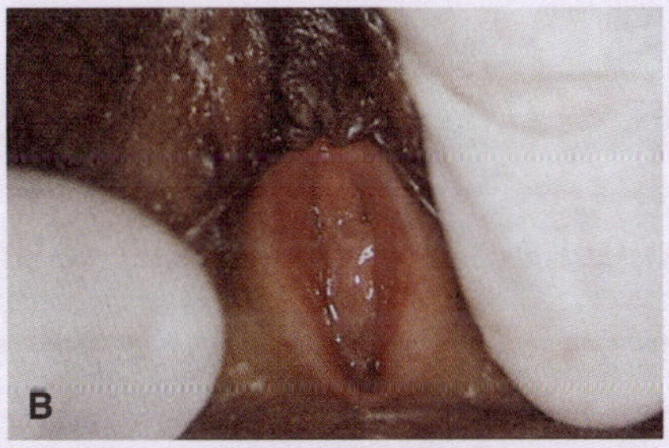

Erythema and superficial abrasions to the labia minora (5-year-old)

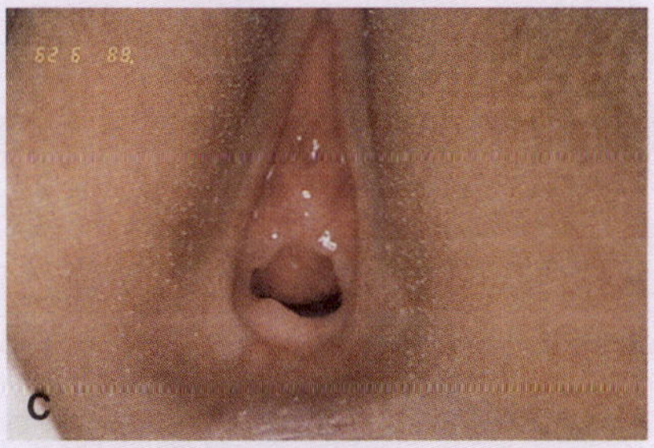

Healed interruption of hymenal membrane at 9 o'clock (4-year-old)

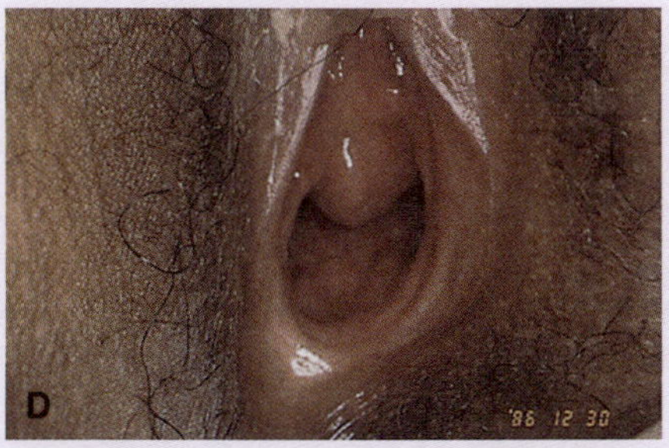

Narrowed posterior ring continuous with floor of vagina (12-year-old)

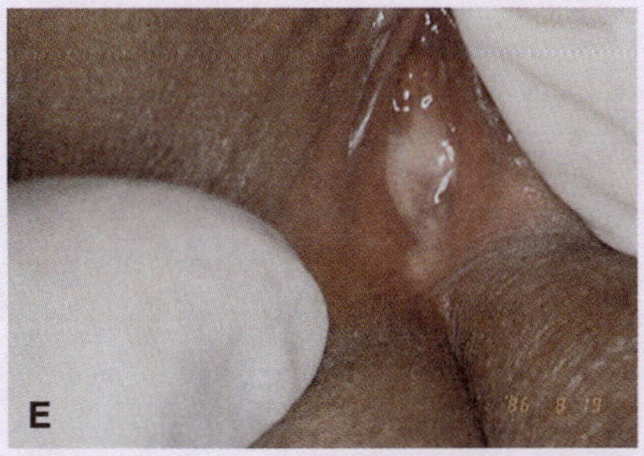

Copious vaginal discharge and erythema (9-year-old)

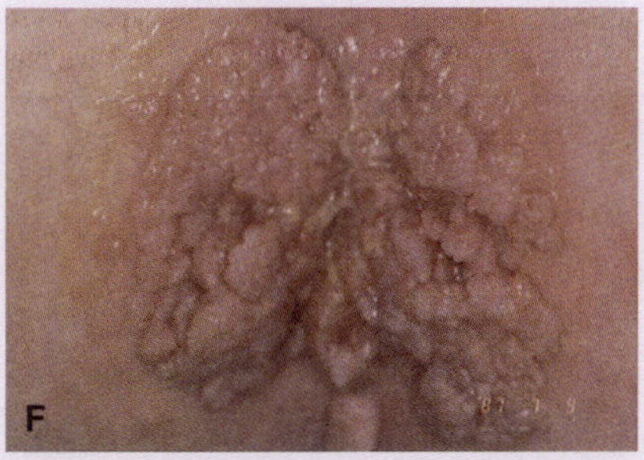

Extensive condylomata around the anus (2-year-old)

Source: Reece R, Ludwig S, eds. *Child Abuse Medical Diagnosis and Management.* 2nd ed. Lippincott Williams & Wilkins; 2001.

TABLE 23-13. Common Abnormalities in the Male Genitourinary System

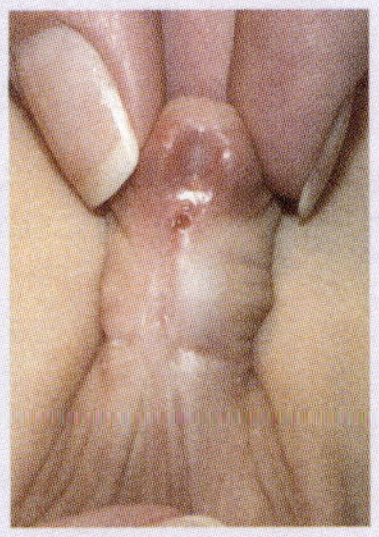

Hypospadias

Hypospadias is the most common congenital penile abnormality. The urethral meatus opens abnormally on the ventral surface of the penis. One form is shown above; more severe forms involve openings on the lower shaft or scrotum.

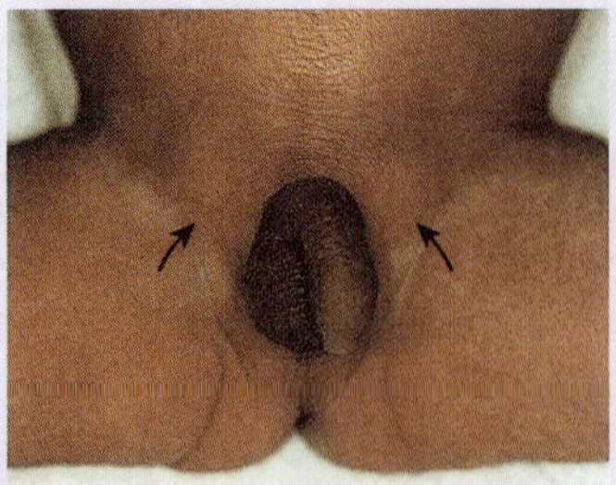

Undescended Testicle

You should distinguish between undescended testes, shown above (with testes in the inguinal canals—see *arrows*), from highly retractile testes from an active cremasteric reflex.

Sources of photos: *Hypospadias*—Courtesy of Warren Snodgrass, MD, Hypospadias Specialty Center; *Undescended Testicle*—Fletcher M. *Physical Diagnosis in Neonatology*. Lippincott-Raven; 1998.

TABLE 23-14. Common Musculoskeletal Findings in Young Children

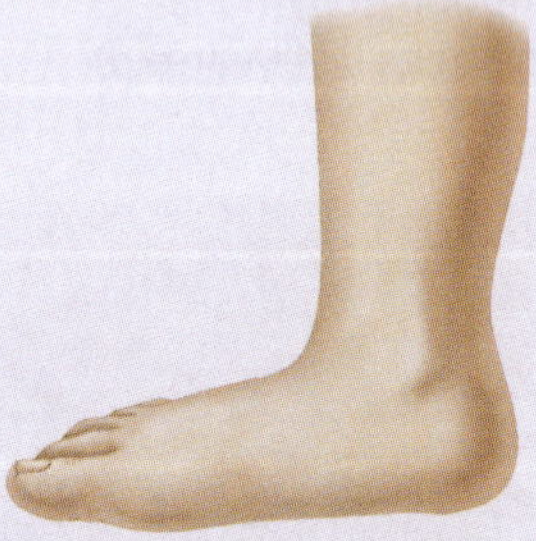

Flat feet or *pes planus* from laxity of the soft tissue structures of the foot

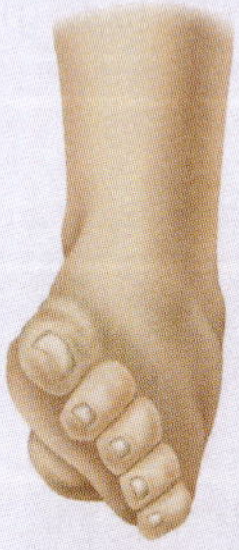

Inversion of the foot (*varus*)

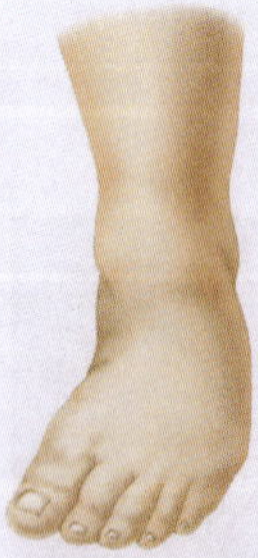

Metatarsus adductus in a child. The forefoot is adducted and not inverted.

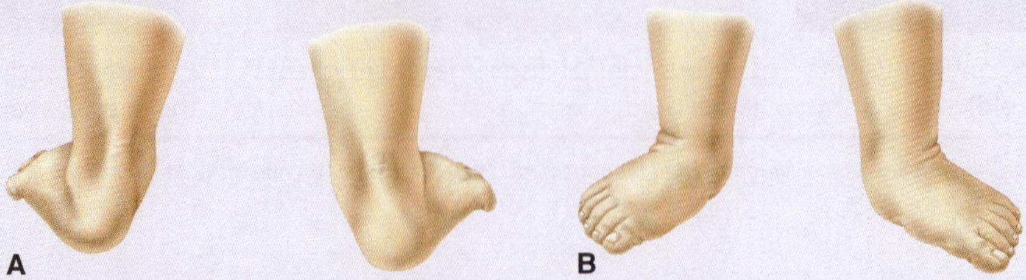

Pronation in a toddler. **A:** When viewed from behind, the hindfoot is everted. **B:** When viewed from the front, the forefoot is everted and abducted.

TABLE 23-15. Power of Prevention: Vaccine-Preventable Diseases

This table shows photographs of children with vaccine-preventable diseases. Childhood vaccines have been named the single most important clinical intervention in the world in terms of influence on public health. Because of vaccinations, we hope you will never see many of these conditions, but you should be able to identify them. Try to identify the diseases before reading the captions.

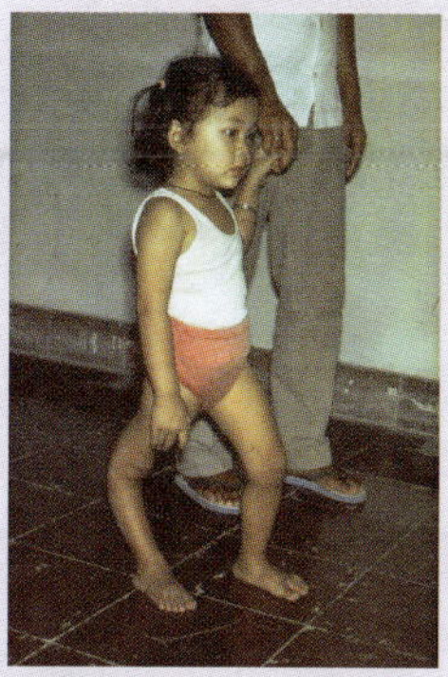

Polio

The deformed leg of this child is from polio

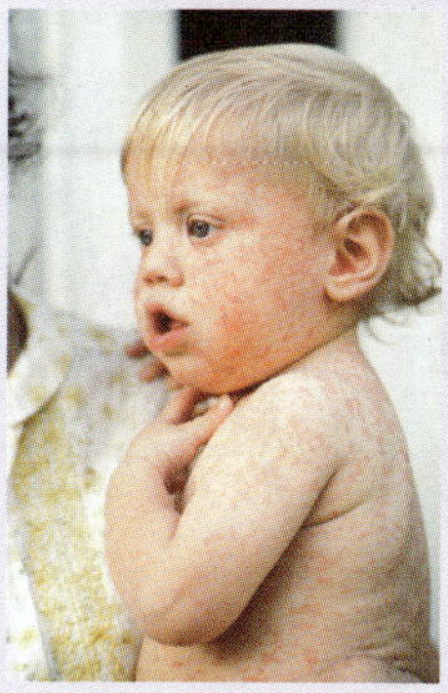

Measles

Characteristic rash of measles, in the presence of a child who also has coryza, conjunctivitis, fever, and this diffuse rash

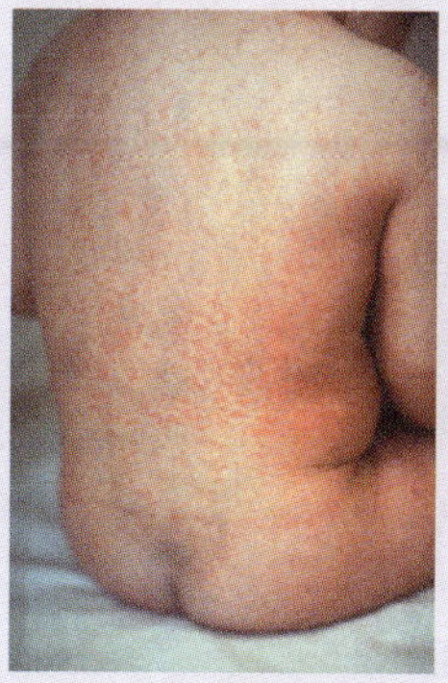

Rubella

Rubella rash on a child's back

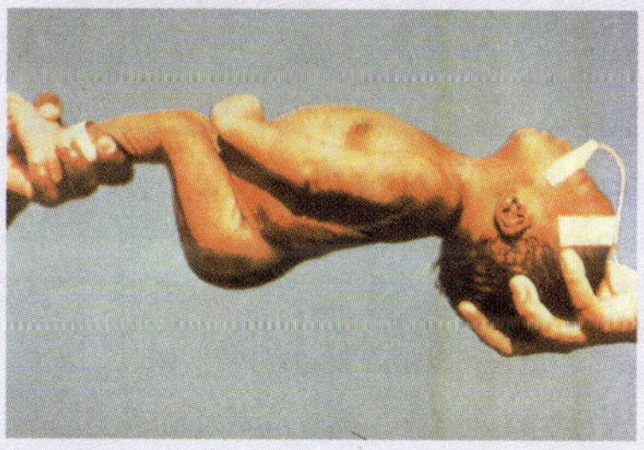

Tetanus

Rigid newborn with neonatal tetanus

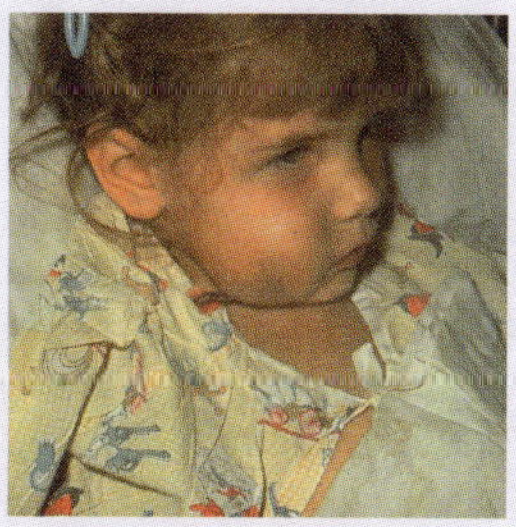

***Haemophilus Influenzae* Type b**

Buccal cellulitis from this invasive bacterial disease

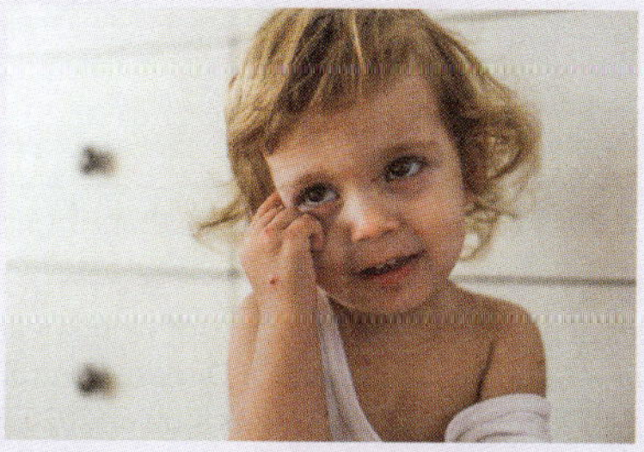

Varicella

An infant with a severe form of varicella.

(continued)

TABLE 23-15. Power of Prevention: Vaccine-Preventable Diseases *(Continued)*

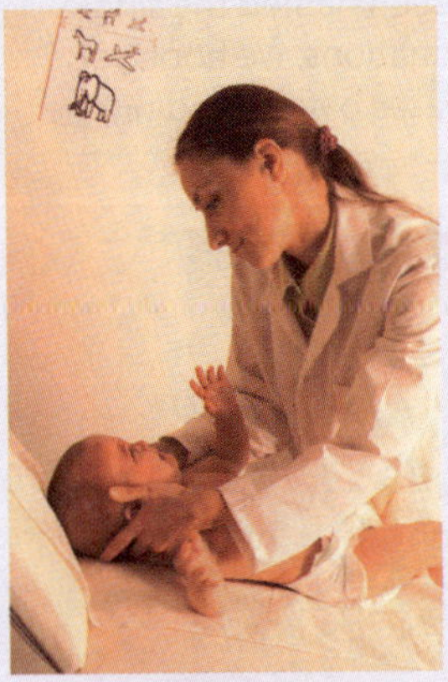

Meningitis

Nuchal rigidity

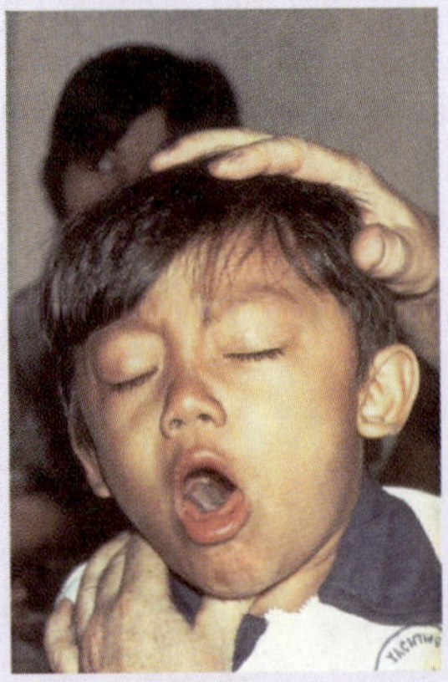

Pertussis

Paroxysmal cough with a "whoop" at the end

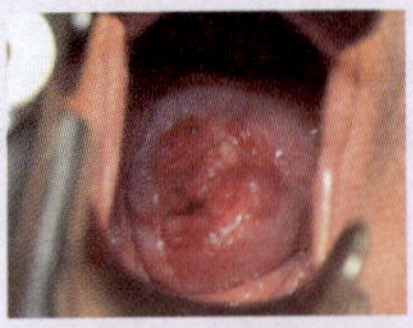

Cervical Cancer

Largely prevented through vaccination with human papillomavirus vaccine.

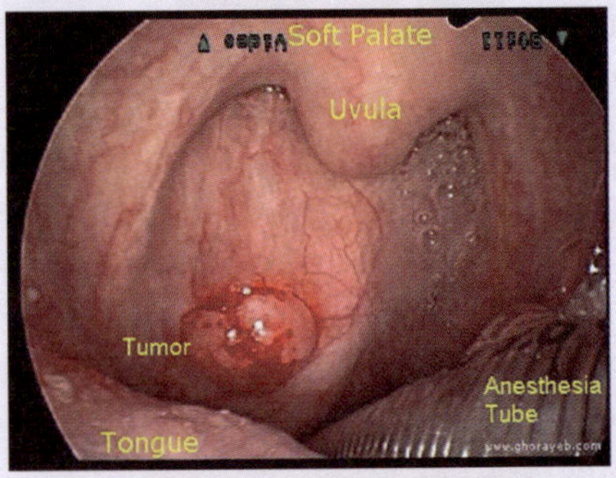

Sequelae of Human Papillomavirus: Oropharyngeal Cancer.

Sources of photos: *Polio*—Courtesy of World Health Organization; *Haemophilus influenzae*—Courtesy of Children's Immunization Project, St. Paul, Minnesota; *Tetanus*—Courtesy of Centers for Disease Control and Prevention. *Pertussis*—Courtesy of Centers for Disease Control and Prevention; *Varicella*—Tagher G, Knapp L. *Pediatric Nursing.* Wolters Kluwer; 2020, Fig. 29-8; *Cervical Cancer*—Berek J. *Berek & Novak's Gynecology.* 16th ed. Wolters Kluwer; 2020, Fig. 38-1; *Oropharyngeal Cancer*—From http://www.ghorayeb.com/OropharyngealCarcinoma.html. Reprinted with permission from Bechara Y. Ghorayeb, MD.

CHAPTER

24

Pregnant Woman

ANATOMY AND PHYSIOLOGY

Physiologic Hormonal Changes

Multiple physiologic changes occur in the setting of normal pregnancy, many mediated by endocrinologic changes. These complex, albeit normal, hormonal variations of pregnancy result in visible changes in anatomy (Fig. 24-1). The basal metabolic rate increases 15% to 20% during pregnancy, increasing daily energy demands by an estimated 85, 285, and 475 kcal/d in the first, second, and third trimesters, respectively.

- *Estrogen* promotes endometrial growth that supports the early embryo. It appears to stimulate marked enlargement of the pituitary gland (by up to 135%) and increased prolactin output from its anterior lobe, which readies breast tissue for lactation. Estrogen also contributes to the hypercoagulable state that puts pregnant women at four to five times higher risk for thromboembolic events, primarily in the venous system.
- *Progesterone* levels increase throughout pregnancy, leading to increased tidal volume and alveolar minute ventilation, though respiratory rate remains constant; respiratory alkalosis and subjective shortness of breath result from these changes. Decreased gastrointestinal motility from progesterone contributes to gastroesophageal reflux, constipation, and biliary diseases in pregnancy (such as cholelithiasis and cholestasis). Progesterone relaxes tone in the ureters and bladder, causing hydronephrosis (in the right ureter more than the left) and an increased risk of bacteriuria.
- *Human chorionic gonadotropin (hCG)* has five variant subtypes. Two are crucial to maintaining the pregnancy, one produced by the corpus luteum in early pregnancy to stabilize the endometrium and prevent loss of the early embryo. The other is produced by the placenta throughout gestation, supporting progesterone synthesis. Serum and urine pregnancy assays test primarily for the two pregnancy-related hCG variants; the other three isoforms are produced by different cancers and the pituitary gland.
- *Placental growth hormone* influences fetal growth and the development of preeclampsia. *Human placental lactogen* (related to the placental growth hormone family) and other hormones contribute to insulin

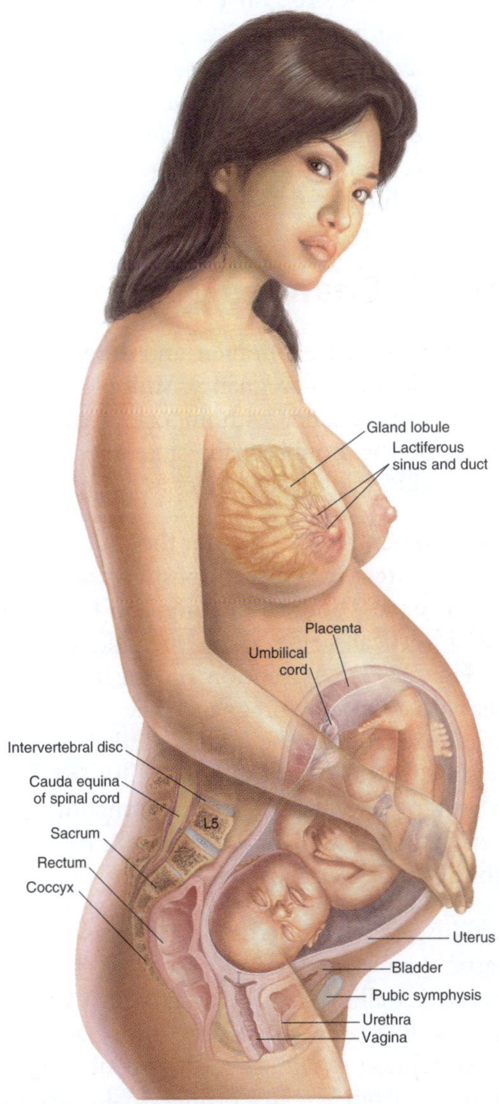

FIGURE 24-1. Pregnant woman with breast and uterine changes. Anatomic relation of uterus with near-term infant to nearby structures also shown.

resistance during pregnancy and the development of gestational diabetes (GDM), which carries a lifetime risk of progressing to type 2 diabetes of up to 60%.

- *Thyroid function* changes include an increase in *thyroid-binding globulin* due to rising levels of estrogen and cross-stimulation of *thyroid-stimulating hormone (TSH)* receptors by beta-hCG. This results in a slight increase, usually in the normal range, in serum concentrations of free T3 and T4, while serum TSH concentrations appropriately decrease. This transient apparent "hyperthyroidism" should be considered physiologic. Normal pregnancy is considered a euthyroid state throughout all trimesters.
- *Relaxin* is secreted by the corpus luteum and placenta and is involved in the remodeling of reproductive tract connective tissue to facilitate delivery, increased renal hemodynamics, and increased serum osmolality. Despite its name, relaxin does not affect peripheral joint laxity during pregnancy.
- *Erythropoietin* increases during pregnancy, which raises erythrocyte mass. Plasma volume increases to a greater extent, causing relative hemodilution and physiologic anemia, which can protect against blood loss during birth.

Anatomic Changes

Changes in the breasts, abdomen, and urogenital tract are the most visible signs of pregnancy. Multiple organ systems are affected in pregnancy with important changes to the physiology of the nonpregnant state (see Table 24-1, Anatomic and Physiologic Changes in Normal Pregnancy.

External Abdomen. As the skin over the abdomen stretches to accommodate the fetus, purplish *striae gravidarum* or "stretch marks" and a **linea nigra**, a brownish black pigmented vertical stripe along the midline skin, may appear (Fig. 24-2). As tension on the abdominal wall increases with advancing pregnancy, the rectus abdominis muscles may separate at the midline, called *diastasis recti*. If diastasis is severe, especially in multiparous women, only a layer of skin, fascia, and peritoneum may cover the anterior uterine wall, and fetal parts may be palpable through this muscular gap.

Uterus. Muscle cell hypertrophy, increases in fibrous and elastic tissue, and development of blood vessels and lymphatics all contribute to growth of the uterus. The uterus increases in weight from approximately 70 g at conception to almost 1,100 g at delivery, when it accommodates from 5 to 20 L of fluid. In the first trimester, the uterus is confined to the pelvis and shaped like an inverted pear; it may retain its prior *anteverted* (forward-leaning), *retroverted* (backward-leaning), or *retroflexed*

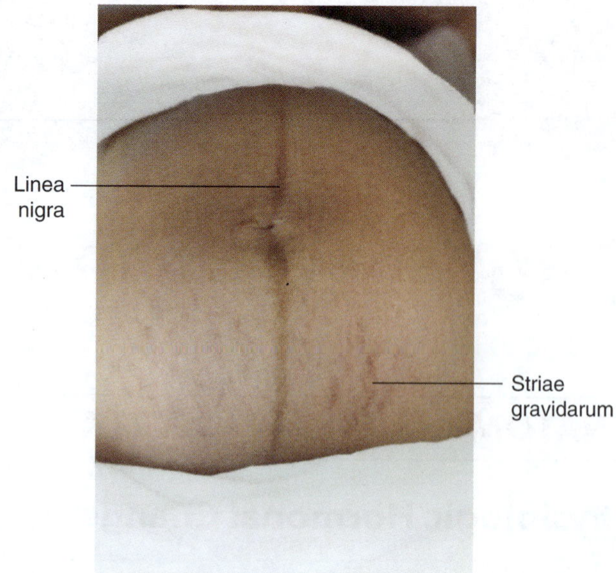

FIGURE 24-2. Striae gravidarum or "stretch marks" and linea nigra in the abdomen.

(backward-bent) position. By the second trimester (12 to 14 weeks), the gravid uterus becomes externally palpable as it expands into a globular shape beyond the pelvic brim. Also, during this time, the enlarging fetus pushes the uterus into an anteverted position that encroaches into the space usually occupied by the bladder, triggering frequent voiding. The intestines are displaced laterally and superiorly. There is also a slight uterine dextrorotation to accommodate the rectosigmoid structures on the left side of the pelvis.

The uterus stretches its own supporting ligaments, causing *"round ligament pain"* in the lower quadrants.

This dextrorotation leads to greater discomfort on the right side as well as increased right-sided hydronephrosis.

Growth patterns of the gravid uterus are shown in Figure 24-3, demonstrating the correlation between gestational age and measurable fundal height. Sagittal

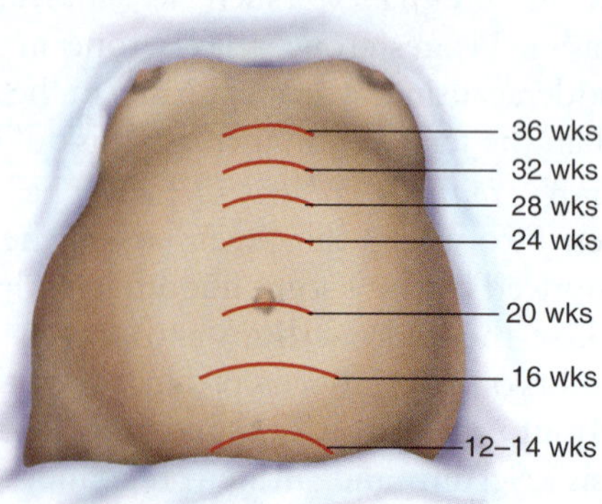

FIGURE 24-3. Uterine fundal height by weeks of pregnancy.

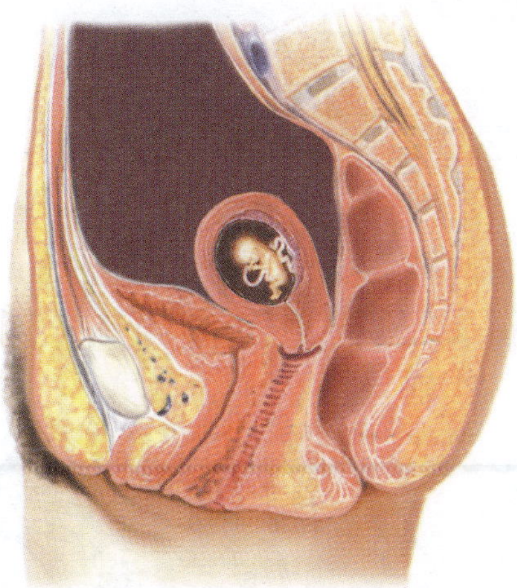

FIGURE 24-4. Sagittal depiction of the gravid abdomen during first trimester (1–12 weeks).

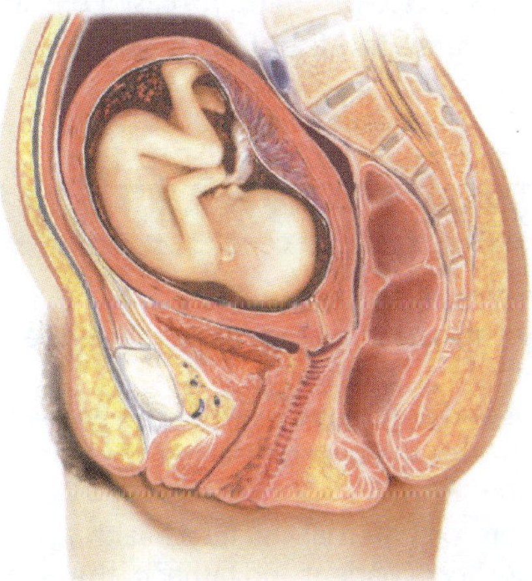

FIGURE 24-5. Sagittal depiction of the gravid abdomen during second trimester (13–26 weeks).

depictions of the gravid abdomen during each trimester appear in Figures 24-4 to 24-6.

Vagina. Increased vascularity throughout the pelvis gives the vagina and cervix a bluish color, known as the **Chadwick sign**. The vaginal walls appear deeply rugated due to thicker mucosa, loosening of connective tissue, and hypertrophy of smooth muscle cells. Normal vaginal secretions may become thick, white, and more profuse, known as **leukorrhea of pregnancy**. Increased glycogen stores in the vaginal epithelium give rise to a proliferation of Lactobacillus acidophilus, which lowers the vaginal pH. This acidification protects against some vaginal infections, but at the same time, increased glycogen may contribute to higher rates of vaginal candidiasis.

Cervix. Approximately 1 month after conception, the cervix softens and also becomes bluish or cyanotic in color,

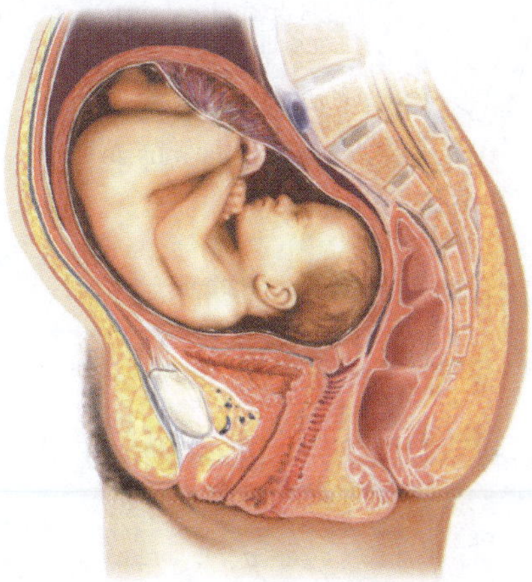

FIGURE 24-6. Sagittal depiction of the gravid abdomen during third trimester (27–40 weeks).

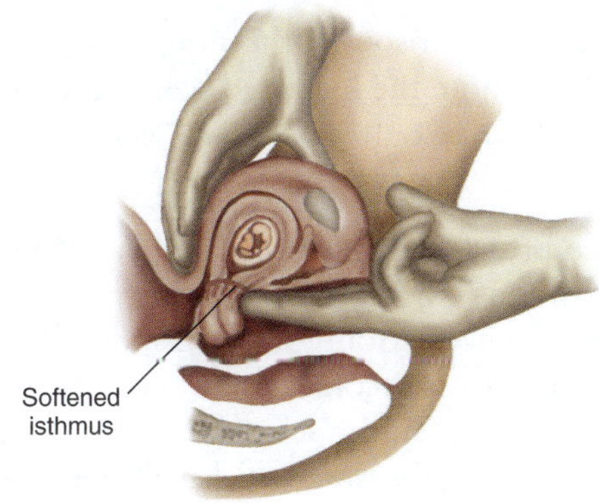

FIGURE 24-7. Hegar sign, palpable softening of the cervical isthmus.

reflecting the increased vascularity, edema, and glandular hyperplasia throughout the cervix. *Hegar sign* is the palpable softening of the cervical isthmus, the portion of the uterus that narrows into the cervix, illustrated in Figure 24-7. This cervical remodeling involves rearrangement of the cervical connective tissue that decreases collagen concentration and facilitates **cervical dilation** during delivery. Copious cervical secretions fill the cervical canal soon after conception with a tenacious mucus plug that protects the uterine environment from outside pathogens and is expelled as bloody show at delivery.

Adnexae. Early in pregnancy, the corpus luteum, which is the ovarian follicle that has discharged its ovum, may be prominent enough to be felt on the affected ovary as a small nodule; this disappears by mid-pregnancy as the placenta takes over hormonal support of the developing pregnancy.

Breasts. The breasts become moderately enlarged due to hormonal stimulation that causes increased vascularity and glandular hyperplasia (Fig. 24-8). By the end of the first

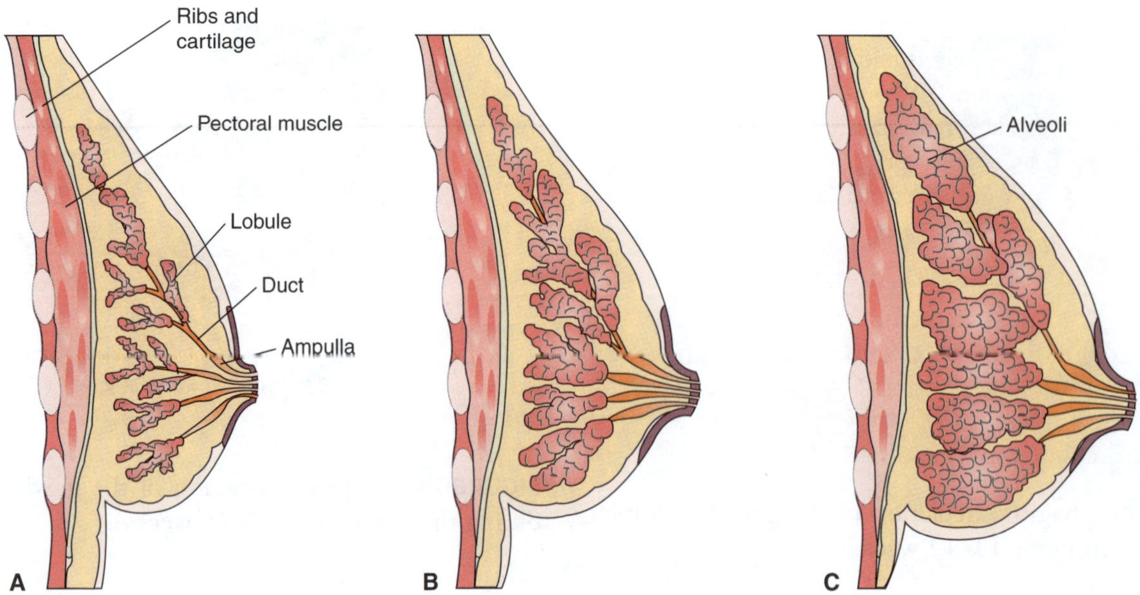

FIGURE 24-8. Comparison of the nonpregnant, nonlactating, adult breast (**A**); pregnant breast (**B**); and lactating breast (**C**). In C, note the increased size of the overall breast, as well as its ducts and lobules. (From Evans RJ et al. *Canadian Maternity, Newborn & Women's Health Nursing*. 2nd ed. Wolters Kluwer; 2015, Fig. 21-3.)

trimester, the breasts become more nodular. The nipples become larger and more erectile, with darker areolae and more pronounced Montgomery glands. The venous pattern over the breasts becomes visibly more prominent as pregnancy progresses. In the second and third trimesters, some women secrete *colostrum*, a thick, yellowish, nutrient-rich precursor to milk. Breast tenderness may make them more sensitive during examination.

HEALTH HISTORY: GENERAL APPROACH

Prenatal visits are an opportunity to engage the pregnant adult in routine medical care and optimize obstetric outcomes for both mother and fetus. In general, the prenatal visit should review symptoms of concern for the pregnant patient, assess maternal and fetal well-being, and provide anticipatory guidance for the upcoming gestational weeks before the next visit. While many pregnant patients will present for care with a family member or partner present, the examiner should also remember to interview the patient privately, as some components of the history and health screening may be unknown to the other people in the room who are present to support the patient. This is particularly true with respect to past obstetric history, attitudes toward the pregnancy, substance use, sexually transmitted infections, and intimate partner violence. During the initial visit, take the health history while she is still clothed.

Components of the Initial Prenatal Visit

- Confirmation of pregnancy
- Determining gestational age and expected date of delivery
- Symptoms of pregnancy
- Concerns and attitudes toward the pregnancy
- Current health and past clinical history
- Past obstetric history
- Risk factors for maternal and fetal health
- Family history of patient and father of the newborn
- Plans for genetic screening and aneuploidy testing
- Plans for breastfeeding
- Plans for postpartum contraception

Initial Prenatal History

Prenatal care focuses on optimizing health and minimizing risk for the mother and fetus.

The goals of the initial prenatal visit are to define the health status of the mother and fetus, confirm the pregnancy and estimate gestational age, develop a plan for continuing care, and counsel the mother about her expectations and concerns. Initial prenatal visits are best timed early in pregnancy but may occur at later in gestation; tailor your history to where it falls during the mother's gestational cycle. During subsequent visits, you should assess any interval changes in the health status of both the mother and fetus, review specific physical examination findings related to the pregnancy, and provide counseling and timely preventive screenings.

Confirmation of Pregnancy. Ask about confirmation of pregnancy: Has the patient had a confirmatory urine pregnancy test, and when? When was her last menstrual period (LMP)? Has she had an ultrasound to establish dates? Explain that serum pregnancy tests are rarely required to confirm pregnancy.

Determining Gestational Age and Expected Date of Delivery. Accurate dating is best done early and contributes to appropriate management of the pregnancy (Box 24-1). Dating establishes the timeframe for reassuring the patient about normal progress, establishing paternity, timing screening tests, tracking fetal growth, and effectively triaging preterm and postdated labor.

Symptoms of Pregnancy. Has the patient had missed periods, breast tenderness, nausea or vomiting, fatigue, or urinary frequency? See Box 24-2 for a list of normal as well as concerning symptoms.

Concerns and Attitudes Toward Pregnancy. Ask how the patient feels about the pregnancy. Is she excited, concerned, or scared? Was the pregnancy planned and desired? If not, does she plan to complete the pregnancy to term, terminate, or consider adoption? Is a partner, father of the baby, or other family support network involved? As you elicit her viewpoints, use open-ended questions and be flexible and nonjudgmental. Respect diverse family structures, such as extended family support, single parenthood, or pregnancy conceived by sperm donation with or without a partner of either gender. Support the patient's choices when unexpected admissions arise, such as a pregnancy resulting from a coerced sexual act, or the wish to end the pregnancy.

Box 24-1. Determining Gestational Age and the Expected Date of Delivery

- **Gestational age.** To establish gestational age, count the number of weeks and days from the first day of the LMP. If the actual date of conception is known (as with in vitro fertilization), a conception age which is 2 weeks less than the menstrual age can be used to calculate *menstrual age* (i.e., a corrected or adjusted LMP dating) to establish dating. Counting this menstrual age from the LMP, although biologically distinct from date of conception, is the standard means of calculating fetal age, yielding an average pregnancy length of 40 weeks.
- **Expected date of delivery (EDD).** The EDD is 40 weeks from the first date of the LMP. Using the *Naegele rule*, the EDD can be estimated by taking the LMP, adding 7 days, subtracting 3 months, and adding 1 year. For example:
  - LMP = November 26, 2020
  - +7 days = December 2, 2020
  - −3 months = September 2, 2020
  - +1 year = September 2, 2021 = EDD
- **Limitations on pregnancy dating.** Patient recall of the LMP is highly variable. Even when this date is accurate, the LMP can be affected by hormonal contraceptives, menstrual irregularities, or variations in ovulation that result in atypical cycle lengths. LMP dating should be checked against physical examination markers such as fundal height, and any wide discrepancies should be clarified by ultrasound evaluation. In clinical practice, dating by ultrasound is widespread, regardless of the certainty of the LMP, even though this approach is not currently endorsed by national guidelines.

Current Health and Past Clinical History. Explore any past or present clinical conditions. Pay particular attention to conditions that affect pregnancy, such as abdominal surgeries, hypertension, diabetes, cardiac disorders including childhood surgery for congenital heart disease, asthma, autoimmune disorders, hypercoagulability states from lupus anticoagulant or anticardiolipin antibodies, mental health disorders such as postpartum depression, human immunodeficiency virus (HIV), sexually transmitted infections (STIs), and abnormal Pap smears.

Past Obstetric History. How many prior pregnancies has the patient had? How many were term deliveries, preterm deliveries, spontaneous and terminated pregnancies, and how many were live births? Were preterm births spontaneous or iatrogenic? Were there any complications from diabetes, hypertension, preeclampsia, intrauterine growth restriction, or preterm labor in any of the prior pregnancies? Were deliveries by vaginal delivery, assisted delivery (vacuum or forceps), or cesarean section? Were there any complications during labor and delivery such as large babies (fetal macrosomia), fetal distress, or emergency interventions? Were prior deliveries complicated by shoulder dystocia or postpartum hemorrhage?

A nomenclature for pregnancy outcomes has been developed and has evolved over time. It is often part of any oral or written communication related to a woman's reproductive history. *Gravidity* refers to the number of times that a woman has been pregnant, and *parity* is the number of times that she has given birth to a fetus to a viable age (≥24 gestational weeks), regardless of whether the child was born alive or was stillborn. For example, a woman who is described as "gravida 2, para 2" (G2P2) has had two pregnancies and two deliveries after 24 weeks, and a woman who is described as "gravida 2, para 0" (G2P0) has had two pregnancies, neither of which survived to a gestational age of 24 weeks.

Parity is further broken down into *term deliveries, preterm deliveries, abortions* (spontaneous abortions and terminated pregnancies), and *living children,* which yields the mnemonic "TPAL" when listed in that order. A woman with two spontaneous losses prior to 20 weeks'

Box 24-2. Common Concerns during Pregnancy and Their Explanations

Common Concerns	Trimester	Explanation
Abdominal pain (lower)	Second	Rapid growth in the second trimester causes tension and stretching of the round ligaments that support the uterus, causing sharp or cramping pain with movement or position change
Abdominal striae	Second or third	Stretching of the skin and tearing of the collagen in the dermis contribute to thin, usually pink, bands, or *striae gravidarum* (stretch marks). These may persist or fade over time after delivery.
Amenorrhea (missed periods)	All	High levels of estrogen, progesterone, and hCG build up the endometrium and prevent menses, causing a missed period, which is often the first noticeable sign of pregnancy.
Backache	All	Hormonally induced relaxation of the pelvic ligaments contributes to musculoskeletal aches. Lordosis required to balance the gravid uterus contributes to lower back strain. Breast enlargement may contribute to upper backaches.
Breast tenderness/ tingling	First	Pregnancy hormones stimulate the growth of breast tissue, which causes swelling and possible aching, tenderness, and tingling. Increased blood flow can make delicate veins more visible beneath the skin.
Constipation	All	Constipation results from slowed gastrointestinal transit due to hormonal changes, dehydration from nausea and vomiting, and the supplemental iron in prenatal vitamins.
Contractions	Third	Irregular and unpredictable uterine contractions (*Braxton Hicks* contractions) are rarely associated with labor. Contractions that become regular or painful should be evaluated for onset of labor.
Edema	Third	Decreased venous return, obstruction of lymphatic flow, and reduced plasma colloid oncotic pressure commonly cause lower extremity edema. However, sudden severe edema and hypertension may signal preeclampsia.
Fatigue	First/Third	Fatigue is related to the rapid change in energy requirements, sedative effects of progesterone, changes in body mechanics due to the gravid uterus, and sleep disturbance. Many women report increased energy and well-being during the second trimester.
Heartburn	All	Progesterone relaxes the lower esophageal sphincter, allowing gastric contents to reflux into the esophagus. The gravid uterus also exerts physical pressure against the stomach with increasing gestational age, contributing to reflux symptoms.
Hemorrhoids	All	Hemorrhoids may be caused by constipation, decreased venous return from increasing pressure in the pelvis, compression by fetal parts, and changes in activity level during pregnancy.
Loss of mucus plug	Third	Passage of the mucus plug is common during labor but may occur prior to the onset of contractions. As long as there are no regular contractions, bleeding, or loss of fluid, loss of the mucus plug is unlikely to trigger the onset of labor.
Nausea and/or vomiting	First	This is poorly understood but appears to reflect hormonal changes, slowed gastrointestinal peristalsis, alterations in smell and taste, and sociocultural factors. Up to 75% of women experience nausea in pregnancy. Hyperemesis gravidarum is vomiting with weight loss of >5% of prepregnancy weight.
Urinary frequency	All	Increases in blood volume and filtration rate through the kidneys result in increased urine production, while pressure from the gravid uterus reduces potential space for the bladder. Dysuria or suprapubic pain should be investigated for urinary tract infection.
Vaginal discharge	All	Asymptomatic milky white discharge, leukorrhea, results from increased secretions from vaginal and cervical epithelium due to vasocongestion and hormonal changes. Any foul-smelling or pruritic discharge should be investigated.

gestation, three living children who were delivered at term, and a current pregnancy, would be referred to as "G6P3023." One common error is to assign a multiple pregnancy, for example, twins, as a count of two for either gravity or parity. In practice, each pregnancy receives only one count in any of the categories regardless of the number of fetuses, except for *living children,* when all are counted. So, for a first pregnancy with twins delivered at term, the correct designation is G1P1002.

Risk Factors for Maternal and Fetal Health. Does she use tobacco, alcohol, or illicit drugs? What about prescription medications, over-the-counter drugs, or herbal preparations? Does she have any toxic exposures at work, at home, or in other settings? Is her nutritional intake adequate, or is she at risk from obesity? Does she have an adequate social support network and source of income? Are there unusual sources of stress at home or work? Is there any history of physical abuse or intimate partner violence?

Family History. Ask about the genetic and family history of the patient and her partner and/or father. What are the ethnic backgrounds of the patient and father? Is there any family history of genetic diseases such as sickle cell anemia, cystic fibrosis, or muscular dystrophy, among others? Have babies in the family had any congenital problems?

Plans for Genetic Testing and Aneuploidy Screening. All pregnant patients should be offered both aneuploidy screening and diagnostic genetic testing to rule out common chromosomal aneuploidies, such as trisomies 21, 18, and 13 and sex-chromosome abnormalities. Additionally, carrier screening for certain autosomal-recessive disorders such as Tay–Sachs disease, spinal muscular atrophy (SMA), cystic fibrosis (CF), and fragile X syndrome is recommended for targeted screening along with hemoglobin electrophoresis to test for hemoglobinopathies.

Plans for Breastfeeding. Breastfeeding protects the baby against a variety of infectious and noninfectious conditions and exerts a protective effect on the mother against breast cancer and other conditions. Education during pregnancy and clinician encouragement increase the subsequent rate and duration of maternal breastfeeding.

Plans for Postpartum Contraception. Initiate this discussion early, as postpartum contraception reduces the risk of unintended pregnancy and shortened interpregnancy intervals, which are linked to increases in adverse pregnancy outcomes. Plans for contraception will depend on the patient's preferences, clinical history, and decision about breastfeeding.

Concluding the Initial Visit. As you conclude the visit, reaffirm your commitment to the woman's health and her concerns during pregnancy. Review your findings, discuss any tests or screenings that are needed, and ask if she has further questions. Reinforce the need for regular prenatal care and review the timing of future visits. Record your findings in the prenatal record.

Subsequent Prenatal Visits

Though the optimal number of prenatal appointments has not been well established, obstetric visits traditionally follow a set schedule: monthly until 28 gestational weeks, then biweekly until 36 weeks, then weekly until delivery. Update and document the history at every visit, especially fetal movement felt by the patient, contractions, leakage of fluid, and vaginal bleeding. The physical examination findings at every visit should include vital signs (especially blood pressure and weight), fundal height, verification of fetal heart rate (FHR), and determination of fetal position and activity, as described in Techniques of Examination to follow. At each visit, the urine should be tested for infection, glucose, and protein.

PHYSICAL EXAMINATION: GENERAL APPROACH

As with history taking, the physical examination in the pregnant woman is primarily focused and problem based. The exception is the first prenatal visit, when a complete physical examination is required and includes a breast and pelvic examination of the gravid patient. Patients may resist any part of this examination. This reluctance may stem from personal circumstances (e.g., sexual assault) or cultural boundaries which should be explored and understood.

Due to both the physiologic changes of pregnancy and the sensitive nature of the examination, priority must be given to the patient's comfort and privacy, considering her individual and cultural sensitivities. If partners or children are present, ask if she wants them to stay during the physical examination. If she has never had a pelvic examination, take the time to explain what is involved and seek her cooperation with each step. Concerns about modesty should be balanced against the need for a complete examination.

To ease examination of the breasts and abdomen, ask the patient to wear a gown with the opening in front. Make sure that the equipment and examining tables accommodate pregnant patients who are obese. Also, this may be the opportune time to ask the patient to empty her bladder prior to starting especially prior to the pelvic examination.

TECHNIQUES OF EXAMINATION

Key Components of the Examination of the Pregnant Woman

- Assess general health, emotional state, nutritional status, and neuromuscular coordination.
- Measure height and weight. Calculate BMI.
- Measure the blood pressure at every visit.
- Inspect the head and neck (facial skin changes or edema, hair condition and distribution, conjunctival pallor, nasal congestion or epistaxis, teeth and gum health, thyroid masses or nodules).
- Inspect, percuss, and auscultate the thorax and lungs.
- Palpate location of the apical impulse.
- Auscultate the heart (S_1 splitting, murmurs, venous hum or mammary souffle).
- Inspect the abdomen (striae, scars, size, shape, and contour).
- Palpate the abdomen (masses, fetal movement, uterine contractility and fundal height).
- Auscultate fetal heart tones (location, rate and rhythm).
- Inspect the external genitalia (labial varicosities, cystoceles, rectoceles, lesions, sores, Bartholin and Skene gland tenderness and cysts).
- Inspect the internal genitalia by performing speculum and bimanual examinations.
  - *Speculum examination:* Inspect the cervix (color, shape, os closure) and vaginal walls (color, relaxation, rugae, and discharge). Perform a Pap smear if indicated.
  - *Bimanual examination:* Palpate the cervix (length, os), uterus (shape, consistency, and position), adnexa (masses, tenderness), pelvic floor strength.
- Inspect the anus (masses or hemorrhoids).
- Examine the extremities (varicosities, edema) and elicit reflexes (hyperreflexia).
- Perform Leopold maneuvers (if indicated).

Positioning

In early pregnancy, the patient can be examined in the supine position. In later trimesters, the patient should adopt the semi-sitting position with the knees bent (Fig. 24-9) or with a slight leftward decubitus position. This position is more comfortable and reduces the weight of the gravid uterus on the descending aorta and inferior vena cava. The pregnant woman should avoid lying supine for long periods. Most portions of the examination (except the pelvic examination) should be done in the sitting or left-side-lying position.

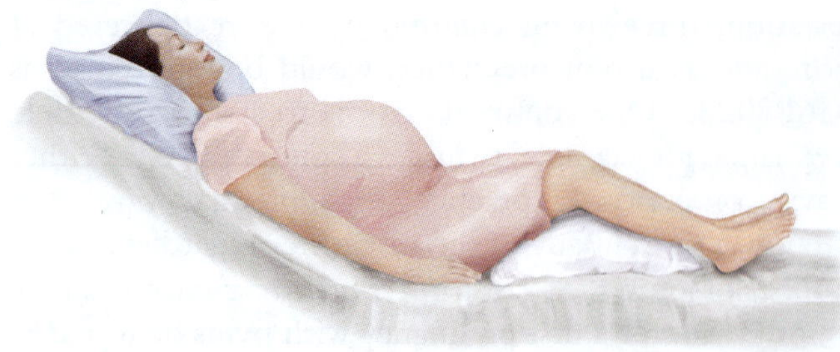

FIGURE 24-9. Semi-sitting position of the pregnant person for examination.

Compression interferes with venous return from the lower extremities and pelvic vessels, causing the patient to feel dizzy and faint, also known as *supine hypotension*.

During the examination, encourage the patient to sit upright if she feels lightheaded; make sure she takes her time if she needs to stand up. Complete your examination relatively quickly.

Examining Equipment

Make your touch and hand motions comforting as you examine the pregnant woman. Warm your hands and use firm yet gentle palpation rather than abrupt pressure or kneading. When possible, keep your fingers flattened together in smooth continuous contact with the skin on the abdominal surface. The palmar surfaces of your fingertips are the most sensitive.

Before beginning the examination, gather the equipment listed in Box 24-3.

General Inspection

Assess the general health, emotional state, nutritional status, and neuromuscular coordination of the patient as she walks into the room and moves onto the examining table.

Height, Weight, and Vital Signs

Measure the height and weight. Calculate the body mass index (BMI) at the first prenatal visit with standard tables, using 19 to 25 as normal.

Weight loss due to nausea and vomiting that exceeds 5% of prepregnancy weight is considered excessive, representing *hyperemesis gravidarum,* and can lead to adverse pregnancy outcomes.

Measure the blood pressure at every visit. Blood pressure parameters in pregnancy follow the recommendations of the Eighth Joint National Committee (JNC8). Baseline prepregnancy readings are important for determining the patient's usual range. In the second trimester, blood pressure normally drops below the nonpregnant state.

Box 24-3. Equipment for Examining the Pregnant Woman

- *Gynecologic speculum and lubrication:* Due to vaginal wall relaxation during pregnancy, a larger-than-usual speculum may be needed in multiparous patients.
- *Sampling materials:* Because of the increased vascularity of vaginal and cervical structures, the cervical brush may cause bleeding that interferes with Pap smear samples, so the "broom" sampling device is preferred during pregnancy. Use additional swabs as needed to screen for STIs, group B strep, and wet mount preparations.
- *Tape measure:* A plastic or paper tape measure is used to assess the size of the uterus after 20 gestational weeks.
- *Doppler fetal monitor and gel:* to assess fetal heart tones after 10 weeks' gestation.

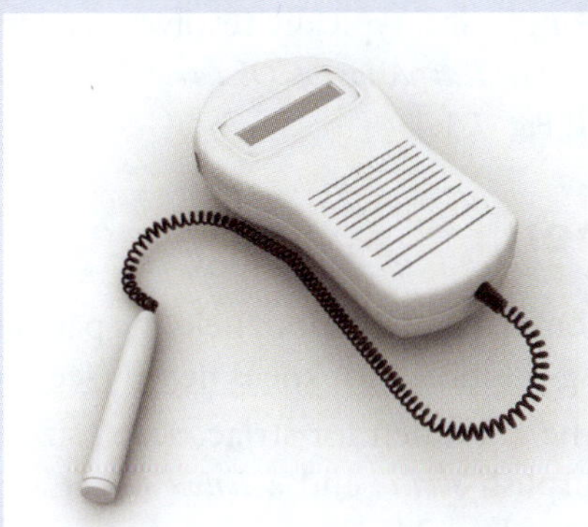

Handheld Doppler monitor.

Hypertensive disorders affect 5% to 10% of all pregnancies and can affect virtually every organ system so all elevations in blood pressure must be closely monitored.

Gestational hypertension is systolic blood pressure (SBP) >140 mm Hg or diastolic blood pressure (DBP) >90 mm Hg first documented after 20 weeks, without proteinuria or other evidence of preeclampsia, that resolves by 12 weeks postpartum.

Hypertension can be both an independent diagnosis and a marker of preeclampsia (Box 24-4). Preeclampsia increases cardiovascular disease risk eight- to ninefold in women with preeclampsia giving birth before 34 weeks' gestation.

Box 24-4. Definition of Preeclampsia

SBP ≥140 or DBP ≥90 after 20 weeks on two occasions at least 4 hours apart in a woman with previously normal BP or BP ≥160/110 confirmed within minutes *and* proteinuria ≥300 mg/24 hours, protein to creatinine ratio ≥0.3, or dipstick 1+;

OR

New-onset hypertension without proteinuria and any of the following: thrombocytopenia (platelets <100,000/µL), impaired liver function (liver transaminase levels more than twice normal), new renal insufficiency (creatinine >1.1 mg/dL or doubles in the absence of renal disease), pulmonary edema, or new-onset cerebral or visual symptoms.

Chronic hypertension is SBP >140 or DBP >90 that predates pregnancy or is diagnosed in the first 20 weeks' gestation.

Count the respiratory rate, which should remain normal throughout pregnancy.

Dyspnea accompanied by increased respiratory rate, cough, crackles, or respiratory distress points to possible infection, asthma, pulmonary embolus, or peripartum cardiomyopathy.

Head and Neck

Face the seated patient and inspect the head and neck, paying particular attention to the following features:

Face. Irregular brownish patches around the forehead, cheeks, nose, and jaw are known as *chloasma* or **melasma**, the "mask of pregnancy," a normal skin finding during pregnancy.

Facial edema after 20 gestational weeks is suspicious for preeclampsia and should be investigated.

Hair. Hair may become dry, oily, or sparse during pregnancy; mild hirsutism on the face, abdomen, and extremities is also common.

Localized patches of hair loss should not be attributed to pregnancy (though postpartum hair loss is common).

Eyes. Assess the conjunctivae and sclera for signs of pallor and jaundice.

Anemia may cause conjunctival pallor.

Nose. Inspect the mucous membranes and septum. Nasal congestion and nose bleeds are more common during pregnancy due to vascular congestion from increased circulating blood volume.

Erosions and perforations of the nasal septum may represent use of intranasal cocaine.

Mouth. Examine the teeth and gums. Gingival enlargement with bleeding is common during pregnancy.

Dental problems are associated with poor pregnancy outcomes, so initiate prompt dental referrals for tooth and gum pain or infections.

Thyroid gland. Modest symmetric enlargement caused by glandular hyperplasia and increased vascularity is normal on inspection and palpation.

Thyroid enlargement, goiters, and nodules are abnormal and require investigation.

Thorax and Lungs

Inspect the thorax for contours and breathing patterns. Percuss to observe diaphragmatic elevation that may be seen as early as the first trimester. Auscultate for clear breath sounds without wheezes, rales, or rhonchi.

Heart

Palpate the apical impulse, which may be rotated upward and to the left toward the fourth intercostal space by the enlarging uterus.

Auscultate the heart. Listen for a *venous hum* or a continuous *mammary souffle* ("a puff of air," pronounced *soo-fuhl*) often found during pregnancy due to increased blood flow through the breast vasculature. The mammary souffle is commonly heard during late pregnancy or lactation, is strongest in the second or third intercostal space at the sternal border bilaterally, and is typically both systolic and diastolic, though only the systolic component may be audible. There may be increased splitting of S_1 due to increased circulating blood volume and 90% of patients will have an audible systolic murmur.

Assess dyspnea and signs of heart failure for possible peripartum cardiomyopathy, particularly in the late stages of pregnancy.

Auscultate for murmurs.

Murmurs may signal anemia but may also be related to the physiologic increase in circulating blood volume. A diastolic murmur in pregnancy is never normal and should be investigated further.

Breasts

The breast examination is similar to that of a nonpregnant woman but with some notable differences.

Inspect the breasts and nipples for symmetry and color. Normal changes include a marked venous pattern, darkened nipples and areolae, and prominent Montgomery glands which typically resolve postpartum (Fig. 24-10).

Inverted nipples need attention at the time of birth if breastfeeding is planned.

Palpate for masses and axillary lymph nodes. Normal breasts may be tender and nodular during pregnancy.

Pathologic masses may be difficult to isolate but warrant immediate attention. Severe focal tenderness with erythema in mastitis requires immediate treatment.

Compress each nipple between your thumb and index finger; colostrum may express from the nipples during later trimesters. Reassure the patient that this is normal and that she may also experience *"let down,"* a spontaneous mild leakage often accompanied by a cramping sensation in the breast during a hot shower or orgasm in the third trimester.

Bloody or purulent discharge should not be attributed to pregnancy.

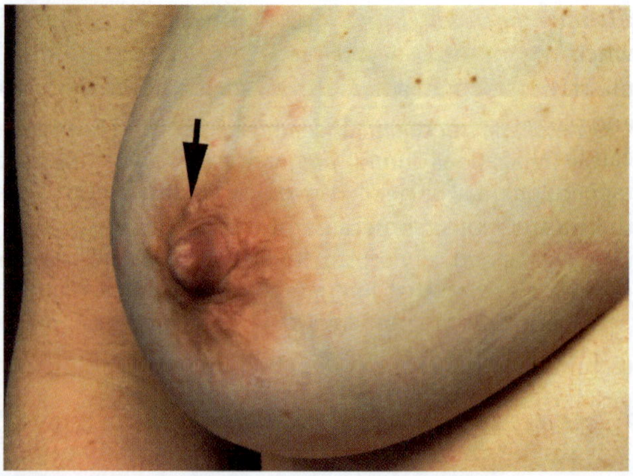

FIGURE 24-10. Hypertrophic areolar sebaceous glands (Montgomery glands). These can be seen in up to 36% of pregnant women and typically resolve postpartum. (From Kroumpouzos G. *Text Atlas of Obstetric Dermatology.* Wolters Kluwer; 2014, Fig. 7-1.)

Abdomen

For the abdominal examination, help the patient move into a semi-sitting position with knees flexed (see Fig. 24-9).

Inspect the abdomen for striae, scars, size, shape, and contour. Purplish *striae* and a *linea nigra* are normal in pregnancy (see Fig. 24-2).

Cesarean scars on the abdomen may not match the orientation of the scar on the uterus, which is important when evaluating whether vaginal delivery is appropriate after cesarean section.

Palpate the abdomen for:

- *Organs and masses.* The mass of the gravid uterus is expected.
- *Fetal movement.* The examiner can usually feel movements externally after 24 gestational weeks; the mother can usually feel these by 18 to 24 weeks. The maternal sensation of fetal movement is traditionally known as "quickening."

  If fetal movement is not felt after 24 weeks, consider a miscalculation of gestational age, fetal death or severe morbidity, or false pregnancy. Confirm fetal health and gestational age with an ultrasound.

- *Uterine contractility.* Irregular uterine contractions occur as early as 12 weeks and may be triggered by external palpation during the third trimester. During contractions, the abdomen feels tense or firm to the examiner, obscuring the palpation of fetal parts; after the contraction, the palpating fingers sense the relaxation of the uterine muscle.

  Before 37 weeks, regular uterine contractions with or without pain and bleeding are abnormal, suggesting preterm labor.

- *Measure the fundal height* if gestational age is >20 weeks, when the fundus should reach the umbilicus. With a plastic or paper tape measure, locate the pubic symphysis and place the "zero" end of the tape measure where you can firmly feel that bone (Fig. 24-11). Then extend the tape measure to the very top of uterine fundus and note the number of centimeters measured. Though subject to error between 16 and 36 weeks, measurement of the **fundal height** in centimeters should roughly equal the number of weeks of gestation. This widely used technique may underdetect newborns who are small for gestational age.

If fundal height is *4 cm larger* than expected, consider multiple gestation, a large fetus, extra amniotic fluid, or uterine leiomyoma. If fundal height is *4 cm smaller* than expected, consider low-level amniotic fluid, missed abortion, intrauterine growth retardation, or fetal anomaly. These conditions should be investigated by ultrasound.

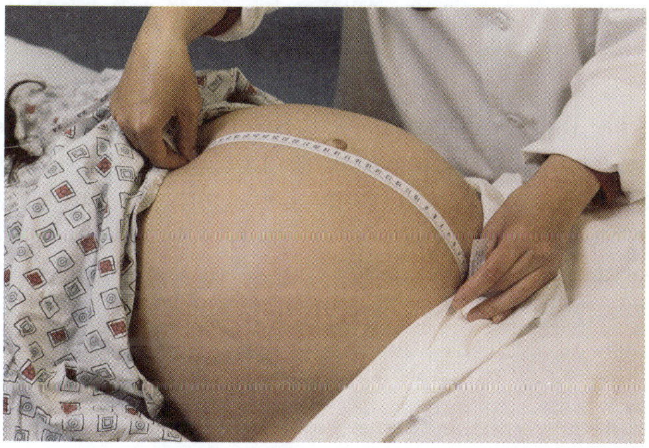

FIGURE 24-11. Measuring the fundal height from the pubic symphysis to the top of the uterine fundus using a tape measure.

- *Auscultate the fetal heart tones.* The Doppler fetal monitor is the standard instrument for measuring **fetal heart tones**, which is normally audible as early as 10 to 12 weeks' gestation. Detection of fetal heart tones may be slightly delayed in patients who are obese.

Inaudible fetal heart tones may indicate fewer weeks of gestation than expected, fetal demise, false pregnancy, or observer error; inability to locate the FHR should always be investigated with formal ultrasound.

- *Location.* From 10 to 18 weeks' gestation, the fetal heart tones are located along the midline of the lower abdomen. After that time, the fetal heart tones are best heard over the back or chest and depend on fetal position; the Leopold maneuvers can help identify the position.

After 24 weeks, auscultation of more than one fetal heart tone in different locations with varying rates suggests multiple gestation.

- *Rate.* The *FHR* ranges between 110 and 160 beats per minute (BPM). A heart rate of 60 to 90 BPM is usually maternal, but an adequate FHR should be confirmed.

Sustained dips in FHR, or *"decelerations,"* have a wide differential diagnosis but always warrant investigation, at least by formal FHR monitoring.

- *Rhythm.* FHR should vary 10 to 15 BPM from second to second, especially later in the pregnancy. After 32 to 34 weeks, the FHR should become more variable and increased with fetal activity. This subtlety can be difficult to assess with a Doppler but can be tracked with an FHR monitor if any questions arise.

Lack of beat-to-beat variability is difficult to discern with a handheld Doppler, so this finding warrants formal FHR monitoring.

Genitalia

For this portion of the examination, the patient will need to be supine with her feet placed in foot rests. Assemble the needed equipment in advance and minimize the time she spends in this position to avoid dizziness and hypotension from uterine compression of the major abdominal vessels.

External Genitalia. Inspect the external genitalia. Relaxation of the vaginal introitus and enlargement of the labia and clitoris are normal changes of pregnancy. In multiparous women, scars from perineal lacerations or episiotomy incisions may be present.

Inspect for labial varicosities, cystoceles, rectoceles, and any lesions or sores.

Labial varicosities that arise during pregnancy can become tortuous and painful. Cystoceles and rectoceles may be pronounced due to the muscle relaxation of pregnancy. Lesions and sores occur with herpes simplex infection.

Palpate the Bartholin and Skene glands for tenderness and cysts.

Internal Genitalia. Prepare for both a speculum and bimanual examination.

Speculum Examination. Relaxation of the perineal and vulvar structures during pregnancy may minimize, but not eliminate, discomfort from the speculum examination. The increased vascularity of vaginal and cervical structures promotes friability, so insert and open the speculum gently to prevent tissue trauma and bleeding. During the third trimester, perform this examination only when necessary as descent of the fetal parts into the pelvis can make the examination very uncomfortable.

- *Inspect the cervix for color, shape, and closure.* Typically, the external os in a nulliparous cervix appears as a circular dot, and in a parous cervix more like an arc or "slit-like." A parous cervix may also look irregular due to healed lacerations from prior deliveries (Fig. 24-12). The inner portion of the cervix everts slightly during pregnancy, called *ectropion*, and appears as a glandular friable darker pink or red area inside the os.

A pink cervix suggests a nonpregnant state. Cervical erosion, erythema, discharge, or irritation suggests cervicitis, and warrants investigation for STIs.

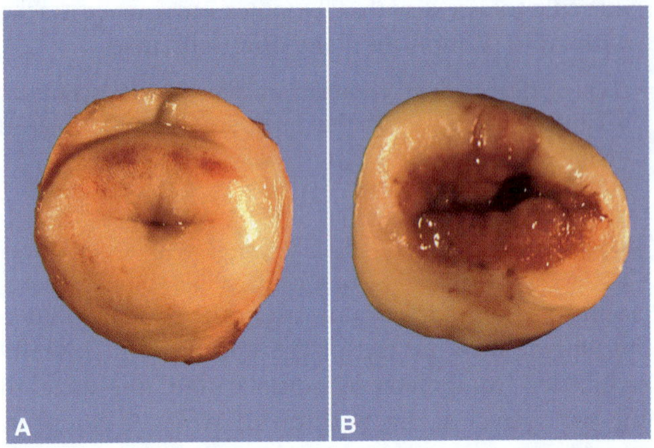

FIGURE 24-12. Typically, the external os in a nulliparous cervix appears as a circular dot (**A**), and in a parous cervix, the opening is wider and more slit-like and gaping (**B**). (From Reichert RA. *Diagnostic Gynecologic and Obstetric Pathology*. Wolters Kluwer; 2012, Fig. 3-1.)

- *Perform a Pap smear if indicated,* and collect other vaginal specimens such as STI cultures, wet mount samples, or group B strep swabs as appropriate.
- *Inspect the vaginal walls* as you withdraw the speculum. Check for color, relaxation, rugae, and discharge. Normal findings include bluish color, deep rugae, and increased milky white discharge, or *leukorrhea*.

Investigate abnormal vaginal discharges for possible candida or bacterial vaginosis, which can affect pregnancy outcome.

Bimanual Examination. Performing the bimanual examination is often easier during pregnancy due to pelvic floor relaxation. Avoiding sensitive urethral structures, insert two lubricated fingers into the introitus, palmar side down, with slight pressure downward on the perineum. Maintaining downward pressure on the perineum, gently turn the fingers palmar side up.

Cervix. Because of softening during pregnancy, or *Hegar sign* (see Fig. 24-7), the cervix may be difficult to identify. If there are nabothian cysts or healed lacerations from prior deliveries, the cervix may feel irregular.

- *Estimate cervical length.* Palpate the lateral surface of the cervical tip to the lateral fornix. Prior to 34 to 36 weeks' gestation, the cervix should retain its initial length of 3 cm or greater.
- *Palpate the cervical os.* This may be easier if the patient moves her heels as close to her buttocks as possible, which shortens the vagina, and places her closed fists under her buttocks to tip the pelvis upward, which makes posterior cervices easier to palpate. The *external os* may be open to admit a fingertip in multiparous women. The *internal os*, the narrow passage between the endocervical canal and the uterine cavity, should be closed until late pregnancy, regardless of parity. The internal os may only be palpable by reaching behind or past the fetal parts.

Cervical opening or shortening (**cervical effacement**) prior to 37 weeks may indicate preterm labor.

- As with the speculum examination, in late pregnancy, examine the cervix only when necessary because palpation is very uncomfortable. Warn patients that it may cause cramping and pressure.

Uterus. With your internal fingers placed at either side of the cervix and the external hand on the patient's abdomen, use the internal fingers to gently lift the uterus upward toward the abdominal hand. Capture the fundal portion of the uterus between your two hands and assess the uterine size, keeping in mind the contours of the gravid uterus at various gestational intervals, depicted in Figure 24-3. Palpate for shape, consistency, and position.

An irregularly shaped uterus suggests uterine leiomyomata, or fibroids, or a bicornuate uterus, one with two distinct cavities separated by a septum.

Adnexa. Palpate the right and left adnexa. The corpus luteum may be palpable as a small nodule on the affected ovary during the first weeks after conception. After the first trimester, adnexal masses become difficult to feel.

Adnexal tenderness or masses early in gestation require ultrasound evaluation to rule out ectopic pregnancy. Acute pelvic inflammatory disease is rare in pregnancy, especially after the first trimester, because the adnexa are sealed by the gravid uterus and mucus plug.

Pelvic floor. Evaluate pelvic floor strength as you withdraw your examining fingers.

Anus, Rectum, and Rectovaginal Septum

Inspect for external hemorrhoids. If present, note their size, location, and any evidence of thrombosis.

Hemorrhoids often become engorged late in pregnancy; they may be painful, bleed, or thrombose.

The rectal examination is not standard in prenatal care unless there are concerning symptoms like rectal bleeding or masses or conditions that compromise the rectovaginal septum. Rectal examination may help you assess the size of a retroverted or retroflexed uterus, but transvaginal ultrasound provides superior information.

Extremities

Ask the patient to resume sitting or to lie on her left side. Inspect the legs for varicose veins.

Varicose veins may begin or worsen during pregnancy.

Palpate the extremities for edema in the pretibial, ankle, and pedal distributions. Although several scales exist based on the extent of edema or the time it takes for a skin indentation to rebound, it is more prudent to describe and record your observation as you would any skin examination finding. Physiologic edema is common in advanced pregnancy, during hot weather, and in women who stand for long periods of time due to decreased venous return from the lower extremities.

Unilateral severe edema with calf tenderness warrants prompt evaluation for DVT. Hand or facial edema after 20 gestational weeks is nonspecific for preeclampsia but should be investigated.

Elicit the *knee* and *ankle deep tendon reflexes.*

Hyperreflexia may signal cortical irritability from preeclampsia, but clinical accuracy is variable.

SPECIAL TECHNIQUES

Leopold Maneuvers

Leopold maneuvers are used to determine the fetal position in the maternal abdomen beginning in the second trimester; accuracy is greatest after 36 weeks' gestation (Fig. 24-13). Although less accurate for assessing fetal growth, these examination findings help determine readiness for vaginal delivery by assessing:

- Upper and lower fetal pole, namely, the proximal and distal fetal parts
- Maternal side where the fetal back is located
- Descent of the presenting part into the maternal pelvis
- Extent of flexion of the fetal head
- Estimated size and weight of the fetus (an advanced skill that will not be addressed further here)

Common deviations include *breech presentation* (when parts other than the head, such as buttocks or foot, present at the maternal pelvis), and lack of engagement of the presenting part in the maternal pelvis at term. If discovered prior to term, breech presentations may sometimes be corrected by rotational maneuvers.

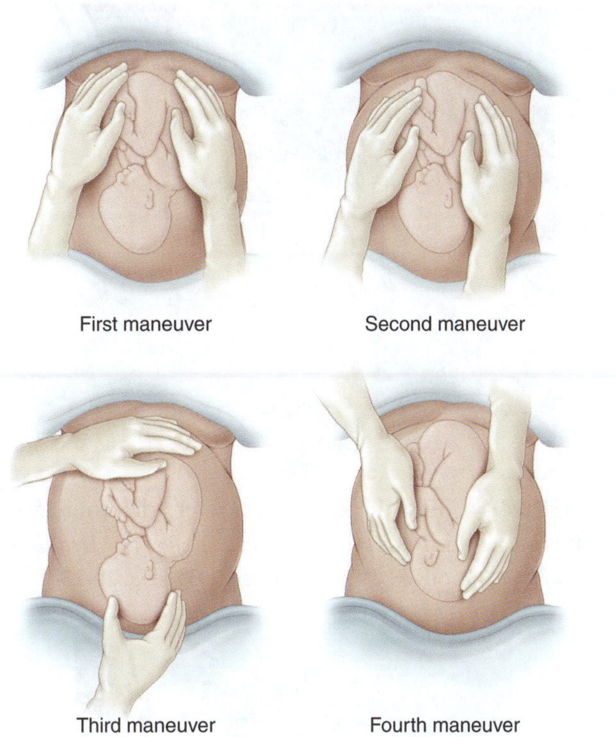

FIGURE 24-13. Leopold maneuvers for determining fetal position after 36 weeks' gestation. (From Casanova R. *Beckmann and Ling's Obstetrics and Gynecology.* 8th ed. Wolters Kluwer; 2019, Fig. 9-7.)

It is important to note that all findings are not truly diagnostic, and as such ultrasound may be required to conclusively determine the fetal position.

First Maneuver (Upper Fetal Pole). Stand at the woman's side, facing her head. Palpate the uppermost part of gravid uterus gently, with the fingertips together, to determine what fetal part is located at the fundus, which is the "upper fetal pole" (Fig. 24-14).

The fetal buttocks are usually at the upper fetal pole; they feel firm but irregular, and less globular than the head. The fetal head feels firm, round, and smooth. Occasionally, neither part is easily palpated at the fundus, as when the fetus is in a transverse lie.

Second Maneuver (Sides of the Maternal Abdomen). Place one hand on each side of the woman's abdomen, capturing the fetal body between them (Fig. 24-15). Steady the uterus with one hand and palpate the fetus with the other, looking for the back on one side and extremities on the other.

By 32 weeks' gestation, the fetal back has a smooth, firm surface as long or longer than the examiner's hand.

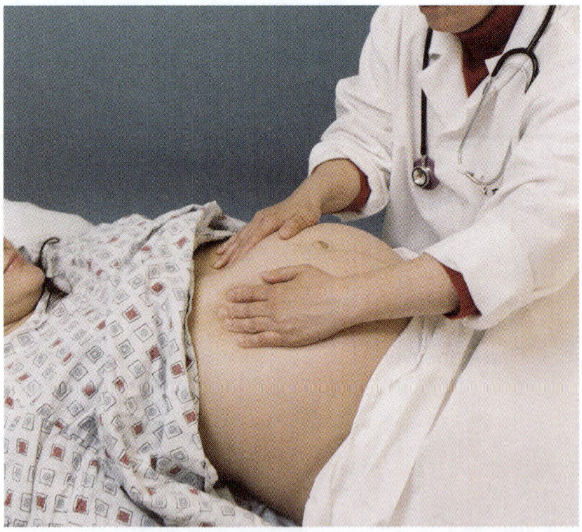

FIGURE 24-14. First Leopold maneuver: determination of what is in the fundus. (From Weber JR, Kelley JH. *Health Assessment in Nursing*. 6th ed. Wolters Kluwer; 2018, Fig. 29-13.)

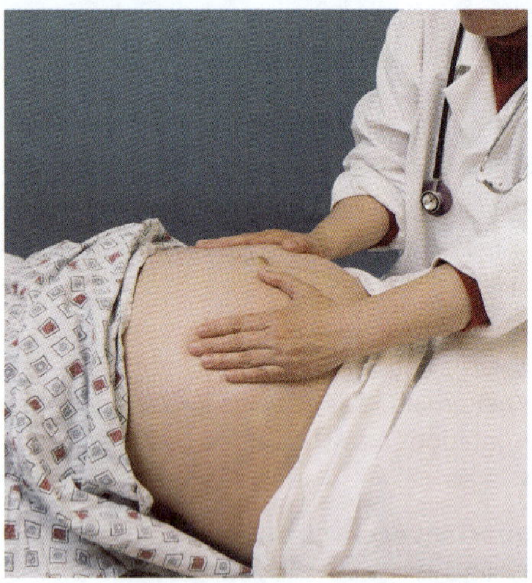

FIGURE 24-15. Second Leopold maneuver: evaluation of the fetal back and extremities. (From Weber JR, Kelley JH. *Health Assessment in Nursing*. 6th ed. Wolters Kluwer; 2018, Fig. 29-14.)

The fetal arms and legs feel like irregular bumps. The fetus may kick if awake and active.

Third Maneuver (Lower Fetal Pole and Descent into Pelvis). Place the flat palmar surfaces of the fingertips on the fetal pole just above the pubic symphysis (Fig. 24-16). Palpate the presenting fetal part for texture and firmness to distinguish the head from the buttock. Judge the descent, or engagement, of the presenting part into the maternal pelvis.

Again, the fetal head feels very firm and globular; the buttocks feel firm but irregular, and less globular than the head. In a *vertex* or *cephalic* presentation, the fetal head is the presenting part. If the most distal part of the lower fetal pole cannot be palpated, it is usually engaged in the pelvis. If you can depress the tissues over the maternal

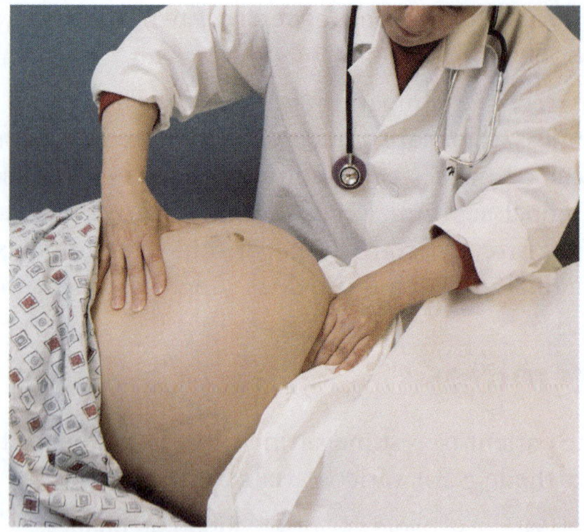

FIGURE 24-16. Third Leopold maneuver: palpation of the presenting part above the symphysis. (From Weber JR, Kelley JH. *Health Assessment in Nursing*. 6th ed. Wolters Kluwer; 2018, Fig. 29-15.)

bladder without touching the fetus, the presenting part is proximal to your fingers.

Fourth Maneuver (Flexion of the Fetal Head). This maneuver assesses the flexion or extension of the fetal head, presuming that the fetal head is the presenting part in the pelvis. Facing the woman's feet, with your hands positioned on either side of the gravid uterus, identify the fetal front and back sides (Fig. 24-17). Using one

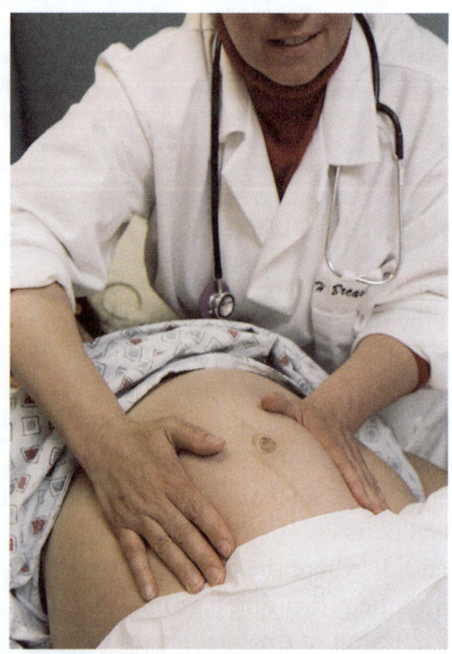

FIGURE 24-17. Fourth Leopold maneuver: determination of the direction and degree of flexion of the head. (From Weber JR, Kelley JH. *Health Assessment in Nursing*. 6th ed. Wolters Kluwer; 2018, Fig. 29-16.)

hand at a time, slide your fingers down each side of the fetal body until you reach the "cephalic prominence," that is, where the fetal brow or occiput juts out.

If the cephalic prominence juts out along the line of the fetal back, the head is extended. If the cephalic prominence juts out along the line of the fetal anterior side, the head is flexed.

RECORDING YOUR FINDINGS

Typically, the record for a pregnant patient follows a standard order: age, Gs and Ps, weeks of gestation, means of determining gestational age (ultrasound vs. LMP), followed by chief complaint, chief pregnancy complications, then important history and examination findings. Two sample write-ups are given below.

Recording the Physical Examination of the Pregnant Woman

"32-year-old G3P1102 at 18 weeks' gestation by LMP presents to establish prenatal care. Pregnancy complicated by closely spaced pregnancies, prior iatrogenic preterm birth for preeclampsia, and prior cesarean delivery. Patient does not yet note fetal movement; denies contractions, vaginal bleeding, and leakage of fluids. On external examination, low-transverse cesarean scar is evident; fundus is palpable just below umbilicus. On internal examination, cervix is open to fingertip at the external os but closed at the internal os; cervix is 3 cm long; uterus enlarged to size consistent with 18-week gestation. Speculum examination shows leukorrhea with positive Chadwick sign. FHR by Doppler is between 140 and 145 BPM."

These findings describe the examination of a healthy pregnant woman at 18 weeks' gestation.

OR

"21-year-old G1P0 at 33 weeks' gestation as determined by 19-week ultrasound presents with chief complaint of decreased fetal movement. Pregnancy complicated by rare prenatal visits and homelessness. Patient reports minimal fetal movement over the last 24 hours; denies contractions, vaginal bleeding, or leakage of fluid. On external exam, a nontender gravid abdomen with no scars is noted; fundus is measured at 32 cm; fetus is vertex but not engaged in pelvis by Leopold maneuvers. On internal examination, cervix is closed, long, and high; speculum examination shows thin gray discharge with clue cells on wet mount. FHT by Doppler are between 155 and 160 BPM."

These findings describe the examination of a more complex presentation of a pregnant woman at 33 weeks' gestation.

HEALTH PROMOTION AND COUNSELING: EVIDENCE AND RECOMMENDATIONS

Important Topics for Health Promotion and Counseling

- Nutrition
- Weight gain
- Exercise and physical activity
- Substance use including tobacco, alcohol, and illicit drugs
- Intimate partner violence screening
- Screening for perinatal depression
- Immunizations
- Prenatal laboratory screening
- Genetic testing and aneuploidy screening
- Prenatal supplementation
- Unintended pregnancy

Nutrition

Evaluate the nutritional status of the pregnant woman during the first prenatal visit. Assess for inadequate nutrition as well as for obesity.

- *Take a diet history.* What does she typically eat for each meal? How often does she eat? Does she have nausea that limits her eating? Does she have any history of conditions that affect food intake like diabetes, eating disorders, or past bariatric surgery?
- *Review the BMI and laboratory findings.* Measure height and weight, then calculate the BMI; note that later in pregnancy, the BMI reflects the gravid uterus. The hematocrit is a screen for anemia, which may reflect nutritional deficiency, underlying clinical issues, or the expected hemodilution seen later in pregnancy.
- *Caution pregnant women about foods to avoid.* Pregnant women are especially vulnerable to listeriosis. To help prevent listeriosis, encourage pregnant women to avoid:
    - Unpasteurized milk and foods made with unpasteurized milk
    - Raw and undercooked seafood, eggs, and meat
- *Regarding fish and shellfish,* some nutrients like omega-3 fatty acids and dehydroepiandrosterone (DHEA) may enhance fetal brain development. Intake should include 8 to 12 oz a week of fish lower in mercury such as salmon, shrimp, pollock, tuna (light canned), tilapia, catfish, and cod. White tuna consumption should be limited to 6 oz a week. Pregnant women should avoid fish higher in mercury like tilefish, shark, swordfish, and king mackerel.

Make a nutritional plan. Review goals for weight gain that are tailored to the woman's BMI. Small frequent meals may help with mild nausea. Consider a team-based approach involving dieticians or behavioral health specialists in complex cases such as gestational diabetes mellitus (GDM) or eating disorders.

Weight Gain

Weight gain should be closely monitored during pregnancy as poor birth outcomes are associated with both excessive and inadequate weight gain. Ideally, women should begin pregnancy with a BMI as close to the normal range as possible. Women with a normal BMI should gain 25 to 35 lb during pregnancy. In 2013, ACOG affirmed the revised 2009 weight gain recommendations by the National Institute of Medicine (Box 24-5).

Obtain weights at each visit and plot the results on a graph so that they are easy for you and your patient to review and discuss.

Exercise and Physical Activity

Physical activity during pregnancy has a number of psychological benefits and reduces risk of excessive gestational weight gain, GDM, preeclampsia, preterm birth, varicose veins, and deep vein thrombosis (DVT). It may reduce the length of labor and complications during delivery. In contrast, excess activity is associated with low birth weight, so educating your patients about recommended guidelines is important.

Pregnant women should engage in ≥30 minutes of moderate exercise on most days of the week unless there are contraindications. Women initiating exercise during pregnancy should be cautious and consider programs developed specifically for pregnant women. Water-based exercises can temporarily help alleviate musculoskeletal aches, but immersion in hot water should be avoided. After the first trimester, women should avoid exercise in the supine position, which compresses the inferior vena cava and can cause dizziness and decreased placental blood flow. Because the center of gravity shifts in the third trimester, advise against exercises that cause loss of balance. Contact sports or activities that risk abdominal trauma are contraindicated throughout pregnancy. Pregnant women also should avoid overheating, dehydration, and any exertion that causes notable fatigue or discomfort.

Substance Use including Tobacco, Alcohol, and Illicit Drugs

Women should abstain from substance abuse during pregnancy. Provide universal screening, which can uncover subtle issues, and address these topics in a neutral and constructive manner. Incarceration, confrontation, and criminalization of substance abuse have all been shown to worsen outcomes of pregnancy for women and their children.

Tobacco. Tobacco use increases the risk of spontaneous abortion, fetal death, and fetal digit anomalies. Cessation is the goal, but any decrease in use is favorable. Tobacco use is implicated in 13% to 19% of all low–birth-weight babies and many other poor pregnancy outcomes, including a twofold risk of placenta previa, placental abruption, and preterm labor.

Alcohol. No safe dose of alcohol has been established. Women should abstain throughout pregnancy. Fetal alcohol syndrome, the neurodevelopmental sequelae of alcohol exposure during fetal development, is the leading cause of preventable mental disability.

Illicit Drugs. Illegal drugs have significant detrimental effects on fetal development; pregnant women with addiction should be referred for treatment immediately and screened for HIV and hepatitis C infection.

Box 24-5. Recommendations for Total and Rate of Weight Gain during Pregnancy, by Prepregnancy BMI, 2009

Prepregnancy BMI[a]	Total Weight Gain (Range in pounds)	Rates of Weight Gain Second and Third Trimesters (pounds/week)	Mean Range
Underweight, or <18.5	28–40	1	1.0–1.3
Normal weight, or 18.5–24.9	25–35	1	0.8–1.0
Overweight, or 25.0–29.9	15–25	0.6	0.5–0.7
Obese, or >30.0	11–20	0.5	0.4–0.6

[a]To calculate BMI, go to Calculate Your Body Mass Index, National Heart, Lung, and Blood Institute at http://www.nhlbi.nih.gov/health/educational/lose_wt/BMI/bmicalc.htm.

Abuse of prescription drugs. Ask about the unusual use of narcotics, stimulants, benzodiazepines, and other commonly abused prescription drugs.

Herbal and unregulated supplements. Herbal supplements during pregnancy may harm the developing fetus. Unregulated supplements or vitamins, especially if formulated outside the United States, may contain lead and other toxins. Review and discuss any intake of supplements and consider pregnancy toxicology screening to determine the extent of fetal exposure, particularly for lead.

Intimate Partner Violence Screening

Pregnancy is a time of increased risk from intimate partner violence. Pre-existing patterns of abuse may intensify from verbal to physical abuse or from mild to severe physical abuse. Up to one in five women experiences some form of abuse during pregnancy, which has been associated with delayed prenatal care, low birth weight, or even death of the mother and fetus.

Universal screening of all women for domestic violence without regard to socioeconomic status, including pregnant women at the first prenatal visit and at least once each trimester should be undertaken. For a direct nonjudgmental approach, use simple questions as listed in Box 24-6.

Watch for nonverbal clues of abuse such as frequent last-minute appointment changes, unusual behavior during visits, partners who refuse to leave the patient alone during the visit, and bruises or other injuries. It may take several visits for the patient to admit to being abused due to fear about safety and reprisal.

Once the patient acknowledges abuse, ask about the best way for you to help her. She may set limits on sharing information. Accept her decisions about how to handle her situation safely, with the caveat that if children are involved, you may be required to report harmful behaviors to the authorities. Maintain an updated list of shelters, counseling centers, hotline numbers, and other trusted local referrals (Box 24-7). Plan future appointments at more frequent intervals. Finally, complete as thorough a physical examination as the patient permits and document all injuries on a body diagram.

Box 24-6. Screening Approach for Intimate Partner Violence

Initial Framing Statement

"Because violence is so common in many women's lives and because there is help available for women being abused, I now ask every patient about domestic violence."

Screening Questions

- "Within the past year—or since you have been pregnant—have you been hit, slapped, kicked, or otherwise physically hurt by someone?"
- "Are you in a relationship with a person who threatens or physically hurts you?"
- "Has anyone forced you to have sexual activities that made you feel uncomfortable?"

Box 24-7. Types of Contraception Methods

Methods	Types of Contraception
Natural	Fertility awareness/periodic abstinence, withdrawal, lactation
Barrier	Male condom, female condom, diaphragm, cervical cap, sponge
Implantable	Intrauterine devices (IUD), subdermal implant of levonorgestrel
Pharmacologic/ hormonal	Spermicide, oral contraceptives (estrogen and progesterone; progestin only), estrogen/progesterone injectables and patch, hormonal vaginal contraceptive ring, emergency contraception
Surgery (permanent)	Tubal ligation; transcervical sterilization; vasectomy

Screening for Perinatal Depression

Screen women at least once during the perinatal period for depression and anxiety symptoms using a standardized, validated tool. Additionally, provide or refer pregnant and postpartum persons who are at increased risk of perinatal depression to counseling interventions. Commonly used depression screening tools for the pregnant or peripartum adult include the Edinburgh Postnatal Depression Scale (EPDS) or the Patient Health Questionnaire-9 (PHQ-9).

The *Edinburgh Postnatal Depression Scale (EPDS)* consists of 10 self-reported items, takes less than 5 minutes to complete, has a low required reading level, and is easy to score. The EPDS includes anxiety symptoms, which are a prominent feature of perinatal mood disorders, and excludes constitutional symptoms of depression, such as changes in sleeping patterns, that are common in pregnancy and the postpartum period. The EPDS has relatively high sensitivity and specificity. The *Patient Health Questionnaire 9 (PHQ-9)* is a brief nine-item questionnaire focused on the nine diagnostic criteria for *Diagnostic and Statistical Manual of Mental Disorders*, 4th edition (DSM-IV) depressive disorders. It is one of the most validated tools in mental health and can be a powerful tool to assist clinicians with diagnosing depression and monitoring treatment response).

Immunizations

Given the persistent increase in pertussis infection it is recommended that Tdap be administered during each pregnancy, ideally at 27 to 36 weeks' gestation, regardless of the prior immunization history. Caretakers in direct contact with the infant should also receive Tdap. *Inactivated influenza vaccination* is indicated in any trimester during the influenza season. The following vaccines are safe during pregnancy: pneumococcal, meningococcal, and hepatitis B. Hepatitis A, meningococcal polysaccharide and conjugate, and pneumococcal polysaccharide vaccines can be given, if indicated. The following vaccines are not safe during pregnancy: measles/mumps/rubella, live attenuated influenza, polio, zoster, and varicella. All women should have rubella titers drawn during pregnancy and be immunized after birth if found to be nonimmune.

Prenatal Laboratory Screenings

Routine laboratory testing is recommended in early pregnancy to identify possible conditions which could impact the health of the mother or the outcome of the pregnancy.

Rh(D) Incompatibility Screening. The ABO blood type and Rh(D) type are recommended for all pregnant women. ABO type may be important in the case of urgent transfusion need in late pregnancy or with delivery. This may also be important to communicate to the pediatric provider if there is a risk of ABO incompatibility between the mother and neonate. Rh(D) type is recommended due to the risk of developing isoimmunization in Rh-negative women. Rh(D) isoimmunization increases the risk of fetal anemia, hydrops fetalis, and fetal death.

A type and screen should be sent from the first prenatal visit. If the antibody screen is positive, the antibody should be identified, and a titer obtained. Rh(D) screening is typically performed at the first prenatal visit, at 28 weeks, and at delivery. Women who are Rh-negative should be given anti-D immunoglobulin at 28 weeks' gestation and again within 3 days of delivery to prevent alloimmunization (if the infant is Rh-positive).

Screening for Syphilis. Congenital syphilis occurs when *Treponema pallidum*, a spirochete, infects the fetus in utero. Universal screening is recommended as identification of infection and appropriate treatment usually prevents adverse outcomes for both mother and infant. Due to the risk of fetal demise with syphilis infection in pregnancy, any woman who gives birth to a stillborn fetus should be tested for syphilis.

A nontreponemal test is recommended, such as the Venereal Disease Research Laboratory (VDRL) test or the Rapid Plasma Reagin (RPR) test. A reactive VDRL or RPR test should be followed up with a treponemal test, such as fluorescent treponemal antibody absorption (FTA-ABS), to confirm the diagnosis of syphilis, as false-positive screening is relatively common in pregnancy. All pregnant women should be screened at the initial prenatal visit. Women who are at high risk of infection (commercial sex work, drug use, multiple sexual partners, or STI diagnosis during pregnancy) should be re-screened at 28 weeks' gestational age and again at delivery.

Bacteriuria Screening. Send a urine culture at the first prenatal visit to screen for asymptomatic bacteriuria in all pregnant women. High-risk patients include those with history of urinary tract infection (UTI), urinary tract anomalies, diabetes mellitus, hemoglobin S, or preterm labor in the current pregnancy.

A clean-catch urine culture should be sent as a screening test in early pregnancy. Patients with a positive screening urine culture should be treated with antibiotics for 3 to 7 days. For low-risk patients, repeat testing is typically not recommended if the first screening urine culture is negative. High-risk patients may be rescreened at a later point in gestation, though ACOG does specify an optimal timeframe for re-screening. A test of cure should be sent for those patients who were treated for asymptomatic bacteriuria in early pregnancy, typically 1 week after completion of antibiotic therapy.

Hepatitis B Screening. Determining hepatitis B immunity status is important to identify women who are at risk for hepatitis B infection in pregnancy. Patients who lack immunity to hepatitis B should be vaccinated during pregnancy. Patients who have evidence of hepatitis B infection in pregnancy should be counseled about maternal health risks, including liver dysfunction, cirrhosis, and hepatocellular carcinoma. The risk of mother-to-child transmission is as high as 90% when active and passive immunization is not used. Patients with active hepatitis B infection in pregnancy are eligible for treatment to decrease viral load and, subsequently, lower the likelihood of in utero maternal-to-child transmission. Patients with positive hepatitis B infection in pregnancy should be identified by the pediatric team in order to treat the neonate with hepatitis B vaccination and hepatitis B immune globulin (HBIG) to prevent vertical transmission.

Hepatitis B surface antigen should be sent for all pregnant women at the first prenatal visit, even if previously vaccinated or tested. Women with positive screening should have further testing for hepatitis B e antigen (HBeAg), hepatitis B e antibody (anti-HBe), HBV DNA, and aminotransferase levels, which may guide further care and treatment in pregnancy. High-risk patients (multiple sexual partners, STI treatment in pregnancy, injection drug use, or a sexual or household contact with chronic HBV) should be retested at the time of delivery.

HIV Infection Screening. Human immunodeficiency virus (HIV) screening is recommended because HIV is a serious health disorder that can be easily diagnosed, treated, and the cost of screening is low. Universal screening for pregnant women is more effective than risk-based screening to detect unsuspected maternal HIV and to prevent vertical transmission. Certain high-risk populations should be identified, which includes women with injection drug use, those who exchange sex for money or drugs, women with STIs diagnosed in pregnancy, those with multiple sexual partners, certain high HIV-prevalence populations, or a woman with an HIV-infected partner. Treatment with antiretroviral therapy (ART) has significantly reduced the rate of perinatal transmission, with maternal-to-child transmission rates now <2% with the combination of universal screening and prophylactic ART administration. Due to the risk of maternal-to-child transmission of untreated HIV in pregnancy, all women should be screened for HIV in pregnancy, regardless of screening in previous pregnancies.

HIV antibody testing with a fourth-generation HIV-1/HIV-2 immunoassay should be sent as permitted by local and state regulations (e.g., some states require verbal consent for HIV testing). If the screen is positive, confirmatory testing with an HIV-1/HIV-2 antibody differentiation immunoassay is performed, along with a plasma HIV RNA level. HIV screening should be performed at the initial prenatal visit, with patient refusal of HIV testing documented in the health record (i.e., an "opt-out" approach). High-risk populations should be re-screened in the third trimester, ideally before 36 weeks' gestation. For women who were not screened during pregnancy, rapid HIV testing is recommended during the delivery admission.

Iron Deficiency Screening. Iron deficiency is the second most common cause of anemia in pregnancy, affecting up to 50% of pregnant women worldwide. Increased iron turnover, along with increased erythrocyte production and fetoplacental growth, can lead to worsening iron deficiency in pregnancy. Iron deficiency is characterized by a microcytic anemia, which can have serious consequences in pregnancy such as fetal growth restriction, premature birth, and low birth weight. Maternal iron deficiency reduces iron stores in the fetus. Perinatal iron deficiency, particularly in the third trimester, has been shown to impact fetal neurogenesis, development, and myelination.

Screen all pregnant women for anemia during pregnancy. Ideally, iron deficiency should be identified and treated before the third trimester, which will allow for ample time to replete iron stores and decrease the risk of neonatal iron deficiency.

A complete blood count (CBC) is sent, which also includes the mean corpuscular volume (MCV). In patients with anemia (hemoglobin <11 g/dL or hematocrit <33%) and low MCV, iron studies should be sent to evaluate for iron deficiency. Typically, screening is performed in nonpregnant adults with serum ferritin levels (with <30 ng/mL confirming a diagnosis of iron deficiency). However, for pregnant women, those with chronic medical conditions or borderline ferritin levels, complete iron studies may be required. These additional tests include serum iron, total iron binding capacity (TIBC), and transferrin saturation. For patients with microcytic anemia without evidence of iron deficiency, hemoglobin electrophoresis should be sent to rule out sickle cell disease or thalassemia. a CBC should be sent during the initial prenatal visit. Repeat screening for anemia may be considered between 24 and 28 weeks, with further evaluation and treatment.

Gestational Diabetes Screening. GDM is abnormal glucose tolerance in the setting of pregnancy, which is mediated by diabetogenic hormones secreted by the placenta. GDM is associated with maternal risks, including cesarean delivery, preeclampsia, postpartum hemorrhage, and higher-order perineal laceration. Fetal and neonatal risks of GDM include excessive fetal growth, polyhydramnios, stillbirth, shoulder dystocia, birth injury, NICU admission, neonatal hypoglycemia, and neonatal hyperbilirubinemia. Due to the significant morbidity associated with impaired glucose tolerance in pregnancy and GDM, screen all pregnant women for diabetes.

The most common screening test performed is two-step screening. A 50-g oral glucose tolerance test (OGTT) is administered and venous glucose checked 1 hour after the glucose load, with screening thresholds of 130 to 140 mg/dL used at various institutions. Patients with a positive 50-g screen then undergo a 100-g, 3-hour diagnostic OGTT. Patients are diagnosed with gestational diabetes when two or more values are abnormal on the 3-hour OGTT. Screening for GDM is recommended between 24 and 28 weeks' gestation for all pregnant women. early screening is recommended for women who are overweight/obese (BMI >25) with one or more additional risk factor, including high-risk ethnicity, gestational diabetes in a prior pregnancy, hypertension, hypercholesterolemia, or first-degree relatives with diabetes mellitus.

Genetic Testing and Aneuploidy Screening

Offer aneuploidy screening and diagnostic testing (with chorionic villus sampling or amniocentesis) to all pregnant women, regardless of maternal age. If indicated, pursue additional tests related to the mother's risk factors, such as screening for Tay–Sachs disease or other genetic disorders.

Prenatal Supplementation

Multivitamin and Mineral Supplementation. Daily prenatal vitamin and mineral supplements should include 600 IU of vitamin D and at least 1,000 mg of calcium. If not present in the prenatal vitamins, recommend 150 to 290 µg of daily iodine in pregnant and breastfeeding women, as iodine deficiency is widespread. Women should be advised that excess amounts of fat-soluble vitamins like vitamins A, D, E, and K can cause toxicity.

Folic Acid Supplementation. Folate deficiency in pregnancy has a well-documented association with neural tube defects (NTDs), and multiple studies have shown that folic acid supplementation reduces the risk of recurrent NTDs. Folate requirements increase from 50 to 400 µg daily in pregnancy. Folic acid is obtained from dietary sources such as leafy greens, legumes, and meat consumption.

Iron Supplementation. Iron requirements increase dramatically during pregnancy, with increasing amounts of iron needed with advancing gestation to support maternal erythrocyte mass, fetal RBC production, and fetoplacental growth. Cumulatively, 500 mg of iron is required to support maternal RBC production, and an additional 300 to 350 mg is needed for fetoplacental growth. Although studies have not directly demonstrated a benefit to maternal and fetal/neonatal health, there are documented risks of iron deficiency in pregnancy.

The CDC recommends 30 mg/day of oral iron supplementation be started at the first prenatal visit, which is the dose typically available in iron-containing prenatal vitamins. Additionally, women should be encouraged to ingest iron-rich foods. Patients with anemia should increase oral iron supplementation doses to 60 to 120 mg/day. For patients with profound iron-deficiency anemia, lack of response to oral supplementation, or advanced gestational age, intravenous iron supplementation may be required.

TABLE 24-1. Anatomic and Physiologic Changes in Normal Pregnancy

Organ System	Organ of Interest	Change in Normal Pregnancy	Clinical Relevance
Vital signs	Heart rate	↑ (Progresses throughout gestation)	
	Blood pressure	↓ (Nadir in second trimester)	
	Respiratory rate	↔	
	Oxygen saturation	↔	
Skin	Skin	Increased cutaneous blood flow	Dissipation of excess heat due to increased metabolism
		Hyperpigmentation	
		Spider angiomata and palmar erythema	Unclear clinical significance, likely related to hyperestrogenemia
	Hair	Scalp hair thickening	
		Hirsutism	Unclear clinical significance. Severe hirsutism with signs of virilization should be investigated.
Respiratory	Lungs	↑ Oxygen consumption 20%	Shifts CO_2 from fetus to maternal circulation
		↓ Arterial pCO_2	
		↑ Ventilation	ABG will demonstrate respiratory alkalosis
		↓ TLV, RV, FRC	
		↑ TV, minute ventilation	Aids in CO_2 removal
		↓ Pulmonary vascular resistance	
		←→ Lung compliance	
	Diaphragm	Diaphragm elevated 4 cm	Diaphragmatic elevation and increased minute ventilation contribute to sensation of dyspnea in pregnancy
Cardiovascular	Heart	↑ Cardiac output up to 50%	Related to both increased pulse and stroke volume. Further augmented by almost 20% in multifetal gestations.
		Heart displaced left and upward	Appearance of cardiomegaly on imaging
		Exaggerated split S1	Systolic murmurs are common, in up to 90% of pregnant patients
		Hyperdynamic LV function	
	Peripheral vasculature	↓ Systemic vascular resistance	↑ Venous pooling and postural hypotension.
		↓ BP (diastolic > systolic)	
		↓ Venous flow in the lower extremities due to compression by the gravid uterus	↑ Dependent edema and varicose veins. Predisposes to thrombosis.
Gastrointestinal	Stomach	↓ Gastric emptying	Contributes to nausea, acid reflux
		↓ Esophageal sphincter tone	
	Intestinal tracts, large and small	Displaced superiorly and laterally	Appendicitis may present atypically.
		↓ Motility	Contributes to hemorrhoids, constipation
	Hepatobiliary tree	←→ Liver size	
		↑ Hepatic blood flow	
		↓ Serum albumin concentration	
		↓ Gallbladder motility	↑ biliary stasis and incidence of cholesterol gallstones, cholecystitis. ↑ risk of cholestasis

(continued)

TABLE 24-1. Anatomic and Physiologic Changes in Normal Pregnancy *(Continued)*

Organ System	Organ of Interest	Change in Normal Pregnancy	Clinical Relevance
Hematologic	Plasma	↑ Circulating volume 40–45%	Provision of nutrients to the fetus/placenta, protection against impaired venous return
	Blood	↑ Erythrocyte production and volume	Protection against blood loss during parturition
		↑ Reticulocyte count	Unclear clinical significance—related to hemodilution and ↑ consumption
		↑ Iron turnover	Leads to iron deficiency anemia, pica
		↓ Hemoglobin and hematocrit	
		↑ Leukocytosis	
		↓ Platelets	Increased risk of epistaxis, nasal congestion
		↑ Inflammatory markers (CRP, ESR)	Unreliable markers of inflammation
	Coagulation	↑ Clotting factors (except factors XI and XIII)	
		↑ Fibrinogen	Maintains balance of coagulation and fibrinolysis—overall hypercoagulable state
		↓ Protein C and total protein S	
		↑ Fibrinolysis and ↑ D-dimer	D-dimer is an unreliable marker of thrombotic risk
Urinary	Bladder	Hyperplasia of bladder muscle and connective tissue	↑ urinary frequency and incontinence
		Elevation of trigone	
		↑ Bladder pressure	
	Ureters	Laterally displaced and compressed	Contributes to hydronephrosis, more commonly right-sided
		↑ Dilation and relaxation	
	Kidneys	↑ Renin–angiotensin–aldosterone system	Maintains BP in the first trimester. Hypertension does not result in normal pregnancy due to angiotensin II refractoriness as pregnancy progresses.
			Contributes to urinary frequency
		↑ Kidney size	
		↑ GFR and plasma flow	
		↓ Serum creatinine	Cr >0.9 mg/dL should be evaluated
		↑ Creatinine clearance 30%	
Musculoskeletal	Spine	Lumbar lordosis	Shifts center of gravity to accommodate the gravid uterus. May contribute to low back pain.
		Pelvic joint relaxation—symphysis pubis, sacroiliac and sacrococcygeal joints	Pubic symphysis separation >1 cm may cause significant pain and gait disturbance

CRP, c-reactive protein; ESR, erythrocyte sedimentation rate; VTE, venous thromboembolism; LV, left ventricle; BP, blood pressure; TLV, total lung volume; RV, residual volume; FRC, functional residual capacity; TV, tidal volume; CO_2, carbon dioxide; GFR, glomerular filtration rate.

CHAPTER 25

Older Adult

The World Health Organization has recognized the aging of the population in many countries around the world as one of the most significant challenges of the 21st century. It has been estimated that by the year 2050, the number of people older than 60 years worldwide will exceed 2 billion. In the United States, life span at birth is currently 81 years for women and 76 years for men. In several countries in Asia and Europe, the average life expectancy has already exceeded 80 years, particularly among women. Hence, the "*demographic imperative*" to societies worldwide is to maximize not only life span but also "health span," so that older adults maintain full function as long as possible, enjoying rich and active lives in their homes and communities (Fig. 25-1).

Although statistics group aging by decades, aging is hardly chronologic, measured by time in years, but encompasses the complex interplay of health and illness. Studies show that *healthy* or "*successful*" aging is not strictly clinical but rests on variables such as positive cognition and mental health, physical activity, and social networks. Promoting healthy aging thus leads to interactive goals in clinical care—"an informed activated patient interacting with a prepared proactive team, resulting in high-quality satisfying encounters and improved outcomes" and a distinct set of clinical attitudes and skills. This approach individualizes decision making and allows patients to express preferences about which "health states are important to them and their relative priority" (Box 25-1).

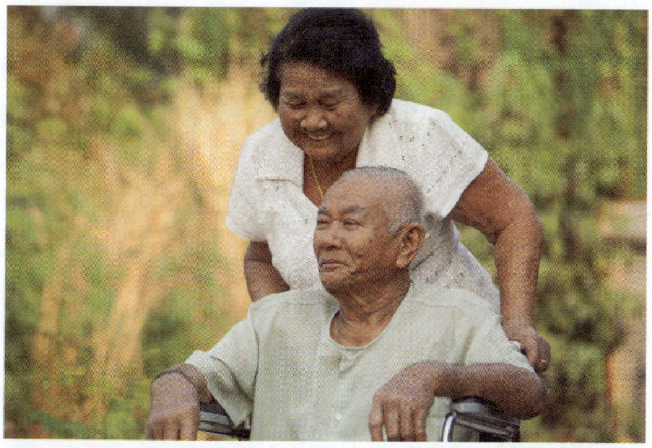

FIGURE 25-1. Older adults maximizing health span can enjoy rich, active lives. (Used with permission form Shutterstock. By WitthayaP.)

This chapter uses the term "older adult" for persons 65 years and older over terms such as "senior," "aged," or "elderly."

Box 25-1. Key Points in the Care of the Older Adult in the Primary Care Setting

- It is crucial to recognize geriatric syndromes, multifactorial conditions occurring primarily in older adults, in the primary care setting.
- The most important geriatric syndromes in primary care are falls, urinary incontinence, frailty, and cognitive impairment.
- Elements of ideal geriatric primary care include assessment of functional status, frequent medication review, careful evaluation of the benefits and burdens of any new test or treatment, and frequent assessment of goals of care and prognosis.
- Innovative delivery systems—either comprehensive care, consulting assessment or hospital-level care for acute conditions at home—can improve geriatric primary care. High-value features of geriatric care systems include ensuring 24/7 access to care, providing a team-based approach in performing medication reconciliation and comprehensive geriatric assessments, and integrating palliative care into treatment planning.

ANATOMY AND PHYSIOLOGY

Primary aging reflects changes in physiologic reserves over time that are independent of changes from disease.

However, these changes can lead to the development of multiple impairments, decline in overall functional capacity, and associated morbidity and mortality. These significant alterations in physiology tend to have the most impact during periods of stress, such as exposure to fluctuating temperatures, dehydration, or even shock. For example, decreased cutaneous vasoconstriction and sweat production can impair responses to heat; declines in thirst may delay recovery from dehydration; and the physiologic drops in maximum cardiac output, left ventricular filling, and maximum heart rate may impair the response to shock.

See Table 25-1, Selected Normal Anatomic and Physiologic Changes with Aging and Related Disease Outcomes.

Vital Signs

Blood Pressure. Systolic blood pressure (SBP) tends to rise with aging. The aorta and large arteries stiffen and become atherosclerotic. As the aorta becomes less distensible, a given stroke volume causes a greater rise in SBP. Diastolic blood pressure (DBP) stops rising at approximately the sixth decade.

With the greater rise in SBP, systolic hypertension with a widened pulse pressure (PP) often ensues.

At the other extreme, many older adults develop *orthostatic (postural) hypotension*.

Heart Rate and Rhythm. In older adults, resting heart rate remains unchanged, but there are declines in the pacemaker cells of the sinoatrial node and the maximal heart rate, which affect the response to exercise and physiologic stress. Older adults are more likely to have abnormal heart rhythms such as atrial or ventricular ectopy.

Asymptomatic rhythm changes are generally benign. However, some rhythm changes cause *syncope*.

Respiratory Rate and Temperature. Respiratory rate and temperature are unchanged, but changes in temperature regulation lead to a susceptibility to hypothermia.

Skin, Nails, and Hair

With age, the skin wrinkles, becomes lax, and loses turgor. The dermis is less vascular, causing lighter skin to look paler and opaquer. Skin on the backs of the hands and forearms appears thin, fragile, loose, and transparent. There may be purple patches or macules, termed **actinic purpura**, that fade over time. These spots and patches come from blood that has leaked through poorly supported capillaries and spread within the dermis (Fig. 25-2).

Nails lose luster with age and may yellow and thicken, especially on the toes. Hair undergoes a series of changes. Scalp hair loses its pigment, changing hair color to gray. Hair loss on the scalp is genetically determined. As early as 20 years, a man's hairline may start to recede at the temples and then at the vertex. In women, hair loss follows a similar but less severe pattern. In both sexes, the number

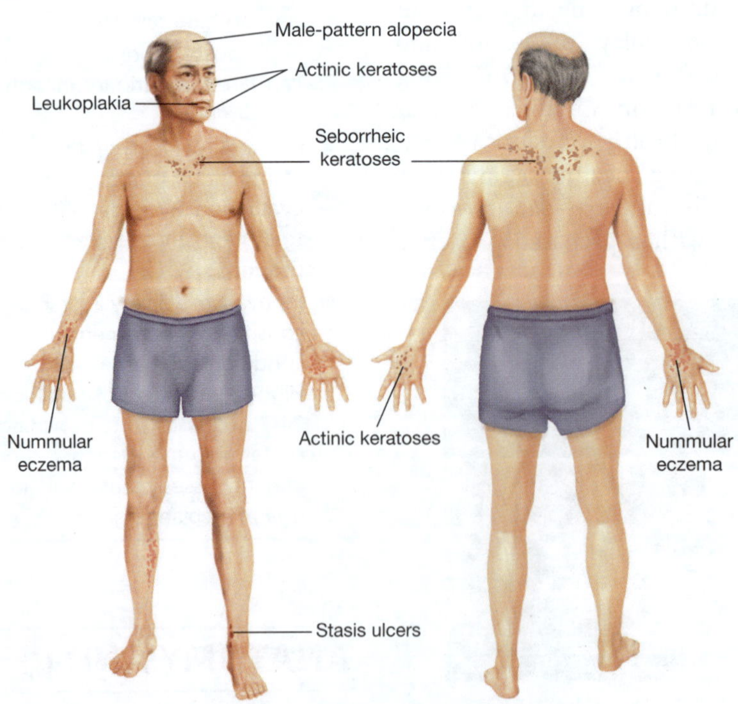

FIGURE 25-2. Skin and hair changes in older adults.

of scalp hairs decreases in a generalized pattern, and the diameter of each hair gets smaller. There is also normal hair loss elsewhere on the body—the trunk, pubic areas, axillae, and limbs. Women over 55 years may develop coarse facial hairs on the chin and upper lip.

Many of these changes are more common in lighter-skinned patients and may not apply to patients with darker skin tones.

Eyes

The eyes, ears, and mouth show more visible changes of aging. The fat that surrounds and cushions the eyes within the bony orbit may atrophy, making the eyeballs appear to recede. The skin of the eyelids becomes wrinkled and may hang in looser folds. Fat may push the fascia of the eyelids forward, creating soft bulges, especially in the lower lids and the inner third of the upper lids. Because of fewer lacrimal secretions, older patients may complain of dry eyes. The corneas lose some of their luster.

The pupils become smaller, making it more difficult to examine the ocular fundi. The pupils may also become slightly irregular but should continue to respond to light and show the near reaction.

Visual acuity remains fairly constant between ages 20 and 50 years. It diminishes gradually until approximately 70 years and then more rapidly. Nevertheless, most older adults retain good to adequate vision (20/20 to 20/70 as measured by standard charts). Near vision, however, begins to blur noticeably for virtually everyone. From childhood on, the lens gradually loses its elasticity, with progressive loss of accommodation and the ability to focus on nearby objects. Ensuing **presbyopia** usually becomes noticeable during the fifth decade (Fig. 25-3). Thickening and yellowing of the lens impairs the passage of light to the retina, requiring more light for reading and doing fine work.

Aging increases the risk of developing cataracts, glaucoma, and macular degeneration.

Cataracts affect 10% of patients in their 60s and over 30% in their 80s.

Because the lens continues to expand with aging, it may push the iris forward, narrowing the angle between iris and cornea and increasing the risk of narrow-angle glaucoma.

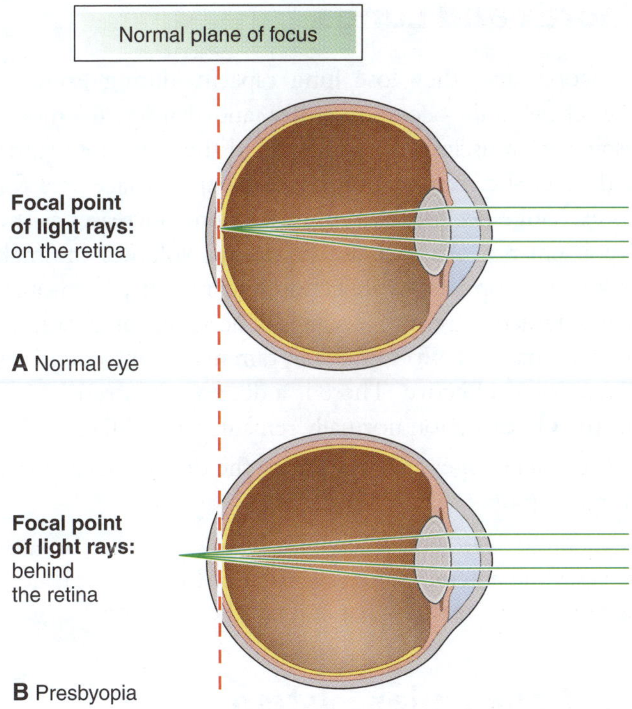

FIGURE 25-3. Refractive changes with aging. **A.** Normal. **B.** Presbyopia. With age, the lens stiffens and can no longer cause rays from near objects to converge on the retina. Rays converge behind the retina. (From McConnell TH. *The Nature of Disease: Pathology for the Health Professions.* 2nd ed. Jones & Bartlett Learning; 2014, Fig. 25-5.)

Ears

Hearing acuity usually declines with age. Early losses, which start in young adulthood, involve primarily the high-pitched sounds beyond the range of human speech and have relatively little functional significance. Gradually, loss extends to sounds in the middle and lower ranges. Hearing loss associated with aging, known as **presbycusis**, becomes increasingly evident, usually after age 50 years.

Nose, Mouth, Teeth, and Lymph Nodes

With aging, there are decreased salivary secretions and loss of taste; medications and various diseases can exacerbate these changes. Decreased olfaction and increased sensitivity to bitterness and saltiness also affect taste. Teeth may wear down, become abraded, or fall out due to dental caries or periodontal disease. In patients without teeth, the lower portion of the face looks small and sunken, with accentuated "purse-string" wrinkles radiating from the mouth. The bony ridges of the jaws that once surrounded the tooth sockets are gradually resorbed, especially in the lower jaw. With aging, the cervical lymph nodes become less palpable. In contrast, the submandibular glands become easier to feel.

Overclosure of the mouth may lead to maceration of the skin at the corners, or *angular cheilitis.*

Thorax and Lungs

As people age, they lose lung capacity during exercise. The chest wall becomes stiffer and harder to move, respiratory muscles may weaken, and the lungs lose some of their elastic recoil. Lung mass and the surface area for gas exchange decline, and residual volume increases as the alveoli enlarge. An increase in closing volumes of small airways predisposes to atelectasis and risk of pneumonia. Diaphragmatic strength declines. The speed of breathing out with maximal effort gradually diminishes, and coughing becomes less effective. There is a decrease in arterial pO_2, but the O_2 saturation normally remains above 90%.

Skeletal changes can accentuate the dorsal curve of the thoracic spine.

Osteoporotic vertebral collapse produces *kyphosis,* which increases the anteroposterior diameter of the chest. However, the resulting "barrel chest" has little effect on function.

Cardiovascular System

A number of changes occur in the neck vessels, cardiac output, heart sounds, and murmurs.

Review the effects of aging on blood pressure and heart rate described on p. 220.

Neck Vessels. Lengthening and tortuosity of the aorta and its branches occasionally result in kinking or buckling of the carotid artery low in the neck, especially on the right. The resulting pulsatile mass, occurring chiefly in women with hypertension, may be mistaken for a carotid aneurysm. A tortuous aorta occasionally raises the pressure in the jugular veins on the left side of the neck by impairing their drainage within the thorax.

In older adults, systolic bruits heard in the middle or upper portions of the carotid arteries indicate stenosis from atherosclerotic plaque. Cervical bruits in younger people are usually innocent.

Cardiac Output. Myocardial contraction is less responsive to stimulation from β-adrenergic catecholamines. There is a modest drop in resting heart rate, but a significant drop in the maximum heart rate during exercise. Although heart rate drops, stroke volume increases, so cardiac output is maintained. Diastolic dysfunction arises from decreased early diastolic filling and greater dependence on atrial contraction. There is increased myocardial stiffness, notably in the left ventricle, which also hypertrophies.

Risk of heart failure increases with loss of atrial contraction and onset of atrial fibrillation due to decreased ventricular filling.

Extra Heart Sounds—S_3 and S_4. As a person ages, decreased ventricular compliance and impaired ventricular filling result in a *fourth heart sound,* often auscultated in otherwise healthy older people. In contrast, auscultating a *third heart sound,* is strongly suggestive of heart failure from volume overload of the left ventricle in conditions like heart failure and valvular heart disease (e.g., mitral regurgitation).

An S_4 is seldom heard in young adults other than well-conditioned athletes.

A physiologic S_3 is commonly heard in children and may persist as late as age 40 years, especially in women.

Cardiac Murmurs. Middle-aged and older adults commonly have a *systolic aortic murmur.* This murmur is detected in approximately one-third of people at age 60 years, and in more than half of those reaching 85 years. With aging, fibrotic changes thicken the bases of the aortic cusps. Calcification follows, resulting in audible vibrations. Turbulence produced by blood flow into a dilated aorta may further augment this murmur. In most older adults, the process of fibrosis and calcification, known as *aortic sclerosis,* does not impede blood flow.

The aortic valve leaflets can become calcified and immobile, resulting in *aortic stenosis* and outflow obstruction. Clinically distinguishing aortic sclerosis from aortic stenosis is difficult. Both carry increased risk for cardiovascular morbidity and mortality.

Similar changes alter the mitral valve, but usually about one decade later than the aortic valve. Calcification of the mitral valve annulus, or valve ring, impedes normal valve closure during systole, causing the systolic murmur of *mitral regurgitation.*

This change in the configuration of the mitral valve may become pathologic as volume overload increases in the left ventricle.

Peripheral Vascular System

The peripheral arteries tend to lengthen, become tortuous, and feel harder and less resilient. There is increased arterial stiffness and decreased endothelial function.

Although arterial and venous disorders, especially atherosclerosis, are more common in older adults, these are not normal changes of aging. Loss of arterial pulsations is not typical and demands careful evaluation.

Abdominal or back pain in older adults raises the important concern of possible abdominal aortic aneurysm, especially in male smokers over age 65 years.

Rarely, after age 50 years but especially after age 70 years, the temporal arteries may develop giant cell, or temporal, arteritis, leading to loss of vision in 15% of patients and headache and jaw claudication.

Breasts and Axillae

The normal adult female breast is soft but may be granular, nodular, or lumpy. This uneven texture represents physiologic nodularity, palpable throughout or only in parts of the breasts. With aging, the female breasts tend to get smaller, more flaccid, and more pendulous as glandular tissue atrophies and is replaced by fat. The ducts surrounding the nipple may become more palpable as firm stringy strands. Axillary hair diminishes. Males may develop gynecomastia or increased breast fullness due to obesity and hormonal changes.

Abdomen

During the middle and later years, the abdominal muscles tend to weaken, there is decreased activity of lipoprotein lipase, and fat may accumulate in the lower abdomen and near the hips even when the weight is stable. These changes often produce a softer, more protruding, abdomen which patients may interpret as fluid or evidence of disease.

The change in abdominal fat distribution increases the risk of cardiovascular disease.

Aging can blunt the manifestations of acute abdominal disease. Pain may be less severe, fever is often less pronounced, and signs of peritoneal inflammation, such as guarding and rebound tenderness, may be diminished or even absent.

Male and Female Genitourinary System; Prostate

As men age, sexual interest appears to remain intact, although frequency of intercourse appears to decline after age 75 years. Several physiologic changes accompany decreasing testosterone levels. Erections become more dependent on tactile stimulation and less responsive to erotic cues. The penis decreases in size, and the testicles drop lower in the scrotum. Pubic hair may decrease and become gray.

Protracted illnesses, more than aging, lead to decreased testicular size.

Erectile dysfunction (**ED**), or the inability to maintain an erection, affects approximately 50% of older men. Vascular causes are the most common, from both atherosclerotic arterial occlusive disease and corpora cavernosa venous leak.

Chronic diseases such as diabetes, hypertension, dyslipidemia, and smoking, as well as medication side effects, all contribute to the prevalence of ED.

In women, ovarian function usually starts to decline during the fifth decade; on average, menstrual periods cease between age 45 and 52 years. As estrogen stimulation falls, many women experience hot flashes, sometimes for up to 5 years. Symptoms range from flushing, sweating, and palpitations to chills and anxiety. Sleep disruption and mood changes are common. Women may report vaginal dryness, urge incontinence, or dyspareunia. Several vulvovaginal changes occur: Pubic hair becomes sparse as well as gray, and the labia and clitoris become smaller. The vagina narrows and shortens, and the vaginal mucosa becomes thin, pale, and dry, with loss of lubrication. The uterus and ovaries diminish in size. Within 10 years after menopause, the ovaries are usually no longer palpable. The suspensory ligaments of the adnexa, uterus, and bladder may also relax. Sexuality and sexual interest are often unchanged, particularly when women are untroubled by partner issues, partner loss, or unusual work or life stress.

Age-related changes to the urinary system include decreased innervation and contractility of the detrusor muscle, loss of bladder capacity, urinary flow rate, and the ability to inhibit voiding.

The prevalence of urinary incontinence increases with age due to these age-related changes.

In men, there is androgen-dependent proliferation of prostate epithelial and stromal tissue, termed *benign prostatic hyperplasia (BPH)*, that begins in the third decade, continues to the seventh decade, then appears to plateau.

Only half of men will have clinically significant enlargement and only half of those will report symptoms such as urinary hesitancy, dribbling, and incomplete emptying. These symptoms can often be traced to other causes like coexisting disease, use of medications, and lower urinary tract abnormalities.

Musculoskeletal System

Both men and women lose cortical and trabecular bone mass throughout adulthood; men more slowly, and women more rapidly after menopause.

These changes lead to increased risk of fracture.

Calcium resorption from bone, rather than diet, increases with aging as parathyroid hormone levels rise. Subtle losses in height begin soon after maturity; significant shortening is obvious by old age. Most loss of height occurs in the trunk and reflects thinning of the intervertebral discs leading to *kyphosis* and an increase in the anteroposterior diameter of the chest (Fig. 25-4).

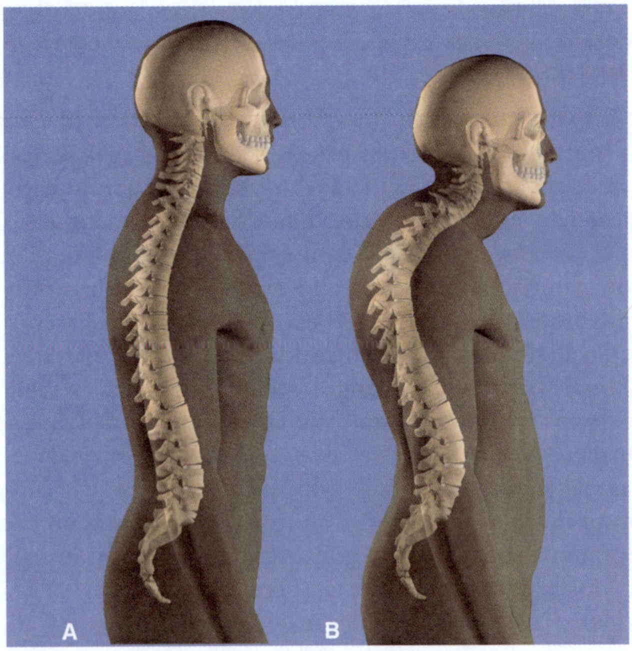

FIGURE 25-4. Aging changes in the vertebral column. **A.** Normal spinal column. **B.** Kyphosis. (Source: LifeART image copyright (c) 2019 Lippincott Williams & Wilkins. All rights reserved.)

Added flexion at the knees and hips also contributes to shortened stature. These changes cause the limbs of an older adult person to look long in proportion to the trunk.

The kyphosis can be further aggravated and made more pronounced by shortening or even collapse of the vertebral bodies from osteoporosis.

With aging, there is a 30% to 50% decline in muscle mass in relation to body weight in both men and women, and ligaments lose some of their tensile strength. *Sarcopenia* is the loss of lean body mass and strength with aging. The causes of muscle loss are multifactorial, including inflammatory and endocrine changes as well as sedentary lifestyle.

Substantial evidence shows that strength training in older adults can slow or reverse this process.

Range of motion diminishes, in part due to osteoarthritis.

Nervous System

Aging affects all aspects of the nervous system, from mental status to motor and sensory function and reflexes. Brain volume, cortical brain cells, and intrinsic regional connecting networks decrease, and both microanatomical and biochemical changes have been identified. Nevertheless, most older adults maintain their self-esteem and adapt well to their changing capacities and circumstances.

Mental Status. Although older adults generally perform well on mental status examinations, they may display selected impairments, especially at advanced ages. Many older people complain about memory problems. This is usually from "*benign senescent forgetfulness*," which can occur at any age. This common phenomenon usually manifests as difficulty recalling the names of people or objects or details of specific events.

Identifying benign senescent forgetfulness can allay fear of Alzheimer disease.

Older adults also retrieve and process data more slowly and take longer to learn new information. Their motor responses may slow and their ability to perform complex tasks may diminish. Diagnosis can be difficult because both mood disturbances and cognitive changes can alter the patient's ability to recognize or report symptoms. It is important to recognize these conditions promptly to delay functional decline. Older patients are also more susceptible to *delirium*, a temporary state of confusion and inattention that may be the first clue to infection, problems with medications, or an underlying cognitive impairment.

Try to distinguish these age-related changes from manifestations of mental disorders that are prevalent in older adults like depression and dementia.

Mood. Older adults experience the death of loved ones and friends, retirement from valued employment, diminution in income, and often growing social isolation in addition to physiologic changes and decreased physical capacity. Including the impact of these significant life events in the assessment of mood and affect and addressing these issues may improve the patient's quality of life.

Motor System. Changes in the motor system are common. Older adults move and react with less speed and agility and skeletal muscles decrease in bulk. The hands of an older patient often look thin and bony due to atrophy of the interosseous muscles that leaves concavities or grooves. Muscle wasting tends to appear first between the thumb and the hand (first and second metacarpals), then affects the other metacarpals. It may also flatten the thenar and hypothenar eminences of the palms. Arm and leg muscles can show signs of atrophy, exaggerating the apparent size of adjacent joints. Muscle strength, though diminished, is relatively well maintained.

Occasionally, older adults develop a benign essential tremor in the head, jaw, lips, or hands. These benign tremors are faster, disappear at rest, and without muscle rigidity.

Benign tremors may be confused with parkinsonism. Parkinsonian tremors are slightly slower and persist at rest, and with associated muscle rigidity.

Position and Vibratory Sense; Reflexes. Aging can also affect vibratory and position sense and reflexes. Older adults frequently lose some or all vibration sense in the feet and ankles (but not in the fingers or over the shins). Less commonly, position sense may diminish or disappear. The gag reflex may be decreased or absent. Abdominal reflexes may diminish or disappear. Ankle reflexes may be symmetrically decreased or absent, even when reinforced. Less commonly, knee reflexes are similarly affected. Partly because of musculoskeletal changes in the feet, the plantar responses become less obvious and more difficult to interpret.

If there are associated abnormal neurologic findings, or if atrophy and reflex changes are asymmetric, search for an explanation other than aging.

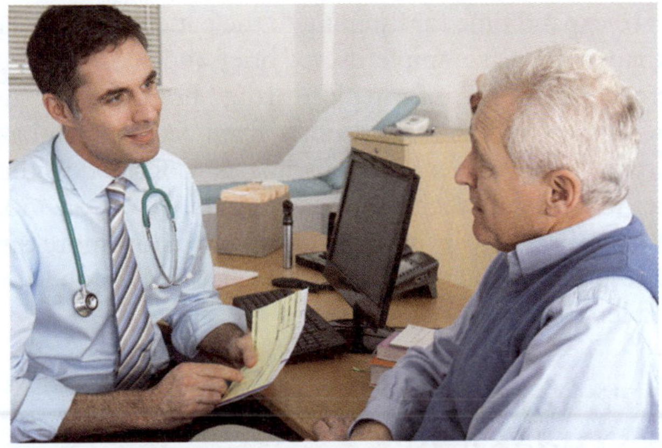

FIGURE 25-5. Conducting the health interview fully facing the patient and at eye level.

HEALTH HISTORY: GENERAL APPROACH

As you interview older adults, you will need to modify your usual approach to obtaining the Health History. It calls for enhanced interviewing techniques and a special emphasis on certain topics not often emphasized or discussed with younger adults. As with all patients, your demeanor should convey respect, patience, and cultural awareness. Be sure to elicit from older patients their preferred way of being addressed.

Communicating Effectively with Older Adults

First, take the time to adjust the environment of the office, hospital, or nursing home to put your patient at ease. Recall the physiologic changes in temperature regulation, and make sure that the environment is neither too cool nor too warm. Bright lighting helps compensate for changes in lens proteins and allows the older patient to see your facial expressions and gestures more clearly. Older adults require 30% more light for equivalent vision, and up five times brighter light in areas for reading and task completion. However, ensure that no glare is emitted from light sources especially on highly polished surfaces. If possible, create gradual changes of light levels when coming in from outdoors. Face the patient directly, sitting at eye level (Fig. 25-5). Patients with quadriceps weakness benefit from chairs with higher seating and a wide stool with a handrail leading up to the examining table.

More than 50% of older adults have hearing deficits, especially for higher frequency tones (presbycusis), so choose a quiet room that is free of distractions or noise. Speak in low tones, and make sure the patient is using glasses, hearing aids, and dentures to assist with communication (Box 25-2).

Box 25-2. Tips for Communicating Effectively with Older Adults

- Provide a well-lit, moderately warm setting with minimal background noise, chairs with arms, and access to the examining table.
- Face the patient and speak in low tones; make sure the patient is using glasses, hearing devices, and dentures, if needed.
- Adjust the pace and content of the interview to the stamina of the patient; consider two visits for initial evaluations.
- Allow time for open-ended questions and reminiscing; include family and caregivers when indicated, especially if the patient has cognitive impairment.
- Make use of screening instruments, the clinical record, and reports from other health disciplines.
- Provide written instructions and make sure they are in large print and easy to read.
- Always give the patient an updated medication list that includes the name of the medication, dosage instructions, and why the medication is being prescribed.

Shaping the Content and Pace of the Visit

With older adults, rethink the traditional format of the visit. Older patients often measure their lives in terms of years left rather than years lived. They may reminisce about the past and previous experiences. By listening to these life reviews, you gain important insights that help you understand and support them as they work through painful feelings or recapture joys and accomplishments. At the same time, it is important to weigh the need to assess complex problems against the patient's endurance and possible fatigue.

To expand time for listening to the patient but prevent exhaustion, make ample use of brief and well-validated screening tools, information from home visits and the clinical record, and reports from family members, caregivers, and other health disciplines. Consider dividing the initial assessment into two visits. Two or more shorter visits may be more productive to allow more time to respond to questions since explanations may be slow and lengthy.

Eliciting Symptoms from the Older Adult

Eliciting the history calls for an astute clinician: patients may accidentally or intentionally underreport symptoms; the presentation of acute illnesses may differ from younger patients; common symptoms may mask a geriatric syndrome; or patients may have cognitive impairment. Use simple sentences with prompts to elicit necessary information. For patients with severe cognitive impairments, confirm key symptoms with family members or caregivers in the patient's presence and with his or her consent. To avoid invalid assumptions, explore how older patients view themselves and their situations. Listen for their priorities and coping skills. These insights strengthen your partnerships with both patients and families as you evolve plans for care and treatment.

Underreporting. Older patients tend to give more positive ratings to their overall health than younger adults, even when affected by disease and disability. Some are reluctant to report their symptoms. Some are afraid or embarrassed; others try to avoid clinical expenses or the discomforts of diagnosis and treatment. Still others overlook their symptoms, thinking they are merely part of aging, or they may simply forget about them. To minimize delayed diagnosis and treatment, ask direct questions, use the well-validated geriatric screening tools, and consult with family members and caregivers.

Atypical Presentations of Illness. Acute illnesses present differently in older adults. Older patients with infections are less likely to have fever. Older patients having a myocardial infarction are less likely to report chest pain and may commonly report symptoms atypical of myocardial infarction such as shortness of breath, palpitations, syncope, and confusion. One-third of older adults with hyperthyroidism present with fatigue, weight loss, and tachycardia in lieu of the classic features of heat intolerance, sweating, and hyperreflexia. Up to 35% present with new-onset atrial fibrillation.

In older adults, the prevalence of hyperthyroidism is 0.5% to 4% and of hypothyroidism, ~10% in men and 16% in women.

Hyperthyroidism increases the risk of osteoporosis, and, in affected women, the risk of hip and vertebral fractures increases threefold.

In older adults, hypothyroidism is most commonly caused by autoimmune thyroiditis (Hashimoto thyroiditis); fatigue, weakness, constipation, dry skin, and cold intolerance are often attributed to other conditions, medication side effects, or aging.

Geriatric Syndromes. Managing an increasing number of interrelated conditions calls for recognizing the symptom clusters of different *geriatric syndromes.*

A **geriatric syndrome** is "a multifactorial condition that involves the interaction between identifiable situation-specific stressors and underlying age-related risk factors, resulting in damage across multiple organ systems," as shown in Figure 25-6. These syndromes are strongly linked to functional decline. Examples include *functional impairment, frailty, delirium, depression, cognitive impairment, falls,* and *urinary incontinence.*

Experts state that "evaluating functional status, frailty, and other geriatric syndromes while simultaneously addressing individual disease processes is at the heart of geriatric approach to primary care." It is especially important to recognize these syndromes because symptoms may cluster in patterns unfamiliar to the patient.

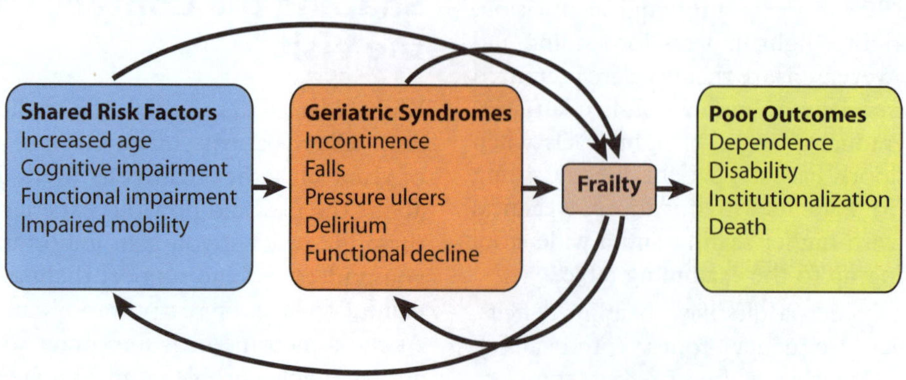

FIGURE 25-6. Interaction between geriatric syndromes and age-related risk factors resulting in poor outcomes.

Addressing Cultural Dimensions of Aging

As the older population grows larger, it will also grow more diverse. Knowledge and skills about the cultural dimensions of aging are the cornerstone to improving health care for the rapidly growing number of older adults of diverse ethnic backgrounds.

The changing demographics of aging only hint at how older adults of different ethnicities experience suffering, illness, and decisions about their health care. Culture and socioeconomic attributes affect the epidemiology of illness and mental health, the process of acculturation in families, individual concerns about aging, choices about healers and when to pursue symptoms, the potential for misdiagnosis, and disparities in health outcomes. Culture shapes beliefs about the entire spectrum of aging: work and retirement, perceptions of health and illness, the utility of medications, use of health care proxies, and preferences about dying, to name just a few. Improving competence in care for diverse older populations is a critical step in improving health outcomes.

Aging racial/ethnic minority populations have poorer health outcomes in cardiovascular disease, diabetes, cancer, asthma, and human immunodeficiency virus/acquired immunodeficiency syndrome as well as shorter life spans.

Experts recommend letting patients establish their cultural identity by exploring four key areas during the interview:

- the individual's cultural identity;
- cultural explanations of the individual's illness;
- cultural factors related to the psychosocial environment and levels of function; and
- cultural elements in the clinician–patient relationship.

Learn to convey respect to older adults through culturally specific nonverbal communication. Direct eye contact or handshaking, for example, may not be culturally appropriate. Identify critical life experiences from the country of origin or migration history that affect the patient's outlook and psyche. Ask about family decision making, spiritual advisors, and traditional healers and practices. Cultural values particularly affect decisions about the end of life.

Older adults, family, and even an extended community group may make these decisions with or for the older patient. Such group decision making is quite different from the focus on individual autonomy and informed consent featured in contemporary health care settings. Eliciting the stresses of migration and acculturation, using medical interpreters effectively, enlisting "patient navigators" from the family and community, and accessing culturally validated assessment tools will help you provide empathic care of older adults.

Special Areas of Concern When Assessing Older Adults

- Functional impairments in activities of daily living and instrumental activities of daily living
- Medication management
- Smoking
- Alcohol
- Nutrition

Other areas of concern among older adults are addressed in more detail in the following sections:

- Acute and persistent pain
- Cognitive impairment
- Urinary incontinence
- Falls

Symptoms in the older adult can have many meanings and interconnections, as seen with the geriatric syndromes. Approach these areas with extra thoroughness and sensitivity, always with the goal of helping your older patients to maintain their optimal level of function and well-being.

Functional Impairments in Activities of Daily Living and Instrumental Activities of Daily Living

The daily activities of older adults, especially those with chronic illness, provide an important baseline for future evaluations. First, ask about how well the patient performs the **activities of daily living (ADLs)**, which consist of six basic self-care abilities—bathing, dressing, toileting, transferring, continence, and feeding. Then, move on to higher level functions, the **instrumental activities of daily living (IADLs)**—using the telephone, shopping, preparing food, housekeeping, laundry, transportation, taking medicine, and managing money.

Can the patient perform these activities independently, does he or she need some help, or is the patient entirely dependent on others?

Start with open-ended questions like "Tell me about your typical day" or "Tell me about your day yesterday." Then probe for more detail... "You got up at 8 AM? How is it getting out of bed?... What did you do next?" Ask if activity levels have changed, who is available for help, and what helpers or caregivers actually do. Remember that assessing the patient's safety is a clinical priority.

Medication Management

The magnitude of adverse drug events leading to hospitalization and poor patient outcomes underscores

Box 25-3. Improving Medication Safety among Older Adults

- Perform a thorough *medication history* includes name, dose, frequency, and the *patient's view* of the reason for taking each drug. Ask the patient to bring in all medication bottles and over-the-counter products to develop an accurate medication list.
- Complete a *medication reconciliation* at every visit especially after care transitions.
- Explore all components of *polypharmacy*—a major cause of morbidity—including suboptimal prescribing, concurrent use of multiple drugs, underuse, inappropriate use, and nonadherence.
- Ask specifically about over-the-counter products; vitamin and nutritional supplements; and mood-altering drugs such as opioids, benzodiazepines, and recreational substances.
- Assess medications for drug interactions.

the importance of a thorough medication history (Box 25-3). Adults over age 65 years receive approximately 30% of all prescriptions. Almost 40% take five or more prescription drugs daily. Older adults have more than 50% of all reported adverse drug events causing hospital admission, reflecting pharmacodynamic changes in the distribution, metabolism, and elimination of drugs that place them at increased risk. Medications are the single most common modifiable risk factor associated with falls.

Review strategies for avoiding **polypharmacy**. Keep the number of drugs prescribed to a minimum and "start low and go slow" with respect to dosing. Learn about drug–drug interactions and consult the *2019 AGS Beers Criteria*, widely used by health care providers, educators, and policymakers. In addition to a list of hazardous drugs for older adults, this new criteria now include lists of select drugs that should be avoided or have their dose adjusted based on the individual's kidney function and select drug–drug interactions documented to be associated with harms in older adults.

Smoking

Smoking is harmful at all ages. At each visit, advise smokers, approximately 9.5% of older adults, to quit. The commitment to stop smoking may take time, but quitting is crucial for reducing the risk of heart disease, pulmonary disease, malignancy, and loss of daily function.

Alcohol

Recommended drinking limits are lower for adults over age 65 years due to physiologic changes that alter alcohol metabolism, frequent comorbid illness, and risk of drug

Box 25-4. Clues to Alcohol-Use Disorders in Older Adults

- Memory loss, cognitive impairment
- Depression, anxiety
- Neglect of hygiene, appearance
- Poor appetite, nutritional deficits
- Sleep disruption
- Hypertension refractory to therapy
- Blood sugar control problems
- Seizures refractory to therapy
- Impaired balance and gait including falls
- Recurrent gastritis and esophagitis
- Difficulty managing warfarin dosing
- Use of other substances that may lead to addiction such as sedatives or opioid analgesics, illicit drugs, nicotine

interactions. Older adults should have no more than 2 drinks on any one day or 7 drinks a week. More than 40% of adults over age 65 years drink alcohol, about 4.5% are binge-drinkers, and 2% to 4% may have abuse or dependence. More than 14% of older adults exceed the recommended limits. When health status is taken into account, more than 53% have harmful or hazardous drinking. From 10% to 15% of older patients in primary care practices and up to 38% of hospitalized older adults are reported to have problem drinking. Despite the high prevalence of alcohol-related problems, rates of detection and treatment are low. Screening all older adults for harmful alcohol use is especially important due to adverse interactions with most medications and exacerbation of comorbid illnesses, including cirrhosis, gastrointestinal bleeding or reflux disease, gout, hypertension, diabetes, insomnia, gait disorders, and depression in up to 30% of older patients.

Watch for clues of excess alcohol consumption (Box 25-4) especially in patients with recent bereavement or losses, pain, disability or depression, or a family history of alcohol disorders.

Nutrition

Taking a dietary history and using nutritional screening tools often reveal nutritional deficits. Prevalence of undernutrition increases with age, affecting up to 10% of nursing home residents and up to 50% of older patients at hospital discharge. Recent data suggest that only 30% to 40% meet recommended guidelines for daily intake of fruit and vegetables. Older adults with chronic diseases are particularly vulnerable, especially those with poor dentition, oral or gastrointestinal disorders, depression or other psychiatric illness, and drug regimens that affect appetite and oral secretions.

SPECIAL TOPICS IN OLDER ADULT CARE

Frailty

Frailty is a multifactorial geriatric syndrome characterized by an age-related lack of adaptive physiologic capacity occurring even in the absence of identifiable illness. Frailty typically signifies loss of muscle mass, decreased energy and exercise intolerance, and decreased physiologic reserve, with increasing vulnerability to physiologic stressors.

Advance Directives and Palliative Care

Many older patients are interested in discussing end-of-life decisions and would like providers to initiate these discussions *before* the onset of serious illness. *Advance care planning* involves several tasks: providing information, clarifying the patient's preferences, and identifying the surrogate decision maker. You can begin this discussion by linking these decisions to a current illness or experiences with relatives or friends. Ask the patient about "Do Not Resuscitate" orders specifying life support measures "if the heart or lungs were to stop or give out." Also encourage the patient to designate in writing a health care proxy or durable power of attorney for health care, "someone who can make decisions reflecting your wishes in cases where you are unable to or in an emergency."

Roughly half of hospitalized older adults require surrogate decision making within 48 hours of admission. Common topics include life-sustaining care, surgeries and procedures, and discharge planning. Conversations about life care choices help patients and their families prepare openly and in advance for a peaceful death. Pursue these discussions during office visits rather than in the stressful environment of the emergency department or intensive care unit.

Experts note that *advance care directives* can be more flexible, depending on the situation. These directives "may range from general statements of values to such specific orders as do not resuscitate (DNR), do not intubate (DNI), do not hospitalize, do not provide artificial hydration or nutrition, or do not administer antibiotics. Different situations, including different stages of health and illness, demand different types of advanced care directives, and thus require both different conversations and different training in leading such discussions." Moreover, always consult patients with capacity about current options because their decisions supersede prior written instructions.

For patients with advanced or terminal illnesses, include the review of advanced directives in an overall plan for *palliative care*. **Palliative care** encompasses the alleviation of pain and suffering and the promotion of optimal quality of life across all phases of treatment, including curative interventions and rehabilitation (Fig. 25-7). Its goals are "to consider the physical, mental, spiritual, and social well-being of patients and

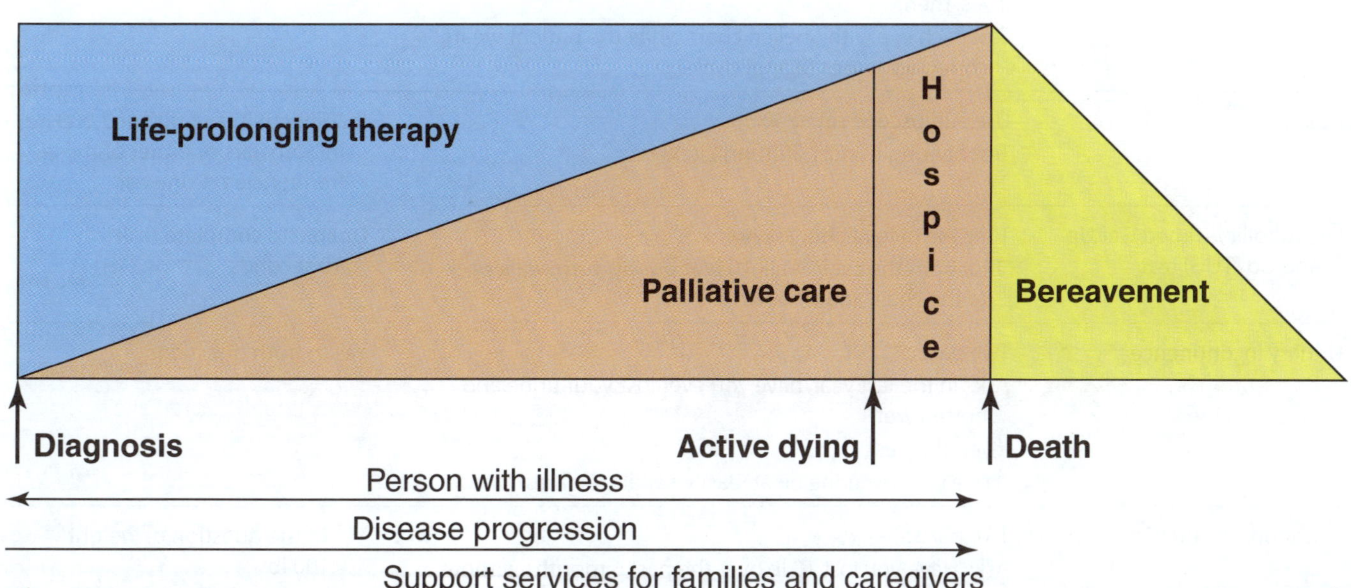

FIGURE 25-7. The place of palliative care within the course of illness. (From Burggraf V et al. *Healthy Aging: Principles and Clinical Practice for Clinicians.* Wolters Kluwer; 2015, Fig. 29-1.)

their families in order to maintain hope while ensuring patient dignity and respecting autonomy" both for patients with serious illnesses and for patients considering hospice care at the end of life. To ease patient and family distress, use effective communication skills: Make good eye contact; ask open-ended questions; respond to anxiety, depression, or changes in the patient's affect; show empathy; and be sure to consult caregivers.

PHYSICAL EXAMINATION: GENERAL APPROACH

As you have observed in the previous sections, the assessment of the older adult has several unique features compared to the customary format of gathering the health history. Because of its importance to older adult health, the physical examination has a distinct focus on functional assessment. Therefore, the Techniques of Examination section will start with the functional assessment. Following this are the components of the "head-to-toe" examination, tailored to the older adult.

TECHNIQUES OF EXAMINATION

Assessing Functional Status

All visits are opportunities to promote the patient's independence and optimal level of function. Although the specific goals of care vary from patient to patient, preserving the patient's functional status is of primary importance. *Functional status* is the ability to perform tasks and fulfill social roles associated with daily living across a wide range of complexity. Establishing functional status provides a baseline for making interventions that optimize the patient's level of function and for identifying geriatric syndromes that can be treated or delayed.

Your assessment of functional status begins as the patient enters the room. The *10-Minute Geriatric Screener* is one of several validated and time-efficient performance-based assessment tools (Box 25-5). It is brief, has high interrater agreement, and can be easily used by office staff. It covers three important areas: cognitive, psychosocial, and physical functions. It includes vision, hearing, and questions about urinary incontinence, an often-hidden source of social isolation and distress.

Box 25-5. 10-Minute Geriatric Screener

Problem	Screening Measure	Positive Screen
Vision	Two parts: Ask: "Do you have difficulty driving, or watching television, or reading, or doing any of your daily activities because of your eyesight?" If yes, then: Test each eye with Snellen chart while the patient wears corrective lenses (if applicable).	Yes to question and inability to read >20/40 on Snellen chart
Hearing	Use audioscope set at 40 dB Test hearing using 1,000 and 2,000 Hz.	Inability to hear 1,000 or 2,000 Hz in both ears or either of these frequencies in one ear
Leg mobility–Timed Get Up and Go (TUG) test	Time the patient after asking: "Rise from the chair. Walk 10 feet briskly, turn, walk back to the chair, and sit down."	Unable to complete task in 10 seconds
Urinary incontinence*	Two parts: Ask: "In the last year, have you ever lost your urine and gotten wet?" If yes, then ask: "Have you lost urine on at least 6 separate dates?"	Yes to both questions
Nutrition/weight loss	Two parts: Ask: "Have you lost 10 lb over the past 6 months without trying to do so?" Weigh the patient.	Yes to the question or weight <100 lb

(*continued*)

Box 25-5. 10-Minute Geriatric Screener (*continued*)

Problem	Screening Measure	Positive Screen
Memory	Three-item recall	Unable to remember all three items after 1 minute
Depression	Ask: "Do you often feel sad or depressed?"	Yes to the question
Physical disability	Six questions: Are you able to . . .: "Do strenuous activities like fast walking or bicycling?" "Do heavy work around the house like washing windows, walls, or floors?" "Go shopping for groceries or clothes?" "Get to places out of walking distance?" "Bathe, either a sponge bath, tub bath, or shower?" "Dress, like putting on a shirt, buttoning and zipping, or putting on shoes?"	No to any of the questions

*For identifying causes of transient incontinence, the DIAPPERS mnemonic may be helpful:

- *D*elirium,
- *I*nfection (e.g., urinary tract infection),
- *A*trophic urethritis or vaginitis,
- *P*harmaceuticals (e.g., diuretics, anticholinergics, calcium channel blockers, opioids, sedatives, alcohol),
- *P*sychological disorders (e.g., depression),
- *E*xcessive urine output (e.g., heart failure, uncontrolled diabetes),
- *R*estricted mobility (e.g., hip fracture, environmental barriers, restraints),
- *S*tool impaction.

General Survey

As the patient enters the room, how does the patient walk to the chair? Move onto the examining table? Are there changes in posture or involuntary movements? Note the patient's hygiene and dress. Assess the patient's apparent state of health, degree of vitality, and mood and affect. As you talk with the patient, decide if screening for cognitive changes is needed.

Undernutrition, slowed motor performance, loss of muscle mass, or weakness suggests frailty.

Kyphosis or abnormal gait can impair balance and increase risk of falls.

Flat or impoverished affect is seen in depression, Parkinson disease, and Alzheimer disease.

Vital Signs

Measure blood pressure using recommended techniques, checking for increased SBP and *widened pulse pressure.* With aging, SBP and peripheral vascular resistance increase, whereas DBP decreases. For adults aged ≥60 years, the eighth Joint National Committee (JNC8) recommends blood pressure targets of ≤150/90 but notes that if treatment results in SBP <140 and is "well tolerated and without adverse effects to health or quality of life, treatment does not need to be adjusted."

However, in the "oldest old," those aged 80 years and older, other experts cite studies showing that blood pressure targets of 140 to <150/70 to 80 appear optimal for notable reductions in stroke, cardiovascular events, and all-cause mortality.

Isolated systolic hypertension (SBP ≥140 mm Hg with DBP <90 mm Hg) after age 50 years and pulse pressure ≥60 increase risk of stroke, renal failure, and heart disease.

Assess the patient for *orthostatic* or *postural hypotension*, defined as a drop in SBP of ≥20 mm Hg or DBP of ≥10 mm Hg within 3 minutes of standing. Measure blood pressure and heart rate in two positions: supine after the patient rests for up to 10 minutes; then within 3 minutes after standing up.

Orthostatic hypotension occurs in 20% of older adults and in up to 50% of frail nursing home residents, especially when they first get up. Symptoms include lightheadedness, weakness, unsteadiness, visual blurring, and, in 20% to 30% of patients, syncope. Causes include medications, autonomic disorders, diabetes, prolonged bed rest, volume depletion, amyloidosis, postprandial state, and cardiovascular disorders.

Measure heart rate, respiratory rate, and temperature. The apical heart rate often allows better detection of arrhythmias in older patients than does the radial pulse. Use thermometers accurate for lower temperatures. Obtain oxygen saturation using a pulse oximeter.

Respiratory rate ≥25 breaths per minute points to lower respiratory infection, heart failure, and chronic obstructive pulmonary disease exacerbation.

Hypothermia is more common in older patients.

Weight and height are especially important among older adults and are needed for calculation of the BMI. Weight is also a key clinical measure for patients with heart failure and chronic kidney disease. Weight should be measured at every visit, preferably with footwear removed.

Low weight is a key indicator of poor nutrition, seen in depression, alcoholism, cognitive impairment, malignancy, chronic organ failure (cardiac, renal, pulmonary), medication use, social isolation, poor dentition, and poverty. Rapidly increasing daily weights occur in fluid overload.

Skin, Hair, and Nails

Note physiologic changes of aging, such as thinning, loss of elastic tissue and turgor, and wrinkling. Skin may be dry, flaky, rough, and often itchy (*asteatosis*), with a latticework of shallow fissures that creates a mosaic of small polygons, especially on the legs.

Observe any patchy changes in color. Check the extensor surface of the hands and forearms for white depigmented patches, or *pseudoscars,* and for well-demarcated vividly purple macules or patches, *actinic purpura,* that may fade after several weeks (Fig. 25-8).

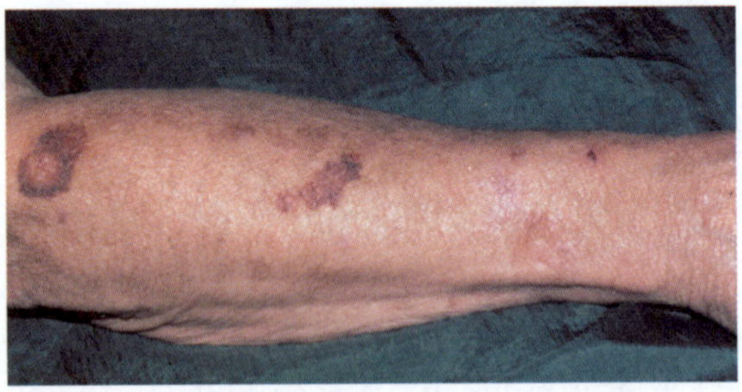

FIGURE 25-8. Actinic purpura on forearm.

Look for changes from sun exposure. Areas of skin may appear weather beaten, thickened, yellowed, and deeply furrowed; there may be *actinic lentigines,* or "liver spots," and *actinic keratoses,* superficial flattened papules covered by a dry scale (Fig. 25-9).

Distinguish such lesions from a basal cell carcinoma, a translucent nodule that spreads and leaves a depressed center with a firm elevated border, and squamous cell carcinoma, a firm reddish-appearing lesion often emerging in a sun-exposed area. A dark raised asymmetric lesion with irregular borders may be a melanoma.

Inspect for the benign lesions of aging, namely *comedones,* or blackheads, on the cheeks or around the eyes; *cherry angiomas,* which often appear early in adulthood; and *seborrheic keratoses,* raised yellowish lesions that feel greasy and velvety or warty.

Vesicular lesions occurring in a dermatomal distribution are suspicious for herpes zoster from reactivation of latent varicella-zoster virus in the dorsal root ganglia. Risk increases with age and impaired cell-mediated immunity.

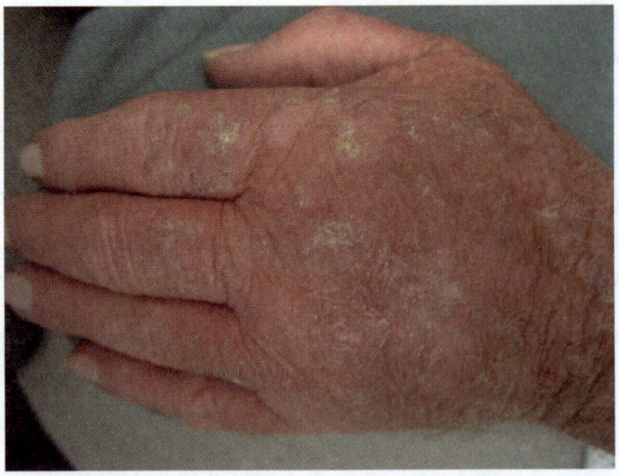

FIGURE 25-9. Actinic keratoses on dorsum of hand. (Image provided by Stedman's.)

In older bed-bound patients, especially those emaciated or neurologically impaired, inspect the skin for damage or ulceration on the sacral and perianal areas, the lower back, heels, and elbows where pressure ulcers commonly occur.

Pressure ulcers arise from obliteration of arteriolar and capillary blood flow to the skin or from shear forces during movement across sheets or when lifted upright incorrectly.

Examine the hair and scalp. Note the distribution, texture, and quantity of hair. Also assess the nails for color or thickening.

Alopecia, or hair loss, can be diffuse, patchy, or total. Male and female pattern hair loss are normal with aging.

Eyes

Inspect the eyelids, the bony orbit, and the eye. The eye may appear recessed from atrophy of fat in the surrounding tissues. Observe any *senile ptosis* arising from weakening of the levator palpebrae, relaxation of the skin, and increased weight of the upper eyelid. Check the eyelashes in the lower lids to see whether they are directed toward the eye (**entropion**). This causes the eyelashes and skin of the eyelid to rub against the cornea and conjunctiva causing irritation. Also describe any sagging and outward turning of the lower eyelid and eyelashes (**ectropion**) which can lead to excessive tearing, crusting of the eyelid, mucous discharge, and irritation of the eye. Note yellowing of the sclera, and *arcus senilis,* a benign whitish ring around the limbus.

Test the best-corrected visual acuity in each eye, using a pocket Snellen chart or wall-mounted chart. Note any *presbyopia,* the loss of near vision arising from decreased elasticity of the lens related to aging.

One in three adults suffers some form of visual loss by age 65 years.

Test pupillary constriction to light, both the direct and consensual response and during the near response. Then swing the light beam several times between the right and left eyes. Test the six directions of gaze. Except for possible impairment in upward gaze, extraocular movements should remain intact.

If the pupil dilates as the light swings over, a relative afferent pupillary defect is present, which is suspicious for optic nerve disease. Refer to an ophthalmologist.

Using your ophthalmoscope, carefully examine the lenses and fundi.

The prevalence of cataracts, glaucoma, and macular degeneration all increases with aging.

Using the ophthalmoscope beam, check at 1 to 2 ft for a red reflex. With the ophthalmoscope lens at +10 diopters, inspect each lens close to the eye for opacities. Do not depend on the flashlight alone because the lens may look clear superficially.

Retinal microvascular disease is linked to cerebral microvascular changes and cognitive impairment.

In older adults, the fundi lose their youthful shine and light reflections, and the arteries look narrowed, paler, straighter, and less brilliant. Assess the cup-to-disc ratio, usually 1:2 or less.

An increased cup-to-disc ratio suggests primary open angle glaucoma (POAG), caused by irreversible optic neuropathy and leading to loss of peripheral and central vision and blindness (Fig. 25-10). Prevalence of POAG is four to five times higher in adults with African and Latino ancestry. People of Asian descent are more prone to develop angle-closure glaucoma and normal-tension glaucoma.

Inspect the fundi for colloid bodies causing alterations in pigmentation, called *drusen*. Drusen may be hard and sharply defined, or soft and confluent with altered pigmentation.

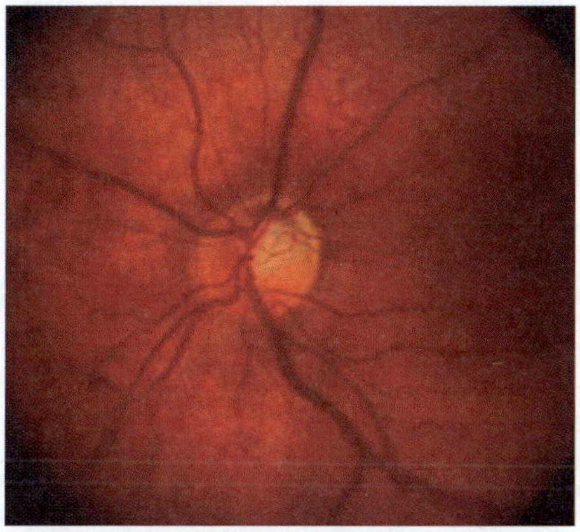

FIGURE 25-10. Fundus with increased cup-to-disc ratio ("disc cupping") due to glaucoma.

Macular degeneration causes poor central vision and blindness (Fig. 25-11). Types include dry atrophic (more common but less severe) and wet exudative, or neovascular.

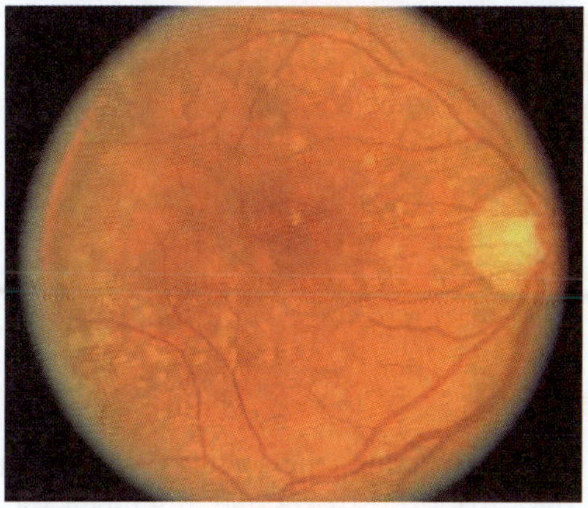

FIGURE 25-11. Fundus with age-related macular degeneration. Notice the "drusen spots" located centrally.

Ears

Test hearing by occluding one ear and using the whispered voice technique or an **audioscope**. Be sure to inspect the ear canals for cerumen because removal can quickly improve hearing. Asking if hearing loss is present is an effective screening method. Proceed to audiometry for those saying yes; check acuity to whispered voice for saying no.

Mouth and Teeth

Examine the oral cavity for odor, appearance of the gingival mucosa, any caries, mobility of the teeth, and adequacy of saliva. Inspect closely for lesions on any of the mucosal surfaces. Ask the patient to remove dentures so that you can check the gums for denture sores.

Malodor points to poor oral hygiene, periodontitis, and caries. Gingivitis accompanies periodontal disease. Dental plaque and cavitation may cause caries. For increased tooth mobility from abscesses or advanced caries, consider removal to prevent aspiration. Decreased salivation results from medication effects, radiation, Sjögren syndrome, or dehydration. Oral tumors can cause lesions, usually on the lateral margins of the tongue and floor of the mouth.

Neck

Continue with your usual examination of the thyroid gland and lymph nodes.

In older adults, common causes of hyperthyroidism are Graves disease and toxic multinodular goiter. Causes of hypothyroidism include autoimmune thyroiditis, followed by drugs, neck radiotherapy, thyroidectomy, or radioiodine ablation.

Thorax and Lungs

Complete the usual examination, observing for subtle signs of changes in pulmonary function.

Increased anteroposterior diameter, purse-lipped breathing, and dyspnea with talking or minimal exertion suggest chronic obstructive pulmonary disease.

Cardiovascular System

Review your findings from measurement of the blood pressure and heart rate.

Isolated systolic hypertension and a widened PP are cardiac risk factors, prompting a search for left ventricular hypertrophy (LVH).

Begin by inspecting the jugular venous pressure. Palpate the carotid upstrokes and auscultate for carotid bruits.

A tortuous atherosclerotic aorta can raise pressure in the left jugular veins by impairing emptying into the right atrium. A tortuous aorta can also cause kinking of the carotid artery low in the neck on the right, chiefly in women with hypertension, which can be mistaken for a carotid aneurysm.

Carotid bruits can occur in aortic stenosis. The presence of bruits from carotid stenosis increases risk of ipsilateral stroke.

Assess the point of maximal impulse (PMI), then auscultate S_1 and S_2. Listen also for the extra sounds of S_3 and S_4.

A sustained PMI is present in LVH; a diffuse PMI and an S_3 signal left ventricular dilatation from heart failure or cardiomyopathy. An S_4 often accompanies hypertension.

Beginning in the second right interspace, listen for cardiac murmurs in all areas of auscultation. Describe the timing, shape, location of maximal intensity, radiation, intensity, pitch, and quality of each murmur you detect.

A systolic crescendo–decrescendo murmur in the second right interspace suggests aortic sclerosis or aortic stenosis, seen, respectively, in up to 40% and 2% to 3% of community-dwelling older adults. Both are associated with an increased risk of cardiovascular disease and death.

A harsh holosystolic murmur at the apex radiating to the axilla suggests mitral regurgitation, the most common murmur in older adults.

Breasts and Axillae

Palpate the breasts carefully for lumps or masses. Include palpation of the tail of Spence that extends into the axilla. Examine the axillae for lymphadenopathy. Note any scaly, vesicular ulcerated lesions on or near the nipple.

Any lumps or masses in older women, and, more rarely, in older men, mandate further investigation for possible breast cancer.

Peripheral Vascular System

Carefully palpate the brachial, radial, femoral, popliteal, and pedal pulses. Confirm diminished or absent pulses findings with an ankle–brachial index (ABI).

Diminished or absent pulses are present in peripheral arterial disease (PAD) with an ABI <0.9. The ABI has a sensitivity of 70% and specificity of 90%. In patients with PAD, 30% to 60% report no leg symptoms.

Abdomen

Inspect the abdomen for masses or visible pulsations. Auscultate for bruits over the aorta and the renal and femoral arteries. Palpate to the right and left of the midline for aortic pulsations. Try to assess the width of the aorta by pressing more deeply on each of its lateral margins.

Abdominal bruits are suspicious for atherosclerotic vascular disease.

A widened aorta of ≥3 cm and pulsatile mass occur in abdominal aortic aneurysm, especially in older male smokers.

Female Genitalia and Pelvic Examination

Take the time to explain your plans for the examination and arrange for careful patient positioning. You may need help from an assistant to move the older woman onto the examining table, then into the lithotomy position. Raising the head of the table may make her more comfortable. For the woman with arthritis or spinal deformities who cannot flex her hips or knees, an assistant can gently raise and support the legs, or help the woman into the left lateral position.

Inspect the vulva for changes related to menopause such as thinning of the skin, loss of pubic hair, and decreased distensibility of the introitus. Identify any labial masses.

Bluish swellings may be varicosities. Bulging of the anterior vaginal wall below the urethra may be an urethrocele or urethral diverticulum.

Benign masses include condylomata, fibromas, leiomyomas, and sebaceous cysts.

Inspect for any vulvar erythema.

Erythema with satellite lesions results from Candida infection; erythema with ulceration or a necrotic center is suspicious for vulvar carcinoma. Multifocal reddened lesions with white scaling plaques occur in extramammary Paget disease, a form of intraepithelial adenocarcinoma.

Inspect the urethra for caruncles or prolapse of fleshy erythematous mucosal tissue at the urethral meatus. Note any enlargement of the clitoris.

Clitoral enlargement may accompany androgen-producing tumors and use of androgen creams.

Spread the labia, press downward on the introitus to relax the levator muscles, and gently insert the speculum after moistening it with warm water or a water-soluble lubricant. If you find severe vaginal atrophy, a gaping introitus, or an introital stricture from estrogen loss, you will need to change the size of the speculum.

The thin patchy atrophic white plaques of lichen sclerosus are more common in postmenopausal women and may be precancerous.

Inspect the vaginal walls, which may be atrophic, and the cervix. Note any thin cervical mucus or vaginal or cervical discharge.

Estrogen-stimulated cervical mucus with ferning is seen in use of hormone replacement therapy, endometrial hyperplasia, and estrogen-producing tumors.

If indicated, use an endocervical brush (or less commonly, a wooden spatula) to obtain endocervical cells for the Pap smear. Consider using a blind swab if the atrophic vagina is too small.

After removing the speculum, ask the patient to bear down to detect uterine prolapse or a cystocele, urethrocele, or rectocele.

Perform the bimanual examination. Check the motion of the cervix and palpate for any uterine or adnexal masses.

Mobility of the cervix is restricted with inflammation, malignancy, or surgical adhesion.

Enlarging uterine fibroids, or leiomyomas, can be normal or malignant leiomyosarcoma; ovarian masses or enlargement are seen in ovarian cancer.

Perform the rectovaginal examination if indicated. Assess for uterine and adnexal irregularities through the anterior rectal wall and check for rectal masses. Change gloves after the bimanual examination so that no blood is present on your gloves when you obtain the stool sample.

A uterus that is enlarged, fixed, or irregular may have adhesions or contain a malignancy. Rectal masses are found in colorectal cancer.

Male Genitalia and Prostate

Examine the penis, retracting the foreskin, if present. Examine the scrotum, testes, and epididymis.

Findings include smegma, penile cancer, and scrotal hydroceles.

Proceed with the rectal examination. Assess rectal tone. Palpate for any rectal masses or nodularity or masses of the prostate. The anterior and central lobes of the prostate are inaccessible to palpation, which limits your ability to detect prostate enlargement or malignancy.

A loss of rectal tone can result in fecal incontinence. Rectal masses suggest colorectal cancer.

Rule out prostate cancer if nodules or masses are present.

Musculoskeletal System

Your evaluation of this system began with leg mobility testing during the 10-Minute Geriatric Screener (see Box 25-5) at the outset of the visit. Leg mobility is routinely tested by the "*Timed Get up and Go*," or *TUG, test* for gait and balance, an excellent screen for risk of falling (Box 25-6).

Box 25-6. Timed Get Up and Go Test

Performed with patient wearing regular footwear, using usual assistive device if needed, and sitting back in an armless chair. After instructing the patient on what to do, on the word "Go," the patient should:

1. Get up from the armless chair
2. Walk 3 m (in a line)
3. Turn around
4. Walk back to the chair
5. Sit back down

Time the second effort. Observe patient for postural stability, steppage, stride length, and sway.

Scoring:

- Normal: completes task in <10 seconds
- Abnormal: completes task in >20 seconds

If the patient has joint deformities, deficits in mobility, pain with movement, or a delayed "get up and go" perform a more thorough examination of individual joints and a more comprehensive neurologic examination.

Look for degenerative joint changes in osteoarthritis and joint inflammation from rheumatoid or gouty arthritis.

Low scores correlate with good functional independence; high scores correlate with poor functional independence and higher risk of falls.

Nervous System

As with the musculoskeletal examination, your evaluation began with the 10-Minute Geriatric Screener (see Box 25-5). Carefully assess memory and affect.

Pay close attention to gait and balance, particularly standing balance; timed 10-foot walk; stride characteristics like width, pace, and length of stride; and careful turning. When gait abnormalities are detected, pursue a more detailed neurologic examination.

Abnormalities of gait and balance, especially widening of base, slowing and lengthening of stride, and difficulty turning, are correlated with risk for falls.

Examine for evidence of *T*remor, *R*igidity, *A*kinesia, and *P*ostural instability, or TRAP.

These are several of the most common features of Parkinson disease. The tremor in Parkinson disease is slow frequency, occurs at rest, has a "pill-rolling" quality, and is aggravated by stress and inhibited during sleep or movement.

Also look for bradykinesia, the most characteristic clinical sign, and micrographia, shuffling "freezing" gait, and difficulty rising from a chair.

RECORDING YOUR FINDINGS

Note that initially you may use sentences to describe your findings; later you will use phrases. The style below contains phrases appropriate for most write-ups. As you read through this physical examination, you will notice some atypical findings. Try to test yourself. See if you can interpret these findings in the context of all you have learned about the examination of the older adult.

Recording the Physical Examination of the Older Adult

Mr. J is an older adult who appears healthy but overweight, with good muscle bulk and tone. He is alert and interactive, with good recall of his life history. He is accompanied by his son.

Vital Signs: BP 145/88 mm Hg right arm, supine; 154/94 mm Hg left arm, supine. Heart rate (HR) 98 and regular. Respiratory rate (RR) 18/min. Temperature (oral) 98.6°F. Ht. (without shoes) 5′ 10″. Wt. (dressed) 195 lb, BMI 28.

10-Minute Geriatric Screener:

Vision: Patient reports difficulty reading. Visual acuity 20/60 on both eyes on Snellen chart.

Hearing: Cannot hear whispered voice in either ear. Cannot hear 1,000 or 2,000 Hz with audioscope in either ear.

Further evaluation for glasses and possibly a hearing aid is needed.

Leg Mobility: Able to walk 10 ft briskly, turn, walk back to chair, and sit down in 9 seconds.

Urinary Incontinence: Has lost urine and gotten wet on 20 separate days.

Further evaluation for incontinence, including "DIAPPERS" assessment, prostate examination, and postvoid residual (requires bladder scan or catheterization) is needed.

Nutrition: Has lost 15 lb over the past 6 months without trying.

Evaluate and monitor weight loss. Needs nutritional screen.

Memory: Can remember three items after 1 minute.

Depression: Does not often feel sad or depressed.

Physical Disability: Can walk fast but cannot ride a bicycle. Can do moderate but not heavy work around the house. Can go shopping for groceries or clothes. Can get to places out of walking distance. Can bathe each day without difficulty. Can dress, including buttoning and zipping, and can put on shoes.

Consider an exercise regimen with strength training.

Physical Examination:

Skin. Warm and moist. Nails without clubbing or cyanosis. Hair thinning at crown.

Head, Eyes, Ears, Nose, Throat (HEENT). Scalp without lesions. Skull NC/AT. Conjunctiva pink, sclera muddy. Pupils 2 mm constricting to 1 mm, round, regular, equally reactive to light and accommodation. Extraocular movements intact. Disc margins sharp, without hemorrhages or exudates. Mild arteriolar narrowing. TMs with good cone of light. Weber midline. AC ≥ BC. Nasal mucosa pink. No sinus tenderness. Oral mucosa pink. Dentition fair. Caries present. Tongue midline, slight beefy redness. Pharynx without exudates.

Neck. Supple. Trachea midline. Thyroid lobes slightly enlarged, no nodules.

Lymph Nodes. No cervical, axillary, epitrochlear, or inguinal lymph nodes.

Respiratory. Thorax symmetric. Kyphosis noted. Lungs resonant with good excursion. Breath sounds vesicular. Diaphragms descend 4 cm bilaterally.

Cardiovascular. JVP 6 cm above the left atrium. Carotid upstrokes brisk, without bruits. PMI tapping, in the 5th ICS, 9 cm lateral to the midsternal line. II/VI harsh holosystolic murmur at the apex, radiating to the axilla. No other murmurs. No S_3, faint S_4 noted.

Abdomen. Flat, with active bowel sounds. Soft, nontender. No masses or hepatosplenomegaly. Liver span 7 cm in right midclavicular line; edge smooth and palpable at the RCM. No CVAT.

Genitourinary. Circumcised male. No penile lesions. Testes descended bilaterally, smooth without masses or tenderness.

Rectal. Good rectal sphincter tone. Rectal vault without masses. Stool brown, negative for occult blood.

Extremities. Warm and without edema. Calves supple.

Peripheral Vascular. Pulses 2+ and symmetric.

Musculoskeletal. Mild degenerative changes at the knees, with quadriceps wasting. Crepitation felt in both knees. Good range of motion in all joints.

Neurologic. Oriented to person, place, and time. Montreal Cognitive Assessment (MoCA): score 29. Cranial nerves II–XII intact. Motor: Decreased quadriceps bulk. Tone intact. Strength 4/5 throughout. RAMs, finger-to-nose intact. Gait with widened base. Sensation intact to pinprick, light touch, position, and vibration. Romberg negative. Reflexes 2+ and symmetric, with plantar response downgoing.

(continued)

HEALTH PROMOTION AND COUNSELING: EVIDENCE AND RECOMMENDATIONS

Important Topics for Health Promotion and Counseling in the Older Adult

- When to screen
- Screening for visual and hearing impairments
- Exercise and physical activity
- Household safety and fall prevention
- Immunizations
- Cancer screening
- Detecting the "3 Ds": delirium, dementia, and depression
- Elder mistreatment and abuse

When to Screen

As more adults live into their 80s and beyond, decisions about screening become more complex, and the evidence base for screening decisions becomes more limited. The aging population is physiologically heterogeneous, many with numerous chronic diseases and also many with delayed or absent disability. Moreover, level of function in "successful aging" does not always parallel the number of chronic ailments, and there are substantial regional gaps in availability and use of preventive services. Although there is relative consensus about immunization recommendations and falls prevention, screening for specific diseases remains more controversial. In general, individualized screening decisions should be based on each older adult's health and functional status, including presence of comorbidity, rather than age alone. This approach is depicted in Figure 25-12. The vertical axis shows the health status distribution of the population age 65 years and older, and the horizontal bars show the variation in importance of specific measures.

The American Geriatrics Society recommends a five-step approach to screening decisions:

1. Assess patient preferences
2. Interpret the available evidence
3. Estimate prognosis
4. Consider treatment feasibility
5. Optimize therapies and care plans

If life expectancy is short, give priority to treatment that benefits the patient in the time that remains. Consider avoiding screening if it overburdens the older adults who have multiple clinical problems, shortened life expectancy, or dementia. Tests that help with prognosis and planning may still be warranted even if the patient does not want to pursue treatment.

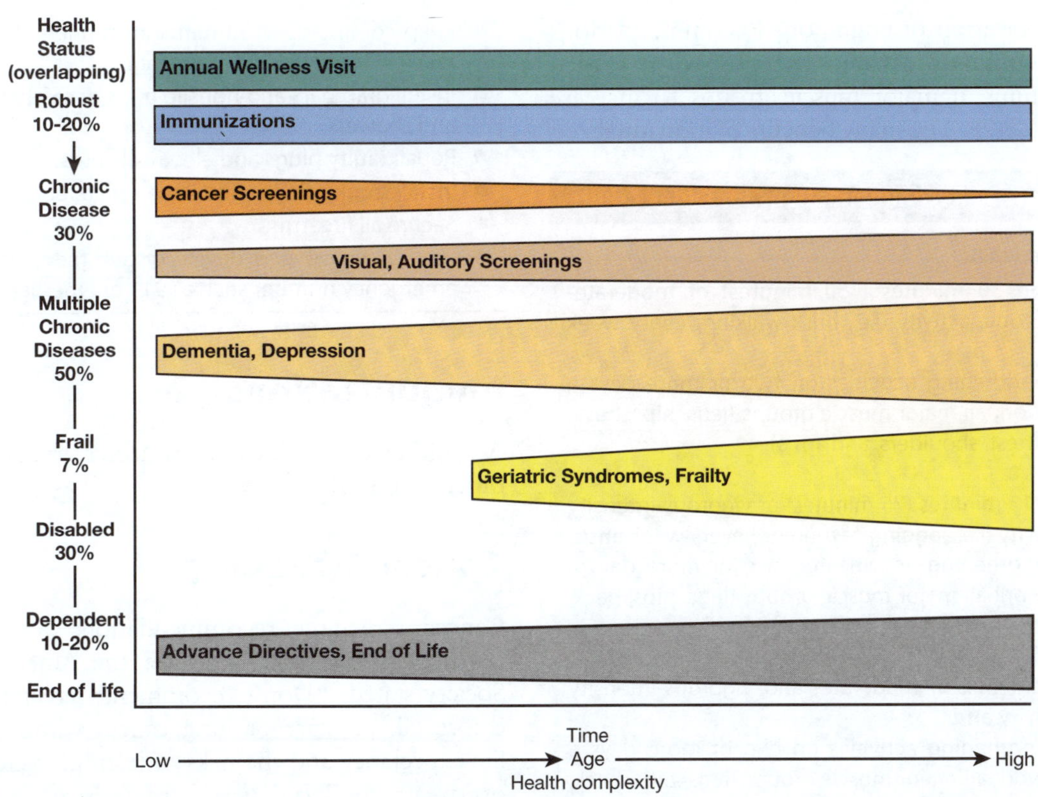

FIGURE 25-12. Older adults: relative role of screening and preventive services according to functional status.

Screening for Visual and Hearing Impairments

Among adults aged 65 to 69 years, 1% have visual impairment, increasing to 17% of those over age 80 years. About a third of adults over age 65 years have hearing loss, increasing to 80% in those over age 80 years.

Geriatricians recommend screening for *vision* and *hearing* as they are vital sensory modalities for daily living. They are key items in the *10-Minute Geriatric Screener.*

- Test vision objectively using an eye chart.
- Ask the patient whether they feel they have hearing impairment. If the patient says yes or gives an equivocal response, then they should be referred for audiometric testing. If the patient says no then proceed to the whisper test and more formal testing, if indicated.

Exercise and Physical Activity

Exercise is one of the most effective ways to promote healthy aging. Abundant literature documents the many benefits of physical activity in older adults, even in those who are frail. These include a "decrease in all-cause mortality; reduced risk of functional limitation and role limitation, falls, hypertension, diabetes, colorectal cancer, and breast cancer; and improvement in cognitive function, physical function . . . quality of life . . . gait speed, balance, and performance of activities of daily living" as well as preservation of cognition. Recommendations emphasize combining aerobic exercise with graded resistance training in major muscle groups to increase strength (Box 25-7). The many benefits of individualized supervised exercise plans usually outweigh the risks of joint pain, falls, and cardiac events.

Box 25-7. Exercise Recommendations for Older Adults

Adults need at least:

- 2 hours and 30 minutes (150 minutes) of moderate-intensity aerobic activity (i.e., brisk walking) every week **and**
- muscle-strengthening activities on two or more days a week that work all major muscle groups (legs, hips, back, abdomen, chest, shoulders, and arms)

OR

- 1 hour and 15 minutes (75 minutes) of vigorous-intensity aerobic activity (i.e., jogging or running) every week **and**
- muscle-strengthening activities on two or more days a week that work all major muscle groups (legs, hips, back, abdomen, chest, shoulders, and arms)

OR

- an equivalent mix of moderate- and vigorous-intensity aerobic activity **and**
- muscle-strengthening activities on two or more days a week that work all major muscle groups (legs, hips, back, abdomen, chest, shoulders, and arms)

Household Safety and Fall Prevention

Approximately 30% of adults aged 65 and older fall each year. Many have hip fractures and traumatic brain injuries that impact daily function and independence. Emergency room visits and deaths are most likely to involve yard and garden equipment, ladders and stepstools, personal-use items like hair dryers and flammable clothing, and bathroom and sports injuries. Encourage older adults to adopt corrective measures for poor lighting, chairs at awkward heights, slippery or irregular surfaces, and environmental hazards (Box 25-8).

Box 25-8. Household Safety Tips for Older Adults

- Install bright lighting and lightweight curtains or shades.
- Install handrails and lights on all staircases. Pathways and walkways should be well-lit.
- Remove items that cause tripping like papers, books, clothes, and shoes from stairs and walkways.
- Remove or secure small throw rugs and other rugs with double-sided tape.
- Wear shoes both inside and outside the house. Avoid bare feet and wearing slippers.
- Store medications safely.
- Keep commonly used items in cabinets that are easy to reach without using a step stool.
- Install grab bars and nonslip mats or safety strips in baths and showers.
- Repair faulty plugs and electrical cords.
- Install smoke alarms and have a plan for escaping fire.
- Secure all firearms.
- Have a clinical alert device/system for calling a universal emergency number such as 911 or emergency contacts.

Immunizations

A number of vaccines are routinely recommended for older adults (Box 25-9).

Cancer Screening

Cancer screening recommendations for older adults remain controversial. In 2015, the American Geriatrics Society stated: "Don't recommend screening for breast, colorectal, prostate or lung cancer without considering life expectancy and the risks of testing, overdiagnosis and overtreatment." *Individualized decision making* based on the principles outlined in "When to Screen" discussed

Box 25-9. Older Adult Immunizations, 2018

- *Influenza vaccination:* One high-dose vaccine annually
- Tetanus, diphtheria, and acellular pertussis (Tdap) vaccination: Administer 1 dose to older adults who previously did not receive a dose of tetanus toxoid, reduced diphtheria toxoid, and acellular pertussis vaccine (Tdap) as an adult or child
- *Tetanus and diphtheria toxoids (Td):* One dose Td booster every 10 years
- *Varicella vaccination:* Administer 2 doses to older adults without evidence of immunity to varicella 4 to 8 weeks apart
- *Zoster vaccination:* Administer 2 doses of recombinant zoster vaccine (RZV) 2 to 6 months apart to adults ≥50 years regardless of past episodes of herpes zoster or receipt of zoster vaccine live (ZVL)
- *Pneumococcal vaccination:* Administer to immunocompetent older adults 1 dose of *13-valent pneumococcal conjugate vaccine* (PCV13, Prevnar13) at age 65 years or older then followed by 1 dose of *23-valent pneumococcal polysaccharide vaccine* (PPSV23, Pneumovax23) at least 1 year after PCV13. Once a dose of PPSV23 is given at age 65 years or older, no additional doses of PPSV23 should be administered.

earlier should be advocated since "guidelines become less robust and evidence-based as individuals age and/or develop declining health status and disabilities."

The recommendations of the USPSTF that target straightforward age cutoffs are summarized in Box 25-10.

Recent more complex published frameworks include "weighing quantitative information, such as risk of cancer death and likelihood of beneficial and adverse screening outcomes, as well as qualitative factors, such as individual patients' values and preferences." The American College of Physicians has developed high- and low-value screening strategies that factor in health benefits, frequency of screening, and harms and costs (Box 25-11).

Box 25-10. Screening Recommendations for Older Adults

- **Breast cancer (2016):** Recommends mammography every 2 years for women aged 50 to 74 years (grade B) and cites insufficient evidence for screening women aged ≥75 years (I statement).
- **Cervical cancer (2018):** Recommends *against* routine screening for women over age 65 years if they have had adequate recent screening with normal Pap smears and are not otherwise at high risk for cervical cancer, based on fair evidence (grade D).
- **Colorectal cancer (2016):** Recommends screening adults age 50 years through 75 years (grade A). The USPSTF in its new recommendation highlighted the evidence of reduction in mortality rather than emphasizing the specific screening approaches since no head-to-head studies exist demonstrating one strategy to be more effective than others. Available strategies and screening intervals include colonoscopy every 10 years, CT colonography every 5 years, annual fecal immunochemical test, annual high-sensitivity fecal occult blood test (FOBT), fecal DNA test every 1 or 3 years, or flexible sigmoidoscopy every 5 years. Recommends that routine screening for adults aged 76 to 85 years be individualized, considering the patient's overall health and prior screening history due to moderate certainty that the net benefit is small (grade C).
- **Prostate cancer (2018):** Recommends that decisions about prostate-specific antigen testing for men aged 55 to 69 years be individualized, taking into account the patient's values and preferences in the decision due to moderate certainty that the net benefit is small (grade C). Before deciding to screen, men should discuss the potential benefits and harms of screening with their clinician. Recommends *against* PSA-based screening for prostate cancer in men 70 years and older due to evidence that expected harms are greater than expected benefits.
- **Lung cancer (2013):** For adults aged 55 to 80 years with a 30 pack-year smoking history, and those who currently smoke or have quit within the past 15 years, recommends annual screening with low-dose computed tomography (grade B). Screening should be *discontinued* once a person has not smoked for 15 years or develops a health problem that substantially limits life expectancy or the ability to or willingness to undergo invasive diagnostic procedures or to have curative treatment.
- **Skin cancer (2016):** States that evidence is insufficient to balance the benefits and harms of whole-body skin examination by a clinician (I statement).

Detecting the "3 Ds": Delirium, Dementia, and Depression

Delirium and dementia are increasingly common conditions in clinical practice and can present with subtle findings. Keep them in mind as you assess cognition and mental status. Differentiating depression, cognitive impairment, and altered consciousness can be challenging.

Delirium. Delirium is an acute confusional state characterized by sudden onset, fluctuating course, inattention, and at times alteration of consciousness. Upon hospital admission, approximately 11% to 25% of older adult patients will have delirium and an additional 29% to 31% of older adult patients admitted without delirium will develop delirium. Risk for developing delirium depends on both predisposing conditions that increase susceptibility and the immediate precipitating factors. The Confusion Assessment Method (CAM)

Box 25-11. Low-Value Screening for Five Types of Cancer in Adults >65 Years

Cancer Type	Screening Strategy	Low Value (not recommended)
Breast	Any screening	Older adult women ≥75 years or older adult women ≥65 years not in good health and with life expectancy <10 years
Cervical	Any screening	Older adult women >65 years with previous recent negative screening results
Colorectal	Any screening	Older adults >75 years or older adults ≥65 years not in good health and with life expectancy <10 years
	Colonoscopy	Older adults 65–74 years with normal colonic examination results (i.e. without adenomatous polyps) within the last 10 years or normal flexible sigmoidoscopy results within the last 5 years
Prostate	PSA testing	Older adult men 65–69 years who have not had an informed discussion and have not expressed a clear preference for testing after the discussion Older adult men >69 years or older adult men 65–69 years and not in good health and with a life expectancy <10 years

is recommended for screening at-risk patients. It is important to note that cognitive impairment is the most consistently observed vulnerability factor for development of delirium.

Dementia. Dementia is characterized by declines in memory and cognitive ability that interfere with activities of daily living. In the DSM-5, delirium and dementia fall under the new category of *neurocognitive disorders.* One of the aims of this reclassification is to reduce the stigma associated with dementia. The most common types are Alzheimer disease (affecting 5 million Americans over age 65 years), Lewy body dementia, and frontotemporal dementia. Diagnosing dementia requires exclusion of delirium and depression. Teasing out age-related changes in cognition from *mild neurocognitive disorder* (also termed *mild cognitive impairment* or *prodromal dementia*) is also challenging. Less than 2% of patients with dementia have potentially reversible causes, such as hypothyroidism, medication side effects, normal pressure hydrocephalus, or major depression.

Once you identify cognitive changes, a number of steps are helpful for planning patient care (Box 25-12).

Depression. *Depression* affects 5% to 7% of community-dwelling older adults and approximately 10% of older

Box 25-12. Caring for Patients with Altered Cognition

- **Collateral information:** Obtain collateral information from family members and caretakers.
- **Neuropsychological testing:** Consider formal neuropsychological testing.
- **Contributing factors:** Investigate contributing factors such as medications; metabolic abnormalities; depression; delirium; substance abuse; and other clinical and psychiatric conditions, including vascular risk from diabetes and hypertension.
- **Caregivers:** Counsel families about the challenges for caregivers. The National Institute on Aging website: https://www.nia.nih.gov/health/topics/caregiver-health/ is especially helpful about "Alzheimer caregiving." Review household safety measures.
- **Drivers with dementia:** Learn the laws about reporting *drivers with dementia* in your state. Consult the American Academy of Neurology evidence-based practice parameters for drivers with dementia, updated in 2010, and guidelines from numerous professional organizations, including the American Medical Association. Note, however, that underlying quantitative evidence linking assessment to road safety is limited. A 2013 Cochrane review details the pitfalls of disqualifying impaired drivers, which can lead to depression and social withdrawal if disqualification is premature. The review concludes that for drivers with dementia, there is no good evidence that neuropsychological or on-road assessment will maintain mobility and improve safety. The authors call for more research to develop assessment tools "that can reliably identify unsafe drivers with dementia in an office setting" and determine what changes in function provide a threshold for disqualification, as no single validated test is available.
- **Advance directives:** Encourage patient and family discussion of appointing a health care proxy and arranging for power of attorney, health care power of attorney, and advance directives while the patient can still contribute to active decision making.

men and 18% of older women, but is often undiagnosed, untreated, or undertreated. Prevalence rises in those with multiple comorbidities and hospitalizations. Depressed men over age 65 years are at increased risk for suicide and require particularly careful evaluation. Effective treatment for older adults both reduces morbidity and extends life, and includes exercise, supportive and group therapy, and medication. Screening for the general adult population is recommended and should be implemented with adequate systems in place to ensure accurate diagnosis, effective treatment, and appropriate follow-up. Commonly used depression screening instruments include the Patient Health Questionnaire (PHQ) and the Geriatric Depression Scale in older adults.

Elder Mistreatment and Abuse

Screen vulnerable older adults for possible *elder mistreatment,* which includes abuse, neglect, exploitation, and abandonment. Prevalence ranges from 5% to 10%, depending on the population studied, and is even higher among older adults with depression and dementia. Many cases are undetected due to the patient's fear of reprisal, physical or cognitive inability to report abuse, and unwillingness to expose the abuser, of whom 90% are family members. **Self-neglect**, or "the behavior of an older adult person that threatens his/her own health and safety," is also a growing national concern and represents more the 50% of adult protective service referrals.

TABLE 25-1. Selected Normal Anatomic and Physiologic Changes with Aging and Related Disease Outcomes

Normal Changes in Anatomy and Physiology	Clinical Manifestations and Disease Outcomes
Cardiovascular	
■ Increase in thickness of left ventricular wall, involving both myocyte hypertrophy and increase in collagen deposition secondary to decreased turnover of these cells ■ Myocardial thickening combined with lipofuscin deposits, fatty infiltration, and fibrosis ■ Dilation of left atrium ■ Loss of about 10% of pacemaker cells every decade ■ Increased fibrosis, myocyte hypertrophy, and calcium deposition ■ Increase in dilation, elasticity and rigidity of arterial walls, with decrease in sensitivity to receptor-mediated agents ■ Increase in peripheral resistance and decrease in central arterial compliance	1. Decrease in early diastolic cardiac filling, increase in cardiac filling pressure and lower threshold for dyspnea 2. Left ventricular stiffness and thus a fourth heart sound 3. Lone atrial fibrillation 4. Sinus arrest or tachy–brady syndrome 5. Prolonged PR and QRS intervals and right bundle branch block 6. Atherosclerosis 7. Systolic hypertension 8. Stroke
Respiratory	
■ Decrease in number and elasticity of parenchymal elastic fibers, the latter in part because of decrease in collagen levels ■ Less effective ciliary action ■ Less compliant and stiffer chest wall ■ Weaker respiratory muscles and diaphragm, the latter by about 25% ■ Decrease in forced expiratory volume and forced vital capacity (30% by age 80) ■ Increase in residual volume by about 20 mL/year	1. Gradual loss of elastic recoil of lungs 2. Smaller airway size, with airway collapse in lower lung zone 3. Increase in susceptibility to respiratory infections 4. Decrease in both quiet breathing (effort-independent) 5. Decrease in forced breathing (effort-dependent) 6. Decrease in PaO_2 due to ventilation–perfusion mismatching (acceptable $PaO_2 = 100 - [0.32 \times \text{age}]$) 7. Decrease in pulmonary reserve and exercise tolerance
Gastrointestinal	
■ Increase in tongue varicosities ■ Decrease in saliva production ■ Increase in nonperistaltic spontaneous contractions of esophagus ■ Decrease in stomach acid production ■ Decreased gastric acid clearance ■ Slowed gastric emptying after fatty meal, prolonging gastric distention ■ Decrease in gut-associated lymphoid tissue ■ Atrophy of large intestine mucosa ■ Decrease in tensile strength of colonic smooth muscle ■ Decrease in effectiveness of colonic contractions and sensitivity of rectal wall ■ Decrease in calcium absorption ■ Atheromata in large intestine vessels ■ Decrease in liver size and blood flow ■ Decrease in pancreatic mass and enzyme reserves ■ Hyperplasia of pancreatic duct ■ Increase in pancreatic cyst formation, fatty deposition and deposition of lipofuscin granules in acinar cells	1. Increase in oral infections and gum disease 2. Dysphagia 3. Atrophic gastritis (in those >70 years, the incidence of atrophic gastritis is 16%) 4. Decrease in vitamin B_{12} and iron absorption 5. Gastroesophageal reflux disease 6. Increasing meal-induced satiety 7. Impaired response to gastric mucosal injury, thus increasing risk of both gastric and duodenal ulcers 8. Increase in diverticulosis 9. Frequent constipation 10. Bone loss 11. Chronic intestinal ischemia 12. Impaired clearance of drugs requiring phase I metabolism 13. Decrease in insulin secretion and increase in insulin resistance

(continued)

TABLE 25-1. Selected Normal Anatomic and Physiologic Changes with Aging and Related Disease Outcomes *(Continued)*

Normal Changes in Anatomy and Physiology	Clinical Manifestations and Disease Outcomes
Urinary ■ Decrease in number and length of functional renal tubules ■ Increase in tubular diverticula and basement membrane thickness ■ Altered vascular pattern, atherosclerotic changes, altered arteriole-glomerular flow and focal ischemic lesions ■ Decrease in creatinine clearance and glomerular filtration rate, the latter by about 10 mL/decade ■ Decrease in concentrating and diluting capacity of kidneys ■ Decrease in serum renin and aldosterone by about 30–50% ■ Decrease in vitamin D activation	1. Impairs permeability and decreased ability to resorb glucose 2. Decreased renal blood flow with a selective loss of cortical vasculature 3. Decrease in elimination of drugs and toxins (Given a decrease in renal drug elimination among older adult patients, clinicians must dose drugs for these patients with care. When hepatic clearance of drugs requiring phase I metabolism is also impaired, these drugs must be dosed with particular care) 4. Fluid and electrolyte abnormalities causing increased volume depletion and dehydration, hyperkalemia and decrease in sodium and potassium excretion and conservation 5. Vitamin D deficiency
Immunologic/Hematologic ■ Average decline in function, including more stimulus and time required for activation ■ Decrease in T-cell function ■ Decrease in naive T cells and increase in memory T cells ■ Gradual decrease in B-cell function ■ Decrease in response of naive B cells to new antigens ■ Atrophy of thymus ■ Loss of ability of hematopoietic stem cells to self-renew ■ Decrease in rate of erythropoiesis and incorporation of iron into red blood cells	1. Less primary and secondary responses to infection 2. Reduced body's ability to mount immune response to new pathogens 3. Production of abnormal antibodies 4. Decrease in production and functioning of T lymphocytes 5. Decrease in proliferation of natural killer cells 6. Decrease in production of cytokines needed for maturation of B cells 7. Dysfunctional immune system 8. Slight decrease in average values of both hemoglobin and hematocrit
Sensory Organs Vision ■ Loss of periorbital fat ■ Laxity of eyelids ■ Thickening and yellowing of lens combined with lipid infiltrate accumulations (arcus senilus) ■ Increase in fibrosis of iris ■ Increase in lens size and rigidity due to constant formation of central epithelial cells at front of lens ■ Progressive increase in annular layers of lens ■ Compression of central components that become hard and opaque ■ Decrease in lacrimation Hearing ■ Thickening of tympanic membrane and loss in its elasticity as well as in efficiency of its ossicular articulation ■ Decrease in the elasticity and efficiency of ossicular articulation ■ Increasing deficit in central processing Smell and Thirst ■ Decrease in smell detection by about 50% ■ Decrease in thirst drive ■ Impaired control of thirst by endorphins	1. Sunken eyes 2. Senile entropion and ectropion 3. Increase in vulnerability to conjunctivitis 4. Decrease in transparency of cornea 5. Decreases accommodation and slows dark adaptation (as dark adaptation decreases with age, a person's continuing recognition of objects in subdued light requires double the illumination every 13 years) 6. Presbyopia 7. Increase in rate of cataract formation 8. Dry eye syndrome 9. Conductive deafness affecting low-frequency sounds 10. Sensorineural hearing loss of high-frequency sounds 11. Difficulty discriminating source of sound 12. Impaired discrimination of target from noise 13. Diminished ability to enjoy food and decrease in appetite 14. Dehydration

(continued)

TABLE 25-1. Selected Normal Anatomic and Physiologic Changes with Aging and Related Disease Outcomes *(Continued)*

Normal Changes in Anatomy and Physiology	Clinical Manifestations and Disease Outcomes
Dermatologic ■ Decrease in skin elasticity ■ Decrease in barrier function ■ Slower cell replacement ■ Ineffective DNA repair ■ Altered mechanical protection and decrease in sensory perception ■ Decrease in immunologic and inflammatory responses ■ Decrease in sweating and effectiveness of thermoregulation ■ Decrease in vitamin D production ■ Loss of melanocytes at base of hair follicles ■ Slowing of linear nail growth	1. Lax skin 2. Dry skin 3. Rough skin with delayed healing 4. Increase in rate of photocarcinogenesis 5. Greater susceptibility to injury 6. Chronic low-grade infections and impaired wound healing, with persistent wounds and weak scars 7. Tendency toward hyperthermia and greater vulnerability to both heat and cold 8. Osteomalacia 9. Gray hair 10. Nails thicker, duller and more brittle, opaque and yellow, with development of longitudinal ridges
Nervous System Central Nervous System ■ Decrease in weight of brain and cerebral blood flow by about 20% ■ Decrease in number and functioning of nerve cells ■ Less fluid and stiffer cell membranes in brain neurons ■ Irregularity in structure of internal membranes ■ Accumulation of lipofuscin and tangled neurofibrils ■ Decrease in ability of neuron to grow branches of both axons and dendrites Peripheral Nervous System ■ Age-related changes in somatic motor function ■ Slower action potentials and spreading of muscle cell contraction ■ Lower peak strength of muscle contractions, with slower relaxation	1. After age 70, gradual decrease in vocabulary, with increase in semantic errors and abnormal prosody 2. Increased forgetfulness in noncritical areas, which does not affect function or impair recall of important memories 3. After age 80, slower central processing, which prolongs time to complete tasks 4. Decrease in fine motor control 5. Decrease in cells that can be stimulated and decrease in maximum strength of muscular contractions 6. Prolonged time required for impulses to arrive, muscle cells to contract and movements to be initiated 7. Decrease in maximal muscle strength when performing quick movements
Musculoskeletal Muscle ■ Decrease in muscle fibers (mainly type II—fast switch) ■ Replacement of lost muscle tissue with tough fibrous tissue Bone ■ Decrease in vitamin D absorption, which decreases osteoblasts ■ Decrease in bone formation and modeling by osteoblasts and osteoclasts, impairing bone microarchitecture Joints ■ Decrease in thickness of articular cartilage, though not in nonarticular cartilage ■ Stiffer collagen, resulting in disordered cartilage matrix	1. Decrease in muscle mass (sarcopenia), leading to lean body mass 2. Thin, bony appearance to hands 3. Brittle bone 4. Greater susceptibility to fracture, with slower healing 5. Osteoporosis 6. Dorsal kyphosis 7. Less ability to handle mechanical stresses 8. Joint breakdown, including inflammation, pain, stiffness, and deformity 9. Overall decrease and limitation in movement 10. Decrease in arm swing and steadiness of walking

(continued)

TABLE 25-1. Selected Normal Anatomic and Physiologic Changes with Aging and Related Disease Outcomes *(Continued)*

Normal Changes in Anatomy and Physiology	Clinical Manifestations and Disease Outcomes
Endocrine	
Pituitary gland ■ Minimal changes but on average, decrease in pulsatile secretion pattern, including nocturnal pulsatile secretion of prolactin	1. Decrease in size of various structures 2. Decrease in lean body mass to fat ratio 3. Insomnia 4. Deficit in free-radical defenses
Pineal gland ■ Decrease in diurnal melatonin rhythm	5. Increase in rate of hypo-and hyperthyroidism 6. Vitamin D deficiency
Thyroid gland ■ Atrophy, with increased fibrosis and nodule formation ■ Decrease in T4 production in the very old (if aging is normal, blood thyroxine concentration continues unchanged even though T4 production decreases)	7. Orthostatic hypotension 8. Masculinization of postmenopausal women 9. Decrease in immune function increasing the risk of infection and cancer 10. Changes in skin, hair, muscle and bone and decrease in body fat, despite increase in leptin
Parathyroid glands ■ In women over 40 years of age, increase in parathyroid hormone and decrease in metabolism, with associated decrease in 1,25 (OH) vitamin D levels and changes in bone mineral homeostasis	11. Skin changes, increase in LDL and decrease in bone minerals 12. Decrease in body fat
Adrenal gland ■ Moderate decrease in aldosterone secretion ■ In postmenopausal women, Increase In androgen secretion	
Thymus ■ Decrease in immune function	
Male gonads ■ Large decrease in estrogen and progesterone ■ After age 70, decrease in leptin	

UNIT 4

Case-Based Learning

We do not learn from experience…
We learn from reflecting on experience.

~John Dewey

Case 1: A 22-Year-Old Female with Hypertension and Obesity

A 22-year-old nulliparous female, married for 2 years, presented with complaints of weight gain, increased pigmentation, increased facial hair, acne, and oligomenorrhea. She also had a history suggestive of proximal myopathy, easy bruisability, and abdominal striae and is on antihypertensive treatment since the past 1 year. There was no history of any type of contraceptive use.

Examination revealed increased blood pressure, proximal myopathy, purple striae over abdomen, and medial aspect of both thighs. She was obese with BMI of 26.49 kg/m^2 and abdominal circumference 92 cm.

Investigations revealed hypokalemia with metabolic alkalosis, impaired fasting glucose, dyslipidemia, 8 AM cortisol 23 µg/dL, 11 PM cortisol 22.29 µg/dL, overnight dexamethasone suppression test (ONDST) 18.17 µg/dL, low-dose dexamethasone suppression test (LDDST) 15.95 µg/dL, high-dose dexamethasone suppression test (HDDST) 14.34 µg/dL, and ACTH 115 pg/mL. MRI pituitary revealed 13 × 11 mm adenoma.

Q1. What are we dealing with?

A On the basis of history, clinical examination, biochemical, and hormonal evaluation, she is a case of ACTH-dependent Cushing syndrome.

Q2. What is Cushing syndrome?

A Cushing syndrome is a disease that is characterized by chronic glucocorticoid excess. Clinically, it manifests by features of protein catabolism along with varying signs and symptoms. The most common cause of Cushing syndrome is exogenous intake of glucocorticoids.

Q3. What are the most discriminatory clinical features of Cushing syndrome?

A Clinical findings such as obesity, hypertension, and diabetes are not helpful in discriminating the patients with Cushing syndrome from general population as they are highly prevalent among the general population. However, if hypertension, diabetes, or osteoporosis occurs at a younger age, then one should suspect Cushing syndrome. But the most discriminatory features are easy bruisability, proximal muscle weakness, striae (especially if purplish and > 1 cm wide), facial plethora, and cuticular/pulp atrophy.

Q4. Who should be screened and when should screening for Cushing syndrome be done?

A When the discriminatory features are present in patients, then they should be evaluated for the presence of Cushing syndrome.

Q5. What are the causes of Cushing syndrome?

A One of the very important parts of evaluation is a good history regarding drug intake, because exogenous corticosteroid use is the most common cause of Cushing syndrome. After ruling out exogenous cause, the most common cause is ACTH-secreting pituitary adenoma in 70% of patients; 10% of patients have ectopic source of ACTH such as small cell carcinoma of the lung. Twenty percent of patients have an ACTH-independent cause, mainly adrenal adenoma.

Q6. How is Cushing syndrome diagnosed?

A After initial clinical suspicion and ruling out exogenous cause, we need to proceed to establish the diagnosis and etiology of Cushing syndrome in a stepwise manner. Prior to proceeding, one should remember that cortisol has diurnal rhythm, highest level early in the morning while the nadir levels during midnight. First, we need to establish that the patient is suffering from hypercortisolemia. Hypercortisolemia, demonstrated by loss of the normal circadian rhythm of cortisol secretion, and disturbed feedback of the hypothalamic–pituitary–adrenal (HPA) axis are the cardinal biochemical features of Cushing syndrome. Two abnormal first-line test results should be required for the diagnosis of Cushing syndrome. For screening 24-hour urinary free cortisol, midnight salivary cortisol and LDDST (both 1 mg, overnight, or 2 mg, 2 days) are used. At least two of them should be positive. All the three screening tests have excellent sensitivity (> 90%), but 2-day LDDST has the highest specificity if the cutoff used is 50 nmol/L. After initial screening, if two of the three tests are positive, then 8 AM ACTH should be measured; values > 20 pg/mL are suggestive of ACTH-dependent Cushing syndrome while ACTH < 10 pg/mL is suggestive of ACTH-independent Cushing syndrome; values between 10 and 20 pg/mL are intermediate and need further evaluation with corticotropin-releasing hormone (CRH). In case of ACTH-dependent Cushing syndrome, 8 mg 2-day high-dose dexamethasone and pituitary MRI should be done. In case of ACTH-independent Cushing syndrome, adrenal CT scan should be done. Inferior petrosal sinus sampling (IPSS) may be necessary to localize the lesion in case of ACTH-dependent Cushing syndrome.

Q7. What is the treatment and prognosis?

A After establishing the diagnosis, treatment of choice is surgery. For pituitary lesion that is a microadenoma, in majority of patients, transsphenoidal surgery is the preferred approach. Remission rate for pituitary microadenoma varies from 65% to 90%.

Case 2: A Short-Statured Female with Headache and Unconsciousness

An 18-year-old, short-statured female was brought unconscious to the accident and emergency department by her mother. She had a history of mild, frequent occipital headaches, not interfering with daily activities, for the past several years. The day before, she had a severe headache and also vomited twice before becoming unconscious the following morning. According to her mother, she had not attained menarche. There was no history of fever, trauma, and use of illicit drugs, alcohol, or tobacco. There was no family history of hypertension or diabetes. No other significant family history was forthcoming.

On examination, she was found to be short statured with height 112 cm and weight 40 kg. Her upper body was developed better than the lower. Her pulse rate was 126/min with radiofemoral delay. Her respiratory rate was 28/min with Cheyne–Stokes pattern of breathing. Her BP was 200/140 mmHg in the left upper limb and she was febrile (100°F).

General physical examination also revealed cubitus valgus, shield-like chest, and a midsternal keloid. Her external genitalia and breasts were normal but she was found to have sparse axillary and pubic hair. She also had a midsystolic murmur over the precordium. The lung fields were clear. The abdomen revealed no masses and the neurological examination revealed a GCS of 6/15 with neck stiffness and Kernig sign positive. Her left pupil was dilated and nonreactive with ipsilateral ptosis. Ophthalmoscopy showed bilateral subhyaloid hemorrhages with papilledema.

Laboratory test revealed hyponatremia of 119 mEq/L. The electrocardiogram showed prolonged QT interval and T-wave inversion with a "J" hump (Osborne wave).

A chest roentgenogram revealed bilateral notching of the posteroinferior surface of the 7th, 8th, 9th, and 10th ribs with the cardiac shadow having "figure of 3" or "inverted E appearance." Lung fields were normal.

USG abdomen revealed bilateral streak gonads and a hypoplastic uterus. Kidneys, liver, and spleen were normal.

Q1. What is the primary diagnosis and why do you say so?

A Short stature with primary amenorrhea points to a diagnosis of Turner syndrome with a chromosomal karyotype of XO. Cubitus valgus, shield-like chest, and a midsternal keloid are additional features of Turner syndrome present in her. She also had sparse axillary and pubic hair indicating delayed secondary sexual characteristics.

Q2. What is the cardiovascular anomaly in her?

A Turner syndrome is usually associated with coarctation of aorta, which is characterized by radiofemoral delay and high blood pressure in the upper limbs. The upper part of the body is well developed compared with the lower since the defect is mostly "postsubclavian." In addition to the presence of midsystolic precordial murmur, collateral vessels are formed and cause pulsations over the back. These vessels are best visualized when the patient bends forwards (Suzman sign). A bruit may also be heard over them at times.

Coarctation of aorta may be associated with ventricular septal defect and congenital bicuspid aortic valve in a case of Turner syndrome.

Q3. What is the cause of her present unconscious state?

A She had subarachnoid bleeding secondary to ruptured berry aneurysm. Berry aneurysms are associated with coarctation of aorta. The subarachnoid bleed is responsible for her neck stiffness, Kernig sign, subhyaloid hemorrhages in ocular fundi, and papilledema. The severe headache and signs of meningeal irritation are due to chemical inflammation of the pia and arachnoid layers of the brain by the blood degradation products.

Her neurological signs favor the diagnosis of a ruptured left posterior communicating artery aneurysm, with the bleed causing compression of the ipsilateral cranial nerve III.

Q4. What is the cause of her mild, frequent occipital headaches?

A Lesser headaches are caused by intermittent aneurysmal subarachnoid hemorrhage or "sentinel bleed." These usually precede the "worst headache" (thunderclap headache) that occurs with the rupture of aneurysm.

Q5. What is hyponatremia due to?

A Hyponatremia is due to elevation of atrial natriuretic factor, cerebral salt wasting, and syndrome of inappropriate antidiuretic hormone secretion (SIADH).

Q6. What are the ECG changes due to?

A Prolonged QT, T-wave inversion, and J hump (Osborne waves) are seen in subarachnoid hemorrhage, hypothermia, and metabolic acidosis. In addition, features of LVH may occur in coarctation of aorta.

Q7. Interpret the chest X-ray findings.

A Bilateral notching of the posteroinferior surface of the 7th, 8th, 9th, and 10th ribs, also called *Dock sign*, corresponds to the enlarged collaterals connecting internal mammary or intercostal vessels with superior epigastric vessels. Rib notching only on the right side suggests presence of an anomalous right subclavian artery. Rib notching only on the left side suggests coarctation proximal to the left subclavian artery. The figure of "3" or inverted "E" sign is due to indrawing of the lateral wall of the aortic arch with poststenotic dilatation. Lung fields here are normal but may at times suggest ARDS.

Q8. What does the ultrasound suggest?

A The ultrasound findings of bilateral streak gonads and a hypoplastic uterus suggest the diagnosis of Turner syndrome.

Q9. What is the next diagnostic step?

A The patient should be further investigated by a plain CT head (without contrast) to look for blood in the subarachnoid space and ventricles.

Q10. What is the next step in management?

A The next step in management would be cerebral angiography to look for location of berry aneurysms and subjecting them to procedures such as aneurysmal clipping and endovascular coiling.

Q11. What will a lumbar puncture reveal?

A A lumbar puncture in this case would reveal a uniformly blood-stained CSF with supernatant xanthochromia on centrifugation. Examination of the supernatant under microscope would reveal crenated RBCs, thus distinguishing it from a traumatic tap.

Q12. What are the sites of intracerebral hemorrhages?

A These are as follows:

- Putamen—commonest
- Thalamus
- Pons
- Along corona radiata close to the internal capsule
- Cerebellum
- Lobar hemorrhages (amyloid angiopathy)—atypical sites
- Berry aneurysms, in and around the circle of Willis

Case 3: A 46-Year-Old Female with Acral Enlargement

A 46-year-old female, P6, amenorrhic for the past 6 years, had her last childbirth 7 years back and presented with complaints of acral enlargement, increased sweating, and change in shoe size noticed 1 year back. She is a known case of hypertension since 5 months. She also gives a history of mild to moderate headache off and on, which is present all over cranium, but not associated with vomiting. She also complains of pain in both knee joints and snoring. There is no history of diminution of vision, decreased appetite, nausea, vomiting, recurrent pain in abdomen, constipation, cold intolerance, proximal myopathy, easy bruisability, polyuria, polydipsia, and spontaneous galactorrhea.

On examination, the patient is fully conscious and oriented, and has normal vitals with features of frontal bossing, prominent supraorbital ridge, acral enlargement, macroglossia, large fleshy nose, acanthosis nigricans, and thyromegaly. No prognathism is present but there is expressive galactorrhea. Systemic examination is within normal limits.

Laboratory findings are as follows: blood sugar fasting 102 mg/dL, postprandial 124 mg/dL, HbA1c 5.5%, LH 1.06 IU/mL, FSH 5.95 IU/mL, prolactin >200 ng/mL, T4 8.6 µg/dL, TSH 1.6 mIU/mL, cortisol 5.22 µg/dL, and post-glucose growth hormone >33.8 ng/mL. CBC and renal and liver function tests are normal. MRI was suggestive of 31 × 20 × 20 mm. T2 heterogeneous FLAIR isointense mass lesion seen in sellar and suprasellar regions, forming figure-of-eight pattern, lifting and compressing optic chiasma, invading the right cavernous sinus with encasement of right internal carotid artery (ICA), and abutting the left ICA. Perimetry revealed bitemporal hemianopia.

Q1. What is the diagnosis?

A Here, we have a patient who is 46 years of age and has amenorrhea for the past 6 years. She also has complaints of acral enlargement, hyperhidrosis, and headache. In view of these clinical features, acromegaly should be a possibility.

Q2. What is acromegaly?

A Acromegaly is derived from a Greek word meaning "akros" (extremity) and "megalos" (enlargement). Acral is a term pertaining to the outermost parts of the extremities (i.e., hands and feet) and face (i.e., supraorbital ridges, chin, nose, lips, and ears). It represents enlargement of soft as well as bony tissue in acral region.

Clinically active acromegaly is characterized by worsening headache, hyperhidrosis, progressive soft tissue swelling, new-onset visual deficits, difficult to control hyperglycemia, and resistant hypertension.

Q3. What is pseudoacromegaly?

A Pseudoacromegaly is an appearance similar to acromegaly but without growth hormone excess. It occurs in patients with morbid obesity (severe insulin resistance), pachydermoperiostitis, hypothyroidism, insulin-like growth factor 2 (IGF-2)-secreting tumors, and drugs such as minoxidil and phenytoin.

Q4. What are the causes of acromegaly?

A Over 95% of patients with acromegaly harbor a GH-secreting pituitary adenoma. Rare causes are GH-secreting pancreatic islet cell tumor and lymphoma, primary growth hormone–releasing hormone excess, or both.

Q5. Who should be screened for acromegaly?

A Screening for acromegaly should be considered in patients with typical signs and symptoms of acromegaly or those patients having clustering of multiple comorbidities such as type 2 diabetes mellitus, hypertension, sleep apnea syndrome, debilitating arthritis, carpal tunnel syndrome, and hyperhidrosis, even in the absence of typical features of acromegaly.

Q6. How is acromegaly diagnosed?

A Screening test for acromegaly is measurement of serum IGF-1 level. IGF-1 is mainly secreted from liver under the influence of growth hormone. Unlike growth hormone that has episodic secretion, IGF-1 has a constant level. Once IGF-1 is found to be raised, it should be further confirmed by measuring growth hormone after 75 g of glucose given orally. Growth hormone value >1 ng/mL after glucose load is diagnostic of acromegaly. After biochemical confirmation of growth hormone excess, pituitary imaging is required. Most sensitive and specific imaging modality of pituitary imaging is contrast-enhanced dynamic magnetic resonance imaging.

Q7. What is the treatment and prognosis?

A Most common cause of acromegaly is a pituitary macroadenoma (>1 cm in diameter). Treatment of choice is surgery. Transsphenoidal surgery is preferred. However, recurrence rate is about 50% in cases of macroadenoma while it is 10–20% in microadenoma. Treatment of recurrence is variable depending on various factors and this includes resurgery, medical therapy in the form of somatostatin analogues, or gamma knife surgery.

Case 4: A 28-Year-Old Female with Heat Intolerance and Proptosis

A 28-year-old female married for the past 3 years, having primary infertility, presented with heat intolerance, increased sweating, anxiety, tremor, palpitation, weight loss, decreased sleep, and increased appetite for 1 year. She also complained of oligomenorrhea, hyperdefecation, and swelling in front of the neck. There was history of proptosis with grittiness in eyes for the past 1.5 years. There was no family history of thyroid disorder or autoimmune disease.

On examination, she appeared anxious and restless. Her pulse rate was 124/min and regular, blood pressure was 140/60 mmHg, and she had fine tremors with warm and moist palms. She had grade II soft and diffuse goiter with presence of a bruit. Ophthalmic examination revealed proptosis. There was no dermopathy or acropachy. On investigation, serum T3 was 5.4 ng/mL (0.8–1.8), T4 23.4 µg/dL (4.8–13), and TSH 0.001 µIU/mL (0.3–5.5). Ultrasonography of neck revealed diffusely enlarged thyroid gland with increased blood flow on color Doppler. Thyroid uptake scan with technetium showed diffusely increased uptake.

Q1. What are we dealing with?

A In view of the presence of infertility, hyperadrenergic symptoms, neck swelling, and proptosis, we are probably dealing with Graves' disease.

Q2. What is thyrotoxicosis and what is hyperthyroidism?

A Thyrotoxicosis is a condition characterized by symptoms and signs associated with augmented metabolism and increased adrenergic sensitivity secondary to high circulating levels of thyroid hormones. This high level of thyroid hormones can be due to increased production or uncontrolled release of preformed hormones; sometimes, overzealous use of levothyroxine can also lead to thyrotoxicosis.

It should be noted that thyrotoxicosis refers to increased circulating levels of thyroid hormone, irrespective of thyroid gland functioning, while hyperthyroidism is a state of increased circulating levels of thyroid hormones with hyperfunctioning of thyroid gland. Thus, "all patients with hyperthyroidism are thyrotoxic, while all patients with thyrotoxicosis are not hyperthyroid." Graves' disease, the most common cause of hyperthyroidism, is associated with ophthalmopathy in nearly 50% of patients. Goiter in Graves' disease is characterized by diffuse enlargement of thyroid, soft on palpation, nodularity is usually absent, and a bruit can be present over thyroid.

Biochemically, thyrotoxicosis is characterized by increased T3 and T4 levels along with suppressed levels of TSH. Ratio of T3:T4 (ng/dL:µg/dL) >20 is suggestive of hyperthyroidism while ratio of <20 is suggestive of thyroiditis. But these two conditions are best differentiated on the basis of nuclear imaging where hyperthyroidism is characterized by increased uptake of radiotracers while thyroiditis is associated with reduced uptake.

Q3. What are the causes of thyrotoxicosis?

A Etiology of thyrotoxicosis includes Graves' disease, toxic multinodular goiter, toxic adenoma, subacute de Quervain thyroiditis (virus infection), painless thyroiditis/postpartum thyroiditis (autoimmune), acute bacterial thyroiditis, and drug-induced thyroiditis (amiodarone, interferon-γ, tyrosine kinase inhibitors).

Q4. What are the treatment modalities available for hyperthyroidism?

A There is no consensus regarding the best treatment, because of the fact that none is ideal. There are three effective treatment options that exist; however, the physician and patient preference and availability of treatment option often dictate the choice. Radioiodine is preferably used in the United States when compared with Europe or Japan where the antithyroid drugs are utilized as first-line therapy. Surgery as a first-line therapy is used much less often as it demands significant surgical expertise.

Q5. What are the available antithyroid drugs?

A Thyroiditis is usually self-limiting condition and it requires symptomatic treatment in the form of beta-blockers and NSAIDs. Carbimazole, methimazole, and propylthiouracil (PTU) are the available antithyroid drugs. PTU is used only during the first trimester of pregnancy because of shorter half-life and increased chances of hepatic failure. PTU is used during pregnancy because of low placental transfer. Neo-Mercazole is used at the dose of 1 mg/kg body weight initially in two to three divided doses; once T3 and T4 are normalized, then maintenance dose of 5–10 mg/day is required. TSH normalization usually takes longer time so initially patients are monitored with T3 and T4 levels. Fifty to sixty percent of patients achieve remission after 12–18 months of therapy and the drugs can be stopped in this subgroup of patients. Those who do not achieve remission can continue antithyroid drugs lifelong, or undergo surgery or radioiodine ablation.

Q6. What is thyroid-associated orbitopathy?

A Thyroid-associated orbitopathy (TAO) is the orbital manifestation of Graves' disease characterized by immune-mediated inflammation of the extraocular muscles and retro-orbital tissue. It consistently occurs in the presence of autoimmune thyroid disease, irrespective of the functional status of thyroid function. Ninety percent of patients with TAO have Graves' disease, 10% are euthyroid, and 3–4% have hypothyroidism.

Case 5: A 34-Year-Old Male with Chronic Cough and Recent Hemoptysis

A 34-year-old male presented with a complaint of hemoptysis for 2 days. He gave a history of chronic cough with expectoration of copious mucopurulent sputum on and off for the past 6 years, at times with fever. The sputum often used to have an offensive odor. He had consulted several doctors in the past and was given antibiotics frequently after which the cough used to subside only to flare up after 1 or 2 months. Chest X-ray taken twice at intervals of 2 years revealed no abnormalities. The patient also complained of increasing breathlessness on exertion but there was no chest pain. He worked as a bus driver and found it difficult to carry on with his work. He was married but had no children. There was no family history of similar illnesses.

Physical examination revealed a thin-built individual with clubbing and a respiratory rate of 30/min but with no cyanosis.

Respiratory examination revealed bilateral coarse basal crackles. Other systems were clinically normal.

Q1. What will be your approach to the patient?

A Fever and cough with expectoration of copious, offensive, mucopurulent sputum on and off for 6 years suggest a chronic parenchymal/airway disease. Pleural disorders present initially with pleuritic chest pain (absent in this patient). Presence of clubbing and bilateral coarse crackles supports the clinical diagnosis of bronchiectasis. Bronchiectasis may present with hemoptysis due to the rupture of bronchial arteries. In this patient, hemoptysis, of late, with worsening breathlessness suggests an exacerbation of the illness warranting investigations and intervention.

At times, chest roentgenography may not reveal any gross abnormality and a high-resolution CT scan (HRCT) may be required. After sputum culture and sensitivity reports are obtained, appropriate antibiotics can be decided. However, postural drainage is the hallmark of therapy. Serum immunoglobulin levels, serum alpha-1-antitrypsin (AAT) levels, *Aspergillus* precipitins, and serum total IgE levels should be ordered along with autoimmune screening tests such as ANA and rheumatoid factor.

Q2. What is bronchiectasis?

A Bronchiectasis refers to abnormal, irreversible dilatation of terminal bronchioles to a size greater than 2 mm in diameter.

Q3. What are the classical clinical features of bronchiectasis?

A The classical features are copious sputum production, clubbing, and coarse leathery crepitations. Bronchial breathing in bronchiectasis may occur if there is development of pneumonic consolidation or enlargement of a bronchiectatic cavity.

Q4. Why does the sputum smell foul?

A The sputum is foul smelling due to infection by anaerobic organisms such as *Bacteroides fragilis* and *Fusobacterium* species.

Q5. What are the usual organisms that can be cultured from the sputum of a patient with bronchiectasis?

A These are *Klebsiella*, *Haemophilus influenzae*, *Streptococcus pneumoniae*, *Staphylococcus aureus*, anaerobic organisms such as *Pseudomonas aeruginosa*, *Rhodococcus equi*, and *Nocardia*, and fungi (*Aspergillus*). These organisms can also be cultured in lung abscess.

Remember: KISS A PROF

Q6. Why did the patient not have children?

A At times, bronchiectasis is part of primary ciliary dyskinesia (immobile cilia syndrome). Such patients have loss of ciliary function in seminiferous tubules and bronchi.

Q7. What are the types of bronchiectasis?

A
- Saccular or cystic
- Cylindrical or fusiform
- Varicose
- Traction

Q8. What are the complications of bronchiectasis?

A Rupture of bronchial vessels resulting in massive hemoptysis is an important complication.

Infection in bronchiectasis may spread to neighboring structures such as pleura, lung parenchyma, pericardium, and endocardium leading to empyema, pneumonia, pericarditis, and endocarditis, respectively.

In some cases, bronchiectasis may have a distant spread resulting in cerebral abscess. Amyloidosis is a rare complication.

Q9. What are the special types of bronchiectasis?

A
- *Nodular bronchiectasis*: Commonly associated with *Mycobacterium avium-intracellulare* infection
- *Central (proximal) bronchiectasis*: Is pathognomonic of allergic bronchopulmonary aspergillosis (ABPA)
- *Bronchiectasis sicca*: Dry form of bronchiectasis in which no sputum is expectorated but only hemoptysis occurs. It usually affects upper lobes and etiology is tuberculosis

Q10. What is the investigation of choice in bronchiectasis?

A HRCT is the investigation of choice in bronchiectasis. It has an advantage over conventional CT in that it can take as little as 2-mm slice cuts. In earlier times, bronchography was the investigation of choice in such cases.

Q11. What are the indications for surgery in bronchiectasis?

A
- Failure of medical treatment
- Involvement of a particular segment or lobe
- Massive hemoptysis

Q12. What are the antibiotics of choice in bronchiectasis?

A Second- or third-generation cephalosporins with additional cover for *Pseudomonas* and respiratory quinolones such as levofloxacin are the antibiotics of choice in a case of bronchiectasis.

Q13. What is the mainstay of therapy?

A The mainstay of therapy is postural drainage, that is, drainage of sputum by placing the patient in appropriate posture and percussing his back to facilitate cough.

Q14. What are the chest X-ray features of bronchiectasis?

A Chest X-ray shows the presence of multiple cystic spaces called *cluster of grapes* or *honeycomb appearance* in a case of bronchiectasis.

Q15. What are the CT chest findings in bronchiectasis?

A
- *Cylindrical bronchiectasis*: Parallel tram-track lines or signet-ring appearance composed of a dilated bronchus cut horizontally with pulmonary artery (a diameter of bronchus greater than 1.5 times that of the adjacent vessel suggests bronchiectasis)
- *Varicose bronchiectasis*: Beaded bronchi, with alternate areas of dilatation and constriction
- *Cystic bronchiectasis*: Large cystic spaces and a honeycomb appearance (emphysema has thinner walls)

Case 6: A 57-Year-Old Male with Chronic Cough and Recent Breathlessness

A 57-year-old man presented with shortness of breath of 3-year duration, more so for the past 2 days. He took his regular inhalers but was not relieved. He also complained of fever with chills associated with yellowish sputum for the past 4 days. There was no history of chest pain. Over the past 3 years, he had been suffering from chronic cough with expectoration of mucoid sputum. He was admitted twice in the past due to worsening of symptoms. After discharge, he was given inhalers and was told to quit smoking. However, he could not give up the habit that he acquired 16 years back and only reduced the number of cigarettes to 3 or 4 per day from a previous 15–20 per day. He noticed that the symptoms did not subside completely and some degree of cough and breathlessness always remained. There was no history of loss of appetite, loss of weight, or hemoptysis. There was no family history of similar illnesses. He had no known food or drug allergies. He worked at a palm oil estate and found it difficult to carry on with his work lately. He was married and had four children.

On physical examination, he was found to be breathless at rest with an audible wheeze and a respiratory rate of 30/min. There was no cyanosis. Pursed lip breathing was seen during prolonged expiration. His chest was barrel shaped with increased anteroposterior diameter. Respiratory examination revealed vesicular breath sounds with prolonged expiratory phase and generalized rhonchi. Other systems were clinically normal.

Chest X-ray on admission revealed hyperinflated lung fields.

Q1. What will be your approach to the patient?

A The patient is likely to suffer from chronic obstructive pulmonary disease (COPD) as suggested by a history of cough with expectoration of mucoid sputum on and off for 3 years. Recently, he presented with worsening breathlessness not relieved by regular inhalers indicating acute exacerbation. There was also fever with yellowish sputum for 4 days, likely due to some chest infection that might be responsible for this exacerbation of COPD.

As immediate management, the patient should be given controlled oxygen therapy, nebulized bronchodilators (salbutamol and ipratropium bromide), systemic corticosteroids (IV hydrocortisone or oral prednisolone), and antibiotics for pneumonia. He needs to be closely monitored for his vital signs, respiratory signs, arterial blood gases, and electrolytes, especially for hypokalemia. If he deteriorates with features of respiratory failure or evidence of hypercapnia and respiratory acidosis on ABG, he should be considered for ventilatory support, noninvasive ventilation (NIV) being the first line of treatment. Intubation and mechanical ventilation should be considered if NIV is contraindicated or if the patient is unable to tolerate NIV. If he improves, nebulizing drugs should be gradually tapered off and changed to inhalers.

Before discharge, the patient must be checked to ensure that he is following correct inhaler technique. He must also be strictly advised to quit smoking. This can be with the help of support groups or special programs where available.

For long-term management, the patient should be put on regular inhaled bronchodilators and inhaled corticosteroids too if there are frequent exacerbations. He should also be assessed for the need of long-term oxygen therapy.

Q2. How do you assess airflow obstruction clinically?

A Airflow obstruction is assessed clinically by measuring the forced expiratory time (FET).

Normal individuals can empty their chest from a state of full inspiration in 4 seconds or less. The end point of FET is detected by auscultating over the trachea in the suprasternal notch. Prolongation of the FET to more than 6 seconds indicates airflow obstruction.

Q3. How do you assess airflow obstruction by spirometry?

A If FEV_1/FVC ratio <70%, it indicates an obstructive airway defect.

Further assessment of severity of airflow obstruction according to postbronchodilator FEV_1 as a percentage of predicted value is as follows:

Severity	FEV_1
Mild	≥80% predicted
Moderate	50–80% predicted
Severe	30–49% predicted
Very severe	<30% predicted or <50% + chronic respiratory failure

Q4. What are the risk factors for development of COPD?

A Tobacco smoke is a major risk factor in the pathogenesis of COPD. Chemicals, occupational exposures, and indoor and outdoor air pollution are also recognized risk factors.

Q5. What are the components of COPD?

A These are chronic bronchitis and emphysema.

- *Chronic bronchitis* is a clinical diagnosis. There should be presence of cough with mucoid expectoration for at least 3 months in a year for 2 successive years.
- *Emphysema* is a pathological diagnosis. There is abnormal permanent enlargement of the airways distal to the terminal respiratory bronchioles with destruction of their walls without obvious fibrosis.

Q6. What are the complications of COPD?

A These are acute exacerbations, pulmonary hypertension, cor pulmonale, secondary polycythemia, type 2 respiratory failure, and pneumothorax.

Q7. What are the organisms cultured from the sputum of a patient with exacerbation of COPD?

A
- *Common*: Haemophilus influenzae, Streptococcus pneumoniae, Moraxella catarrhalis
- *Less common*: Chlamydia pneumoniae, Pseudomonas aeruginosa

Q8. Why does COPD cause polycythemia and what is the treatment?

A Polycythemia occurs due to long-standing hypoxemia, which stimulates erythropoietin production from the kidney. It is treated by venesection.

Q9. What are the clinical features of type 2 respiratory failure?

A In addition to hypoxia, there is carbon dioxide retention in type 2 respiratory failure. It manifests with drowsiness, central cyanosis, bounding peripheral pulses (due to vasodilatation), warm extremities (due to vasodilatation), and flapping tremors (asterixis).

Q10. What are the characteristic CXR features of COPD?

A Chest X-ray typically shows hypertranslucency; hyperinflated lung fields with flattened diaphragm; long, narrow, tubular-shaped heart; and emphysematous bullae.

Q11. What is the treatment of acute exacerbation of COPD?

A
- *Controlled oxygen therapy*: 24% or 28% oxygen should be used with the aim of maintaining PaO_2 >8 kPa (60 mmHg) (or SaO_2 >90%) without worsening acidosis
- *Nebulized bronchodilators*: Short-acting β_2-agonists combined with an anticholinergic agent (ipratropium bromide)

- *Systemic steroids*: IV hydrocortisone or oral prednisolone for 10 days
- *Antibiotic therapy*: To cover chest infection; penicillin and macrolide
- *Noninvasive ventilation (NIV)*: In patients with hypercapnic respiratory failure despite optimal medical therapy (early noninvasive ventilation in patients with mild-to-moderate respiratory acidosis during an acute exacerbation of COPD reduces the need for endotracheal intubation, the length of hospital stay, and the in-hospital mortality)
- *Mechanical ventilation* if the patient is intolerable to NIV

Q12. Should high-concentration oxygen be given in acute exacerbation of COPD? Why?

A No. High-concentration oxygen is avoided in severe cases of COPD exacerbation because it may cause respiratory depression, carbon dioxide retention, and worsening acidosis.

Q13. What are the therapeutic options for stable COPD?

A Management of stable COPD is multidisciplinary, with options such as smoking cessation, education, vaccination for influenza and pneumococcal infections, breathing exercises, pulmonary rehabilitation, pharmacotherapy with inhaled bronchodilators, inhaled corticosteroids for selected patients, phosphodiesterase-4 inhibitors, long-term domiciliary oxygen therapy, and surgery.

Case 7: A 52-Year-Old Male with Progressive Breathlessness

A 52-year-old male driver presented to the accident and emergency department with progressive breathlessness since 3 months. There was no cough but the patient complained of mild fever on and off for the same period. Three months ago, he had a pleuritic chest pain on the right side that disappeared after a week. The patient did not have hemoptysis and had reportedly worked in a company dealing with insulation of wires 30 years ago for about 7 years.

Examination revealed an individual with signs of respiratory distress, respiratory rate of 34/min, pulse of 88/min, and a BP of 122/78 mmHg. His JVP was normal and there was clubbing with no pedal edema or cyanosis. Right axillary lymph nodes were enlarged and palpable.

Respiratory examination revealed a gross tracheal shift to the left and decreased VF and VR on the right, with stony dullness on percussion. Breath sounds were diminished in intensity on the right side.

After a chest X-ray and CT that revealed evidence of massive right pleural effusion, the patient was drained of the pleural fluid. Laboratory analysis of the pleural fluid revealed that it was an exudate with a high hyaluronic acid content. A pleural biopsy confirmed the diagnosis.

Q1. What is your diagnosis?

A This is a case of pleural mesothelioma with massive right pleural effusion.

Q2. What could be the predisposing factor for its development?

A The predisposing factor is working in asbestos industry (asbestos roofing, shipbuilding, insulation of wires, etc.). It may develop even 30–40 years after the exposure to asbestos.

Q3. Can pleural fluid analysis suggest mesothelioma?

A A high hyaluronic acid in pleural fluid can suggest pleural mesothelioma, which needs to be confirmed by a pleural biopsy. Pleural biopsy can confirm mesothelioma in 80% of cases.

Q4. What are Light criteria?

A These are criteria to decide whether pleural fluid is an exudate or transudate. Pleural fluid is said to be an exudate in the presence of following:

- Pleural fluid protein/serum protein >0.5
- Pleural fluid LDH/serum LDH >0.6
- Pleural fluid LDH more than two-third of normal upper limit for serum LDH

A drawback of these criteria is that they do not take into account the presence or absence of inflammatory cells.

Q5. How does a pleural effusion manifest in chest X-ray?

A A curvilinear shadow is seen if a minimum of 300 mL of pleural fluid is present. If the amount is between 150 and 300 mL, a radiograph in the lateral decubitus position on the side of effusion would show a straight line opacity. Minimal blunting of costophrenic angle indicates the presence of about 100 mL of fluid. If the amount of pleural fluid is suspected to be even less than this, USG is essential.

Q6. What are the clinical features of an effusion?

A
- Tracheal shift to the opposite side
- Decreased VF and VR
- Stony dullness on percussion, which goes high up in axilla due to capillary suction

- Diminished breath sounds
- A bronchial breathing may at times be heard just above the effusion (at the air-fluid interspace) with egophony

Effusion is an Enemy of the trachea—it pushes it away from its side!

Q7. What is artificial pleurodesis?

A Artificial pleurodesis refers to the adhesion of visceral and parietal layers of pleura by injection of doxycycline, *Corynebacterium parvum*, kaolin, etc., to prevent reaccumulation in refractory cases.

Q8. What is hepatic hydrothorax?

A Hepatic hydrothorax refers to right-sided transudative pleural effusion in a patient with cirrhosis of liver.

Q9. Mention some special conditions where the pleural fluid is altered.

A
- Rheumatoid effusions have high cholesterol, low glucose, and high protein content in pleural fluid.
- Effusions in SLE have ANA and LE cells in pleural fluid.
- Effusions in acute hemorrhagic pancreatitis are high in amylase content.
- Pulmonary infarction may be an exudate (80%) or a transudate (20%).

Q10. What is the significance of increased adenosine deaminase in pleural fluid?

A Level of adenosine deaminase greater than 32 IU/L in pleural fluid is suggestive of tuberculosis. It also occurs in rheumatoid disease.

Case 8: A 35-Year-Old Chronic Smoker with Right Chest Pain

A 35-year-old man presents to the medicine OPD with a 7-day history of mild fever, dry cough, and right-sided chest pain. The chest pain is described as sharp, stabbing in character and increases on deep inspiration or coughing. On examination, the patient looks thin built, the chest looks slightly asymmetrical, and the trachea is deviated toward the left. On percussion and auscultation, he had a dull note and absent breath sounds in right basal lung fields and right infra-axillary region. There is a history of an acute febrile episode 2 weeks back for which the patient took over-the-counter medications. The patient claims to have taken paracetamol for fever and a 5-day course of an antibiotic; however, this is undocumented. The patient is a chronic smoker and smokes an average of three to four cigarettes every day for the past 25–30 years. He has also been consuming alcohol occasionally for the past 10 years and is a vegetarian by diet. Otherwise, his past history is unremarkable.

Q1. What is the most probable diagnosis?

A The chest pain is sharp and stabbing and increases on inspiration and coughing, characteristics typical of pleural inflammation. The patient has a history of a recent acute febrile episode that was treated (insufficiently?) using over-the-counter medications. Bacterial (e.g., pneumonia) and viral (e.g., influenza) infections are an important cause of pleuritis. The inflammatory response due to pleuritis and/or pneumonia can lead to fluid accumulation between the visceral and parietal layers of the pleura. A large number of patients with pneumonia develop parapneumonic pleural effusions especially if they are inadequately treated for pneumonia. The trachea is deviated toward the left; this means that the trachea is being pushed by something on the right or pulled by something on the left. Left-sided percussion and auscultation are normal, whereas there is a dull note and absent breath sounds in right basal lung fields; this is NOT due to air (pneumothorax) because presence of air will be percussed as a resonant note. Therefore, the most probable diagnosis is right-sided pleural effusion.

Q2. If the patient also gives a history of evening rise of temperature, night sweats, and a gradual loss of weight, will your diagnosis change?

A These symptoms are characteristic of tuberculosis. Remember, tuberculosis can affect any part of the body. However, a combination of the patient's clinical picture along with the three characteristic symptoms points to a diagnosis of tuberculous pleural effusion (TPE). TPE is one of the most common forms of extrapulmonary tuberculosis especially in developing countries. It usually presents as an acute illness with complaints of fever, cough, and pleuritic chest pain accompanied with evening rise of temperature, night sweats, and a gradual loss of weight.

Q3. What is trail sign? What are the conditions that can cause deviation of the trachea?

A Trail sign is the prominence of sternal head of sternocleidomastoid due to the shift of trachea to the same side. Conditions that can cause tracheal deviation include pneumothorax, pleural effusion, atelectasis, pleural fibrosis, pulmonary fibrosis, and mediastinal lymphoma.

Q4. In what other conditions will you get a dull note on chest wall percussion?

A Dull note is heard normally over the liver and the spleen at the base of the right and left lungs, respectively. A dull note on percussion is also heard in lung consolidation and pleural thickening.

Q5. Name one condition each due to chronic smoking and chronic alcohol consumption that can lead to a similar presentation.

A
- Chronic smoking—lung cancer
- Chronic alcohol consumption—acute pancreatitis

Q6. What investigations will you order next for this patient?

A A chest X-ray should be done. Pleural fluid should be obtained by thoracentesis. Gross characteristics of the sample must be noted. Further testing should include pleural fluid and serum protein and LDH levels, pleural fluid glucose, pleural fluid differential cell counts, and pleural fluid culture/cytology. CT chest and pleural fluid biopsy are done only if indicated.

Q7. What are Light criteria?

A The fluid is considered an exudate if any of the following is found:
- Ratio of pleural fluid to serum protein greater than 0.5
- Ratio of pleural fluid to serum LDH greater than 0.6
- Pleural fluid LDH greater than two-thirds of the upper limits of normal serum value

Q8. How will you manage this patient?

A Once the diagnosis is confirmed, treat the underlying cause. Therapeutic thoracentesis may be useful if the patient is severely dyspneic but be careful not to cause a pneumothorax. Complicated parapneumonic effusions and empyemas usually need to be drained by tube thoracostomy. Pleurodesis may be helpful in cases of recurrent pleural effusions. Indwelling tunneled pleural catheters offer an alternative to pleurodesis especially in recurrent malignant pleural effusions.

Q9. What are the likely complications of pleurocentesis?

A Pain, dry tap, subcutaneous hematoma, pneumothorax, hemothorax, and injury to the diaphragm/liver/spleen are the likely complications of pleurocentesis.

Q10. What are the dangers of self-medication with over-the-counter medicines?

A Incorrect diagnosis, adverse drug reactions and interactions, inadequate treatment leading to chronicity, development of resistance of pathogens, and delay in seeking professional medical advice are the dangers of self-medication with over-the-counter medicines.

Case 9: A 45-Year-Old Male with History of Treated Pulmonary Tuberculosis

A 45-year-old male, who was treated for pulmonary tuberculosis 5 years ago, attended the medical outpatient department with complaints of breathlessness on exertion since 3 months, cough with expectoration since 1 month, and mild fever on and off. There was no history of hemoptysis, orthopnea, or palpitations. The patient felt that he was losing weight of late. He was a diabetic on glimepiride 4 mg/day and metformin 500 mg twice daily. There was no family history of tuberculosis. The patient's mother died of end-stage renal failure due to diabetic nephropathy.

General examination revealed a poorly nourished individual with a body temperature 99°F, pulse rate 88/min, BP 110/80 mmHg, and a respiratory rate 20/min. JVP was normal. There were no signs of respiratory distress, cyanosis, clubbing, icterus, lymphadenopathy, and pedal edema. The patient was mildly anemic.

Systemic examination revealed drooping of right shoulder with hollowing of right supraclavicular and infraclavicular fossae, crowding of ribs with narrow intercostal spaces on the right side, and restriction of right-sided chest movements on respiration. Trail sign was positive with the prominence of right sternocleidomastoid muscle. There were no engorged vessels over the chest wall and the vocal fremitus was decreased over right apical region. Percussion note was dull over right supraclavicular and infraclavicular regions. On auscultation, breath sounds were decreased over the right supraclavicular and infraclavicular regions and there was bronchial breathing in the right infraclavicular region. There were no crepitations or rhonchi. Vocal resonance was also decreased over the right apical region. Breath sounds were increased on the left side but there was no bronchial breathing or other adventitious sounds.

CVS, CNS, and abdominal examinations were normal.

ESR was 20 mm/h and the total leukocyte count was 10,000 cells/mm^3. Acid-fast bacilli (AFB) were absent in sputum sample on three consecutive occasions.

Chest roentgenogram showed tracheal shift to the right, drooping of the right shoulder, crowding of ribs, and narrow intercostal spaces in the right apical region. No pulmonary infiltrates were detected. There was no tenting of diaphragm. The left lung was hyperlucent and appeared to be hyperinflated.

Q1. What is your interpretation of the patient's status?

A The patient suffered from pulmonary tuberculosis in the past and had been treated for the same. He is also a diabetic on treatment. Of late, he has developed some symptoms that trouble him, making one think of a reinfection with tuberculosis bacilli, but he is not in respiratory distress, neither cyanosed nor clubbed, and his body temperature is also normal.

Examination findings such as diminished chest movements on the right, drooping of right shoulder with hollowing of supraclavicular and infraclavicular fossae, crowding of the ribs, narrowing of intercostal spaces, and a positive Trail sign indicate lung volume loss in right apical region, most likely secondary to *fibrosis due to past pulmonary tuberculosis.*

The diagnosis of fibrosis is also supported by the findings of dullness on percussion and decreased VF/VR along with decreased breath sounds over the same region.

Q2. What is Trail sign (sternomastoid sign)?

A It is the prominence of sternomastoid on the side of tracheal shift. The trachea and the sternomastoid muscle are enclosed rigidly by the pretracheal fascia, an extension of the deep cervical fascia. Any shift of trachea exerts traction on the fascia and hence the sternomastoid becomes prominent due to the relaxant effect.

Trail sign should always be confirmed by palpation. When the index finger is pushed between the trachea and the sternomastoid, the angle/gap is narrower on the affected side.

Remember: FIBROSIS is trachea-FRIENDLY! It pulls the trachea to its side

Q3. How do you make out whether the patient has reinfection with tubercle bacilli and requires treatment again or whether fibrosis is a result of old pulmonary tuberculosis?

A Presence of the following suggests reinfection:

- *Symptoms*: Fever, cough with expectoration, and loss of weight may suggest a reinfection.
- *Signs*: Moist, fine crepitations usually indicate reinfection.
- *Investigations*: Elevated ESR and presence of acid-fast bacilli (AFB) in sputum indicate reinfection.

Treatment of reinfection requires a course of antituberculous drugs to be administered again. In this patient, reinfection is unlikely as the temperature is normal, there is no respiratory distress, and there are no moist, fine crepitations. The mild loss of weight warrants checking the diabetic status of the patient. However, sputum for AFB, CXR, and ESR are warranted to confirm reinfection. Here, sputum for AFB was negative and ESR was normal.

Q4. Can you get bronchial breathing in fibrosis?

A Yes.

- It may be due to an *associated cavity* within the area of fibrosis. In this case, the bronchial breathing would be low pitched (cavernous) and localized, and the patient would have post-tussive suction* that is pathognomonic of a cavity. Crack pot resonance over a cavity is rarely elicited. Post-tussive crepitations indicate liquefaction necrosis.
- In *pulled trachea syndrome*, the trachea is pulled to the side of fibrosis and a gross shift of trachea results in bronchial breathing over the affected infraclavicular region. It is not due to the cavity but due to auscultation over the pulled trachea.

Q5. How do you differentiate cavity from a pulled trachea syndrome?

A Cavity can be differentiated from pulled trachea syndrome by:

- Presence of post-tussive suction
- Presence of bronchial breathing in the axillary region

In the axilla, auscultatory events in all the lobes can be heard. In pulled trachea syndrome, the bronchial breathing is heard in the infraclavicular region due to tracheal shift, but not heard in the axilla.

*Following a bout of coughing which is an expiratory process and empties the cavity, air gushes in rapidly to fill the empty cavity during the next succeeding inspiration. This is post-tussive suction.

Q6. Why are breath sounds increased on the left side in this case?

A When the whole lung or part of it is destroyed on one side, the lung on the other side has to do additional work to compensate for the diseased lung and therefore it undergoes compensatory hypertrophy. This condition is called *compensatory emphysema*.

In this condition, percussion note is resonant (as in emphysema) but breath sounds are louder on auscultation in contrast to emphysema where they are diminished. Compensatory emphysema is unilateral, whereas emphysema is bilateral.

Q7. What pulmonary function tests will be useful in fibrosis?

A FEV_1/FVC will be normal in fibrosis, which is a restrictive lung disease. (FEV_1 and FVC are proportionately reduced.)

FEV_1/FVC will be reduced in obstructive lung diseases. (FEV_1 is more reduced than FVC.)

Case 10: A 60-Year-Old Diabetic Female with Foot Lesion

A 60-year-old lady, a known case of type 2 diabetes for 4 years, on triple combination of oral antidiabetic drugs but with poor glycemia control, was admitted with fever, pain, and swelling of left big toe and foot of 1-week duration. There was no history of trauma to the foot. There was a history of tingling and pain in both lower limbs for 2 years. There was no family history of diabetes.

Examination revealed a conscious, oriented patient, with a BP of 130/80 mmHg, PR of 88/min, bilateral nonpalpable posterior tibial arteries, presence of bruit over right carotid, acanthosis nigricans, skin tags, pitting pedal edema, and absent ankle and knee reflexes. Left foot had blisters and pus discharge over big toe. It was also swollen and the local temperature was increased.

Investigations revealed leukocytosis, neutrophilia, and normal renal and liver function tests. Pus c/s from left foot revealed growth of MRSA. X-ray of foot revealed osteomyelitis of left distal phalanx of big toe.

Q1. What is diabetic foot?

A Diabetic foot can be described as aberrations of nerve supply, vascular supply, bones, joints, or soft tissues of foot, resulting from persistent hyperglycemia, with or without infection or breach in continuity of skin in a patient with diabetes.

Approximately 20% of hospital admissions among patients with diabetes are the result of diabetic foot. The rate of lower limb amputation in patients with DM is 15 times higher than that in patients without diabetes. It is estimated that approximately 50–70% of all lower limb amputations are due to diabetic foot ulcers.

Q2. What are the risk factors for diabetic foot?

A The risk factors for diabetic foot are as follows:

General or systemic factors	Local factors
■ Uncontrolled hyperglycemia ■ Duration of diabetes ■ Peripheral vascular disease ■ Blindness or visual loss ■ Chronic renal disease ■ Older age	■ Peripheral neuropathy ■ Structural foot deformity ■ Trauma and improperly fitted shoes ■ Callus ■ History of prior ulcer amputation ■ Prolonged elevated pressures ■ Limited joint mobility

Q3. How is diabetic foot ulcer classified?

A There are many different classifications for diabetic foot ulcer such as Wagner-Meggitt, University of Texas, and PEDIS (perfusion, extent, depth, infection, and sensation). Wagner's classification is frequently used in clinical practice because of its simplicity. It is based on depth of ulcer, but it does not include the etiopathogenesis or the size of the ulcer. Although the Texas classification includes infection and ischemia as the criteria, it does not take neuropathy or gangrene into account. The PEDIS classification is helpful in the treatment as it distinguishes between a limb-threatening and a life-threatening diabetic foot ulcer.

Q4. What are the tests to assess diabetic peripheral neuropathy and loss of protective sensation?

A Ankle reflex, vibration perception, and monofilament test are used bedside to assess neuropathy and at-risk feet. Pain, touch, and temperature sensation are used to assess small fiber neuropathy. Five simple clinical tests, each with evidence from well-conducted prospective clinical cohort studies, are considered useful in the diagnosis of loss of protective sensation (LOPS) in the diabetic foot. Ideally, two of these should be regularly performed during the screening exam—normally the 10-g monofilament and one other test. One or more abnormal tests would suggest LOPS, while at least two normal tests (and no abnormal test) would rule out LOPS. The five tests include 10-g monofilament, ankle reflex, pinprick, vibration perception using 128-Hz tuning fork, and biothesiometer for assessing vibration perception threshold.

Q5. How is a diabetic foot ulcer managed?

A Management of diabetic foot includes good glycemic control, control of infection, thorough debridement by removing all the necrotic tissues, and strict off-loading, meaning that the patient should not bear weight on the ulcerated limb. If ischemia is present, then restoration of good blood supply should be done. Use of growth factors, maggot therapy, and negative-pressure therapy can also be done in selected patients.

Case 11: A 48-Year-Old Male with Splenomegaly

A 48-year-old male presented with complaints of pain and fullness in left hypochondrium for 6 months. He experienced vague ill health, easy fatigability, and early satiety, which were progressively increasing. There was no history of regurgitation, vomiting, hematemesis, melena, jaundice, distension of abdomen, high-grade fever, night sweats, significant weight loss, bone pains, and bleeding tendency.

On examination, he had mild pallor; icterus and lymphadenopathy were absent. The abdomen was soft with fullness in left hypochondrium. Spleen was enlarged and palpable 10 cm below left costal margin. It was firm and nontender. Splenic notch was easily palpable. Fluid thrill and shifting dullness were absent.

Q1. What is the normal size and location of a spleen?

A A normal spleen is < 250 g in weight and maximum 12 cm in length and/or width of 7 cm assessed by radionuclide scan. It lies entirely within the rib cage and is not palpable normally. By ultrasonography, the normal size of spleen in adults is 13 cm (cephalocaudal).

Q2. How do you percuss the spleen?

A The percussion of the spleen can be accomplished by three methods: Nixon's method, Castell's method, and percussion of Traube's semilunar space (see p. 479).

- *Castell's method*: Percuss in the lowest left intercostal space in the anterior axillary line (usually the eighth or ninth IC space). This space should remain resonant during full inspiration. Dullness on full inspiration indicates possible splenic enlargement (a positive Castell's sign).
- *Nixon's method (optional)*: Place the patient in right lateral decubitus. Begin percussion midway along the left costal margin. Proceed in a line perpendicular to the left costal margin. If the upper limit of dullness extends > 8 cm above the left costal margin, this indicates possible splenomegaly.

Q3. When do you say spleen is massively enlarged? What are the causes?

A The spleen is labeled as massively enlarged when it is palpable more than 8 cm below left costal margin or its drained weight is more than 1000 g. The common causes of massive splenomegaly are chronic myeloid leukemia, chronic lymphocytic leukemia, lymphoma, hairy cell leukemia, myelofibrosis with myeloid metaplasia, autoimmune hemolytic anemia, polycythemia vera, and Gaucher disease.

Q4. What is hypersplenism?

A Hypersplenism is a tetrad characterized by splenomegaly, cytopenia(s), hyperplastic or normal bone marrow, and response to splenectomy. The sluggish flow of blood through the congested cords and immune mechanisms may be responsible for cytopenias.

Q5. What are the complications of removal of spleen? How can you prevent them?

A Splenectomy predisposes individual to infections by capsulated bacteria such as *Streptococcus pneumoniae* and *Haemophilus influenzae*, some Gram-negative enteric bacteria, and parasitic infections such as babesiosis. This is because of failure to remove opsonized bacteria and also formation of antibodies against polysaccharide capsule. Although splenectomized patients are at risk throughout their life, the risk is highest in the first 3 years. The most common sites are lung, skin, and blood and it may be polymicrobial infection in 15% of individuals. The case fatality rate of pneumococcal sepsis in the absence of spleen is 50–80%. Therefore, pneumococcal vaccine should be administered to patients 2 weeks before splenectomy is scheduled, with repeat vaccination 5 years thereafter. Vaccination against *H. influenzae* and *Neisseria meningitides* is also advocated.

Q6. Name an absolute contraindication to splenectomy.

A Splenectomy is absolutely contraindicated in bone marrow failure as spleen is the site for extramedullary hematopoiesis.

Q7. What is tropical malarial spleen?

A Tropical splenomegaly or hyperactive malarial splenomegaly (HMS) is a consequence of abnormal immune response to chronic or repeated malarial infections in individuals living in endemic regions. It is characterized by massive splenomegaly, hepatomegaly, and increased titer of serum IgM malarial antibody. Malarial parasite may not be found in peripheral blood smear in some patients. Most of the individuals respond to antimalarial chemoprophylaxis but some may be refractory and may develop malignant lymphoproliferative disorder.

Case 12: A 35-Year-Old Jaundiced Male with Hematemesis and Melena

A 35-year-old male presented to the emergency department at 1 PM with a history of vomiting fresh blood several times since morning. He did not complain of abdominal pain or change in the color of his stools but had passed dark tarry stools on two previous occasions within a span of 6 months. He had been a chronic alcoholic and a heavy smoker for the past 14 years. He also admitted having frequent extramarital affairs.

General examination revealed a pale, jaundiced individual with a regular pulse rate of 108/min and a blood pressure of 90/60 mmHg. Other findings were mild clubbing, palmar erythema, spider nevi, and bilateral gynecomastia.

Cardiovascular and respiratory system examinations were unremarkable. Abdominal examination revealed a moderately distended abdomen with positive shifting dullness. Fluid thrill was absent. Spleen was palpable by the dipping method of palpation. There were several distended tortuous veins radiating from the umbilicus. The external genitalia and rectal examination was normal. Neurological examination revealed asterixis.

Q1. What are the causes of blood in vomiting?

A
- Ulcers (peptic)
- Gastric antral vascular ectasia (watermelon stomach)
- Iatrogenic—aspirin intake
- Alcohol intake
- Blood dyscrasias
- Linear tear in the gastroesophageal junction (unassociated with liver disease and characterized by severe retching) called Mallory-Weiss syndrome
- Esophageal varices rupture
- Connective tissue disorders such as Ehlers–Danlos syndrome and pseudoxanthoma elasticum
- Arteriovenous malformation—Dieulafoy lesion
- Inherited disorders such as Osler–Weber–Rendu syndrome (autosomal dominant)
- Neoplasms of stomach and esophagus
- Prolapse of the part of gastric mucosa into esophagus
- Portal hypertensive gastropathy

Q2. What is hematemesis? When does it occur?

A *Hematemesis* is vomitus of red blood or "coffee-grounds" material. Stomach should contain at least 120 mL of blood for hematemesis to occur. It indicates upper gastrointestinal source of bleed.

Q3. What is melena? When does it occur?

A *Melena* is black, tarry, sticky, foul-smelling stool. It occurs when blood remains in the GI tract for more than 14 hours. At least 60 mL of blood is required to produce one melenic stool.

Q4. How do you differentiate a melenic stool from the stool of a patient consuming iron capsules?

A The stool of a patient taking iron is black but not sticky or malodorous.

Q5. How do you differentiate upper and lower GIT anatomically?

A Anatomically, the upper GIT lies above the attachment of the ligament of Treitz at the second part of duodenum. Lower GI lies below this attachment.

Q6. What is the significance of abdominal pain in a patient with GI bleed?

A A patient with GI bleed may have abdominal pain secondary to a superimposed peptic ulcer or pancreatitis secondary to alcoholism.

Q7. When is hematemesis said to be massive?

A Hematemesis is said to be massive when the amount of blood vomited is between 150 and 500 mL/day.

Q8. What are the consequences of chronic alcohol consumption on the GIT?

A
- Acute pancreatitis
- Cirrhosis of liver
- Peptic ulcer
- GERD
- Alcoholic hepatitis
- Fatty liver

Q9. What is the significance of sexual promiscuity in this patient?

A Sexual promiscuity can lead to hepatitis B and C, which can cause cirrhosis.

Q10. What are the signs of liver cell failure from head to toe?

A
- Alopecia
- Madarosis (loss of eyelashes)
- Jaundice
- Parotid enlargement*
- Fetor hepaticus (due to accumulation of methyl mercaptans)
- Clubbing
- Terry's nails
- Palmar erythema
- Dupuytren contracture*
- Asterixis
- Loss of axillary hair
- Spider nevi
- Gynecomastia (painless)
- Ascites
- Loss of pubic hair
- Testicular atrophy
- Pedal edema

Q11. What are spider nevi? Where are they found?

A Spider nevi are pulsatile telangiectasias with centrally dilated arteriole and radiating branches.

In cirrhosis, they are seen in the area of drainage of superior vena cava, that is, above a line joining the two nipples (intermammary line).

Q12. What are the signs in ascites?

A
- Tanyol sign—increased epigastrium–umbilicus distance compared with umbilicus–symphysis pubis distance (reverse occurs in pelvic pathology such as ovarian cyst in females)
- Shifting dullness (1000–1500 mL free fluid should be present to elicit this)
- Fluid thrill—seen in massive/tense ascites
- Puddle sign—detects as little as 120 mL of free fluid, now replaced by USG
- Divarication of recti—weakness of rectus abdominis
- Dipping method of palpation for organomegaly—displaces the fluid and hits the organ
- Abdominojugular reflux—absent in hepatic venous occlusion (Budd–Chiari syndrome)

Q13. What is the significance of examination of external genitalia and rectum in this case?

A External genitalia and rectum should be examined to look for gonadal atrophy and hemorrhoids in this case. These are seen in cases of cirrhosis with portal hypertension.

Q14. What are the clinical features of portal hypertension?

A These include ascites, bleeding esophageal varices (hematemesis and melena), dilated and tortuous veins radiating from umbilicus with the flow of blood away from umbilicus (caput medusae), bruit heard over collaterals (Cruveilhier–Baumgarten syndrome), and splenomegaly.

Q15. What is the significance of a palpable spleen becoming nonpalpable in portal hypertension?

A It signifies that the patient had a massive UGI bleed.

Q16. What are the sites of portosystemic anastomosis?

A
- Coronary vein and short gastric veins ⇔ veins of the lesser curve of the stomach and the esophagus, leading to the formation of varices
- Inferior mesenteric vein ⇔ rectal branches that, when distended, form hemorrhoids
- Umbilical vein ⇔ epigastric venous system around the umbilicus (caput medusae)
- Retroperitoneal collaterals ⇔ gastrointestinal veins through the bare areas of the liver being another site of anastomosis

Q17. What are the investigations done in UGI bleed?

A These are endoscopy, angiography, USG abdomen, and LFT.

Q18. How do you treat UGI bleed?

A Variceal bleeding:
- Fluid resuscitation with colloids/albumin with or without blood transfusion is done in cirrhosis.
- Octreotide IV, a somatostatin analogue, is given.
- Vasopressin intravenously (or terlipressin) acts to vasoconstrict splanchnic vasculature and secondary reduction in portal venous pressure.
- Nadolol and nitrates also reduce portal venous pressure and are more useful for rebleeding.
- Endoscopic banding and sclerotherapy for varices (agents: ethanolamine oleate, sodium morrhuate) are performed in addition.
- If bleeding persists, mechanical balloon tamponade with Sengstaken–Blakemore or Minnesota tube is resorted to followed by a

*Only in alcoholic cirrhosis.

transjugular intrahepatic portosystemic shunt (TIPS).

Nonvariceal bleed:

- Resuscitation with fluids—crystalloids or colloids/blood—is done.
- Proton pump inhibitors such as omeprazole or pantoprazole reduce mortality in severe disease.
- Tranexamic acid—an inhibitor of fibrinolysis—is promising.
- There is no indication for the use of somatostatin or octreotide.

Remember: Vomiting Blood for treatment of UGI bleed

- *V*asopressin intravenously acts to vasoconstrict splanchnic vasculature
- *O*ctreotide—a somatostatin analogue
- *M*echanical tamponade—Sengstaken–Blakemore tube
- *I*nhibitors of proton pump (Omeprazole)
- *T*erlipressin (a derivative of vasopressin)
- *I*nfusion of blood/blood products
- *N*adolol, nitrates
- *G*elfoam embolization
- *B*anding of varices
- *L*iver transplantation
- *O*esophagoscopic sclerotherapy (ethanolamine oleate, sodium morrhuate, sodium tetradecyl sulphate)
- *O*thers–TIPS, proximal gastric vagotomy
- *D*istal splenorenal and portosystemic shunts

Q19. What are the causes of lower gastrointestinal (LGI) bleed?

A
- *A*mebiasis
- *B*acillary dysentery (shigellosis)
- *C*arcinoma colon
- *D*iverticulitis
- *E.* coli (EHEC) infection
- *F*issure-in-ano
- *G*ranulomatous (Crohn) and ulcerative colitis
- *H*emorrhoids (piles)
- *I*schemic colitis

Q20. How does it present?

A *Hematochezia* is the passage of bright red or maroon blood from the rectum. *Occult GI bleeding* (GIB) may be identified in the absence of overt bleeding by a fecal occult blood test or the presence of iron deficiency. Patients may present only with *symptoms of blood loss or anemia* such as light-headedness, syncope, angina, or dyspnea.

Q21. What are the investigations done in LGI bleed?

A
- Endoscopy/newer endoscopic techniques
- Sigmoidoscopy/colonoscopy
- Angiography of splanchnic vasculature
- Occult blood in stools (FOBT)
- USG abdomen

Case 13: A 28-Year-Old Female with Breathlessness and Palpitations

A 28-year-old female attended the medical outpatient department with complaints of breathlessness on exertion and orthopnea for the past 5 years and palpitations for the past 5 months. She also had a history of recurrent respiratory infections and two episodes of hemoptysis a year ago and had sought medical help for the same. She was diagnosed to have some heart ailment and was prescribed long-term medications for it. She also complained of swelling of legs on and off for the past 3 years. She gave a history of recurrent sore throat and joint pains and swelling in childhood that involved knee, ankle, and elbow but did not produce deformities. Her pregnancy 2 years ago was uneventful.

General examination revealed a thin-built individual who was afebrile and had an irregularly irregular pulse with a rate of 122/min. Her BP was 100/70 mmHg and her JVP was raised 5 cm above the clavicle with prominent "cv" waves. She was mildly anemic and had bilateral pitting pedal edema. There was no clubbing or cyanosis.

Examination of the cardiovascular system revealed a tapping apical impulse in the fifth intercostal space in the midclavicular line. There was marked left parasternal heave and P2 was palpable. A diastolic thrill was palpable in the mitral area. Auscultation revealed irregular heart sounds with a loud P2. S1 was variable in intensity and there was an opening snap heard best between the mitral and tricuspid areas. A mid-diastolic murmur that had no presystolic accentuation was heard best in the mitral area along with a pansystolic murmur that was conducted to the left axilla and inferior angle of left scapula. There was another pansystolic murmur best heard in the tricuspid area and increasing with inspiration.

Lung fields revealed bilateral basal crackles. Abdominal examination revealed no organomegaly. CNS was normal.

Q1. What is your provisional diagnosis?

A This appears to be a case of rheumatic heart disease (RHD) with mitral stenosis (MS) (dominant lesion), mitral regurgitation (MR), tricuspid regurgitation (TR) (functional), pulmonary hypertension, atrial fibrillation (AF), and congestive heart failure (CHF).

Q2. Why do you say MS?

A Presence of mid-diastolic murmur in the mitral area with opening snap favors the diagnosis of MS. The absence of presystolic accentuation is due to atrial fibrillation. Moreover, there was left parasternal heave indicative of RVH or left atrial enlargement (LAE) due to MS. The systolic BP is only 100 mmHg and favors a stenotic lesion.

Q3. What are the auscultatory features of MS?

A The auscultatory features of MS are as follows:

- Loud S1 (variable in this patient due to AF): It is due to increased left atrial pressure that keeps valve cusps widely apart at the beginning of systole so that when they close, they do so with a forcible shut. It is absent when the valve is calcified. Tapping apical impulse is due to a palpable loud S1.
- Opening snap: It is a high-pitched sound that occurs due to increased left atrial pressure that forces the valve cusps to open but there is abrupt halting of the valve cone when the valve cusps are forced apart. It is best heard at the apex or along a line drawn from mitral to tricuspid area and can be absent in calcification of valve when it is not pliable.
- Low-pitched rough and rumbling mid-diastolic murmur with a presystolic accentuation in the mitral area (heard best with the bell of the stethoscope), with the patient in the left lateral position and the breath held in expiration.
- Absent S3 in pure MS—S3 indicates rapid ventricular filling, which is not a feature of MS.

Q4. Why do you say MR?

A Presence of a pansystolic murmur in the mitral area conducted to the axilla favors the diagnosis of MR. Only an MR murmur can be conducted to the left axilla and also to the inferior angle of left scapula.

Q5. What are the other features of MR?

A Other features of MR include attenuation of S1 due to ineffective closure of mitral valves and features of LVH (apical impulse being displaced down and out). However, these are not seen in the index case as MS appears to be the dominant lesion. The dominant MS is also substantiated by the low systolic BP of 100 mmHg.

The pansystolic murmur of MR is conducted to axilla if anterior mitral valve leaflet is involved and to the pulmonary area if the posterior mitral valve leaflet is involved. The murmur is best heard in expiration as it is a left-sided murmur. Sometimes S3 can be heard due to rapid ventricular filling.

Q6. Why do you say that the patient has functional TR?

A Presence of a pansystolic murmur in the tricuspid area that is nonradiating and increasing in intensity with inspiration (Carvallo sign) favors the diagnosis of functional TR. Moreover, there is a loud and palpable P2 suggestive of pulmonary hypertension. The large "cv" wave in JVP is diagnostic of TR. All TR murmurs are functional (secondary to pulmonary hypertension) except in rare cases of Ebstein anomaly and infective endocarditis in IV drug abusers.

Q7. What is the cause of pulmonary hypertension? Why is the "a" wave in JVP absent in this case?

A Presence of MS and MR increases left atrial pressure that is transmitted backwards through the pulmonary veins to the lungs and then through the pulmonary arteries to the right ventricle leading to the development of pulmonary hypertension, left atrial enlargement, and right ventricular hypertrophy.

There is no prominent "a" wave in JVP in spite of pulmonary hypertension as there is no effective atrial contraction due to atrial fibrillation in this patient.

Q8. Why do you say that the patient has AF?

A We say so because the patient's pulse is irregularly irregular and there are no "a" waves in JVP in spite of pulmonary hypertension. S1 is also variable and presystolic accentuation of the mid-diastolic murmur of MS is absent. It is always prudent to determine the pulse deficit, calculated as heart rate – pulse rate. If it is more than 10, it is suggestive of AF; otherwise, it could be due to ventricular ectopics.

Q9. How do you assess the severity of MS?

A Severity of MS is assessed on the basis of the following:

- A2–OS interval (the shorter the A2–OS interval, the more severe is the stenosis)
- Duration of mid-diastolic murmur (the longer the murmur, the more severe is the stenosis)
- Character of S1—soft, indicating immobile cusps
- Presence of pulmonary hypertension

- Narrow pulse pressure
- Diameter of mitral valve orifice on ECHO—<1 cm^2, severe, tight, critical MS; 1–1.5 cm^2, moderate MS; and >1.5 cm^2, mild MS (normal diameter is 4–6 cm^2).

Q10. What are the causes of mid-diastolic murmurs in the mitral area?

A
- Austin Flint murmur of aortic regurgitation—due to the regurgitant stream impinging on the anterior mitral valve leaflet
- Carey Coombs murmur of acute rheumatic valvulitis—disappears on treatment
- Ritan's murmur of complete heart block
- Left atrial myxoma—murmur varies with posture
- Ball valve thrombus—murmur varies with posture
- Functional mid-diastolic murmurs—mitral regurgitation, ventricular septal defect

Q11. What are the ECG manifestations of mitral valve diseases?

A
- Mitral stenosis—P mitrale (see Fig. C-1) in several leads, best appreciated in LII, bifid "P" in V1, features of right-axis deviation and right ventricular hypertrophy
- Mitral regurgitation—may cause features of LVH with left-axis deviation

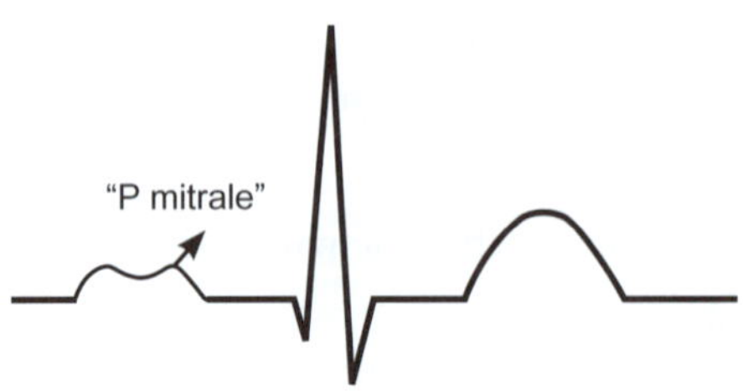

FIGURE C-1. P mitrale in mitral stenosis.

Q12. What are the chest roentgenogram findings in mitral stenosis?

A
- Mitralization or straightening of the left heart border
- Double contour of the right border of the heart—outer being left atrium and inner being right atrium (this is called "shadow within shadow" appearance)
- Dilated pulmonary arteries with peripheral narrowing or pruning suggestive of pulmonary hypertension (this is preceded by dilatation of the upper lobe pulmonary veins)
- Elevated and horizontal left upper lobe bronchus caused by left atrial enlargement
- Calcification of the valve at times

Case 14: A 70-Year-Old Male with Stroke

A 70-year-old obese male, diabetic and hypertensive on treatment, and a chronic smoker for the past 25 years, was brought to the emergency department at 12 noon with complaints of inability to use the right upper and lower limbs and slurring of speech for the past 6 hours. There was no history of convulsions. The wife of the patient said that he suffered two similar episodes in the past but on both occasions had complete recovery within a day.

On examination, he was conscious with a blood pressure of 180/110 mmHg. His pupils were equal and reactive to light and there was preferential gaze to the left. He was able to close his eyes normally but had deviation of the angle of the mouth to the left on talking and drooling of saliva from the right angle of the mouth. His left nasolabial fold was prominent. Sensations and vision were intact. Babinski sign was present on the right side. Deep tendon jerks were brisk and ankle clonus was present on the right side. There was no carotid bruit.

A CT of head showed evidence of a translucent lesion in the left internal capsule with minimal cerebral edema and no midline shift.

Q1. What is the diagnosis? What is the site and nature of the lesion in this patient?

A This is a case of partial anterior circulation stroke (PACS). The patient has recovered from the stage of spinal shock.

The lesion is present in the left internal capsule. The vascular event that led to this condition is thrombosis causing right hemiplegia and dysphasia.

Q2. How do you differentiate stroke due to thrombosis from that due to embolism and hemorrhage?

A The differentiating features are as follows:
- *Embolism*: It occurs at any time of the day.
- *Thrombosis*: It usually occurs early in the morning after a period of inactivity at night. A classical history of getting up early in the morning to go to the toilet, falling down due to weakness of limbs, and calling for help favors a thrombotic etiology.
- *Hemorrhage*: It usually occurs late in the evening or night after a hard physical labor or mental strain in a patient with uncontrolled severe hypertension. There is leakage of blood into the brain substance causing convulsions and loss of consciousness (extravascular event).

In this particular case, the preferential gaze of the patient to the left (toward the site of the lesion in the brain) indicates a thrombotic etiology. In an irritative lesion (hemorrhage), the preferential gaze would be to the right (away from the site of lesion in the brain).

Q3. What are TACS, PACS, LACS, and POCS? What are their features?

A TACS, or total anterior circulation stroke, occurs due to large artery involvement (middle cerebral artery [MCA] and anterior cerebral artery [ACA]) giving rise to all the following clinical features:

- Affection of speech (if dominant hemisphere is involved) or hemispatial neglect (if nondominant hemisphere is involved)
- Homonymous hemianopia
- Contralateral extremity and facial weakness

In PACS, or partial anterior circulation stroke, the patient has any two of the above-mentioned features.

In POCS, or posterior circulation stroke, there is involvement of vertebral artery, basilar artery, and posterior cerebral artery giving rise to diplopia, dysphagia, visual disturbances, vertigo, nystagmus, and ipsilateral cranial nerve palsy with crossed hemiplegia.

In LACS, or lacunar stroke, small arteries are involved giving rise to focal/minor deficit. Lacunes are small (<1.5 cm^3) infarcts and some of the features are ataxic hemiparesis, dysarthria, and clumsy hand syndrome.

Q4. What is stroke-in-evolution?

A Stroke-in-evolution is a progressively increasing stroke in terms of both the area of involvement and severity. It is always due to thrombosis.

Q5. How do you differentiate capsular stroke from a cortical stroke and a brainstem stroke?

A

- *Cortical stroke*: Results in monoplegia
- *Capsular stroke*: Results in hemiplegia (dense)
- *Brainstem stroke*: Results in ipsilateral cranial nerve palsies with contralateral hemiplegia

All produce hemiplegia on the opposite side due to crossing of corticospinal (pyramidal) tract at the lower border of medulla (pyramid).

Q6. What is the type of facial palsy in this patient? Why do you say so?

A This patient suffers from right upper motor neuron (UMN) facial palsy.

The clinical points in favor of this include involvement of the right lower half of the face with sparing of upper half as suggested by the patient being able to close his eyes, prominence of left nasolabial fold, and ipsilateral hemiplegia.

Q7. How do you differentiate UMN from LMN facial palsy?

A UMN facial palsy involves contralateral lower half of the face, whereas LMN facial palsy involves ipsilateral upper and lower halves of the face. Upper half of the face is spared in UMN facial palsy due to bilateral innervation by the corticobulbar fibers.

Q8. Why is the seventh cranial nerve always involved in a case of hemiplegia?

A This is because the nucleus of the seventh cranial nerve supplying lower half of the face has unilateral cortical control. All other cranial nerves have bilateral representation in cerebral cortex.

Q9. What is Babinski sign? What are its other causes?

A Babinski sign refers to the extensor plantar response that occurs along with fanning of other toes on stroking the lateral aspect of sole. It is typically seen in a patient with UMN lesion.

It is also seen in infants younger than 1 year (due to nonmyelination of the spinal cord). Other causes include deep sleep and coma.

Q10. How do you look for plantar response in an amputated limb?

A To elicit plantar response in an amputated limb, we scratch the lowermost amputated part of the limb and look for contraction of tensor fascia lata.

Q11. What is crossed hemiplegia? Explain its basis.

A Crossed hemiplegia refers to ipsilateral cranial nerve palsies with contralateral hemiplegia. It occurs in a brainstem lesion.

The nuclei of cranial nerves in the brainstem are involved ipsilaterally as the corticospinal tract passes through them. The hemiplegia is contralateral as the corticospinal tract crosses at the lower end of the medulla in the pyramid to the opposite side.

Q12. Why are sensations intact in this patient?

A The sensory fibers are situated in the posterior-most part of the posterior limb of internal capsule and not in the anterior two-third of the posterior limb. They convey the fibers from thalamus to parietal cortex. Since this area is spared, the sensations are intact in this patient.

Q13. How would you manage this patient?

A
- Reduction of cerebral edema—IV 20% mannitol (fast drip), oral glycerol, and IV furosemide for 4–5 days (anticerebral edema measures given for more than 5 days carry a risk of inducing rebound cerebral edema by breaking down the integrity of the blood–brain barrier)
- Avoidance of dexamethasone because of high BP
- Administration of thrombolytic rTPA (alteplase) within 4.5 hours of the onset of stroke if CT head does not show evidence of hemorrhage (it would not be effective in this patient as 6 hours had already passed when he was brought to the hospital)
- Care of bed sores—frequent turning of the patient and applying powder on the back
- Care of bowel and bladder
- Nutrition
- Physiotherapy

Case 15: A 25-Year-Old Female with Off-and-On Headache

A 25-year-old female presents to medicine OPD with a chief complaint of on-and-off headache. Each episode of headache lasts for a few hours, is severe and throbbing in character, and is accompanied by nausea and vomiting. The headache is always unilateral and is aggravated by even the slightest movement. The patient's mother reports that her daughter has been having similar episodes of headache for the past 2–3 years and symptomatic treatment offers only mild relief. The episodes have been gradually increasing in frequency. There is no history of any visual or sensory symptoms before or during the episode of headache. Physical examination is normal and no other reasonable cause of headache can be found. There is no history of any systemic illness in the patient or similar complaints in any other family member. Ophthalmic, otorhinolaryngological, and neurological examinations are also normal.

Q1. What is the most probable diagnosis? Why?

A The most probable diagnosis is migraine because there is a history of multiple similar episodes without any neurological deficit. The headache is associated with nausea and vomiting.

Q2. What are the alarming/red flag signs of headache?

A
- First severe headache
- Worst headache ever
- Interferes with sleep or early morning headache
- Associated with fever or vomiting
- Onset after age 55
- Abnormal neurological examination
- Induced by bending, coughing
- Known systemic illness
- Local tenderness over temporal artery
- Subacute worsening over days and weeks

Q3. The patient does not give a history of any visual or sensory aura. Can a diagnosis of migraine be made in the absence of aura symptoms?

A Yes. The presence of aura is not required for diagnosing migraine. In fact, only 25–30% of patients with migraine experience any aura-like symptoms.

Q4. What is the role of CGRP in migraine?

A CGRP stands for calcitonin gene-related peptide. It is synthesized in neurons, is a potent vasodilator, and is thought to play a role in the transmission of pain. Recent research suggests that CGRP levels are elevated during acute migraine attacks. CGRP receptor antagonists, anti-CGRP, antibodies and anti-CGRP receptor antibodies are thought to be effective in treating or preventing migraine episodes. However, the benefit of these drugs in migraine and their potential side effects are still under research.

Q5. What are the treatment options for this patient?

A Nonpharmacological options should be tried first, including maintaining a headache diary, healthy diet, regular exercise, and stress reduction. Maintaining a headache diary will help the patient in identifying the trigger factor(s) and subsequent avoidance of these factors, if possible. Pharmacological options include NSAIDs for mild to moderate headache and Triptans (selective 5-HT 1B/1D agonists) for moderate to severe headache. Sometimes certain antiepileptics, antidepressants, and antihypertensives are used for prophylactic therapy; however, definitive data regarding their efficacy in migraine prophylaxis are lacking. Novel therapies involving CGRP antagonism are under trial. The patient is a female of reproductive age and should be counseled that OCPs may also act as a trigger for migraine. If there is a history of OCP use, the patient should be advised to either change the OCP or discontinue its use for some time and use alternative contraceptive methods.

Case 16: A 32-Year-Old Female with Bilateral Lower Limb Weakness

A 32-year-old female presented to the emergency department with weakness of both lower limbs for 5 days. The weakness was symmetrical in onset, initially distal but had progressed to involve the proximal muscles so that she now had difficulty in climbing stairs and getting up from squatting position. She also complained of paresthesia in both lower limbs since onset. The bladder and bowel were unaffected. There was no history of low backache, root pains, trauma, band-like sensation, myalgias, headache, altered sensorium, cranial nerve involvement, or a similar episode in the past. The patient suffered from gastroenteritis 10 days prior to this episode.

On examination, the patient was conscious, oriented, and cooperative. She had symmetrical lower motor neuron (LMN) weakness in both lower limbs, more proximal than distal, with mild impairment of pain and temperature sensations. Rest of the neurological and systemic examination was normal.

Q1. What is the probable clinical diagnosis of this case?

A The classical presentation of an ascending, symmetrical limb weakness with areflexia and minimal sensory impairment with an antecedent infection suggests Guillain–Barre syndrome as the most probable diagnosis. *Campylobacter jejuni* and CMV infections are the most common preceding infections but fever and systemic features should be absent at the time weakness is evolving.

Q2. What are the features of LMN lesion?

A Decreased muscle tone and reflexes go in favor of LMN lesion.

Q3. How will you confirm your diagnosis?

A GBS is a clinical diagnosis, confirmed by nerve conduction studies that show slowing of nerve conduction, prolonged distal latencies, and conduction blocks in acute inflammatory demyelinating polyneuropathy (AIDP). It also helps in classifying the various subtypes of GBS and monitoring treatment response. CSF analysis done at the end of the first week of illness shows elevated CSF protein without pleocytosis (albuminocytological dissociation).

Q4. What are the variants of the disease?

A The clinical spectrum of GBS includes AIDP, which is the commonest variant, acute motor axonal neuropathy (AMAN), acute motor sensory axonal neuropathy (AMSAN), and Miller Fisher syndrome (MFS) characterized by ataxia, areflexia, and ophthalmoplegia.

Q5. How will you manage the patient?

A Specific treatment of GBS is either high-dose IVIG (2 g/kg body weight given over 5 days) or plasmapheresis (40–50 mL/kg PE four to five times).

Q6. How will you assess for the need for mechanical ventilation?

A Mechanical ventilation is required in 30% of patients. Even in the absence of respiratory distress, $PaCO_2$ >48 mmHg, PaO_2 <56 mmHg on room air, FVC (forced vital capacity) <15 mL/kg, impaired swallowing, inefficient cough, and basal atelectasis are predictors for the need of mechanical ventilation.

Q7. What is the prognosis of the patient?

A GBS is monophasic illness, reaching a plateau within 4 weeks of onset. The mortality rate is 5% usually due to secondary respiratory complications.

Case 17: A 28-Year-Old Male with Unilateral Knee Pain

A 28-year-old male presents to the emergency department with a 2-week history of worsening left knee pain, subjective fever, and chills. He sustained a gunshot wound to his right proximal tibia 8 months ago and was treated surgically with bullet removal and a course of oral antibiotics. He now notes purulent drainage and ulceration of his wound with marked erythema and tenderness. On examination, he is afebrile with normal vital signs. The patient is comfortable in bed and has a 1-cm wound just inferolateral to his right knee with mild focal tenderness, surrounding erythema, and purulent drainage. He is neurovascularly intact, but has severe pain with active range of motion of his knee. Radiographs of the knee are normal: his WBC is $12.5 \times 10^3/mm^3$, ESR is 78 mm/h, and CRP is 38.8 mg/L. The patient does have elevated inflammatory markers and a purulent wound. Despite the absence of fever and normal radiographs, we cannot exclude osteomyelitis or septic arthritis. Blood cultures should be taken and he should be admitted for further workup and started on intravenous antibiotics. The X-ray of left knee is given in Figure C-2.

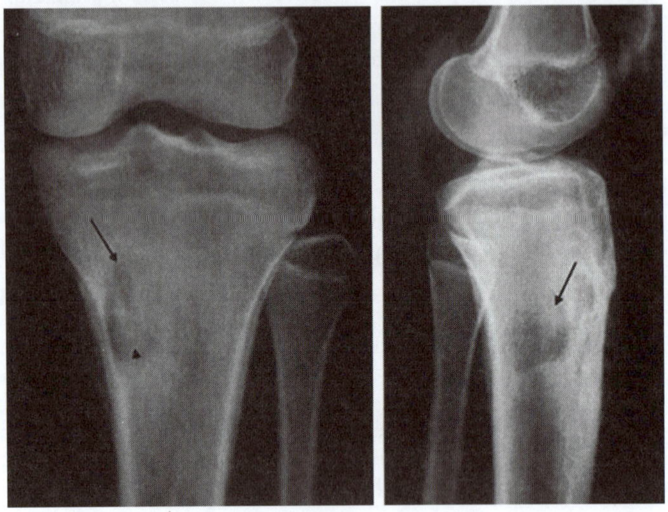

FIGURE C-2. X-ray of left knee.

Q1. What is your differential diagnosis for this patient's knee pain?

A This patient's symptoms of subjective fever, erythema, and tenderness over a gunshot wound suggest an infectious etiology. Musculoskeletal infections can involve the bone, joints, or the soft tissues.

In this patient, we should consider osteomyelitis, septic arthritis, surgical wound infection, and necrotizing fasciitis.

Q2. Which radiographic or laboratory tests will you order?

A
- Laboratory investigations
  - Hemoglobin
  - Complete blood count—TC (total count), DC (differential count), and ESR (erythrocyte sedimentation rate)
  - C-reactive protein analysis
- Radiological investigations
  - Plain X-ray of left knee with proximal leg
  - MRI of left knee with leg

Q3. What are the characteristic features of chronic osteomyelitis?

A
- *Sequestrum*: Avascular piece of bone surrounded by granulation tissue with persistent neutrophilic discharge
- *Involucrum*: Dense sclerotic new bone surrounding the sequestrum
- *Cloacae*: Multiple perforation in involucrum

Types of Sequestrum

Black sequestrum	Actinomycosis and calcaneal fractures
Bombay sequestrum	Overlying skin loss
Button sequestrum	Pheochromocytoma
Coke sequestrum	Tuberculosis
Granular sequestrum	*Salmonella*
Ivory sequestrum	Syphilis
Rice grain/sandy/feathery sequestrum	Tuberculosis
Ring sequestrum	Amputation stump and around pin tracts
Tubular sequestrum	Segmental fractures

Q4. MRI of the right knee reveals findings consistent with osteomyelitis of the proximal tibia. What would you expect to find on MRI? Why were the original radiographs negative?

A
- Osteomyelitis is an infection of the bone most commonly associated with a sinus tract from previous surgery, trauma, decreased vascular flow, or a wound (as in our patient).
- A minority of cases arise from bacteremia by hematogenous osteomyelitis. Patients will often present with focal pain, fever, and erythema around the site of infection. Inflammatory markers such as ESR and CRP are often elevated.
- MRI is the imaging modality of choice, approaching 100% sensitivity.
- Changes on MRI: Increase in *edema and water content* within the bone, so we would expect a *decrease in T1 and an increase in T2 marrow signal* in this patient's left proximal tibia.
- CT and technetium bone scans are useful adjuncts in patients with a contraindication to MRI.
- Radiographs often take 1–2 weeks to show any change and at least 30% of bone loss must be present to identify osteomyelitis on X-ray.

Q5. What is your treatment plan?

A Blood cultures are negative in about half of all cases of osteomyelitis. Therefore, we must rely on surgical cultures to help dictate appropriate antibiotic therapy. Patients are often given at least 4 weeks of antibiotics postoperatively. Prognosis depends on the patient's medical comorbidities and nutritional status, location of the lesion (metaphyseal infections do better than diaphyseal lesions), and the severity of bone loss.

Q6. What are the treatment options available for chronic osteomyelitis?

A
- Sequestrectomy or saucerization of the cavity
- Organism identification and infection control
- Cavity filling with bone cement or bone graft
  - Antibiotic polymethyl methacrylate (PMMA) beading (penicillin/cephalosporin/clindamycin/vancomycin) with occlusive dressing
  - Bone transplant with Ilizarov technique

Q7. What is Garre's sclerosing osteomyelitis?

A
- A unifocal form of chronic recurrent multifocal osteomyelitis (CRMO)
- Nonsuppurative sclerosing chronic osteomyelitis
- MC site: Mandible or diaphysis of tubular bone
- Features: Thickened and distended bony segment without abscess or sequestra
- Treatment: Excision of the involved fragment

Case 18: A 76-Year-Old Male with Polyarthritis

A 76-year-old retired general practitioner presented to the rheumatology department with polyarthritis, which had developed insidiously over the previous 18 months. He had been a lifelong asthmatic with a 10-year history of hypertension. He was a heavy smoker and a heavy social drinker. He used to take diclofenac, enalapril, and prednisolone 5 mg daily, and salbutamol and beclometasone inhalers. He admitted to self-medicating with oral steroids for most of his life to control his chest symptoms.

On examination, he had atrial fibrillation and a barrel-shaped chest. He had bilateral swelling of his MCP joints, a left knee effusion, a right olecranon bursa, Dupuytren's contractures, and signs consistent with right carpal tunnel syndrome. Investigation results were as follows:

- Hb 16 g/L; TLC 7 × 10^9/L; platelets 232 × 10^9/L
- Liver function normal; creatinine 135 µmol/L; glomerular filtration rate (GFR) 55; fasting glucose 5.5 mmol/L; urate 642 mmol/L
- CRP 10; rheumatoid factor (RF) latex screen positive; ELISA equivocal; anticitrullinated C-peptide (ACCP) negative

X-ray of both hands is given in Figure C-3.

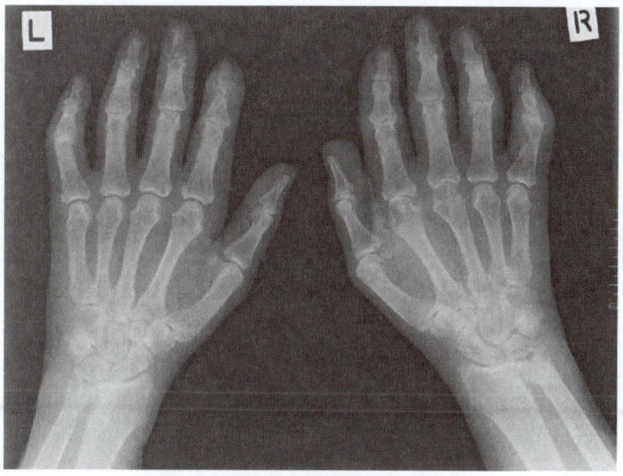

FIGURE C-3. X-ray of both hands.

Q1. What is the likely diagnosis and why?

A The most likely diagnosis is chronic gout. The differential diagnosis is between an acute inflammatory arthritis such as rheumatoid arthritis and chronic gout. The radiograph shows asymmetrical swelling with "punched-out" erosions away from the joint surface with no osteopenia (Fig. AII-3). The long-term steroid use is likely to have masked early episodic attacks of gout. Gout often affects osteoarthritic joints. Tophi over Heberden's or Bouchard's nodes can ulcerate and discharge, mimicking septic arthritis. This patient could have developed an acute inflammatory arthritis in addition to long-standing chronic gout, which had been masked by long-term steroid use. This is an important differential diagnosis to be considered as the management of the two conditions is very different.

Q2. Aspirate from the knee helped confirm the diagnosis. What are the likely findings?

A Knee aspirate revealed negatively birefringent monosodium urate crystals. A diagnosis of gout is confirmed by the presence of uric acid crystals in a joint bursa or tophus. Aspirate from his olecranon bursa was thick, chalky, and rich in urate crystals. Ideally, affected joints should be aspirated. However, if there are no actively inflamed joints, aspirate and washout from unaffected joints can aid diagnosis. The most common joint used in this situation is the knee. Diagnosis is confirmed if uric acid crystals are present in macrophages.

Q3. What is the significance of the rheumatoid factor and uric acid levels?

A The rheumatoid factor is positive in approximately 10% of patients over the age of 60, and the percentage increases with age. The ACCP antibody is more specific for rheumatoid arthritis, and can help to differentiate between the two conditions. However, negative ACCP antibodies do not help to differentiate between gout and rheumatoid arthritis.

Hyperuricemia does not equate to a diagnosis of gout. Furthermore, serum urate levels fall, and may be misleadingly low during attacks of gout. However, hyperuricemia is the most important risk factor for developing acute gout, with a 5-year cumulative risk of one-third for patients with serum urate > 0.6 mmol/L.

Q4. What are the clinical manifestations of hyperuricemia?

A The clinical manifestations of hyperuricemia are as follows:

- Asymptomatic hyperuricemia
- Acute gout
- Recurrent gout
- Chronic tophaceous gout
- Renal stone
- Rarely urate nephropathy

Q5. What management strategies will you suggest?

A Gout is associated with hypertension, metabolic syndrome, insulin resistance, diabetes, and chronic renal failure. Once a diagnosis of gout is established, the aim of management is to control symptoms, prevent future attacks, and prevent structural damage of joints and kidneys. The management strategies are as follows:

- NSAIDs should be stopped as they can exacerbate hypertension and decrease renal perfusion. Simple analgesics should be used for pain relief. Intra-articular or intramuscular steroids can help settle the acute inflammatory symptoms.
- Oral colchicine in a dose of 500 μg twice to four times daily is an alternative treatment for inflammatory joint symptoms.
- Lifestyle advice is important. Patients with early or mild gout can prevent future attacks by altering their lifestyle. In general, patients are advised to drink plenty of water to prevent renal stones. Overproducers of uric acid and those taking uricosuric agents are particularly prone to renal stones. Sweetened soft drinks and drinks high in fructose are associated with increased risk of gout in men. Dietary advice is the same as the general advice given for the associated metabolic syndrome. In addition, patients should avoid foods rich in purines such as red meat, game, offal, and shellfish.
- Alcohol enhances urate production, decreases renal urate clearance, decreases solubility of urate crystals, and can be relatively dehydrating. Patients are advised to avoid beer and binge drinking.
- It is important to monitor renal function and general metabolic state. The lipid-lowering drugs atorvastatin and fenofibrate, and the antihypertensives losartan and amlodipine, have mild uricosuric effects. This may be helpful when treating the comorbid conditions associated with gout.
- For long-term control of joint symptoms, the serum urate needs to be lowered and maintained below the saturation point for monosodium urate (<0.38 mmol/L). Target levels for serum urate are <0.30 mmol/L (BSR [British Society for Rheumatology]) and <0.36 mmol/L (European League Against Rheumatism [EULAR]). Long-term treatment using uricostatic or uricosuric therapies is needed if patients are unable to lower their serum urate sufficiently to prevent attacks of gout with lifestyle modification. This is especially so in patients with renal failure with symptomatic gout.
- The long-term treatment of choice is prevention of urate production using allopurinol, which is a xanthine oxidase inhibitor and inhibits production of urate from hypoxanthine and xanthine. Allopurinol should be started once the acute symptoms have been settled for 2–6 weeks using colchicines (or NSAIDs if the patient is not in renal failure); otherwise, there is a significant risk of acute gouty flare.
- Patients who are intolerant or allergic to allopurinol can use a uricosuric agent to enhance urate renal clearance. These drugs inhibit the urate anion exchange in the proximal nephron (URAT-1). Sulfinpyrazone (200–800 mg/day in divided doses), probenecid (0.5–2.0 g/day), and benzbromarone (50–200 mg/day) are used as second-line agents. Febuxostat (40–80 mg/day) is a recently developed nonpurine selective xanthine oxidase inhibitor, which is available to patients who are allergic to allopurinol and have failed uricosuric therapy. Enzyme therapy with urate oxidase is now licensed for intravenous infusion treatment for allopurinol-intolerant patients. However, its use is limited by antibody formation and cost.

Case 19: A 67-Year-Old Male with Low Backache

A 67-year-old man with a 26-year history of AS presented to the rheumatology clinic with increased pain in his back. Four months back, he had been admitted in hospital under the general medicine team after collapsing at home. A diagnosis of pulmonary embolism was made and confirmed on a computed tomography pulmonary angiogram (CTPA). The patient was discharged home on warfarin, but continued to have severe pain in his back. The pain was not alleviated by exercise, prevented sleep, and was very debilitating.

There was no history of weight loss or systemic features of infection, and the patient had no prior treatment with immunosuppressive therapy. His analgesia included diclofenac 50 mg three times daily and morphine sulfate tablets 10 mg twice daily. Examination revealed a moderate kyphosis. He was tender to palpation over T12–L3 with restricted hip movement and no evidence of peripheral synovitis. The patient was afebrile and system examination was unremarkable, including intact neurology. His Bath Ankylosing Spondylitis Disease Activity Index (BASDAI) score was 6/10 and his spinal pain Visual Analogue Score (VAS) was 9/10 cm.

Investigations showed the following—Hb 13.5 g/dL, TLC 7.7 × 10^9/L, platelets 192 × 10^9/L, creatinine 110 µmol/L, CRP 8 mg/L, ESR 4 mm/h.

MRI spine of this patient is shown in Figure C-4.

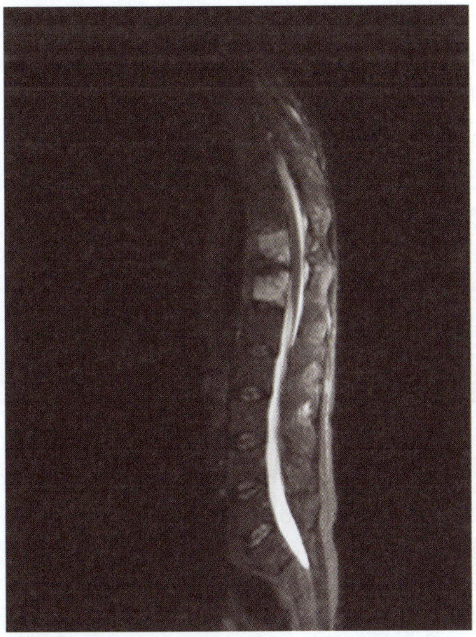

FIGURE C-4. MRI of the spine.

Q1. What is your differential diagnosis of the back pain?

A The patient has a raised BASDAI and spinal VAS, which could indicate a flare in his inflammatory back pain. However, the pain is more mechanical in nature, i.e., it does not settle with exercise and there is point tenderness over the spine. A recent pulmonary embolism may suggest an undiagnosed malignancy with secondary metastases in the spine. Other differentials include an acute discitis or osteomyelitis, although the normal CRP and lack of fever would argue against this. Finally, the patient sustained a fall when he collapsed at home, so he should be investigated for a fracture.

Q2. What does the MR scan show?

A The MRI of the spine demonstrates high signal in the vertebral bodies of T11 and T12 extending into the posterior elements, with collapse of the superior end plate of T12 and the inferior end plate of T11. The findings would be in keeping with a traumatic Andersson lesion, or pseudoarthrosis, involving the posterior elements. The lack of high signal in the disc space itself makes infection unlikely. There is extrusion of the disc material anteriorly and the anterior longitudinal ligament is displaced. There is no evidence of spinal canal stenosis and the cord signal is normal. The diagnosis of AS is confirmed by the partial fusion of the lumbar and thoracic vertebrae. Standard CT allows better evaluation of fractures and destructive vertebral lesions than MRI of the spine and was subsequently performed in this case (Fig. C-5). This confirmed AS with a T11/12 Andersson lesion as the cause of the sudden-onset back pain in this patient.

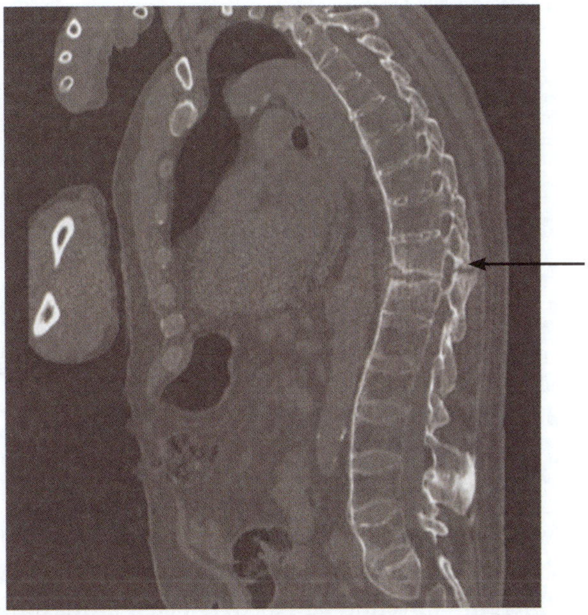

FIGURE C-5. Sagittal CT image of spine showing Andersson lesion.

Q3. How would you manage this patient?

A This patient's spine is unstable with an increased risk of spinal cord compression if left untreated. Surgical fixation is the treatment of choice. The possible complications of spinal surgery include damage to the spinal cord or spinal nerves in addition to general risks including anesthetic complications, bleeding, thrombosis, dural tear, infection, and persistent pain.

Q4. Would you consider this patient for biological therapy?

A Although this patient has raised BASDAI and spinal VAS scores, these can be attributed to the pseudoarthrosis rather than reflecting inflammatory disease activity. This patient would be unlikely to benefit from biological therapy and treatment should focus on surgical correction, appropriate analgesia, and physiotherapy postoperatively.

Q5. What are the current NICE guidelines for the treatment of ankylosing spondylitis (AS) with biological therapy?

A NICE guidance recommends the use of the TNF inhibitors adalimumab and etanercept as treatment options in adults with severe active AS. There are three elements that should be satisfied before a patient is eligible for anti-TNF therapy. First, the modified New York criteria for the diagnosis of AS must be satisfied, including the radiological criterion and at least one clinical criterion.

- Clinical criteria
  - Low back pain present for >3 months, improved by exercise but not relieved by rest
  - Limitation of lumbar spine motion in sagittal and frontal planes
  - Limitation of chest expansion relative to normal values for age and sex
- Radiological criterion
- Sacroiliitis on radiographs

Furthermore, there must be evidence of sustained active spinal disease, which is confirmed by:

- Score of ≥4 units on BASDAI
- Score of ≥4 cm on the 0–10 cm spinal pain VAS

These scores must be measured twice, at least 12 weeks apart, on stable treatment. Lastly, patients should have failed treatment with at least two different conventional NSAIDs taken at maximum tolerated or recommended dosages for 4 weeks, respectively.

Case 20: A 30-Year-Old Male with Vertigo and Ear Discharge

A 30-year-old IT professional presented to the OPD with a history of recurrent episodes of vertigo, with white, mucoid discharge from his right ear for the past 10 years. The discharge started with an episode of acute rhinosinusitis and has gradually progressed, aggravating and becoming yellowish in color with each episode of upper respiratory infection and on swimming. He has also noticed reduced hearing in the right ear for the past 5 years, such that he is having trouble with telephonic communication, which worsens during episodes of active ear discharge. He also gives a history of having had right-sided nasal obstruction for almost 15 years and frequent upper respiratory infections with heaviness of head and postnasal discharge, which gets relieved to some extent with medications.

On examination, he is well built and nourished, and no abnormalities were found on general physical examination. On ENT examination, white, mucoid discharge was found in the right external auditory canal, and a medium-sized central perforation was revealed in the tympanic membrane after aural toileting. Hearing assessment showed evidence of moderate conductive hearing loss in the right ear. Nasal examination showed a deviation of the nasal septum to the right side with tenderness over right frontal sinus area.

Q1. What is the likely diagnosis?

A The most likely diagnosis is right chronic otitis media, mucosal type, active with moderate conductive hearing loss, with deviated nasal septum to the right with acute rhinosinusitis.

Here, the septal deviation and history of frequent upper respiratory infections are contributory to the development of chronic otitis media. Reduced airflow on the side of deviation would cause impaired ventilation of the paranasal sinuses, leading to rhinosinusitis. Nasal infection spreads via the eustachian tube to the ear, causing acute otitis media. Frequent upper respiratory infections prevent spontaneous closure of a resultant perforation leading to squamous epithelial overgrowth over its margins, when it is called a permanent perforation.

Q2. What are the two types of chronic otitis media and mention the differentiating points between the two?

A Chronic otitis media is a chronic inflammation of part or whole of the middle ear cleft (eustachian tube, tympanic cavity, attic, aditus, and mastoid air cell system), characterized by the presence of ear discharge and a permanent perforation of the tympanic membrane.

It is classified into two types—mucosal or safe disease (previously called tubotympanic variety) and squamosal or unsafe variety (previously, atticoantral).

Features	Mucosal COM	Squamosal COM
Discharge	Profuse, mucoid discharge, colorless and odorless	Scanty, purulent discharge, foul smelling, and blood stained
Perforation	Central perforation in the tympanic membrane (a perforation that is surrounded by tympanic membrane on all sides)	Marginal perforation (wherein at least one of the sides of the perforation is not bordered by the TM or annulus)
Complications	Lesser chances for complications (hence, called safe variety)	More chances for complications (hence, unsafe). Complications arise in the presence of cholesteatoma, which erodes the surrounding bones and causes spread of infection into the deeper aspects of the temporal bone or into the cranial cavity
Granulations	Granulations are uncommon, and polyp, if present, appears pale	Granulations are common and polyp may be red and fleshy looking
Deafness	Mild-to-moderate conductive deafness	Conductive or mixed hearing loss

Q3. What results do you expect on tuning fork testing in this patient? Name three tuning fork tests that can be done to detect malingering.

A The tuning fork tests that are routinely done in the OPD for patients complaining of reduced hearing are Rinne test, Weber test, and absolute bone conduction test. These tests are carried out using a Gardiner Brown tuning fork, preferably in a quiet environment.

- *Rinne test*: Rinne test is carried out using 256-, 512-, and 1024-Hz tuning forks, so as to give an approximate idea about the degree and type of hearing loss. The patient is explained about the procedure. The prongs of the tuning fork are struck against a firm surface, at the junction of its upper one-third and lower two-thirds. The vibrating tuning fork is held at its stem and the base is placed over the mastoid bone; the patient is instructed to raise his or her hand as soon as the sound stops. The tuning fork is then immediately brought forward and positioned parallel to the external auditory canal, a little away from the external auditory meatus. Now, if the patient can still hear the sound produced by the vibrating prongs of the tuning fork, then it means that air conduction is better than bone conduction (Rinne positive), whereas if he hears the sound longer when placed over the mastoid bone, it means that the bone conduction is better than air conduction (Rinne negative).
  - *Rinne positive*: Normal and sensorineural hearing loss (SNHL). In SNHL, the air and bone conduction is equally reduced, but the patient is able to appreciate some sound when the tuning fork is brought closer to the pinna, hence giving an impression of air conduction being better than bone conduction.
  - *Rinne negative*: Conductive hearing loss. Any obstruction to sound conduction to the inner ear via the external auditory canal (wax/foreign body), tympanic membrane (perforation), and ossicles (erosion/dislocation) can cause conductive hearing loss (CHL). Here, air conduction is impeded due to the above-mentioned causes, but sound is conducted freely through the bone to the cochlea, giving negative Rinne.
  - *False-negative Rinne*: Severe unilateral SNHL. Here, the patient is unable to hear by both air and bone conduction in the affected ear, but when the tuning fork is placed over the mastoid, sound is conducted through the skull to the opposite cochlea (transcranial conduction), and the patient is able to hear. But he or she hears nothing when the tuning fork is in front of the pinna. Hence, it gives a false impression of his or her bone conduction being better than air conduction.
  - *False-positive Rinne*: In case of a patient who has a cholesteatoma that has eroded the ossicles, he or she is ideally supposed to show a CHL pattern on Rinne testing, but if the cholesteatoma is bridging the gap formed by eroded ossicles and conducts the sound to the cochlea, then Rinne may be positive.
- *Weber test*: After properly explaining the test to the patient, a vibrating tuning fork is placed over a midline bony prominence of the face (vertex/forehead/glabella/chin) and the patient is asked

to indicate the side of the ear that hears the sound better. The Weber test shows lateralization only if there is a difference in hearing of more than 5 dB between the two ears. In conductive deafness, it lateralizes to the poorer hearing ear, whereas in SNHL, the sound is better heard in the normal/ better hearing ear.

- *Absolute bone conduction test*: The vibrating tuning fork is placed over the patient's mastoid, and as soon as he or she stops hearing the sound, the tuning fork is brought to the mastoid process of the examiner for comparison (assuming that the examiner has normal hearing). If the examiner is able to hear the sound even after it has stopped for the patient, then it means that the patient has a SNHL. In normal ears and conductive deafness, ABC is equal to that of the examiner.

Type of deafness	Rinne	Weber	ABC
Conductive	Negative (BC > AC)	Lateralized to affected ear	Same as examiner
Sensorineural	Positive (AC > BC)	Lateralized to better ear	Shorter duration

The tests for malingering are Stenger test, Teal test, and Chimani Mooss test.

In this patient, we expect a conductive hearing loss in the right ear and the tuning fork tests are expected to give the following results:

Conduction lists	Right	Left
Rinne test		
256 Hz	Negative	Positive
512 Hz	Negative	Positive
1024 Hz	Positive	Positive
Weber test	Lateralized to the right ear	
Absolute bone conduction test	Same as examiner on both sides	

Q4. If this patient develops malaria-like fever, with headache and progressive pallor, what complication would you suspect? Briefly describe the tests that are positive in this condition.

A One should suspect lateral sinus thrombophlebitis in such a scenario. The following signs are positive in this condition:

- *Griesinger sign*: Erythema, edema, and tenderness over mastoid (due to thrombosis of mastoid emissary vein) occur.
- *Tobey-Ayer test*: Compression of IJV on the normal side raises the pressure of cerebrospinal fluid (measured by lumbar puncture and manometer), but when the IJV on the side of disease is compressed, there is no rise in CSF pressure. This is because the lumen is already occluded by thrombus on the affected side and, hence, compression will not make any difference to the blood column.
- *Crowe-Beck sign*: Pressure on IJV of the normal side results in engorgement of retinal vessels and papilledema, due to obstruction to the other side due to thrombophlebitis.
- *Radiology*: This includes CT and MRI—delta sign.

Q5. What is a cholesteatoma?

A Cholesteatoma, in simple terms, is an epidermal sac, in which keratin debris accumulates. This sac has the capacity for expansion, by eroding the underlying bone (usually the ossicles) by liberation of osteolytic enzymes, hence forming a channel for spread of infection into the intracranial cavity or deeper parts of the temporal bone. Patients with cholesteatoma have a characteristic fishy odor to their ear discharge, due to osteitis.

Q6. Mention the investigations and surgical management.

A
- Investigations
  - Examination of the ear under microscope and sending any discharge, if present, for culture and sensitivity
  - Routine blood investigations (CBC, RBS, LFT, RFT, serology, urine microscopy)
  - Pure tone audiometry (for type and degree of hearing loss, and also for documentation)
  - X-ray bilateral mastoids Schuller's view (to get an idea about pneumatization of mastoid, extent of disease, and the presence of anatomical variations in the position of sigmoid sinus and middle cranial fossa dura)
  - HRCT of the temporal bone not routinely recommended in all cases of COM, but advisable in squamosal disease, especially with extensive cholesteatoma or inability to visualize the tympanic membrane, to accurately determine the extent of bony destruction and complications due to cholesteatoma
- Surgical management
  - *Myringoplasty*: Simple closure of the perforation in the tympanic membrane when the ossicular chain is intact

- *Tympanoplasty*: A surgical procedure that is aimed at eradication of the disease in the middle ear and reconstruction of the hearing mechanism (i.e., the perforation of TM is closed, and along with that the ossicular chain is also repaired)
- *Mastoidectomy*: A surgical procedure that addresses the disease in the mastoid air cell system, so that chances of recurrence are reduced by eliminating a source of the disease (this is usually combined with a tympanoplasty)

For an unsafe variety of COM, always a mastoid exploration with tympanoplasty is done, to ensure complete removal of the disease.

Case 21: A 4-Year-Old Female Child with Fever and Headache

A 4-year-old girl was brought to the emergency department with a history of fever and headache for the past 15 days. The fever was moderate grade and had no specific pattern or diurnal variation. The headache was however debilitating and the child became restless and often had projectile vomiting, which brought some relief. The headache and vomiting were usually most severe on waking up in the morning. On the day she presented, the child had an epileptic seizure in the form of tonic spasms of the whole body followed by clonic movements. The whole episode lasted for around 10 minutes after which the child became unresponsive for about 1 hour. While the child was being rushed to the hospital and regaining consciousness, the mother noticed that she was not moving the left side of her body well.

Past history revealed a history of fever with catarrhal symptoms followed by maculopapular eruption 6 months back. At that time, other children in the neighborhood also suffered from a similar illness, suggesting a strong possibility of measles.

On examination, the child was found to have BP above 99th centile. The response to verbal commands was absent; she however could localize the painful stimulus (coma grade 2). On cranial nerve examination, the pupils were sluggishly reacting to light bilaterally with no restriction of eye movements. There was facial nerve palsy of the left side, upper motor neuron type; the muscle power on the left side was decreased (2/5). There was hypertonia and hyperreflexia in all four limbs and bilateral planters were extensors. The signs of meningeal irritation in the form of neck stiffness and Kernig sign were evident.

Q1. What is the condition the child is suffering from?

A The presence of fever points toward infective pathology, headache and projectile vomiting toward increased intracranial tension, and features of meningeal irritation toward likely meningitis. The child also has hemiparesis along with facial nerve involvement of the same side referred to as complete hemiparesis. This suggests a lesion above the brainstem. (Hemiparesis on one side with cranial nerve involvement of the other side is referred to as crossed hemiparesis and is seen with lesions involving the brainstem.) The long duration of fever is suggestive of chronic infection of the brain (acute illness is usually of 1-week duration).

Q2. What are the differential diagnoses?

A The likely differential diagnoses for the child with chronic infection of the brain include tubercular meningitis, partially treated pyogenic meningitis, enteric encephalopathy, and brain abscess. The uncommon causes may be fungal or protozoal infection of the brain.

Chronic infection of the brain in the presence of past history of measles and family history of tuberculosis raises the strong possibility of it being tubercular meningitis.

Q3. What are clinical grades of coma?

A The clinical grades of coma are defined as follows:

- *Grade 1*: Drowsy or irritable with inconsistent response to verbal stimuli
- *Grade 2*: Purposeful response (localization or withdrawal) to painful stimulus
- *Grade 3*: Non-purposeful response (posturing) to painful stimulus
- *Grade 4*: No response to painful stimulus

Q4. How will you differentiate upper motor neuron lesion from the lower motor neuron lesion? Give examples of each. What is the type of facial nerve involvement in this case?

A In an upper motor neuron lesion, the upper face is spared due to bilateral representation in the cortex. Upper motor neuron involvement is due to corticonuclear fibers to facial nucleus being affected. The site of involvement could be anywhere from cortex to the nerve nucleus.

In a lower motor neuron lesion, the whole face is affected (ipsilateral side); the site of involvement is nucleus or direct injury to the facial nerve.

The facial nerve involvement in this case is an upper motor neuron lesion.

Q5. How will you confirm the diagnosis? What is the role of CBNAAT and line probe assay in the diagnosis of tuberculosis?

A The diagnosis requires index of suspicion backed by examination findings and the results of investigations. Presence of suggestive symptoms, family history of contact with an adult patient with tuberculosis, positive Mantoux test with CSF, and neuroimaging findings help in establishment of diagnosis.

The imaging findings in a case of neurotuberculosis include basilar meningitis, communicating hydrocephalus, infarcts/calcification especially in the basal ganglia region, and tuberculomas. The latest recommendation is for the cartridge-based nucleic acid amplification test (CBNAAT) for demonstrating the nuclear material of *Mycobacterium tuberculosis* in the patient's saliva or body fluid.

Q6. What are the likely complications?

A Advanced cases of neurotuberculosis may be fatal. The complications in the survivors may range from cognition problems and motor or sensory deficits to endocrinological and seizure disorders.

Q7. How will you manage a case of tuberculous meningitis (TBM)?

A The treatment consists of four-drug treatment for the intensive phase and three-drug treatment for the maintenance phase. Prednisolone in a dose of 1–2 mg/kg is utilized for the initial 4–6 weeks for reducing the chances of complications.

Q8. How will you protect the susceptible children in the household with an adult with tuberculosis?

A The susceptible children below 5 years of age should receive prophylaxis. The dose of Isoniazid (INH) for chemoprophylaxis is 10 mg/kg (instead of currently recommended dosage of 5 mg/kg) administered daily for 6 months. TB preventive therapy should be provided to:

- All asymptomatic contacts (under 6 years of age) of a smear-positive case, after ruling out active disease and irrespective of their BCG or nutritional status
- All HIV-infected children who either had a known exposure to an infectious TB case or are tuberculin skin test (TST) positive (≥5 mm induration) but have no active TB disease
- All TST-positive children who are receiving immunosuppressive therapy (e.g., children with nephrotic syndrome, acute leukemia)
- A child born to mother who was diagnosed to have TB in pregnancy (in this case, the child should receive prophylaxis for 6 months, provided congenital TB has been ruled out; BCG vaccination can be given at birth even if INH chemoprophylaxis is planned)

Case 22: An 8-Year-Old Male Child with History of Off and On Diarrhea

An 8-year-old male child was brought to the outpatient department with a history of off and on diarrhea for the past 6 years. According to the mother, the child would pass loose stools most of the days, the frequency and consistency temporarily improved by treatment from various private practitioners. The child had been dewormed on multiple occasions in the past. There was also a history of pica. According to the mother, the child was doing well when he was on predominant milk-based diet and developed these loose stools as well as faltering growth with the introduction of complementary food items. There were no significant neonatal events. There was no history of allergy, especially cow milk protein allergy, tuberculosis, or inflammatory bowel disease in the family members.

On examination, the child was found to be a thin and small-looking child for his age. There was no apparent facial dysmorphism. He also showed moderate pallor but no clubbing or edema. There were no features of vitamin and mineral deficiency.

Q1. What are you dealing with?

A The child is a case of chronic diarrhea that needs evaluation.

Q2. What are the types of diarrhea in children?

A Diarrhea is classified into acute, persistent, or chronic diarrhea based on the onset and duration of symptoms. An insidious-onset diarrhea lasting for more than 14 days fulfills the criteria for chronic diarrhea.

Q3. Name some causes of chronic diarrhea in children.

A The common causes to be evaluated include celiac disease, giardiasis, cow milk protein allergy, abdominal tuberculosis, inflammatory bowel disease, and immunodeficiency.

Q4. What is the classical presentation of celiac disease? Are there some comorbid conditions to identify?

A Celiac disease is the most common cause of chronic diarrhea in children in north India. The onset of diarrhea with the introduction of complementary feeds (and likely gluten-containing cereals too) is a strong marker toward celiac disease. The children with celiac disease lack the ability to digest and assimilate gluten, which is typically found in wheat and some other grains too. Children with IDDM (insulin-dependent diabetes mellitus) type 1, Down syndrome, Turner syndrome, autoimmune thyroid disorder, and selective IgA deficiency are at increased risk.

Celiac disease classically presents as chronic diarrhea. The other manifestations may be failure to thrive, short stature, or unexplained anemia.

Q5. How do you confirm the diagnosis?

A The diagnosis rests on clinical features backed by serology in the form of raised tissue transglutaminase antibody or antiendomysial antibody. Upper duodenal biopsy with characteristic gross and histopathological examination finding clinches the diagnosis.

Q6. What is the treatment for a case of celiac disease?

A The treatment consists of elimination of all sources of gluten from the diet—gluten-free diet (GFD). This is therapeutic as well as diagnostic. The response to GFD consists of disappearance of symptoms as well as weight and height gain assessed after 3 months of commencement of GFD. Other therapies consist of supplementation of iron and folic acid as well as other micronutrients.

Case 23: A 20-Month-Old Female Child with Increasing Pallor

A 20-month-old girl was brought to the outpatient department with complaints of increasing paleness of body for 1 month and fast breathing and mild difficulty in breathing for the past 2 days. She had received two blood transfusions at the age of 8 and 15 months for similar complaints and was sent home on oral iron supplementation, which she was regularly taking. She was the only child of parents having consanguineous marriage and the mother had a history of three miscarriages. Antenatal, natal, and postnatal history was uneventful.

On examination, the child was found to be tachycardic and tachypneic. She was irritable with evidence of severe pallor in the form of paleness of palmar creases. She had slight facial puffiness with prominence of malar bones unlike any of her parents. There was no icterus, skin or mucosal bleed, significant lymphadenopathy, or bone tenderness. The abdominal examination revealed distended abdomen; liver was palpable 5 cm below the costal margin, soft and tender; spleen was 4 cm below costal margin, firm and nontender. No fluid thrill or shifting dullness was elicited. On cardiovascular examination, S3 gallop was audible. There were occasional fine crackles at the bases of lungs.

Q1. What is your diagnosis? What are the differential diagnoses?

A Most probable diagnosis in this case with anemia, hepatosplenomegaly, characteristic facies, and repeated blood transfusion is beta thalassemia major. Differential diagnoses may be other causes of hemolytic anemia such as hereditary spherocytosis, red cell membrane defect, sickle cell disease, and infections such as chronic malaria.

Q2. What is the cause of this morbidity?

A Thalassemia major is an inherited disorder that results from decreased production of beta chains of hemoglobin. As a result, other normally formed chains are not able to pair with beta chains to form normal hemoglobin and get accumulated in cell as unstable product leading to early destruction of red blood cell. The pallor usually presents at around 6 months when fetal hemoglobin (comprising two alpha and two gamma chains) gets replaced by adult hemoglobin (comprising two alpha and two beta chains). Severe pallor and hepatosplenomegaly are seen in all cases.

Q3. What type of anemia is seen in such case?

A Anemia of microcytic hypochromic type not responding to iron therapy is suggestive of thalassemia.

Q4. What may be the cause of breathing difficulty seen in this case?

A Breathing difficulty may be because of severe anemia or pulmonary infection or congestive heart failure.

Q5. How will you confirm the diagnosis?

A The diagnosis requires complete blood count with general blood picture, which shows anemia with microcytosis, narrow red cell distribution width (RDW, unlike iron deficiency anemia), shift to left, and basophilic stippling. The reticulocyte count is elevated. The confirmatory test is hemoglobin electrophoresis, which shows elevated HbF and absence of HbA.

Q6. What is the definitive treatment?

A Hematopoietic stem cell transplantation is the definitive treatment for thalassemia major.

Q7. What is the side effect of chronic blood transfusion?

A Chronic blood transfusions can lead to iron overload, which subsequently leads to organ toxicity.

Q8. What is chelation therapy? Name some drugs used for chelation therapy.

A Chelation therapy involves introduction of chelation drugs such as deferoxamine, deferiprone, or deferasirox to remove excess iron from the body.

Q9. What is role of genetic counseling in this case?

A Genetic counseling can be done for prenatal testing of thalassemia in the fetus.

Case 24: A 6-Month-Old Infant with Difficulty in Breathing

A 6-month-old infant was brought with complaints of gradually worsening breathing and feeding difficulty for the past 2 days. On the day of presentation, the child developed chest indrawing and could suckle only intermittently while feeding. The child was having moderate fever, cough, and runny nose for 5 days. Some other members in the household also suffered from flu-like symptoms in the preceding few days. Birth and perinatal events were uneventful and the child was appropriately immunized for age. There was no past history of chest infections or suck rest cycle while feeding. There was history of atopyin the family. The father and paternal aunt suffered from episodic attacks of asthma and rhinitis, respectively.

When seen in the emergency department, the child was irritable and fussy. He ran moderate fever of 102°F and had tachypnea as well as increased work of breathing in the form of chest indrawing and nasal flaring. SpO_2 at room air was 92%. The chest was symmetrical with equal movements bilaterally. Breath sounds were equally heard on both sides and fine crackles and rhonchi were auscultated. The heart sounds were normal without any muffling. On abdominal examination, the liver and spleen were palpable below the costal margin.

Q1. What are the possibilities?

A The presence of fever along with respiratory symptoms suggests infection of the respiratory tract. The possibilities are bronchiolitis and pneumonia. Bronchiolitis is more likely because there is preceding history of viral prodrome followed by features of respiratory distress. Pneumonia on the other hand usually follows an acute onset.

Q2. What are the likely organisms causing this illness?

A The most common cause for bronchiolitis is respiratory syncytial virus (RSV). Other likely pathogens may be adenovirus, parainfluenza virus, influenza virus, or *Mycoplasma pneumoniae*.

Q3. How will you investigate this case?

A The investigations may show leukocytosis with lymphocytic predominance. A rapid diagnostic test utilizing monoclonal antibodies can identify RSV in the nasopharyngeal aspirate.

Q4. What is the radiological finding in this case?

A The chest X-ray shows evidence of air trapping in the form of hyperinflated lung fields, which are hyperlucent with pushed-down diaphragm. The infiltrates may follow interstitial pattern.

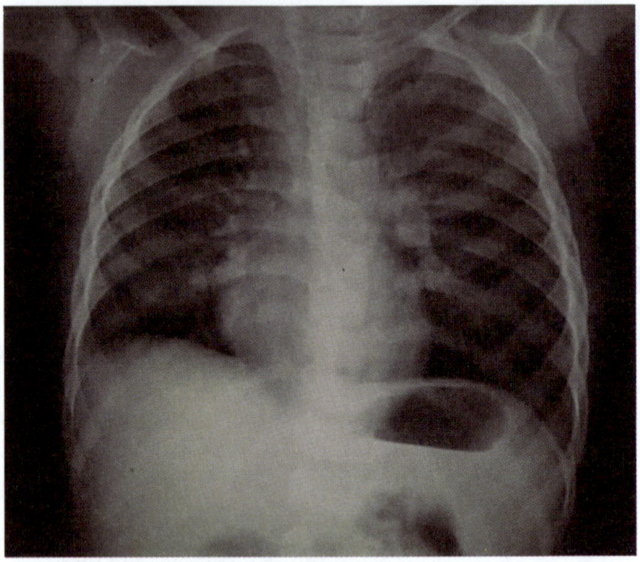

Q5. What are the complications to look at?

A Bronchiolitis is usually a self-limiting disease. A minority may develop severe respiratory compromise with respiratory acidosis, which may even turn fatal.

Q6. How will you treat such a case?

A The treatment consists of moist oxygen inhalation with maintenance of fluid, electrolyte, and sugar balance. There is no role of antibiotics. Bronchodilators may be beneficial especially for children above 6 months of age. Antiviral in the form of ribavirin may be beneficial only for children with underlying congenital heart disease, chronic lung disease, or immunodeficiency.

Q7. What are the predisposing factors?

A The risk factors include male sex, family history of atopy, and significant respiratory problem in the neonatal period.

Q8. Are there some long-term complications to worry about?

A Bronchiolitis in early childhood increases the risk of future asthma.

Case 25: A 3-Year-Old Male Child with Delayed Motor Milestones

A mother brought her 3-year-old boy to the outpatient department due to the child's inability to walk independently as well as stiffness of legs that was gradually worsening. The child was able to walk with support of parents or furniture but usually walked on his toes. He was able to perform almost all activities with his hands expected for his age. He was born prematurely at 34 weeks weighing 1.73 kg as a result of preterm premature rupture of membranes. The baby required some assistance for breathing at birth and had an NICU stay for 6 days. During infancy, the child showed delay in attainment of milestones more so for the motor ones such as head control and sitting. Tightness of the limbs was first noted during infancy as the mother had difficulty in changing diapers.

On examination, the boy was conscious and alert, and interacted normally. Intelligence and speech were normal for his age and all the cranial nerves were intact. Tone was found to be increased in lower limbs with the presence of adductor spasm and scissoring of lower limbs on being held in arms. Power was 5/5 in upper limbs and 4/5 in both the lower limbs. Deep tendon reflexes (DTR) were exaggerated in the lower limbs. Babinski sign was positive.

Q1. What is your diagnosis?

A This is case of spastic diplegia, which is a type of cerebral palsy usually seen as sequelae of preterm delivery.

Q2. What is cerebral palsy?

A Cerebral palsy is a nonprogressive disorder of posture, movement, and tone due to static encephalopathy acquired during brain growth in fetal life, infancy, or early childhood.

Q3. What is classification of cerebral palsy?

A Cerebral palsy (CP) can be categorized as follows:

- Spastic (pyramidal) CP: Most common, accounting for two/third of cases characterized by increased tone. It is further classified into the following:
  - Diplegia: All limbs are affected but involvement of lower limbs is more than that of upper limbs. It is commonly seen in preterm babies associated with periventricular leukomalacia, which mainly involves the part of brain controlling lower limbs. Mentation is usually preserved and seizures are uncommon.
  - Hemiplegic: There is unilateral involvement but hands are more involved than legs. Seizures may be seen.
  - Quadriplegic: All limbs are affected. Mental retardation and seizures are common.
- Extrapyramidal/athetoid/dyskinetic CP: Presence of involuntary movements or fluctuating tone, choreoathetoid being most common (usually following kernicterus)
- Mixed type

Q4. What are Levine (POSTER) criteria for diagnosis of cerebral palsy?

A The Levine (POSTER) criteria for diagnosis of cerebral palsy are abnormalities in four of the following six categories: Posturing or abnormal movements/Oropharyngeal problems/Strabismus/Tone (hypertonia/hypotonia)/Evolutional maldevelopment (persistence of primitive reflexes)/Reflexes (increased DTR or persistent Babinski reflex).

Q5. What are some causes of cerebral palsy? What proportion of cerebral palsy is related to birth asphyxia?

A The causes of cerebral palsy may be prenatal/perinatal/postnatal (infection/metabolic/genetic/asphyxia/trauma/prematurity/toxin/kernicterus). Contrary to the popular belief, birth asphyxia is the cause of cerebral palsy in only 10–20% of cases.

Q6. What symptoms during infancy can lead to suspicion of cerebral palsy?

A Symptoms suggestive of cerebral palsy in infancy are stiffening during dressing or washing, persistent fisting or cortical thumb, delayed motor milestones such as head lag, inability to sit or stand at an appropriate age, and early feeding difficulties.

Q7. Discuss the management of cerebral palsy.

A Management of cerebral palsy is multidisciplinary consisting of physiotherapy, occupational therapy, speech therapy, early stimulation program, medications, and surgery. Brain is very plastic in the first decade of life so there is good prognosis with early intervention; hence, early diagnosis is also necessary.

Case 26: A 4-Year-Old Male Child with Anasarca

A 4-year-old boy was brought with the complaints of swelling over the body and decreased urine output for the past 20 days. The swelling was first noticed around the eyes and mostly observed when the child woke up in the morning. It gradually progressed to involve trunk and limbs and persisted for the whole day. Along with this, there was decrease in the amount of urine passed. There was however no change in the color of urine observed. There was no history of breathlessness or headache. There was no history of preceding fever, skin infection, photosensitive eruptions, or jaundice in the recent past.

The child was found to be a dull-looking, bloated child. The vitals were normal for his age. Facial puffiness was striking. Generalized edema was present, pitting type. Systemic examination revealed a distended abdomen with transversely stretched umbilicus. No organomegaly was detected on palpation or by dipping method. Shifting dullness was present, suggesting free fluid in the peritoneum. Rest of the systems were found to be normal.

Q1. What are the causes of anasarca in children? What is the likely cause in this child?

A The causes of anasarca or generalized swelling in children include anemia with hypoproteinemia, congestive heart failure, nephrotic syndrome (NS), cirrhosis of liver, and protein-losing enteropathy.

Swelling commencing from the face, most prominent in the morning and associated with decreased urine output, suggests likely renal cause, most probably NS.

Q2. What is the hallmark of nephrotic syndrome? Why is the present case less likely to be nephritic syndrome?

A NS is characterized by heavy proteinuria, hypoalbuminemia, and edema. There may be associated hyperlipidemia. The presence of hypertension and hematuria goes more in favor of nephritic syndrome or significant lesion nephritic syndrome.

Q3. What are the types of NS based on etiology and histopathology?

A NS may be primary (idiopathic) in almost 90% of the cases. In the rest, it may be secondary to amyloidosis, SLE, postinfectious glomerulonephritis (GN), or hepatitis B nephropathy.

Based on histopathological findings, most of the cases do not show significant changes on light microscopy and they are labeled as minimal change disease. Majority of the children with NS fall in this category. The other group has significant lesions seen on routine microscopy.

Q4. Enlist the investigations you will order for this case.

A The investigations include urine examination for protein, RBCs and casts, CBC, RFT (renal function tests), LFT (liver function tests), TSP (total serum proteins) with A:G ratio, and MTX (CXR [chest X-ray], C3 and ASO titer, HBs antigen, and urine culture if indicated).

Q5. How will you treat such a case?

A Treatment includes no added salt diet, diuretics, and steroids, usually prednisolone (for the first attack—6 weeks daily followed by 6 weeks alternate-day treatment).

Q6. What are the long-term complications of treatment to look at?

A Long-term complications include cushingoid facies, hirsutism, hypertension, early fusion of epiphysis causing arrest in growth, subcapsular cataract, and depressed immunity causing flaring up of latent infections, especially tuberculosis.

Q7. When do you go for other drugs? Name alternative drugs used in NS.

A The children with repeated relapses while on long-term therapy are the candidates for alternative drugs (as steroid-sparing agents). Alternate drugs include the following: Cyclophosphamide, levamisole, mycophenolate mofetil, cycloserine, and rituximab.

Q8. What are the likely complications of nephritic syndrome?

A Complications include increased risk of infections, especially cellulitis, pneumonia, peritonitis, and meningitis. There is increased risk of thrombosis of deep veins of legs and renal, pulmonary, and cerebral veins.

Q9. Name some vaccinations you will advise for children with NS.

A Vaccines to be advised include pneumococcal and varicella.

Q10. What are the indications of kidney biopsy in patients with nephritic syndrome?

A The indications of kidney biopsy include young age at presentation (below 1 year), gross or persistent microscopic hematuria, hypertension, deranged renal function, low C3 level, or nonresponse to steroid therapy.

Case 27: A 20-Year-Old Pregnant Female with Headache and Swelling Over Legs

A 20-year-old woman in her first pregnancy at 36 weeks of gestation has come to the emergency room (ER) with complaints of epigastric pain and headache over the past 2 hours with increasing swelling of legs over a week, currently up to midthigh. She has no past medical history of significance. She has been perceiving fetal movements well with no leaking or bleeding per vaginum. Examination in ER revealed a BP of 170/110 mmHg and urine dipstick protein 3+ with brisk knee jerk. There is no pallor or icterus. There is no history of any decreased urine output. Abdominal examination showed a relaxed uterus corresponding to the period of gestation with adequately grown fetus with reactive nonstress test (NST). Ultrasound showed a single fetus in cephalic presentation with amniotic fluid index (AFI) 4.5 with estimated fetal weight of 2.7 kg with placenta in upper segment and no evidence of retroplacental clots. A diagnosis of preeclampsia was made and the patient was admitted for further management.

Q1. How do you classify hypertensive disorders of pregnancy?

A

Gestational hypertension	Systolic BP ≥140 mmHg or diastolic BP ≥90 mmHg, at least two measurements 4 hours apart after 20 weeks in a previously normotensive woman with BP resolving to normal within 12 weeks postpartum
Preeclampsia–eclampsia	BP ≥140/90 mmHg and proteinuria (>300 mg/day or urine protein creatinine ratio ≥0.3 or urine dipstick ≥1+) In the absence of proteinuria, hypertension with any of the following: ■ Thrombocytopenia <1 lakh/mm^3 ■ Renal insufficiency (Sr creatinine >1.1 mg/dL or doubling in the absence of other renal disease) ■ Impaired liver function (elevated transaminases to twice the normal) ■ Pulmonary edema ■ Cerebral or visual symptoms
Eclampsia	Convulsion (generalized tonic clonic seizure [GTCS]) that cannot be attributed to another cause in a woman with preeclampsia
Chronic hypertension	BP ≥140/90 mmHg before pregnancy or before 20 weeks of pregnancy or persisting beyond 12 weeks postpartum
Chronic hypertension with superimposed preeclampsia	Chronic hypertension with additional features for preeclampsia or increasing quantity of preexisting proteinuria

Q2. What are the risk factors for preeclampsia?

A

- Teenage pregnancy
- Elderly >35 years
- Lower socioeconomic status
- Primigravida
- New paternity
- Hypertensive disorder in previous pregnancy
- Family history of hypertension or preeclampsia
- Obesity
- Chronic hypertension
- Renal, vascular, immunological, and connective tissue disorders
- Gestational diabetes mellitus
- Multifetal pregnancy

Q3. What are the complications of preeclampsia?

A

Maternal	**Fetal**
Antepartum hemorrhage	Preterm labor
Eclampsia	Prematurity
Pulmonary edema/ARDS	Oligohydramnios
HELLP syndrome	Fetal growth restriction
Renal and hepatic failure	Low birth weight
Coagulopathy/DIC	Respiratory distress
Intracranial hemorrhage	Perinatal asphyxia
Abruptio placentae	Intrauterine death
Postpartum hemorrhage	Maternal death

Q4. What are the investigations to be performed in this case?

A

- Laboratory
  - Hemoglobin, platelets
  - Urine protein, routine examination and microscopy
  - Renal function and liver function tests
  - Coagulation test (if coagulopathy is suspected)
- Nonstress test (NST)/cardiotocogram (CTG)
- Ultrasound: Number of fetus, presentation, biometry, estimated fetal weight, liquor, Doppler, placental position with presence/absence of retroplacental clots
- Chest X-ray—if suspected pulmonary edema

Q5. What is the plan of management in this case?

A

- Admission
- Controlling blood pressure—antihypertensives (labetalol—first choice)
- Magnesium sulfate prophylaxis
- BP charting, urine input and output charting
- Laboratory investigations
- NST/USG

- Counseling the patient about the risks and complications
- Induction of labor (if pregnancy <34 weeks—delivery can be delayed for 24–48 hours to cover a course of corticosteroids if maternal and fetal condition remains stable)

Q6. What is the mechanism of action of magnesium sulfate and what is Pritchard regimen?

A
- Mechanism
  - It is a potent vasodilator that reduces ischemia caused by cerebral vasospasm.
  - It blocks the entry of calcium into synaptic endings, altering neuromuscular transmission.
  - It antagonizes the excitatory NMDA receptor.
- Pritchard regimen
  - Loading dose: 4 g of 20% $MgSO_4$ intravenous over 3–5 minutes, 10 g of 50% $MgSO_4$ deep intramuscular (5 g in each buttock)
  - Maintenance dose: 5 g of 50% $MgSO_4$ deep intramuscular every 4 hours in alternate buttock

Q7. What is HELLP syndrome?

A
- Hemolysis (elevated LDH and peripheral smear)
- Elevated liver enzymes
- Low platelets

Case 28: A 31-Year-Old Pregnant Female with Shortness of Breath

A 31-year-old woman G3P2L2 at her 32 weeks of gestation has been having increasing frequency of shortness of breath over the past 1 month. She has had similar complaints in the previous two pregnancies but the onset in this pregnancy has been earlier than before. She has no significant past medical or family history. She had two vaginal deliveries 3 years and 1 year 5 months back. Examination showed a pale conjunctiva and palate with cheilitis. There were no nail or hair changes. Vitals: BP, 100/60 mmHg; PR, 104/min; and RR, 18/min. Abdominal examination revealed a relaxed uterus corresponding to 28 weeks of gestation with good fetal heart. On enquiry, the patient gives a history of noncompliance with iron tablets as she was intolerant and had problems such as nausea, constipation, and heartburn. Her CBC revealed the following: Hb, 7.2 g%; TLC, 12,000; DLC, N70 L25 E4 M1; and platelets, 1.67 lakh/mm^3 with normocytic-microcytic hypochromic peripheral smear.

Q1. How do you grade anemia based on severity?

A ICMR grading:
- *Mild*: 10–10.9 g%
- *Moderate*: 7–9.9 g%
- *Severe*: 4–6.9 g%
- *Very severe*: <4 g%

WHO grading:
- *Mild*: 9–10.9 g%
- *Moderate*: 7–8.9 g%
- *Severe*: <7 g%

Q2. What is physiological anemia of pregnancy?

A This is due to increase in plasma volume (40%), which is more than the rise in RBC (30%) resulting in hemodilution. It reaches maximum by 32 weeks. However, Hb does not fall below 11 g% in the first trimester and 10 g% in the second and third trimesters. Peripheral smear would mostly show normocytic normochromic picture.

Q3. What are the investigations to be done in this patient?

A
- CBC with peripheral smear
- Urine: Routine examination and microscopy
- Stool: Ova, cyst
- Urine c/s
- Renal and liver function test
- Iron studies: Sr iron, Sr ferritin, transferrin saturation, TIBC
- Screen for thalassemia in high-risk cases

Q4. What are the complications of severe anemia in pregnancy?

A
- Maternal
  - Infection
  - Cardiac failure
  - Preterm labor
  - Abruption
  - Postpartum hemorrhage
  - Sepsis
  - Subinvolution
  - Lactation failure
  - Wound dehiscence
  - Deep vein thrombosis
- Fetal
  - Abortions
  - Prematurity
  - Low birth weight
  - IUGR
  - Fetal anemia

Q5. How will you manage this patient?

A
- Admission and investigations
- Ascertaining the cause of anemia (iron deficiency in this case)
- Deworming the patient (albendazole 400 mg stat)

- Calculating the iron requirement by Ganzoni formula:

  Total iron dose (mg) = body weight (kg) × (target – actual hemoglobin) (g/L) × 0.24 + iron for iron stores (mg)*
- Parenteral iron therapy (number of doses based on the requirement)
- Monitoring weekly for improvement in hemoglobin levels
- Advice regarding iron-rich foods and high-protein diet
- NST for fetal well-being
- USG and Doppler for IUGR and to monitor serially for growth and liquor

Q6. What are the stages of iron deficiency anemia?

A
- Storage iron depletion
  - Insufficient dietary iron intake
  - Decrease in iron stores to maintain serum ferritin levels
  - No physical symptoms
  - Low serum ferritin levels
- Iron-deficient erythropoiesis
  - Lower hemoglobin and hematocrit levels
  - Possible reduction in hemoglobin levels but not beyond normal values
- Frank iron deficiency anemia
  - Low MCV and hemoglobin levels
  - Increased physical symptoms such as dyspnea, increased fatiguability, lassitude, palpitation

Q7. What are the causes of nonimprovement of anemia?

A
- Noncompliance to treatment
- Malabsorption
- Continuation of blood loss (may be occult)
- Associated vitamin/mineral deficiency
- Infection
- Wrong diagnosis of iron deficiency anemia

Case 29: A 70-Year-Old Male with Bradykinesia

A 70-year-old male presented to the outpatient department with slowness of movements and tremors in right upper limb for 3 months. These complaints were insidious in onset and gradually progressive, in the absence of weakness of any limb or sensory complaints. There was no history of fever, headache, altered behavior/sensorium, trauma, cognitive decline, and postural instability.

The patient was conscious, oriented, and cooperative, with a Mini-Mental State Examination (MMSE) score of 27. He had decreased facial expression with a staring look and infrequent eye blinking. The speech was monotonous and hypophonic. The bulk and nutrition of all limbs was normal. There was rigidity in right upper limb interspersed with tremors. The power and sensations were normal in all limbs. There were no signs of cerebellar or autonomic dysfunction.

Q1. What is the clinical diagnosis of the patient?

A The presence of bradykinesia, rigidity, and rest tremors gradually developing over months to years in an elderly patient suggests Parkinson disease as the probable diagnosis. These three features along with postural instability and gait disturbance are regarded as the "cardinal motor features" of the disease. The other motor features such as micrographia, hypophonia, hypomimia, *serpentine stare*, and dysphagia are attributed to bradykinesia or akinesia.

Q2. What are the components of MMSE?

A MMSE is a questionnaire used for assessing cognitive impairment. It has 30 questions pertaining with orientation, registration, attention and calculation, recall, language, and praxia. Any score greater than or equal to 24 points (out of 30) indicates a normal cognition.

Q3. Describe the characteristic gait in parkinsonism.

A The characteristic gait of Parkinson disease (PD) is festinant gait. The patient has a stooped posture with start hesitation. He has short, shuffling steps with slow turns and reduced arm swing. Later, he may develop freezing of gait and frequent falls.

Q4. Name some nonmotor features of Parkinson disease.

A In addition to motor symptoms, patients with PD have nonmotor symptoms such as anosmia, depression/anxiety, sleep disturbances, autonomic dysfunction, sensory disturbance, and restless leg syndrome. They appear before the onset of motor symptoms and are also known as prodromal premotor symptoms.

Q5. What are atypical parkinsonism and secondary parkinsonism?

A Parkinson disease must be differentiated from atypical and secondary parkinsonism. Atypical parkinsonism is also a neurodegenerative disorder but with more widespread involvement. It includes multiple system atrophy, progressive supranuclear palsy, corticobasal degeneration, and frontotemporal dementia. These

*Iron stores: 15 mg/kg if body weight <35 kg; 500 mg if body weight >35 kg.

are characterized by absence of rest tremor, no motor asymmetry, early gait impairment and falls, rapid clinical course, and poor response to levodopa.

Secondary parkinsonism is attributed to drugs, toxins (Cu, Mn), tumor, infections, and stroke.

Q6. Which drugs and toxins have been implicated in the development of parkinsonism?

A Among the drugs, neuroleptics are the most common cause of parkinsonism, along with calcium channel blockers, lithium, and amiodarone.

Q7. How will you manage the patient?

A The most effective treatment of PD is levodopa (combined with peripheral decarboxylase inhibitor) and all patients eventually need it. The other drugs are dopamine agonist (ergot—bromocriptine, pergolide; nonergot—pramipexole, ropinirole), MAO-B inhibitor (selegiline, rasagiline), COMT inhibitor (entacapone, tolcapone), and amantadine.

Q8. What are the complications of chronic levodopa therapy?

A About 10% of patients per year on levodopa therapy develop motor complications—dyskinesia (choreiform movements, dystonia) and motor fluctuations (on–off phenomenon).

Case 30: A 65-Year-Old Female with Knee Pain

A 65-year-old woman presents with a 2-year history of right knee pain. The pain is exacerbated by activity and improves with rest. She denies constitutional complaints, such as fever, weight loss, and fatigue. The patient is moderately obese with a body mass index (BMI) of 32 kg/m^2. Her right knee is not warm or swollen, but there is crepitus and medial joint line tenderness. Range of motion of the right knee is from 5° to 90°. Plain films of the right knee demonstrate narrowing of the medial joint space (Fig. C-6), subchondral sclerosis, and osteophyte formation. The patient has failed 6 months of nonoperative therapy, including attempts at weight loss and activity modification, physical therapy, bracing, and pain medication. Her right knee pain has become progressively more severe and her range of motion has worsened (5–80°).

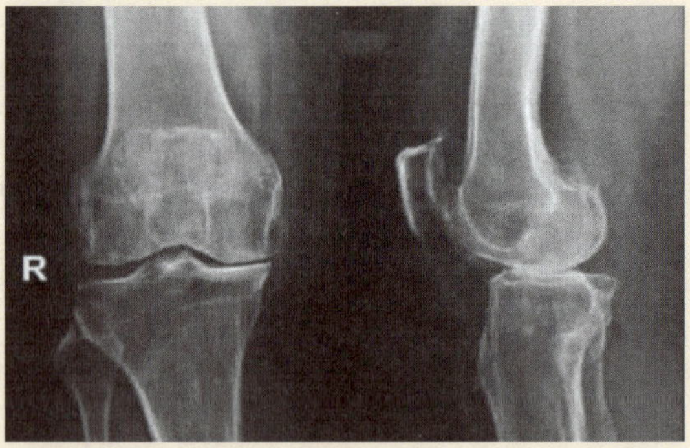

FIGURE C-6. X-rays of right knee.

Her laboratory values are as follows:

- Hb: 11.2 g/dL
- TLC: 6000 cells/mm^3
- Blood urea: 34 mg/dL
- Serum creatinine: 0.9 mg/dL
- Serum uric acid: 5.3 mg/dL

Q1. What is the differential diagnosis?

A The possible differential diagnosis can be as follows:
- Osteoarthritis
- Rheumatoid arthritis
- Crystalline arthropathies such as gout or pseudogout
- Seronegative spondyloarthropathies such as ankylosing spondylitis, psoriatic arthritis
- Septic arthritis

Q2. What is the likely diagnosis?

A Given the patient's age and clinical presentation, osteoarthritis is the most likely diagnosis. Osteoarthritis is the most common form of joint disease. It is characterized by loss of articular cartilage, which results in damage to the underlying bone. The process results in pain, stiffness, and loss of joint mobility. The pain is typically worse with use of the joint and improves with rest. Loss of the smooth articulating surface accounts for the finding of crepitus when the joint is moved. Joints affected in osteoarthritis are the hips, knees, and PIP and DIP joints. The most common joint involvement in osteoarthritis is knee joint.

Radiographs of the affected joint typically show joint space narrowing, subchondral sclerosis, osteophyte formation, and subchondral cysts. The patient's symptoms, physical exam findings, and radiographs are most consistent with osteoarthritis.

Q3. What is the pathogenesis of osteoarthritis?

A Osteoarthritis is characterized by degeneration of articular cartilage and often is associated with overuse or trauma to the joint. The pathogenesis in osteoarthritis is failure of chondrocytes to repair damaged articular cartilage. When the articular cartilage is not properly maintained, the joint space narrows, and the bones in the diarthrodial knee joint may come in direct contact with one another, which results in wear and tear and leads to bony proliferation, with the formation of subchondral sclerosis and osteophytes. Subchondral cysts arise secondary to microfractures and may contain amorphous gelatinous material.

Q4. What changes occur in the cartilage of osteoarthritic joints?

A Osteoarthritic cartilage is characterized by the following:

- Increased water content
- Alterations in proteoglycans
- An increase in the chondroitin/keratin sulfate ratio
- Collagen abnormalities

Q5. What are the risk factors associated with developing osteoarthritis?

A

- Obesity, joint trauma, and muscle weakness increase the mechanical forces to which the articular cartilage is subjected.
- Gender, hormones, metabolic disorders, and genetics also play a role.
- Elderly populations are affected by this disease more frequently and more severely than younger populations.
- Obesity is the strongest modifiable risk factor for osteoarthritis.

Note: Osteoarthritis can be classified as primary (idiopathic disease caused by intrinsic defect, the most common form) or secondary, with an underlying cause (e.g., trauma, infection, congenital deformity).

Q6. What are the initial treatment options for osteoarthritis of the knee?

A

- Supportive measures: Weight loss and activity modification; bracing, including compartmental unloader bracing, and/or ambulatory assistive devices
- Physiotherapy
  - Wax bath
  - Active quadriceps strengthening exercises
  - Active ankle pump exercises
- Medical management
  - Oral pain medications (such as NSAIDs)
  - Corticosteroid injections
  - Viscosupplementation
  - Topical analgesics
  - May try supplements such as glucosamine and chondroitin sulfate
- Surgical management
  - Proximal fibular osteotomy in case of grades 1 and 2
  - High tibial osteotomy (HTO) for grades 2 and 3
  - Unicompartmental knee replacement
  - Total knee replacement for grade 4 and varus knees
- Newer biological treatment: Platelet-rich plasma therapy, adipocyte-rich stromal cell injections, autologous chondrocyte implantation

Q7. What is the next appropriate treatment option?

A The most common and effective treatment for end-stage degenerative joint disease of the knee is total knee arthroplasty (TKA). Other surgical treatment options include arthroscopic debridement, HTO for treatment of varus deformity, distal femoral osteotomy for treatment of valgus deformity, unicompartmental knee arthroplasty, and patellofemoral arthroplasty.

Glossary

abnormal uterine bleeding bleeding between menses; includes infrequent, excessive, prolonged, or postmenopausal bleeding

acanthosis nigricans deeply pigmented velvety axillary skin

accessory muscle use using muscles that assist, but do not play a primary role, in tidal breathing; sign of respiratory distress

acoustic blink reflex blinking of the eyes in response to a sudden sharp sound used as a crude test of hearing among infants

actinic purpura purple patches or macules that come from blood that has leaked through poorly supported capillaries and spread within the dermis; associated with normal aging

active range of motion degree of movement around a single joint that a patient can perform without assistance

activities of daily living (ADLs) functions that are necessary, but not sufficient, for maintaining an independent living status; consist of six basic self care abilities: bathing, dressing, toileting, transferring, continence, and feeding

acute diarrhea painless loose or watery stools that last less than 14 days' duration

acute pain normal, predicted physiologic response to an adverse chemical, thermal, or mechanical stimulus that typically lasts less than 3 to 6 months and is commonly associated with surgery, trauma, and acute illness

adenomyosis endometrial glands and stroma that occur within the myometrium

affect fluctuating pattern of observable behaviors that expresses subjective feelings or emotions through tone of voice, facial expression, and demeanor; the external representation of emotional state

afferent pupillary defect medical sign observed during the swinging flashlight test in which the affected pupil constricts less and therefore appears to dilate when the bright light stimulus moves from the unaffected to the affected eye; also known as *Marcus Gunn pupil*

Allen test physical examination maneuver performed to assess the integrity of the circulation of the palmar arterial arches done by compressing the ulnar and radial arteries simultaneously for at least 5 seconds, followed by the sequential release of compression of each artery while observing the hand for arterial filling

ambulatory blood pressure monitoring (ABPM) blood pressure monitoring that provides 24-hour average blood pressures and averages of daytime (awake), nighttime (asleep), systolic, and diastolic blood pressures; considered to be the reference standard

amenorrhea absence or cessation of menstrual bleeding for 3 months or more in the setting or normal menstrual cycles or for 6 months or more in the setting of irregular menstrual cycles

anal fissure tear in the skin distal to the dentate line typically caused by increased sphincter tone

anal fistula complication of anorectal abscesses that results in an abnormal connection between internal mucosal and external skin

anal verge junction between the outside of the anus with skin with hair and hairless skin

aneroid sphygmomanometer blood pressure measuring device that uses mechanical parts to transmit the pressure in the cuff to a dial; aneroid means "without fluid"

anisocoria difference of >0.4 mm in the diameter of one pupil in comparison to the other; seen in healthy individuals but could also be an important indication of CN III palsy or Horner syndrome

anisocoria unequal pupil size, which may be physiologic (seen in 20% of population) or pathologic

anterior fontanelle area where the major sutures intersect in the anterior portion of the skull, which measures 4 to 6 cm in diameter at birth; in ~80% of infants, closes by age 18 months and in ~90% by 22 months

anterior superficial cervical lymph node group located anterior and superficial to the sternocleidomastoid

anxiety abnormality of thought content manifesting as apprehensive anticipation of future danger or misfortune accompanied by feelings of worry, distress, and/or somatic symptoms of tension

apex of the prostate distalmost portion of the prostate felt during a rectal examination

Apgar score assessment of the newborn immediately after birth; its five components classify the newborn's neurologic recovery from the stress of birth and immediate cardiopulmonary adaptation to extrauterine life, and scoring is based on a 3-point scale (0, 1, or 2) for each component

aphasia disorder in speech fluency; see also *Broca aphasia* and *Wernicke aphasia*

aphthous ulcer painful, shallow whitish gray oval ulceration surrounded by a halo of reddened mucosa in the oral cavity also known as "canker sore"

apocrine sweat glands found chiefly in the axillary and genital regions and usually open into hair follicles. Bacterial decomposition of apocrine sweat is responsible for adult body odor

appropriate for gestational age newborn classification based on the Ballard Score that places the newborn at 10th to 90th percentile for gestational age and birth weight on the intrauterine growth curve

arthralgia joint pain without evidence of arthritis or inflammation

asterixis intermittent, brief, irregular loss of muscle tone to sustain posture when attempting to hold the arms outstretched with the wrists and fingers held in extension; commonly seen with hepatic encephalopathy

ataxia loss of control of coordinated voluntary movements

atrophy loss of muscle bulk

attention ability to focus or concentrate over time on a particular stimulus or activity

audioscope lightweight, handheld instrument that combines a pure-tone screening audiometer and otoscope into a single unit used for screening hearing impairment

Barlow maneuver performed on newborn and infant hips to detect signs of dislocation or hip instability; tests the ability to sublux or dislocate an intact but unstable hip

barrel chest increased anterior–posterior diameter of the chest wall resembling the shape of a barrel, most often associated with lung hyperinflation due to emphysema

base of the prostate most proximal portion of the prostate felt during a rectal examination; prostatic tissue located near the seminal vesicles

blanchable quickly regains redness when pressure is lifted from skin (2 to 3 seconds)

blocking disturbance in thought process wherein a patient has sudden interruptions of speech in mid-sentence or before the idea is completed; may be striking in schizophrenia

body mass index (BMI) measure of body fat based on weight in relation to height and applies to most adult men and women

bradykinesia slowness of movement

Broca aphasia expressive aphasia with preserved comprehension but slow, nonfluent speech

bronchial breath sound soft, nonmusical sound heard on both phases of the respiratory cycle that mimics tracheal sound; indicates airway patency surrounded by consolidated lung tissue (e.g., pneumonia) or fibrosis

bronchophony sign in which spoken words are louder over an area of consolidated lung

bruit abnormal high-pitched sound resulting from turbulent blood flow, usually heard during systole during the auscultation of an artery; commonly heard in patients with a dialysis arteriovenous fistula or an atherosclerotic plaque resulting in severe arterial narrowing

bulla circumscribed elevation of the epidermis containing clear fluid >1 cm in diameter

bullous myringitis sequela of otitis media that presents with painful hemorrhagic vesicles on the tympanic membrane and may involve the ear canal.

bursitis inflammation of a bursa, often with pain, erythema, and swelling

cannon A waves regular or irregular rhythmic elevations in the jugular venous pressure resulting from atrial contraction against a closed tricuspid valve or noncompliant right ventricle; usually seen in complete heart block or tricuspid stenosis

caput succedaneum swelling over the occipitoparietal region of a newborn from capillary distention and extravasation of blood and fluid resulting from the vacuum effect of rupture of the amniotic sac; swelling typically crosses suture lines and resolves in 1 to 2 days

cataract opacification of the lens

cervical dilation opening of the internal os of the cervix, assessed with an internal digital examination and reported in centimeters; progressive cervical dilation is suggestive of labor

cervical effacement thinning of the uterine cervix during labor, with 0% effacement being least effaced to 100% effacement, at which point the cervix is as thin as the adjacent lower uterine segment

Chadwick sign bluish discoloration of the cervix and vagina due to increased vascular congestion in early pregnancy

chemosis swelling of the conjunctiva

chronic diarrhea painless loose or watery stools that last more than 30 days' duration

chronic pain pain not associated with cancer or other medical conditions that persists for more than 3 to 6 months; pain lasting more than 1 month beyond the course of an acute illness or injury; or pain recurring at intervals of months or years

circumlocution abnormality in fluency of speech in which phrases or sentences describing a word are substituted in place of the word

circumstantiality disturbance in thought process wherein a patient's speech has unnecessary detail, indirection, and delay in reaching the point; occurs in people with obsessions

clanging disturbance in thought process wherein a patient's speech has choice of words based on sound, rather than meaning, as in rhyming and punning; occurs in schizophrenia and manic episodes

clonus rhythmic, beating movement of a joint in alternating directions that may be provoked by testing the muscle stretch reflexes; seen most commonly at the ankle, where there is alternative dorsiflexion and plantarflexion; indicates abnormal hyperreflexia

cognition mental processes involved in gaining knowledge and comprehension, which include orientation, attention, memory, and higher cognitive functions (information and vocabulary, calculations, abstract thinking, and constructional ability)

compulsions abnormality of thought content manifesting with repetitive behaviors that the person feels driven to perform in response to an obsession, aimed at preventing or reducing anxiety or a dreaded event or situation; these behaviors are excessive and unrealistically connected to the provoking stimulus

condyloma manifestation of human papillomavirus infection; anal warts

confabulation disturbance in thought process wherein a patient fabricates facts or events in response to questions to fill in the gaps from impaired memory; seen in Korsakoff syndrome from alcoholism

configuration shape of single lesions and the arrangement of groups of lesions

constipation inability to pass bowel movements with normal passage of flatus; should be present for the last 3 months with symptom onset at least 6 months prior to diagnosis and meet at least two of the following conditions: <3 bowel movements per week; ≥25% or more defecations with either straining or sensation of incomplete evacuation; lumpy or hard stools; or manual facilitation

constitutional symptoms patient concerns that accompany many disease processes whose underlying etiologies are often not confined to a specific organ system but rather broadly affecting a patient's physical state with regard to vitality, health, and strength; may include fatigue, weakness, fever, chills, night sweats, weight loss or weight gain, and pain

Cooper ligaments suspensory ligaments of the breast

corneal ulcer often painful, infection of the cornea with epithelial defect

crackles discontinuous, nonmusical, short, explosive lung sounds that arise from small distal airways popping open during inspiration; fine crackles are softer, higher pitched, and more frequent per breath than coarse crackles

crepitus audible or palpable crunching during movement of tendons or ligaments over bone or areas of cartilage loss

cryptorchidism testis is atrophied and lies outside the scrotum in the inguinal canal, abdomen, or near the pubic tubercle; it may also be congenitally absent; there is no palpable testis or epididymis in the unfilled scrotum

cuticle part of the fingernail that extends from the nail fold and functions as a seal that protects the space between the fold and the plate from external moisture

cyanosis bluish discoloration of the skin that can indicate decreased oxygen in the blood or decreased blood flow in response to a cold environment

deep cervical chain lymph node group located deep in the sternocleidomastoid and often inaccessible to examination

delirium multifactorial syndrome, characterized by an acute confusional state marked by sudden onset; fluctuating course; inattention; and, at times, changing levels of consciousness

delusion abnormality of thought content wherein the patient has fixed, false belief that does not change in the face of conflicting evidence

dentate line divides the upper two-thirds of the anal canal with the distal third, between the transition zone of the anoderm and columnar mucosal tissue

depersonalization abnormality of thought content wherein the patient's sense of self or identity is different, changed, unreal, lost, or detached from the mind or body

derailment (loosening of associations) disturbance in thought process wherein a patient shifts topics in a loosely connected or unrelated way without awareness of doing so; seen in schizophrenia, manic episodes, and other psychotic disorders

derealization abnormality of thought content wherein the patient's sense of self or identity is different, changed, unreal, or remote

dermis dense layer of interconnecting collagen and elastic fibers containing epidermal appendages, hair follicles, and most of the terminals of the cutaneous nerves; inferiorly, merges with subcutaneous adipose tissue

dermoscope handheld device that provides cross-polarized or unpolarized light to visualize patterns of pigmentation or vascular structures

dextrocardia abnormal condition in which the apex of the heart is located in the right hemithorax, due to abnormal folding of the heart tube during embryologic development; may be associated with the anatomic reversal of the atria and the abdominal viscera (dextrocardia with situs inversus)

digital sphygmomanometer blood pressure measuring device that uses oscillometric techniques to measure blood pressure

diplopia double vision

direct inguinal hernia less common than indirect hernia, usually seen in older men, and originating from above the inguinal ligament near the external inguinal ring; hernia contents are rarely palpated in the scrotum, and it does not course down the inguinal canal

distension physical examination finding that is the result of increased air trapped in the lumen of the bowel from an ileus or mechanical obstruction; the abdomen will feel tight like a balloon filled with air

distribution how skin lesions are scattered or spread out

dynamic stabilizers components of a joint that are capable of movement (e.g., muscles)

dysarthria impaired articulation of speech

dysdiadochokinesia clumsy, disorganized, irregular performance of rapid alternative movements that is seen with cerebellar disease

dysmenorrhea pain with menses, often with bearing down, aching, or cramping sensation in the lower abdomen or pelvis

dysmetria manifestation of ataxia in which a movement over- or undershoots the intended target; most commonly used to describe inaccuracy on finger-to-nose testing but can refer to coordinated movement of any body part, even eye movements

dysphagia difficulty swallowing

dysphonia abnormality in word articulation resulting in impaired quality, tone, or pitch of the voice

ecchymoses nonblanchable, larger areas of purpura

eccrine sweat gland widely distributed epidermal appendage that opens directly onto the skin surface; helps control body temperature by sweat production

echolalia disturbance in thought process wherein a patient repeats the words and phrases of others; occurs in manic episodes and schizophrenia

ectopic pregnancy pregnancy located outside of the uterus

ectropion age-associated change that causes sagging and outward turning of the lower eyelid and eyelashes that can lead to excessive tearing, crusting of the eyelid, mucus discharge, and eye irritation

edema clinically relevant interstitial fluid that develops as a result of increased venous pressure, decreased capillary osmotic pressure, or decreased lymphatic drainage

effusion pathologic joint fluid that may be visible or palpable

egophony sign in which spoken "ee" is heard as "ay" when auscultating an area of consolidation (e.g., pneumonia)

endometrial polyp sessile or pedunculated projection from the surface of the endometrium as a result of localized hyperplastic overgrowths of endometrial glands and stroma around a vascular core

endometriosis endometrial glands and stroma that occur outside the uterus

entropion age-associated change in the eyelids that causes the eyelashes in the lower lids to be directed toward the eye, which, in turn, causes them to irritate the cornea and conjunctiva

epidermis most superficial layer of the skin composed of thin avascular keratinized epithelium

episcleritis painful inflammation of the sclera, which does not blanch with phenylephrine

erectile dysfunction (ED) inability to maintain an erection

erosion loss of epidermal or mucosal epithelium

erythema redness of the skin or mucous membranes, caused by *hyperemia* (increased blood flow) in superficial capillaries

erythroplakia area of erythema or redness of the mucus membrane; lesions should be biopsied as they are associated with an increased risk of malignancy

eschar dead tissue appearing black or brown dry, thick, and leathery

exophthalmos axial bulging of the eye anteriorly out of the orbit

exostosis benign bony overgrowth of the osseous external auditory canal, often circumferential, secondary to exposure to cold wind or water; also known as "surfer's ear"

extinction condition in which sensory stimuli (visual, tactile, or otherwise) can be correctly detected on one side of the body when it is presented individually, but not when it is presented simultaneously with a similar stimulus on the other side of the body

failure to thrive defined as (a) growth <5th percentile for age; (b) drop >two quartiles in 6 months; or (c) weight for length <5th percentile

fasciculations small irregular twitching movements affecting small groups of muscle fibers that cause movement of the overlying skin; in contrast to myoclonus, they do not cause movement across the joint; sign of lower motor neuron pathology

femoral hernia least common type of hernia, originating below the inguinal ligament and more lateral than an inguinal hernia; no hernia contents can be palpated in the scrotum, and it can be difficult to differentiate from lymph nodes

fetal heart tones audible sounds made by the fetal heart, assessed with bedside Doppler, and reported as a fetal heart rate (FHR); normal FHR is between 110 and 160 beats per minute

fibroid (leiomyoma, myoma) benign tumors arising from smooth muscle cells of the myometrium

flight of ideas disturbance in thought process wherein a patient has a continuous flow of accelerated speech with abrupt changes from one topic to the next based on poorly connected but understandable associations, plays on words, or distracting stimuli; most frequently noted in manic episodes

food fear state in which patients avoid food intake, usually in the setting of chronic mesenteric ischemia, because eating provokes abdominal pain as the arterial supply to the intestines is not enough to adequately provide oxygenation during food ingestion

frailty multifactorial geriatric syndrome characterized by an age-related lack of adaptive physiologic capacity occurring even in the absence of identifiable illness; typically signifies loss of muscle mass, decreased energy and exercise intolerance, and decreased physiologic reserve, with increasing vulnerability to physiologic stressors

fundal height measured distance from the symphysis pubis to the top of the uterine fundus, in centimeters; after 20 weeks, the fundal height should approximate the gestational age in weeks

galactorrhea milky nipple discharge unrelated to breastfeeding

gangrene advanced stage of peripheral arterial disease whereby arterial occlusion provokes ulceration and tissue necrosis of the extremity perfused by the compromised artery

gel phenomenon brief periods of daytime stiffness following inactivity that usually last from 30 to 60 minutes then get worse again with movement

general survey series of observations regarding the patient's overall general health and obvious physical characteristics based on certain parameters, such as appearance, consciousness, level of distress or discomfort, dress, personal hygiene, facial expression, odors, posture, gait, and motor activity

genu valgum knock-kneed

genu varum bowed legs

geographic tongue benign but chronic condition in which a portion of the tongue has a rough, unusual appearance (looking like a map) that can vary over time and is thought to be a benign inflammatory process

geriatric syndrome multifactorial condition that involves the interaction between identifiable situation-specific stressors and underlying age-related risk factors, resulting in damage across multiple organ systems

gingivitis inflammation of the gingiva that presents with erythema and edema of the gums with swollen interdental papillae

goiter enlargement of the thyroid gland to twice its normal size

guarding involuntary flexion of muscles at the site of inflammation upon palpation, sign of intra-abdominal infection

gynecomastia glandular proliferation of the male breast

hallucination abnormality of perception wherein the patient perceives disturbances that seem real but lack actual external stimuli

heart murmur heart sound heard during systole or diastole that represents turbulent blood flow, usually due to blood rapidly moving from a high pressure to a lower pressure chamber; common examples include: (1) pulmonary flow murmurs during high cardiac output states such as pregnancy, adolescence, anemia, or thyrotoxicosis; (2) stenotic aortic valve or pulmonic valve (systolic murmurs); (3) regurgitant mitral or tricuspid valve (systolic murmurs); (4) stenotic mitral or tricuspid valves (diastolic murmurs); or (5) regurgitant aortic or pulmonic valves (diastolic murmurs); (6) congenital murmurs, such as that of a ventricular septal defect (harsh, holosystolic murmur) or a patent ductus arteriosus (continuous murmur)

heave abnormally strong precordial impulse lasting the entire duration (or slightly less) of systole, discovered during palpation of the precordium; if found in the left parasternal area, it usually represents right ventricular hypertrophy or pulmonary hypertension, and if found in the midclavicular to anteroaxillary area, it usually represents a left ventricular aneurysm

HEEADSSS assessment valuable tool for assessing the physical, emotional, and social well-being of adolescents analogous to the Review of Systems; acronym stands for **H**ome environment, **E**ducation and employment, **E**ating, peer-related **A**ctivities, **D**rugs, **S**exuality, **S**uicide/depression, and **S**afety from injury and violence

hemiparesis weakness of one side of the body (*hemiplegia* refers to paralysis of one side of the body; *paraplegia* means paralysis of the legs; *quadriplegia* means paralysis of all four limbs)

hemorrhoid vascular cushions that help maintain resting anal pressure and tone

hernia abnormal outpouching of bowel, fat, or organs through the wall of a cavity where they normally reside; seen in the ventral, inguinal, and femoral areas

home blood pressure monitoring (HBPM) regular self-monitoring measurements of blood pressure by a patient outside the clinic setting

hydrocele nontender, fluid-filled mass within the tunica vaginalis that transilluminates, and the examining fingers can palpate above the mass within the scrotum

hyperopia farsightedness

hyperpyrexia extreme elevation in temperature, >41.1°C (106°F)

hypertrophic obstructive cardiomyopathy common genetic cardiomyopathy associated with a harsh systolic murmur created by turbulent blood flow through the left ventricular (LV) outflow tract during systole; characteristic murmur is made louder with LV volume depletion (standing after squatting or after ingesting a large fatty meal) and is made softer with increased LV volume or with increased afterload (isometric handgrip)

hyphema pooling of blood in the anterior chamber of the eye

hypospadias congenital displacement of the urethral meatus to the inferior surface of the penis; meatus may be subcoronal, midshaft, or at the junction of the penis and scrotum (penoscrotal)

hypothermia abnormally low temperature, <35°C (95°F) rectally

illusion abnormality of perception wherein the patient misinterprets external stimuli

incoherence disturbance in thought process wherein a patient's speech is incomprehensible and illogical, with lack of meaningful connections, abrupt changes in topic, or disordered grammar or word use; seen in severe psychotic disturbances (usually schizophrenia)

indirect inguinal hernia most common type of hernia, originating from above the inguinal ligament at the internal inguinal ring; hernia contents can be palpated coming down the inguinal canal, touching the fingertip

insight awareness that symptoms or disturbed behaviors are normal or abnormal

instrumental activities of daily living (IADLs) complex functions necessary to maintain independent living, including using the telephone, shopping, preparing food, housekeeping, laundry, transportation, taking medicine, and managing money

jaundice yellowing of the skin resulting from increased bilirubin

joint symmetry observation of whether a joint change is present on both sides of the body or just one

judgment process of comparing and evaluating alternatives when deciding on a course of action; reflects values that may or may not be based on reality and social conventions or norms

Korotkoff sounds auscultatory sounds heard through a stethoscope during measurement of blood pressure; phase I is the first appearance of faint, repetitive, clear tapping sounds that gradually increase in intensity for at least two consecutive beats in the systolic blood pressure, and phase V is the point at which all sounds finally disappear completely, which corresponds to the diastolic pressure

lagophthalmos inability to close the eyes completely leading to ocular exposure

large for gestational age newborn classification based on the Ballard Score that places the newborn at >90th percentile for its gestational age and birth weight on the intrauterine growth curve

Leopold maneuvers four maneuvers used to palpate the fetus through the maternal abdomen to identify fetal position and determine a clinical estimate of the fetal weight

lesion any single area of altered skin

leukoplakia painless white patch on a mucous membrane that does not easily scrape off, lesions should be biopsied as they are associated with an increased risk of malignancy

leukorrhea of pregnancy asymptomatic milky white discharge due to increased cervical and vaginal secretions from hyperestrogenemia and vascular congestion

ligamentous laxity excess mobility of joint ligaments

linea nigra hyperpigmentation of the linea alba, located along the midline of the maternal abdomen

lymphadenopathy abnormal enlargement of lymph nodes from bacterial infection, viral infection, malignancy, or lymphoma

lymphedema nonpitting edema caused by lymphatic obstruction that usually occurs after radiation therapy, lymph node dissection, or rare parasitic infections

macule circumscribed flat area of change in color of the skin <1 cm in diameter

major neurocognitive disorder condition characterized by cognitive impairment as the most prominent and defining feature with acquired deficits, which represent a decline from previous functioning

masked hypertension office blood pressure <140/90 mm Hg, but an elevated daytime blood pressure of >135/85 mm Hg on home or ambulatory testing

mastodynia (or mastalgia) pain of the breast

McBurney sign tenderness at deep palpation at McBurney point (1/3 the distance between the anterior superior iliac spine and the umbilicus), associated with appendicitis

median sulcus groove on the surface of the prostate palpable during a rectal examination that separates the left and right prostatic lobes

melanoma least common skin cancer but the most lethal due to its high rate of metastasis and high mortality at advanced stages

melasma hyperpigmentation of the face seen in approximately half of pregnant women, typically distributed along the cheeks, and sometimes including the forehead, chin, and bridge of the nose; colloquially called the "mask of pregnancy"; also known as *chloasma*

menarche age at onset of menses

menometrorrhagia heavy menstrual bleeding with intermenstrual bleeding

menopause absence of menses for 12 consecutive months, usually occurring between ages 48 and 55 years

menorrhagia heavy or prolonged menstrual bleeding

menstrual cycle most ovulatory menstrual cycles last 21 to 35 days with 7 or fewer of bleeding

metrorrhagia intermenstrual bleeding

miosis small, constricted pupillary diameter

monoarticular one joint affected

Montgomery glands sebaceous glands of the areola

mood pervasive and sustained emotion that colors the person's perception of the world; the internal experience of emotional state

Murphy sign associated with acute cholecystitis; deep palpation of the right upper quadrant resulting in inspiratory halt upon deep inspiration; result of the diaphragm pushing the gallbladder down toward the point of deep palpation, causing tenderness

myalgias generalized muscle "aches and pains"

mydriasis large, dilated pupillary diameter

myoclonus intermittent, brief, irregular jerking movements that may be generalized or affect a single muscle or body segment

myopia nearsightedness

neologism disturbance in thought process wherein a patient has invented or distorted words or words with new and highly idiosyncratic meanings; observed in schizophrenia, psychotic disorders, and aphasia

neuropathic pain unpleasant sensory and emotional experience as a direct consequence of a lesion or disease affecting the somatosensory system; often described as electric shock-like, stabbing, burning, or "pins and needles"

nociceptive (somatic) pain unpleasant sensory and emotional experience linked to tissue damage to the skin, musculoskeletal system, or viscera (visceral pain), but the sensory nervous system is intact; usually described as dull, pressing, pulling, throbbing, boring, spasmodic, colicky

nodule solid elevation of the skin >1 cm in diameter that usually extends into the deeper skin layers

nuchal rigidity increased resistance to passive flexion of the head and neck seen in patients with meningeal inflammation from meningitis or subarachnoid hemorrhage

nystagmus involuntary, rapidly repetitive eye movements that may be horizontal, vertical, or rotary; may be physiologic or associated with either a peripheral or central cause of vertigo

obsessions abnormality of thought content manifesting as recurrent, persistent thoughts, images, or urges experienced as intrusive or unwanted that the person tries to ignore, suppress, or neutralize with other thoughts or actions

obstipation inability to pass flatus or bowel movement

occipital lymph node group located at the base of the skull posteriorly

odynophagia pain with swallowing

oligoarticular or pauciarticular involvement of two to four joints

oligomenorrhea cycle length >35 days or fewer than nine cycles per year

optic blink reflex blinking in response to bright light used to indirectly assess vision in newborns

oral candidiasis thick white coating in the mouth from *Candida* infection; lesions can be scrapped off, in contrast to leukoplakia; also known as "thrush"

orientation awareness of personal identity, place, and time, which requires both memory and attention

orthopnea shortness of breath while lying flat that most commonly develops in patients with left ventricular failure and results from the redistribution of pulmonary edema to the most dependent portion of the lung; most easily assessed by querying how many pillows a patient uses to sleep

orthostatic hypotension sustained reduction in systolic blood pressure of at least 20 mm Hg or in diastolic blood pressure of at least 10 mm Hg within 3 minutes of standing

Ortolani test performed on newborn and infant hips to detect signs of dislocation or hip instability; detects the presence of a posteriorly dislocated hip

otitis externa inflammation or infection of the external auditory canal that may involve the auricle. Exam reveals tragal tenderness and pain with movement of the pinna. The ear canal appears edematous, tender, and often with erythema and associated discharge or debris

otitis media inflammation of the middle ear, with evidence of an erythematous and bulging tympanic membrane, and possibly a purulent effusion visualized behind the tympanic membrane

ovarian torsion complete or partial rotation of the ovary on its ligamentous supports, resulting in impedance of its blood supply, often presenting with pain

Paget disease of the breast rare type of breast cancer that involves the skin of the nipple and areola

pain unpleasant sensory and emotional experience associated with tissue damage

palliative care encompasses the alleviation of pain and suffering and the promotion of optimal quality of life across all phases of treatment, including curative interventions and rehabilitation

pallor abnormal coloration of an extremity seen in the setting of decreased blood flow

palpitations abnormal sensation of feeling one's own heart beat; may be rapid, slow, regular, or irregular and is a common symptom of many arrhythmias as well as anxiety associated with those arrhythmias

papilledema optic nerve head swelling, which may represent elevated intracranial pressure

papule small solid elevation of the skin <1 cm in diameter

paraphasia abnormality in fluency of speech resulting in words being malformed, wrong, or invented

paraphimosis tight prepuce that, once retracted, cannot be returned; edema ensues

paroxysmal nocturnal dyspnea sudden onset of shortness of breath occurring at night when patients with heart failure become recumbent that results when extracellular fluid (usually lower extremity edema) is resorbed into the vasculature, raising intracardiac pressure and causing the sudden onset of pulmonary edema

passive range of motion degree of movement around a single joint that the examiner can achieve without the assistance of the patient

patch circumscribed flat area of change in color of the skin >1 cm in diameter

peau d'orange dimpled texture that resembles an orange peel

pelvic inflammatory disease (PID) infection involving the uterus, fallopian tubes, and ovaries

Pemberton sign flushing during neck hyperextension and arm elevation from compression of the thoracic inlet from the thyroid gland itself or from clavicular movement

perceptions sensory awareness of objects in the environment and their interrelationships (external stimuli)

periodic respiration alternating pattern of periods rapid and slow breathing in newborns, especially those born prematurely; also known as *periodic breathing*

peritonitis sign of intra-abdominal sepsis, abdominal will be rigid and board-like upon palpation with marked diffuse tenderness with palpation; patients will also report significant pain with deep breathing and coughing as the result of irritation of the inflamed peritoneal cavity

perseveration disturbance in thought process wherein a patient has persistent repetition of words or ideas; occurs in schizophrenia and other psychotic disorders

persistent diarrhea painless loose or watery stools that last between 14 and 30 days' duration

petechiae nonblanchable, punctate foci of hemorrhage

phimosis tight prepuce that cannot be retracted over the glans

phobia abnormality of thought content manifesting as persistent, irrational fear accompanied by rigid avoidance of provoking stimulus

pilosebaceous gland (oil gland) epidermal appendage that produces a fatty substance secreted onto the skin surface through the hair follicles; present on all skin surfaces except the palms and soles

plaque large flatter elevation of the skin, sometimes formed by papules coalescing

pleural friction rub discontinuous, nonmusical, low-frequency, grating sound heard during inspiration and expiration (biphasic) often best heard in the axilla and bases of the lungs; arises from inflammation and roughening of the visceral pleura as it slides against the parietal pleura (e.g., pleuritis, malignancy)

poikilothermia decrease in temperature of one extremity as compared symmetrically with the other extremity that signifies arterial obstruction; when occurring acutely, it suggests an occlusive arterial thrombus

point of maximal impulse strongest impulse noticed during palpation of the precordium, which is usually the left ventricular apical impulse; however, in the setting of pulmonary hypertension or right ventricular hypertrophy, the point of maximal impulse may be located over the right ventricle in the left parasternal area

polyarticular involvement of more than four joints

polypharmacy use of a large number of medications usually >5; use of potentially inappropriate medications; medication underuse and medication duplication

posterior auricular lymph node group located behind the ear and superficial to the mastoid process

posterior cervical lymph node group located along the anterior edge of the trapezius

posterior fontanelle area where the major sutures intersect in the posterior portion of the skull measuring 1 to 2 cm at birth and usually closes by 2 months

postmenopausal bleeding bleeding occurring 6 months or more after cessation of menses

preauricular lymph node group located in front of the ear

premature ovarian failure menopause before 40 years old

premenstrual syndrome (PMS) cluster of emotional, behavioral, and physical symptoms occurring 5 days before menses for three consecutive cycles

presbycusis gradual loss of high-pitched sounds that extends to sounds in the middle and lower ranges; associated with normal aging

presbyopia progressive loss of accommodation and the ability to focus on nearby objects due to the gradual loss of lens elasticity; associated with normal aging

pressure injury or ulcer results from sustained compression that obliterates arteriolar and capillary blood flow to the skin and from shear forces created by body movements

primitive reflexes infantile automatisms that develop during gestation, are generally demonstrable at birth, and disappear at defined ages; evaluation of these reflexes is used to assess the newborn's and infant's developing central nervous system (abnormality suggests neurologic disease); examples include palmar and plantar grasp, rooting, startle or Moro, parachute, and stepping

pruritis ani itching and irritation of the skin at the anus; can be the result of poor hygiene or external hemorrhoids

ptosis drooping of the upper eyelid seen in CN III palsy, Horner syndrome, myasthenia gravis, or mechanical problems with the muscles that lift the eyelid

pulsus alternans abnormal pulse characterized by an alternating "strong" and "weak" pulse quality found in patients with significant left ventricular dysfunction thought to originate due to abnormal contractility in the failing heart; may be detected by palpation, while auscultating the blood pressure, or by Doppler echocardiography

pulsus paradoxus abnormal pulse characterized by exaggerated swings in systolic pressure due to increased ventricular interdependence, usually found in cardiac tamponade or severe asthma exacerbations; normally, systolic pressure decreases by 2 to 4 mm Hg, but, in pulsus paradoxus, systolic pressure decreases by >10 to 12 mm Hg with inspiration, as the filling of the right ventricle impedes filling of the left ventricle

pulsus parvus abnormally weakened pulses, suggesting peripheral vascular disease when symmetric, decreased intravascular volume when asymmetric

pulsus tardus abnormally sluggish pulses, usually observed in aortic stenosis or low cardiac output states

purpura nonblanchable, raised and palpable violaceous lesion

pustule small circumscribed elevation of the epidermis filled with purulent fluid

pyrexia elevated body temperature

quickening maternal sensation of fetal movement

rash widespread eruption of lesions

rebound tenderness pain with release of tension from palpation, associated with intra-abdominal infection

rhonchi considered a variant of wheeze arising from the same mechanism but lower in pitch, similar to snoring; may be heard on inspiration, expiration, or both; may be affected by cough, implicating secretions in the mechanism (unlike wheeze)

rigidity increase in muscle tone that remains the same throughout the range of motion; it is not velocity dependent and is seen in central disorders affecting the basal ganglia, such as *Parkinson disease*

Rinne test hearing test utilizing a tuning fork (typically 512 Hz) used to evaluate primarily unilateral hearing loss. Compares air (AC) and bone conduction (BC) in each ear. In a normal ear or one with sensorineural hearing loss, AC = BC. In conductive hearing loss, BC > AC.

Rotter nodes interpectoral nodes in between the pectoralis major and minor muscles

Rovsing sign palpation of the left lower quadrant resulting in pain in the right lower quadrant, suggestive of appendicitis

sciatica radicular gluteal and posterior leg pain usually caused by impingement of nerve roots at the L4–S1 levels

scoliosis abnormal curvature or vertebral rotation of the spine

sensory neglect impairment in the perception of and attention to stimuli on one side of the body that is not due to a deficit in primary sensory modalities (e.g., a patient may not be aware of objects in the left visual field even though the visual apparatus is completely normal)

serous effusion serous amber fluid behind the tympanic membrane, often secondary to viral upper respiratory infections or sudden changes in atmospheric pressure; an air-fluid level or air bubbles may be seen

shotty lymph nodes small, mobile, discrete, nontender nodes found normally

significant weight loss defined as loss of 5% or more of usual body weight over a 6-month period

slough inflammatory exudate composed of proteinaceous tissue, fibrin, neutrophils, and bacteria, rather than nonviable tissue; usually light yellow/cream colored and moist and soft

small for gestational age newborn classification based on the Ballard Score that places the newborn at <10th percentile for its gestational age and birth weight on the intrauterine growth curve

smegma cheesy, whitish material; may accumulate normally under the foreskin

spasticity increase in muscle tone seen in central diseases affecting the corticospinal tract that is velocity dependent and worsens at the extremes of range of motion; resistance increases with more rapid movement

sphygmomanometer device for measuring blood pressure

stadiometers devices specifically designed for the accurate measurement of height

static stabilizers components of a joint that are incapable of movement (e.g., bones and ligaments)

stiffness perceived tightness or resistance to movement

Still murmur most common benign murmur found in children described as a grade I–II/VI, musical, vibratory, early, and midsystolic murmur with multiple overtones located over the mid or lower left sternal border; it may also be heard over the carotid arteries

strabismus condition in which the eyes are not aligned and can move independently

stridor continuous, musical, high-pitched sound heard over the upper airways or at a distance without a stethoscope; results from airflow across a narrowed upper respiratory tract

subconjunctival hemorrhage benign, bright red patch representing a small bleed underneath the conjunctiva

submandibular lymph node group located midway between the angle and the tip of the mandible

submental lymph node group located in the midline behind the tip of the mandible

supernumerary nipples accessory nipples that develop along the embryonic milk line

supraclavicular lymph node group located deep in the angle formed by the clavicle and the sternocleidomastoid

syncope sudden onset of loss of consciousness due to lack of adequate perfusion to the brain; when resulting from innate cardiac pathology, such as a fatal or near-fatal arrhythmia, syncope is often associated with injury to the face, dentition, major joint dislocation, or fractures

tactile fremitus palpable vibratory transmission felt on the chest wall during speaking; intensity changes depending on the characteristics of the airways and lung parenchyma

tendinitis inflammation of a tendon, often with pain and focal swelling

tenosynovitis inflammation and swelling of a tendon sheath

terminal hair coarse, thick, pigmented hair such as scalp hair and eyebrows

testicular torsion twisting of the testicle on its spermatic cord produces an acutely painful, tender, and swollen organ that is often retracted upward in the scrotum; cremasteric reflex is nearly always absent on the affected side

thoracoabdominal paradox inward movement of the chest and outward movement of the abdomen during inspiration, which is a normal finding in newborns but not older infants; also known as *paradoxical breathing*

thought content themes that occupy the patient's thoughts and perceptual disturbances including level of insight and judgment

thought process logic, coherence, and relevance of the patient's thought as it leads to selected goals (how people think)

thrill abnormal vibratory impulse palpated over areas of turbulent blood flow, most commonly observed in patients with a dialysis arteriovenous fistula, a stenotic aortic valve, or a ventricular septal defect

tonsillar (jugulodigastric) lymph node group located at the angle of the mandible

tonsillitis inflammation of the tonsils; tonsils appear enlarged and erythematous and may have exudates

tracheal breath sound hollow, nonmusical sound heard clearly in both phases of the respiratory cycle and is best appreciated by listening over the neck; transports intrapulmonary sounds thus indicating airway patency

transmitted voice sounds sounds generated in the larynx heard when auscultating the thorax; resonance changes depending on characteristics of the airways and/or parenchyma

Trendelenburg sign test for severe hip disease with its associated weakness of the gluteus medius muscle

trichiasis aberrant growth of eyelashes in which the hair turns inward toward the eye

tubo-ovarian abscess abscess involving the fallopian tube; ovary; and, occasionally, adjacent organs

tympanosclerosis deposition of hyaline material within the layers of the tympanic membrane that may be associated with ear infections; appears as a chalky white patch with irregular borders on the otherwise translucent tympanic membrane

ulcer lesion with deeper loss of the epidermis and at least the upper dermis

Valsalva maneuver provocative examination maneuver wherein a patient performs a forced exhalation with a closed glottis; significantly reduces venous return to the heart, which has diagnostic utility in heart failure, hypertrophic obstructive cardiomyopathy, and pulmonary hypertension

varicocele gravity-mediated varicose veins of the spermatic cord, usually found on the left; feels like a soft "bag of worms" in the spermatic cord above the testis, and, if prominent, appears to distort the contours of the scrotal skin (note: varicocele collapses in the supine position, so examination should be both supine and standing)

vellus hair short, fine, inconspicuous, and relatively unpigmented hair

venous hum soft, hollow, continuous benign murmur, louder in diastole, heard just below the right clavicle found in preschool or school-aged children; can be completely eliminated by maneuvers that affect venous return, such as lying supine, changing head position, or jugular venous compression

vernix caseosa cheesy white material present at birth composed of water, proteins, and lipids, which covers the body and forms a barrier against maceration and infection and moisturizes the fetus to pass through the birth canal

vesicle small circumscribed elevation of the epidermis containing clear fluid less than 1 cm in diameter

vesicular (normal) breath sound soft, nonmusical sound heard best on inspiration and early expiration across all lung fields; considered a normal breath sound

Virchow node enlargement of a supraclavicular node, especially on the left, suggesting possible metastasis from a thoracic or an abdominal malignancy

vital signs collective term for blood pressure, heart rate, respiratory rate, and temperature

Weber test hearing test utilizing a tuning fork (typically 512 Hz) used to evaluate primarily unilateral hearing loss. The tuning fork is placed midline on the forehead. Normally the sound is heard equally on both sides. A patient with conductive hearing loss will hear the sound louder on the affected side. A patient with sensorineural hearing loss will hear the sound louder on the unaffected side.

Wernicke aphasia receptive aphasia with impaired comprehension but fluent speech

wheal circumscribed, raised lesion consisting of dermal edema, typically lasting <24 hours; also known as *hives* or *urticaria*

wheeze continuous, musical, high-pitched lung sounds heard on inspiration, expiration, or both; arise from rapid and turbulent airflow across airways narrowed almost to the point of closure

whispered pectoriloquy sign in which whispered words are heard louder and clearer over an area of consolidated lung

white coat hypertension (isolated clinic hypertension) blood pressure ≥140/90 mm Hg in medical settings and mean awake ambulatory readings of <135/85 mm Hg

Index

Note: Page numbers followed by *t*, *f*, and *b* indicate table, figure, and box respectively.

B

D

H

P

Q

R